TEXTBOOK OF
PHARMACOLOGY

TEXTBOOK OF
PHARMACOLOGY

CEDRIC M. SMITH, M.D.

Professor, Department of Pharmacology and Therapeutics
State University of New York
School of Medicine and Biomedical Sciences
Buffalo, New York

ALAN M. REYNARD, Ph.D.

Professor, Department of Pharmacology and Therapeutics
Director, Office of Information Systems
State University of New York
School of Medicine and Biomedical Sciences
Buffalo, New York

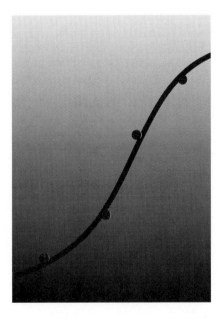

W. B. SAUNDERS COMPANY
Harcourt Brace Jovanovich, Inc.
Philadelphia   London   Toronto   Montreal   Sydney   Tokyo

W. B. SAUNDERS COMPANY
Harcourt Brace Jovanovich, Inc.

The Curtis Center
Independence Square West
Philadelphia, PA 19106

Library of Congress Cataloging-in-Publication Data

Textbook of pharmacology / [edited by] Cedric M. Smith,
    Alan M. Reynard.
            p.   cm.
    ISBN 0-7216-2442-1
    1. Pharmacology.   I. Smith, Cedric M.
    II. Reynard, Alan M.
    [DNLM: 1. Pharmacology.   QV 4 T355]
    RM300.T48 1991
    615'.1 — dc20
    DNLM/DLC
    for Library of Congress   91-13831

Editor: Martin J. Wonsiewicz

Developmental Editor: Lawrence J. McGrew

Designer: Karen O'Keefe

Production Manager: Peter Faber

Manuscript Editors: Mimi McGinnis and Pam Wight

Illustration Coordinator: Peg Shaw

Page Layout Artist: Dorothy Chattin

Indexer: Richard Lehne

Cover Designer: Ellen Bodner-Zanolle

Textbook of Pharmacology   ISBN 0-7216-2442-1

Last digit is the print number: 9   8   7   6   5   4   3   2   1

Contributors

Margaret A. Acara, Ph.D. ▪ Professor, Department of Pharmacology and Therapeutics, School of Medicine and Biomedical Sciences, State University of New York at Buffalo, Buffalo, New York

Ann M. Arvin, M.D. ▪ Professor of Pediatrics, Stanford University School of Medicine; Medical Staff, Stanford University Medical Center; Medical Staff, Children's Hospital at Stanford, Stanford, California

Thomas R. Beam, Jr., M.D. ▪ Associate Professor, Departments of Medicine and Microbiology, School of Medicine and Biomedical Sciences, State University of New York at Buffalo; Associate Chief of Staff for Education, Buffalo Veterans Administration Medical Center, Buffalo, New York

Joseph R. Bertino, M.D. ▪ Professor of Pharmacology and Medicine, Cornell University School of Medicine; Chairman, Program of Molecular Pharmacology and Therapeutics; Attending Physician, Memorial Sloan-Kettering Cancer Center, New York, New York

Richard E. Bettigole, M.D. ▪ Associate Professor, Department of Medicine; Clinical Associate Professor, Department of Pathology, School of Medicine and Biomedical Sciences, State University of New York at Buffalo; Attending Physician, Erie County Medical Center; Consultant, Veterans Administration Medical Center; Consultant, Buffalo General Hospital; Consultant, Roswell Park Cancer Institute, Assistant Attending Physician, Sisters of Charity Hospital, Buffalo, New York

Katherine R. Bonson, Ph.D. ▪ Instructor, Department of Pharmacology and Therapeutics, State University of New York at Buffalo, Buffalo, New York

Oliver M. Brown, Ph.D. ▪ Associate Professor, Department of Pharmacology, College of Medicine, State University of New York, Health Science Center at Syracuse, Syracuse, New York

Alexander C. Brownie, Ph.D., D.Sc. ▪ Professor, Department of Biochemistry, Research Professor of Pathology, Research Professor of Medicine, School of Medicine and Biomedical Sciences, State University of New York at Buffalo, Buffalo, New York

Daniel S. Camara, M.D. ▪ Associate Professor, Department of Medicine, School of Medicine and Biomedical Sciences, State University of New York at Buffalo; Clinical Director of Gastroenterology, Hepatology, and Nutrition; Head, Endoscopy Unit, Buffalo General Hospital, Buffalo, New York

Edward A. Carr, Jr., M.D. ▪ Professor, Department of Pharmacology and Therapeutics; Professor, Department of Medicine, School of Medicine and Biomedical Sciences, State University of New York at Buffalo; Consultant, Buffalo Veterans Administration Medical Center; Consultant, Erie County Medical Center, Buffalo, New York

David B. Case, M.D. ▪ Clinical Associate Professor, Department of Medicine, Cornell University Medical College; Associate Attending Physician, The New York Hospital–Cornell University Medical Center, New York, New York

Arthur W. K. Chan, Ph.D. ▪ Research Associate Professor, Department of Pharmacology and Therapeutics, School of Medicine and Biomedical Sciences, State University of New York at Buffalo; Research Institute on Alcoholism, Buffalo, New York

Robert M. Cooper, Pharm.D. ▪ Associate Professor, Department of Pharmacy; Associate Dean, School of Pharmacy, State University of New York at Buffalo, Buffalo, New York

Peter S. Creticos, M.D. ▪ Medical Director, Johns Hopkins Centers for Asthma and Allergic Diseases, Baltimore, Maryland

Roger K. Cunningham, Ph.D. ▪ Associate Professor, Department of Microbiology, School of Medicine and Biomedical Sciences, State University of New York at Buffalo, Buffalo, New York

Paul J. Davis, M.D. ▪ Professor and Chairman, Department of Medicine, Albany Medical College, Albany, New York

Jill G. Dolgin, Pharm.D., D.A.B.A.T. ▪ Assistant Clinical Professor of Pharmacy and Pediatrics, Schools of Pharmacy and Medicine and Biomedical Sciences, State University of New York at Buffalo; Director, Western New York Regional Poison Control Center; Adjunct Faculty, Department of Pediatrics, Childrens Hospital of Buffalo, Buffalo, New York

Peter K. Gessner, Ph.D. ▪ Professor, Department of Pharmacology and Therapeutics, School of Medicine and Biomedical Sciences, State University of New York at Buffalo, Buffalo, New York

Linda A. Hershey, M.D., Ph.D. ▪ Associate Professor, Department of Neurology; Research Associate Professor, Department of Pharmacology and Therapeutics, School of Medicine and Biomedical Sciences, State University of New York at Buffalo; Chief, Neurology Service, Department of Veterans Affairs, Veterans Administration Medical Center, Buffalo, New York

Dennis M. Higgins, Ph.D. ▪ Associate Professor, Department of Pharmacology, School of Medicine and Biomedical Sciences, State University of New York at Buffalo, Buffalo, New York

Peter J. Horvath, Ph.D. ▪ Assistant Professor, Nutrition Program, School of Health-Related Professions, State University of New York at Buffalo, Buffalo, New York

Shyam D. Karki, Pharm.D. ▪ Assistant Clinical Professor, School of Pharmacy, State University of New York at Buffalo, Buffalo; Director, Department of Pharmacy, Monroe Community Hospital, Rochester, New York

Shigihiro Katayama, M.D., Ph.D. ▪ Associate Professor of Medicine, The Fourth Department of Medicine, Saitama Medical School, Saitama, Japan

Paul J. Kostyniak, Ph.D., D.A.B.T. ▪ Associate Professor, Department of Pharmacology and Therapeutics, School of Medicine and Biomedical Sciences; Director, Toxicology Research Center, State University of New York at Buffalo, Buffalo, New York

Claire M. Lathers, Ph.D., F.C.P. ▪ Associate Professor, Department of Pharmacology, Medical College of Pennsylvania, Philadelphia, Pennsylvania; Pharmacologist, Food and Drug Administration, Rockville, Maryland; Visiting Scientist, Universities Space Research Association, National Aeronautics and Space Administration, Houston, Texas, and Uniformed Services University of the Health Sciences, Bethesda, Maryland

Suzanne G. Laychock, Ph.D. ▪ Professor, Department of Pharmacology and Therapeutics, School of Medicine and Biomedical Sciences, State University of New York at Buffalo, Buffalo, New York

James B. Lee, M.D. ▪ Professor, Department of Medicine; Chief, Hypertension Program Unit, Department of Medicine, State University of New York at Buffalo; Attending Physician, Erie County Medical Center; Academic in Medicine, Buffalo General Hospital; Consultant in Medicine, Veterans Administration Medical Center, Buffalo, New York

D. Lynn Loriaux, M.D., Ph.D. ▪ Clinical Director, National Institute of Child Health and Human Development, National Institutes of Health, Bethesda, Maryland; Chief, Division of Endocrinology, Oregon Health Sciences University, School of Medicine, Portland, Oregon

Robert J. McIsaac, Ph.D. ▪ Emeritus Professor, Department of Pharmacology and Therapeutics, State University of New York at Buffalo, Buffalo, New York

K. S. Nair, M.D., Ph.D., M.R.C.P.(U.K.) ▪ Associate Professor of Medicine, Endocrinology and Metabolism Unit, Department of Medicine, University of Vermont College of Medicine; Attending Physician, Medical Center Hospital of Vermont, Burlington, Vermont

Lynnette K. Nieman, M.D. ▪ Expert, National Institute of Child Health and Human Development; Ward Chief, 10 West Endocrine Unit, Clinical Center, National Institutes of Health, Bethesda, Maryland

Daniel K. O'Rourke, M.D. ▪ Department of Pharmacology, Medical College of Pennsylvania, Philadelphia, Pennsylvania; Clinical Associate, National Institutes of Health, Bethesda, Maryland

Ralph J. Parod, Ph.D. ▪ Gradient Corporation, Cambridge, Massachusetts

Alan M. Reynard, Ph.D. ▪ Professor, Department of Pharmacology and Therapeutics; Director, Office of Information Systems, School of Medicine and Biomedical Sciences, State University of New York at Buffalo, Buffalo, New York

Jerome A. Roth, Ph.D. ▪ Professor, Department of Pharmacology and Therapeutics, School of Medicine and Biomedical Sciences, State University of New York at Buffalo, Buffalo, New York

Robert Scheig, M.D. ▪ Professor, Department of Medicine, School of Medicine and Biomedical Sciences, State University of New York at Buffalo; Chief of Medicine, Buffalo General Hospital, Buffalo, New York

Steven M. Simasko, Ph.D. ▪ Assistant Professor, Department of Physiology, School of Medicine and Biomedical Sciences, State University of New York at Buffalo, Buffalo, New York

F. Estelle R. Simons, M.D., F.R.C.P.C. ■ Professor and Head, Section of Allergy and Clinical Immunology; Deputy Chairman, Department of Pediatrics and Child Health, University of Manitoba Faculty of Medicine; Head, Section of Allergy and Clinical Immunology, Children's Hospital of Winnipeg, Winnepeg, Manitoba, Canada

Keith J. Simons, B.Sc.(Pharm.), M.Sc., Ph.D. ■ Professor, Faculty of Pharmacy, Department of Pediatrics and Child Health; Professor, Faculty of Medicine, Department of Chemistry, Faculty of Science, University of Manitoba, Winnepeg, Manitoba, Canada

Cedric M. Smith, M.D. ■ Professor, Department of Pharmacology and Therapeutics, School of Medicine and Biomedical Sciences, State University of New York at Buffalo, Buffalo, New York

Stephen W. Spaulding, M.D., C.M. ■ Professor, Department of Medicine, School of Medicine and Biomedical Sciences, State University of New York at Buffalo; Associate Chief of Staff for Research and Development, Veterans Administration Medical Center, Buffalo, New York

Ronald S. Swerdloff, M.D. ■ Professor of Medicine, University of California at Los Angeles School of Medicine, Los Angeles; Chief, Division of Endocrinology and Metabolism, Harbor–University of California at Los Angeles Medical Center, Torrance, California

Kathleen M. Tornatore, Pharm.D., B.S.Pharm. ■ Assistant Professor, Department of Pharmacy, School of Pharmacy, State University of New York at Buffalo; Pharmacokinetic Consultant, Veterans Administration Medical Center, Buffalo, New York

James W. Tracy, Ph.D. ■ Associate Professor, Departments of Comparative Biosciences and Pharmacology, University of Wisconsin Medical School, Madison, Wisconsin

David J. Triggle, Ph.D. ■ Dean, School of Pharmacy, University Distinguished Professor, State University of New York at Buffalo, Buffalo, New York

Elizabeth A. Vande Waa, Ph.D. ■ Assistant Scientist, Departments of Comparative Biosciences and Pharmacology, University of Wisconsin Medicine School, Madison, Wisconsin

Robert L. Volle, Ph.D. ■ President, National Board of Medical Examiners, Philadelphia, Pennsylvania

Christina Wang, M.D. ■ Professor of Medicine, University of California at Los Angeles School of Medicine; Director of Andrology, Divisions of Endocrinology, Metabolism, and Reproductive Endocrinology/Infertility, Cedars-Sinai Medical Center, Los Angeles, California

Alan Winkelstein, M.D. ■ Professor, Division of Hematology and Bone Marrow Transplantation, Department of Medicine, University of Pittsburgh School of Medicine; Montefiore University Hospital, Pittsburgh, Pennsylvania

Jerrold C. Winter, Ph.D. ■ Professor, Department of Pharmacology and Therapeutics, School of Medicine and Biomedical Sciences, State University of New York at Buffalo, Buffalo, New York

Preface

Pharmacology is the study of drugs—what they are, what effects they have, what happens to them, and how they work. The *Textbook of Pharmacology* reflects the "essential knowledge which every medical student . . . must have," as identified by the Association of Medical School Pharmacology. It includes such topics as the mechanisms of action of drugs on molecular and systemic levels as well as how drugs are absorbed and distributed in the body, metabolized, and excreted.

The book is designed to serve, not as a reference source, but as a readable text for the initial course in medical pharmacology. Because it will be used by the medical student and eventual medical practitioner, it emphasizes the agents commonly prescribed in the diagnosis and treatment of disease, as well as the substances involved in poisoning and toxic reactions. References have been limited to recent articles and reviews judged to be useful to medical students with an interest in more detailed information.

A number of chapters on topics not usually found in pharmacology texts are included: diagnostic drugs; drug effects on sensory systems; psychiatric symptoms produced by drugs; drug-food interactions. In addition, we review the rapidly expanding print and computer-based information resources about drugs, computer-assisted learning, as well as adverse drug effects and interactions.

Rational medical therapy requires the judicious selection and application of knowledge about drugs. *Textbook of Pharmacology* will assist students in making such therapeutic decisions regarding the drugs they will encounter in the future. Nevertheless, it is neither a therapeutic manual nor a reference source for dosages or treatment regimens; examples of dosages are provided on a selective basis to illustrate the context for the medical use of specific drugs.

We acknowledge the important contributions of Rachel Byron Moore of bioGraphics, Inc., for the many new and redrawn illustrations and of William Pudlack for drawings of chemical structures. We wish to thank Ronald Rubin, Ph.D., chairman of this pharmacology department, for his encouragement; Martin Wonsiewicz, our editor (formerly of Saunders), for his sustained guidance and encouragement; and our many colleagues for their helpful reviews and suggestions. In addition, we acknowledge the pioneering efforts of the authors of previous pharmacology textbooks.

Contents

General Principles

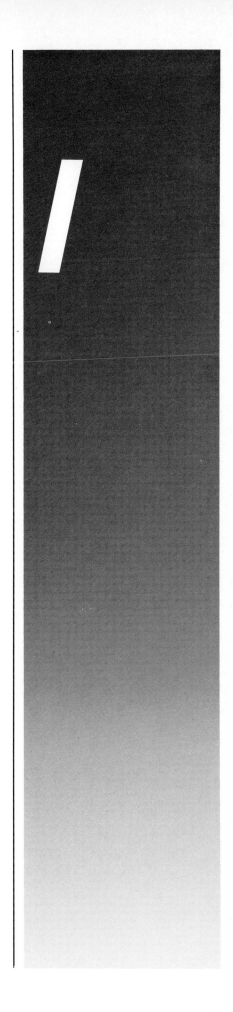

Introduction to Pharmacology: Receptors

1

Jerrold C. Winter

Pharmacology is concerned with all facets of the interaction of chemicals with biological systems. When such interactions are applied to the cure or amelioration of disease, the chemicals are usually called drugs. This chapter gives a rational basis for the classification of that body of facts and details that composes medical pharmacology. This is accomplished by providing a basic pharmacological vocabulary and by presenting the fundamental principles that govern encounters between drugs and living tissues.

Most drugs produce effects by combining with biological receptors. The chemical bonds that form between drug molecule and receptor are usually reversible. The ease with which drug and receptor interact is influenced by the degree of complementarity of their respective three-dimensional structures. For this reason, minor chemical modification of a drug may produce profound changes in its pharmacological activity.

Multiple Receptors/Selective Toxicity

Pharmacology is a hybrid science. It freely draws upon the intellectual resources of all the basic medical sciences and contributes to every aspect of clinical medicine. It is appropriate, therefore, that the concept of *receptors,* a central theorem of pharmacology, should have arisen from the work of John Newport Langley, a physiologist, and Paul Ehrlich, a polymath best remembered for his work in immunology and in the chemotherapy of syphilis.

While still an undergraduate in the department of physiology at Cambridge University, Langley studied the antagonism by atropine of the contractile effects of pilocarpine on smooth muscle. Describing his results in 1878, he made the assumption "that there is a substance or substances in the nerve endings or gland cells with which both atropine and pilocarpine are capable of forming compounds. On this assumption then the atropine and pilocarpine compounds are formed according to some law of which their relative mass and chemical affinity for the substance are factors."

Over the next three decades a clearer picture of the nature of these "substances" evolved slowly in Langley's mind. Based upon his experiments with isolated nerve-muscle preparations, he concluded that the drugs did not act directly on the nerve endings or on the muscle. He observed that nicotine causes contraction of muscle whether or not the muscle is innervated. Furthermore, curare, a drug then commonly thought to act upon nerve endings, blocks the effects of nicotine even in denervated muscle. Finally, a muscle paralyzed by curare still contracts when stimulated electrically. Langley concluded that nicotine and curare must combine with something that is neither nerve nor muscle; in 1905 he called it "receptive substance."

Two drugs can compete with each other.

Drugs compete for a "receptive substance."

The subject of Ehrlich's M.D. thesis in 1878 was the histological utility of certain vital dyes. Impressed by the specificity with which dyes interact with tissues, he postulated that a drug can have a therapeutic effect only if it has "the right sort of affinity." However, his first application of this idea was to immunology rather than to pharmacology. In his side-chain theory, Ehrlich suggested that there is binding between toxins and antitoxins via chemically specific functional groups. Later he expanded this idea to include chemoreceptors located in parasites; these receptors could serve as targets for chemically aimed "magic bullets." Despite the appeal that such ideas have for modern pharmacologists, Ehrlich long resisted the application of his theory to drug-tissue interactions in general. There was simply too great a conceptual gap between the firm binding of an arsenical poison to a trypanosome and the evanescent effects of many drugs. But the passage of time, the accumulation of data, and in particular, a careful consideration of Langley's experiments eventually caused Ehrlich's "doubts to disappear and made the existence of chemoreceptors seem probable."

Receptors can serve as targets for drugs.

Today receptor theory serves as a unifying concept for the explanation of the effects of chemicals on biological systems, whether these chemicals be of exogenous (pharmacological) or endogenous (physiological) origin. A modern statement of the receptor theorem is that of Goldstein, Aronow, and Kalman: in general, a drug produces a particular effect by combining chemically with some specific molecular constituent (receptor) of the biological system upon which it acts. The function of the receptor molecule in the biological system is thereby modified to produce a measurable effect.

Drugs modify the biological function of receptors.

In searching for chemicals that would kill trypanosomes, Ehrlich discovered that arsanilic acid was quite effective. When injected into infected mice, soon the blood was completely free of parasites. Unfortunately, the mice died shortly thereafter of arsanilic acid poisoning. Arsanilic acid was not an effective therapeutic agent because it was not *selectively toxic* to trypanosomes. Albert (1979) provides the following definition: a remedy is said to have selectivity when it can influence one kind of living cell without affecting others, even when these cells are close neighbors.

Drugs need to act selectively on specific receptors, otherwise they may damage the host.

In Ehrlich's time and no less so today, it is a goal of pharmacology to discover drugs that are highly selective in their actions. In the context of receptors, a drug may be intended to act upon a single type of receptor, and no others, to produce its therapeutic effect. In some areas of therapeutics, that goal has been approximated; many antibacterial drugs are remarkably free of effects upon mammalian cells. In other areas, the goal is still far distant; drugs used in an attempt to kill cancer cells often produce toxicity at unintended sites.

Binding Forces in the Drug-Receptor Complex

A variety of chemical forces are involved in drug-receptor binding.

If drug and receptor interact via chemical forces, then our understanding of drug-receptor interactions will be limited by our knowledge of the chemical forces involved. At the beginning of this century, Ehrlich's reluctance to apply the notion of chemoreceptors to all drug-tissue interactions was in part due to an incomplete knowledge of possible binding forces between drug and receptor. Thus, covalent bonds would readily explain the interaction of arsanilic acid with a trypanosome but would fail to account for the fleeting nature of the interaction between acetylcholine and a muscle. Today, we are reasonably confident that the range of known chemical bonds is adequate to rationalize all known drug-receptor interactions.

COVALENT BONDS

The sharing of valence electrons between two atoms constitutes a covalent bond. Because of their considerable bond energy, ranging from 50 to 150 kcal/mol, covalent bonds are usually irreversible at body temperature in the absence of a catalyst. Examples include the interaction of an alkylating agent with a cancer cell, monoaminoxidase inhibitors that act irreversibly, and certain organophosphorus insecticides that form covalent bonds with the enzyme cholinesterase. However, the formation of covalent bonds between a drug and its receptor is relatively uncommon in pharmacology.

NONCOVALENT BONDS

In the absence of covalent bonds, a reversible interaction occurs between drug and receptor. Nonetheless, the interaction must be of sufficient duration and stability to initiate the chain of events leading to a pharmacological effect. These reversible chemical bonds are of several types, and more than one type would be expected to act at the same time. In general the precise contribution of individual bond types is not known. However, the structural features of a drug provide insight into the nature of the bonds it is likely to form with receptors.

Ionic Bonds

Ions are chemical entities that carry a net negative or positive charge. A physiologically significant example is provided by acetylcholine, which permanently carries a positive charge by virtue of its quaternary ammonium group. Any model of the interaction between acetylcholine and its receptors must include ionic bonds. The strength of such bonds has been variously estimated at between 5 and 10 kcal/mole — highly significant in initiating biological effects but readily reversible at body temperature. Ionic bonds are coulombic in nature; thus their force diminishes with the square of the distance between interacting groups. Although some drugs are, like acetylcholine, permanently charged, many more are weak acids and bases, ionized to varying degrees at the pHs found in biological fluids (see later in this chapter).

Hydrogen Bonds

A number of relatively weak interactions between drug and receptor are due to nonuniformities in electron distribution within molecules. The best known of these is the hydrogen bond. First described in detail by Linus Pauling, hydrogen bonds arise between hydrogen atoms covalently linked to highly electronegative atoms, such as oxygen, nitrogen, and fluorine. For example, in the water molecule, a shift of electrons away from hydrogen and toward oxygen yields a polar molecule; we can imagine the oxygen having a fractional negative charge that is balanced by the relative positive nature of the hydrogens. In the presence of other water molecules, interactions occur between these electron-rich and electron-poor areas. Hydrogen bonding accounts for the high boiling point of water relative to comparable molecules in which such bonds cannot form. Their energy is about 2–5 kcal/mole.

In addition to hydrogen bonds, other coulombic forces of attraction will arise between any molecules that are not fully symmetrical in their distribution of electrons. Thus, complementary areas of electron excess and deficiency will attract one another in what are called dipole-dipole interactions. The energy of these interactions is comparable to that of hydrogen bonds.

Van der Waals Bonds

Deviations from the ideal gas law, $PV = nRT$, caused the Dutch physicist J. D. van der Waals to postulate attractive forces between uncharged molecules that are brought close to one another. Van der Waals forces (also called Heitler-London forces or electron correlation attractions) are due to the mutual interaction of the electrons and nuclei of adjacent molecules. The strength of the attraction is critically dependent upon the distance between the molecules. The maximal force occurs when the molecules are separated by their so-called van der Waals radii. If they come closer, there are strong repulsive forces between the electron shells. As the molecules separate beyond the van der Waals radii, the force diminishes as the seventh power of the distance. Van der Waals bonds are relatively weak and contribute about 0.5 kcal/mole. Groups such as benzene rings, with their homogeneous distributions of electron density, are likely contributors to van der Waals interactions.

The Hydrophobic Effect

The formation of hydrogen bonds between water molecules confers sufficient stability that liquid water can be regarded as highly structured. When any solute is dissolved in water, that structure is disturbed. If nonpolar groups are added to water, they will arrange themselves to minimize disturbance of the hydrogen-bonded water structure. Thus, in an aqueous medium hydrophobic groups on receptor and drug may be forced into close contact. The increased stability provided by the most appropriate arrangement of nonpolar groups in aqueous media gives rise to a weak noncovalent bond, the hydrophobic bond. In the polar world of hydrogen-bonded water, nonpolar groups are more likely to be found together than apart.

Stereocomplementarity: The Lock and Key Analogy

Although a single covalent bond is adequate to maintain contact between drug and receptor, the low energy conferred by noncovalent bonds requires that larger numbers be formed. The fact that the force of coulombic interactions diminishes as the square of the distance between interacting groups suggests that interacting groups must have structures that permit close approximation of their surfaces. Even more dramatic is the decrease of van der Waals forces as the seventh power of the distance. These factors lead directly to a consideration of the three-dimensional structure of drugs and receptors.

In its common tetravalent state, carbon forms four sp-hybridized bonds with adjacent atoms. The carbon atom can be imagined to be at the center of a tetrahedron with the four bonds directed toward the corners. An interchange of any two groups yields a second structure, nonsuperimposible with the first; such isomers are referred to as *enantiomorphs*. Louis Pasteur recognized that the crystalline enantiomorphic forms of tartaric acid rotate polarized light in opposite directions. This fact, together with the observation that certain molds selected only one of the enantiomers for use, led him to conclude that molecular asymmetry "constitutes perhaps the only sharply defined difference between the chemistry of dead and living matter."

The German chemist and enzymologist Emil Fischer applied Pasteur's concept to the subject of enzyme-substrate interactions. He compared the action of two different enzymes, emulsin from bitter almonds and maltase from yeast, on enantiomeric methyl-glucosides. He found that emulsin hydrolyzed the one form but not the other, whereas maltase had an opposite action. In 1895, Fischer wrote the following: "[the enzymes'] specific effect on the glucosides might thus be explained by assuming that the intimate contact between the molecules necessary for the release of the chemical reaction is possible only with similar geometrical configurations. To use a picture, I would say that the enzyme and the substrate must fit together like lock and key . . ." Fischer's lock and key analogy has had great influence upon the course of modern pharmacology.

STRUCTURE-ACTIVITY RELATIONSHIPS

Imagine that you have been presented with a lock and an elaborately notched and grooved key and asked to determine the features essential to opening the lock. If you now proceed to have cut a set of keys that incorporate each feature in isolation and in every possible combination with every other feature and test each key in the lock, you will soon know what is essential and what is not. Within limits, much the same approach can be taken with drugs.

Morphine provides an interesting example of what may be learned from studies of structure-activity relationships. The pharmacological properties of opium, of which morphine is a major active principle, have been known for several thousand years. Morphine was isolated in pure form from opium by Serturner in 1806, its structure was determined in 1925 by Gulland and Robinson, and it was totally synthesized by Gates and Tschudi in 1952.

Morphine has an elegant structure. An immediate question is whether simpler forms might be more or less efficacious, might be agonists or antagonists, might be more or less toxic, and so on. In fact, thousands of morphine congeners have been examined for their pain-relieving properties, and it has been found that drugs such as meperidine and methadone are efficacious. Such findings suggest that the essential features for analgesic activity are an electron-rich area (the benzene ring) joined by a three-carbon bridge to a tertiary amino group. Structure-activity studies of this nature have been done with a wide variety of drugs in an attempt to identify better therapeutic agents.

THE STEREOSELECTIVITY OF RECEPTORS

By identifying the structural and geometric features of a molecule that produce a specific pharmacological effect, we may not only get a new drug but we may also learn much about the structure of the receptor upon which it acts. For example, humans have physiological receptors that, when occupied by various chemicals, lead to the sensation of sweetness. Saccharin is an intensely sweet substance that a simple molecular modification renders tasteless. Examination of the structures of saccharin and N-methylsaccharin suggests complementary structural features in the "sweetness" receptor.

There are many drugs that contain an asymmetric carbon atom, and if there is any validity to our lock and key analogy, at least some optical isomers should interact quite differently with receptors. Indeed, this is certainly the case with the optical isomers levorphanol and dextrorphan; the former is comparable to morphine in its properties, whereas the latter is inactive as an analgesic. (In modern terminology, a center of asymmetry is sometimes called a chiral center or center of chirality from the Greek *kheir*, hand.)

Despite obvious examples of stereospecificity in drug action, therapeutic agents often are available only as the racemate, an optically inactive equimolar mixture of optical isomers. Although racemic mixtures are commonly regarded as single drugs, this is not true. The two components may have similar or quite different receptor specificities; they may interact or they may exert quite independent pharmacological effects. It has been recognized that the use of racemates hopelessly confounds pharmacokinetic investigations.

Although the majority of the pharmacological effects considered in this book are best accounted for in terms of an interaction between a drug and a macromolecular receptor, there are exceptions. For example, some diuretics work by changes they effect in osmolality rather than by interaction with a

Morphine

Meperidine

Methadone

Saccharin

N-methylsaccharin

Pharmacological Effects Not Mediated by Specific Receptors

specific receptor. They are filtered in the kidney but are not reabsorbed, which leads to a decrease in back diffusion of water and a resultant diuresis. Drugs such as ammonium chloride and sodium bicarbonate may be used to alter the pH of bodily fluids. In toxicology, chelating agents are used to bind toxic heavy-metal ions. In cancer chemotherapy, a group of so-called unnatural analogs substitutes for biologically essential chemicals with resulting cell death. Although we do not understand the way in which drugs such as general anesthetics work, some believe that they have a nonspecific effect on lipid membranes. In none of these instances can we properly speak of a macromolecular receptor. Exceptions such as these do not detract from the utility of the receptor concept, but each is noted in subsequent chapters.

References

Albert A: Selective Toxicity, The Physico-Chemical Basis of Therapy. 6th ed. London: Chapman & Hall, 1979.

Goldstein A, Aronow L, Kalman SM: Principles of Drug Action: The Basis of Pharmacology. 2nd ed. New York: John Wiley & Sons, 1974.

Pratt WB, Taylor P: Principles of Drug Action. The Basis of Pharmacology, 3rd ed. [Revised edition of Goldstein A, Kalman SM, Aronow L, 2nd ed, 1973, 1974.] New York: Churchill Livingstone, 1990.

Dose-Effect Relationships, Interactions, and Therapeutic Index

2

Jerrold C. Winter

The receptor concept proposed by Ehrlich and by Langley had little immediate impact upon pharmacology. Textbooks in the first decades of this
century were little more than compilations of verbal descriptions of the
effects of drugs. A quantitative and analytical base was needed. In the years
following World War I, Alfred Joseph Clark provided that base. Clark
assumed that the interaction between drug and receptor was analogous to
the adsorption of gases by a metal surface, i.e., a reversible reaction governed by the law of mass action.

Beginning with the assumption that drug and receptor interact in a
reversible chemical reaction governed by the law of mass action, the nature
of the relationship between the dose of a drug and its effects can be predicted. Prediction and reality are often quite similar: when pharmacological
effect is plotted versus the logarithm of the dose, a sigmoid curve results.
Such dose-effect curves provide the basis for the terms affinity and intrinsic
activity in isolated systems and for the terms potency and efficacy in patients.

Herbal and drug recipes have practical
utility but no explanatory power.

The interaction between drug and receptor can be represented by the
following equation:

$$[R] + [X] \rightleftharpoons [RX]$$

where [R] is the concentration of free receptors, [X] is the concentration of
drug in the vicinity of the receptors, and [RX] is the concentration of the
drug-receptor complex. The law of mass action states that the velocity of a
chemical reaction is proportional to the active masses of the reacting substances. Thus, the dissociation constant, K_x, of the drug-receptor complex is
given by the following equation:

$$K_x = [R][X]/[RX] \qquad (1)$$

If we now assume that we can account for all the receptors as being
either free or bound, then the concentration of free receptors, [R], is equal to
the total concentration of receptors, $[R_T]$, minus that fraction occupied by
drug, [RX], or

$$[R] = [R_T] - [RX]$$

Substituting into equation 1, we obtain

Drug-Receptor Interactions and the Law of Mass Action

$$K_x = ([R_T] - [RX]) [X]/[RX],$$
$$K_x[RX] = [R_T] [X] - [RX] [X],$$
$$[RX] (K_x + [X]) = [R_T] [X], \text{ and}$$
$$[RX]/[R_T] = [X]/(K_x + [X]) \qquad (2)$$

Thus, the fraction of all receptors that is combined with drug is a function of the concentration of drug in the vicinity of the receptor and the dissociation constant of the drug-receptor complex.

Equation 2 assumes practical importance if we make what is generally called the "occupancy assumption" regarding the interaction of drugs with receptors. Specifically, we will assume that (1) the magnitude of the pharmacological effect, E, is directly proportional to [RX], the concentration of the drug-receptor complex, and that (2) the maximal pharmacological effect, E_{max}, occurs when all receptors are occupied by drug. Equation 2 may now be rewritten as follows:

$$E/E_{max} = [X]/(K_x + [X]) \qquad (3)$$

Although Clark himself expressed reservations about the validity of the occupancy assumption, equation 3 has been found over the years to be in accordance with a remarkable variety of pharmacological observations.

Graphical Representation

In pharmacology it is conventional to plot E or E_{max} versus dose expressed on a log scale. Figure 2–1 shows the effects of acetylcholine as determined by Clark in the 1920s. With such data it is possible to estimate K_x directly. Thus, when

$$E/E_{max} = \tfrac{1}{2} = [X]/(K_x + [X]),$$
$$K_x = [X]$$

Receptor theory can explain relationships between dose and response (D-R).

It must be kept in mind that this estimate of K_x is valid only to the extent that our assumptions regarding the interaction between drug and receptor are valid. Later, we consider a few of the modifications to Clark's theory that have been necessitated by pharmacological fact. For more advanced treatments of the subject, see Black and Leff (1983) and Kenakin (1984).

Drug-Receptor Versus Enzyme-Substrate Interactions

Recalling that Emil Fischer's lock-and-key analogy was based upon enzyme-substrate interactions, it should not surprise us that there are many

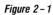

Figure 2–1

Dose-response relationships for acetylcholine. *(A)* Inhibition of isometric response of frog ventricle. *(B)* Contraction of frog rectus abdominis. Abscissa: Log molar concentration. Ordinate: Percent of maximal response. (Redrawn from Clark AJ: General Pharmacology. Vol 4 of Handbuch der experimentellen Pharmakologie, 66. Berlin: Springer-Verlag, 1937.)

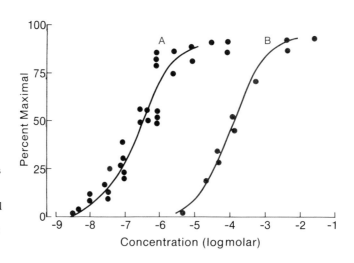

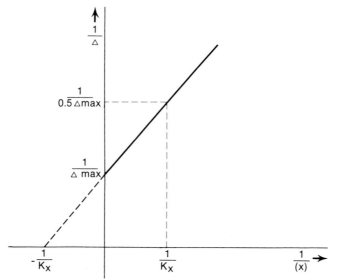

Figure 2-2

The double-reciprocal or Lineweaver-Burke plot.

analogies between enzyme-substrate and drug-receptor interactions. However, in biochemistry it is conventional to rearrange equation 3.

$$E/E_{max} = [X]/(K_x + [X])$$
$$E = [X]E_{max}/(K_x + [X])$$
$$1/E = (K_x + [X])/[X]E_{max}$$
$$1/E = (K_x/E_{max})\,(1/[X]) + 1/E_{max} \tag{4}$$

As seen in Figure 2-2, the so-called double-reciprocal or Lineweaver-Burke plot yields a straight line with slope $= K_x/E_{max}$ and intercept $= 1/E_{max}$.

The Dose-Effect Relationship in Isolated Systems: Affinity and Intrinsic Activity

Much of what is presumed to be known about drug-receptor interactions has been derived from experiments using "isolated systems." For example, a classical experiment involves removing a piece of smooth muscle from the ileum of a guinea pig, suspending the tissue in a bathing solution, and observing contractions or relaxations of the muscle in response to drugs added to the bath. In an isolated system we assume that a direct relationship exists between the calculated drug concentrations in the bath and the concentration to which the relevant receptors are exposed.

AFFINITY

Affinity

Figure 2-3 shows the contractile effects of acetylcholine and propionylcholine on a piece of guinea pig ileum. Two features of the figure are obvious: both drugs produce the same maximal effect, but a higher concentration of propionylcholine is required for any given degree of contraction. According to the occupancy assumption, fewer receptors are occupied by propionylcholine than by acetylcholine when the two drugs are present in equal concentrations. In this situation, we say that acetylcholine has a higher *affinity* for the receptor than does propionylcholine. Affinity is a measure of the probability that a drug molecule will interact with its receptor to form the drug-receptor complex. Affinity is inversely proportional to K_x, the dissociation constant of the drug-receptor complex.

Figure 2-3

Dose-response relationships for acetylcholine and propionylcholine in causing contraction of isolated guinea pig ileum. Abscissa: Drug concentration expressed on a log scale. Ordinate: Percent of maximal response. (Redrawn from Burgen AS, Mitchell JF (eds): Gaddum's Pharmacology. 6th ed, 3. New York: Oxford University Press, 1968, by permission of the Oxford University Press.)

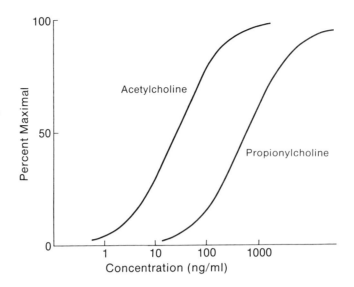

Intrinsic activity

INTRINSIC ACTIVITY

If mere occupancy of a receptor were sufficient to produce a pharmacological effect, then all drugs acting upon a common receptor would produce the same maximal effect. The data in Figure 2–4 indicate that this is not always the case. A group of drugs acting upon a common receptor produces clearly different maximal effects. To explain observations such as this, the Dutch pharmacologist E. J. Ariens proposed that a drug must not only have affinity for a receptor but must also possess a second property that he called *intrinsic activity*.

Intrinsic activity is a measure of the biological effectiveness of a drug-receptor complex. It is a proportionality constant, here termed k_{ia}, which relates the quantity of complex formed to the magnitude of the pharmacological effect produced. Thus,

$$E \text{ is proportional to } [RX] \text{ or}$$
$$E = k_{ia}[RX]$$

For example, if we imagine two drugs, one with an intrinsic activity of 1 (a full agonist) and the other with an intrinsic activity of 0.5 (a partial agonist), the pharmacological effects we can expect for the two drugs are given by

$$E_A = 1[RX] \text{ and}$$
$$E_B = 0.5[RX].$$

The Dose-Effect Relationship in Intact Organisms: Potency and Efficacy

As useful as isolated systems have been and will continue to be, we often must consider the effects of drugs not in isolated bits of tissue but in the whole animal. Here we must deal with the effects of drugs in what we will refer to as the intact organism or, when the intact organism in question is a human being, the patient. In this situation, no direct relationship can be assumed to exist between drug dose and concentration of drug at receptors.

POTENCY

Figure 2–5 depicts the dose-effect relationship in human subjects for two opioid analgesics, morphine and dihydrocodeine. They have comparable maximal effects in providing pain relief, but their dose-response curves are

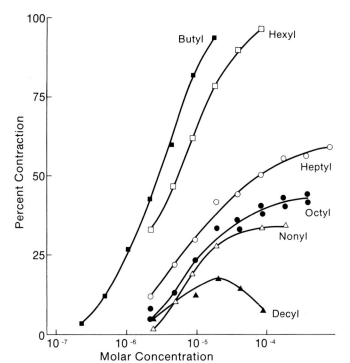

Figure 2-4

Dose-response relationships for a homologous series of compounds presumed to act upon a common receptor. Abscissa: Percent of maximal response. Ordinate: Molar concentration plotted on a log scale. (Redrawn from Stephenson RP: A modification of receptor theory. Br J Pharmacol 11:379–393, 1956.)

Potency

at different points on the dose axis. We say that the drugs differ in *potency;* the lower the dose required to produce a given degree of analgesia, the higher the potency of the drug. Thus, morphine is more potent than dihydrocodeine.

Dose-effect curves for drugs of differing potencies in intact organisms can be deceptively similar to those for drugs of differing affinities in isolated systems. However, there are a number of reasons why we should expect no constant relationship between affinity for an isolated receptor and potency in a patient. Most of these have to do with the absorption, distribution, metabolism, and excretion of drugs. For example, a drug that is poorly absorbed following oral administration will be far less potent than one that is readily absorbed, even if the two drugs have equal affinities for a common receptor.

It is conventional to express potency in producing a given therapeutic effect in terms of milligrams of drug per kilogram of body weight (mg/kg) or milligrams per patient to produce that effect. For example, only micro-

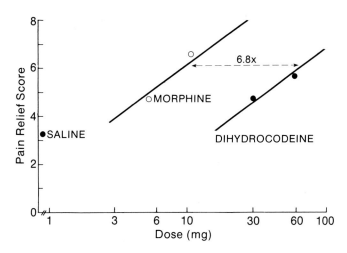

Figure 2-5

Dose-response relationships for morphine and dihydrocodeine in relieving pain in human subjects. Abscissa: Dose plotted on a log scale. Ordinate: Pain relief expressed in arbitrary units. (Redrawn from Goldstein A, Aronow L, Kalman SM: Principles of Drug Action: The Basis of Pharmacology. 2nd ed, 388. New York: John Wiley & Sons, copyright © 1974, John Wiley & Sons.)

grams per kilogram of a "high-potency" antipsychotic drug may be effective, whereas hundreds of milligrams of a "low-potency" drug are needed for the same effect.

EFFICACY

Efficacy

The ability of a drug to produce a desired therapeutic effect is called *efficacy*. The two drugs shown in Figure 2–5 are approximately equally efficacious; despite their obvious differences in potency, both produce the same maximal therapeutic effect. In Figure 2–6 two analgesic drugs are shown, oxycodone and nefopam, that differ in their efficacies. The property of efficacy has legal as well as therapeutic importance. The 1962 Kefauver-Harris amendments to the Federal Food, Drug, and Cosmetics Act require *proof of efficacy* of a drug before it can be marketed. Before that time only *evidence of safety* was needed.

POTENCY VERSUS EFFICACY

Consistent usage of the terms potency and efficacy as they are defined previously is recommended. However, confusion may arise when either speaker or listener attaches to potency the common English definition of potent as "the capability of causing strong physiological or chemical effects, as medicines or alcoholic beverages." Occasionally, the intent is to deceive, e.g., a salesperson may impute greater efficacy to a drug that is merely more potent; more often it is simple ignorance. For example, heroin is approximately three times as potent as morphine. This has at various times been misinterpreted to the general public as meaning that heroin is three times as effective as morphine in the relief of pain and that pain-sufferers are being denied a dramatically more effective analgesic because of the unapproved status of heroin in the United States. In fact, heroin and morphine are of approximately equal efficacy.

Few drugs are of such low potency that the sheer physical bulk of the administered drug presents a problem. Thus, potency *per se* is rarely of clinical significance.

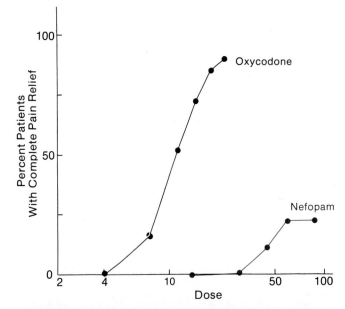

Figure 2–6

Dose-response relationships for oxycodone and another analgesic (nefopam) in relieving pain in human subjects. Abscissa: Dose plotted on a log scale. Ordinate: Percent of patients responding with complete relief of pain. (Redrawn from Tigerstedt I, Tammisto T, Leander P: Comparison of the analgesic dose-effect relationships of nefopam and oxycodone in postoperative pain. Acta Anaesthesiol Scand 23:555–560, 1979.)

Pharmacology was defined in Chapter 1 as dealing with the interactions of chemicals with biological systems. However, concomitant with actions on biological systems, two drugs may interact with each other. Drug *interaction* is the term applied to this phenomenon. Although the possible mechanisms by which drug interactions may arise are quite varied, the consequences of such interactions are rather simply categorized. Two drugs may interact in a variety of ways to produce a change in the effects of one or the other or both. When the effects are additive or supra-additive, the terms *summation* and *potentiation* are used. The phenomenon in which the effects of two drugs are less than predicted from their effects alone is called *antagonism*. The previously introduced concepts of affinity and intrinsic activity together with a consideration of possible bonds formed between drug and receptor provide a rational basis for the several types of antagonism that have been observed.

SUMMATION OR ADDITIVITY

When the effects of two drugs given at the same time are exactly as would have been predicted from the sum of their effects when given alone, we speak of summation or, alternatively, additivity. In effect, summation occurs only when drugs do not interact. Although summation is conceptually simple, this phenomenon is less common than one might expect, and it should never be assumed to occur.

POTENTIATION

The observation that the effects of two drugs are greater than would have been predicted from their effects in isolation is called potentiation or, alternatively, synergism. A classic example of potentiation is provided by the sympathomimetic effects of tyramine in the presence of a monoamine oxidase (MAO) inhibitor. Tyramine acts on presynaptic storage sites to release norepinephrine, which then causes an increase in blood pressure. Because MAO is a major regulator of the presynaptic stores, inhibition of the enzyme causes more norepinephrine to be available for release by tyramine. In addition, there is evidence that MAO inhibitors decrease the metabolic inactivation of tyramine. Thus, in patients treated with an MAO inhibitor for depression, a warning must be given against eating foods high in tyramine.

ANTAGONISM

The phenomenon in which the effects of two drugs are less than predicted from their effects when given alone is called *antagonism*. The term *pharmacological antagonism* usually refers to diminution of a drug's effects at a common receptor site. Clearly, the effects of a drug may be diminished in a number of other ways. In principle, any antidote may be regarded as an antagonist. Examples include diminution of *absorption* of a toxin by its *adsorption* on activated charcoal or the inactivation of heavy metals by chelating agents. In addition, a drug that produces a pharmacologically opposite effect, but at a different site, may be regarded as an antagonist. For example, norepinephrine and acetylcholine are mutually antagonistic in terms of heart rate by effects at pharmacologically distinct sites in the sinoatrial node. Similarly, histamine and norepinephrine produce opposite effects on blood pressure through their effects on independent adrenergic and histaminergic receptors on smooth muscle of blood vessels. The phenomenon in which two drugs are antagonistic because of opposing effects arising at distinct sites is sometimes called *physiological antagonism*.

Drug Interactions: Summation, Potentiation, Antagonism

Adsorption is not absorption and vice versa.

Agonist
Antagonist

Both agonists and antagonists may bind to a receptor.

Although both physiological antagonism and the use of agents such as activated charcoal are of clinical significance, they are not representative of true *pharmacological antagonism*. This term is reserved for the phenomenon in which two drugs interact either directly or indirectly with a common receptor to produce a diminished total effect. The concepts of affinity and intrinsic activity allow us to rationalize such interactions.

An *agonist* is a drug that has affinity for a receptor and intrinsic activity at that receptor. In contrast, an *antagonist* is a drug that has affinity for the receptor but is devoid of intrinsic activity; formation of the antagonist-receptor complex does not directly produce a pharmacological response. Several types of antagonist-receptor interaction are known and provide the basis for subtypes of pharmacological antagonism.

Surmountable Antagonism

The interaction of closely related analogs provides an illustration of *surmountable antagonism* (Fig. 2–7). The agonist succinylcholine has both an affinity for the receptor and intrinsic activity at the receptor, as evidenced by the dose-related contraction of frog muscle that it produces. In the presence of a specific antagonist the agonist is still able to cause contraction, but a higher concentration of the agonist is required for any given degree of contraction. We may assume that the antagonist functions by virtue of its affinity for the acetylcholine receptor together with its lack of intrinsic activity at that receptor. Furthermore, we may assume that the relationship of agonist and antagonist at the receptor is strictly competitive; at any instant the proportion of receptors occupied by the agonist and by the antagonist is a function of the concentrations of each of the two agents in the vicinity of the receptor. Hence, the effects of the antagonist may be reversed simply by increasing the concentration of agonist to a sufficient degree.

The terms *reversible antagonism* and *competitive antagonism* are sometimes regarded as being synonymous with surmountable antagonism. However, because "reversible" and "competitive" have had associated with them a variety of mechanistic implications, the purely phenomenological term *surmountable* is preferred.

Figure 2–7

Surmountable antagonism. The dose-response relationship for succinylcholine alone and in the presence of its ethyl analog. Abscissa: Molar concentration expressed on a log scale. Ordinate: Percent of maximal contraction of frog rectus abdominis. (Data from Ariens EJ, Simonis AM, Van Rossum JM: *In* Ariens EJ (ed): Molecular Pharmacology: The Mode of Action of Biologically Active Compounds. Vol 1, 151. New York: Academic Press, 1964.)

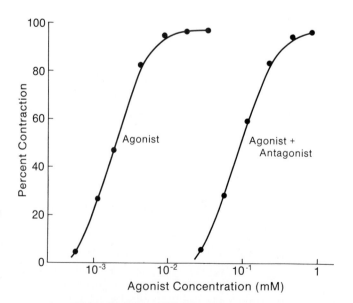

Insurmountable Antagonism

A classic example of this type of antagonism is provided by the interaction of epinephrine and dibenamine. In Figure 2–8 it is seen that epinephrine causes contraction of an isolated strip of cat spleen. However, in the presence of dibenamine, the maximal possible degree of contraction is reduced. This type of interaction may be rationalized on the basis of the occupancy assumption and the irreversible inactivation of the receptor by the antagonist. Thus, if dibenamine interacts with the epinephrine receptor in such a fashion that it is removed from the pool of receptors available to epinephrine, the occupancy assumption predicts that the maximal effect will be reduced.

Partial Agonists

So far we have assumed that an agonist produces the maximal possible effect, i.e., its intrinsic activity (i.a.) is 1.0. On the other hand, antagonists have been assumed to produce no agonistic effects; their intrinsic activity is 0.0. Such drugs are sometimes called *full agonists* (i.a. = 1.0) and *pure antagonists* (i.a. = 0.0), respectively. These qualifying terms are used because, as we saw in Figure 2–4, some drugs — those with intrinsic activities intermediate between 0.0 and 1.0 — produce less than full agonistic effects,

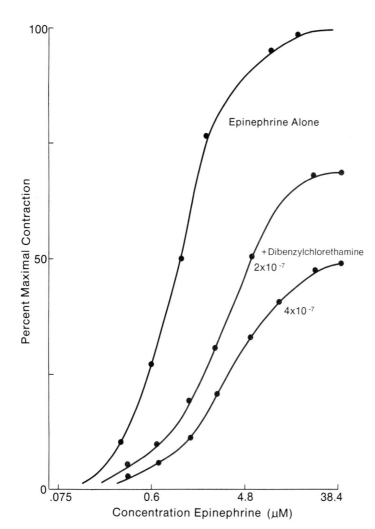

Figure 2–8

Insurmountable antagonism. The dose-response relationship for epinephrine alone and in the presence of Dibenamine. Abscissa: Concentration plotted on a log scale. Ordinate: Percent of maximal contraction of isolated cat spleen. (Redrawn from Bickerton RK: The response of isolated strips of cat spleen to sympathomimetic drugs and their antagonists. J Pharmacol Exp Ther 142:99–110, 1963, © by American Society for Pharmacology and Experimental Therapeutics.)

Figure 2–9

Hypothetical dose-response relationships for a full agonist (A), a mixed agonist/antagonist (B), and the two drugs in combination. Abscissa: Concentration expressed on a log scale. Ordinate: Percent of maximal effect.

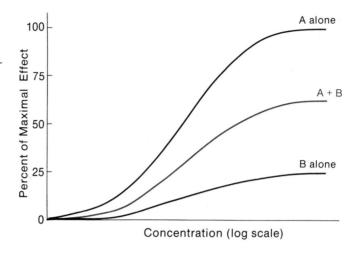

Partial agonist

hence the term *partial agonist.* In addition, consideration of Figures 2–9 and 2–10 reveal that such drugs not only are partial agonists but may serve as *partial antagonists* as well.

For simplicity's sake, the drugs shown in Figure 2–9 are assumed to bind reversibly to a common receptor. They are further assumed to have equal affinity for the receptor and intrinsic activities of 1.0 and 0.25, respectively. Thus, drug A will produce 100% of the maximal response when given alone and drug B will produce 25% of the maximal. However, when both are present at the same time in maximally effective concentrations, the modified occupancy assumption predicts that less than the maximal effect will result. The reason is that one half of the receptors will be occupied by drug A yielding 50% of the maximal effect and one half of the receptors will be occupied by drug B, which contributes 12.5% of the maximal effect. The sum of the two is 62.5% response. In this situation, drug B partially antagonizes drug A.

Figure 2–10 provides experimental evidence in support of the preceding interpretation of the action of partial agonists. The data shown were obtained in drug interaction experiments in rats trained to discriminate

Figure 2–10

The effects of a partial agonist alone and in combination with a full agonist. Rats were trained to discriminate the effects of 3.0 mg of morphine from those of saline solution. *Closed circles:* Nalorphine alone. *Open squares:* Nalorphine in the presence of 3.0 mg of morphine. Ordinate: Trials to the morphine lever as morphine-appropriate responses. Abscissa: Dose of nalorphine. (Redrawn from Holtzman SG: Discriminative stimulus properties of opioid agonists and antagonists. *In* Cooper SJ (ed): Theory in Psychopharmacology. Vol 2. London: Academic Press, 1983.)

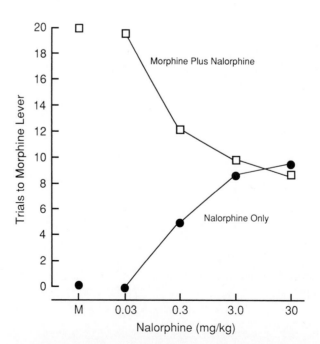

between saline solution and 3 mg/kg morphine. When a range of doses of nalorphine is given, partial agonist activity is evident. However, when nalorphine is administered in combination with a fully effective dose of morphine, antagonism of morphine is observed.

As is discussed in detail in Chapter 18, considerable clinical significance attaches to partial agonists of the opioid, narcotic analgesic type. When opioid partial agonists are administered alone, they are effective pain relievers; when given in the presence of a complete opioid agonist, however, antagonistic effects may be observed.

The Therapeutic Index

A goal of pharmacological science is to discover drugs that possess efficacy but produce no adverse effects. That goal is but rarely achieved; undesired effects occur with all drugs at some dose. The relationship between adverse and beneficial effects is expressed by the *therapeutic index*. The response of an individual patient to a drug is influenced not only by the essential features of the drug but also by factors, especially genetic and immunological factors, peculiar to the patient.

SELECTIVITY

A drug is often classified in terms of its most prominent effect or the first effect attributed to it. Such descriptions should not obscure the fact that every drug produces multiple effects. Selectivity refers to the degree to which a drug acts upon a given site relative to all possible sites of interaction (Albert, 1979). Thus, a drug is characterized adequately only when its full spectrum of activities — pharmacological, therapeutic, and toxic — is considered.

THERAPEUTIC INDEX

A simple means to provide a quantitative assessment of the relative benefits and risks of a drug is to divide the dose that produces toxic effects by the dose that produces the desired therapeutic effect. Thus, for a drug that induces sleep in 50% of the treated population at a dose of 1.5 mg/kg and induces death at a dose of 1500 mg/kg, we get a ratio of 1500/1.5, and the drug is said to have a therapeutic index of 1000. The 50%-effective dose is often chosen because this represents the most reliable portion of the dose-response curves. For the therapeutic effect, the 50%-effective dose is called the ED_{50} (the median effective dose) and, for the median toxic effect, the TD_{50}. Thus, in our example, the therapeutic index (T.I.) = TD_{50}/ED_{50}. Where the toxic effect is lethal, the TD_{50} is alternatively designated the LD_{50}. (For example, the LD_{50} is a commonly determined measure of toxicity in experimental animals.)

Therapeutic index, margin of safety, and benefit/risk ratio reflect the same general concept.

MULTIPLE THERAPEUTIC INDICES

Textbooks of pharmacology will be searched in vain for a table listing the therapeutic indices for a series of drugs; such a table does not exist. The reason is simple: no drug has but a single toxic effect, and many drugs have more than one therapeutic effect. Every drug, then, has not one but many possible therapeutic indices, each one of which considers a specific therapeutic effect and a specific toxic effect and perhaps each of these in a specific patient population. For example, Figure 2–11 shows a therapeutic and a toxic effect of digitoxin. It is obvious that such data do not permit neat, single-value expressions of a therapeutic index for digitoxin. In this light we see the therapeutic index not as a single, unchanging number but

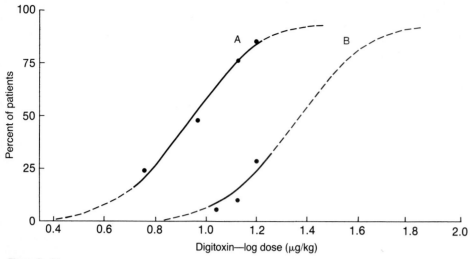

Figure 2–11

Therapeutic index. Dose-response relation-ships for a therapeutic effect *(A)* and a toxic effect of vomiting *(B)* of digitoxin in patients with auricular fibrillation. Abscissa: Dose expressed on a log scale. Ordinate: Percent of patients responding. (Redrawn from Marsh DF: Outline of Fundamental Pharmacology, 28, 1951. Courtesy of Charles C Thomas, Publisher, Springfield, Illinois.)

Figure 2–12

Log dose-response curve as a cumulative normal frequency distribution of sensitivities of the individual responsive units. (Reprinted with permission of Macmillan Publishing Company from Biostatistics by Avram Goldstein. Copyright © 1964 Avram Goldstein.)

as a more general expression of the relation between the good (desirable) and the bad (undesirable) effects of drugs. Other terms expressing relationships between desirable and toxic effects are the *benefit/risk ratio* and the *margin of safety.*

HETEROGENEITY OF THE PATIENT POPULATION

Students are familiar with the practice of "grading on a curve"; the frequency of occurrence of specific numerical values is plotted versus the range of possible values, and letter grades are assigned to various parts of the distribution. If a smooth line connecting the points is bell-shaped, the data are said to follow a normal or gaussian distribution. In nature it is observed often that a normal distribution is more closely approximated

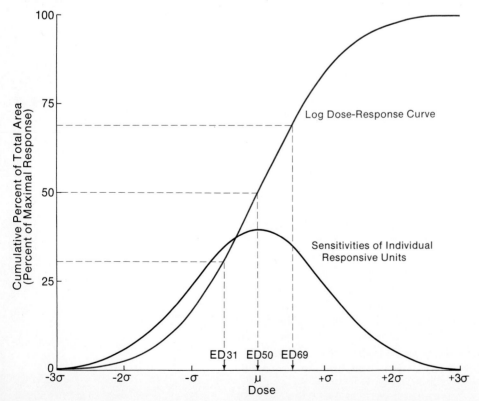

when a logarithmic rather than an arithmetic scale is employed; the data are then said to be *log-normally* distributed.

As shown in Figure 2–12, dose-response curves so far considered may be regarded as cumulative frequency curves for a log-normally distributed population. The practical consequence is that the response of isolated tissues to drugs is proportional to the logarithm of drug concentration (e.g., Fig. 2–1). Furthermore, it is observed often that the data that express the pharmacological response of subjects within a patient population are normalized when dose is expressed on a log scale (e.g., Fig. 2–5). However, therapeutically significant exceptions are known in which sensitivity to drugs follows neither a normal nor a log-normal distribution.

Pharmacogenetics

The variation in drug sensitivity within a population is assumed to be largely genetic in origin. Often these sources of variation are sufficiently subtle that no subpopulations can be discerned and the sensitivity distribution is represented adequately by a log-normal curve. Pharmacogenetics is concerned, in general, with genetic influences upon drug sensitivity and, in particular, with those instances where distinct subpopulations can be identified.

Drug Allergy

A particularly important form of nonhomogeneous sensitivity to drug effects is mediated by the immune systems of the body. The manifestations of drug allergy range from mild skin irritation to lethal anaphylactic shock. Drug allergy is discussed in detail in Chapter 64.

References

Albert A: Selective Toxicity, The Physico-chemical Basis of Therapy. 6th ed. New York: Halsted, 1979.

Black JW, Leff P: Operational models of pharmacological agonism. Proc R Soc Lond [Bibl] 220:141–162, 1983.

Clark AJ: General Pharmacology. Vol 4 of Handbuch der experimentellen Pharmakologie. Berlin: Springer-Verlag, 1937.

Holtzman SG: Discriminative stimulus properties of opioid agonists and antagonists. *In* Cooper SJ (ed): Theory in Psychopharmacology. Vol 2. London: Academic Press, 1983.

Kenakin TP: The classification of drugs and drug receptors in isolated tissues. Pharmacol Rev 36:165–222, 1984.

3

Drug Absorption, Distribution, and Termination of Action

Jerrold C. Winter

Drug Absorption

The movement of a drug from its site of application into the blood is called drug absorption. In general, the process may be diffusion or active transport and the barriers to that movement are largely lipid in nature. For this reason, the degree of solubility of a drug in lipid is an important factor in its absorption. The lipid solubility of many drugs, so-called weak acids and bases, is influenced by the pH of the aqueous media that they encounter. Drug absorption may be influenced also by the way in which the drug is formulated. Thus, when therapeutically indicated, a low rate of release and a prolonged period of absorption may be achieved.

In some therapeutic situations, drugs are applied directly to the sites at which they are to act. For example, an antibiotic-containing ointment may be spread over a break in the skin. More often, the receptors to which drugs are directed are located at a distance from the site of application of the drug. For example, the acetylsalicylic acid contained in a swallowed aspirin tablet must somehow make its way to the brain and tissues of the head if headache is to be relieved. The two general processes involved are *absorption*, the movement of drug into the blood from its site of application, and *distribution*, the movement of drug from the blood to its site(s) of action or storage.

PHYSIOLOGICAL FACTORS IN DRUG ABSORPTION

For purposes of considering drug absorption, the human body may be regarded as a series of water-filled sacks made of fat, or put another way, a series of aqueous media separated by lipid barriers. Figure 3–1 provides a general scheme.

Consider again an aspirin tablet taken by mouth. The solid tablet must dissolve in the aqueous environment of the stomach and small intestine, i.e., water solubility is required. Molecules in solution now encounter a lipid barrier to absorption, the epithelial lining of the gastrointestinal (GI) tract. Because there is no active transport system for aspirin, passage of the drug through that barrier requires lipid solubility. Having passed the epithelial barrier, drug molecules again encounter an aqueous medium, the extracellular fluid, which in turn bathes the endothelial barrier presented by the capillary wall. In fact, capillary walls in the peripheral circulation are so porous that even lipid-insoluble materials can pass through into the blood. At this point, molecules of acetylsalicylic acid have passed from the mouth to the blood; they have been absorbed.

PHYSICOCHEMICAL FACTORS IN DRUG ABSORPTION

The influence of physicochemical factors on drug absorption depends to a significant degree upon the site to which the drug is applied. For drugs that

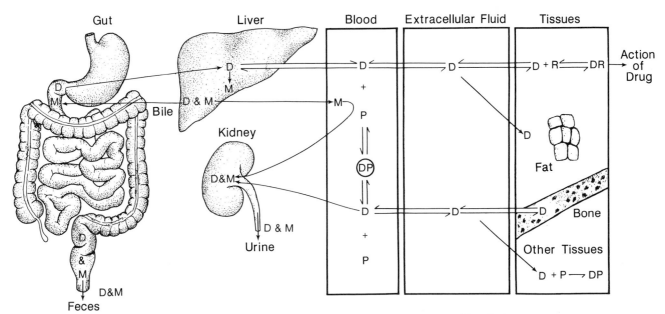

Figure 3-1

Schematic representation of what may happen to a drug, D, in the body. (M = metabolites; P = plasma protein; R = receptor.) (Courtesy of DS Riggs.)

must cross the skin or the epithelial lining of the GI tract, lipid solubility is of great importance. For drugs placed in the vicinity of the peripheral capillary beds of muscles or other tissues, lipid solubility is of minor importance; even most ionized species cross with ease. Indeed, the capillary wall is of sufficient porosity that even drugs with molecular weights as great as 60,000 may be absorbed by passive diffusion.

Lipid-Water Partition Coefficient

A measure of the distribution of a drug between a lipid and an aqueous phase is provided by the lipid-water partition coefficient. Thus, a coefficient of 1 means that a drug is as soluble in a nonpolar solvent, such as heptane, as in water, a polar solvent. Highly lipid-soluble materials, such as the barbiturate thiopental, have coefficients much greater than 1 and readily cross lipid barriers. In contrast, materials that are quite insoluble in both polar and nonpolar media are pharmacologically inert. For example, barium sulfate is a highly toxic material if absorbed, but because of its poor solubility it can be introduced into the GI tract as an x-ray contrast medium without hazard.

Ionization of Drugs

In general, the ionized form of a drug is less lipid-soluble and more water-soluble than the nonionized form. The degree to which many drugs are ionized is influenced by the hydrogen ion content (pH) of any aqueous medium in which they are placed. In a limited but significant number of instances in pharmacology and toxicology, the distribution of a drug between its ionized and nonionized forms can be influenced by manipulation of the pH of bodily fluids. Such drugs are referred to as weak acids and weak bases.

Most are accustomed to regarding as acids those substances that yield hydrogen ions (protons) upon dissociation, and as bases those substances that yield hydroxyl ions. In considering drugs as acids and bases, we define an acid as a substance that in its uncharged form is a proton donor. A base, in contrast, is a substance that in its uncharged form is a proton acceptor. Thus, both acids and bases may exist in a proton donor and in a proton acceptor form.

The dissociation of an acid is given by

$$AH \rightleftharpoons A^- + H^+$$

and of a base by

$$BH^+ \rightleftharpoons B + H^+$$

For each, the proton donor or acid form is written on the left.

A distinction must also be made between "strong" acids and bases and "weak" acids and bases. The degree of dissociation of a strong acid like hydrochloric acid or of a strong base like sodium hydroxide is not influenced by the pH changes normally encountered in physiological systems. Thus, weak acids and bases are defined as those whose dissociation can be altered by pH differences compatible with the function of biological systems.

Weak acids
Weak bases

The Henderson-Hasselbalch Equation. Problems regarding the influence of pH upon weak acids and bases may be solved using the Henderson-Hasselbalch equation, which is derived as follows:

$$acid \rightleftharpoons base + H^+$$

The acid dissociation constant is expressed as

$$K_a \rightleftharpoons [base]\,[H^+]/[acid]$$

Thus,

$$H^+ = K_a\,\{[acid]/[base]\}$$
$$pH = pK_a - \log[acid]/[base]$$
$$pH - pK_a = \log[base]/[acid]$$

When $pH = pK_a$, $\log[base]/[acid] = 0$. Because antilog $0 = 1$, the ratio of the concentrations of base to acid is unity, i.e., equal concentrations of each.

The Intuitive Approach. Although the Henderson-Hasselbalch equation may be used directly to solve problems involving weak acids and weak bases, many students prefer an alternative procedure. One simply writes the equation for the acid dissociation of the weak acid or base and applies the principle of Le Chatelier: if the conditions of a system, originally in equilibrium, are changed, the equilibrium will shift in such a direction as to tend to restore the original conditions.

For example, a weak acid

$$AH \rightleftharpoons A^- + H^+$$

Some pK_as of common drugs:
  morphine (base) 9.85
  barbital (acid) 7.43
  cocaine (base) 5.59

when $pH = pK_a$, $[AH] = [A^-]$ (our initial equilibrium). However, when $pH < pK_a$, i.e., when the concentration of H^+ is greater at equilibrium, the reaction will shift to the left and AH will be greater than A^-. The numerical value of the ratio is given by the antilog of the absolute value of the difference between pH and pK_a, i.e.,

$$AH/A^- = antilog\,|pH - pK_a|$$

Similarly, when pH > pK_a, i.e., when the concentration of H^+ is less at equilibrium, the reaction will shift to the right and A^- will be greater than AH. The ratio of A^-/AH is then

$$A^-/AH = \text{antilog} \, |pH - pK_a|$$

The same reasoning applies to weak bases, but the starting equilibrium is given by

$$BH^+ = B + H^+$$

When pH is less than pK_a, the equilibrium is shifted to the left and $BH^+ > B$. Conversely, when pH is greater than pK_a, $B > BH^+$. Again the numerical values of the ratios are given by the antilog of the differences between pH and pK_a.

Consideration of these facts makes it clear that the consequences of a shift in pH away from equilibrium conditions are opposite for weak acids and weak bases. Thus, at a pH less than pK_a, the nonionized, more lipid-soluble form of a weak acid is favored, whereas it is the ionized, less lipid-soluble form of a weak base that is present in excess.

However, it must be kept in mind that the degree of ionization is but one factor in absorption. For example, a drug whose lipid-soluble form is favored in the acidic conditions of the stomach may nonetheless be absorbed almost entirely in the small intestine because of the much greater absorptive area of the latter organ.

CONTROL OF RATE OF ABSORPTION IN POISONING AND THERAPEUTICS

Rate of perfusion is a factor in drug absorption. When bitten on the hand by a poisonous snake, it is prudent to apply a tourniquet to the affected limb. The pertinent pharmacological principle is that the rate of absorption of a drug from its site of injection is proportional to the rate of blood flow past that site. In contrast to the physical application of a tourniquet, a pharmacological means to control blood flow is provided by vasoconstricting substances. Thus, for example, local anesthetic agents are administered often in combination with epinephrine. Local constriction of arterial vessels by epinephrine diminishes blood flow in the area, diminishes the amount of anesthetic absorbed, and thus diminishes the risk of systemic toxic effects.

Local blood flow and drug absorption

Drug Formulation

Often adequate therapeutic effects are critically dependent upon maintenance of appropriate blood and tissue levels of a drug. Because it is sometimes inconvenient or impractical to administer drugs on a schedule best suited to ensuring adequate blood levels, means of extending the period of absorption of drugs have been sought. In general these attempts have taken two forms: (1) chemical alteration of the drug itself and (2) the use of a supporting medium. An example of the former is provided by haloperidol. Intramuscular (IM) injection of the decanoate ester of the antipsychotic drug haloperidol provides a drug depot. Slow hydrolysis of the ester and release of the active drug permits a 4-week dosing interval.

Physical forms of drugs influence their pharmacological properties.

An alternative approach to sustained absorption of drugs is to place the drug in a medium from which the drug will diffuse slowly. A common site of application is the skin. Figure 3–2 shows a skin patch designed to deliver nitroglycerine over a period of 24 hours.

Figure 3-2

A cross-sectional diagram of a transdermal drug administration system for nitroglycerin. The trade-marked system, TRANSDERM-NITRO, is depicted. It consists of four layers. Proceeding from the top, externally visible surface toward the bottom surface that is attached to the skin: the Backing layer of aluminized plastic that is impermeable to nitroglycerin; the Drug Reservoir containing nitroglycerin adsorbed on lactose, colloidal silicon dioxide, and silicone medical fluid; an ethylene/vinyl acetate copolymer Semipermeable Membrane that is permeable to nitroglycerin; and a silicone Adhesive surface covered until use by a Protective Peel Strip.

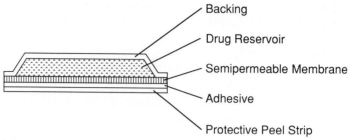

Backing

Drug Reservoir

Semipermeable Membrane

Adhesive

Protective Peel Strip

DRUG DISTRIBUTION

The general circulation carries drug molecules to every cell in the body.

Upon reaching the general circulation, either by direct injection or following absorption from another site, a drug is distributed throughout the body. The rate at which the drug leaves the blood and reaches extravascular locations and receptors is dependent upon a number of pharmacological and physiological factors. In general, capillary walls are sufficiently porous that lipid solubility is not a limiting factor in the passage of drugs into extracellular water. The capillaries of the brain are an exception; drugs with low lipid solubility and the ionized forms of drugs can cross the blood-brain barrier only slowly if at all.

Once a drug is absorbed into the general circulation, it can be expected to reach every cell in the body. This fact is often brought to our attention by the occurrence of adverse effects in tissues far removed from the intended site of therapeutic action. However, before a drug can act upon specific drug receptors, it must exit the blood. (An exception to this statement would be drugs intended to act upon receptors on the luminal side of blood vessels or on cells or proteins of the blood.) The factors that earlier were considered with respect to drug absorption will again be of importance.

GENERAL FACTORS IN DRUG DISTRIBUTION

Concentration Gradient

The rate at which a drug leaves the circulation is proportional to the concentration gradient of unbound drug from plasma to extracellular water.

Blood Flow

The quantity of drug that enters a given tissue is proportional to the rate of blood flow through that tissue.

Physicochemical Factors

For drugs with molecular weights less than about 60,000, the capillary wall presents no barrier to passage of drugs even if their lipid solubility is inherently low or they are in the ionized state. Capillaries of the central nervous system (CNS) are an exception (see The Blood-Brain Barrier.)

BINDING OF DRUGS TO PLASMA PROTEINS

A drug bound to plasma protein is pharmacologically inert.

Albumin is the principal protein of plasma in terms of drug binding. The molecular weight of plasma albumin is approximately 69,000. At pH 7.4, albumin is capable of interacting with both anions and cations. The interaction between drug and albumin is characterized in the same way as the drug-receptor interaction discussed above:

$$X + P \rightleftharpoons XP$$

Although the interaction is nearly always reversible, the half-life of the complex may range from less than a second to more than a year. Because the molecular weight of the complex exceeds 69,000, the complex cannot cross the capillary wall. While bound to plasma protein, a drug does not contribute to the concentration gradient, cannot be filtered by the kidney, and in general is pharmacologically inert. It should be noted, however, that the reversible binding of a drug to plasma protein may function as a reservoir that slowly releases the active agent.

RELATIVE PERMEABILITIES OF CAPILLARY BEDS

All capillary beds, with the exception of those found in the CNS, are sufficiently "leaky" to permit the passage of most unbound drug molecules even in the ionized state. Nonetheless, there are differences. The relative order of rates of permeability is generally taken to be as follows:

$$\text{liver} > \text{kidney} > \text{muscle} = \text{fetus (placental)} \gg \text{brain}$$

Without reliable evidence to the contrary, the existence of a "placental barrier" to drug distribution should never be assumed; drugs administered to pregnant women should be expected to reach the embryo or fetus.

Assume that drugs administered to a pregnant woman are given as well to her developing child.

THE BLOOD-BRAIN BARRIER

Capillaries in the CNS differ from all other capillaries in that cerebral endothelial cells have tight junctions between them. This is the morphological basis for what is termed the *blood-brain barrier.* In a few areas of the brain the barrier is absent. These include the lateral nuclei of the hypothalamus, the area postrema of the fourth ventricle, the pineal body, and the posterior lobe of the hypophysis.

The blood-brain barrier has the properties of a lipid barrier without pores. The consequences for drug distribution are that agents with inherently low lipid solubility as well as ionized forms of drugs are unable to exit the circulation and enter extracellular water of the brain. It must be noted, however, that for highly lipid-soluble drugs there is, in effect, no blood-brain barrier.

For lipid-soluble drugs, there is no blood-brain barrier.

Termination of Drug Action

It is to be expected that the effects of a drug upon the body will diminish with the passage of time. Any mechanism that diminishes drug concentration at its receptors will contribute to termination of drug action. Principal among these mechanisms are drug excretion, which may occur via several different routes, and drug metabolism to inactive products. Significant interactions may occur between disease states and the rates of drug metabolism and of drug excretion.

Earlier in this chapter, we assumed that most pharmacological effects are the consequence of a reversible interaction between a drug and its receptor and that the magnitude of the effect is proportional to the concentration of the drug-receptor complex. Thus, any process that diminishes the concentration of a drug in the vicinity of its receptor will contribute to the termination of the effects of the drug. Three major contributing factors must be considered: (1) drug redistribution or storage, (2) drug excretion, and (3) drug metabolism.

DRUG REDISTRIBUTION OR STORAGE

A prime example of the consequences of redistribution is provided by the short-acting barbiturate sodium thiopental. The nonionized form of this drug is highly lipid-soluble. When administered intravenously, the drug rapidly crosses the blood-brain barrier and produces anesthesia. However, as more thiopental enters poorly perfused tissues, such as subcutaneous fat, the blood levels of thiopental decline and a new equilibrium is established. As this slow loss to fat tissues occurs, the thiopental concentration gradient between blood and brain soon favors passage from brain to blood, and anesthesia is reversed.

It should be noted that body fat is not an unfillable sink and that with continuous administration of thiopental a new equilibrium will be achieved in which anesthetic levels of the drug will be maintained in the blood for an extended period of time. Other examples include fat-soluble agents, such as the insecticide DDT and the psychoactive drug tetrahydrocannabinol, which are detectable in the body long after a single exposure or administration.

The binding of drugs to plasma proteins is a form of drug storage in that bound drug is pharmacologically inert. Disease states such as hypoalbuminemia, in which the concentration of plasma protein is severely depressed, may contribute to elevated blood levels of drugs that are normally bound extensively to plasma protein.

Bone may provide a storage site for drugs as well as for toxic agents. When administered to children during the period of enamel formation, tetracyclines may be deposited in the bone and produce permanent discolorations of the teeth. Of more profound toxicological consequence is the deposition in bone of strontium 90, a product of nuclear fission reactions. A high-energy beta emitter with a half-life of 28 years, strontium 90 is a significant radiation hazard primarily because of its ability to mimic calcium in bone.

DRUG EXCRETION

Elimination of a drug from the body is an obvious means to terminate its pharmacological actions. Indeed, the effects of some drugs are diminished as a direct function of their rate of excretion. The major routes of excretion are considered briefly here.

> Some drugs and toxins are detectable in body fat for years after a single exposure.

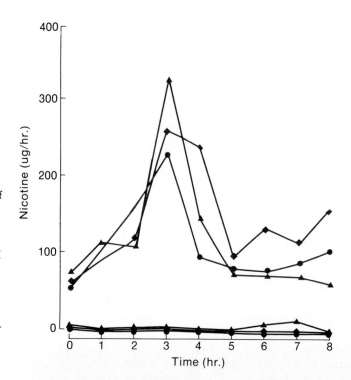

Figure 3-3

The effect of urinary pH on the excretion of nicotine when smoking a cigarette *(circles)* or chewing a gum containing 2 mg *(triangles)* or 4 mg *(squares)* of nicotine. The top graphs are for a urinary pH of 4.7–5.3, and the bottom graphs are for a urinary pH of 7.4–8.0. Abscissa: Time in hours. Ordinate: Micrograms of nicotine excreted per hour. (Redrawn from Feyerabend G, Russell MAH: Effect of urinary pH and nicotine excretion rate on plasma nicotine during cigarette smoking and chewing nicotine gum. Br J Clin Pharmacol 5:295, 1978, by permission of Blackwell Scientific Publications, Ltd.)

Renal Excretion

This is the major route by which drugs exit the body. Nearly all unbound drugs enter the glomerular filtrate. However, net renal excretion depends upon a complex interplay between active or passive reabsorption and tubular secretion. These are discussed in greater detail in Chapter 34.

The kidney as an organ of drug elimination

In general, the rate of renal excretion of a drug is a function of its pharmacological properties and its concentration in the blood together with the rate of urine production. The presence of impaired renal function necessitates a re-evaluation of drug dosages deemed appropriate for normal individuals.

The renal excretion of some weak acids and bases can be influenced significantly by alteration of the pH of the urine. This is illustrated in Figure 3–3. Acidification of the urine results in an increase in the rate of urinary excretion of nicotine, a weak base. The explanation is that a more acidic environment favors formation of the ionized, less lipid-soluble form of nicotine with a resultant decline in the amount that is passively reabsorbed following filtration. Conversely, renal excretion of weak acids is favored by more alkaline conditions.

Acidification of the urine favors the elimination of weak bases.

Biliary Excretion

Drugs present in the liver may be secreted along with bile into the duodenum. However, like the bile acids, drugs thus excreted may be reabsorbed along the length of the gut. Thus, net biliary excretion will depend upon the rate of subsequent reabsorption through the enterohepatic circulation.

Excretion by the Lungs

Detectable quantities of many drugs appear in expired air. Of greatest importance are the anesthetic gases (see Chapter 16). Successful inhalation anesthesia depends upon the passage of the gas from inspired air to the blood and thence to the brain and other sites of action. Reversal of this process results in recovery from anesthesia.

With the exception of the gaseous anesthetics, excretion of drugs by the lungs does not represent a major means of termination of drug *action*. However, analysis of the concentration of ethanol in expired air provides a noninvasive, widely used means to assess blood levels and, by inference, degree of intoxication with the drug.

Excretion in Other Fluids

All drugs, especially those with a high degree of water solubility, are excreted in tears, sweat, and breast milk. Loss of drugs in these fluids is not a significant factor in the termination of drug action. However, there is concern that toxic effects may arise in breast-fed infants. For this reason, all medications taken by nursing women should be regarded as potential hazards to their babies.

DRUG METABOLISM

Although some drugs are excreted unchanged, most undergo some degree of metabolic alteration in the body. Whereas drug metabolism occurs at many sites throughout the body, the most significant area quantitatively is the liver. In general, the product of metabolism is more water-soluble, hence more readily excreted through the kidney, and less active pharmacologically than is the parent drug.

The liver as an organ of drug metabolism

A few drugs are converted metabolically from inactive to active forms.

The classic example of such activation was provided by Gerhard Domagk. He found that PRONTOSIL, inactive against streptococci *in vitro,* was an effective antistreptococcal agent *in vivo.* The active metabolic product of PRONTOSIL was later shown to be sulfanilamide. For his discoveries, Domagk received the Nobel Prize in Medicine for 1939.

Drug metabolism is discussed in detail in Chapter 6.

Routes of Administration

Jerrold C. Winter

4

Drugs may be introduced into the body in a variety of ways; among the more common methods of administration are by swallowing the drug and by injection. The route of administration that is chosen may have a profound effect upon the speed and efficiency with which the drug acts. In addition, adverse effects due both to the drug itself and to the medium of administration are influenced by route. For example, the risk of viral and bacterial infection is maximized when drugs are administered intravenously.

The relative importance of the various physiological and physicochemical factors outlined previously may be profoundly influenced by the way in which a drug is introduced into the body. Traditionally, the so-called routes of administration have been divided into two major classes: enteral, referring to the intestine, and parenteral, meaning other than the intestine. As we shall see, a dichotomous classification of the possible routes of drug administration is simplistic and may be misleading.

For the purposes of this discussion, the gastrointestinal (GI) tract will be assumed to run from mouth to rectum. A major advantage of administering drugs through the GI tract is that the concomitant risk of viral and bacterial infection is minimized. The precise route that a drug follows from the GI tract to the general circulation is influenced significantly by the site within the GI tract from which the drug is absorbed.

The Gastrointestinal Tract

ORAL ADMINISTRATION

Drugs placed in the mouth and swallowed are said to have been taken "by mouth" or in Latin, *per os*. Hence, the abbreviation p.o. refers to the oral route. It should be noted that swallowing the drug is implicit in oral administration. Drugs that are simply placed in the mouth and held there are absorbed in a significantly different fashion (see later in this chapter). Although the stomach is not usually regarded as a major organ of absorption, significant amounts of small, lipid-soluble molecules may be absorbed across the stomach wall. Ascorbic acid is an example. The acidic conditions typical of the stomach favor the uncharged, lipid-soluble, proton-donor form of ascorbic acid.

ORAL ADMINISTRATION AND THE FIRST-PASS EFFECT

Drugs absorbed from the small intestine following oral administration enter the hepatic portal circulation and thus may be acted upon by hepatic enzymes prior to reaching the general circulation. The alteration of a drug by liver enzymes is commonly referred to as the *first-pass effect*. Occasion-

The first-pass effect

ally, the inactivation of drugs in the first-pass effect is of such magnitude that an alternative route of administration is required. Although the first-pass effect specifically refers to hepatic inactivation, the concept is sometimes extended to include gastric and intestinal inactivation as well.

OTHER ENTERAL ROUTES OF ADMINISTRATION

Sublingual Administration

Passage of drugs across mucosal membranes

Drugs placed in the mouth and held beneath the tongue are said to be administered *sublingually*. The mucosal lining of the oral cavity presents a lipid barrier to absorption. However, for drugs with high lipid solubility, the sublingual route is appropriate. For example, nitroglycerin tablets placed beneath the tongue quickly produce plasma levels of the drug adequate for the relief of the chest pain of angina pectoris. In addition, absorption is not through the hepatic portal circulation, so that the first-pass effect is avoided. More recently, morphine has been formulated for what has been called *buccal administration* (Latin *bucca:* cheek). Absorption of the drug, placed between the cheek and the gum, is prolonged and the first-pass effect avoided.

Rectal Administration

The mucosal lining of the rectum provides a relatively convenient site for drug administration. The principles involved are similar to those described previously for the oral mucosa. The first-pass effect is avoided to a significant degree, but the exact extent depends on the area of the rectal mucosa from which the drug is absorbed. The inferior and middle rectal veins drain directly to the general circulation, but the superior rectal vein enters the hepatic portal circulation. Rectal administration of drugs is often employed in infants and young children, in patients unable to take drugs by mouth, and in situations in which protracted vomiting makes oral administration ineffective.

Drug Administration by Injection

Although humans have taken crude drugs by mouth throughout history, administration by injection was made possible only in the last century by the invention of the hypodermic needle. With the availability of thin, hollow needles, drugs could be deposited in various tissues as well as into the general circulation. Such routes are commonly referred to as *parenteral*.

INJECTION INTO THE BLOOD

The invention of thin, hollow needles made possible the injection of drugs directly into the blood.

By direct injection of drugs into the general circulation, all barriers to absorption are bypassed. The onset of drug action is rapid, and between-patient variability associated with absorption is reduced to a minimum. Unfortunately, these advantages are offset to a significant degree by an increased probability of adverse effects, including infection (see later in this chapter).

Intravenous Administration

The close control of plasma levels made possible by this route are such that an intravenous (IV) line is established routinely in many emergency and inpatient situations. In addition, discrete IV injection is performed often when rapid onset of drug action is essential or in patients in whom a drug is especially irritant to tissue when given by other parenteral routes.

Intra-arterial Administration

This route is chosen much less commonly than the IV. Its use is restricted almost entirely to regional perfusion of an area with a particularly toxic agent, a not uncommon situation in cancer chemotherapy, and to diagnostic procedures. In the latter case, a radiopaque material is injected intra-arterially to visualize the vascular system of the brain, heart, or other organ.

INJECTION INTO OTHER SITES

In addition to direct placement of drugs in the general circulation, injections into muscle or beneath the skin are common. In contrast with IV or intra-arterial administration, all barriers to absorption are not bypassed and, as a result, considerable variation in the magnitude and time of onset of drug effects is to be expected. Contrary to popular belief, the rate and efficiency of drug absorption following intramuscular or subcutaneous injection may be greater than, equal to, or less than that following oral administration, depending on the drug under consideration.

Subcutaneous Injection

Because the drug has direct access to skin capillaries, absorption is usually quick and efficient. However, the rate of absorption is proportional to blood flow in the area of injection. A number of drugs are specifically formulated for subcutaneous (SC) injection.

Intramuscular Injection

A large muscle such as the deltoid or gluteus maximus is chosen usually. As is the case with SC administration, blood flow in the area of injection is a major factor in rate of absorption. Ready access to muscle capillaries is generally assumed, but more recent studies indicate that this is not necessarily the case. Thus, for example, in grossly obese patients, presumed intramuscular (IM) injections may in fact be intralipomatous. Because of the relatively low rate of perfusion of fat by the blood, a lower rate of absorption is predicted from fat than from muscle. In addition, there is some evidence that rate of drug absorption may be influenced by the particular muscle chosen for injection. However, the clinical consequences of these and other variables are poorly defined. For example, massage or muscle activity can sometimes significantly increase the rate of absorption.

It was noted previously that drugs are not necessarily more rapidly or more efficiently absorbed following IM injection than when given by mouth. The clearest example of this fact is provided by certain of the benzodiazepines, such as diazepam and chlordiazepoxide. The most likely explanation is poor solubility in water coupled with drug-induced irritation at the site of injection. This interpretation is supported by reports by patients of significant pain at the site of injection.

Some drugs are delivered more efficiently by mouth than by IM injection.

Epidural and Intrathecal Injection

Induction of spinal anesthesia by injection of drugs in the vicinity of the spinal cord has a long history. However, the discovery of opiate receptors in the spinal cord has led to a greatly expanded use of the epidural and intrathecal routes in the treatment of pain. For example, one anticipated advantage of intrathecal administration of morphine is the ability to use doses sufficiently small that only insignificant amounts of the drug reach other areas of the central nervous system (CNS).

Other Routes of Drug Administration

THE RESPIRATORY TRACT

A number of drugs are used for their local effects upon the lungs. For example, an acute asthmatic attack may be treated by inhalation of an aerosol containing a beta-adrenergic agonist. However, because of their large surface area and proximity to the pulmonary circulation, the lungs also provide an efficient means for drug absorption. Lipid-soluble, readily volatilized drugs rapidly reach pharmacologically significant levels in the blood after introduction into the lungs. The anesthetic gases represent the most common class of therapeutic agent administered in this way (see Chapter 16). In addition, however, a number of drugs used primarily in a nonmedical setting for their pleasurable effects may be inhaled after volatilization. Included in the latter group are the free-base forms of nicotine, tetrahydrocannabinol, phencyclidine, cocaine, and heroin. As is the case with nicotine-containing cigarettes, significant pathological effects on lung tissue may be caused by tars and other substances inhaled together with the desired pharmacological agent.

THE SKIN

The skin is not an impermeable barrier to drug absorption.

Although the stratum corneum provides an effective barrier to the absorption of many drugs, it has long been known that systemic toxic effects may arise following exposure of large areas of the skin to agents such as the organophosphate insecticides. In more recent years, therapeutic use has been made of the ability of lipid-soluble drugs to reach capillaries beneath the skin. When administered in this way, the route of administration is referred to as *transdermal, transcutaneous,* or *percutaneous.* Drugs available at present for transdermal delivery include nitroglycerin, scopolamine, clonidine, and some beta-adrenergic antagonists.

Comparative Advantages and Disadvantages of Enteral, Parenteral, and Other Routes of Administration

No single method of drug administration is ideal for all drugs in all circumstances. Because of the chemical and pharmacological properties of some drugs, certain methods of administration are ineffective, inefficient, or hazardous. Examples include insulin and other readily digested drugs for which a parenteral route is required; in contrast, a number of drugs are not available in parenteral form and must be given by mouth. When the use of a specific route of administration is contraindicated, that fact will be specified in the prescribing information provided by the manufacturer.

In many instances, drugs are available in a variety of formulations that provide the opportunity to employ several different routes of administration. Selection of the most appropriate route must take into account a number of factors, some general in nature, others specific to an individual patient.

COMPLIANCE

There are many reasons why drugs are not taken as prescribed.

It is assumed often that once a drug is prescribed, it will be taken faithfully as directed. Studies of patient compliance with prescribed directions have found this expectation to be unfulfilled in a significant proportion of the patient population. A low rate of compliance is particularly likely when (1) the patient is impaired by mental retardation, dementia, or psychiatric illness; (2) the patient is impaired by paralysis, arthritis, or other physical conditions; (3) the drug provides no readily perceived beneficial effect as, for example, the prophylactic use of antibiotics; (4) the drug must be taken frequently or at odd times during the day or night (once-a-day administration is preferable when possible); and (5) the immediate adverse effects of the drug make the patient feel worse despite a beneficial therapeutic effect. Factor 5 is illustrated by some antihypertensive agents currently in use and, most dramatically, by a number of drugs used in the treatment of cancer.

The probability of patient compliance with a prescribed drug regimen is enhanced by systematic education of the patient with respect to the expected benefits of a given drug as well as the adverse effects that may be expected. Too often it is erroneously assumed either that the patient is already aware of the relevant facts regarding her or his pharmacological treatment or that the patient is incapable of understanding simple explanations and instructions.

In those instances when adequate compliance is deemed unlikely, drugs may be administered by mouth in the presence of a health professional, or more commonly, the drug is administered by injection. An example of the latter case is provided by the outpatient maintenance of schizophrenic patients in which a slowly absorbed form of an antipsychotic drug is injected intramuscularly or subcutaneously at 2-week or longer intervals. Conversely, when the probability of compliance is high, the oral route of administration is unsurpassed in terms of convenience and safety.

RISK OF INFECTION

The degree to which barriers to absorption are bypassed is correlated positively with the risk of bacterial or viral infection. Thus, the oral route rarely presents a hazard in this regard, whereas IV administration requires strict adherence to sterile technique. Extensive information regarding infection following parenteral administration has gratuitously been provided by some groups of drug abusers: a SC or IV route is often employed; unsterile drugs, syringes, and needles commonly are used; and there is a tradition of sharing among users.

Nonmedical injection of drugs presents a high risk of infection.

In addition to infection at or in close proximity to the site of injection, bacterial endocarditis and viral hepatitis have long been recognized. More recently, transfer of the human immunodeficiency virus (HIV) and subsequent development of the acquired immunodeficiency syndrome (AIDS) have been demonstrated.

EFFICIENCY OF ABSORPTION

Multiple factors contribute to variation in rate and extent of drug absorption between individuals. The degree of variation is influenced by the route of administration that is chosen. It is reasonable to assume that variation is greatest for drugs taken by the oral route and that variation is reduced to zero by IV administration.

Variability in absorption of drugs

For drugs taken by mouth, sources of intrapatient and interpatient variability include pH of the stomach and intestine, gastric emptying time, and the presence or absence of food in the GI tract. Manufacturer's prescribing information stipulates usually the most appropriate relationship among meals, fluids, and the taking of specific drugs (see Chapter 64 regarding food-drug interactions). This information should diligently be passed on to the patient, because this is a common source of uncertainty, confusion, and anxiety.

It previously was noted that IM injection of drugs does not eliminate variability in absorption. Gauge and length of the needle chosen, depth of injection, site of injection, and ratio of fat to muscle are all significant factors.

HAZARDS PECULIAR TO INTRAVENOUS ADMINISTRATION

In addition to the risk of infection associated with the IV route, other potential hazards must be considered as well. These may be summarized as follows: (1) Once injected, distribution of the drug cannot be altered significantly. (2) IV injection is sometimes associated with cardiac, vascular, or circulatory disturbances that may be fatal. Although such effects are presumed to be more common when highly adulterated drugs of abuse are used, there is some risk even under the best of conditions. The probability of occurrence of such reactions appears to be related, among other factors, to the rapidity of injection. IV injections should be made slowly, preferably over a period of 1 minute or more. (3) Anaphylactoid reactions may be especially severe (see Chapter 64). As with all such reactions, death may occur within a few minutes. (4) Inadvertant injection of air may result in air embolism in the pulmonary or other vasculature.

Rapid IV injections are associated sometimes with sudden death.

5

Tolerance, Physical Dependence, and Drug Abuse

Jerrold C. Winter

Chronic administration of drugs may lead to tolerance, a state of diminished responsiveness to the drug, and to physical dependence, a state in which continued presence of the drug is required for normal function. Tolerance and physical dependence may accompany the use of therapeutic agents as well as of drugs of abuse. The withdrawal syndrome characteristic of physical dependence on some drugs is potentially fatal. Every physician must be aware of the types of physical dependence and their medical implications.

TOLERANCE

Drug tolerance refers to a state of diminished responsiveness to a drug as a consequence of prior exposure. This phenomenon is sometimes called *acquired tolerance* to distinguish it from *innate tolerance*. The latter term refers to relative insensitivity to drug action, which is independent of prior exposure. In its simplest form, drug tolerance is reflected in a parallel shift of the dose-response curve to the right as is illustrated in Figure 5–1. The degree of drug tolerance, i.e., the extent to which the dose-response curve is shifted, is quite variable and depends on the effect being measured and on the specific drug. For example, the degree of tolerance to a drug such as ethanol (a factor of about 2) is modest, whereas the dose-response curves for opiates may shift by a log unit or more.

The phenomenon in which tolerance to one drug confers tolerance to another is called *cross-tolerance*. Depending upon the specific mechanism by which tolerance arises, cross-tolerance may or may not reflect similar therapeutic effects (see later in this chapter). However, it is not unusual for drugs of a given class, e.g., opioid analgesics, to display cross-tolerance.

PHYSICAL DEPENDENCE

The phenomenon in which, as a consequence of prior exposure to a drug, the continued presence of that drug is required for normal function is called *physical dependence*. Physical dependence is defined in terms of the signs and symptoms that occur following termination of the drug of dependence. Collectively, the signs and symptoms following cessation of drug administration make up the *abstinence syndrome* or the *withdrawal syndrome*. Proof of physical dependence on a given drug is provided by the ability of that drug to relieve the abstinence syndrome. Drug tolerance is correlated generally with physical dependence, and it is commonly assumed that drug tolerance is a necessary prerequisite for the development of physical de-

Definition of Terms

Innate tolerance/acquired tolerance

Physical dependence is defined in terms of an abstinence syndrome.

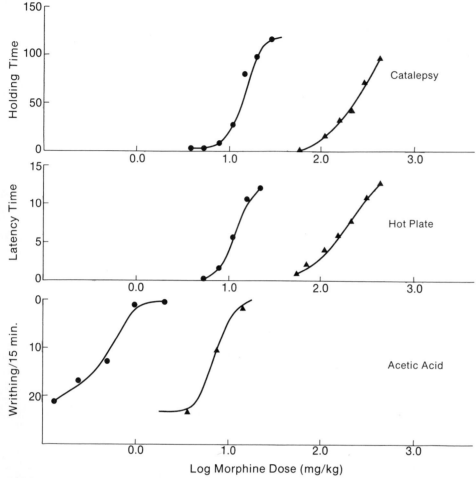

Figure 5-1

Tolerance to the analgesic effects of morphine in rats. Dose-response curves on the left side of each panel were obtained prior to chronic treatment with morphine. Twice daily administration of 16 mg/kg of morphine for 20 days causes each of the curves to shift to the right. Abscissa: Dose expressed on a log scale. Ordinate: Measures of catalepsy, hot-plate latency, and writhing induced by acetic acid, respectively. (Redrawn from Fernandes M, Kluwe S, Coper H: The development of tolerance to morphine in the rat. Psychopharmacology 54:197–201, 1977.)

Drug abuse cannot be defined in purely pharmacological terms.

pendence. However, the converse is not true; physical dependence need not accompany drug tolerance.

As noted previously, tolerance to one drug of a pharmacological class often confers tolerance to others of the class. A similar phenomenon, *cross-physical dependence*, is observed with respect to physical dependence. Thus, termination of the abstinence syndrome is afforded not only by the primary drug of dependence but also by other drugs of the same class.

DRUG (SUBSTANCE) ABUSE

Drug tolerance and physical dependence are pharmacological phenomena whose parameters may be expressed fully in scientific terms. In contrast, drug abuse is commonly defined as the use, usually by self-administration, of any drug in a manner that deviates from the approved medical or social patterns within a given culture. Although drug tolerance and physical dependence may be elements in some forms of drug abuse, they are neither necessary nor sufficient conditions for drug abuse. For example, patients treated with opiates for the relief of pain often display both tolerance and physical dependence; such patients are not drug abusers. (See also Chapter 67.)

The Origins of Drug Tolerance

Events responsible for drug tolerance may be divided into two categories. First are those that reduce the effective concentration of drug at receptor sites; in general these occur at a distance from the receptor. For example, a drug-induced increase in the rate of its own metabolism will result in less drug reaching its pharmacological receptors. Second are those adaptive changes that take place either at the receptor or in systems closely connected with the drug's action; this is referred to as *cellular tolerance.*

DISPOSITIONAL AND METABOLIC TOLERANCE

Any process that results in fewer drug molecules reaching their receptors will contribute to tolerance. Thus, for example, tolerance would be expected to arise as a consequence of changes in absorption, metabolism, excretion, or rate of passage across membranes. Of these possible mechanisms, clear evidence has been obtained only for altered metabolism following chronic exposure to drugs. Tolerance as a result of metabolic changes is called *metabolic tolerance* or *pharmacokinetic tolerance.*

Metabolic tolerance will be observed for any drug able to induce the synthesis of enzymes responsible for its inactivation. The best-documented site of origin of metabolic tolerance is the hepatic microsomal enzyme system. If the enzymes thus induced are responsible for the inactivation of other drugs, cross-tolerance will be observed. The example that follows shows the effects of chronic exposure of humans to high doses of pentobarbital (600–1200 mg/day) on the rate of metabolism of antipyrine, a drug used often as an indicator of the activity of hepatic mixed-function oxidase. (This is discussed further in Chapter 6.)

Group	N	Antipyrine Half-Life
control	61	12.5 hours
		($P < 0.001$)
barbiturate	8	5.3 hours

CELLULAR TOLERANCE

For many drugs acting upon the CNS, it is not possible to explain drug tolerance in terms of metabolic adaptation. Either blood levels of the drug are unchanged in the tolerant state or changes in blood levels are inadequate to explain the degree of tolerance observed. In these situations, it is commonly assumed that adaptation has occurred either at the receptor site or in the transduction system linking receptor occupation with pharmacological effect. Tolerance in the presence of unchanged concentrations of drug in the vicinity of its receptor is called *cellular tolerance* or *pharmacodynamic tolerance.*

Metabolic factors cannot explain all forms of drug tolerance.

Behavioral tolerance is a form of cellular tolerance that arises as a consequence of adaptive behavioral mechanisms. It develops most commonly when a drug-induced effect has adverse consequences; behavioral tolerance then tends to be specific for that effect. For example, a physician-alcoholic may become quite adept at masking the ataxic effects of ethanol while other actions of the drug are unaltered.

CROSS-TOLERANCE AS AN INDICATION OF ACTION UPON A COMMON RECEPTOR

Although it is certainly true that a group of drugs acting on a common receptor may exhibit cross-tolerance, it is not safe to assume that drugs cross-tolerant to one another act upon a common receptor. For example, barbiturates may induce hepatic enzymes responsible for the metabolism of drugs acting on diverse receptors in the CNS.

Tachyphylaxis

TACHYPHYLAXIS (ACUTE TOLERANCE)

Because of the influence of dose and frequency of administration upon tolerance, it is seldom possible to define precisely for a given drug the time course over which tolerance develops. Thus, in a clinical setting tolerance may be apparent only after several weeks of treatment with divided oral doses or may arise much more quickly following continuous IV administration. Nonetheless, it is observed generally that the development of tolerance is a relatively slow process, perhaps, as in metabolic tolerance, corresponding to the rate of synthesis of metabolic enzymes.

In those exceptional instances when tolerance develops rapidly, the term *acute tolerance* or *tachyphylaxis* (rapid protection) is used. A classic example is provided by the sympathomimetic agent tyramine. Closely spaced infusions of tyramine are at first followed by a pronounced pressor effect, which is then quickly decreased in magnitude. Tyramine tachyphylaxis is attributed to rapid depletion by tyramine of presynaptic stores of norepinephrine. Acute tolerance is manifested by many sedative-hypnotics, such as ethanol and benzodiazepines (see Chapters 19 and 20).

Physical Dependence

Physical dependence is of various types.

TYPES OF PHYSICAL DEPENDENCE

It was stated previously that physical dependence is defined in terms of the signs and symptoms that occur following termination of the drug of dependence and that these signs and symptoms are collectively termed the abstinence or withdrawal syndrome. Based upon observation of their respective withdrawal syndromes, several types of physical dependence are evident.

Depressant-type Physical Dependence

This form of physical dependence is also called the ethanol-barbiturate type. Convulsions are a prominent component of this type of physical dependence, and largely for this reason, untreated withdrawal has a significant mortality. Although there are sufficient subtle differences between depressants to suggest subtypes of depressant-type physical dependence, the withdrawal syndrome to ethanol is suppressed significantly by barbiturates and by benzodiazepines. (See Chapters 19, 20, and 67 for details.)

Opiate-type Physical Dependence

This, the second major form of physical dependence, is also called *dependence of the narcotic-analgesic type.* The classic reference drug for opiate dependence is morphine. The withdrawal syndrome is characterized by autonomic hyperactivity. Cross-physical dependence as manifested by suppression of the abstinence syndrome is exhibited by a large number of drugs that share morphine's pharmacological activities. (See Chapter 67 for details.)

Other Forms of Physical Dependence

Dependence of the depressant and opiate types has long been recognized. In addition, it is clear now that a variety of nondepressant, nonopiate drugs can induce other forms of physical dependence. Indeed, it can be argued that chronic administration of every drug induces adaptive changes that will be evident upon termination of drug treatment.

Whether we judge physical dependence to be present is largely a matter of what we are willing to accept as a withdrawal syndrome. For example, clonidine is a widely used antihypertensive agent that, upon abrupt termination of administration, is associated with rebound hypertension. Likewise, withdrawal of caffeine is associated with headache, nicotine with anxiety, cocaine with depression. Most authorities now accept these more subtle signs of abstinence syndromes as indications of true physical dependence.

An abstinence syndrome is relieved by readministration of the drug of dependence.

RATIONAL TREATMENT OF WITHDRAWAL SYNDROMES

It has been noted that the various types of physical dependence are differentiated by the characteristics of their withdrawal syndromes and that cross-physical dependence is defined by the ability of one drug to relieve the withdrawal syndrome of another. Thus, reinstitution of the primary drug of dependence or substitution of a drug that exhibits cross-physical dependence to it represents rational drug therapy. Often, the choice of a specific agent is influenced by local, regional, or national customs. For example, whereas those experiencing withdrawal from ethanol are seldom treated in a medical setting with ethanol, drugs as diverse as barbiturates, benzodiazepines, and chloral hydrate are often employed. Although there are a number of factors that influence the decision to provide pharmacological treatment for a specific withdrawal syndrome, the primary consideration is the hazard to the patient. (See Chapter 67 for details regarding specific drugs of dependence.)

6

Drug Metabolism

Jerome A. Roth

Metabolism of lipid-soluble drug to water-soluble products facilitates excretion.

The activity and duration of action of drugs are regulated *in vivo* by a number of factors, including the rate at which they are metabolically inactivated by various enzyme systems. A number of different and specific enzymatic processes throughout the body are responsible for the degradation and subsequent inactivation of drugs and other toxic agents. Although many of these processes are required for the homeostatic regulation of endogenous compounds, they function also to catabolize a variety of pharmacologically and toxicologically active agents. The end result of this catabolic process is the conversion of lipid-soluble xenobiotics to metabolic products that are considerably more water-soluble. This increased solubility in water facilitates their elimination in the urine or bile.

The majority of foreign substances that are taken into the body, regardless of the route of administration, are converted to metabolites that are excreted more rapidly than the original agent. During periods of impaired drug metabolism, elimination of drugs can be greatly reduced and, if not appropriately detected and subsequently prevented, can lead to excessive drug levels and subsequent toxic manifestations. Thus, the activity of the enzyme systems involved in drug metabolism can greatly influence the biochemical or pharmacological activity and toxic characteristics of any foreign substance taken into the body.

Before the different biochemical systems that are involved in the inactivation of drugs are described, it must be understood how drug metabolism influences the regulation and the pharmacological properties of drugs.

Duration of Drug Action

Drug metabolism influence on drug action:

1. Duration of drug action
2. Drug interactions
3. Drug activation
4. Drug toxicity or side effects

For many drugs the duration of action is inversely proportional to the rate at which they are metabolically inactivated. In other words, the more rapidly a drug is converted *in vivo* to inactive metabolites, the shorter its duration of action will be; conversely, the slower its rate of degradation, the longer its duration of action. Although these appear to be obvious relationships, it is an extremely important consideration because dosing regimens of many drugs are designed primarily on the basis of this factor alone. Factors that influence the levels or activity of the drug-metabolizing enzyme systems will subsequently alter duration of drug action as well as the rate at which the drug will accumulate. The differences observed in the duration of action of many drugs within the human population are due in large part to the variation in the levels of the drug-metabolizing enzyme systems.

The relationship between drug metabolism and duration of drug action has been investigated extensively and is exemplified by the drug hexobarbital. As demonstrated in Table 6–1, there is an inverse relation-

Table 6–1 SPECIES DIFFERENCES IN METABOLISM OF HEXOBARBITAL*			
Species	Sleeping Time (minutes)	Hexobarbital Half-Life (minutes)	Enzyme Activity (μg/g • hour)
Mice (12)	12 ± 8	19 ± 7	598 ± 184
Rabbits (9)	49 ± 12	60 ± 11	196 ± 28
Rats (10)	90 ± 15	140 ± 54	134 ± 51
Dogs (8)	315 ± 105	260 ± 20	36 ± 30

Reprinted with permission from Biochem Pharmacol 1:152, Quinn GP, Axelrod J, Brodie BB: Species, strain and sex differences in metabolism of hexobarbitone and amidopyrine, antipyrine, and aniline, copyright 1958, Pergamon Press plc.
* Dose of barbiturate 100 mg kg^{-1} (50 mg kg^{-1} in dogs). Figures in parentheses refer to number of animals in each species. Data are given in mean $\pm$ standard deviation.

ship between the rate of hepatic metabolism of hexobarbital and sleeping time in the various animal species listed. As indicated, the more rapidly hexobarbital is metabolically inactivated, the shorter the duration of its action. These data reveal that the duration of action of hexobarbital is regulated by the rate at which it is enzymatically degraded.

Although this relationship holds true for many drugs, it is important to stress that duration of drug action can be influenced also by a number of other factors, such as transport and redistribution of a drug from one compartment in the body to another. Similarly, drug metabolism does not lead necessarily to the formation of inactive catabolites; thus, duration of drug action may not always be related directly to its rate of degradation. Therefore, it is difficult often to predict *a priori* which factor will be the primary determinant regulating the duration of drug action.

Inverse relationship between rate of metabolism and duration of drug action

Drug Interactions

It is not an uncommon medical practice to prescribe more than one medication at a time to treat multiple symptoms or ailments of patients. Therefore, there is a real potential hazard for any two drugs to influence each other not only at the pharmacologically active site but also at the enzyme system involved in drug detoxification. In regard to the latter interaction, there are two possible mechanisms by which one drug can alter the rate of metabolism and utlimately the inactivation of another drug.

The first of these involves a direct competition for binding of the drugs at the enzyme responsible for their inactivation.

$$A \xrightarrow{\text{Enzyme}} A_{\text{inact}}$$

$$B \xrightarrow{\text{Enzyme}} B_{\text{inact}}$$

$$A \xrightarrow{\text{B present}} \text{decrease metabolism of A}$$

$$B \xrightarrow{\text{A present}} \text{decrease metabolism of B}$$

In this case, the two drugs simply act as competitive inhibitors, each decreasing the extent of metabolism of the other. The degree of inhibition of each drug is influenced by their concentration at the enzyme site in relation to their respective Michael-Menten constant (Km). The drug having the higher ratio between the concentration at the enzyme site and the Km value will produce the greatest inhibitory effect. Inhibition of the metabolism of one or both drugs can lead to toxic manifestations, resulting in potentially serious or possibly lethal side effects of one or both drugs. There are numerous examples in the literature demonstrating the direct interaction of drugs at the site of metabolism. (Clinical aspects of drug interactions are discussed further in Chapters 64 and 67.)

Drug interaction may involve competitive inhibition.

Drug interaction may be caused by induction of drug-metabolizing enzyme systems.

The second mechanism by which drugs can influence each other's metabolism has to do with an important property of the major enzyme system involved in the metabolism of many drugs. As discussed in greater detail later in this chapter, many drugs are metabolized by the mixed-function oxidase enzyme system. This enzyme system is unique because drugs can *induce the levels of the mixed-function oxidase* within the liver and thus increase not only their own metabolism but that of other pharmacological agents as well.

$$\text{Drug} \xrightarrow{\text{Enzyme}} \text{Drug}_{\text{inact}}$$

$$\text{Drug} \xrightarrow{\text{Enzyme}} \text{Drug}_{\text{inact}} \text{ (increase metabolism)}$$

For example, barbiturates have been shown experimentally to increase their own rate of metabolism and that of a variety of other drugs by a factor of two or three. The induced metabolism has been shown experimentally to be caused by an increased synthesis of the mixed-function oxidase enzyme system. This process of enzyme induction is one of the major mechanisms responsible for *metabolic tolerance* that is observed with many drugs.

It is generally accepted that all agents that are metabolized by the mixed-function oxidase are capable also of inducing this enzyme. However, in some cases the toxicity of the inducing agent is greater than that for induction of the enzyme system, and thus induction is not always observed. Induction of drug metabolism can occur also with ingestion of certain foods or with exposure to a variety of environmental agents that are oxidized by the mixed-function oxidase. Thus, the rate at which drugs are inactivated may be influenced and regulated by a variety of different environmental factors that ultimately effect the levels of this enzyme *in vivo*.

The physiological consequence of the two types of drug interaction are of course different. Direct competitive inhibition of drugs can lead to elevated concentrations of either of the two agents, potentially leading to drug toxicity or side effects. In direct contrast, drug induction of the mixed-function oxidase enzyme system can result in the increased metabolism of drugs, thus decreasing the duration of drug action as well as the concentration of the drug required to produce a therapeutic response.

Drug Activation

Drug activation involves prodrug metabolism to biologically active agent.

In the preceding discussion, drug metabolism is represented as a necessary process required for the termination of the action of drugs. Although this is true for the majority of drugs used clinically, in certain instances metabolism can actually lead to drug activation. The exploitation of drug activation is one of the newer approaches in therapeutics by which drug efficacy can be maximized by selectively generating pharmacologically active metabolites at specific target sites *in vivo*. A variety of methods have been employed to produce this selectivity, including the regulation of drug transport and the selective metabolism of drugs by enzymes localized in specific cells in the body.

An example of drug activation is the use of the drug levodopa for treatment of the symptoms of Parkinson's disease. This disorder is characterized biochemically by a degeneration of the dopaminergic nerve tracts leading from the substantia nigra to the striatum, resulting in an insufficient production of dopamine in the dopaminergic nerve terminals in the striatum. The neurotransmitter itself, dopamine, cannot be administered directly to these patients because of the serious side effects it would produce in the periphery, and also because it cannot cross the blood-brain barrier. In addition, it would be rapidly inactivated by monoamine oxidase and catechol-O-methyltransferase in the periphery. Thus, the amino acid precursor of dopamine, L-dihydroxyphenylethylamine, levodopa, is used as treatment of Parkinson's disease. Levodopa is transported across the blood-brain barrier into the brain, whereupon it is taken up into the dopaminergic neurons and decarboxylated by the enzyme, L-aromatic amino acid decarboxylase, to form dopamine, as illustrated in Figure 6–1. (See also Chapter 24.)

Figure 6–1

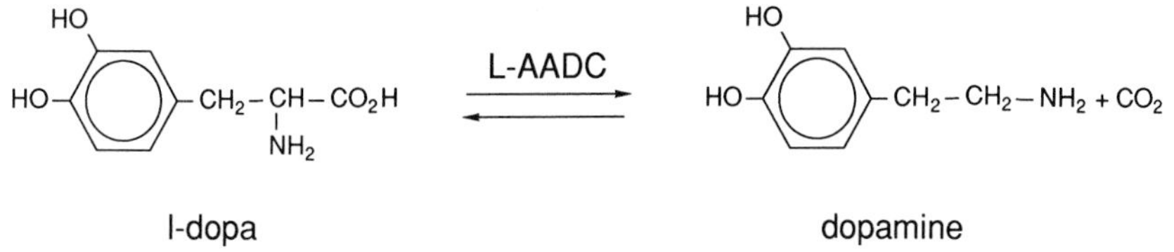

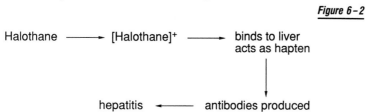

l-dopa   dopamine

Drug Toxicity and Side Effects

As described previously, it is generally assumed that metabolism of drugs and other xenobiotics results in their detoxification. In other words, in most cases metabolism results in the formation of biochemically inactive products that are usually more hydrophilic and thus are more readily excreted in the urine. However, metabolism of certain drugs and xenobiotics, instead of leading to formation of inactive compounds, in fact leads to formation of toxic and even carcinogenic catabolites. The toxicity or carcinogenicity results usually from the formation of highly reactive intermediates that are capable of reacting with specific cellular components to produce their toxic effects.

Metabolites of drugs can be toxic or produce side effects.

For example, the widely used anesthetic agent halothane can lead to hepatitis and subsequent death in appropriately sensitized individuals. It is believed that during the degradation of halothane, a reactive free radical is produced that can bind to specific sites within the liver and thereupon act as a hapten. Antibodies are produced subsequently to the hapten, thus precipitating halothane hepatitis upon subsequent exposure to susceptible individuals. The frequency of halothane hepatitis increases with an increased number of exposures to halothane (Fig. 6–2).

Figure 6–2

Halothane ⟶ [Halothane]⁺ ⟶ binds to liver acts as hapten

hepatitis ⟵ antibodies produced

Another important example whereby drug metabolism leads to toxicity involves the carcinogenic polycyclic aromatic hydrocarbons, such as 3,4-benzpyrene. As illustrated in Figure 6–3, 3,4-benzpyrene is metabolized to a highly reactive epoxide intermediate that has been shown to be the active carcinogenic agent. This reactive intermediate is presumed to be

Figure 6–3

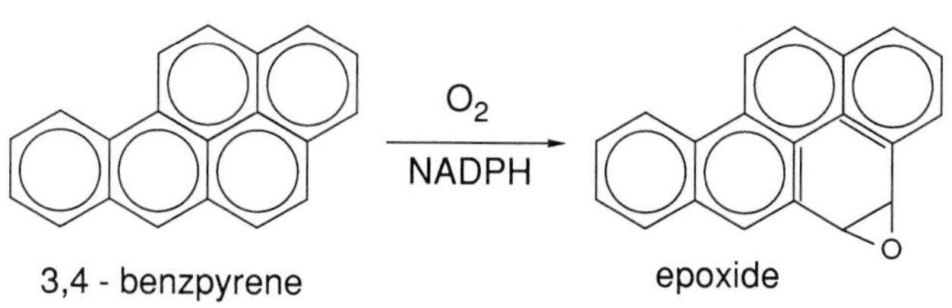

3,4 - benzpyrene   epoxide

capable of forming adducts with DNA within the nucleus, thus leading to production of tumors.

There are also examples in which formation of toxic metabolites may be of practical importance and beneficial to humans. The pesticide parathion is metabolized within the liver to form the potent and toxic acetylcholinesterase inhibitor paraoxon (Fig. 6–4). Paraoxon in humans is hydrolyzed rapidly to inactive catabolites by a variety of esterases. In general, insects lack these detoxifying esterases, and therefore, toxic levels of paraoxon build up within the insects. These selective detoxifying reactions within humans permit these compounds to be effectively employed as selective toxins of insects.

Figure 6–4

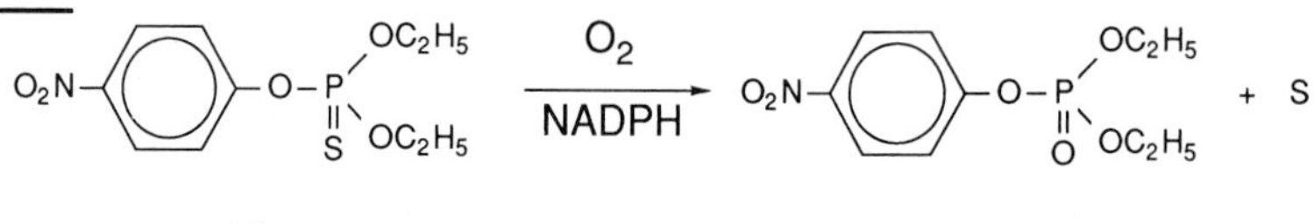

parathion   paraoxon

Pathways of Drug Metabolism

As a practical approach to studying and classifying the enzymatic pathways involved in drug metabolism, it has proved useful to divide the degradative processes into two separate stages or phases.

$$\text{Drug} \xrightarrow{\text{Phase I}} \begin{array}{c}\text{introduction of}\\ \text{polar group}\end{array} \xrightarrow{\text{Phase II}} \begin{array}{c}\text{conjugation of}\\ \text{polar group}\end{array}$$

Phase I drug metabolism involves the mixed-function oxidase enzyme system.

Phase I involves *oxidation of the drug* and is catalyzed by the *mixed-function oxidase enzyme system.* The mixed-function oxidase is considered to be the principal drug-metabolizing enzyme system in the body because it has a broad substrate specificity (i.e., it catalyzes the oxidation of a wide variety of substances) and, in addition, can catalyze a variety of different reactions. As discussed later, there are multiple forms of the mixed-function oxidase, each of which possesses unique but overlapping substrate specificity. The reactions catalyzed by this enzyme system increase the *hydrophilicity* (water solubility) of drugs and thus facilitate their elimination by the kidney.

Phase II drug metabolism involves a variety of transferases.

Phase II of drug metabolism consists of a number of enzymes that catalyze the formation of conjugates with the oxidized drug. The enzymes catalyzing these reactions are classified as *transferases,* and in all cases the conjugates that are produced are ionized at physiological pH. A variety of transferases exist, including the glucuronyl transferases, sulfotransferases, and glutathione transferases, as well as several specific amino acid transferases. Conjugation of drugs leads ultimately to the generation of highly water soluble, ionic compounds, which are readily excreted in the urine. Therefore, the net effect of Phases I and II is the conversion of lipid-soluble drugs to ionically charged water-soluble agents that are removed efficiently from the body.

MIXED-FUNCTION OXIDASE ENZYME SYSTEM

As noted earlier, the mixed-function oxidase system is considered to be the major enzyme system responsible for the metabolism of drugs and other xenobiotics. High levels of the mixed-function oxidase are present in the liver, which is generally considered to be the major site of drug metabolism. However, this enzyme system is present in almost all organs, and thus drug metabolism can occur throughout the body.

The mixed-function oxidase is present predominantly on the smooth endoplasmic reticulum of liver cells, although activity is associated also with the rough endoplasmic reticulum. The enzyme system has been purified, and three distinct components have been isolated: cytochrome c reductase (cytochrome P-450 reductase), cytochrome P-450, and a phospholipid.

As illustrated in Figure 6–5, the first component, cytochrome c reductase, catalyzes the initial transfer of an electron from nicotinamide-adenine dinucleotide phosphate (NADPH) to the cytochrome. The enzyme has an absolute requirement for NADPH and requires Mg^{2+} for activity. The enzyme contains one molecule each of flavin adenine dinucleotide (FAD) and flavin mononucleotide (FMN) as cofactors. This reductase is capable of donating two electrons to the cytochrome, the first of which reduced the heme iron to the ferrous form and the second to oxidized oxygen to the superoxide anion.

The second component, cytochrome P-450, is the terminal electron acceptor and is the *binding site* of drugs. The designation cytochrome P-450 is actually a generic term that denotes a family of cytochromes that are immunologically and biochemically distinct, although all accept an electron from NADPH cytochrome c reductase. Specific antibodies have been raised to the different forms of cytochrome P-450, demonstrating specific structural differences between the different species of this cytochrome. At least 16 different species of the cytochrome have been identified to date. The unique substrate specificities of the different forms of cytochrome P-450 are imparted by the structure of the apoprotein. The cytochromes contain iron that is chelated to a porphyrin ring system that is identical to that of hemoglobin, protoporphyrin IX. Because sex steroid hormones have been shown to induce different forms of this cytochrome, males and females possess different ratios of several cytochrome P-450 species. Selective induction of specific forms of cytochrome P-450 with various drugs and other exogenous agents has been used in the purification and characterization of the different species of this cytochrome.

The last essential component of the mixed-function oxidase system is a phospholipid that is required to act as a membrane surface to allow for the exchange of electrons from the reductase to the iron of the cytochrome.

The second electron that oxidizes oxygen to the superoxide anion can come also from cytochrome b_5 and cytochrome b_5 reductase, a nicotinamide-adenine dinucleotide (NADH)-specific reductase (Fig. 6–5). Under conditions in which NADPH is limiting, it is believed that the second electron can be donated by the cytochrome b_5 system. This latter enzyme system cannot take the place of NADPH cytochrome c reductase as a donor of the first electron.

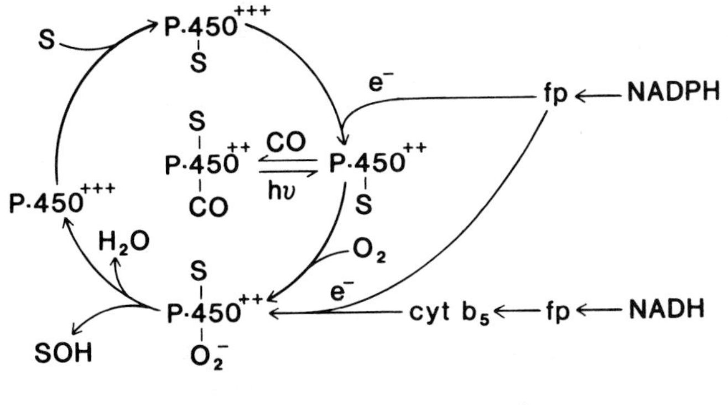

Mixed-function oxidase is located predominantly in smooth endoplasmic reticulum.

Mixed-function oxidase components:

1. NADPH cytochrome C (P-450) reductase donates electrons to Fe^{3+} of cytochrome.
2. Cytochrome P-450 drug binds to cytochrome P-450
3. NADH cytochrome b_5 and cytochrome b_5

Figure 6–5

As noted in the reaction, for every molecule of oxygen consumed in the reaction, one atom is utilized to oxidize the substrate, whereas the other atom of oxygen results in the production of one molecule of water. NADPH is capable of donating two electrons in the reaction: the first is utilized to oxidize iron to the ferrous state after substrate binds, whereas the second electron from a second molecule of NADPH reacts with oxygen to produce a highly reactive superoxide anion, which reacts with substrate to produce product. The reduced cytochrome is capable of complexing with carbon monoxide, resulting in a complex that absorbs light at approximately 450 mμ. The wavelength for the absorbance of light observed is specific for the different forms of P-450 and normally varies between 447 and 553 mμ. Because carbon monoxide is capable of binding to the reduced cytochrome, it can act as a potent inhibitor of the mixed-function oxidase, and this interaction is used often to determine experimentally whether a drug is oxidized by this enzyme system.

Reactions Catalyzed by the Mixed-Function Oxidase

The mixed-function oxidase is a relatively unique enzyme system because it can catalyze the oxidation of a variety of different types of reactions, as indicated here.

Aromatic Ring Hydroxylation. The example given in Figure 6–6 is for the oxidation of benzene to phenol. Almost all drugs or xenobiotics that contain an aromatic ring system will undergo ring hydroxylation. In some cases, hydroxylation can occur on a given aromatic ring more than once. Ring hydroxylation may or may not lead to the total inactivation of the drug.

Reactions catalyzed by mixed-function oxidase:

1. Aromatic ring hydroxylation
2. Side-chain hydroxylation
3. *N*-dealkylation
4. *O*-dealkylation
5. *S*-dealkylation
6. Sulfoxidation
7. Desulfuration
8. Deamination
9. Dehalogenation

Figure 6–6

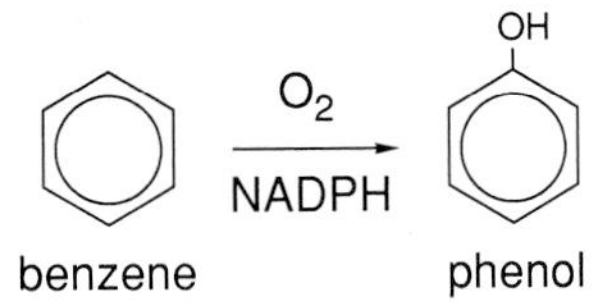

benzene   phenol

Figure 6–7

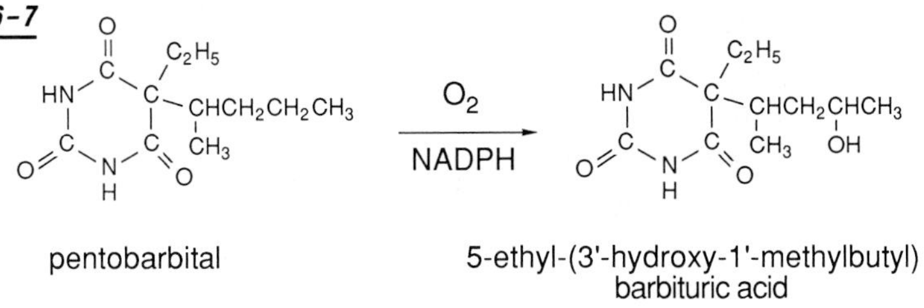

pentobarbital

5-ethyl-(3'-hydroxy-1'-methylbutyl) barbituric acid

Side-Chain Hydroxylation. The example presented in Figure 6–7 is for the side-chain hydroxylation of pentobarbital. In general, side-chain hydroxylation is not as common an occurrence as ring hydroxylation, although when it does occur it often results in the inactivation of the parent drug.

***N*-dealkylation.** Figure 6–8 presents the *N*-demethylation of the antipressant drug imipramine. In this case, the tertiary amine is demethylated to form the secondary amine along with production of one molecule of formaldehyde. *N*-dealkylation reactions are relatively common in that numerous other drugs that contain a tertiary or secondary amine also undergo *N*-dealkylation reactions. Other examples of drugs undergoing *N*-dealkylation reactions include several of the phenothiazine antipsychotic and

Figure 6–8

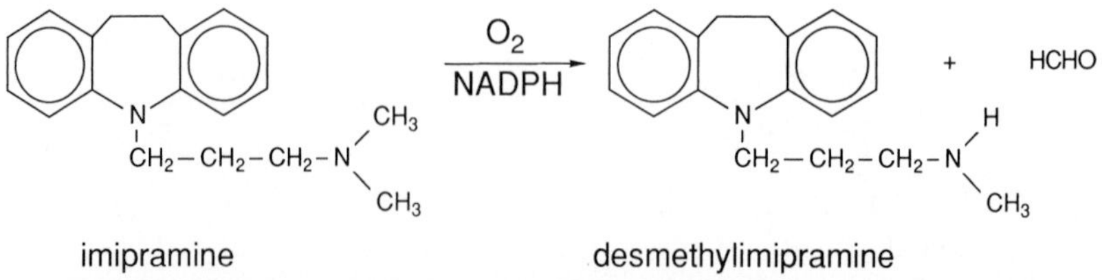

imipramine   desmethylimipramine

tricyclic antidepressant agents, diazepam (VALIUM), and *N*-substituted barbiturates. *N*-dealkylation does not necessarily result in the inactivation of the parent drug because the product may have either more or less pharmacological activity than the parent agent.

O-dealkylation. This reaction is similar to that for *N*-dealkylation but in this case involves the oxidation of an ether. The example given in Figure 6–9 is for the drug codeine.

Figure 6–9

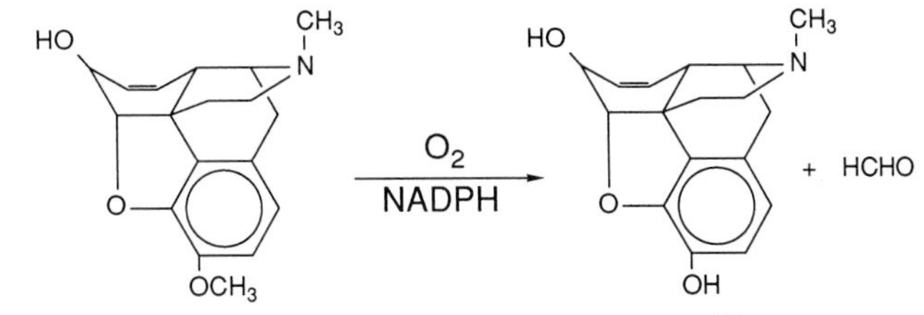

codeine (methylmorphine)   morphine

S-dealkylation. The reaction shown in Figure 6–10 is for the drug 6-methylthiopurine. This reaction is involved in the activation of this drug to the pharmacologically active form.

Figure 6–10

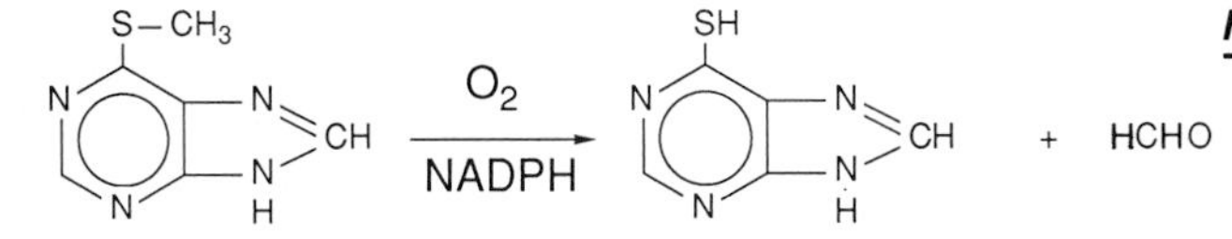

6-methylthiopurine   6-mercaptopurine

Sulfoxidation. Many drugs that contain a thioether linkage can undergo oxidation to form the sulfoxide. As illustrated in Figure 6–11, the phenothiazines undergo sulfoxidation to form the inactive catabolite. Formation of the sulfoxide of the vitamin biotin can also be catalyzed by the mixed-function oxidase enzyme system.

Figure 6–11

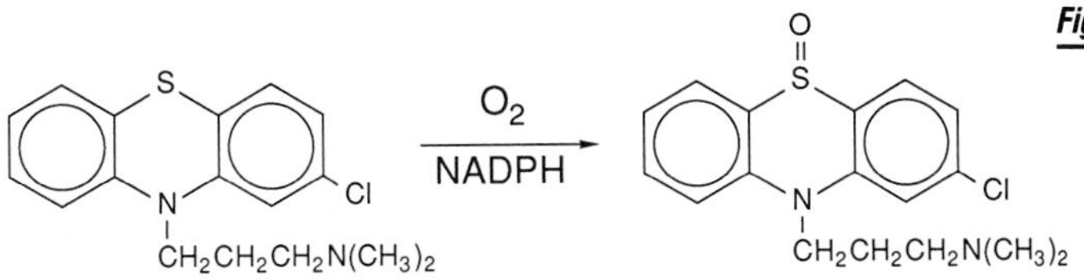

chlorpromazine   chlorpromazine sulfoxide

Desulfuration. The example of desulfuration presented in Figure 6–12 is for the barbiturate thiopental. For the thiobarbiturates, desulfuration does not result in inactivation of the parent drug but leads to production of the oxy-derivative, which possesses lower pharmacological activity. As illustrated in Figure 6–4, parathion also undergoes a desulfuration reaction. Desulfuration of parathion leads to formation of the acetylcholinesterase inhibitor paraoxon.

Figure 6–12

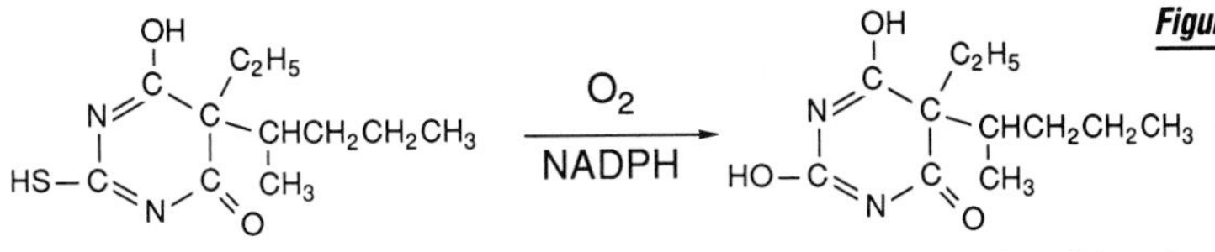

thiopental   pentobarbital (enol form)

Deamination. There are a number of enzymes that catalyze the deamination of endogenous and exogenous amines. These include monoamine oxidase (MAO), diamine oxidase (DAO), plasma amine oxidase, and the mixed-function oxidase. MAO, as well as plasma amine oxidase, catalyzes the deamination of biogenic amines and structurally related monoamine drugs, whereas DAO is specific for compounds containing diamines such as cadaverine and spermine (discussed later). The mixed-function oxidase is responsible primarily for the deamination of sympathomimetic amines that contain an α-methyl group on the carbon atom adjacent to the primary amine as shown in Figure 6–13 for amphetamine.

Figure 6–13

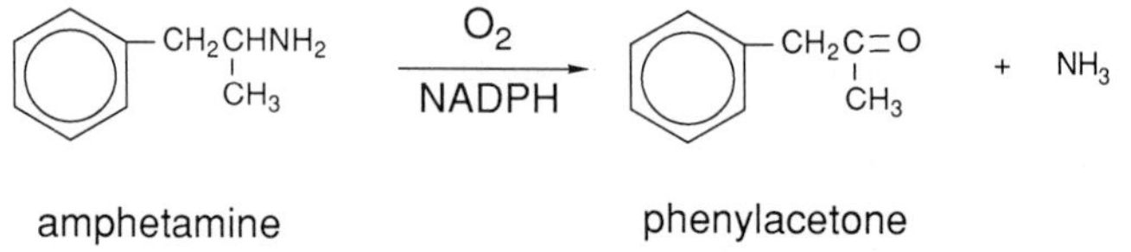

amphetamine   phenylacetone

Amphetamine is a structural analog of phenylethylamine, a compound that is readily deaminated by MAO. The presence of the α-methyl group on phenylethylamine causes this compound to no longer be a substrate for MAO, and thus its deamination occurs exclusively through the mixed-function oxidase. This latter reaction is a slow reaction compared with the deamination of phenylethylamine by MAO.

Dehalogenation. There are a number of enzymes responsible for the dehalogenation of drugs *in vivo*. The mixed-function oxidase reaction responsible for the dehalogenation of several aromatic ring and aliphatic halogens is illustrated in Figure 6–14 for the anesthetic agent halothane. Halothane undergoes a dehalogenation reaction that leads to the production of an unstable free radical intermediate. The majority of this intermediate is converted into trifluoroacetaldehyde and subsequently trifluoroacetic acid. However, a small percentage of the free radical binds to components within the liver and acts as the hapten, which ultimately leads to hepatitis as explained earlier.

Figure 6–14

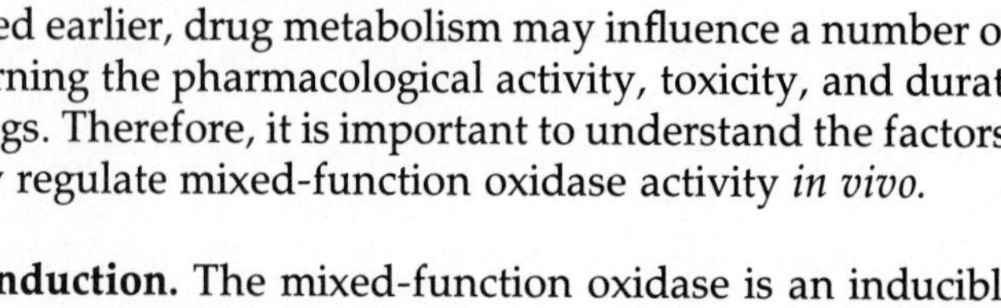

halothane   free radical

Factors Regulating Mixed-Function Oxidase

As indicated earlier, drug metabolism may influence a number of parameters concerning the pharmacological activity, toxicity, and duration of action of drugs. Therefore, it is important to understand the factors that may potentially regulate mixed-function oxidase activity *in vivo*.

Enzyme Induction. The mixed-function oxidase is an inducible enzyme system because exposure to a drug or a variety of other endogenous or exogenous agents has the potential to promote an increase in enzyme activity. This can be observed experimentally in the laboratory when exposing rats to a number of different drugs or chemicals. The exposure of rats to phenobarbital or 3-methylcholanthrene will cause a selective increase in the rate of metabolism of hexobarbital, 3,4-benzpyrene, and aminopyrine (Table 6–2). Phenobarbital induces the metabolism of hexo-

Factors regulating mixed-function oxidase activity:

1. Enzyme induction
2. Age
3. Sex
4. Genetic differences

Table 6–2 EFFECT OF PRETREATMENT OF RABBITS WITH PHENOBARBITAL AND 3-METHYLCHOLANTHRENE

Substrate	Pretreatment*	Enzyme Activity (μmoles/mg protein/hour)
Hexobarbital	Control	0.69
	PB	1.21
	3-MC	0.27
3,4-benzpyrene	Control	0.19
	PB	0.21
	3-MC	0.34
Aminopyrine	Control	1.07
	PB	3.40
	3-MC	1.38

From Gram TE, Rogers LA, Fouts JR: Effect of pretreatment of rabbits with phenobarbital or 3-methylcholanthrene on the distribution of drug-metabolizing enzyme activity in subfractions of hepatic microsomes. J Pharmacol Exp Ther 157:435–437, 1967, © by American Society for Pharmacology and Experimental Therapeutics.
* PB = phenobarbital; 3-MC = 3-methylcholanthrene.

barbital and aminopyrine but has little effect on the oxidation of 3,4-benzpyrene. In contrast, 3-methylcholanthrene induces the metabolism of 3,4-benzpyrene but fails to increase the oxidation of either hexobarbital or aminopyrine. This experiment demonstrates that the mixed-function oxidase enzyme system is inducible and that different agents will selectively induce the formation of specific forms of the cytochrome P-450 possessing unique substrate specificities. Which form or forms of the cytochrome are selectively induced by any given agent is dependent on the substrate specificity of the different cytochromes. Thus, often induction of mixed-function oxidase activity involves the increased synthesis of several different forms of the cytochrome. Current research has focused on the cytosolic biochemical receptors for the inducing agents and the structure of the genes regulating production of these cytochromes.

Induction of the mixed-function oxidase activity may not only involve an increased production of the cytochrome but may also involve an increased production of the NADPH-cytochrome c reductase. It is difficult to predict *a priori* which drugs will induce reductase activity as well as that of the cytochrome. In general, the polycyclic aromatic hydrocarbons, such as 3-methylcholanthrene and 3,4-benzpyrene, do not increase NADPH-cytochrome c reductase activity *in vivo*.

Age. The specific activity of liver mixed-function oxidase normally reaches adult levels within 3–8 weeks after birth. This rapid production of the oxidase is most likely caused by the exposure of infants to environmental pollutants that stimulate mixed-function oxidase activity. The livers of human fetuses contain appreciable mixed-function oxidase activity and thus are capable of oxidizing a variety of drugs that cross the placental membranes. In contrast, laboratory animals, for whom the environment is carefully controlled, often have little if any mixed-function oxidase activity in the liver of the fetus, although as in the human, animal mixed-function oxidase activity increases rapidly to adult levels within several weeks after birth.

This difference in fetal liver mixed-function oxidase between humans and laboratory animals is extremely important in testing the teratogenic properties of drugs. For example, the hypnotic drug thalidomide was suspected of producing severe limb malformations (phocomelias) in humans, although initial testing of this drug in laboratory animals failed to demonstrate this teratogenic property. It was determined subsequently that a metabolite of the drug that could not cross the placental membrane was, in fact, the teratogenic agent. Because the fetuses of many laboratory animals lack mixed-function oxidase activity and are unable to produce the teratogenic metabolite *in utero,* initial studies failed to demonstrate that thalidomide was teratogenic. However, the livers of human fetuses are capable of degrading thalidomide to the teratogenic catabolite, thus resulting in the severe limb malformations observed in children born to pregnant women exposed to thalidomide.

There is also evidence in the literature to suggest that hepatic mixed-function oxidase activity is decreased in the geriatric population, thus accounting, in part, for the increased half-life of some drugs observed in this population.

Sex. Males have higher mixed-function oxidase activity than females because testosterone induces mixed-function oxidase activity whereas estradiol decreases activity. The difference in the content of the different forms of cytochrome P-450 observed in the livers of males and females is most likely caused by these sex steroid hormones.

Genetic Differences. The most important factor regulating mixed-function oxidase activity is the genetic variation in the human population. This can be clearly observed experimentally in laboratory animals in which different strains of rats possess different levels of activity of this oxidase.

PHASE II (CONJUGATION REACTIONS)

Phase II of the drug-metabolizing enzyme system consists of a variety of enzymatic reactions, all of which involve conjugation of either the parent or the oxidized drug. These reactions are catalyzed by several different transferases, all of which generate an end product that is ionized at physiological pH. With few exceptions, conjugation results in inactivation of the parent drug or its active catabolites and also facilitates its excretion within the kidney. Thus, conjugation reactions represent an important process involved in inactivation of drugs *in vivo.* The following sections describe some of the important conjugation reactions.

> Phase II of drug metabolism involves various transferases that conjugate drug with an ionizable compound.

Glucuronide Conjugation

Formation of the glucuronide conjugate represents one of the major degradative processes involved in drug detoxification and inactivation. The reac-

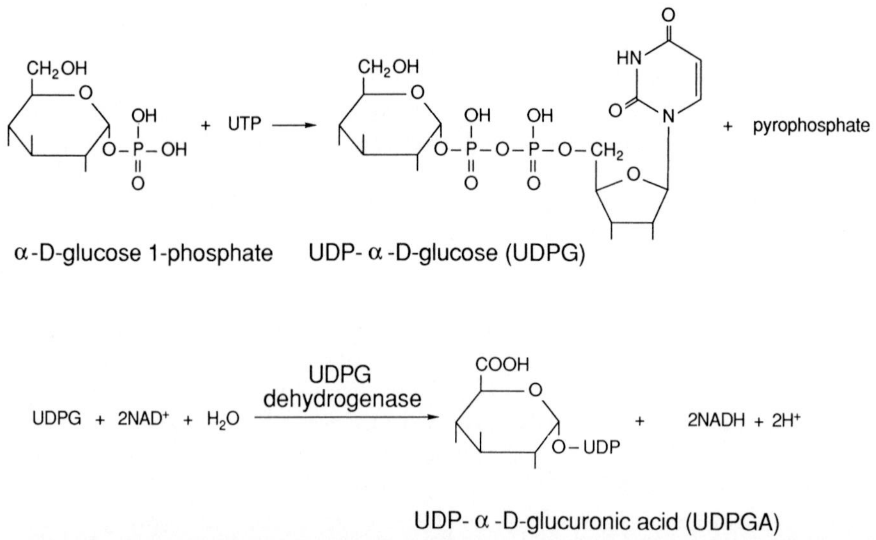

α-D-glucose 1-phosphate   UDP-α-D-glucose (UDPG)

UDPG + 2NAD⁺ + H₂O →(UDPG dehydrogenase)→ + 2NADH + 2H⁺

Figure 6–15

UDP-α-D-glucuronic acid (UDPGA)

tions involved in synthesis of the glucuronide donor uridine diphosphate (UDP)–glucuronic acid are presented in Figure 6–15.

UDP–glucuronic acid transferase represents a family of enzymes that is located in the endoplasmic reticulum of the cell. Like the mixed-function oxidase, this transferase is inducible upon exposure to certain drugs. These enzymes can catalyze the conjugation of hydroxy groups, sulfhydryl groups, and primary amines as well as carboxylic acids. The end product of these reactions is the formation of the ionized glucuronide drug conjugate (Fig. 6–16). (Although most glucuronide conjugates are less active than the parent compound, some, such as a morphine-glucuronide conjugate, discussed in Chapter 18, are more active than morphine itself.)

Glucuronide conjugate is a major Phase II metabolizing reaction.

Figure 6–16

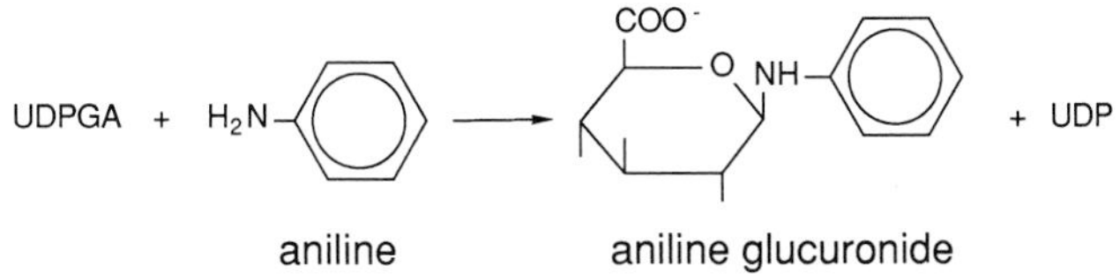

UDPGA + H₂N—⟨benzene ring⟩ → aniline glucuronide + UDP

aniline   aniline glucuronide

Sulfate Conjugation

Sulfate conjugation and glucuronide conjugation are the two major Phase II conjugation reactions. The enzymatic steps involved in sulfate conjugation are presented in Figure 6–17.

The first step in the reaction catalyzed by the enzyme sulfurylase thermodynamically favors the reverse reaction. However, this reaction

Sulfate conjugation is a major Phase II metabolizing reaction.

Figure 6–17

$ATP + SO_4^=$ →(sulfurylase) adenosine 5'-phosphosulfate (APS) + pyrophosphate

adenosine 5'-phosphosulfate (APS)

$APS + ATP$ →(APS-kinase) 3'-phosphoadenosine 5'-phosphosulfate (PAPS) + ADP

3'-phosphoadenosine 5'-phosphosulfate (PAPS)

PAPS + p-hydroxyacetanilid →(sulfotransferase) p-hydroxyacetanilid sulfate + 3'-phosphoadenosine 5'-phosphate

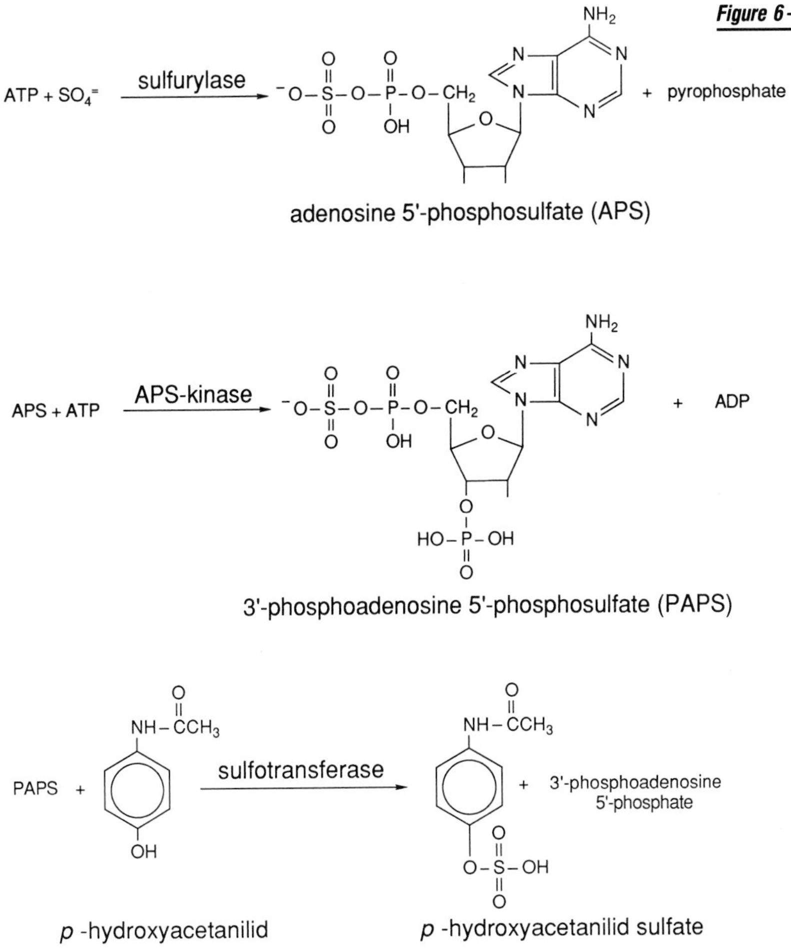

p-hydroxyacetanilid   *p*-hydroxyacetanilid sulfate

proceeds in the forward direction because the enzyme is coupled to APS-kinase, which subsequently converts adenosine-5'-phosphosulfate (APS) to the sulfate donor 3'-phosphoadenosine-5'-phosphosulfate (PAPS). In addition, a number of pyrophosphatases are present that rapidly break down inorganic pyrophosphate formed by the sulfurylase reaction and thus prevent the reverse reaction from occurring.

Similar to the glucuronide transferases, the sulfotransferases also represent a family of enzymes. More recent studies have identified two functionally distinct forms of phenol sulfotransferase that possess distinct but overlapping substrate specificity. These enzymes are involved in the conjugation of a wide variety of drugs and other xenobiotics. Sulfoconjugation can occur on both phenolic compounds and aromatic amines. The end product of this reaction is the ionized sulfate ester of the drug.

A variety of other sulfotransferases have been identified that appear to selectively sulfate steroids. These steroid sulfotransferases also utilize PAPS as the sulfate donor.

In general, both glucuronide and sulfate conjugation result in the formation of a biologically inert catabolite. Although this is usually the case for most drugs, in several instances conjugation has been reported to promote the biological response of drugs and other agents. For example, the sulfate ester of minoxidil produced *in vivo* appears to be the active form of the parent drug, because minoxidil sulfate is both an antihypertensive agent and a hair growth–promoting factor. Similarly, the sulfate conjugates of N-hydroxy-2-acetylaminofluorene and structurally related compounds have been reported to be potent carcinogens (Fig. 6–18). In the absence of formation of the sulfate ester within the cell, these unconjugated compounds have been shown not to be carcinogenic.

Figure 6–18

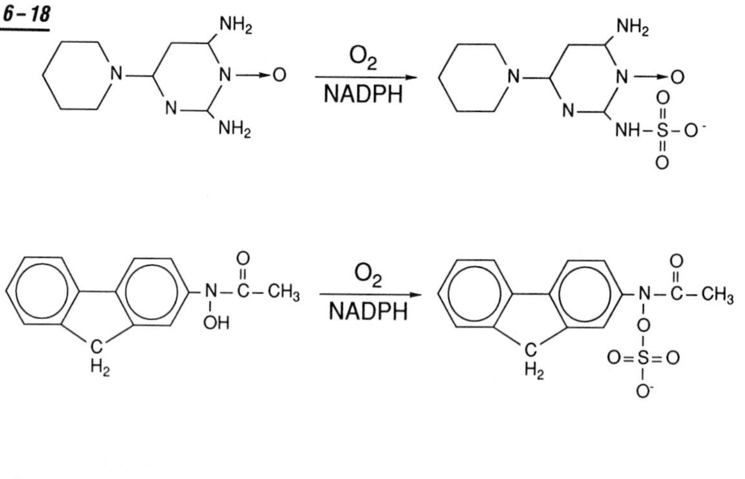

Other Conjugation Reactions

A variety of other compounds are also capable of serving as esterifying agents for a variety of drugs. These conjugating substrates include glutathione and a variety of amino acids. In all cases, the conjugate that is formed is ionized at physiological pH, thus assuring that the esterified drug or other exogenous agent will be excreted rapidly by the kidney.

Other enzymatic pathways involved in drug metabolism:

1. Acetylation
2. Transulfuration
3. O,N,S-methylation
4. Alcohol and aldehyde oxidations
5. Reduction reactions
6. Ester or amide hydrolysis
7. Deamination

OTHER PATHWAYS INVOLVED IN DRUG METABOLISM

Acetylation

Aromatic amines and hydrazines undergo acetylation reactions. The reaction is catalyzed by the enzyme N-acetyltransferase, which proceeds by a double-displacement (ping-pong) reaction mechanism as illustrated for isoniazid (Fig. 6–19).

Figure 6–19

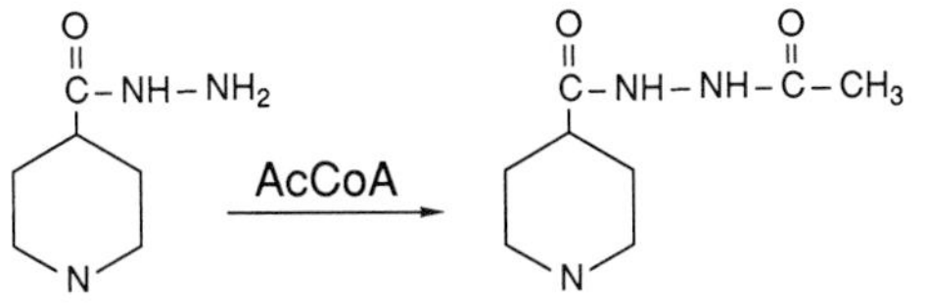

$$\text{enzyme} + \text{AcCoA} \rightleftharpoons \text{Ac-enzyme} + \text{CoA}$$
$$\text{Ac-enzyme} + \text{isoniazid} \rightleftharpoons \text{Ac-isoniazid} + \text{enzyme}$$
$$\text{AcCoA} + \text{isoniazid} \xrightarrow{\text{enzyme}} \text{Ac-isoniazid} + \text{CoA}$$

In the human population the enzyme displays genetic polymorphism and can be divided into "fast" and "slow" acetylators. The half-life of the reaction for isoniazid in fast acetylators is approximately 70 minutes, whereas in the slow acetylators this value is greater than 3 hours (Fig. 6–19). The structure of the enzyme is identical in the two groups, and only the concentration of the enzyme is different. From a genetic standpoint, fast acetylation is an autosomal dominant trait. In the United States the distribution between the two groups is about 50:50. Eskimos are in general fast acetylators, whereas Jews and North African Caucasians are slow acetylators.

Because of the rather large differences in the rate of degradation of drugs between the two populations, it is mandatory that individuals who are prescribed drugs that are known to be inactivated by acetylation be tested to determine whether they are fast or slow acetylators. Numerous examples in the literature have described toxicity in slow acetylators caused by administration of an inappropriately high dose that is prescribed normally for fast acetylators.

Transulfuration Reactions (Detoxification of CN⁻)

There are two reactions important in the detoxification of CN^-. The first reaction, as illustrated in Figure 6–20, is catalyzed by a mitochondrial sulfotransferase (rhodanase; transsulfuralase) that utilizes thiosulfate as the donor molecule. The second reaction utilizes β-mercaptopyruvic acid as the sulfur donor and is catalyzed by a cytosolic sulfotransferase. Either thiosulfate or β-mercaptopyruvic acid can be used clinically to treat individuals exposed to toxic levels of cyanide (Fig. 6–20).

Figure 6–20

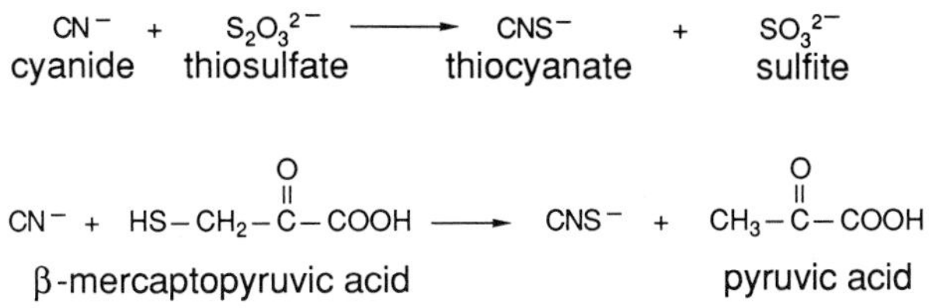

O, N, and S Methylation Reactions

A variety of methyltransferases exist that are capable of methylating hydroxyl, amine, or free sulfhydryl groups on drugs and other xenobiotics. These methyltransferases utilize *S*-adenosylmethionine (SAM) as the methyl donor. An example of O-methylation by the enzyme catechol-O-methyltransferase is presented in Figure 6–21.

Figure 6-21

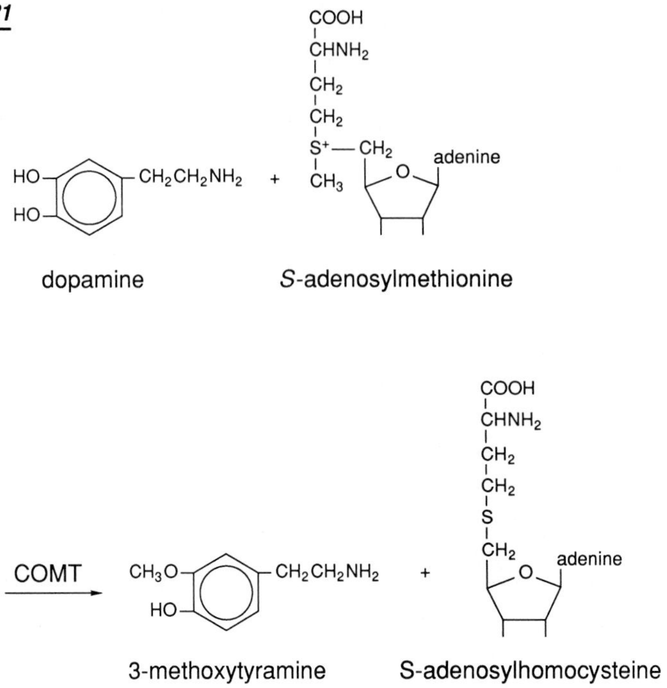

Alcohol and Aldehyde Oxidations

Alcohols and aldehydes are normally oxidized *in vivo* by alcohol dehydrogenase and aldehyde dehydrogenase. Both enzymes require nicotinamide-adenine dinucleotide (NAD) as the cofactor and have a broad substrate specificity. The oxidation of chloral hydrate to trichloroacetic acid is illustrated in Figure 6-22.

Figure 6-22

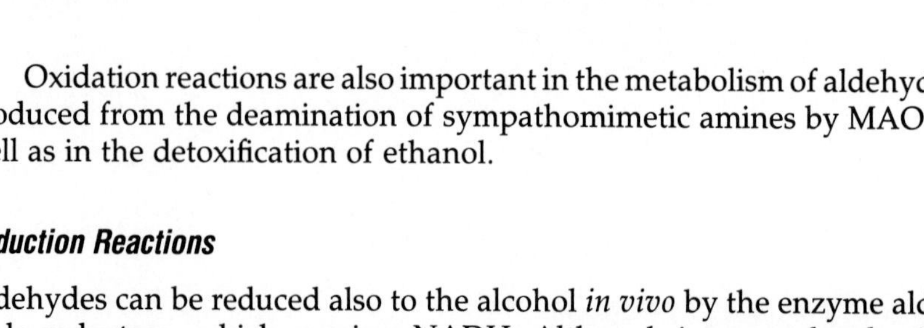

Oxidation reactions are also important in the metabolism of aldehydes produced from the deamination of sympathomimetic amines by MAO as well as in the detoxification of ethanol.

Reduction Reactions

Aldehydes can be reduced also to the alcohol *in vivo* by the enzyme aldehyde reductase, which requires NADH. Although in general reduction reactions are not as common as oxidation, they do occur in specific cases. For example, the aldehyde product of norepinephrine, 3-methoxy-4-hydroxyphenyl-β-hydroxyacetaldehyde, is preferentially reduced to form 3-methoxy-4-hydroxyphenylglycol (MHPG) in brain (Fig. 6-23), whereas in the periphery the major metabolite of this aldehyde is the oxidized acidic product.

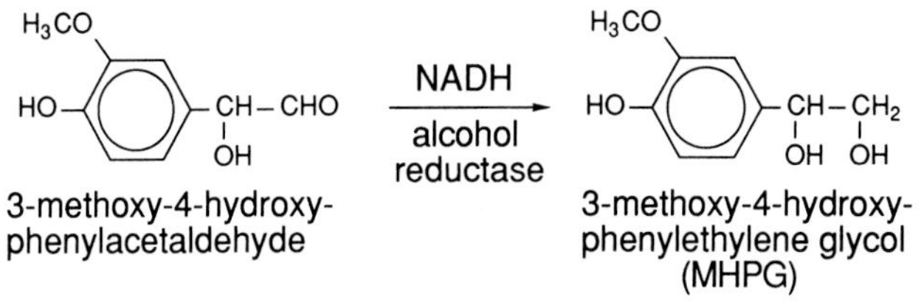

Figure 6-23

3-methoxy-4-hydroxy-phenylacetaldehyde → (NADH, alcohol reductase) → 3-methoxy-4-hydroxy-phenylethylene glycol (MHPG)

Hydrolysis (Esterases and Amidases)

A variety of substrate specific and nonspecific esterases and amidases are present *in vivo*, for example the ester hydrolysis of procaine (Fig. 6-24).

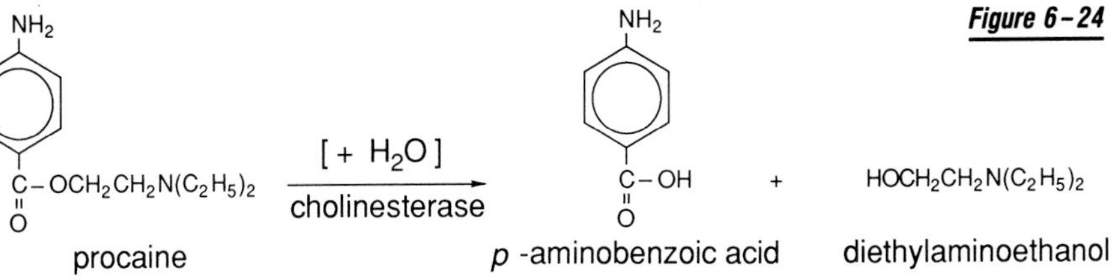

Figure 6-24

procaine → $[+ H_2O]$, cholinesterase → p-aminobenzoic acid + diethylaminoethanol

Deamination

As mentioned earlier, there are several enzymes catalyzing the deamination of amines. These are MAO, plasma amine oxidase (benzylamine oxidase), DAO, and the mixed-function oxidase. A brief description of the properties and specificities of these enzymes follows.

Monoamine Oxidase. Two forms of MAO, Type A and Type B, are found on the outer mitochondrial membrane (Fig. 6-25). These enzymes have different substrate specificities and are responsible for the deamination of catechol and phenolic amines *in vivo*. The substrate specificities of the two enzymes are presented below.

Type A MAO	*Type B MAO*
norepinephrine	norepinephrine
dopamine	dopamine
tyramine	tyramine
5-hydroxytryptamine	phenylethylamine

The enzyme is somewhat unique in that the apoenzyme is bound covalently to the 8-methyl group of FAD by a thioether linkage. In the brain the A form is localized to neurons, whereas the B form predominates in astroglia with the exception of B MAO in some serotonergic neurons.

Figure 6-25

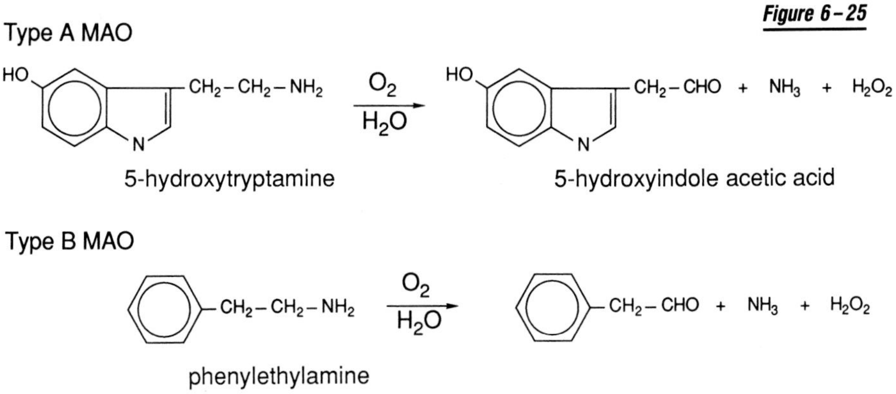

Type A MAO

5-hydroxytryptamine → (O_2, H_2O) → 5-hydroxyindole acetic acid + NH_3 + H_2O_2

Type B MAO

phenylethylamine → (O_2, H_2O) → CH_2-CHO + NH_3 + H_2O_2

Studies have identified several human subjects (Norrie's disease) in which the genes for both MAO A and MAO B are deleted. These studies suggest that the genes that code for the two species of MAO are located near each other.

As discussed in Chapter 22, inhibitors of MAO were the first class of drugs used clinically to treat depression. The drugs that are used clinically are irreversible nonselective inhibitors of both forms of the oxidase.

Plasma Amine Oxidase (Benzylamine Oxidase). The function of plasma amine oxidase is unknown, although it has a substrate specificity similar to that of the B form of MAO. It is a soluble enzyme and is found predominantly in the plasma and blood vessel walls. There is some debate in the literature as to whether this enzyme contains pyridoxal phosphate as a cofactor. The rate of deamination by plasma amine oxidase is extremely slow compared with that with MAO, and thus its role *in vivo* is uncertain.

Diamine Oxidase. As the name implies, DAO is responsible for the deamination of diamines, such as putrescine and cadaverine (Fig. 6–26). The enzyme has an absolute specificity for diamines and will not deaminate monoamines. The enzyme is soluble and contains FAD as a cofactor.

Figure 6–26

$$H_2N-(CH_2)_5-NH_2 \xrightarrow[\substack{\text{diamine}\\ \text{oxidase}}]{O_2} H_2N-(CH_2)_4-CHO + NH_3$$
cadaverine

This chapter serves as a general outline describing the different biochemical reactions that are involved in the detoxification of drugs. Which pathway ultimately plays a role in the inactivation of any drug can be determined only by experimental measurements. Many drugs can be degraded by several different enzymes or pathways within the body. For example, there are over 128 different metabolites that have been isolated in patients receiving the antipsychotic drug chlorpromazine. Some of the known metabolites of this antipsychotic agent are pharmacologically active, whereas others are inactive. Details of the specific routes of metabolism for the different classes of drugs are presented in the appropriate chapters.

References

Kappas A, Alvares AP, Anderson KE, et al: Effect of charcoal-broiled beef on antipyrine and theophylline metabolism. Clin Pharmacol Ther 23:445–450, 1978.
Guengerich FP: Characterization of human microsomal cytochrome P-450 enzymes. Annu Rev Pharmacol Toxicol 29:241–264, 1989.
Mulder GJ, Caldwell J, Van Kempen GMJ, Vonk RJ (eds): Sulfate Metabolism and Sulfate Conjugation. London: Taylor and Francis, 1982.
Roth JA: Phenol Sulfotransferase. Neuromethods 5:575, 1986.
Quinn GP, Axelrod J, Brodie BB: Species, strain and sex differences in metabolism of hexobarbitone and amidopyrine, antipyrine, and aniline. Biochem Pharmacol 1:152, 1958.
Caldwell J, Davies S, Boots D, O'Gorman J: Interindividual variation in the sulfation and glucuronidation of paracetamol and salicylamide in human volunteers. *In* Mulder GJ, Caldwell J, VanKempen GMS, Vonk RJ (eds): Sulfate Metabolism and Sulfate Conjugation. London: Taylor and Francis, 1982.
Dutton G: Glucuronidation of Drugs and Other Compounds, p 7. Boca Raton, FL: CRC Press, 1980.
Guengerich FP: Mammalian Cytochromes P-450. Boca Raton, FL: CRC Press, 1987.
Singer TP, Von Korff RW, Murphy DL: Monoamine Oxidase: Structure, Function, and Altered Functions. New York, Academic Press, 1979.

7

Pharmacokinetics

Paul J. Kostyniak

Pharmacokinetics is a quantitative approach to the behavior of drugs or chemicals in the body. Mathematical models based on certain assumptions and data collected on the absorption, distribution, and excretion of the drug are used to predict the quantitative pattern and time course of drug disposition in the body.

When one knows the basic mathematical model that a drug follows after being given to a patient, the quantitative aspects of drug disposition may be followed over the time course of drug therapy by measurements of drug levels in suitable representative media, such as biological fluids (blood, plasma, cerebrospinal fluid [CSF]), elimination products (urine, feces), or expired air.

There are two basic approaches to studying drug and chemical disposition: the "simplest model" approach and the "physiologically based modeling" approach. Both approaches can be useful in certain situations.

Traditionally, investigators have strived toward modeling the disposition of drugs and chemicals by applying the *simplest* mathematical compartmental model that would adequately fit experimentally derived data. The goal of this approach is to use samples from an easily accessible body compartment (i.e., blood, urine, saliva, and the like) as an indicator of therapeutically relevant drug concentrations at specific drug target sites, in an effort to maintain drug levels in a therapeutically effective range without significant toxic side effects. This approach has served the needs of the clinical pharmacologist and physician for some years.

Another approach to pharmacokinetics has gained popularity lately, especially in agencies such as the Environmental Protection Agency that are responsible for the risk assessment necessary in the regulation of human chemical exposures. This approach, termed *physiologically based pharmacokinetic modeling*, strives to model exactly the disposition of chemicals in defined physiologically identifiable *compartments*. In concept it tends toward larger, more complicated mathematical models that will predict tissue concentrations within specific organs, tissues, fluids, or cellular compartments. Although this is a more phyiologically defined, purist approach that can in fact be of considerable use in risk assessment of chemical exposures, it provides little more clinically useful information to the physician concerned with effective drug therapy than the traditional simplest model approach. Thus, the increased complexity inherent in this more exact approach is not needed to be able to understand the kinetic behavior of a specific drug within the body. For this reason the discussion here is limited to the simplest model approach.

The route of administration and the chemical formulation of the drug

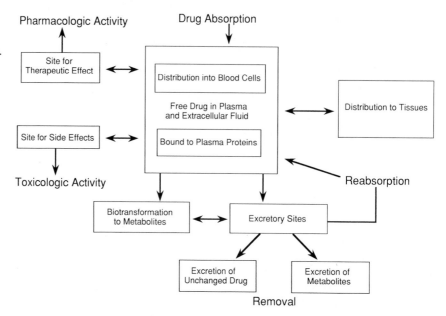

Drugs undergo compartmentalization within
the body.

or chemical determine the amount and rate at which the chemical gains
access to the systemic circulation. Once the drug or chemical has been
absorbed it can be modified within the organism into various states, as
indicated in Figure 7-1, including

1. *Compartmentalization*—the distribution of the drug or chemical
from the administration site into particular compartments. These may be
actual physically identifiable compartments or may be mathematically
defined entities. Movement of the drug among compartments is a dynamic,
ongoing function whereby drug concentrations within a given compartment are constantly changing.

2. *Metabolism*—chemical or enzymatic transformation of the parent
compound into chemically distinct metabolites, transformations which
occur at varying rates. These biotransformed metabolites may have greater
or lesser activity (therapeutic or toxic) than the parent compound.

3. *Excretion*—the appearance of parent compound or metabolites in
elimination products, such as urine, feces, expired air, or hair.

Thus, transformations are occurring constantly from one state of the
drug to another. The transformations diagrammed here are generally first-
order processes, and the rate at which a particular transformation occurs
can be described by a coefficient or rate constant k. Thus, being first order,
the rate of change from one drug state (A) to another drug state (B) bears a
direct relation to the quantity or concentration of the substance in the first
state (A) or for

$$A \longrightarrow B$$

$$dA/dt = -kA \tag{1}$$

or stated directly, the rate of change of A with respect to time is directly
proportional to the amount of A present. Similarly, the build-up of product
is also a function of the amount of reactant present, or

$$dB/dt = kA \tag{2}$$

Oftentimes the net result of these numerous first-order dispositional patterns result in a kinetic profile within a central compartment (blood or plasma) that mimics a first-order process or a series of summed first-order processes. Therefore, we will begin by considering a simple one-compartment, first-order kinetic model and build upon that model in an attempt to provide the tools necessary to understand the kinetic modeling of drugs and chemicals within the body. We will go through the step-by-step derivation of the various functions that we will use in our modeling approach, because an understanding of where equations come from is essential in their proper application in the appropriate situation.

The simplest model of drug disposition considered here depicts the body as a single homogeneous compartment with a constant volume (V), which is diagrammatically illustrated in Figure 7–2.

Just as we relate concentration to the absolute amount of solutes in a given chemical solution, the concentration of drug in the body (C) is related to the absolute amount of drug (S) by the relationship

$$C = \frac{S}{V} \tag{3}$$

Therefore, we can easily calculate the concentration resulting from a known amount of drug (S) if we know the volume of distribution (V) of the drug. This relationship is used frequently in pharmacokinetic problem solving. The volume of distribution can be determined easily by determining the extrapolated blood concentration experimentally (C_0) soon after a bolus dose of the drug (D). Equation 3 then becomes

$$C_0 = \frac{D}{V}$$

where V can be calculated knowing the dose and concentration of drug.

The rate of change in the absolute amount of drug (S) in the body is described by equation 4

$$dS/dt = -kS \tag{4}$$

which on rearrangement gives

$$dS/S = -kdt \tag{5}$$

which on integration yields

$$S = S_0 e^{-kt} \tag{6}$$

This relationship in equation 6 allows us to calculate the expected amount of drug (S) in the compartment at any time (t) when the dose (S_0) and rate constant for drug elimination (k) are known.

Equation 6 may be written also in terms of concentration of drug (C) in the compartment rather than absolute amount (S). By substituting for S in equation 6 from equation 3 we get

$$C = C_0 e^{-kt} \tag{7}$$

The One-Compartment Open Model With Rapid Intravenous Injection

Drug disposition is a dynamic process with drug concentrations changing constantly.

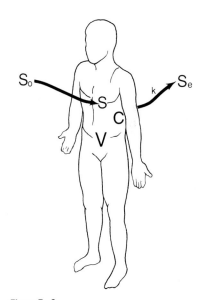

Figure 7–2

Diagrammatic representation of the one-compartment first-order kinetic model, where S_0 is the amount of drug injected (dose) at time = 0. It is assumed that there is *instantaneous mixing* throughout the volume of the compartment (V). S is the instantaneous amount of drug in the body at any time (t). C is the instantaneous concentration of drug in the body (i.e., blood level of drug) at any time (t). S_e is the cumulative amount of drug excreted at any time (t). k is the first-order rate constant of elimination of drug from the body and has the units of time^{-1}.

Figure 7–3

The concentration of drug in plasma is plotted against the time after a single bolus dose of the drug injected intravenously. The figure assumes instantaneous mixing. On linear coordinates, the blood concentration falls exponentially. The rate constant for the function plotted is 0.3465/hour.

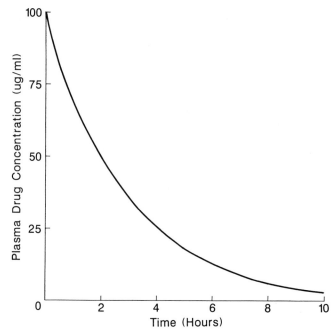

In first-order kinetics, the amount of drug excreted is dependent upon the plasma concentration or body burden.

Thus, this equation indicates that a plot of drug concentration against time would produce a first-order exponential decay function with an intercept on the y axis at C_0, as indicated in Figure 7–3.

Exponential function and graphical representations are not particularly amenable to rapid derivation of clinically useful pharmacokinetic parameters. Therefore, a further log transformation of this function (equation 7) results in a *linear* function, whereby

$$\ln C = \ln C_0 - kt \tag{8}$$

As indicated in equation 8, the natural log of C declines as a linear function of time with a slope of k and an intercept of $\ln C_0$. Thus, a plot of drug concentration versus time on a semilog paper yields a linear function, as indicated in Figure 7–4.

By rearranging equation 8, the amount of drug in the body (S) at any

Plotting first-order kinetic data on semilog paper yields a linear function.

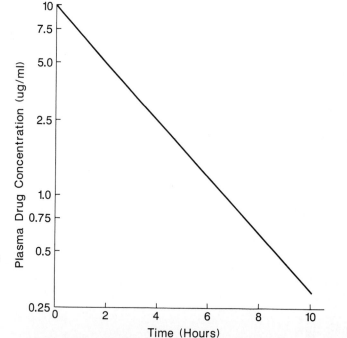

Figure 7–4

The concentration of drug in plasma is plotted against the time after a single bolus dose of the drug injected intravenously. The figure assumes instantaneous mixing. On semilog paper the first-order function is a straight line. This linear plot allows for the direct graphical determination of the half-time of the function. The function plotted has a rate constant of 0.3465/hour.

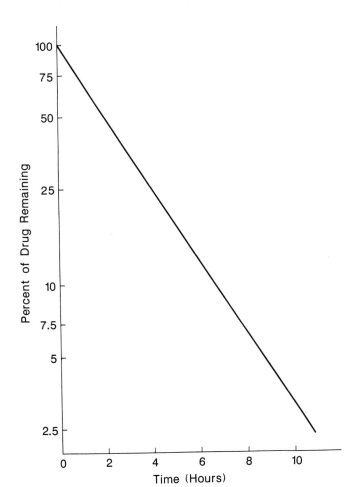

Figure 7–5

Normalized plot of percent of drug remaining (S/S_0 or C/C_0) against the time after a single bolus dose of the drug injected intravenously. The figure assumes instantaneous mixing. The function plotted has a rate constant of 0.3465/hour.

time (t) can be expressed as a function of the initial dose by plotting $\ln S/S_0$ as a function of t, where

$$\ln S/S_0 = -kt \qquad (9)$$

This normalized function of the log of the percent of initial dose of drug remaining at any time t is depicted in Figure 7–5.

From this relationship several additional clinically useful parameters may be derived. One such parameter is the half-time for this function.

Biological Half-Time

The one-compartment open model is analogous to other first-order processes with which the student should already have some familiarity. The first-order decay of radionuclides and first-order chemical reaction kinetics may be expressed by the same equations already derived (i.e., equation 9). The half-time is a parameter common to all these processes, which is convenient to describe the rate at which the process proceeds. It is defined as the time required for S to decline by a factor of ½. For the single-compartment open model of elimination of a drug or chemical from the body, the biological half-time of the drug or chemical is the time required to reduce the body burden of the drug or chemical by ½.

One half of the body burden of drug is eliminated in 1 half-time.

The relationship of the half-time to the rate constant k is easily demonstrated. Taking equation 9, we can substitute one specific time for (t), namely the biological half-time ($t_{1/2}$) for that drug, and the equation becomes

$$\ln \tfrac{1}{2}S_0/S_0 = -kt_{1/2} \qquad (10)$$

The value of S was changed to ½S_0, because by definition the half-time is the time it takes for S to decrease by ½.

Rearrangement of this equation yields the relationship of the rate constant to the half-time:

$$t_{1/2} = \frac{\ln 2}{k} \qquad (11)$$

or

$$t_{1/2} = \frac{0.693}{k} \qquad (12)$$

Thus, when we know the rate constant for elimination of a drug or chemical, equation 12 allows us to easily calculate the half-time. Similarly, as indicated in Figure 7–5, graphical data on the concentration of the drug in plasma (or other suitable biofluid) allow for the graphical determination of the half-time from which the rate constant may be easily calculated.

The amount of drug remaining in the body is depicted as a function of its half-life in Figure 7–6.

Thinking of drug kinetics in terms of the drug's half-life is an easy way to approximate drug levels in time after dosing. Because the process is first order, with the decline in drug being proportional to the instantaneous body burden, the absolute amount of drug being excreted continues to decrease in time. As indicated in Table 7–1, nearly 94% of the initial dose of drug is eliminated in a time period equivalent to four half-times. At this point the absolute change in body burden of drug becomes diminishingly small relative to the initial body burden.

For practical purposes we consider a first-order reaction to have

Drug body burden and concentration exhibit the same rate of decline.

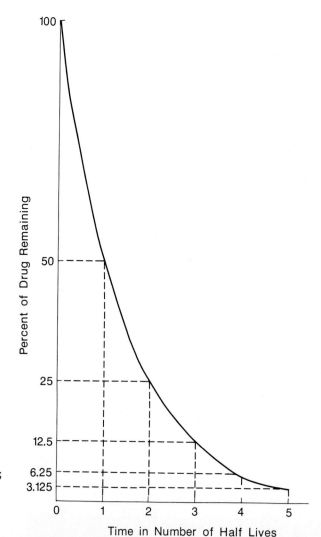

Figure 7–6

The percent of drug remaining (S/S₀ or C/C₀) is plotted against the number of drug half-lives after a single bolus dose of drug injected intravenously. The drug plotted has a biological half-time ($t_{1/2}$) of 1 hour, which corresponds to a rate constant of 0.693/hour.

Table 7-1. THE FRACTIONAL AMOUNTS REMAINING OR THE PERCENTAGE OF DRUG REMAINING AFTER A GIVEN NUMBER OF HALF-LIVES

Number of Half-Lives	% of Drug Remaining	Proportion of Drug Remaining
0	100	1
1	50	½
2	25	¼
3	12.5	⅛
4	6.25	1/16
5	3.125	1/32

reached completion in four to five half-lives (in actuality this is equivalent to 94–97% completion). In the case of the one-compartment open model, we will also consider a single dose to have been nearly completely excreted after four to five half-lives, realizing that as with any first-order reaction, although the drug concentration changes become negligible at infinite times (four to five half-lives) they only approach, but never become, zero.

A ONE-COMPARTMENT OPEN MODEL WITH CONSTANT DOSE RATE

Taking the same single-compartment model, we will alter the single dose at time zero to a continuous-dosing model similar to the clinical situation in which a patient receives a continuous intravenous (IV) infusion of drug. In this case first-order kinetics of drug elimination still prevail. However, with a continuous zero-order input, rather than starting off at a peak concentration as in the single-dose model, we begin at low drug concentrations that tend to increase as the infusion continues. A typical plot of drug concentration versus time for the continuous infusion model is given in Figure 7–7.

In looking at the change in drug body burden over time, we can write the following mass balance equation where

rate of drug change = rate of drug input − rate of drug output or

$$dS/dt = I - E \tag{13}$$

where I = rate of zero-order input of drug into the patient, and E = summation of excretion of the drug by all pathways expressed as a rate.

As indicated earlier, a first-order excretion process is assumed to be in effect as in equation 4 such that the rate of drug excretion will be proportional to the instantaneous body burden (S) or

$$E = kS \tag{14}$$

where k is the same rate constant for excretion described earlier. Equation 13 then becomes

$$dS/dt = I - kS \tag{15}$$

Because the input rate is constant or zero order, it can be described by a rate constant (m). Assume that a constant fraction (f) of a dose rate (m) is absorbed such that I = fm and equation 15 then becomes

$$dS/dt = fm - kS \tag{16}$$

A Variation of the Single-Compartment Model

Drugs administered at a fixed continuous dose rate will reach a plateau or steady state concentration.

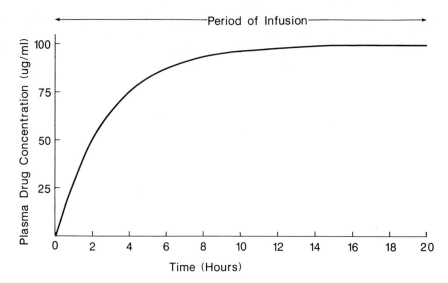

At termination of a continuous infusion,
plasma concentration will undergo a
first-order decline.

Upon integration of this function we obtain the exponential expression

$$S = fm/k(1 - e)^{-kt} \qquad (17)$$

During the period of continual dosing, the body burden approaches its
steady state value. When dosing is stopped, a simple exponential decline in
body burden results, as depicted in Figure 7–8. Steady state may be defined
as a time of no net change in S when rate of input = rate of output, (I = E),
of the drug or chemical. This occurs when e^{-kt} is negligibly small. At $t = \infty$,
esu.$-kt \approx 0$ and

$$S_\infty = \frac{fm}{k} \qquad (18)$$

If f and k are constant properties of the subject for a given drug, then

$$S_\infty \approx m \qquad (19)$$

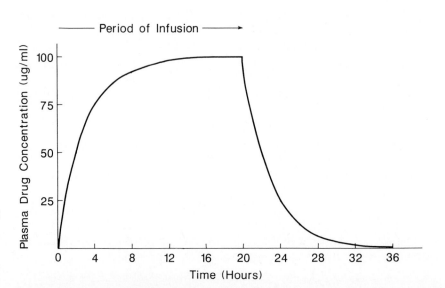

Figure 7–8

The plasma concentration of drug is plotted
against the time from initiation of a
continuous infusion of drug at a zero-order
input rate (m). At 20 hours, the infusion is
stopped and a first-order decline in plasma
drug concentration prevails.

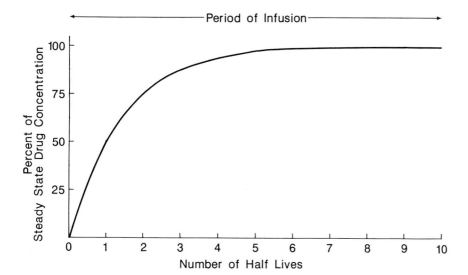

Figure 7–9

The plasma drug concentration expressed as the percent of steady-state drug concentration is plotted against the time measured in half-times from the time of initiation of a continuous infusion of drug at a zero-order input rate (m). Steady state or equilibrium is established within 4–5 half-lives (equivalent to approximately 94% and 97% completion, respectively).

Approach to Steady State

How long does it take to reach steady state? The answer to this question can be put in terms of the kinetic constant already discussed for our first-order model.

Taking equation 17, which describes the first-order constant infusion model, we substitute for fm/k from equation 18. Equation 17 then becomes

$$S = S_\infty (1 - e^{-kt}) \qquad (20)$$

Upon rearrangement expression we obtain the following:

$$S_\infty - S = S_\infty e^{-kt} \qquad (21)$$

This equation states that the difference between the equilibrium body burden (S_∞) and any instantaneous body burden we choose to look at (S_t) declines exponentially as a function of time with the *same* rate constant, k, which governed the first-order excretion of that drug. Because this function is first order, its rate is essentially identical to the first-order process for drug elimination that was already described (equation 6). Thus, as with any first-order function, the process also reaches completion in four to five half-lives. Thus, the rate of approach to steady state is easily described in terms of the half-time of the drug of interest. This is represented diagrammatically in Figure 7–9.

> The approach to steady state is first order.

Because the exponent has only a rate constant and a time parameter, the rate of approach to steady state is *independent* of dose. As a result, an increase in the dose rate results in a proportional change to the steady state concentration of drug (equation 18) but does not affect the time it takes to reach steady state. This is depicted graphically in Figure 7–10.

> An increase in dose rate yields a proportional increase in the steady state plasma concentration or body burden.

Multiple-Dose Case

One of the most common ways to administer drugs is in divided doses separated by some time interval; for example, this is common in oral antibiotic therapy.

Figure 7-10

Body burden in milligrams is plotted against the time from initiation of a continuous infusion of drug at three different rates; m = 10 mg/hour, 2m = 20 mg/hour, and 4m = 40 mg/hour. The drug depicted here has a biological half-life of 2 hours. All three infusion rates result in similarly shaped curves, indicating that the approach to steady state is the same in each case. The drug concentrations reached at steady state are directly proportional to the rate of drug input.

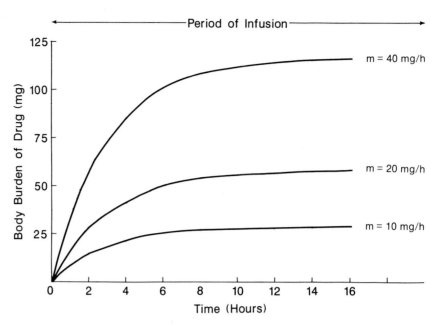

An intermittent-dosing regimen results in peak and trough plasma concentrations and body burdens.

We can treat this case as being analogous to the constant dose rate model discussed previously. In this case equation 20 can be applied with only a modification of the dose rate function. Instead of a continuous infusion we have altered the input of drug into individual doses (D) separated by a dosing interval (τ), and the rate of drug input m becomes D/τ. Substituting for m = D/τ in equation 20 we arrive at the relationship

$$\bar{S} = fD/k\tau \, (1 - e^{-kt}) \qquad (22)$$

The graphical depiction of this function in given in Figure 7-11. Rather than the smooth curve approaching equilibrium as seen in the continuous-infusion model, this intermittent-dosing model results in a saw-toothed curve that depicts a rise in drug concentration that results immediately following each dose, followed by the first-order decline that predominates until the next dose is given. At steady state, the drug concentration varies between a maximal (C_∞^{max}) and a minimal value (C_∞^{min}). These values are also referred to as *peak* and *trough* drug concentrations.

The steady state assumption can be used also to calculate the average steady state value of the drug at equilibrium, just as we did for the continuous-infusion model. Because the exponential function is the same in both equations and becomes diminishingly small at large time points or as the process is near completion (i.e., four to five half-times), equation 22 becomes

$$\bar{S}_\infty = fD/k\tau \qquad (23)$$

The minimal and maximal body burden for each dose can be calculated also to the nth dose using the following relationships,

$$S_n^{max} = D \, \frac{1 - e^{-nk\tau}}{1 - e^{-k\tau}} \qquad (24)$$

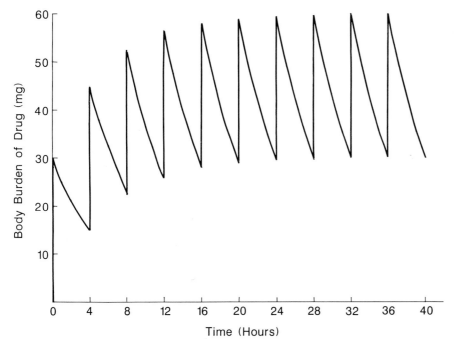

Figure 7–11

The body burden of drug (S) is plotted against time for an intermittent drug dosing regimen of 30 mg of drug (D) given at time 0 and at each 4-hour interval (τ) thereafter. Following each successive dose, first-order excretion kinetics prevail. As with the continuous infusion model, a steady state is reached after 4–5 biological half-lives. The difference between the peak and the trough body burden is equal to the individual drug dose (D).

$$S_n^{min} = D \frac{1 - e^{-nk\tau}}{1 - e^{-k\tau}} e^{-k\tau} \qquad (25)$$

where

S_n^{max} is the amount in the compartment after the nth dose

S_n^{min} is the amount in the compartment τ hours after the nth dose.

At steady state (t = ∞) the values of S_∞^{max} and S_∞^{min} can be calculated as follows:

$$S_\infty^{max} = D \frac{1}{1 - e^{-k\tau}} \qquad (26)$$

$$S_\infty^{min} = D \frac{e^{-k\tau}}{1 - e^{-k\tau}} \qquad (27)$$

At steady state (t = ∞), the input of the drug is equal to the output of drug over the dosing interval and

$$S_\infty^{max} - S_\infty^{min} = D \qquad (28)$$

This occurs at approximately five half-lives after dosing is initiated (see equation 22). Thus S_∞^{max} and S_∞^{min} may be easily calculated for a drug or chemical with a known biological rate constant of excretion (k) for any dose (D) over any dosing interval (τ). At steady state, minimal sampling would be required to monitor the range of drug concentration in plasma.

As indicated in Figure 7–9, it takes a finite time to reach the steady state drug concentration, and the length of this latent period is determined by the half-time of the drug. This has implications regarding the therapeutic effects that the drug is intended to elicit. Conceptually there must be a threshold concentration of drug in plasma above which one could get the

Steady state concentrations may be reached faster by using an initial priming dose of the drug.

Figure 7 – 12

The blood concentration of a drug is plotted in arbitrary units against time on the abscissa. The dashed lines are placed at the blood concentrations that bracket the minimal therapeutic drug concentration and the maximal tolerated drug concentration. After the initial *priming dose,* the peak concentration rises into the effective therapeutic, but not toxic, range of blood concentrations. The administration of *maintenance doses* of the appropriate dose and frequency keeps the blood concentration out of the ineffective zone and below the level associated with toxic effects.

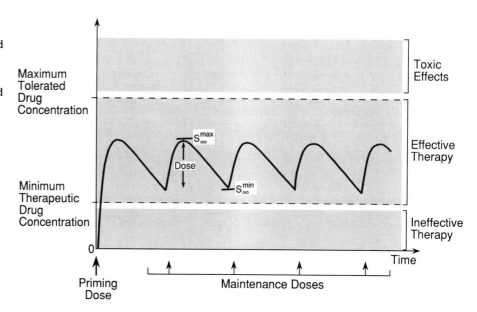

expected outcome, and below which there would be no therapeutic effect (Fig. 7 – 12).

Similarly, as drug concentration increases, the potential for development of adverse or toxic effects increases, and some maximal tolerated drug concentration represents a threshold for developing toxic effects. For effective therapy without serious side effects, the pharmacokinetic challenge is to maintain the drug concentration within a therapeutic range of concentration that is delineated by the threshold for effective therapy (minimal therapeutic drug concentration) and the threshold for toxic effects (maximal tolerated drug concentration).

As indicated earlier, specific steady state concentrations can be readily achieved by selecting appropriate drug dose rates. However, the latent period for reaching steady state results in an initial period during which therapy is ineffective in spite of initiating the drug administration as either the continuous- (IV) or intermittent-dosing models. In order to diminish this latency period an initial priming dose of the drug can be utilized to rapidly increase blood concentrations into the therapeutic range. This is illustrated in Figure 7 – 12, in which an initial large priming dose (i.e., S_∞^{max}) is given. Caution is advised in administration of initial large priming doses, because it is well recognized that with drugs having a low therapeutic index there is a narrow range of blood concentrations of drug that separate effective therapy from toxic effects.

Drug Clearance

The foregoing discussion focused on either the rate of change in total drug on board (body burden) or the rate of change in plasma concentration of drug, both of which follow identical kinetic patterns for the ideal one-compartment model. Drug changes within the body can be viewed also in terms of drug clearance, a concept that mirrors certain physiological elimination processes such as renal or biliary elimination of drugs.

Clearance in the ideal one-compartment model can be thought of as the relative volume of the total compartment cleared over a given time period. A simple equation for clearance can be written as follows:

$$Cl = Vk \tag{29}$$

where clearance (Cl) has the units of volume time^{-1}, V is the volume of distribution, and k is the first-order rate constant described earlier having the units of time^{-1}.

To understand how the concept of clearance fits into the one-compartment pharmacokinetic model derived previously, we will start with the plasma concentration curve for a single bolus dose of drug given at zero time (see Fig. 7–3). This plasma concentration curve is described by equation 7. The area under this curve is simply the integral of that equation, or

$$AUC^{0 \to \infty} = \int_0^\infty C = C_0 \int_0^\infty e^{-kt}dt \qquad (30)$$

$$AUC^{0 \to \infty} = -\frac{C_0}{k}(e^{-k\infty} - e^{-k0}) \qquad (31)$$

$$AUC^{0 \to \infty} = -\frac{C_0}{k}(0 - 1) \qquad (32)$$

$$AUC^{0 \to \infty} = \frac{C_0}{k} \qquad (33)$$

From this relationship one can relate $AUC^{0 \to \infty}$ to clearance by initially substituting for C_0

$$AUC^{0 \to \infty} = D/Vk \qquad (34)$$

and subsequently substituting for Vk, whereby equation 34 becomes

$$AUC^{0 \to \infty} = D/Cl \qquad (35)$$

This approach, which utilizes the concept of clearance to model drug elimination kinetics, relies on data obtained through serial monitoring of plasma drug concentrations after a single bolus dose of the drug. It is described here because many papers in the literature use this convention. This is not a different kinetic model, but rather another way of looking at first-order pharmacokinetic modeling.

References

Bourne DWA, Triggs EJ, Eadie MJ: Pharmacokinetics for the Non-mathematical. Boston: MTP Press Limited, 1986.

Gladtke E, von Hattingberg HM: Pharmacokinetics. New York: Springer-Verlag, 1979.

Hug CC: Pharmacokinetics of drug administered intravenously. Anesth Analg 57:704–723, 1978.

Notari RE: Biopharmaceutics and Clinical Pharmacokinetics. New York: Marcel Dekker, 1987.

Welling PG: Pharmacokinetics. Processes and Mathematics. ACS Monograph 1985. Washington, DC: American Chemical Society, 1986.

Drugs Acting at Synaptic and Neuroeffector Sites

Principles of Neuroeffector Systems

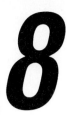

Robert J. McIsaac

The basic understanding of the mechanisms involved in synaptic transmission in the nervous system has been developed primarily through investigations on peripheral neuroeffector systems. The first clear evidence that a chemical substance serves as the transmitter of excitation from nerve to muscle was presented by Otto Loewi in 1921. He demonstrated that a substance was released when the vagus nerve was stimulated and this substance was "active" because it acted on the heart to slow the rate of its beating. This substance was later shown to be the rather simple chemical ester acetylcholine.

Although it was known in the early 1900s that an epinephrine-like substance appeared to be a transmitter released by the sympathetic nerves, it was not until 1946 that von Euler established that the active material released from most sympathetic nerves was norepinephrine.

With the synthesis of radioactively labeled transmitters and their precursors, as well as the discovery and synthesis of relatively specific antagonists to each of the major transmitters, great strides have been made in understanding the mechanisms underlying nerve to nerve communication and nerve to effector cell communication over the past 40 years.

It is now known that many different amines, amino acids, and peptides act as specific excitatory or inhibitory transmitters of information from nerve to nerve, nerve to gland, or nerve to muscle. Furthermore, the concept that transmitters interact with specific receptors consisting of macromolecular proteins has been developed and considerable advance has been made in characterizing and purifying a variety of these receptors.

In this and subsequent chapters, drugs that act principally at one or more sites within the peripheral neuroeffector systems, the autonomic system, and motor nerve–skeletal muscle system are described.

AUTONOMIC NERVOUS SYSTEM

An understanding of the structure and function of the peripheral nervous system is important for a number of reasons:

1. The activity of major organ systems are controlled or regulated by one or both branches of the autonomic nervous system. The activity of these systems (i.e., the gastrointestinal [GI] smooth muscle, smooth muscles of the eye, smooth muscle of the urinary tract, and the cardiovascular system) can be altered pharmacologically. Thus, pathologic conditions that involve these organ systems directly or indirectly can be treated with selectively acting drugs.

2. The autonomic nervous system and the organs it innervates may be the site of side effects also, usually unwanted, of drugs whose principal site is elsewhere. For example, the antipsychotic drug chlorpromazine, in addition to its central effect, can block a norepinephrine receptor and thus cause orthostatic hypotension in some patients. Therefore, in order to understand all the actions of many drugs, it is necessary to be aware of the principles of peripheral synaptic transmission.

3. Lastly, theories developed for synaptic transmission and drug-receptor occupancy have been formulated from studies on the peripheral nervous system and the end-organs and cells they innervate. The principles developed through such studies apply to neuronal transmission within the central nervous system (CNS). Indeed, many of the same neurotransmitters involved in the peripheral nervous system are also some of the important neurotransmitters of the CNS.

Major Components of the Autonomic Nervous System

The autonomic system has two neurons outside the CNS.

The autonomic system is characterized by having two neurons outside the CNS. A preganglionic neuron arises from specific areas in the brain or spinal cord and sends an axon to a collection of neurons outside the spinal cord. The preganglionic nerve is myelinated usually and terminates on a dendrite or soma of a ganglion cell. The postganglionic, unmyelinated nerve may course in a nerve bundle or in a plexus to the effector cell (Figs. 8–1 and 8–2).

Central origins of parasympathetic nerves

Parasympathetic Nervous System (Cranial-Sacral Nervous System). Preganglionic parasympathetic neurons are located in specific areas of the midbrain, medulla, and sacral part of the spinal cord. Parasympathetic nerves leave the brain with the III, VII, IX, and X cranial nerves; the preganglionic fibers terminate within or close to the organs they innervate. Sacral parasympathetic nerves arise from neurons in the sacral spinal cord and leave with spinal nerves to innervate the genitourinary system, colon, and lower GI tract.

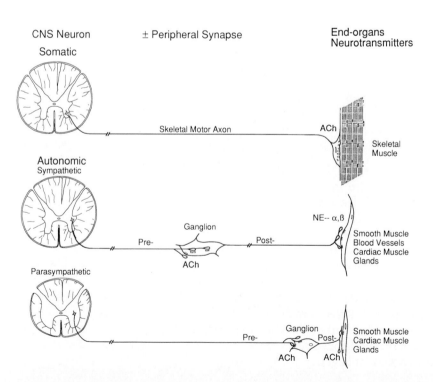

Figure 8–1

Diagrammatic representation of the neuroeffector system. Cholinergic receptors depicted include skeletal neuromuscular nicotinic, ganglionic nicotinic, and postganglionic muscarinic. Adrenergic receptors illustrated are alpha (α) and beta (β). (Pre- = preganglionic nerve; Post- = postganglionic nerve.)

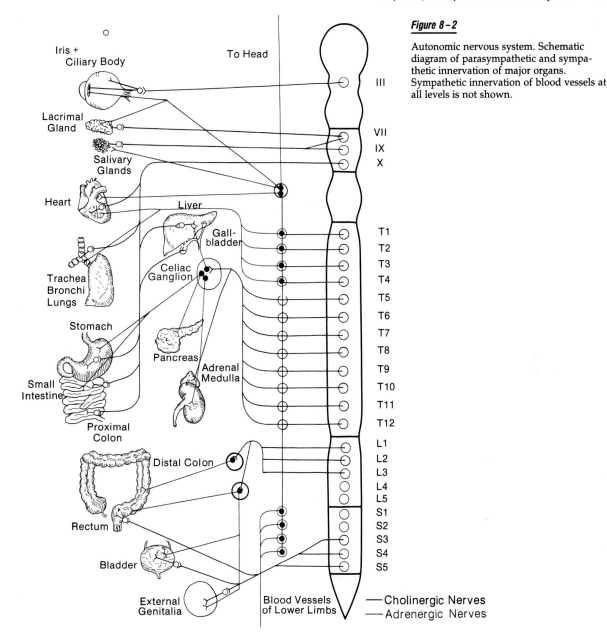

Figure 8-2

Autonomic nervous system. Schematic diagram of parasympathetic and sympathetic innervation of major organs. Sympathetic innervation of blood vessels at all levels is not shown.

——Cholinergic Nerves
——Adrenergic Nerves

Preganglionic parasympathetic nerves terminate on ganglion cells that are on or close to the organ innervated. For example, the vagus nerve arises from cell bodies in the medulla. The cardioinhibitory nerves of the vagus extend from the medulla to the heart and terminate on ganglion cells located on the heart. When a propagated electrical disturbance, the action potential, arrives at the terminal of the parasympathetic nerve, a chemical, acetylcholine, is released from the nerve terminal. The acetylcholine (ACh) diffuses across the narrow synaptic gap and combines with a specific ACh receptor located on the ganglion cell membrane. The combination of ACh with the receptor opens ion channels, allowing sodium to enter the cell and potassium to leave. This change in permeability leads to depolarization of the ganglion cell; the magnitude of this depolarization is graded and regulated by the amount of the ACh-receptor complex formed.

If this cellular depolarization of the ganglion cell is large enough, an action potential is generated on the axon hillock and traverses nondecre-

Acetylcholine is the transmitter released from preganglionic and postganglionic parasympathetic nerves.

mentally to the terminal of the postganglionic parasympathetic axon. When the postganglionic parasympathetic nerve terminal depolarizes, ACh is released, diffuses to a specific receptor on the effector cell, combines with this receptor, and elicits a response. The response elicited by ACh may vary with the anatomical site under consideration, ranging, for example, from depolarization of smooth muscle of the bronchi or gut to hyperpolarization of cardiac pacemaker cells.

Nerves that synthesize and release ACh are designated *cholinergic nerves.* Both preganglionic and postganglionic parasympathetic nerves are cholinergic nerves. Drugs that interact with ACh receptors and have intrinsic activity, i.e., cause an effect similar to ACh, are called *cholinomimetic drugs* (sometimes referred to as parasympathomimetic drugs). Examples of cholinomimetic drugs are bethanechol and pilocarpine. Some drugs may complex also with the ACh receptor but have little or no intrinsic activity, and these drugs are called *cholinolytic* (or parasympatholytic drugs). By occupying the receptor site, cholinolytic drugs prevent the binding of ACh to the receptor and prevent its action and, therefore, reduce the influence of parasympathetic nerve activity on the effector organ.

Sympathetic Nervous System (Thoracic-Lumbar Nervous System). Sympathetic neurons originate in the intermediolateral columns of the thoracic and lumbar spinal cord. Preganglionic nerves leave the spinal cord with spinal nerves and most synapse in vertebral ganglia located on each side of the vertebral column. Some preganglionic sympathetic nerves pass through a vertebral ganglion without synapsing to prevertebral ganglia located in the abdomen (e.g., the coeliac or mesenteric ganglia); a few sympathetic preganglionic nerves synapse on ganglia located on or close to the organs innervated, such as the terminal ganglia on the urinary bladder.

Preganglionic sympathetic nerves are cholinergic, that is, ACh is released as the neurotransmitter from preganglionic sympathetic nerves. Thus, all preganglionic nerves, both parasympathetic and sympathetic, are cholinergic.

An action potential arriving at the terminals of postganglionic sympathetic nerves causes the release of norepinephrine at most sites. The norepinephrine diffuses to the effector cell and combines with a specific receptor to elicit an effect. This effect varies from tissue to tissue.

Nerves that synthesize and release norepinephrine are called *adrenergic nerves.* The term *adrenergic* was coined years ago when it was postulated that adrenaline (epinephrine) was the sympathetic neurotransmitter. An *adrenomimetic drug* (sometimes referred to as a sympathomimetic drug) is one that combines with norepinephrine receptors and has a pharmacological effect similar to stimulation of sympathetic nerves. An adrenolytic drug is one that combines with the norepinephrine receptor but has no intrinsic activity. An *adrenolytic drug* (or sympatholytic drug) will reduce the effect of an adrenomimetic drug or the influence of sympathetic nerve activity on a tissue.

One exception to the statement that postganglionic sympathetic nerves release norepinephrine is the sympathetic nerves to the sweat glands. Although these nerves are anatomically sympathetic nerves, they release ACh as the neurotransmitter (thus, they are cholinergic). This illustrates the necessity for distinguishing autonomic systems on anatomical bases (sympathetic, parasympathetic, preganglionic, postganglionic, and so on) from biochemical and physiological functions, such as cholinergic and adrenergic.

Sympathetic nerves originate in the thoracic and lumbar spinal cord.

Acetylcholine is the transmitter released from preganglionic sympathetic nerves.

Norepinephrine is the transmitter released from most postganglionic sympathetic nerves.

Adrenal Medulla. Certain of the preganglionic sympathetic nerves pass through vertebral ganglia without synapsing to terminate on chromaffin cells of the adrenal medulla. These nerves are cholinergic, i.e., release ACh that acts on specific receptors on chromaffin cells to release epinephrine and norepinephrine into the blood stream. Because the epinephrine/norepinephrine is distributed in blood to all organs, there are widespread effects on a number of tissues and organs whenever the adrenal medulla is activated by the sympathetic system. Because chromaffin cells are derived from the same embryonic tissue that gives rise to autonomic ganglion cells, it should not be surprising, therefore, that they respond pharmacologically similarly to autonomic ganglion cells.

MOTOR NERVES TO SKELETAL MUSCLES

Although motor nerves to the skeletal muscles are not components of the autonomic nervous system, drugs that affect transmission between nerve and skeletal muscle are considered in this unit because the principles involved in synaptic transmission and drug action at this junction are the same as those in the autonomic system, and the transmitter and receptor system involved is similar to that in autonomic ganglia.

Motor nerves to skeletal muscles are cholinergic.

The motor nerve passes without synapse from the motor neuron in the spinal cord to end on a specialized part, the end-plate, of the skeletal muscle fiber. Motor nerves release ACh, which acts on a specific receptor in the end-plate, resulting in depolarization of the end-plate. If the depolarization is of sufficient magnitude, an action potential is generated on the sarcolemma of the muscle cell and is conducted over the muscle membrane initiating the contractile process.

STEPS OF NEUROEFFECTOR TRANSMISSION

Steps in the activation of the neuroeffector system follow a common general pathway:

1. An action potential is conducted over the nerve to its terminal.
2. Depolarization of the presynaptic nerve terminal initiates the release of transmitter. This process requires calcium entry into the nerve terminal. An increase in intracellular calcium initiates the release process, which involves fusion of the storage vesicles with the terminal membrane and exocytosis of the contents into the synaptic gap.

There is evidence that ACh, and possibly other transmitters, is released as discrete amounts, called *quanta*. It is hypothesized that one quanta may be the amount of ACh contained in one storage vesicle.

3. Transmitter combines with its postsynaptic receptor. The transmitter-receptor complex causes a change in the conformation of the receptor, which produces an effect such as activation of an enzyme or increase in permeability of the membrane leading to its depolarization or hyperpolarization, depending on the ion(s) involved.
4. Transmitter action terminates. This may be accomplished by diffusion away from the receptor, re-entrance of the transmitter into the nerve terminal or other cell (uptake), or enzymatic alteration of the transmitter to biologically inactive products.
5. Responsiveness of the postjunctional membrane changes. The sensitivity of the postjunctional membrane may be altered in a number of ways. The response of an effector cell to drugs may be enhanced by denervation or chronic blockade of transmitter release (denervation supersensi-

tivity), reduction in the rate of metabolism or uptake of transmitter, or up-regulation (increase in number) of receptors. A response may be decreased by prolonged depolarization of the membrane or down-regulation of receptors (decrease in number). For example, it has been observed that patients withdrawn abruptly from propranolol (an antagonist for noradrenaline beta receptors) may suffer exacerbation of anginal pain or a rebound hypertension. This supersensitivity is postulated to be related to adaptive increases in the number of beta-adrenergic receptors. Withdrawal from beta receptor antagonist therapy should be accomplished by a gradual reduction in dosage.

6. Multiple transmitters—when the neurohumoral transmission theory described previously was developed, Sir Henry Dale suggested that a nerve would contain only a single specific transmitter substance. However, evidence suggests that this hypothesis may not always be correct, because biologically active peptides have been found to coexist with the more classical neurotransmitters in some nerve terminals. The function of the additional active substances, which in some cases have been shown to be released (coreleased transmitters) during nerve activity, is not clear. It has been suggested that these peptides may modify the action of the primary transmitter or may modify the release of the primary transmitter. For a long time it was observed that stimulation of parasympathetic nerves to salivary glands caused an increase in salivation as well as vasodilation in the gland, but only the salivation was reduced by an ACh antagonist, atropine. This observation may be explained by experiments that indicate two transmitters may be involved: ACh and vasoactive intestinal polypeptide (VIP). Immunofluorescent analysis has demonstrated VIP in cholinergic nerves. VIP causes vasodilation in the submaxillary gland, and both ACh and VIP cause vasodilation; VIP is most important at faster rates of stimulation. An antibody against VIP antagonizes stimulus-induced vasodilation. These results are interpreted to indicate that cholinergic nerves contain both ACh (most important for stimulating secretion) and VIP (important for glandular vasodilation).

IDENTIFICATION OF TRANSMITTERS

The identification of a chemical as a physiological neurotransmitter substance requires rigorous proof, including

1. its presence in the nerve together with a synthetic pathway;
2. its release upon nerve stimulation;
3. a response to exogenously applied substance equal to the response with nerve stimulation;
4. a mechanism for termination of the action of the postulated substance, the putative transmitter;
5. identification of specific antagonists that block the effect of nerve stimulation as well as the effect of exogenously administered chemical.

RECEPTOR CONCEPT

A receptor is defined as a macromolecular molecule with which a neurotransmitter (or drug) interacts to produce its characteristic biological response. In general, the transmitter has an affinity for a specific receptor molecule, and the combination of transmitter with receptor modifies the system to produce a measurable effect. Transmitters have a specificity for their receptors; for example, norepinephrine has little or no affinity for the

ACh receptor, and ACh has little or no affinity for the norepinephrine receptor. (See also discussions in Chapters 1, 2, and 15.)

The capacity of a drug to elicit an effect for a given receptor occupancy is referred to as *intrinsic activity;* the drug must have an affinity for the receptor also. Antagonist drugs have an affinity for the receptor but little or no intrinsic activity. Therefore, antagonists prevent access of active substances to the receptor site but cause no biological response.

Both the ACh and the norepinephrine receptors have been subdivided into two or more subgroups. The ACh receptor has been classified into two major groups, the *nicotinic* and *muscarinic* receptors. Although ACh itself can interact with both classes, drugs are available that interact relatively specifically with one or the other receptor. Both muscarinic and nicotinic receptors can be divided into at least two subgroups; drugs are available that may have a relative specificity for one of the subgroups of receptors.

Both acetylcholine and norepinephrine receptors exist as at least two distinct subgroups.

The norepinephrine receptor has been divided also into two major classes: alpha (α) and beta (β) receptors. This division was made on the basis of the relative potencies of several adrenergic drugs on different organs and of the action of specific antagonistic drugs. Each of these major classes has been subdivided into two subclasses. A more detailed description of these ACh and norepinephrine receptors is presented in the chapters on cholinergic drugs and adrenergic drugs (Chapters 9, 13, and 14).

MODIFICATIONS OF TRANSMITTER RELEASE

Certain toxins, drugs, or procedures may act on the nerve terminal to alter the amount of transmitter released and, therefore, the physiological response to nerve activity. These drugs or procedures are used sometimes to treat pathological problems or in diagnostic tests.

Drugs or toxins may affect autonomic function by increasing or decreasing transmitter release.

Substances That Increase Transmitter Release

1. Drugs that block the increase in potassium conductance—tetraethylammonium, 4-aminopyridinium, and guanidine—increase transmitter release. These cause a prolongation of the action potential and increase the time that calcium can enter the nerve terminal. More free calcium in the cytoplasm leads to an increase in the amount of transmitter released. Guanidine, among other drugs, has been used to treat a rare disease, myasthenic syndrome (or Eaton-Lambert disease), which is due to a defect in the release of ACh from the motor nerve terminal.

2. Posttetanic potentiation increases transmitter release. A brief tetanic stimulation to a nerve causes an increase in response to a single nerve stimulation following the repetitive stimulation. During the tetanus, calcium enters the nerve terminal at a faster rate than it can be sequestered. Therefore, for a time after the tetanus, an increased free calcium is available for transmitter release.

Substances That Decrease Release

1. Botulinum toxin, a potent toxin produced by *Clostridium botulinum,* binds to prejunctional sites on cholinergic nerves and blocks the exocytosis of ACh. Death usually results from respiratory failure.

2. Increased magnesium in the extracellular fluid blocks the entrance of calcium during depolarization of the nerve terminal, thus preventing the release of transmitter that depends on an increase in cytoplasmic free calcium to initiate the exocytosis process.

3. Black widow spider venom initially causes a massive release of ACh and eventual depletion of the nerve terminal as one of its actions.

PHYSIOLOGICAL FUNCTIONS OF THE AUTONOMIC SYSTEM

The autonomic system exercises important control over the function of heart, smooth muscles, and secretory glands.

The most important organs affected by the autonomic nerves for pharmacological considerations are the heart, vascular smooth muscle, secretory glands, and smooth muscles of the eye, GI tract, and bronchioles (Table 8–1; see Figs. 8–1 and 8–2).

Heart

The heart receives innervation by both parasympathetic and sympathetic nerves, and the effects of each on the heart are opposite. In normal young adults the parasympathetic nerves have the predominant effect on heart rate, and the sympathetic nerves are more important when adjustments have to be made for increased activity, changes in the environment, or stress.

Parasympathetic activity slows and sympathetic activity increases heart rate.

The ventricles receive only sympathetic innervation, and parasympathetic nerves have little effect on the ventricular muscle. Activation of the parasympathetic vagus nerve to the heart slows heart rate (a negative chronotropic action), decreases atrial force of contraction, shortens the atrial action potential, and slows the atrioventricular (A-V) conduction velocity leading to partial or complete heart block. Parasympathetic nerves have little effect on ventricular muscle. Activation of sympathetic nerves to the heart increases heart rate (a positive chronotropic action), A-V conduction velocity, the force of contraction of ventricular muscle (a positive inotropic action), and the automaticity of ventricular muscle.

Table 8–1 TYPICAL RESPONSES OF TISSUES TO PARASYMPATHETIC AND SYMPATHETIC INNERVATION

Tissue	Parasympathetic	Sympathetic
Heart		
S-A node	Decreased rate of discharge	Increased rate of discharge
A-V node	Decreased conduction velocity — partial or complete block	Increased conduction velocity
Ventricles	Negligible effect	Increased force of contraction (+ inotropic action) Increased conduction velocity Increased automaticity
Vascular Smooth Muscle		
Arterioles	Local vasodilation	Vasoconstriction
Veins	—	Venoconstriction
Other Smooth Muscle		
Gastrointestinal	Increased tone and motility	Decreased tone and motility
Urinary bladder	Increased tone	Relaxation
Iris	Contraction of sphincter muscle (miosis)	Contraction of radial muscle (mydriasis)
Ciliary muscle	Contraction	—
Bronchial muscle	Contraction	Relaxation
Secretions		
Saliva	Increase in watery secretion	Increase in viscous secretion
Nasopharyngeal	Increased	—
Gastric	Increased	—
Pancreatic	Increased	—
Sweat	—	Increased (cholinergic)

Vascular Smooth Muscle

Both arterioles and veins receive sympathetic vasoconstrictor nerves, and control of peripheral resistance and blood pressure is mediated through an increase or decrease in sympathetic vasoconstrictor activity. Increased activity of sympathetic vasoconstrictor nerves causes vasoconstriction and increased peripheral resistance, whereas decreased sympathetic nerve activity allows the vascular smooth muscle to relax and the peripheral resistance to decrease. Likewise, venoconstriction or venodilation resulting from an increase or decrease in activity on sympathetic nerves to veins will decrease or increase venous capacity, respectively.

> Sympathetic nerves supply the major innervation of vascular smooth muscle.

Parasympathetic vasodilator nerves are mostly involved in local control of blood flow within specific organs (e.g., the tongue). The parasympathetic system is not involved in the control and regulation of total peripheral resistance and blood pressure. However, there are receptors for a number of vasoconstricting and vasodilating substances located on arterioles. These extrasynaptic receptors do not receive nerve input but may be activated by substances present in the blood stream. For example, in the next chapter we point out that ACh-like drugs, when administered parenterally, may act on vascular receptors to cause vasodilation and consequently unwanted hypotension; this effect of these drugs is the result of their actions on extrasynaptic ACh receptors.

Gastrointestinal Smooth Muscle

The parasympathetic nerves to GI smooth muscle exert extrinsic motor control of the smooth muscle. Activation of parasympathetic nerves induces an increase in muscle tone and motility. In contrast, the sympathetic nerves terminate on both ganglion cells and smooth muscle cells; their activation results in inhibition of ganglionic transmission as well as relaxation of the muscle cells.

> Tone and activity of smooth muscle other than vascular is increased by parasympathetic stimulation.

Urinary Bladder

The detrusor muscle of the urinary bladder receives excitatory parasympathetic innervation, which causes contraction of the muscle and increased pressure on the contents of the bladder. Parasympathetic nerves also cause relaxation of the trigone and external sphincter, so that voiding of the contents of the bladder is facilitated. Sympathetic nerves to the bladder have the opposite effects.

With the exception of vascular smooth muscle and the radial muscle of the iris, sympathetic innervation causes relaxation and parasympathetic innervation causes contraction of smooth muscles.

Eye

The iris of the eye receives both parasympathetic and sympathetic innervation. Parasympathetic nerves innervate the sphincter pupillae muscle and cause contraction of this muscle, which leads to narrowing of the pupil (miosis). Sympathetic nerves innervate the radial muscle of the iris and cause contraction of this muscle, which leads to enlargement of the pupil (mydriasis). The ciliary muscle, which is responsible for adjustment of the lens for distant and near vision, receives only parasympathetic innervation. An increase in neuronal activity causes contraction of the ciliary muscle, which causes the lens to assume the more spherical shape necessary for near vision. A decrease in neuronal activity allows the muscle to relax, and the lens becomes adjusted for more distant vision. If the effect of parasympathetic innervation is blocked by drugs, the lens remains adjusted only for distant vision (cycloplegia).

Secretions

Exocrine gland secretions are increased by parasympathetic activity.

Secretion of fluids by various exocrine organs is controlled by the parasympathetic nerves. Tonic parasympathetic activity is often necessary to maintain basal secretion, and increased secretion is obtained when an increase in parasympathetic nerve activity occurs. The most prominent effects observed are increased secretions of the salivary glands, nasopharyngeal glands, and gastric glands. The influence of the sympathetic innervation is variable, ranging from decreased secretion by bronchial glands to an increase in a viscous amylase-containing secretion from salivary glands (see Table 8–1). In contrast to excitatory parasympathetic innervation of the salivary and gastric glands, the excitatory innervation of sweat glands is by cholinergic sympathetic nerves. Acetylcholine (rather than norepinephrine) is the transmitter released from these sympathetic nerves, and the ACh acts on muscarinic receptors on sweat glands to increase output of sweat.

IMPORTANCE OF THE AUTONOMIC NERVOUS SYSTEM

The autonomic nervous system regulates the functions of many organs that are not under voluntary control and maintains harmonious integrated functioning of many organs. In general, the parasympathetic system exerts a more localized influence on discrete organs, functioning mainly to control essential activities and to conserve energy. The sympathetic system is not absolutely essential for life, but it is essential to permit adjustments to changes in activity, environment, and stresses that often occur in life. The activity of the sympathetic system tends to be more generalized than that of the parasympathetic system. During severe stresses, especially those involving emotional reactions, the sympathetic and adrenal medulla may be activated simultaneously (see Fig. 8–1).

Modifying Reflexes

Reflexes may modify pharmacological responses to drugs.

Although the previous description of autonomic innervation of tissues dealt with efferent nerves to the tissues, it should be kept in mind that there are extensive afferent systems that transmit sensory information to integrative nuclei in the CNS. These important areas within the CNS receive sensory input from the periphery as well as input from other areas within the CNS. Any condition or drug that alters an important function, such as a blood pressure change, often sets off reflex activity that tends to minimize the change. One reflex, the baroreceptor reflex (Table 8–2), is especially important for the understanding of the action of drugs that affect vascular smooth muscle. An increase in blood pressure is detected by sensory receptors in the carotid sinus and aortic arch, causing an increased number and frequency of firing of the carotid sinus and aortic arch nerves to the vasomotor center. This reflex leads to a decrease in heart rate and a decrease in sympathetic vasoconstrictor activity to the resistance and capacitance vessels. Conversely, a decrease in blood pressure causes a reflex increase in heart rate and an increase in sympathetic vasoconstrictor activity to the resistance and capacitance vessels. In this manner, the direct effect of a drug may be modified or overwhelmed by reflexes. (Drug effects directly on these and other sensory systems are discussed in Chapter 26.)

Table 8-2 BARORECEPTOR REFLEX			
Reflex	**Sensory Receptors**	**Stimulus**	**Effect**
Baroreceptor	Carotid sinus and aortic arch	Increased blood pressure	Heart rate decreased Peripheral resistance decreased Venous tone decreased
		Decreased blood pressure	Heart rate increased Peripheral resistance increased Venous tone increased

References

Axelsson J, Thesleff S: A study of supersensitivity in denervated mammalian skeletal muscle. J Physiol (Lond) 147:178–193, 1959.

Bannister R (ed): Autonomic Failure: A Textbook of Clinical Disorders of the Autonomic Nervous System. Oxford: Oxford University Press, 1983.

Bartfai T: Presynaptic aspects of the coexistence of classical neurotransmitters and peptides. Trends Pharmacol 6:331–334, 1985.

Birdsall NJM, Hulme EC: Muscarinic receptor subclasses. Trends Pharmacol 4:459–463, 1983.

Bourdois PS, McCandless DL, MacIntosh FC: A prolonged after-effect of intense synaptic activity on acetylcholine in a sympathetic ganglion. Can J Physiol Pharmacol 53:155–165, 1975.

Ceccarelli B, Hurlbut WP: Vesicle hypothesis of the release of quanta of acetylcholine. Physiol Rev 60:396–441, 1980.

Dunant Y: On the mechanism of acetylcholine release. Prog Neurobiol 26:55–92, 1986.

Furchgott RF: Role of endothelium in response of vascular smooth muscle. Circ Res 53:557–573, 1983.

Higgins CB, Vatner SF, Braunwald E: Parasympathetic control of the heart. Pharmacol Rev 25:119–155, 1973.

Howard BD, Gunderson CB, Jr: Effects and mechanisms of polypeptide neurotoxins that act presynaptically. Annu Rev Pharmacol Toxicol 20:307–336, 1980.

Hubbard JI: Microphysiology of vertebrate neuromuscular transmission. Physiol Rev 53:674–723, 1973.

Jope RS: High-affinity choline transport and acetyl CoA production in brain and their roles in regulation of acetylcholine synthesis. Brain Res Rev 1:313–344, 1979.

McCarthy MP, Earnest JP, Young EF, et al: The molecular neurobiology of the acetylcholine receptor. Annu Rev Neurosci 9:383–413, 1986.

North RA: Electrophysiology of the enteric nervous system. Neuroscience 7:315–325, 1982.

Popot JL, Changeux JP: Nicotinic receptor of acetylcholine. Structure of an oligomeric integral membrane protein. Physiol Rev 64:1162–1239, 1984.

Rahamimioff R: The role of calcium in transmitter release at the neuromuscular junction. *In* Thesleff S (ed): Motor Innervation of Muscle, 117–149. London: Academic Press, 1976.

Reichardt LF, Kelly RB: A molecular description of nerve terminal function. Annu Rev Biochem 52:871–926, 1983.

Simpson LL: The origin, structure, and pharmacological activity of botulinum toxin. Pharmacol Rev 33:115–188, 1981.

9

Cholinomimetic Drugs

Robert J. McIsaac

Biochemistry of Cholinergic Nerves

$$H_3C - \overset{\overset{\displaystyle CH_3}{|}}{\underset{\underset{\displaystyle CH_3}{|}}{\overset{+}{N}}} - CH_2CH_2 - O - \overset{\overset{\displaystyle O}{\|}}{C} - CH_3$$

Acetylcholine

Choline acetyltransferase (ChAT) catalyzes the synthesis of ACh from choline and coenzyme A acetate.

The activity of innervated tissues is continuously modulated and controlled by nerves that possess mechanisms not only for the synthesis, storage, release, and termination of transmitters but also for processes that adjust rapidly according to changing physiological needs. Control at each step of these processes is potentially available with the end result of an almost constant source of transmitter in the face of increased or decreased neuronal activity.

SYNTHESIS OF ACETYLCHOLINE

The synthesis of acetylcholine (ACh) is catalyzed by an enzyme, choline acetyltransferase (ChAT), that is found in all cholinergic nerves. ChAT catalyzes the combination of choline with coenzyme A acetate to form ACh. The intracellular choline concentration is the rate-limiting factor in synthesis of ACh, and because choline does not pass through cell membranes easily, a transport process is necessary to maintain adequate intracellular choline concentration for metabolic processes. Evidence has been presented that there are at least two choline transport systems: a high-affinity transport that primarily provides choline for synthesis of ACh, and a low-affinity choline transport system that makes choline available for incorporation into membrane lipids (Jope, 1979). These processes have been studied with the aid of a chemical, hemicholinium-3, which can block the transport processes and reduce the rate of uptake of choline by the nerve membrane (Fig. 9–1). Hemicholinium-3 can thus deplete cholinergic nerves of ACh by this mechanism when the stored ACh is released by neuronal activity.

Factors that control the rate of ACh synthesis are the level of cholinergic nerve activity and the rate of transport of choline into the nerve. During increased nerve activity, the rate of choline transport is increased markedly. This increase in choline transport results in increased intracellular choline, which is available for synthesis to ACh. The process is rather efficient, so that the concentration of ACh in the nerve terminal remains remarkably constant even during prolonged periods of enhanced nerve activity (Bourdois et al, 1975).

STORAGE OF ACETYLCHOLINE

ACh, which is synthesized primarily in neuronal cytoplasm, is taken up and stored in vesicles that are found concentrated in nerve terminals. The

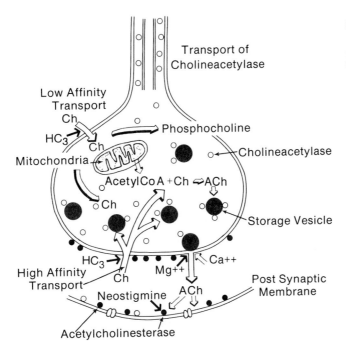

Figure 9-1

Cholinergic nerve terminal showing synthesis, storage, and release of ACh. HC_3 is hemicholinium-3, which antagonizes choline transport.

concentration of ACh in a vesicle is high; the ACh is associated with protein and adenosine triphosphate (ATP). Estimates of the number of ACh molecules per vesicle range from 1 to 50×10^3 for the motor nerve terminal.

RELEASE OF ACh

Evoked release of ACh is triggered by depolarization of nerve terminals. Depolarization allows entry of calcium that is necessary for the release process to occur. By some not yet understood mechanism, the storage vesicle fuses with the nerve membrane, and stored ACh is released by exocytosis.

Depolarization of the nerve terminal triggers release of ACh.

It is hypothesized that ACh, and other transmitters, are released as packets, or quanta (Hubbard, 1973). In the case of ACh, one quanta may be the contents of a single vesicle. With intracellular recording methods, low-frequency spontaneous miniature potentials may be recorded from post-synaptic regions if the recording geometry is correct. These miniature potentials are speculated to be caused by the random spontaneous release of one quanta of ACh. The depolarization of a nerve terminal by an action potential causes the simultaneous release of up to 200–300 quanta, which is sufficient to activate the postsynaptic membrane. Nonquantal mechanisms of ACh release have been proposed also, but their role in synaptic transmission is still in question (Dunant, 1986).

TERMINATION OF ACh ACTION

ACh is hydrolyzed to acetate and choline through the catalytic action of an enzyme, acetylcholinesterase. This enzyme is found associated with cholinergic nerves, and its primary function is to catalyze the hydrolysis of ACh. Choline is about one thousandth as active as a cholinergic agonist than ACh, so the effect of nerve activity is practically terminated. Choline may be transported back then into the nerve terminal to re-enter the synthetic pathway for ACh.

The action of ACh is terminated by enzymatic hydrolysis.

ACh RECEPTORS

Receptors are now identified by either a functional experiment or specific ligand binding techniques. However, in order for proposed receptor nomenclature to be generally accepted, a correlation between functional observations and ligand binding observations must be found. Traditionally the classification of the ACh receptor into two major subdivisions, nicotinic and muscarinic, was based on experiments in the late nineteenth and early twentieth centuries. Otto Schmiedeburg observed that an alkaloid, muscarine, obtained from the mushroom *Amanita muscaria* had pharmacological effects in experimental animals similar to stimulation of postganglionic parasympathetic nerves. Likewise, John N. Langley found that nicotine stimulated, at small doses, and blocked, at larger doses, at autonomic ganglia and neuromuscular junctions. Later, Sir Henry Dale observed that ACh stimulated at autonomic ganglia, neuromuscular junctions, and autonomic neuroeffector junctions. Dale proposed two types of ACh receptors: nicotinic receptors located on ganglia and neuromuscular junctions and muscarinic receptors located on effector cells innervated by postganglionic parasympathetic nerves. The concept was supported by the well-known observations that D-tubocurarine specifically blocked nicotinic receptors and atropine specifically blocked muscarinic receptors.

With the synthesis of numerous congeners of ACh and ACh antagonists, it became apparent that subpopulations of the two types of ACh receptors existed. Decamethonium is a specific antagonist at the neuromuscular junctions but not at ganglia; on the other hand, hexamethonium is a relatively specific antagonist at autonomic ganglia. Furthermore, the agent dimethylphenylpiperazinium (DMPP) is an agonist at ganglia but it has little effect at the neuromuscular junction. More recently, a muscarinic antagonist, pirenzepine, has been found to act selectively at some but not all muscarinic receptors by means of studies of both functional and ligand binding to subgroups of muscarinic receptors.

Ligand binding experiments have the advantage over functional experiments in that studies can be carried out *in vitro* on cells or cell membranes. Although ligand binding techniques are widely used to study receptors and kinetics of ligand binding, definite assignment of a receptor classification requires correlation of functional and binding studies.

Although ACh will complex with receptors at a number of different sites, the concentration of ACh that is required to cause an effect varies with the sites, and different drugs or natural products are available that act more specifically at one cholinergic site than another. On the basis of the specific actions of certain natural products, ACh receptors have been classified into two major groups, nicotinic and muscarinic receptors (Table 9–1).

Table 9–1   TYPES AND LOCATION OF ACh RECEPTORS*

Receptor	Location	Typical Agonist	Typical Antagonist
Muscarinic	Heart Smooth muscle Exocrine glands	Bethanecol Pilocarpine	Atropine
Nicotinic	Autonomic ganglionic neurones End-plate of skeletal muscle	Nicotine Nicotine	Hexamethonium Tubocurarine Pancuronium, Bungarotoxin

* Current classification of ACh receptors is based not on anatomical location but rather on binding and the actions of specific agonists or antagonists. When this method of identifying ACh receptors is used, muscarinic ACh receptors are found in many more tissues than indicated by this historical classification.

Nicotinic Receptors

The characteristic locations of nicotinic receptors are on parasympathetic and sympathetic autonomic ganglia and on the end-plate of skeletal muscles innervated by motor nerves. The name of these receptors derives from the observation that the plant alkaloid nicotine combines with ACh receptors at these sites but not at ACh receptors found on smooth muscles or exocrine glands. Although ACh and nicotine act on receptors at both ganglia and neuromuscular sites, there is even a difference in the receptors at these two sites, because antagonist drugs are available that act relatively specifically only at one site. For example, hexamethonium is an antagonist for ganglionic transmission in usual therapeutic concentrations, but is an antagonist of neuromuscular transmission only at much larger concentrations. Conversely, tubocurarine is an antagonist of neuromuscular transmission in its usual concentrations and causes ganglionic blockade only at larger concentrations.

Structure of the Nicotinic Receptor. The structure of the nicotinic ACh receptor has been studied extensively, and the receptor has been isolated, purified, and crystallized. Although much of the investigations on structure of the nicotinic receptor has been done on receptors isolated from electric fish, which have a rich source of receptor material, there is evidence that the receptors in skeletal muscle and brain are not fundamentally different (Popot and Changeaux, 1984). The receptor is an integral membrane glycoprotein with a molecular weight of about 250,000 daltons. The receptor is composed of four different subunits designated α, β, γ, and δ, which occur in the ratio of $2:1:1:1$, respectively. The four subunits are relatively homogeneous in that they share 35–50% identical amino acid sequences near the NH_2 terminal end and probably derive from a common basic structure. The receptor is inserted in the membrane such that it extends through the membrane and projects into the extracellular space as well as intracellular milieu. The α subunits contain the ACh binding sites (Fig. 9–2).

Nicotinic ACh receptors are found on ganglion cells and the end-plate at motor nerve–skeletal muscle junctions.

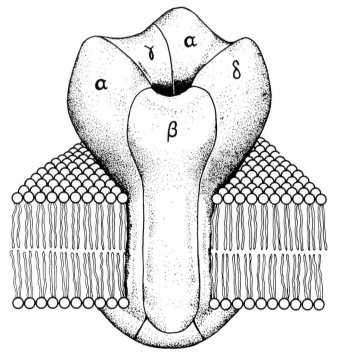

Figure 9–2

Schematic representation of the nicotinic ACh receptor showing the position of four subunits in the membrane (2 α, β, γ, and δ). The center hole represents a channel opened by occupation of the receptor by ACh. (Adapted from Kistler J, Stroud R, Klymrowsky M, et al: Structure and function of an acetylcholine receptor. Biophys J 37:371–373, 1982; and Changeaux J, Devillers-Thiery A, Chemouilli P: Acetylcholine receptor: An allosteric protein. Science 225:1335–1345, 1984.)

Binding of ACh to the receptor causes a conformational change that results in the opening of a pore, 6–7 Å in size, and allows ions to flow. The ionophore occurs in either the closed (resting) or the open (active) state. In the absence of ACh few channels open spontaneously, but in the presence of ACh agonists many channels open. At the neuromuscular junction a presynaptic action potential may cause approximately 2.5×10^5 channels to open transiently generating an end-plate current of about $-400~\mu\text{Å}$ (McCarthy et al, 1986). The interaction of ACh with its receptor is believed to be a two-step process. ACh interacts reversibly with the receptor to form an ACh-receptor complex. This complex then undergoes a reversible conformational change to an active ACh receptor with an open channel.

Muscarinic Receptors

Early pharmacologists discovered that an active ingredient of the mushroom *Amanita muscaria*, muscarine, caused effects similar to that expected from stimulation of postganglionic parasympathetic nerves. So the ACh receptors located on smooth muscle and exocrine glands innervated by postganglionic cholinergic nerves have been designated *muscarinic*. The major locations of muscarinic receptors are on the smooth muscles of the gastrointestinal (GI) and urinary tracts, bronchioles, iris, and cardiac muscle.

Muscarinic ACh receptors are located on smooth muscle cells, exocrine gland cells, and heart cells.

Structure of Muscarinic Receptors. Purification of the muscarinic receptor is currently being accomplished. The muscarinic receptor is a glycoprotein with an amino acid composition different than the nicotinic receptor. One of the major tissue sources for isolation of the muscarinic receptor has been the CNS, and at least two major subgroups of muscarinic receptors have been postulated. Pirenzepine, an antagonist, binds to muscarinic receptors with two affinity states; neuronal receptors bind with high affinity, and peripheral muscarinic receptors bind with low affinity. Receptors binding pirenzepine with high affinity are designated M–1 muscarinic receptors and are found on neuronal tissue and some glands, whereas those binding pirenzepine with low affinity are designated M-2 muscarinic receptors and are found primarily on cardiac tissue, smooth muscle, and some glands. However, most organs contain varying amounts of both receptors. Although many cholinergic agonists (e.g., bethanechol) and antagonists (e.g., atropine) combine nonspecifically with both subgroups, pirenzepine represents a useful pharmacological advance because it is effective in antagonizing vagally mediated acid secretion with a minimal effect on heart rate.

Molecular cloning experiments have produced at least four distinct muscarinic subtypes, which have been designated M-1, M-2, M-3, and M-4. The subtypes M-3 and M-4 exhibit cross-identity with each other and M-1 and M-2 subgroups. The M-1 and M-4 subgroups are closest in identity, and M-2 and M-3 have a similar identity. The various subgroups differ in the number of amino acid residues and the binding of pirenzepine (M-1, M-3, M-4 with high affinity) and binding of AF-DX-116 (11-[2-[(diethylamino) methyl]-1-piperidinyl]acetyl-5-11-dihydro-6H-pyrido [2,3-6][1,4] benzodiazepine-6-one) to M-2 receptors with high affinity. The chemical composition and selective action of muscarinic subgroups are currently under intensive investigation, and this will probably lead to synthesis of useful drugs with selective muscarinic action.

Table 9-2 CHOLINOMIMETIC DRUGS WITH NICOTINIC OR MUSCARINIC ACTIVITY

Drug	Type	Receptor Interaction	Susceptibility to Acetylcholinesterase
Acetylcholine	Ester	Muscarinic and nicotinic	Rapidly hydrolyzed
Carbamylcholine (carbachol)	Carbamate	Muscarinic and nicotinic	Slowly hydrolyzed
Methacholine (Mecholyl)	Ester (β methyl)	Muscarinic	Rapidly hydrolyzed
Bethanechol (Urecholine)	Carbamate (β methyl)	Muscarinic	Slowly hydrolyzed
Pilocarpine	Plant alkaloid	Muscarinic	Not hydrolyzed
Oxotremoxine	Synthetic	Muscarinic	Not hydrolyzed
Nicotine	Plant alkaloid	Nicotinic	Not hydrolyzed

THERAPEUTIC USEFULNESS

Muscarinic agonists that act directly on ACh receptors may be used in situations in which smooth muscle tone has been reduced, such as paralytic ileus following surgery, nonobstructive urinary retention, or where it is necessary to increase smooth muscle tone, for example, in glaucoma to increase the outflow of aqueous humor from the anterior chamber of the eye (Table 9–2). They may be used also, although less frequently, to reduce heart rate during paroxsymal supraventricular tachycardia.

MUSCARINIC (PARASYMPATHOMIMETIC) DRUGS

Although ACh is a prime example of this class of drugs, it is not used clinically because it is so unstable chemically; even when given parenterally it has a brief duration of action because of its rapid hydrolysis by esterases. Nevertheless, when administered parenterally many of the most obvious effects of ACh can be attributed to its interaction with muscarinic (rather than nicotinic) receptors.

The most widely used specific cholinergic muscarinic agonists are *bethanechol* and *pilocarpine.* Both of these drugs exhibit muscarinic actions, but they have no nicotinic effects.

Bethanechol is a carbamate derivative of ACh with a methyl substitution on the beta carbon atom of choline. Methyl substitution on the beta carbon atom confers specificity for the muscarinic receptor. The carbamate substitution makes the molecule less susceptible to enzymatic hydrolysis.

Pilocarpine is an alkaloid obtained from the leaves of a South American plant. The alkaloid was isolated in 1875, and its parasympathomimetic properties were observed soon after.

Although pilocarpine has no obvious chemical relationship to ACh, it has similar pharmacological properties through its agonist action on muscarinic receptors.

Note that the N atoms in pilocarpine are tertiary substituted, unlike ACh, which has the charged quaternary nitrogen, (CH_3)-N^+-R. Therefore, pilocarpine can exist in either the un-ionized or the ionized state, depending on the pH of the biological fluid in which it is dissolved. In the un-ionized form pilocarpine can penetrate biological membranes more readily than the charged ACh molecule. Therefore, it is useful for topical application, for example, to the cornea of the eye where a local effect is desired.

Agonists Acting Directly on Muscarinic Receptors

Bethanechol and pilocarpine are specific muscarinic agonists.

Pilocarpine

Un-ionized pilocarpine can readily cross biological membranes.

MAJOR PHARMACOLOGICAL ACTIONS OF MUSCARINIC AGONISTS

Smooth Muscle

Except for vascular smooth muscle, ACh, bethanechol, and pilocarpine increase the tone, peristaltic activity and contraction of smooth muscles, especially of the GI tract, urinary bladder, and the eye.

Increased tone and contraction of smooth muscle results from the action of agonists on muscarinic receptors to increase membrane permeability to Na^+, K^+, and Ca^{2+}, which results in depolarization of the membrane, an increased frequency of action potentials in smooth muscle membranes, and an increased contraction of the smooth muscle. In part, the effect of ACh on Ca^{2+} permeability is independent of membrane depolarization, because it has been shown that ACh increases Ca^{2+} permeability in depolarized smooth muscle.

Therapeutic Uses. Because pilocarpine is well absorbed from the cornea, it is especially useful for its effects on the sphincter pupillae of the iris and on the ciliary muscle of the eye. By increasing the tone of the sphincter muscle of the iris, pilocarpine causes a constriction of the pupil (miosis). Pilocarpine will increase the tension of the ciliary muscle also, which focuses the lens for near objects. These two effects may be useful in treating patients with increased intraocular pressure, glaucoma, by increasing the outflow of the aqueous humor from the anterior chamber of the eye. In the case of narrow angle glaucoma, pilocarpine probably acts to reduce the blockage of the canal of Schlemm by increasing the contraction of the sphincter muscle of the iris, which pulls the iris away from the canal opening. In open angle glaucoma, pilocarpine probably acts to reduce the restriction to outflow in the trabecular meshwork (Fig. 9–3).

Pilocarpine may be used to treat glaucoma.

Figure 9-3

Schematic drawing of the eye, showing the lens in relation to the ciliary muscles and the muscles of the pupil. The *colored arrows* indicate the flow of the aqueous humor—from the ciliary processes into the posterior chamber, through the pupil into the anterior chamber, leaving at the angle through the trabeculae and through uveoscleral routes. (Modified; Copyright 1989 CIBA-GEIGY Corporation. Reproduced with permission from Atlas of Human Anatomy by Frank H. Netter, M.D. All rights reserved.)

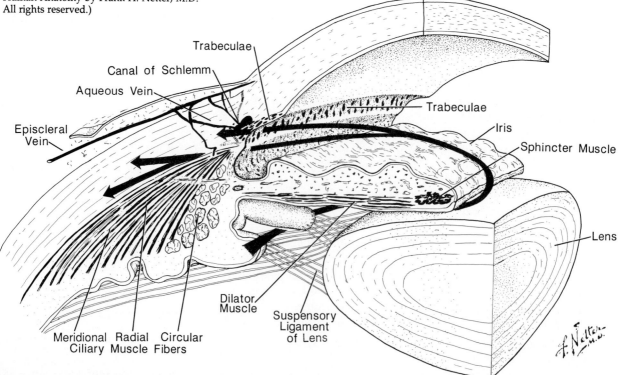

Bethanechol may be used to treat patients who have suffered a loss in tone in the GI tract, for example, postoperatively after abdominal surgery. Bethanechol is also useful to treat urinary retention in the absence of organic obstruction. Cholinomimetics increase the tone of the detrusor muscle and, consequently, decrease bladder capacity. They relax the trigone and external sphincters also, so that voiding is improved in postoperative or postpartum urinary retention.

Bethanechol may be used to increase GI and urinary bladder tone.

Adverse Cholinomimetic Effects on Smooth Muscle. Cholinomimetic drugs may have effects on other smooth muscles that are not useful therapeutically and may be dangerous to some patients.

Blood vessels have muscarinic receptors. These receptors do not receive parasympathetic nerve innervation, but they do respond to circulating cholinomimetic drugs to cause vasodilation leading to a decrease in blood pressure. The muscarinic receptors are located on the vascular endothelium and, when occupied by cholinomimetic drugs, result in the release of an endothelium-dependent relaxing factor that causes relaxation of the smooth muscle (Furchgott, 1983). The decrease in blood pressure is one of the most prominent effects observed upon parenteral administration of ACh. This fall in blood pressure causes a reflex increase in heart rate that may overcome the direct bradycardiac effect of ACh on cardiac pacemaker cells.

Cholinomimetic drugs may increase the tone of bronchiolar smooth muscle. Whereas this increase in tone usually has no significant effect in normal people, it can lead to bronchospasm or asthma in sensitive people. For this reason muscarinic agonists are used with caution or not at all in patients with asthma or a severe allergic condition.

Adverse effects of cholinomimetic drugs on smooth muscle: bronchospasm or asthma

Muscarinic Effects on the Heart

Stimulation of the vagus nerve causes changes in heart rate, cardiac impulse conduction, and the electrical activity of the atrial muscle.

An increase in vagal activity causes a decrease in the rate of Phase 4 depolarization that leads to a decrease in the rate of firing of cardiac pacemaker cells. This action is due to an increase in potassium permeability of the pacemaker's cells elicited by ACh (see also Chapter 32 and 33).

Direct cholinomimetic effects on the heart

ACh causes a shortening of the atrial action potential as well as a depression in its magnitude (Fig. 9–4). These effects of ACh are attributed to an increase in potassium permeability and a reduction in a slow inward current (Ca^{2+}/Na^{+}). The rate of conduction of the atrial action potential is

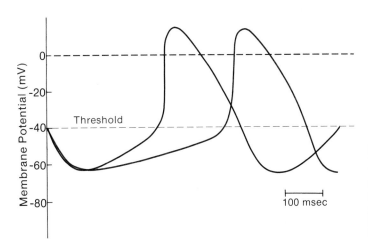

Figure 9-4

Transmembrane potentials of pacemaker cells of mammalian heart illustrating slowing the rate of diastolic depolarization produced by vagus nerve stimulation (color). Threshold is the potential for generation of an action potential.

slowed by ACh, and the strength of atrial contraction may decrease (a negative inotropic effect).

Vagal stimulation delays atrioventricular (A-V) conduction at the A-V node, leading to partial or complete heart block. Cholinomimetic drugs may have all these effects under certain circumstances, but most often the cardiac slowing is modified reflexly because of the drug's effect on blood pressure.

Therapeutic Applications. Stimulation of sensory receptors, for example, in the carotid sinus, is sometimes used to initiate vagal discharge in paroxysmal supraventricular tachycardia. The digitalis glycosides, also used to treat this arrhythmia, act in part by increasing the release of ACh from the vagus nerve (Chapter 32).

MUSCARINIC EFFECTS ON SECRETIONS

The secretions of salivary glands, secretory organs of the upper respiratory tract, and acid-secreting cells of the stomach are increased by cholinomimetic drugs. Pilocarpine causes marked sweating when injected subcutaneously.

ADVERSE EFFECTS OF MUSCARINIC AGENTS

Adverse effects of pilocarpine and bethanechol

The drugs described in this chapter are used only by topical application to the eye (pilocarpine), orally, or by subcutaneous injection (bethanechol) and are never given by intravenous injection. Adverse reactions that may occur include bronchospasm, asthma, nausea, vomiting, GI cramps, and diarrhea. All these unwanted adverse effects are due to predictable dose-related actions of muscarinic agents. Systemic use of drugs of this class are contraindicated in coronary insufficiency, because hypotension may reduce an already inefficient cardiac circulation; in hyperthyroidism, because atrial arrhythmias may be induced; in peptic ulcer, because the drugs increase the secretion of acid gastric juice; and in asthma, because they may cause bronchial constriction.

PREPARATIONS AND DOSES OF MUSCARINIC AGONISTS

Bethanechol is available in tablet form and in injection solution. When used orally for postoperative or postpartum urinary retention or GI paralysis, 5–10 mg is administered hourly until a response or a total dose of 50 mg is attained. When administered subcutaneously, 2.5–5 mg is given initially and repeated at 15–30-minute intervals until a response or four doses have been given.

Pilocarpine is usually used topically, applied to the cornea, to treat glaucoma. Solutions range from 0.5 to 4%, and 1–2 drops are applied up to six times a day.

Summary

Cholinomimetic drugs are useful primarily for their action to increase the tone of smooth muscle, especially of the iris, ciliary muscle, GI tract, and urinary bladder. In contrast, smooth muscle of the vascular bed is relaxed by muscarinic agonists. Muscarinic agonists act directly on cardiac pacemaker cells to slow the rate and depress A-V conduction, but these effects are often overcome by a reflex increase in heart rate and conduction consequent to a drug-induced fall in blood pressure.

Cholinergic agonists that act directly on muscarinic receptors have only limited therapeutic usefulness, because the ones available for therapeutic use at present are rather nonselective. Their actions frequently cause widespread effects in addition to that desired. For example, if bethanecol is used parenterally to increase GI smooth muscle tone, it may also cause hypotension, cardiac rate changes, or bronchial spasm in some patients. If a drug with fewer side effects is available it will be used in preference to a cholinergic agonist.

References

Birdsall NJM, Hulme EC: Muscarinic receptor subclasses. Trends Pharmacol Sci 4:459–463, 1983.

Bourdois PS, McCandlers DL, MacIntosh FC: A prolonged after-effect of intense synaptic activity on acetylcholine in a sympathetic ganglion. Can J Physiol Pharmacol 53:155–165, 1975.

Changeux J, Devillers-Thiery A, Chemouilli P: Acetylcholine receptor: An allosteric protein. Science 225:1335–1345, 1984.

Dunant Y: On the mechanism of acetylcholine release. Prog Neurobiol 26:55–92, 1986.

Furchgott RF: Role of endothelium in response of vascular smooth muscle. Circ Res 53:557–573, 1983.

Hubbard JI: Microphysiology of vertebrate neuromuscular transmission. Physiol Rev 53:674–723, 1973.

Jope JI: High affinity choline transport and acetyl-CoA production in brain and their roles in the regulation of acetylcholine synthesis. Brain Res Rev 1:313–344, 1979.

Kaufman PL, Wiedman T, Robinson JR: Cholinergics. In Sears ML (ed): Pharmacology of the Eye, 149–192. Berlin: Springer-Verlag, 1984.

Kistler J, Stroud R, Klymrowsky M, et al: Structure and function of an acetylcholine receptor. Biophys J 37:371–383, 1982.

McCarthy MP, Earnest JP, Young EF, et al: The molecular biology of the acetylcholine receptor. Annu Rev Neurosci 9:383–413, 1986.

North RA: Electrophysiology of the enteric nervous system. Neuroscience 7:315–325, 1982.

Popot JL, Changeux JP: Nicotinic receptor of acetylcholine: Structure of an oligomeric integral membrane protein. Physiol Rev 64:1162–1239, 1984.

Tuček S: Choline acetyltransferase and synthesis of acetylcholine. In Whitaker VP (ed): The Cholinergic Synapse, Handbook of Experimental Pharmacology, Vol 86, 125–165. Berlin: Springer-Verlag, 1988.

10

Cholinomimetic Drugs—Cholinesterase Inhibitors

Robert J. McIsaac

Acetylcholine (ACh) is metabolized by enzymatic hydrolysis, and if the enzymes involved in its metabolism are inhibited, the rate of hydrolysis is reduced. If the rate of metabolism is reduced, the ACh remains in the vicinity of the receptor for a longer period of time. Therefore, ACh released from cholinergic nerves exerts its effect for a longer period of time and with a greater intensity, and the effect of tonic or reflexly induced neuronal activity is enhanced. Because these drugs act selectively on cholinesterase, their primary effects are exerted on tissues that receive cholinergic innervation.

In addition, any drug whose metabolism is catalyzed by cholinesterases exerts an effect that is intensified and prolonged in patients who have received or been exposed to inhibitors of cholinesterase.

Therapeutic Uses of Cholinesterase Inhibitors

Action and uses of cholinesterase inhibitors

Cholinesterase inhibitors have an advantage over muscarinic agonists that act directly on ACh receptors, because the pharmacological actions of cholinesterase inhibitors are limited to synaptic areas receiving cholinergic nerve input. Therefore, they have the advantage of enhancing the cholinergic control of smooth muscles and the heart without having the potential of the hypotensive effect of muscarinic agonists, because vascular muscarinic receptors are not associated with acetylcholinesterase and are not innervated by cholinergic nerves.

In general, cholinesterase inhibitors are useful for the treatment of the same conditions as muscarinic agonists: glaucoma, nonobstructive urinary retention, and loss of gastrointestinal (GI) tone. In addition, cholinesterase inhibitors have an important action involving nicotinic receptors, because they increase the force of muscular strength, especially when it has been weakened as in myasthenia gravis or competitive neuromuscular block produced by certain drugs used during surgery (see Chapter 13).

Physostigmine can penetrate into the central nervous system (CNS) and is used occasionally for its central action, especially as an antagonist of anticholinergic agents (see Chapter 11).

Major Types of Cholinesterase Enzymes

Two major forms of ChE

There are a number of enzymes that can hydrolyze ACh. Two major types are butyryl-cholinesterase and acetylcholinesterase.

CHOLINESTERASE (ChE)

Butyryl-cholinesterase, known also as plasma cholinesterase or pseudo-cholinesterase, is referred to hereafter as cholinesterase (ChE).

ChE is relatively nonspecific in its substrate requirements and can catalyze the hydrolysis of many esters, but it is not important for the hydrolysis of ACh in the subsynaptic area. Butyrylcholine is used experimentally to identify this enzyme, because butyrylcholine is a substrate for ChE but not for the enzyme that is specific for the hydrolysis of ACh.

ChE is a widely distributed in many organs of the body, including the plasma, liver, kidney, and GI tract. There is no known physiological function for this enzyme, but it may be important for the hydrolysis of ingested esters. It is not important for the termination of the action of ACh released from cholinergic nerves, but it can catalyze the hydrolysis of ACh and related esters that are administered parenterally. The enzyme is important pharmacologically also because it is involved in the metabolism of certain ester drugs, such as succinylcholine and procaine. This action is responsible for the brief lifetime of these drugs in the circulation.

ACETYLCHOLINESTERASE (AChE)

Acetylcholinesterase (AChE) is an enzyme that is relatively specific for the hydrolysis of ACh. The function of AChE is to terminate the action of ACh, and it hydrolyzes ACh at a rapid rate but has little effect on other esters. Methacholine, a congener of ACh, is used experimentally to identify AChE, because it is hydrolyzed by AChE but not by ChE.

AChE is located in and around the terminals of all cholinergic nerves. Red blood cells also contain AChE, but its function in these cells is not known.

Structure of Acetylcholinesterase

AChE is a glycoprotein that exists as a variety of isozymes. The basic building block is a globular monomer of about 80,000 daltons. Six major forms of AChE are possible: three globular forms, and a monomeric, dimeric, and a tetrameric form. The tetrameric form may exist also combined with a collagen tail (Figs. 10–1 and 10–2). The distribution of the various forms varies with tissue and species, but the globular forms are the major fractions in most vertebrate tissues. The collagen-tailed form is found in the basal lamina of the end-plate at skeletal muscles.

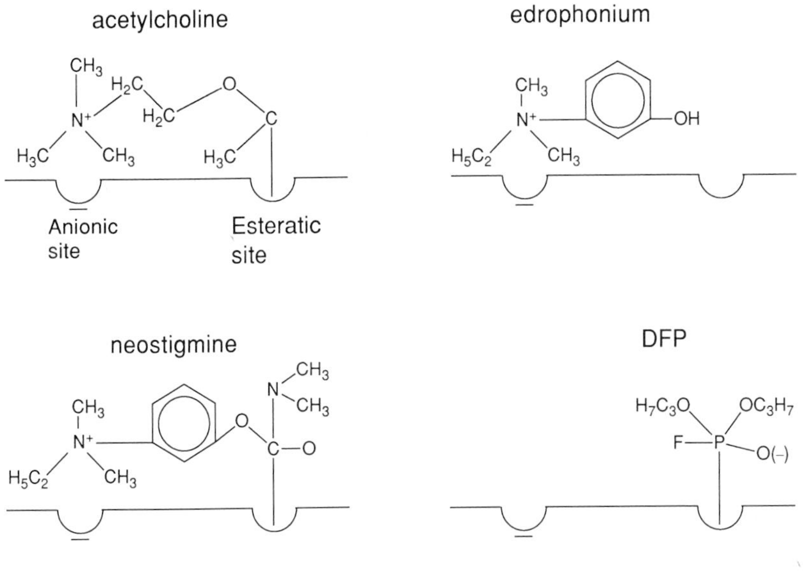

Figure 10–1

Schematic of binding to AChE by acetylcholine and by three AChEIs.

Figure 10–2

Structure of the six main forms of AChE. The globular forms are represented by G, and the collagen-tailed (asymmetrical) forms are represented by A. (Adapted and reprinted with permission from Prog Neurobiol 21:298–322, Brimijoin S: Molecular forms of acetylcholinesterase in brain, nerve and muscle: Nature, localization and dynamics, Copyright 1983, Pergamon Press plc.)

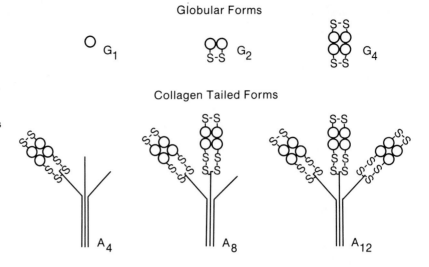

The active site of AChE has an anionic and an esteratic subsite.

The active site on AChE has two subsites: a negatively charged anionic subsite that attracts the charged quaternary nitrogen of choline in ACh molecule through coulombic and hydrophobic forces, and an esteratic subsite that catalyzes the hydrolysis of the ester linkage. A drug that binds to either one or both subsites interferes with the binding of ACh to the active site and decreases the rate of metabolism of ACh (see Fig. 10–1).

Cholinesterase Inhibitors

TRUE REVERSIBLE INHIBITORS

Edrophonium (TENSILON) is attracted to and binds to the anionic subsite. Owing to reversibility of the binding and its rapid renal elimination, the duration of action of edrophonium is short. This is the major advantage of edrophonium, and it is used for diagnostic tests or for therapy when a brief effect is desired.

CARBAMATE ACYLATORS

Physostigmine and neostigmine are carbamate ChE inhibitors.

Physostigmine (ANTILIRIUM, also sometimes called eserine), *neostigmine* (PROSTIGMIN), and *pyridostigmine* (MESTINON) are carbamate acylators. These inhibitors are sometimes called *reversible*, but they actually acylate the subsite and are metabolized slowly by the enzyme. Drugs that contain the carbamate ester linkage (-OCONR'R″) interact at both subsites of the AChE molecule and are hydrolyzed slowly by the enzyme. Cleavage of the alcohol leaves the carbamylated enzyme, which is more stable than the acetylated enzyme: for example, the half-time for regeneration of AChE from the neostigmine carbamylated enzyme is 15–30 minutes.

The major pharmacological difference among physostigmine, neostigmine, and pyridostigmine is that the latter two contain a quaternary nitrogen, whereas physostigmine is a tertiary amine. Thus, physostigmine can exist as a nonionized amine as well as an ionized amine, depending upon the pH of the solution. As physostigmine can more easily penetrate membranes in the un-ionized form than neostigmine, it is used when it is desirable to obtain an effect in the CNS or its absorption on topical administration.

Carbaryl is a carbamate insecticide that inhibits ChEs in a manner similar to neostigmine and other carbamate inhibitors. It is used extensively in garden insecticides.

IRREVERSIBLE ORGANOPHOSPHATE INHIBITORS

Isofluorophate (FLOROPRYL) and *ecothiophate* (PHOSPHOLINE) are irreversible organophosphate inhibitors. A variety of alkoxy- and aryloxy-substituted phosphoric acid compounds acylate ChEs to form rather stable covalent bonds. The inhibitor isofluorophate has two isopropyl groups and a fluoride attached to the phosphorus atom, and in the initial reaction with the enzyme the fluorine is liberated, resulting in formation of a covalent bond between the esteratic site and the phosphorus. With time, an "aging" process occurs that involves the splitting off of an isopropyl group. The chemical aging process is important, because after it has occurred regeneration of the active enzyme is more difficult than after the initial inhibitory reaction.

Isofluorophate is an irreversible organophosphate ChE inhibitor.

The recovery of the phosphorylated enzyme to free enzyme is an extremely slow process, and resynthesis of new enzyme is the principal way of recovery from inhibition by organophosphate inhibitors. Recovery can be hastened with the drug pralidoxime, which reactivates the enzyme (described later in chapter).

With a few exceptions, the organophosphates are lipid-soluble, have a low molecular weight, and are volatile, so they can be absorbed through inhalation, through the skin, and they penetrate easily into the CNS. These characteristics, together with the long duration of action, result in potentially toxic substances

1. Organophosphate insecticides are widely used in agriculture and home garden chemicals. Parathion is a low molecular weight volatile substance that is metabolized *in vivo* to paraoxon, an active ChE inhibitor. An oxygen atom is substituted for the sulfur, a biotransformation reaction that activates rather than detoxifies the parent compound. Parathion is a toxic chemical and has been responsible for many intoxications. Malathion also requires replacement of the sulfur by oxygen for inhibitory activity. Because malathion is metabolized rapidly by plasma carboxylesterases, and the metabolism occurs much more rapidly in vertebrates than insects, it has lower prevalence of toxicity in vertebrates.

2. Nerve gases that are highly volatile and active ChE inhibitors have been prepared for lethal chemical warfare. These chemicals, such as tabun, saran, and soman, are among the most toxic agents ever synthesized.

Pharmacology of Acetylcholinesterase Inhibitors

For the most part the pharmacological properties of these substances can be attributed to an increase in the concentration of ACh at cholinergic receptors due to the inhibition of its enzymatic hydrolysis. Therefore, the properties of acetylcholinesterase inhibitors (AChEIs) can be predicted if one knows what tissues receive cholinergic innervation and the effect of cholinergic nerves on that tissue. In general, the most prominent effects of the AChEIs are those at muscarinic receptors and at the ACh nicotinic receptors on skeletal muscles. It is only with doses larger than the usual therapeutic dose that effects are observed at autonomic ganglia.

Inhibition of AChE potentiates the effect of cholinergic nerves on effector organs.

There are muscarinic ACh receptors in the CNS, and drugs that can penetrate into the CNS (physostigmine and the organophosphate esters) may have a central effect also. The AChEIs that have a quaternary nitrogen group (edrophonium, neostigmine, and pyridostigmine) do not cross membranes easily and do not get into the CNS effectively.

The organophosphate esters are lipid-soluble and many are highly volatile so they are readily absorbed by all routes, including the skin and the lung. Overtreatment with any of the inhibitors allows so much ACh to accumulate at ganglia and neuromuscular synapses that depression of transmission occurs, leading to paralysis of neuromuscular transmission and cardiovascular collapse.

The major uses of AChEI are on eye, GI tract, and neuromuscular junction.

The major useful therapeutic effects of AChEIs are on the smooth muscle of the GI tract and urinary bladder, on the smooth muscles of the eye, and on transmission at the skeletal muscle. Short-acting inhibitors have been used to treat paroxsymal atrial tachycardia.

EYE

ChE inhibitors, usually applied topically to the conjunctiva, cause contraction of the sphincter muscle of the iris leading to miosis (pupillary constriction) and contraction of the ciliary muscle resulting in accommodation of the lens for near vision. The miosis usually lasts longer than the changes in accommodation. These effects are used in the treatment of glaucoma where physostigmine and, to a less extent, the organophosphate isoflurophate are useful for reducing intraocular pressure (see Fig. 9–3).

GASTROINTESTINAL TRACT AND URINARY BLADDER

When there is a loss in tone of the smooth muscles of the small and large bowel, neostigmine is used to increase the tone and motor activity of all parts of the small intestine. Its effect is a result of a combination of actions at the ganglia of Auerbach's plexus and at the smooth muscle fiber. Neostigmine is also effective in facilitating urination when there is a loss in tone of the bladder, e.g., following surgery. Neostigmine increases the tone of the detrusor muscle and decreases the volume of the bladder. This, coupled with a relaxation of the trigone and external sphincter, facilitates urination.

NEUROMUSCULAR JUNCTION

Unlike the direct acting cholinomimetic drugs, the AChEIs have an important action on transmission at the motor nerve–skeletal muscle junction. (By common usage, "neuromuscular junction" most often refers only to the motor nerve junction with skeletal muscle fibers.) Inhibition of AChE at the neuromuscular junction prolongs the lifetime of ACh so that it may recombine with nicotinic receptors at the end-plate repeatedly and cause successive stimulation of ACh receptors. This results in a prolongation of the end-plate potential and generation of multiple action potentials that are propagated over the muscle membrane. The greatest effect of AChE inhibi-

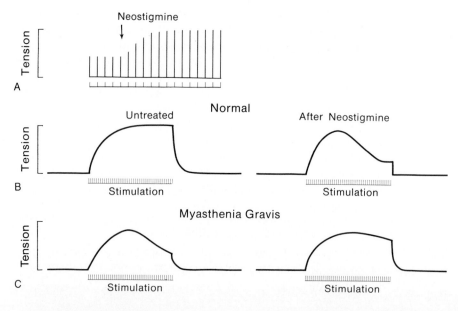

Figure 10–3

Effects of neostigmine on muscle contractions produced by supramaximal nerve stimulation in three different conditions: *(A)* Normal muscle with the nerve stimulated periodically at 10-second intervals. *(B)* Normal muscle with the nerve stimulated repetitively, 25 times per second. *(C)* Myasthenic muscle with the nerve stimulated repetitively 25 times per second.

tion is apparent when neuromuscular transmission has been depressed in some way.

In a normal muscle with the motor nerve stimulated singly at a low frequency, moderate inhibition of AChE causes an increase in twitch strength because of brief repetitive activation of the muscle. However, if the nerve is stimulated at a high frequency, the muscle strength decreases with continued stimulation. This fatigue is due to the excessive build-up of ACh and sustained depolarization of the muscle membrane, resulting in depression of transmission due to depolarization blockade.

Where there is a depression of neuromuscular transmission, such as in myasthenia gravis or during recovery from a competitive neuromuscular blockade after surgery, inhibition of AChE results in an increase in muscle tension at both low- and high-frequency stimulation (Fig. 10–3).

AChEIs increase skeletal muscle strength when it has been depressed.

HEART

Under normal resting conditions, the vagus nerves to the heart exhibit repetitive tonic impulses to the pacemaker cells on the sinoatrial node. When AChE is inhibited, this action of the vagus is enhanced and heart rate slows further. When an AChEI is used for a therapeutic effect on the heart, for example to break a paroxysmal atrial tachycardia, edrophonium may be employed because of its brief duration of action.

OTHER ACTIONS

Central Nervous System

There are muscarinic receptors in the CNS that are innervated by cholinergic nerves, and AChE is as important in terminating the action of ACh in the CNS as in the periphery. Therefore, AChEIs that are able to get into the CNS may have an effect, especially during intoxication with large doses. Small concentrations of physostigmine cause stimulation or facilitation of transmission at various sites, and in larger concentrations depression of transmission occurs. After administration of an AChEI, the electroencephalogram (EEG) is characterized initially by low voltage waves and high frequency, probably due to stimulation of the ascending reticular activating system. Respiratory and other subcortical centers are stimulated at low concentrations but depressed at high concentrations. Many of these central effects of AChEIs are blocked by atropine, a muscarinic antagonist.

Physostigmine and isoflurophosphate can have action in the CNS.

Occasionally, physostigmine is used therapeutically for its CNS effects. Physostigmine can cross the blood-brain barrier, because it can be both un-ionized or ionized at physiological pH. The organophosphate esters are highly lipid-soluble and can gain access also to the CNS; central effects are prominent during intoxication.

Autonomic Ganglia

Inhibition of AChE in autonomic ganglia may lead to repetitive firing of the neurons with either a single stimulation or brief volley. Activation of ganglionic muscarinic receptors is responsible for this firing. Larger concentrations of AChEI cause depression of ganglionic transmission through persistent depolarization mediated by activation of nicotinic receptors.

Secretions

Inhibitors of ChEs may increase secretions, especially of the salivary glands, nasopharyngeal glands, and gastric parietal cells. An increased secretion in the bronchioles as well as constriction of bronchiolar smooth muscle may occur. These effects are prominent during intoxication and may be severe enough to interfere with adequate ventilation.

ABSORPTION AND METABOLISM

Physostigmine is a tertiary amine and can be absorbed from membranes and after oral administration more readily than the charged quaternary nitrogen-containing AChEIs. It is used topically on the conjunctiva because of its absorption characteristics, and it is used when central effects are desired, because it can penetrate into the CNS.

Differences in absorption of AChEIs

Neostigmine and other quaternary nitrogen-containing inhibitors are poorly absorbed by the oral route. Much larger doses of neostigmine are required for oral administration (15–30 mg or more) than after parenteral administration (0.5–2 mg). Both physostigmine and neostigmine are metabolized by plasma esterases, and the metabolic products are excreted in the urine.

Organophosphate inhibitors are highly lipid-soluble and are absorbed well by all routes, including through the skin and the lungs. Organophosphate inhibitors are hydrolyzed by plasma and tissue enzymes. The metabolic products, phosphoric or phosphonic acids, are excreted in the urine.

Adverse and Toxic Effects

ADVERSE EFFECTS

Most adverse effects seen with AChEI are related to an effect on a tissue other than the one for which a pharmacological action is desired or to overtreatment. The most frequent toxic effects are excessive secretions, GI cramps, diarrhea, and slowing of heart rate.

ACUTE INTOXICATION

The organophosphate esters are toxic substances, and in view of their widespread use in both agricultural and residential insecticidal preparations and their bioavailability through the skin and lungs, severe intoxications are reported frequently. The signs and symptoms involve muscarinic effects, nicotinic effects, and effects on the CNS. Fortunately, there are specific antidotes for organophosphate intoxication.

Acute intoxication by organophosphates is potentially lethal.

Intoxication is manifest by copious salivary secretions and secretions of glands in the upper respiratory tract, marked slowing of the heart rate, bronchial muscle constriction, and abdominal cramps and diarrhea. Skeletal muscle may exhibit fasciculations, weakness, and blockade of transmission. Neuromuscular block is most critical, of course, when it involves the respiratory muscles. Central effects include ataxia, confusion, irrational behavior, convulsions, and depression of the respiratory and cardiovascular centers. When death occurs, it is usually due to respiratory failure from both peripheral and central actions. Respiratory depression may be accompanied by circulatory collapse.

Intoxication can be treated specifically by maintaining respiration and by administering a muscarinic receptor antagonist, atropine, plus a drug that reactivates phosphorylated AChE, pralidoxime.

DELAYED NEUROTOXICITY

Certain fluorine-containing organophosphate compounds, such as isofluorophate, can cause a characteristic neurotoxicity that appears several days after exposure to a sufficient single dose or cumulative multiple doses of the toxic chemical. The lesion is characterized by axonal swelling, segmentation, followed by breakdown with secondary demyelination. Initially there are symptoms of mild sensory disturbances, but it may progress to ataxia, fatigue of leg muscles, and muscle paralysis.

This neurotoxicity is not related to anticholinesterase activity, because some inhibitors do not exhibit the toxicity and some organophosphate substances devoid of ChE inhibitory activity cause the neurotoxicity. There is evidence that the initial target of organophosphate-induced delayed neurotoxicity is the phosphorylation of a neurotoxicity protein in the nervous system. The mechanism of development of neurotoxicity is not completely known.

PRALIDOXIME (2-PAM, PROTOPAM)

Normally regeneration of enzyme from the phosphorylated enzyme is an extremely slow process. However, it was observed that nucleophilic reagents, such as hydroxylamine or oxime, increased the rate of regeneration of free enzyme. This led to the synthesis of pralidoxime, which is effective in reactivating phosphorylated AChE and which has found a place in treating organophosphate intoxication in conjunction with atropine. Pralidoxime has a quaternary nitrogen that is attracted to the anionic subsite of the enzyme and places the oxime moiety close to the phosphorus atom. An oxime-phosphonate splits off the enzyme, leaving the regenerated enzyme (Fig. 10–4).

The reactivating action of pralidoxime is most marked at the neuromuscular junction leading to a decrease in neuromuscular block. It has less of an effect at peripheral autonomic sites and is not effective in antagonizing the central effects of intoxication. However, atropine can antagonize the peripheral muscarinic effects (secretions, GI motility, and slow heart

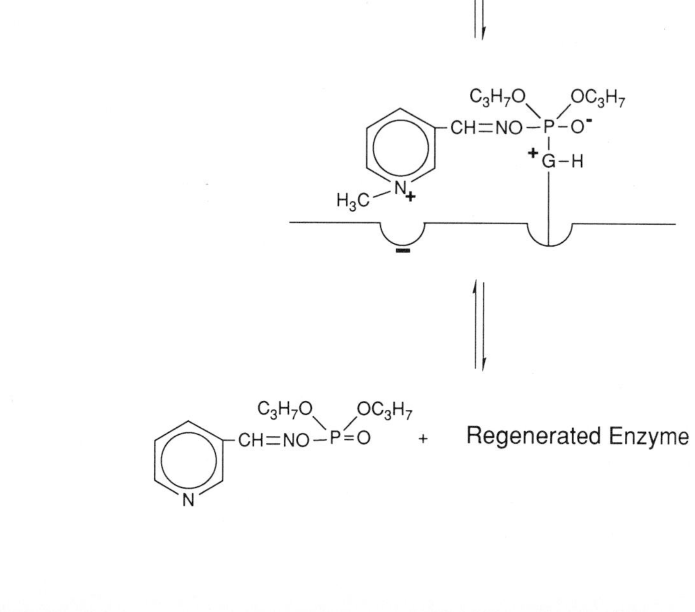

Atropine and pralidoxime are specific antidotes for organophosphate intoxication.

Figure 10–4

Schematic drawing of the reversal of ChE inhibition by oximes.

rate) as well as the central effects of intoxication (described earlier). The pharmacological antidote for organophosphate intoxication includes a combination of both atropine and pralidoxime.

Because pralidoxime does not reactivate carbamylated enzyme and it has weak neuromuscular blocking action itself, pralidoxime is not used for treating intoxication with carbamate ChE inhibitors and, in fact, is contraindicated in this case. The recommended antidote for carbamate intoxication is atropine plus supportive care, including maintenance of a patent airway, oxygen, and artificial respiration if necessary.

Therapeutic Uses

There are four principal areas for which AChEIs are used: disturbances of functions of the GI tract and urinary bladder, the eye, and motor nerve–skeletal muscles. Selected inhibitors may be used occasionally for CNS effects and for cardiac actions.

POSTOPERATIVE PARALYTIC ILEUS AND URINARY RETENTION

Neostigmine may be used for treatment of paralytic ileus and urinary retention.

Neostigmine methylsulfate may be useful in treating postoperative distention of the GI tract or urinary retention after mechanical obstruction has been eliminated as a possible cause. A subcutaneous (SC) dose of 0.5–1.0 mg usually induces peristalsis after 10–30 minutes. The same dose is employed to treat urinary retention. The drug is not used in the presence of a possible mechanical obstruction or in the presence of peritonitis.

GLAUCOMA

An increase in intraocular pressure in primary glaucoma may be caused by an obstruction by the iris to outflow of the aqueous humor at the entrance to the trabecular space (narrow angle or acute congestive glaucoma) or an interference in outflow in the trabecular meshwork (open angle or chronic simple glaucoma) (see Fig. 9–3). Increased intraocular pressure leads to damage of the optic disk and eventually to blindness: glaucoma is a major cause of blindness in adults. Intraocular pressure can be reduced by either facilitating the outflow of aqueous humor or decreasing the production of aqueous humor.

AChEIs used for treatment of glaucoma

The AChEIs may be useful for treating primary glaucoma, either acute or chronic. They decrease intraocular pressure in acute glaucoma by increasing the contraction of the sphincter muscle of the iris and decreasing its obstruction of the canal of Schlemm. In chronic glaucoma they enhance outflow of the aqueous humor by increasing tension of the ciliary muscle, which decreases the obstruction to drainage in the trabecular meshwork (see Fig. 9–3).

Physostigmine salicylate, 0.25–0.5%, is instilled into the conjunctival sac two drops up to four times a day, because physostigmine has a relatively short duration of action. It is sometimes used in combination with the direct-acting parasympathomimetic drug, pilocarpine. Demecarium iodide is an inhibitor that has a somewhat longer duration of action than physostigmine, and one drop of 0.125% solution is used up to twice a day.

Ecothiophate iodide (PHOSPHOLINE IODIDE) is an organophosphate inhibitor that is soluble in aqueous solution. It has a longer duration of action and can be administered in one drop of a 0.03% solution up to twice a day.

Isofluorophate (FLOROPRYL) is unstable in aqueous solutions and is dissolved in oil or as an ointment of polyethene mineral oil gel. It is long acting and is administered once every 8–72 hours. The longer-acting organophosphate inhibitors are used only when other treatments are ineffective, because they have been associated with an increased incidence of lens opacity when used for a prolonged period of time.

Glaucoma can be treated also with adrenergic β-receptor antagonists or by epinephrine. Both of these drugs act by decreasing the production of aqueous humor. The use of adrenergic drugs in glaucoma is covered in later chapters.

MYASTHENIA GRAVIS

Myasthenia gravis is a disease of neuromuscular transmission characterized by weakness and marked fatigue, especially with maintained voluntary muscular effort. Myasthenia gravis is an autoimmune disease that involves the postjunctional end-plate. Antibodies to the ACh receptor can be detected in the serum of 80–90% of patients with myasthenia gravis. Antibodies raised to purified ACh receptor protein cause an experimental myasthenia in animals that resembles in many respects the clinical disease. Antibodies from patients cause a myasthenic syndrome when injected into animals. A decrease in the number of ACh receptors on the end-plate has been observed in myasthenic patients with an increase in the rate of receptor turnover and simplification of the end-plate membrane structure.

ChE inhibitors are used in the diagnosis and treatment of myasthenia gravis. They act by prolonging and increasing the concentration of ACh at the end-plate area, which allows for stimulation of receptors over a greater area of the end-plate membrane, and with the proper use of AChEIs, a marked improvement in muscle strength may be achieved in myasthenic patients.

ChE inhibitors are useful in diagnosis and treatment of myasthenia gravis.

Excessive doses of AChEIs may result in a condition known as a *cholinergic crisis*, characterized by overstimulation of muscarinic receptors as well as muscle weakness due to prolonged depolarization or desensitization of the motor end-plate. Because the muscle weakness of a cholinergic crisis resembles the myasthenic weakness due to insufficient treatment, it is important to identify the cause of the weakness. Excessive therapy with AChEIs is potentially hazardous because it can lead to respiratory distress.

Insufficient treatment of myasthenia gravis may result in a *myasthenic crisis*, a weakness due to a progression of the disease or inadequate treatment with inhibitors. The cause of muscle weakness appearing in a patient, due either to a cholinergic crisis or a myasthenic crisis, can be determined with a test using edrophonium.

Therapy with AChEIs may lead to annoying muscarinic side effects: cramping of GI tract, diarrhea, excessive salivation, visual disturbance, or slow heart rate. These side effects can be reduced or prevented by the addition of atropine, a specific muscarinic antagonist, to the therapeutic regimen. Atropine does not antagonize the action of ACh at nicotinic end-plate receptors (Chapter 11).

Edrophonium chloride (TENSILON) is used for diagnostic purposes because it has a brief duration of action. It can be used to diagnose myasthenia gravis or to test the adequacy of treatment with other longer-acting inhibitors. For diagnosis, 10 mg is drawn into a syringe and 2 mg is injected by the intravenous (IV) route. If no reaction occurs, this is followed by the remaining 8 mg. A patient with untreated myasthenia gravis or undertreated myasthenia responds with an increase in muscle strength without muscle fasciculations and no side effects (salivation, lacrimation, or GI cramps). In a normal person or myasthenic with adequate treatment, no change in muscle strength is observed, fasciculations may be present, and side reactions are minimal. A myasthenic patient overtreated with ChE inhibitors shows decreased muscle strength, fasciculations may be present, and side reactions are severe.

Neostigmine bromide is available for oral administration, and the dosage ranges from 15 to 375 mg/day depending on the patient's response. Neostigmine methylsulfate is available for intramuscular (IM) or SC administration, and the dose starts at 0.5 mg. Neostigmine is a standard for comparing other drugs in the treatment of myasthenia gravis, but *pyridostigmine* (MESTINON), 60–1500 mg/day, is used more often because it has a slightly longer duration of action. *Ambenonium chloride* (MYTELASE) also has a longer duration of action and is used at a dosage level ranging from 5 to 75 mg/day.

Patients may become refractory to ChE inhibitors, especially when large doses are used for a prolonged time. In this case, a 7–10-day drug holiday is effective often in re-establishing drug responsiveness.

Patients who do not exhibit an adequate response to the ChE inhibitors may be benefited by corticosteroid therapy. Thymomas are present in a significant number of myasthenic patients, and thymectomy usually benefits these patients as well as those that do not respond to ChE inhibitors and corticosteroids.

RECOVERY FROM COMPETITIVE NEUROMUSCULAR BLOCKADE

Tubocurarine and similar drugs (see Chapter 13) are used frequently during surgery to ensure adequate neuromuscular relaxation. These drugs act by competing with ACh for the receptor at the end-plate. After surgery is completed it is desirable to obtain rapid recovery from neuromuscular blockade and the accompanying depression of respiration. Neostigmine methylsulfate, 0.5–2 mg, administered by slow IV drip, will hasten recovery of muscle function. It is most effective when given after some muscle response has started to return.

Postsurgical neostigmine may antagonize tubocurarine or pancuronium neuromuscular blockade.

ANTICHOLINERGIC INTOXICATION

Intoxication with atropine and certain other centrally acting drugs, such as the tricyclic antidepressants, includes severe central effects as well as peripheral anticholinergic effects. Physostigmine salicylate is used sometimes to counteract the anxiety, delirium, disorientation, hyperactivity, and seizures that may accompany anticholinergic intoxication. Physostigmine is injected intravenously, 0.5–2 mg, with additional amounts given as necessary. The half-life of physostigmine in plasma is 1–2 hours necessitating additional injections to prevent the return of symptoms. Because physostigmine itself has appreciable toxicity, patients must be monitored carefully in order to prevent either overtreatment or undertreatment.

References

Adou-Donia MB: Organophosphorus ester-induced delayed neurotoxicity. Annu Rev Pharmacol Toxicol 21:511–548, 1981.

Brimijoin S: Molecular forms of acetylcholinesterase in brain, nerve and muscle: Nature, localization and dynamics. Prog Neurobiol 21:298–322, 1983.

Ellin RI: Anomalies in theories and therapy of intoxication by potent organophosphorus anticholinesterase compounds. Gen Pharmacol 13:457–466, 1982.

Grob D: Myasthenia gravis: Pathophysiology and management. Ann NY Acad Sci 377:1–898, 1981.

Hobbiger F: Pharmacology of anticholinesterase drugs. *In* Zaimis E (ed): Neuromuscular Junction, 487–581. Vol 42 of Handbook of Experimental Pharmacology. Berlin: Springer-Verlag, 1976.

Johnson MK: The target for initiation of delayed neurotoxicity by organophosphorus esters: Biochemical studies and toxicological applications. Rev Biochem Toxic 4:141–212, 1982.

Kaufman PL, Wiedman T, Robinson JR: Cholinergics. *In* Sears ML (ed): Pharmacology of the Eye, 149–192. Vol 69 of Handbook of Experimental Pharmacology. Berlin: Springer-Verlag, 1984.

Kerkut GA: Acetylcholinesterase (ACHE) (EC.3.1.1.7). Gen Pharmacol 15:375–378, 1984.

Marquis JK: Non-cholinergic mechanisms in insecticide toxicity. Trends Pharmacol Sci 6:59–60, 1985.

Massoulie J, Bon S: The molecular forms of cholinesterase and acetylcholinesterase in vertebrates. Annu Rev Neurosci 5:57–106, 1982.

Munsat TL: Anticholinesterase abuse in myasthenia gravis. J Neurol Sci 64:5–10, 1984.

Newsom-Davis J: Myasthenia. *In* Crow TJ (ed): Disorders of Neurohumoral Transmission, 7–44. London: Academic Press, 1982.

Takamori M, Kasai M: Experimental myasthenia gravis: A model of receptor disease. Int J Neurol 14:47–60, 1980.

Tautant J-P, Massoulie J: Cholinesterases: Tissue and cellular distribution of molecular forms and their physiological regulation. *In* Whittaker VP (ed): The Cholinergic Synapse, 225–265. Vol 86 of Handbook of Experimental Pharmacology. Berlin: Springer-Verlag, 1988.

Waser PG, Hopff WH, Schaub MC, Hoffman A: Recent advances in identification and isolation of acetylcholinesterase and a cholinergic receptor protein. Adv Biochem Psychopharmacol 36:7–14, 1983.

11

Antimuscarinic Drugs

Robert J. McIsaac

Antimuscarinic drugs are useful to reduce excessive parasympathetic influence on effector organs.

Antimuscarinic drugs have a relatively specific effect at muscarinic receptors to block the effects of acetylcholine (ACh) and related agonists. Most of these drugs have little or no effect on nicotinic receptors in autonomic ganglia or at the neuromuscular junction. However, those antimuscarinic drugs that have a positively charged quaternary nitrogen in their molecule may have a weak ganglionic or neuromuscular action in addition. The drugs in this group are sometimes referred to as *parasympatholytics* or more frequently as *anticholinergic* drugs.

The antimuscarinic drugs are used in conditions requiring a decreased parasympathetic activity. Thus, they find routine use in management of patients with hypermotility of the gastrointestinal (GI) tract, the hyperactive carotid sinus syndrome, and increased gastric acid secretion. They may be used acutely for ophthalmological examination, as an adjunct to general anesthesia, and to treat anticholinesterase poisoning.

Major Prototypic Drugs

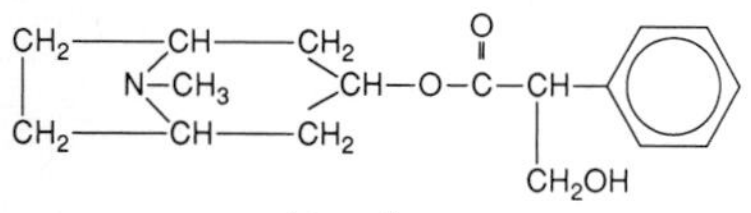

Atropine

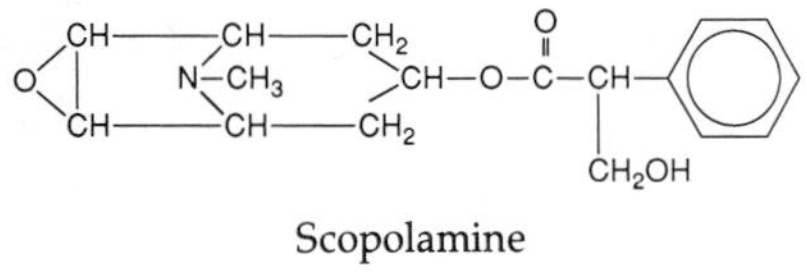

Scopolamine

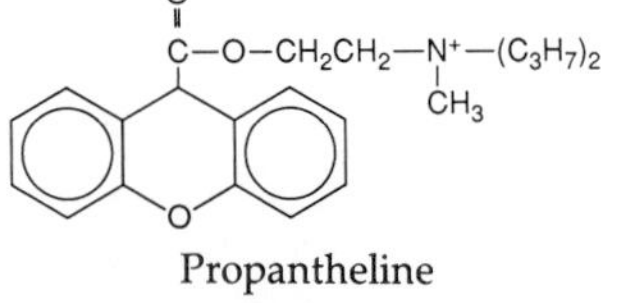

Propantheline

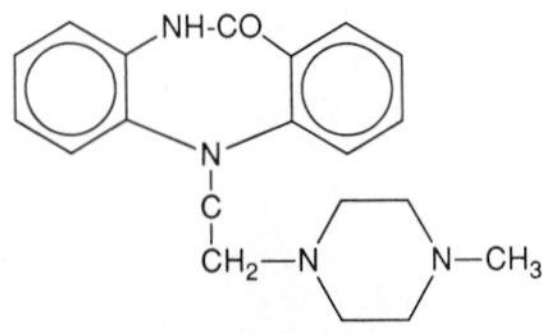

Pirenzepine

The major prototypic drugs in this group are:

Solanacae alkaloids

1. In belladonna extracts the main active ingredient is atropine. Atropine (*dl*-hyoscyamine) is an organic ester of tropic acid and tropine. This alkaloid is isolated from *Atropa belladonna*.

2. Scopolamine (hyoscine) is an organic ester of tropic acid and scopine and is isolated from *Scopolia carniolica* and *Hyoscyamus niger* (henbane).

Synthetic compounds

1. Propantheline (PRO-BANTHINE)
2. Pirenzepine
3. Trihexyphenidyl hydrochloride (ARTANE)

Because of the nonspecificity of the atropine alkaloids (alkaloids = nitrogenous substance from plants) on muscarinic receptors of various tissues, a large number of synthetic substances have been prepared to try to obtain a substance with selective actions on specific tissues; agents that reduce gastric acid secretion without distressing side actions have been sought especially. In general, this has not been achieved, and most of the synthetic antimuscarinic drugs have a spectrum of action similar to that of atropine when used in equally effective doses.

The antimuscarinic drugs act by competing with ACh for muscarinic receptors. Atropine has an affinity for the receptor but has no intrinsic activity, i.e., its combination with the receptor has no agonistic effect. If a sufficient concentration of the drug is in the vicinity of the receptor so that a significant number of receptors are occupied by atropine, ACh can combine with fewer receptors and its effect is reduced. The antimuscarinic drugs have been found to be more effective in blocking the action of circulating cholinergic agonists than in blocking the effects of parasympathetic nerve stimulation.

Atropine and related drugs do not block cholinergic nerve input to all organs at the same dose level, and there is an order of sensitivity to the effect of atropine and related drugs. The block of salivary secretion and nasopharyngeal secretions is most sensitive to atropine; larger doses are required to affect the heart rate; still larger doses are necessary to bring about GI muscle relaxation; and reduction of gastric secretion is least sensitive to atropine. This order of sensitivity to antimuscarinic drugs has important clinical implications, because when they are used to produce smooth muscle relaxation or a decrease in gastric acid, the patient will usually experience distressing side effects, such as severely dry mouth or disturbance of vision.

Mechanism of Action

Antimuscarinic drugs compete with ACh for its muscarinic receptor.

The atropine-like drugs are used primarily for their effect on the eye, GI tract, heart, secretions, and in special circumstances for a central nervous system (CNS) action. Scopolamine is more potent than atropine on the eye, salivary and bronchial secretory glands, and CNS. Atropine is relatively more potent than scopolamine on the heart, the GI tract, and bronchial smooth muscle.

Pharmacology

EYE

Iris

The sphincter muscle of the iris receives innervation by the parasympathetic nerve, and atropine reduces the effect of parasympathetic innervation leading to relaxation of the sphincter muscle. This results in dilation of the pupil or mydriasis. With complete atropinization of the iris, the pupil will no longer respond to light, and photophobia will result (see Fig. 9–3).

In normal eyes, atropine does not have a significant effect on intraocular pressure. In susceptible people, however, atropine may precipitate narrow angle glaucoma through relaxation of the iris so that it obstructs the outflow of the aqueous humor from the anterior chamber.

Atropine produces mydriasis and cycloplegia in the eye.

Ciliary Muscle

The ciliary muscle is controlled only by the parasympathetic nerves. Atropine causes relaxation of the ciliary muscle, and the lens assumes a shape for distant vision. The paralysis of neural control of the ciliary muscle is termed *cycloplegia.*

Atropine is used by topical application to the conjunctiva for an effect on the eye. When it is applied topically to the eye, atropine has a prolonged duration of action, and it may take up to 7–12 days for complete recovery.

The usual therapeutic doses of atropine (0.5 mg) or scopolamine (0.3 mg) administered systemically usually have little effect on the eye in most people. However, larger doses such as those required to control gastric acid secretion or cause smooth muscle relaxation may cause visual disturbances.

HEART

The effect of atropine upon heart rate is complex. With small doses, or initially after usual doses, an initial slowing of heart rate by about 4–8 beats/minute may occur. The slowing is minor and unimportant unless a further slowing of heart rate in patients with bradycardia is not desired. The slowing is believed to be due to stimulation of the central vagal nucleus, and an increased action potential frequency in the vagus has been observed in experimental animals during the slowing phase.

Atropine increases heart rate.

The brief period of slowing is followed by an increase in heart rate due to blockade of the muscarinic receptors of the heart. The increase in rate is most pronounced in young adults where vagal tone is most marked, and the rate may increase by 30–40 beats/minute. Reflex slowing initiated by irritant inhalants, pressure on the carotid sinus, vasopressor drugs, or adrenergic discharge is also reduced or blocked by atropine.

Atropine increases the conduction velocity between the atria and ventricle by blocking the vagal influence on the A-V conducting system.

CIRCULATION

Atropine has a negligible effect on mean systemic blood pressure.

Atropine has no significant effect on systemic blood pressure because parasympathetic innervation of the resistance and capacitance vessels is lacking. However, atropine will antagonize the hypotensive action of systemically administered cholinergic agonists that act on muscarinic receptors found on arterioles. For this reason, atropine should be available whenever direct-acting cholinergic drugs are given systemically.

Toxic doses of atropine cause dilation of cutaneous vessels, and one of the symptoms of atropine intoxication is a reddening of the skin in blush areas. This effect of large toxic doses of atropine is probably due to a direct smooth muscle relaxing action of atropine.

The atropine-like drugs that contain a positively charged quaternary nitrogen atom (such as propantheline) may have weak ganglionic blocking activity. In some patients, especially with larger doses, these drugs may cause hypotension by way of ganglionic blockade.

SECRETIONS

Secretion of saliva, both basal secretion and reflexly stimulated secretion, is one of the functions most sensitive to atropine. The secretion of saliva and of the secretory glands of the nasopharyngeal tract are reduced or blocked by atropine leading to dryness of the mouth and upper respiratory passages. Cold remedies that are available without prescription often contain an antihistamine that has an atropine-like action as well as its histamine antagonistic effect. The dryness resulting from the atropine-like action contributes to the symptomatic relief of nasal congestion and rhinitis accompanying colds.

Dry mouth is an indication of adequate parenteral atropinization.

Theoretically, the antimuscarinic drugs should reduce gastric acid secretion, because the vagus nerve exerts an extrinsic stimulatory influence on gastric secretion. However, experience has shown that with the usual doses of atropine, gastric juice secretion is not altered significantly. Doses of 1 mg or more may reduce the volume of gastric juice and total acid. However, the doses required to affect gastric secretion frequently cause disagreeable side effects. Because there are more effective drugs available for treatment of peptic ulcer, the antimuscarinic drugs are used only as adjunct therapy or when the other drugs are ineffective. The duration of action of atropine upon gastric secretion, even when effective doses are used, is rather brief.

The sweat glands receive innervation by cholinergic sympathetic nerves, and the ACh receptors on the sweat glands are muscarinic. Atropine inhibits the secretion of sweat leading to dryness of the skin. With large doses of atropine the decrease in sweating may lead to an increase in temperature, especially in infants and small children. The hyperthermia is due to a decrease in loss of heat from the skin as well as a central disturbance in temperature control.

GASTROINTESTINAL TRACT

Motility of the GI tract is controlled by an intramural plexus of which the terminal nerves are cholinergic and end on or near muscarinic receptors. The vagus nerve exerts extrinsic motor control on GI smooth muscle and the plexuses. Full doses of atropine lead to an inhibition of motility in the stomach, duodenum, jejunum, ileum, and colon. There is a decrease in tone and amplitude of contractions and a decrease in frequency of peristaltic contractions. Unfortunately, these effects are often accompanied by adverse side effects, such as dry mouth, visual disturbances, and increased heart rate.

Atropine may be used to reduce or block the GI side effects of anticholinesterase inhibitors when they are used for an action on the nicotinic receptors of the neuromuscular end-plate (for example, recovery from competitive neuromuscular blocking drugs or myasthenia gravis).

Atropine may reduce GI motility when hyperactivity is present.

RESPIRATORY TRACT

Atropine blocks secretions of the mucous membranes of the respiratory tract leading to drying of the membrane. The bronchi and bronchioles are relaxed by atropine.

URINARY BLADDER

Atropine can cause a decrease in tone and contraction of the urinary bladder and ureter, but large doses are required. Atropine, or any drug with atropine-like actions, should be used with caution in patients with hyperplasia of the prostate, because it may cause urinary retention in these patients.

CENTRAL NERVOUS SYSTEM ACTIONS OF ATROPINE

Other than the mild vagal stimulation already described, atropine has little effect on the CNS in the normal therapeutic dose. Scopolamine does have effects with normal doses and is usually used when central effects are desired.

Sedation

Scopolamine causes sedation, drowsiness, and amnesia in most patients, but some may react with excitement. The electroencephalogram (EEG) shows a decrease in voltage and frequency of alpha rhythm with a shift to slow activity. The arousal response to photostimulation is depressed. Atropine causes mainly excitement, hallucinations, psychosis, disorientation, and amnesia in toxic doses. All atropine-like drugs have these central effects, and these effects may be particularly troublesome in the elderly (such psychiatric symptoms induced by drugs are discussed in Chapter 27).

Anti-Parkinson's Disease Activity

Parkinson's disease is caused by an imbalance in cholinergic and dopaminergic innervation in the striatal tracts due to a decrease in dopaminergic neurons. In theory a decrease in cholinergic influence or an increase in dopaminergic influence will be beneficial in treating parkinsonism. Levodopa is most effective for treating parkinsonism, but anticholinergic drugs may be used alone or with levodopa to decrease the severity of akinesia, rigidity, and tremor; they have the predictable effect also of decreasing the drooling secondarily (see Chapter 24).

Some of the antipsychotic drugs, such as haloperidol, the phenothiazines, and reserpine, may cause a drug-induced parkinsonian syndrome much like the idiopathic disease. In these patients, anticholinergic drugs are effective in reducing symptoms without interfering with the antipsychotic action of the drugs.

Congeners of atropine, such as procyclidine, trihexyphenidyl, benztropine, and biperiden, which are thought to have a more specific antitremor activity, are used frequently to treat Parkinson's disease or drug-induced parkinsonism (Table 11–1). Although these agents are used for their central actions, they can cause side effects similar to those of atropine, e.g., dry mouth and visual disturbances.

Vestibular Effects

Scopolamine acts centrally to produce sedation, anti-Parkinson's activity, and anti-motion sickness activity.

Scopolamine acts centrally to prevent or reduce salivation, nausea, and vomiting due to motion stresses. It is, in fact, one of the most effective drugs when used prophylactically in preventing motion sickness. The oral administration of the drug has a brief duration of action (4–6 hours), but transdermal patches that provide a more prolonged duration of action are available (see Therapeutic Uses).

Scopolamine probably acts at a number of central sites to prevent motion sickness. Afferent input from the labyrinth to the vestibular nucleus is modulated at the medial ventricular nucleus by ACh (excitatory) and norepinephrine (inhibitory). The ACh receptors in the medial vestibular nucleus are muscarinic, and scopolamine reduces the neuronal output from the vestibular nucleus during natural stimulus (motion) as well as mechanical and electrical stimulation of the labyrinth. The observation that adrenergic amines act synergistically with scopolamine in the prevention of motion sickness is consistent with the hypothesis of an action at the medial vestibular nucleus. Scopolamine has also been postulated to act by blocking muscarinic receptors in the reticular formation and possibly other sites within the CNS. Scopolamine is not effective in preventing nausea and vomiting due to other causes, e.g., pregnancy and drug intoxications.

Table 11–1 CENTRALLY ACTING ANTIMUSCARINIC DRUGS USED IN PARKINSON'S SYNDROME

Drug			
Generic Name	Proprietary Name	Daily Dose Range	Form
Procyclidine	Kemadrin	6–20 mg	5 mg tablets
Trihexyphenidyl hydrochloride	Artane	1–15 mg	2 and 5 mg tablets
Benztropine mesylate	Cogentin	0.5–6 mg	0.5, 1, and 2 mg tablets
Biperiden	Akineton	2–8 mg	2 mg tablets

ADVERSE EFFECTS

With full therapeutic doses the incidence of adverse effects is high. The major adverse effects are attributable to the nonspecificity of action of atropine and its actions on tissues other than the ones for which the drug is being used. The most frequent side effects reported with atropine and related drugs are dry mouth, blurring of vision, photophobia, and rapid heart rate. The incidence of side reactions is high, especially when the drugs are used for the treatment of peptic ulcer or hypermotility of the GI tract.

TOXICITY

Atropine intoxication exhibits a characteristic syndrome, and other drugs, such as antihistamines, phenothiazine antipsychotic drugs, and tricyclic antidepressants, all of which have antimuscarinic activity in addition to their principal actions, exhibit in part a similar toxic syndrome. Infants and children are especially susceptible to atropine intoxication, and most of the few deaths that have occurred were young children. Poisoning has resulted from accidental, excessive ingestion of medicinal preparations or of the many plants containing atropinic alkaloids; in addition, atropinic agents have been taken purposely to induce altered mentation (see Chapter 24). Anticholinergic intoxication is an important cause of memory loss and mental confusion in the elderly, and also one that frequently goes unrecognized.

The symptoms of atropine intoxication are due for the most part to an excessive blockade of muscarinic receptors so that normal functioning of important organs is disrupted. The symptoms include the following:

1. Extremely dry mouth, dry upper respiratory tract, and dry skin.
2. Hallucinations, bizarre behavior, confusion, delirium, and disturbances of memory.
3. Rapid heart rate.
4. Blush, due to vasodilation of the cutaneous blood vessels in the blush areas of the body.
5. Elevation of body temperature, especially in young children and infants. The elevation of temperature is due to a decrease in heat loss from the reduction of sweating as well as a central disturbance of temperature regulation.

Atropine intoxication is rarely fatal except for young children, and it is treated symptomatically. Physostigmine (0.5–2 mg infused slowly IV) is used sometimes to reduce the severity of the central effects resulting from intoxication with atropine or the phenothiazines and tricyclic antidepressants; it is effective in counteracting the confusion, delirium, and coma caused by these drugs. Physostigmine itself is potentially toxic so that it is not without risk, and the patient must be observed carefully. Furthermore, the duration of action of physostigmine is shorter than the duration of the atropine-like drugs, so the administration of physostigmine usually has to be repeated to prevent the reappearance of the symptoms of intoxication.

Atropine and scopolamine are readily absorbed after oral or parenteral administration. They can be absorbed after topical administration, especially from mucous membranes. Because the systemic effects persist for only a few hours, it is often necessary to repeat the usual dosage of 0.4–0.6 mg every 4–6 hours for sustained action. The half-life of a single dose

Adverse and Toxic Effects

Symptoms of atropine toxicity include dry mouth, blush, rapid heart rate, increased temperature, and bizarre behavior.

Absorption and Metabolism

Table 11-2 TIME FOR COMPLETE RECOVERY FROM MYDRIASIS AFTER MAXIMAL EFFECT

Drug	Solution Stength (%)	Mydriasis	
		Peak (Minutes)	Recovery (Days)
Atropine	0.5–3	30–90	7–12
Homatropine	2–5	30–60	1–3
Cyclopentolate	0.5–2	30–60	1
Tropicamide	0.5–1	20–40	0.25

of atropine in humans has been variously reported to be 2.5–6 hours. There is individual and racial variation in atropine excretion. The dose and frequency of administration depend on the severity of need. For example, a large dose of atropine (1–2 mg) repeated often may be necessary to successfully treat anticholinesterase intoxication. On the other hand, atropine-induced mydriasis following topical application to the cornea may last for many hours (Table 11–2).

Most of a single dose of atropine is excreted in the urine within 24 hours; about half of the atropine is unchanged, the remainder are metabolic products.

Therapeutic Uses

Atropine is used topically for refraction of eyes and to treat certain inflammatory diseases of the eye.

EYE

Antimuscarinic drugs are instilled onto the conjunctiva to produce mydriasis and cycloplegia for refraction of the eyes and to treat acute iritis, iridocyclitis, and keratitis. The duration of action of atropine and scopolamine when applied topically to the eye is long (it may take 7–12 days for complete recovery). The shorter-acting drugs, such as homatropine, cyclopentolate, and tropicamide, are often used to produce mydriasis, because recovery occurs faster. However, atropine is more potent in producing cycloplegia than the shorter-acting drugs, so it may be used when cycloplegia is desired (see Table 11–2).

Atropine may be absorbed from the mucous membranes, and it may enter the nasolacrimal duct and be swallowed and absorbed after topical application to the eye in sufficient amounts to cause atropine toxicity, especially in young children. This can be minimized by compression of the lacrimal sac for about 1 minute following application of the solution.

PREANESTHETIC MEDICATION

With the older general anesthetics such as diethyl ether, which was irritating, it was routine to administer atropine prior to general anesthesia to reduce the copious bronchial and salivary secretions caused by the anesthetic agents. Many general anesthetic agents in use now do not cause reflex secretion of fluids, and the routine use of atropine prior to all surgery is not justifiable. However, atropine or scopolamine may be used to reduce secretions during surgery, to prevent reflex bradycardia during surgery, and to prevent drug-induced bradycardia when indicated.

Use of atropine with surgical anesthesia

If a competitive neuromuscular blocking drug is used during surgery, neostigmine is often used postoperatively to hasten recovery from the neuromuscular blockade. In this case, atropine is administered prior to neostigmine to block the muscarinic effects of neostigmine (such as salivary secretions and increased GI motility).

Table 11-3 ANTISPASMODIC/ANTISECRETORY MUSCARINIC ANTAGONISTS			
		Dose	
Generic Name	Proprietary Name	*Oral*	*Parenteral*
Natural Alkaloids			
Belladonna tincture	—	0.6 mL	—
Atropine sulfate	—	0.4–0.6 mg	0.4–0.6 mg
Scopolamine hydrobromide	—	0.3–0.6 mg	0.3–0.6 mg
Quaternary Compounds			
Methscopolamine bromide	Pamine	2.5 mg	—
Glycopyrrolate	Robinol	1–2 mg	0.1–0.2 mg
Propantheline bromide	Pro-Banthine	7.5–15 mg	—
Anisotropine methylbromide	Valpin	50 mg	—
Clindinium bromide	Quarzan	2.5–5 mg	—
Hexocyclium methylsulfate	Tral	25 mg	—
Isopropamide iodide	Darbid	5–10 mg	—
Mepenzolate bromide	Cantil	25–50 mg	—
Methantheline bromide	Banthine	50–100 mg	—
Oxyphenonium bromide	Antrenyl	10 mg	—
Tridihexethyl chloride	Pathilon	25–50 mg	—

If central sedation is also desired in addition to the peripheral effects of atropine, scopolamine is used because it has a more pronounced central effect as well as peripheral actions. An occasional patient reacts to scopolamine with excitement and delirium rather than with sedation.

HYPERMOTILITY OF THE GASTROINTESTINAL TRACT

Atropine and related drugs are more effective in reducing the motility of the hypermotile GI tract than the normal functioning organ. These drugs are useful in a variety of conditions involving increased activity of the GI smooth muscle, including spastic colitis, irritable colon, and functional disorders, such as diarrhea, pylorospasm, and neurogenic colon. Atropine is effective also in reducing the drug-induced hypermotility that may accompany the use of guanethidine, reserpine, and neostigmine. The many drug forms that are available include belladonna tincture, an alcoholic solution of the active ingredients in the leaf. It is inexpensive, and the patient can titrate the dose to his or her needs; the usual dose is 0.6 mL. The main active ingredient is atropine. Another drug form is atropine sulfate, 0.4–0.6 mg, which may be given either orally or parenterally (Table 11–3; see also Chapter 45).

Atropine relaxes the hypermotile GI tract.

PEPTIC ULCER

Theoretically, antimuscarinic agents should be useful for treatment of peptic ulcer, because the parasympathetic vagus nerve is the extrinsic nervous innervation that stimulates the output of gastric acid and is necessary for the action of hormones that act to increase acid output. However, the

Antimuscarinic drugs may be used as adjunct therapy to more effective therapeutic agents in peptic ulcer.

effectiveness of antimuscarinic drugs has been disappointing. Although atropine will decrease total acid, the doses required to have an effect cause disagreeable side effects, and the compliance of patients on antimuscarinic drugs is poor. Atropine also decreases the motility of the stomach and increases emptying time, which permits antacids to remain in the stomach longer. This permits a longer time for neutralization of the acid. Because histamine antagonists and antacids are more effective in the treatment of peptic ulcer and have fewer disagreeable side effects, the antimuscarinic drugs are used only as adjuvants or if other drugs do not work. When atropine or related drugs are used, they are frequently administered at bedtime in order to minimize the disturbance from side effects. The quaternary nitrogen drugs, such as propantheline, are often used in peptic ulcer instead of atropine, because some clinicians feel that they are more effective.

More recent experiments that indicate that there may be at least two subgroups of muscarinic receptors have led to the search for more specific antimuscarinic drugs. Pirenzepine is currently under investigation for its use in the therapy of peptic ulcer. Initial experiments suggest that pirenzepine affects gastric acid secretion at lower doses than other muscarinic responses. Further clinical experience with pirenzepine will have to be obtained before its place in therapy can be established.

HEART

Atropine antagonizes reflex slowing of heart rate.

Atropine does not have pronounced effects on the heart, but it will reduce vagal control of the heart and interfere with vagal depressor reflexes. It is used as a preanesthetic agent to prevent reflex slowing of heart rate or to prevent drug-induced slowing of heart rate. In the rare patient who suffers from hyperactive carotid sinus syndrome, atropine will prevent the bradycardia and syncope that may occur with activation of this reflex. Some clinicians suggest the use of atropine early in acute myocardial infarction accompanied by a severe bradycardia with low cardiac output. The rationale is to increase cardiac output and increase perfusion of the ischemic area of the heart muscle. This use is controversial, because too large an increase in heart rate has been associated with cardiac arrhythmias, and some investigators feel that perfusion of ischemic areas is not improved even with moderate increases in heart rate.

CENTRAL NERVOUS SYSTEM

The use of procyclidine, trihexyphenidyl, benztropine, and biperiden in Parkinson's disease is mentioned in the section on pharmacology of antimuscarinic drugs. Except for drug-induced parkinsonism, these drugs are used only for treatment of Parkinson's disease when the more effective ones are not providing sufficient improvement (see Chapter 24). In drug-induced parkinsonism, levodopa cannot be used and, thus, the antimuscarinic drugs are employed.

Scopolamine, 0.6 mg orally, is useful as a prophylactic agent to prevent motion sickness. In order to avoid oral administration and to obtain a longer duration of effect, a transdermal patch for topical administration of the drug is available. The drug reservoir is separated from the skin by a microporous membrane that meters the drug to the skin. The delivery of active drug occurs over a period of 3 days. The patch is usually placed behind the ear (see Fig. 3–2).

RESPIRATORY TRACT

Many years ago, atropine-containing substances were smoked to relieve asthma. With the introduction of adrenergic amines and theophylline for the treatment of asthma, the use of these crude remedies disappeared. There has been a renewed interest in the parasympathetic innervation of the respiratory tract. It has been found that a motor parasympathetic innervation to the airways is important, especially to the intermediate-sized airways. Thus, there is a recognition that if airway obstruction has a cholinergic basis, atropine should be useful for reducing pulmonary resistance. Atropine sulfate solution has been administered by inhalation to treat bronchitis and asthma. Atropine may have a twofold action: smooth muscle relaxation, and decreased ACh-enhanced mediator release. Atropine is easily absorbed from mucous membranes and may have other systemic effects even when applied locally by inhalation.

An antimuscarinic agent, ipratropium bromide, which has a quaternary nitrogen and is not absorbed easily from mucous membranes, is now being tested clinically for use in bronchitis and asthma. Ipratropium administered by inhalation of a spray causes a decrease in pulmonary resistance in 75–90 seconds. Although it was postulated that side effects would be minimized by use of this drug, it is reported that 20–30% of patients receiving it suffer from dry mouth and throat irritation. One potential disadvantage of antimuscarinic drugs in asthma is that they may cause a reduction in the volume of secretion, leading to an increase in viscosity and formation of plugs in the smaller air passages. Early reports with ipratropium suggest that plug formation may not occur, but more clinical experience with the drug is necessary to determine its place in therapy (see Chapter 62).

ANTICHOLINESTERASE POISONING

Atropine and pralidoxime (PROTOPAM) are specific antidotes for poisoning by organophosphate cholinesterase inhibitors. Atropine, 2–4 mg intravenously (IV) or intramuscularly (IM) given initially, with 2 mg every 5–10 minutes until the symptoms disappear, will reduce the muscarinic manifestations of intoxication. Continuous administration of 1–2 mg every several hours may be necessary as long as symptoms are in evidence. Large doses of atropine are usually required and may be as much as 50 mg the first day. The duration of action of atropine is short compared with the duration of inhibition of cholinesterase, so repeated doses are necessary. Pralidoxime is administered simultaneously with atropine to reduce the neuromuscular block that is present with cholinesterase inhibitor poisoning.

Atropine plus pralidoxime are specific antidotes for organophosphate cholinesterase intoxication.

Pralidoxime is not used with intoxication by carbamate cholinesterase inhibitors, but atropine is effective in suppressing the muscarinic symptoms in carbamate poisoning. Atropine does not reverse any neuromuscular block that may be present, so support of respiration must be maintained during the recovery period.

Certain mushrooms, such as *Amanita muscaria* and selected species of *Inocybe*, contain the alkaloid muscarine that causes rapid development of cholinergic symptoms (salivation, nausea, vomiting, GI cramps, diarrhea, visual disturbances, and bradycardia). Atropine, 2 mg IM, blocks these symptoms. Note that atropine is of no value in the treatment of mushroom poisoning, which has a delayed onset. *Amanita phalloides* and certain other species contain a toxin that damages the liver and kidneys. The intoxication is slow in onset and frequently fatal and not reversible by atropine.

References

Gil DW, Wolfe BB: Pirenzepine distinguishes between muscarinic receptor-mediated phosphoinositide breakdown and inhibition of adenylate cyclase. J Pharmacol Exp Ther 232:608–616, 1985.

Greenstein SH, Abramson DH, Pitts WR III: Systemic atropine and glaucoma. Bull NY Acad Med 60:961–968, 1984.

Gross NJ, Skorodin MS: Anticholinergic, antimuscarinic bronchodilators. Am Rev Respir Dis 129:856–870, 1984.

Hammer R, Giachetti A: Muscarinic receptor subtypes: M-1 and M-2. Biochemical and functional characterization. Life Sci 31:2991–2998, 1982.

Kohl RL, Homick JL: Motion sickness: A modulatory role for the central cholinergic nervous system. Neurosci Biobehav Rev 7:73–85, 1983.

Richman S: Adverse effect of atropine during myocardial infarction. Enhancement of ischemia following intravenously administered atropine. JAMA 228:1414–1416, 1974.

Somerville KW, Langman MJS: Newer antisecretory agents for peptic ulcer. Drugs 25:315–330, 1983.

Vakil DV, Ayiomamitis A, Nizam RM: Use of ipratropium aerosol in long-term management of asthma. J Asthma 22:165–170, 1985.

12

Nicotine and Ganglion-Blocking Drugs

Robert L. Volle

Nicotine is probably the most widely used legal, self-administered substance of abuse available. By behavioral and pharmacological mechanisms not understood, physical and behavioral dependence on nicotine develops, leading to repetitive self-administration. Although there is a trend toward reduced usage, nicotine, tobacco products, and tobacco smoke are major threats to public health. Because safe substitutes are not available and not likely to be developed, an enlightened public health program of education continues to be the best approach toward the goal of improving public health by reducing cigarette and tobacco consumption.

In the U.S. about 33% of males and about 28% of females above the age of 18 can be classified as confirmed smokers. Both figures are down from 1965, when 50% and 32% of the male and female population, respectively, were smokers.

Cigarette smoke when inhaled and nicotine-containing products when chewed or sniffed cause profound complex, acute, and chronic changes in most, if not all, organ systems. Nicotinic receptors are found on axons (sensory and motor) and on many synaptic and neuroeffector junctions (Table 12–1). When activated by nicotine, the receptors initiate prominent excitatory and inhibitory responses by the nerves that modulate the activity of effector organs. Drugs that block nicotinic receptors prevent the neuronal and end organ responses to nicotine.

Attempts have been made to control organ system function by blocking ganglionic nicotinic receptors. For example, the widespread distribution of nicotinic receptors throughout the autonomic nervous system suggests that the interruption of ganglionic transmission by drugs might be useful in the management of some disorders.

Hexamethonium (C_6), a prototypic antagonist of nicotine receptors in autonomic ganglia, was used in the 1950s to control hypertension. However, as revealed by cursory inspection, the usefulness of these drugs to regulate the cardiovascular system is limited by a lack of specificity, i.e., all ganglia are blocked, causing many unacceptable side effects. Ganglionic blocking drugs are used currently only when controlled hypotension is desired and in special cases of autonomic hyperreflexia and hypertensive emergencies.

GANGLIONIC ACTIONS

In some cases, the activation of axonal nicotinic receptors blocks conduction (e.g., vagal "C" fibers) or causes axonal discharges (e.g., Hering's

Nicotine acts by way of receptors located on sensory and motor nerve endings, as well as at many synaptic and neuroeffector junctions.

Nicotine

Table 12-1   EFFECTS OF NICOTINE ON SOME NONJUNCTIONAL AND JUNCTIONAL CELLS BEFORE AND AFTER NICOTINIC RECEPTOR BLOCKADE BY HEXAMETHONIUM (C_6)

Neuronal Substrate	Physiological Response	Nicotine	After C_6	Nicotine After C_6
"C" fiber	Conduction	Axonal blockade	Conduction normal	No block
Carotid body	Sensory nerve discharge to CO_2	Discharge	Discharge normal to CO_2	No discharge
Adrenergic neuron	Norepinephrine release	Norepinephrine release	Norepinephrine release normal	No release
Adrenal medulla	Catecholamine release	Catecholamine release	Block of release	Block of release
Muscle end-plate	End-plate potential (EPP)	Depolarization	EPP normal*	Depolarization*
Ganglia	Synaptic potential	Depolarization	Blocked transmission	Block

*At usual dose of C_6. With higher doses, C_6 has curare-like actions and will block ACh receptor at the skeletal muscle end-plate.

Nicotinic agonists and antagonists are specific for sites of action.

nerve) whereas, in other cases, it stimulates transmitter release (e.g., adrenergic axonal varicosities) (see Table 12-1). These actions can be prevented by nicotine receptors blocking drugs such as hexamethonium (C_6). By contrast, axonal responses to physiological stimulation are unaffected by C_6: thus, it is unlikely that nicotinic receptors are involved in axonal conduction or in transmitter release. The meaning of their presence in axons is not understood.

At junctions where nicotine's actions imitate, albeit crudely, the responses to prejunctional nerve stimulation, receptor block by C_6 prevents

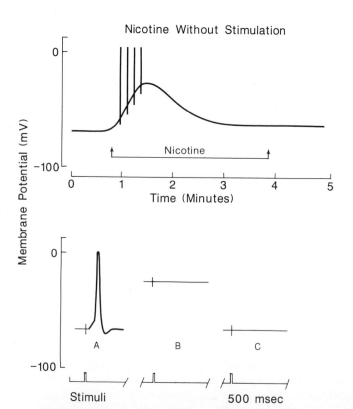

Figure 12-1

Diagrammatic representation of an isolated sympathetic ganglion arranged for preganglionic nerve stimulation (S) and intracellular recording (R) of responses to S and applied nicotine *(top diagram)*.

The *middle diagram* presents the postganglionic responses to nicotine at the 60 mV resting membrane potential, at nicotine-induced depolarization with four action-potential discharges, and at repolarization in the presence of nicotine.

The *bottom recording* is from the same postganglionic cell in response to a single preganglionic stimulus (stimuli) before depolarization (A), during depolarization (B), and during repolarization in the presence of nicotine (C). This sequence illustrates the normal ganglion action potential (A), the depolarization block (B), and the repolarization phase block (C).

responses both to nicotine and to physiological stimulation (see Table 12–1), e.g., splanchnic nerve stimulation and nicotine release catecholamines from the adrenal medulla where both effects are prevented by C_6. Similarly, both the primary response to preganglionic nerve stimulation and nicotine-induced depolarization of autonomic ganglia are blocked by C_6.

The details of how nicotine imitates the actions of acetylcholine at cholinergic junctions has been elucidated best at the neuromuscular junction (see Chapters 8, 9, and 13) and to a lesser extent at autonomic ganglia. At ganglia, nicotine and related drugs cause postjunctional depolarization accompanied initially by repetitive action potentials and later by a block of transmission (Fig. 12–1). During depolarization, the ganglia are insensitive to further stimulation either by nicotinic or nonnicotinic (e.g., 5-hydroxytryptamine, K^+, methacholine) agents. It is surmised that depolarization blockade results from increased sodium inactivation in ganglion cell membrane, hence reduced sensitivity to all ganglionic stimulants. During repolarization, especially in the continued presence of nicotine, responses to a subsequent application of nicotinic agents and to preganglionic nerve stimulation are suppressed (see Fig. 12–1) at a time when responses to nonnicotinic agents are restored. The block of transmission persisting during repolarization results from desensitization of nicotinic receptors (see Chapter 13). Depending on concentration and duration of exposure, nicotine depolarizes ganglia and then blocks transmission by two distinct mechanisms: depolarization and desensitization. The well-known tolerance that develops to the repeated use of nicotine and tobacco products may be due to desensitization of nicotinic receptors at both central and peripheral synapses.

Nicotinic agonists act by initial depolarization followed by desensitization.

Desensitization is one mechanism underlying the acquired tolerance.

ORGAN SYSTEM RESPONSES

In view of the widespread and complex effects of nicotine on most components of the nervous system, it is not surprising that organ system responses to nicotine are variable (Table 12–2). Moreover, tolerance develops to some responses when nicotine is used so that the pattern of response to a single dose may be modified by the extent of previous exposure. Typical

Table 12–2 TYPICAL RESPONSES TO MODERATE* AND TOXIC DOSES OF NICOTINE		
Organ or System	**Moderate**	**Toxic**
Cardiovascular		
Heart rate	Tachycardia	Initial bradycardia followed by tachycardia
Blood pressure	Increased systolic and diastolic	Initial rise followed by hypotension
Circulation	Vasoconstriction of renal and cutaneous beds; vasodilation of skeletal muscle bed	Unpredictable because of shock
Respiration	Stimulation by central action and by activation of chemoreceptors	Irregular; apnea because of block of diaphragm and intercostal muscles
Gastrointestinal	Increase of gastric secretion; increased motility	Nausea, vomiting, diarrhea
Central nervous system	Slight tremor, release of antidiuretic hormone	Mental confusion, convulsions
Salivary gland	Increased secretion	Increased secretion
Eye	Pupil size increased	Miosis, later mydriasis

*Dosage in range obtained with smoking or chewing tobacco.

No specific antagonist is available to treat nicotine poisoning.

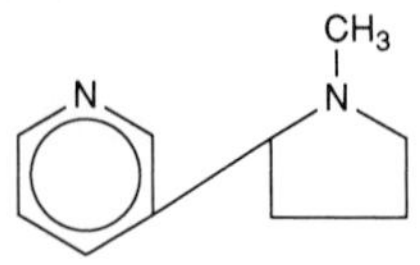

Nicotine

Nicotine itself is absorbed rapidly if applied to skin, oral mucosa, or lung epithelium.

responses to moderate amounts (e.g., nicotine in a cigarette) and toxic concentrations (agricultural and household poisons) of nicotine are listed in Table 12 – 2. Nicotine is deleterious, especially in individuals with cardiovascular and pulmonary diseases, and has no known beneficial pharmacological properties to justify its use.

There is no specific antidote to nicotine. Treatment of acute toxicity depends upon reducing blood levels of nicotine, its elimination from the body, and the symptomatic management of respiratory depression and other signs of toxicity. Nicotinic receptor antagonists are not useful, because toxicity to nicotine results usually in receptor desensitization, a condition not alleviated by drugs that block nicotine receptors. For example, paralysis by nicotine of the diaphragm and respiratory skeletal muscle cannot be reversed by D-tubocurarine (see also Chapter 13).

Chemistry and Products

Nicotine is 1-methyl-2-(3-pyridyl) pyrolidine (see structure) and occurs as a clear oily liquid that turns brown when exposed to air. It is a tertiary amine alkaloid found in all tobacco products and is prepared as a 40% solution for use as an agricultural insecticide and rodenticide.

Nicotine (a weak base with a pKa of 8.0) is absorbed rapidly from the oral, pulmonary, and gastrointestinal (GI) mucosa and accumulates in neurons and other cells. It enters the central nervous system (CNS) rapidly and crosses the placenta and other biological membranes with relative ease. This property is illustrated by the observation that tobacco field workers, especially nonsmokers, may show signs of nicotine poisoning when safeguards are not taken to reduce nicotine intake by way of pulmonary and cutaneous routes. Field workers who are habituated to tobacco products are less likely to manifest the signs and symptoms of nicotine poisoning.

Other Nicotinic Ganglion Agonists

Other nicotinic ganglion agonists include α-lobeline (an alkaloid found in the plant, *Lobelia inflata*), 1,1-dimethyl-4-phenyl-piperazinium iodide, and tetramethylammonium bromide. These compounds possess most of the neuronal actions of nicotine: they are used to study nicotinic receptors but have no clinical applications. The uses of lobeline as a substitute for nicotine to curb tobacco smoking or to stimulate respiration have fallen into disrepute.

Muscarinic Ganglion Agonists

Autonomic ganglia contain a number of receptors — nicotinic, and at least two types of muscarinic cholinergic receptors, catecholamine receptors, and receptors to peptides.

Autonomic ganglion cells, adrenal medullary cells, and adrenergic neurons (see Chapters 8 and 14) possess muscarinic acetylcholine (ACh) receptors that can be activated by ACh and muscarinic agonists (Fig. 12 – 2). In some sympathetic ganglia, preganglionic nerve stimulation evokes a complex series of ganglion potentials consisting of a nicotinic excitatory postsynaptic potential (N), a slow muscarinic inhibitory potential (M_I) and a late-occurring, long-lasting muscarinic excitatory synaptic potential (M_E). The N potential is due to the activation of ganglion nicotinic receptors by ACh and is prevented by C_6. The M_E potential is due to ACh acting upon muscarinic receptors, because it is antagonized by atropine but not C_6. The M_E potential is due to a slowly developing inhibition of an outward current that increases the excitability of the ganglion cell.

There is some controversy about the mechanisms involved in the generation of M_I. Because some ganglia contain dopaminergic small intensely fluorescent (SIF) cells, and some adrenergic and dopaminergic blocking drugs reduce M_I, it has been postulated that M_I is due to a disyn-

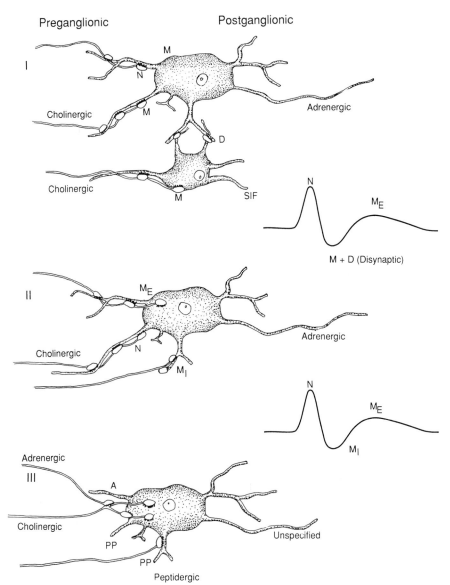

Preganglionic   Postganglionic

Figure 12–2

Semidiagrammatic models of ganglion organization, transmitters, and receptors, depicting preganglionic fibers, the ganglionic cell, and postganglionic activity.

(I) Ganglion with cholinergic nicotinic (N) and muscarinic (M) excitatory ganglionic responses to ACh and inhibitory activity caused by dopamine (D) released from small intensely fluorescent (SIF) cells. The SIF cell is, in turn, activated by ACh through a muscarinic receptor. A possible correspondence of these connections in accounting for the ganglionic potential is presented on the right for models *I* and *II*.

(II) A model ganglionic organization that could account for the complex responses to ACh by an N, excitatory muscarinic (M_E), and inhibitory muscarinic (M_I) receptor.

(III) A model for visceral ganglia showing the presynaptic inhibition by an adrenergic transmitter (A) as well as presynaptic and postsynaptic innervation by a peptide containing (PP, peptidergic) nerve fibers.

aptic process whereby ACh acts on muscarinic receptors on SIF cells to release dopamine that, in turn, acts on the ganglion cell to cause hyperpolarization (see Fig. 12–2). This model accounts for the observation that either atropine or adrenergic blocking agents prevent the hyperpolarization in some sympathetic ganglion cells. Alternatively, a direct action of ACh on ganglionic muscarinic inhibitory receptors can account for the block by atropine (see Fig. 12–2). Careful microapplication of ACh has localized the M_I muscarinic receptor to the ganglion cell. Furthermore, many ganglia do not contain the type of SIF cell required for the disynaptic model of ganglionic transmission.

Finally, differential changes in the complex ganglionic potential caused by the atropine-like drugs pirenzepine and gallamine (see Chapters 11 and 13) suggest that M_E and M_I result from the activation of muscarinic receptor subtypes. Pirenzepine blocks selectively M_E and gallamine blocks M_I.

Muscarinic receptor agonists hyperpolarize and depolarize autonomic ganglia to varying degrees. ACh applied after hexamethonium, or methacholine, to cat superior cervical ganglion (used extensively to study ganglion transmission) causes a delayed onset hyperpolarization and inhibi-

$$H_3C - \overset{+}{\underset{\underset{CH_3}{|}}{\overset{\overset{CH_3}{|}}{N}}} - CH_2CH_2 - O - \overset{\overset{O}{\|}}{C} - CH_3$$

Acetylcholine

Figure 12–3

Ganglion demarcation potentials evoked by ACh before and after nicotinic and muscarinic receptor block by hexamethonium alone and by atropine alone, respectively. When hexamethonium and atropine are applied in combination, all responses to ACh are prevented.

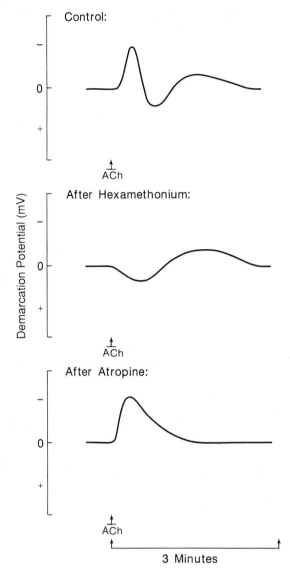

tion of transmission followed by a later-occurring depolarization and excitation (Fig. 12–3). Other experimental agents that stimulate sympathetic ganglia by activation of ganglion muscarinic receptors include 4-[m-chorophenyl-carbamoyloxy]-2-butynyl trimethylammonium chloride (McN-A-343) and N-benzyl-3-pyrrolidyl acetate methobromide (AHR-602). McN-A-343 and AHR-602 increase systemic blood pressure by a ganglionic mechanism blocked by atropine; these drugs have little or no muscarinic activity on smooth muscle or cardiac cells.

Nonnicotinic, Nonmuscarinic Ganglionic Agents

It is possible that polypeptides participate as transmitters in some ganglia. Luteinizing hormone releasing hormone is a putative excitatory transmitter in amphibian sympathetic ganglia. Leu- and met-enkephalins are present in some mammalian ganglia and inhibit ACh release from preganglionic nerve endings by a mechanism that is sensitive to naloxone (see Fig. 12–2). Importantly, adrenergic neurons release catecholamines directly onto preganglionic nerve terminals of pelvic and other visceral ganglia resulting in suppression of ACh release and inhibition of transmission (see Fig. 12–2). These anatomical and pharmacological relationships suggest that some regulation of information exchange between the CNS and the periphery can occur in ganglia.

Table 12-3 GANGLION-BLOCKING DRUGS

Drug	Main Chemical Feature	Special Property
Hexamethonium	Bis-quaternary ammonium	Prototype; erratic absorpton from gut
Tubocurarine	Mono-quaternary	Used to block neuromuscular junction; also blocks ganglia
Trimethaphan	Sulfonium	Short acting; direct vasodilation
Mecamylamine	Secondary amine	Crosses blood-brain barrier; well-absorbed; pH-dependent urinary excretion

These drugs block ganglionic transmission by the antagonism of ACh at the nicotinic ganglion receptor (Table 12–3). They do not prevent ACh release, affect muscarinic ganglion receptors, depolarize ganglion cells, or alter ACh metabolism. Ganglion-blocking drugs inhibit transmission in all autonomic ganglia and the adrenal medulla. Those agents with quaternary ammonium groups do not enter the CNS. (However, if applied directly to central neurons, these drugs block nicotinic receptors, e.g., the Renshaw cell.) The pharmacological responses to ganglion blockade are easy to predict, because they result from the loss of autonomic nervous control of organ activity (Table 12–4).

In general, the organ response depends on the type of innervation (sympathetic, parasympathetic, or both), the pattern of neuronal activity, and organ response to circulating catecholamines. Ganglion blockade and its effect on organ responses are listed in Table 12–4. As can be predicted, the use of these drugs is limited by the occurrence of orthostatic hypotension, blurred vision, dry mouth, constipation, or urinary retention. The therapeutic use of ganglion-blocking drugs is restricted to the management of hypertensive crises, reduction of the effects of sympathetic discharge in autonomic hyperreflexia in patients with spinal cord injury, reduction of blood pressure in aortic dissection, and the induction of controlled hypotension to reduce bleeding in certain surgical procedures.

Trimethaphan camsylate (ARFONAD) is an extremely short-acting sulfonium drug (see structures) that is available only for parenteral use when controlled hypotension is needed. The mechanism whereby trimethaphan blocks ganglion transmission is not known in detail, although the primary effect is due to a block of nicotinic receptors. The hypotensive effect is reversed quickly when the infusion of trimethaphan is terminated. Like hexamethonium and D-tubocurarine, trimethaphan causes histamine release, a factor that contributes to vasodilation and reduced blood pressure.

Ganglion-Blocking Drugs

Ganglion-blocking agents are nearly therapeutically obsolete; they have been largely replaced by more selective and less toxic alternatives.

What would be the consequence of simultaneous interruption of transmission through all autonomic ganglia?

Chapter 8 provides illustrations of the major components of the autonomic nervous system.

Preparations

Hexamethonium (C6)

Trimethaphan

Mecamylamine

Table 12-4 TYPICAL RESPONSES TO GANGLIONIC BLOCKADE

Organ or System	Response
Cardiovascular	
Heart rate	Tachycardia; when heart rate is high, bradycardia may occur.
Blood pressure	Arteriolar vasodilation; venous pooling, decreased venous return, decreased cardiac output. Orthostatic hypotension, a prominent side effect.
Gastrointestinal	Decreased motility leading to constipation; decreased tone leading to gas accumulation.
Urinary bladder	Urine retention.
Eye	Mydriasis and cycloplegia due to loss of cholinergic control.
Salivary gland	Reduced secretion; dry mouth.

Drugs are rarely absolutely specific/selective in their receptor binding—large doses of ganglion-blocking agents may aggravate skeletal neuromuscular blockade by tubocurarine.

Trimethaphan may increase neuromuscular block produced by D-tubocurarine.

Mecamylamine hydrochloride (INVERSINE) is a secondary amine that is well absorbed, penetrates the blood-brain barrier, and crosses the placenta. The mechanism of ganglion blockade is a noncompetitive antagonism of the nicotinic receptor. Excretion by the kidney is dependent upon urinary pH; acid urine promotes the renal clearance of mecamylamine. Side effects referable to central actions of mecamylamine include tremors, mental confusion, seizures, and altered mental states characterized by either depression or mania. In addition to these, the side effects noted earlier for the other ganglion-blocking drugs also apply to mecamylamine; these are the major limitations to its use.

References

See References for Chapters 8 and 35.

Drugs Acting at the Neuromuscular Junction

13

Robert J. McIsaac

Motor nerves pass without synapse from the motor neuron in the spinal cord to the muscle fiber. At the muscle fiber the nerves synapse on a specialized area of a muscle fiber, the end-plate. The membrane of the end-plate is an invaginated structure on which acetylcholine (ACh) receptors as well as the enzyme acetylcholinesterase (AChE) are located. An action potential arriving at the nerve terminal initiates a process that results in the release of the transmitter ACh (Fig. 13–1). Depolarization of the terminal allows calcium to enter, and the increase in ionized calcium in the intracellular cytoplasm stimulates a process resulting in the exocytosis of ACh. The nerve terminals are thought to have receptors with which ACh can combine, and stimulation of these presynaptic receptors can lead to *backfiring* of the nerve and under appropriate circumstances, with some drugs, to multiple muscle responses. ACh is released from the nerve terminals in discrete packets called *quanta,* and it is postulated that one quanta represents the contents of a single storage vesicle of ACh. When a propagated action potential enters the nerve terminal, 200–300 quanta are released simultaneously and the ACh diffuses across the synaptic gap to receptors on the end-plate area.

The invaginations in the end-plate membrane (junctional folds) (see Fig. 13–1) increase the surface area of the membrane. Nicotinic ACh receptors are located on the surface of the end-plate membrane, and AChE is located in the synaptic gap and on the end-plate membrane, especially in the interior of the folds. These nicotinic receptors are somewhat different from those on autonomic ganglia, and the two types can be distinguished by drugs that are relatively specific in their interaction with either ganglionic or end-plate receptors.

Combination of ACh with the receptor causes ion channels to open and sodium and potassium to enter and leave the cell, respectively. This leads to a local, graded depolarization of the end-plate membrane, and the magnitude of the depolarization is proportional to the number of ACh-receptor complexes formed at any one time. This local, graded depolarization is called the *end-plate potential.* The end-plate potential serves as a sink for currents to flow to the adjacent muscle membrane. If the end-plate potential is large enough, an action potential is generated on the adjacent muscle membrane and conducted over the muscle membrane to initiate the muscle contraction. The end-plate potential reaches a maximum within approximately 1 msec and then repolarizes to the resting membrane potential within 5–10 msec. The depolarization and repolarization processes are important for maintaining normal muscle responsiveness to nerve activity,

Physiology of Neuromuscular Transmission

Depolarization of the motor nerve terminal results in ACh release.

ACh combines with end-plate nicotinic receptors to initiate a local, graded depolarization, the end-plate potential.

Figure 13–1

Schematic drawing of a skeletal neuromuscular junction. The inset illustrates the nerve ending cross section at the end-plate area.

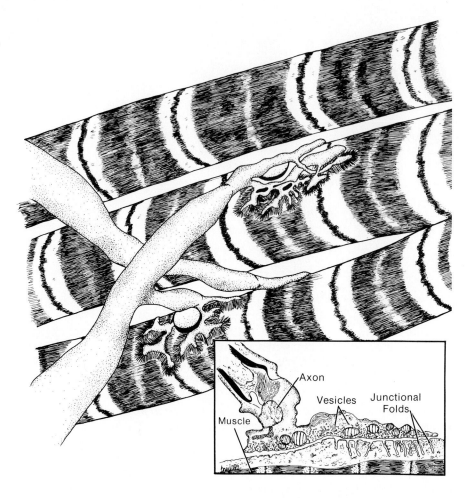

Axon

Vesicles

Junctional Folds

Muscle

and if either process is altered, neuromuscular transmission may be affected.

The amount of ACh released from a nerve terminal by a nerve action potential is appreciably more than enough to elicit an end-plate potential sufficient to cause contraction of the muscle fiber. Thus, normally there is a large margin of safety in neuromuscular transmission. If the amount of ACh released is reduced or the number of postsynaptic ACh receptors is reduced, the margin of safety in transmission is diminished even though transmission may be maintained.

Some drugs interact with ACh receptors and cause a prolonged depolarization of the end-plate that may last minutes rather than milliseconds. This leads to a blockade of transmission because the prolonged depolarization of the end-plate causes inactivation of the immediate surrounding muscle membrane. Drugs and conditions that can lead to this *depolarization block* are nicotine, overtreatment with AChE inhibitors, and succinylcholine (a drug to be discussed later in this chapter).

If the depolarization of the end-plate lasts for a prolonged period, another change called *desensitization* of the receptor occurs. When desensitization occurs, the receptor is altered so that although the transmitter still has an affinity for the receptor, it no longer causes an effect, e.g., opening of ion channels. Thus, during a desensitization period, neuromuscular transmission is blocked, but the end-plate membrane potential returns toward normal, and the block assumes some of the characteristics of a competitive blockade.

DISORDERS OF NEUROMUSCULAR TRANSMISSION

Presynaptic Disorders

Myasthenic Syndrome (Eaton-Lambert Syndrome). Myasthenic syndrome is caused by a defect in the release process of ACh. It is characterized by a generalized muscular weakness and fatigability. In contrast to myasthenia gravis, muscular strength in patients with myasthenic syndrome is weak initially and may improve with continued effort. Since myasthenic syndrome patients may also exhibit dry mouth, constipation, difficulty in micturation, and impotence, the defect in ACh release may involve autonomic cholinergic nerves as well as motor nerves.

ACh release is reduced in myasthenic syndrome and botulinum intoxication.

Botulinum Intoxication. The polypeptide toxin elaborated by *Clostridium botulinum* is the most potent poison known, and only a few molecules of the toxin are required to block a cholinergic synapse. Botulism may be caused by contaminated food or wounds or, in the case of infantile botulism, from organisms growing in the gut. There are eight types of toxins known, but most human intoxications are caused by only two, types A and B.

Botulinum toxin blocks the release of ACh from the nerve terminal without affecting ACh synthesis or storage. The symptoms of intoxication are related to a decrease in cholinergic influences on tissues, but the interference with neuromuscular transmission is the most critical effect because the weakness of muscle contractions can lead to respiratory inadequacy.

Postsynaptic Disorders

Myasthenia Gravis. Myasthenia gravis is an autoimmune disease characterized by the presence of antibodies directed against the ACh receptor. Many myasthenic patients are found to have a decrease in the number of ACh receptors, a simplification of the end-plate structure, circulating antibodies to the ACh receptor, and an increase in the turnover of the ACh receptor. The symptoms include ptosis, weakness of one or more of the muscles initially involving the extraocular muscles or including the bulbar muscles, and in generalized myasthenia, the muscles of the extremities.

Myasthenia gravis is an autoimmune disease directed against ACh receptors on the end-plate.

Muscle strength of myasthenic patients is initially near normal, but fatigue rapidly develops with continued effort. Strength is improved by prolonging the action of ACh with short-acting cholinesterase inhibitors. Patients with myasthenia gravis are much more sensitive to the action of competitive antagonists (such as tubocurarine) acting at the end-plate ACh receptors than are normal people.

Snake Envenomation. Venom from Elapidae (cobras, corals, mambas, and kraits) and Hydrophiidae (sea snakes) have potent neuromuscular effects. One of the components of cobra venom, α bungarotoxin, has been purified and has been employed extensively in the identification and purification of the nicotinic ACh receptor. It is specific for the neuromuscular nicotinic receptor and causes irreversible block of the ACh receptor at the end-plate.

Presynaptic and Postsynaptic Disorders

Neuromuscular weakness can occur from magnesium intoxication, which may occur in renal failure, eclampsia treated with magnesium, and in the use of magnesium-containing cathartics in patients with neuromuscular disorders. An increase in extracellular magnesium leads to antagonism of calcium entrance into the nerve terminal during the action potential and therefore to a decrease in the release of ACh.

Pharmacology of Neuromuscular Block

Neuromuscular blocking drugs are a valuable adjunct for safe surgical anesthesia.

USES OF NEUROMUSCULAR BLOCKERS

Drugs that block neuromuscular transmission are used most frequently as adjuvants to general anesthetics during surgical procedures. They permit the use of less potent but more desirable anesthetics by providing muscular relaxation with lighter planes of anesthesia, and the ability to use lighter planes of anesthesia as well as less irritating anesthetics makes general anesthesia a safer procedure. It is important to note that the neuromuscular blockers discussed in this chapter do not penetrate the central nervous system. They paralyze without affecting consciousness or the perception of pain. Thus, these drugs used alone do *not* provide adequate anesthesia for surgical manipulations on either humans or animals.

Neuromuscular blocking drugs may be used in electroshock therapy to prevent dislocations and fractures of bones during a convulsion. They are also of use in producing muscle relaxation during mechanical respiration.

Tubocurarine has been used as a provocative diagnostic drug for myasthenia gravis, because patients with myasthenia gravis are extremely sensitive to tubocurarine. It is a hazardous procedure, however, because respiration may be severely depressed by the drug. Quantitation of plasma antibodies to the ACh receptor is now the diagnostic procedure more frequently used for myasthenia gravis.

TYPES OF NEUROMUSCULAR BLOCKING AGENTS
(Table 13–1)

Competitive Neuromuscular Blocking Drugs

Competitive neuromuscular blocking drugs compete with ACh for its receptor, combine with the receptor but have no intrinsic activity.

Table 13–1 COMPARISON OF THE MAJOR PROPERTIES OF COMPETITIVE AND DEPOLARIZING NEUROMUSCULAR BLOCKING DRUGS

Response	Competitive Drugs (Tubocurarine or Pancuronium)	Depolarizing Drugs (Succinylcholine)
Effect on resting potential at end-plate	None	Depolarized
Effect on end-plate potential	Reduction	End-plate is depolarized
Effect on tetanic volley to motor nerve	Fatigue during tetanus; posttetanic antagonism	No change during tetanus; no posttetanic antagonism
Inhibition of AChE	Antagonism of block	Enhanced block
Duration of block	Moderate to long depending on dose	Very short
Effect on muscle membrane away from synaptic region	None	None

Depolarizing Block

Agents that interact with the ACh nicotinic receptor on the end-plate and cause a persistent depolarization of the end-plate membrane produce a blockade of neuromuscular transmission. These agents are classed as *depolarizing blockers.*

Two ways of producing neuromuscular block are to compete with ACh for receptor or to depolarize the end-plate.

Order of Blockade

The onset of neuromuscular block exhibits an order of sensitivity with different muscles: the muscles of the eye are most sensitive, followed by mastication, limb, and abdominal muscles; the respiratory muscles are least sensitive to block. Thus, with careful administration of neuromuscular antagonists it is possible to selectively paralyze specific muscle groups without completely depressing respiration.

TUBOCURARINE CHLORIDE

Competitive Neuromuscular Blockers

Curare is a generic term for a number of South American arrow poisons used by Indians of the Amazon and Orinoco river areas. The alkaloids are obtained from species of *Strychnos* and *Chondodenron.* The cellular locus of action and mechanism of action was determined by Claude Bernard in the 1850s, but the first clinical trials of one specific compound, tubocurarine, were not made until 1942.

Pharmacology

Tubocurarine is an antagonist of ACh at the end-plate, with some overlap at autonomic ganglia at higher dosage levels or in particularly susceptible people. Tubocurarine has no intrinsic activity when combined with the ACh receptor, so ACh cannot gain access to the receptor and the end-plate potential is reduced for each nerve stimulus. If the end-plate potential is reduced sufficiently, an action potential is no longer initiated on the surrounding muscle membrane, and contraction of that muscle fiber no longer occurs. With sufficient concentrations of tubocurarine, contraction of the whole muscle may be blocked. The paralysis is not preceded by an initial muscle fiber contraction; rather the block causes a flaccid paralysis.

Tubocurarine competes with ACh for the nicotinic end-plate receptor.

Any procedure that increases the concentration of ACh in the vicinity of the tubocurarine-occupied receptor will tend to reverse the blockade, because the interaction of ACh and tubocurarine with the receptor is competitive. The concentration of ACh at the receptor can be increased by inhibition of AChE with a drug such as neostigmine. A posttetanic antagonism of a curare block is also observed. During the tetanus, an increase in intracellular calcium occurs, and it takes a period of time after the tetanus for the calcium to enter storage sites. The increased intracellular calcium immediately following a brief tetanus results in an increase in ACh released per nerve impulse if the nerve is stimulated at a low frequency (Fig. 13–2).

Neostigmine can antagonize a competitive neuromuscular block.

Tubocurarine chloride is administered by intravenous (IV) injection. A single injection can cause effective neuromuscular paralysis lasting 25–90 minutes. The single dose is followed by additional doses as needed to maintain adequate neuromuscular relaxation. Residual block with tubocurarine may last 2–4 hours. Smaller and smaller amounts of subsequent doses of tubocurarine are required to maintain a constant level of muscular blockade. The cumulative effect with repeated doses is due to the fact that tubocurarine is redistributed to the tissues, which become saturated with repeated doses, and more remains in the extracellular fluid. Hence, larger

Tubocurarine is distributed throughout the extracellular fluid.

Figure 13–2

Reversal of tubocurarine neuromuscular block by repetitive nerve stimulation (top) and a cholinesterase inhibitor (bottom). The motor nerve was stimulated once every 10 seconds during the beginning of recovery from neuromuscular block with tubocurarine, and the muscle response was recorded with a strain gauge. In the top diagram, the nerve was stimulated with a tetanic volley of 50 Hz for 20 seconds. In the bottom diagram, edrophonium was injected intravenously. Both procedures rapidly antagonize tubocurarine-like block.

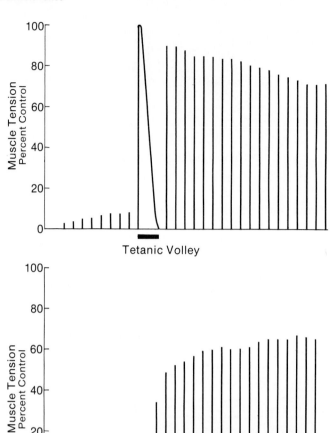

proportions of the dose are present at the receptor compared with the initial dose.

Tubocurarine has two cationic nitrogen moieties in its chemical structure and therefore its distribution is limited to the extracellular fluid. It does not penetrate into the central nervous system and has no central effect. After initial IV administration the drug is redistributed to various tissues. Up to two thirds of the administered dose is excreted in the urine, small amounts are excreted in the bile, and the rest is metabolized. Since renal excretion is the main route of elimination of the drug, patients with renal insufficiency are very sensitive to its action.

Adverse Effects

The major hazard with tubocurarine (and all neuromuscular blocking drugs) is respiratory depression. The drug should not be used without adequate facilities for supporting respiration.

Tubocurarine may cause histamine release and should not be used in patients with severe allergies or patients with a history of asthma because histamine release may cause, in sensitive patients, a severe allergic response or an asthma attack. In addition, circulating histamine may cause a decrease in blood pressure because of the capillary dilation it produces.

The specificity of tubocurarine for receptors at the end-plate is not

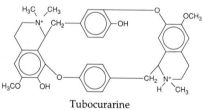

Tubocurarine

Tubocurarine may cause histamine release and hypotension.

absolute, and it can interact with ganglionic nicotinic ACh receptors to cause ganglionic blockade, especially in larger doses. Ganglionic blockade will lead to a decrease in blood pressure. Hypotension during tubocurarine administration may occur through either histamine release or ganglionic blockade.

Reversal of Neuromuscular Block

Recovery from tubocurarine neuromuscular block can be hastened by the administration of a cholinesterase inhibitor such as neostigmine, pyrido-stigmine, or edrophonium. The cholinesterase inhibitors are most effective when given after partial recovery of muscular function has occurred (see Fig. 13–2). Atropine is frequently administered prior to the cholinesterase inhibitors to minimize their muscarinic effects.

METOCURINE IODIDE (METUBINE)

Metocurine is similar in action to tubocurarine but is two to three times as potent. It has a faster onset, but the duration of block is approximately the same as that of tubocurarine. Its major advantage over tubocurarine is that it causes less ganglionic block than does tubocurarine.

GALLAMINE TRIETHIODIDE (FLAXEDIL)

Gallamine is a synthetic curariform drug with the advantage that it does not cause histamine release, bronchospasm, or ganglionic blockade. In doses of more than 0.5 mg/kg, gallamine may cause tachycardia, which reaches a maximum in about 3 minutes and gradually subsides to control rates. Gallamine is excreted by the kidneys.

PANCURONIUM (PAVULON)

Pancuronium is a bis-quaternary steroid with an action similar to that of tubocurarine, with approximately five times the potency. The major advantages of pancuronium are that it has little effect on the circulatory system (although it may cause a slight rise in pulse rate) and it rarely causes histamine release. Pancuronium has replaced tubocurarine in many clinical settings because of these advantages. Its duration of action is roughly similar to that of tubocurarine, and the major route of excretion is by the kidneys.

Pancuronium has, as a side effect, weak anticholinesterase activity and may prolong the action of succinylcholine if it is administered before succinylcholine.

Pancuronium lacks the potential for histamine release and hypotension.

Pancuronium

VERCURONIUM (NORCURON)

Vercuronium is a congener of pancuronium but has less anticholinesterase activity. It is about 33% more potent than tubocurarine, but it has a shorter duration of action than tubocurarine. Like pancuronium, vercuronium causes little circulatory depression. Vercuronium is better tolerated in renal failure; the half-life is 65–75 minutes in normal patients as well as in those in renal failure.

ATRACURIUM (TRACRIUM)

This competitive neuromuscular blocking agent is about one third as potent as pancuronium, but it has an intermediate duration of action. Histamine release is minimal up to a dose of about 0.5 mg/kg. With larger doses, histamine release may occur with a significant decrease in blood pressure, which is usually brief and manageable. Atracurium is spontaneously and enzymatically inactivated and is less dependent on renal excretion than is pancuronium.

Depolarizing Neuromuscular Blocking Agents

MECHANISM OF ACTION

Depolarizing neuromuscular blockers combine with the ACh receptor at the end-plate and act in a manner similar to ACh to cause a conformation change in the receptor and open ion channels. Since depolarizers are not metabolized by AChE, their action at the end-plate continues as long as a sufficient concentration is maintained in the vicinity of the receptor. The prolonged depolarization of the end-plate leads to a rapid block of neuromuscular transmission. The action of these drugs is limited to the receptor at the end-plate, and they do not affect the membrane potential over the muscle membrane.

Prolonged depolarization of the end-plate rapidly blocks transmission.

Since ACh released during a depolarizing block would have the same pharmacological effect, inhibition of AChE does not antagonize the neuromuscular block caused by depolarizing drugs.

CHARACTERISTICS OF DEPOLARIZING BLOCK

Depolarizing agents cause depolarization of the end-plate membrane (Fig. 13-3). The onset of block is frequently accompanied by a fibrillation or fasciculation of muscles. The fibrillation is due to the localized depolarization of the end-plate giving rise to transient fibrillation potentials on individual muscle fibers. The fasciculations are due to repetitive firing of a motor neuron and may be caused by (1) antidromic backfiring of one or more presynaptic nerve terminals and (2) activation of muscle spindles and concomitant reflex activation of a motor neuron due in part to shortening of intrafusal fibers related to an increase of extracellular potassium.

Depolarization block may be initially accompanied by fibrillation or fasciculation of muscle.

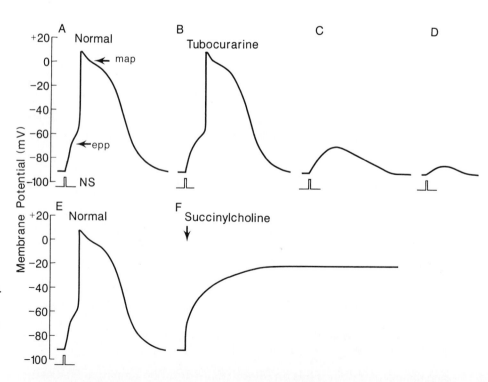

Figure 13-3

Comparison of the effect of tubocurarine and succinylcholine on the intracellular potential recorded from an end-plate of an isolated muscle preparation. In normal muscle (*A* and *E*) the endplate potential (epp) gives rise to a muscle action potential (map). The initial effect of tubocurarine (*B*) is to slow the rate of rise of the epp; the amplitude of the epp is progressively reduced and eventually fails to reach threshold for the initiation of an action potential (*C* and *D*). Note that the resting potential does not change after tubocurarine.

In contrast, the addition of succinylcholine (*F*) results in a prolonged depolarization of the end-plate, even in the absence of any nerve stimulation. (NS and square wave symbols indicate nerve stimulation with single shocks.)

Postoperative muscle pain that may be experienced following the use of succinylcholine is related to the severity of fasciculations during onset of block. Fasciculations can be prevented or minimized by administering a small dose of tubocurarine prior to administering succinylcholine.

Slow skeletal muscle fibers found in nonmammalian species, such as frogs and birds, respond to depolarizing agents with a sustained contracture, and the magnitude of contracture is proportional to the concentration of the drug. One test for depolarizing agents is to observe their effect in chickens. A competitive blocker causes a flaccid paralysis, but a depolarizing drug causes a characteristic contraction of neck and leg muscles drawing the head backward and stiffly extending the legs. (This contracture is a type of muscle shortening associated with graded depolarization of the muscle membrane; it is not, however, associated with repetitive action potentials in either the nerve or the muscle.)

SUCCINYLCHOLINE CHLORIDE (ANECTINE)

Succinylcholine is the only depolarizing blocking agent that is used clinically. Its main advantage is that it has a short duration of action. Succinylcholine may be viewed chemically as two molecules of ACh joined together, and thus it is not surprising that it has some of the actions of ACh.

Succinylcholine has a brief duration of action.

Pharmacology

Succinylcholine combines with the nicotinic receptor at the end-plate and causes the ion channel to open; the resulting ion leakage depolarizes the end-plate membrane.

Initially, this depolarization may be accompanied by fasciculations of the muscle fibers. The fasciculations are transient and followed by neuromuscular block. However, they are significant because postoperative muscle pain seems to be related to the magnitude of the fasciculations, and fasciculations may increase tissue damage in patients with fractures.

In humans the extraocular muscles contain slow fibers that respond with contracture, resulting in a transient increase in intraocular pressure shortly after administration of succinylcholine. Normally this causes no problem, but if the eye is opened prior to succinylcholine the cornea and vitreous humor may be extruded. In addition, in susceptible people acute glaucoma may be induced.

Administration of succinylcholine may cause the extrusion of potassium from tissue, and there may be as much as a 30–50% increase in plasma potassium concentration. This effect is especially marked with prolonged use of succinylcholine or use of this receptor blocker in the presence of extensive soft tissue destruction. The hyperkalemia may result in serious cardiac arrhythmias. An increase in plasma potassium may also antagonize the action of digitalis and cause cardiac failure in susceptible patients.

$$\begin{array}{l} \overset{O}{\overset{\|}{C}}-O-CH_2CH_2-N^+-(CH_3)_3 \\ CH_2 \\ CH_2 \\ \overset{\|}{\underset{O}{C}}-O-CH_2CH_2-N^+-(CH_3)_3 \end{array}$$

Succinylcholine

Metabolism

Succinylcholine is metabolized to succinylmonocholine, and eventually to choline and succinic acid, by plasma cholinesterase. Succinylcholine is not metabolized by AChE. Since cholinesterase inhibitors inhibit the action of both enzymes, the inhibitors will intensify and prolong the action of succinylcholine if given before or during the action of succinylcholine. Therefore, cholinesterase inhibitors are not generally used with succinylcholine.

Succinylcholine is rapidly metabolized by plasma cholinesterase.

One of the major clinical advantages of succinylcholine is its short duration of action, which is a result of its rapid hydrolysis by cholinesterase.

Desensitization

Repeated or large doses of succinylcholine may result in desensitization of the end-plate.

Prolonged administration of succinylcholine or administration of large doses leads to a change in the character of blockade, such that it is no longer a pure depolarizing block, but a type called *desensitization* or *Phase II* block. Characteristics of desensitization are (1) a return of the end-plate membrane potential toward a normal value with a continuation of neuromuscular block, (2) the block is partly reversible with neostigmine, and (3) tetanic stimulation of the nerve is accompanied by fatigue of the response (resembling tubocurarine block). Desensitization is probably due to a change in the conformation of the receptor, such that it exhibits an affinity for succinylcholine, but succinylcholine has no effect on the altered receptor to open ion channels. The onset of desensitization block varies with patients and may vary with muscle groups within one patient, so that some muscles may be desensitized while others are in a depolarizing block (Fig. 13–4).

If recovery of a patient from succinylcholine neuromuscular block is delayed, and there is reason to suspect a desensitization or Phase II block, some anesthesiologists may use neostigmine in an attempt to hasten recovery. The rationale is that if the block is a desensitization blockade, inhibition of AChE may hasten recovery. However, use of neostigmine should be based on the following: (1) a nerve test indicating desensitization block, (2) spontaneous recovery of muscle twitch for at least 20 minutes, reaching a plateau with only slow improvement, and (3) the presence of a mechanism for artificial respiration.

In most clinical situations the mechanism of block with succinylcholine is a depolarizing blockade.

Monitoring Recovery From Neuromuscular Block

Clinical tests can indicate the mechanism of neuromuscular block.

The status of neuromuscular transmission during administration of neuromuscular blocking drugs can be monitored by stimulating a peripheral nerve and recording a muscle response in addition to observing reflexes,

Figure 13–4

Desensitization neuromuscular block. Comparison of the muscle response as a percent of control with the end-plate potential during continuous application of a depolarizing agent, such as succinylcholine. During Phase I, or depolarizing block, the muscle response to nerve stimulation decreases as the end-plate potential is depolarized. During Phase II block, the end-plate potential recovers while the muscle response to nerve stimulation remains blocked. (Also, the Phase II block is partially reversible by a tetanic volley to the nerve or by edrophonium, as shown in Fig. 13–2.)

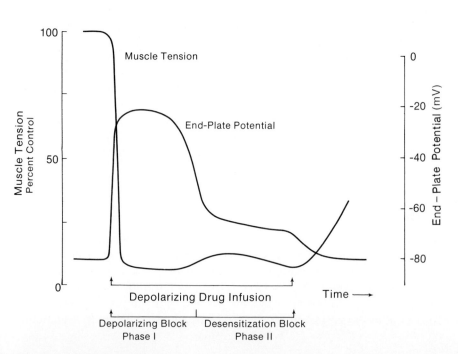

respiration, and gross muscle tension. Tests are often employed when large doses or prolonged administration of depolarizing blockers are necessary, and the possibility of a partial or complete desensitization block is present. The most useful test for determining recovery as well as mechanism of block is the *train-of-four test*. A peripheral nerve, usually the ulnar nerve, is stimulated electrically at the wrist or elbow, and the contraction of a finger (adductor pollicis or flexor digitorum muscle) is measured. The nerve is stimulated at a frequency of 2 Hz for 2 seconds (4 pulses). The volley can be repeated intermittently or periodically every 10–12 seconds. A ratio of the fourth response to the first response is calculated. With competitive drugs, fatigue of the response occurs with successive stimuli and the ratio bears a linear relation to the block of a single twitch. With a depolarizing block by succinylcholine, fatigue of the response does not occur. However, when the succinylcholine block has entered a desensitization phase, fatigue of the response is present (Figs. 13–5 and 13–6). In this way the anesthesiologist can determine when a patient receiving a depolarizing blocker has entered a desensitization or Phase II block. The train-of-four test has the advantage over other nerve-muscle tests because control tests on the unanesthetized patient, frequently uncomfortable, are not necessary.

Genetic-Based Variations in Response

Abnormal Plasma Cholinesterase. A small number of patients have been found to respond to the usual clinical doses of succinylcholine with prolonged neuromuscular blockade and apnea. Analysis of these patients exhibits a familial relationship, and it has been shown that this population had an abnormal gene that gave rise to abnormal plasma cholinesterase. The abnormal cholinesterase is much less effective in hydrolysis of succinylcholine than is normal cholinesterase.

Abnormal responses to succinylcholine

Malignant Hyperthermia. Succinylcholine, halothane, other halogenated inhalational anesthetics, and stress have been associated with an increase in metabolism, muscle rigidity, and rapid increase in body temperature that exceeds 104°F. A familial relationship between these stressors and the appearance of malignant hyperthermia has been shown, and it is believed to be due to a genetic variation found in a very small group of the general population. This condition is a life-threatening emergency and is treated with oxygen, cooling the body, and dantrolene, a drug that blocks calcium

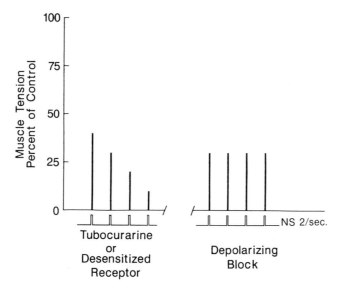

Figure 13–5

Comparison of neuromuscular transmission with repetitive nerve stimulation (2 per second) with tubocurarine and with succinylcholine-induced depolarizing block. Note the rapid increase in the partial block with repeated stimulation in the tubocurarine or desensitized receptor condition.

Figure 13–6

Phases of neuromuscular effects of succinylcholine in one patient. The *upper tracing* depicts the thumb adduction in response to a train of four single shocks applied to the nerve, the train-of-four stimulation. The administration of an intubating dose of succinylcholine (1 mg/kg) resulted in an almost complete paralysis followed by recovery over 8 minutes with nearly complete recovery within another 4 minutes. Note the absence of fade in the response from the first to the fourth twitch.

The *middle tracing* shows single twitches to nerve stimulation every 2 seconds, 2 hours after the top tracing and after a total dose of 10 mg/kg of succinylcholine. Two train-of-four stimulations after additional doses of 40, 20, and 20 mg illustrates the significant fade in the second, third, and fourth responses.

The *lower tracing* presents further recovery with a continuation from the middle tracing with a series of train-of-four stimulations. Note the distinct fade in comparison with equivalent responses in the top tracing; the fourth response is only 37% of the first. The administration of edrophonium results in a rapid increase in twitch height as well as a decrease in the amount of fade. (Adapted and redrawn from Ali HH: Monitoring of neuromuscular function. Semin Anesth 3:284–292, 1984.)

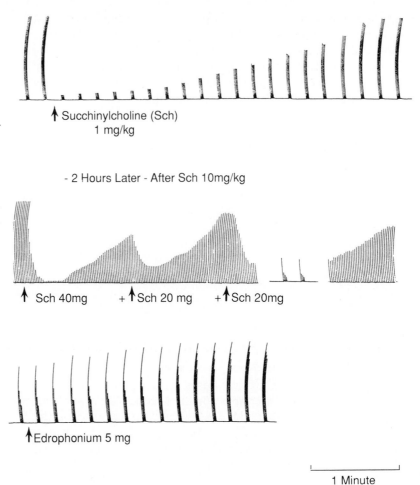

↑ Succinylcholine (Sch)
   1 mg/kg

– 2 Hours Later – After Sch 10mg/kg

↑ Sch 40mg   +↑ Sch 20 mg   +↑ Sch 20mg

↑ Edrophonium 5 mg

|———————————|
    1 Minute

release and reduces muscle rigidity. (Somewhat similar signs and symptoms are observed in the malignant neuroleptic syndrome [Chapter 21] and delirium tremens [Chapter 19].)

Adverse Reactions

As it is with other neuromuscular blocking drugs, depression of respiration is the major hazard with succinylcholine. Occasionally, a bradycardia is observed, especially after a second dose in children. Tachycardia and an occasional arrhythmia may occur. Succinylcholine is never used without a means of supporting respiration mechanically. Postoperative pain may occur, and it is thought to be related to the severity of fasciculations that may appear during onset of neuromuscular block.

Drug Interactions

Some general anesthetics and antibiotics and cholinesterase inhibitors may alter the intensity of neuromuscular blocker action.

WITH COMPETITIVE BLOCKERS

General Anesthetics

With some general anesthetics, such as halothane, enflurane, and methoxyflurane, less tubocurarine is required to produce adequate neuromuscular block.

Antibiotics

A large number of antibiotics may enhance the action of competitive neuromuscular blocking agents. Among the antibiotics are aminoglycosides (streptomycin, neomycin), clinamycin, lincomycin, bacitracin, polymixin B, and colistimethate. These antibiotics have a very weak depressant action on neuromuscular transmission that is not normally observed because there is a large margin of safety in transmission. However, when this safety factor has been reduced by a decrease in number of receptors available to ACh, the effect of these antibiotics may be observed.

Cholinesterase Inhibitors

Cholinesterase inhibitors antagonize the effects of competitive blocking agents. The inhibitors allow ACh to remain in the synaptic region of the receptor for a longer period of time, and the effective ACh concentration is increased, forcing competitive blockers to dissociate from the receptor.

WITH SUCCINYLCHOLINE

Cholinesterase inhibitors prolong the action of succinylcholine. Any other drug that binds to cholinesterase will also prolong its action.

Hexafluorenium is not a neuromuscular blocking drug, but it is a short-acting plasma cholinesterase inhibitor that is occasionally used with succinylcholine to prolong the action of the latter drug. The duration of action of hexafluorenium is 20 – 30 minutes, and it is given at a dose of 2 mg for each 1 mg succinylcholine.

Hexafluorenium Bromide (MYLAXEN)

References

Adams PR: Transmitter action at endplate membrane. *In* Salpeter MM (ed): The Vertebrate Neuromuscular Junction, 317–359. Vol 23 of Neurology and Neurobiology. New York: AR Liss, 1987.

Ali HH: Monitoring of neuromuscular function. Semin Anesthes 3:284–292, 1984.

Ali HH, Utting JE, Gray C: Stimulus frequency in the detection of neuromuscular block in humans. Br J Anaesth 42:967–977, 1970.

Argov Z, Mastaglia FL: Disorders of neuromuscular transmission caused by drugs. New Engl J Med 301:409–413, 1979.

Azar I (ed): Muscle Relaxants: Side Effects and a Rational Approach to Selection. Vol 7 of Clinical Pharmacology. New York: Marcel Dekker, 1987.

Caputy AK, Kim YI, Sanders DB: Neuromuscular block by antibiotics. J Pharmacol Exp Ther 217:369–378, 1981.

Colquhoun D, Dreyer F, Sheridan RE: The actions of tubocurarine at the frog neuromuscular junction. J Physiol (Lond) 293:247–284, 1979.

Cull-Candy SG, Miledi R, Trautmann A, Uchitel OD: 1980. On the release of transmitter at normal, myasthenia gravis, and myasthenic syndrome affected human endplates. J Physiol (Lond) 299:621–638, 1980.

Denborough M: The pathopharmacology of malignant hyperpyrexia. Pharmacol Ther 9:357–365, 1980.

Fambrough D: Control of acetylcholine receptors in skeletal muscle. Physiol Rev 59:165–227, 1979.

Jacobs RS, Burley ES: Nerve terminal facilitatory action of 4-aminopyridine: An analysis of the rising phase of the endplate potential. Neuropharmacology 17:439–444, 1978.

Jenkinson DH: The antagonism between tubocurarine and substances which depolarize the motor end-plate. J Physiol (Lond) 152:309–324, 1960.

Kalow W: Succinylcholine and malignant hyperthermia. Fed Proc 31:1270–1275, 1972.

Lambert JJ, Durant NN, Henderson EG: Drug-induced modification of ionic conductance at the neuromuscular junction. Annu Rev Pharmacol Toxicol 23:505–539, 1983.

Lindstrom J, Dau P: Biology of myasthenia gravis. Annu Rev Pharmacol Toxicol 20:337–362, 1980.

MacLagan J: Competitive neuromuscular blocking drugs. *In* Zaimis E (ed): Neuromuscular Junction, 421–486. Vol 42 of Handbook of Experimental Pharmacology. Berlin: Springer-Verlag, 1976.

Magleby KL: The effect of repetitive stimulation on facilitation of transmitter release at the frog neuromuscular junction. J Physiol (Lond) 234:327–352, 1973.

Simpson LL: Molecular pharmacology of botulinum toxin and tetanus toxin. Annu Rev Pharmacol Toxicol 26:427–453, 1986.

Sokoll MD, Gergis SD: Antibiotics and neuromuscular function. Anesthesiology 55:148–159, 1981.

Speight TM, Avery GS: Pancuronium bromide: A review of its pharmacological properties and clinical application. Drugs 4:163–226, 1972.

Swift TR: Disorders of neuromuscular transmission other than myasthenia gravis. Muscle Nerve 4:334–353, 1981.

Vesell E: Introduction: Genetic and environmental factors affecting drug response in man. Fed Proc 31:1253–1269, 1972.

Viby-Mogensen J: Succinylcholine neuromuscular blockade in subjects heterozygous for abnormal plasma cholinesterase. Anesthesiology 55:231–235, 1981.

Whittaker M: Plasma cholinesterase variants and the anesthetist. Anaesthesia 35:174–197, 1980.

Zaimis E, Head S: Depolarizing neuromuscular blocking drugs. *In* Zaimis E (ed): Neuromuscular Junction, 365–419. Vol 42 of Handbook Experimental Pharmacology. Berlin: Springer-Verlag, 1976.

14

Adrenergic Drugs

Oliver M. Brown

The pharmacology of drugs that have their site of action at cholinergic neuroeffector junctions has been discussed in preceding chapters. This chapter describes drugs that have their primary actions at neuroeffector and synaptic junctions that utilize the other major autonomic neurotransmitter, norepinephrine (NE). Since NE is the transmitter at most postganglionic neuroeffector junctions in the sympathetic nervous system, the agonists at these sites are commonly referred to as *sympathetic, sympathomimetic,* or *adrenergic drugs.*

Selectively acting agents have been discovered that are capable of affecting specific steps involved in the process of adrenergic transmission, analogous to the drugs affecting systems utilizing acetylcholine as the neurotransmitter. Drugs are available that affect the synthesis, the packaging, the release, the interactions with receptors, and the termination of the actions of NE as a neurotransmitter. As is the case for cholinergic drugs, many of the adrenergic drugs have their main site of action at the neurotransmitter receptor either to mimic the action of NE at such receptors (agonists, sympathomimetics) or to impede the access of the neurotransmitters to the receptor binding sites (antagonists, adrenergic blockers).

Since the sympathetic nervous system has an important influence over cardiovascular and respiratory functions, it is obvious that drugs that stimulate or block NE receptors may have profound effects on these two functions. Thus, adrenergic drugs are primarily used to treat several cardiac conditions, blood pressure problems, and asthma. Those drugs that cross the blood-brain barrier will also have effects on the central nervous system (CNS). In addition, the sympathetic nervous system innervates a variety of other organs such as skeletal muscle, intestines, liver, pancreas, and eye.

> Adrenergic drugs act at synapses that use NE as a neurotransmitter.

> Most adrenergic, or sympathetic, drugs either mimic NE or interfere with its action at receptors.

> Adrenergic drugs have important clinical applications in treating conditions of the heart, the eyes, respiration, and blood pressure.

A schematic of the steps involved in the process of chemical transmission involving NE at an autonomic nerve varicosity is shown in Figure 14–1.

Chemical Transmission Involving Norepinephrine

SYNTHESIS OF NOREPINEPHRINE

The synthesis of NE involves a series of biosynthetic steps (Fig. 14–2) that begin with the uptake (active transport) of circulating tyrosine into the nerve varicosity. The rate-limiting step in this series, the hydroxylation of tyrosine to dihydroxyphenylalanine (dopa), is affected by the enzyme tyro-

> The biosynthesis of NE proceeds as follows: tyrosine → dopa → dopamine → NE.

Figure 14-1

Adrenergic neuroeffector transmission.
(NE = norepinephrine; DBH = dopamine-β-
hydroxylase; MAO = monoamine oxidase;
COMT = catechol-O-methyl transferase.)

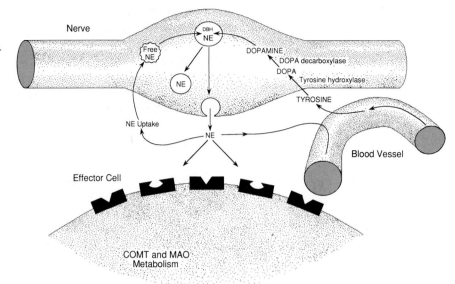

Tyrosine → dopa is the rate-limiting step.

sine hydroxylase. Dopa is then decarboxylated by L-aromatic amino acid decarboxylase to form dopamine. (Note that dopamine is thought to be a neurotransmitter in some parts of the autonomic nervous system.) These two enzymatic conversions take place in the cytoplasm.

The final step in NE synthesis takes place in the synaptic vesicles (sometimes referred to as granules at adrenergic sites). Dopamine is transported into the vesicles, where its hydroxylation to NE is catalyzed by dopamine-β-hydroxylase; thus, there is no synthesis of NE in the cytoplasm. These vesicles not only will take up dopamine but will also package soluble NE that has been taken up by the neuron (see below). The NE packaged in these vesicles (granules) is complexed with adenosine triphosphate (ATP), calcium, and a protein, chromogranin A.

In the adrenal medulla and in other chromaffin cells, there is a further conversion of much of the NE to epinephrine (adrenaline) by the enzyme

Dopamine → NE takes place within synaptic vesicles (granules).

Synaptic vesicles will also take up soluble NE from the cytoplasm.

In chromaffin cells (e.g., adrenal medulla) NE is further methylated to EPI.

tyrosine

DOPA

dopamine

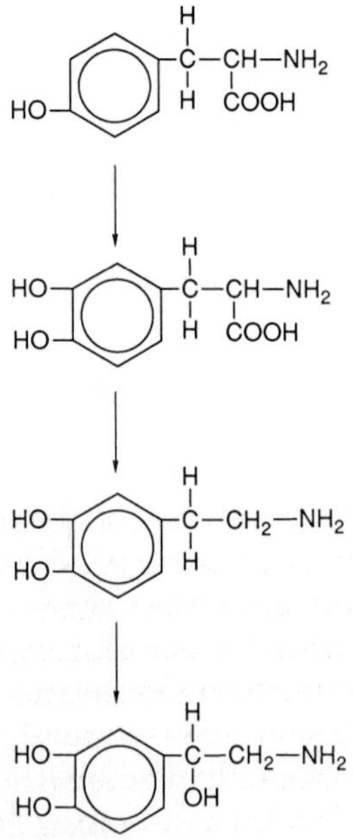

Figure 14-2

Biosynthetic steps leading to the synthesis of NE.

norepinephrine

phenylethanolamine-N-methyltransferase (PNMT). In this case, the newly synthesized NE leaves the vesicles and is methylated to epinephrine in the cytoplasm by PNMT. The epinephrine (EPI) is taken up by a different set of vesicles (chromaffin granules), where it is stored for release. The adrenal chromaffin granules contain EPI and NE in a 4:1 ratio, complexed with ATP, calcium, and chromogranin A.

Note the distinction that NE is primarily a neurotransmitter; i.e., it is released into a synaptic cleft for interaction at the immediately adjacent postjunctional effector cell. In contrast, EPI is primarily a neurohormone; i.e., it is secreted into the blood stream by the adrenal medulla and interacts with effector sites throughout the body.

> NE is primarily a neurotransmitter; EPI is primarily a neurohormone.

RELEASE OF NOREPINEPHRINE

With the arrival of an action potential at nerve varicosities, there are a influx of calcium ions and fusion of synaptic vesicles with the presynaptic plasmalemma, followed by an exocytosis of the vesicle contents into the synaptic cleft (see Fig. 14–1). This exocytosis releases not only the neurotransmitter, NE, but also the other contents of the vesicle, including ATP and dopamine-β-hydroxylase. Once in the synaptic cleft, the released NE is free to diffuse, and it may

> NE is released from nerve varicosity by action potential and influx of calcium.

1. interact with receptors on the postjunctional membrane;
2. interact with receptors on the prejunctional membrane;
3. diffuse out of the cleft and be lost to the circulation;
4. be taken back up through the prejunctional membrane;
5. be taken up through the postjunctional membrane.

> Released NE diffuses and may interact with receptors, be taken up by cells, or continue to diffuse.

Of these possibilities, only number 1 fulfills the neurotransmitter function of the released NE; i.e., NE's interaction with specific synaptic receptors resulting in depolarization of the postsynaptic (effector) cell membrane constitutes successful transmission of the signal from the nerve.

> Nerve signal is successfully transmitted when NE interacts with a receptor on a postsynaptic cell.

Possibility number 2 represents an autoinhibitory control mechanism: stimulation of presynaptic receptors by NE inhibits further release of NE. The remaining three (nos. 3–5) of the possible fates for released NE represent mechanisms for terminating neurotransmission.

> Presynaptic receptors serve a regulatory function.

NOREPINEPHRINE-RECEPTOR INTERACTION

Activation of specific postjunctional adrenergic receptors by NE or other adrenergic agonists causes biochemical and physiological responses that involve "second-messenger" transduction mechanisms (see later in this chapter and Chapter 15). These mechanisms generally either increase available cytosolic calcium concentration, which results in smooth muscle contraction, or decrease available calcium, which results in relaxation of smooth muscle.

> NE interaction with postjunctional receptors triggers various cell responses, mediated by "second messengers."

Both subtypes of β-adrenergic receptors (β_1 and β_2) (see Receptor Types in the Sympathetic System, later in this chapter) are coupled through a G protein (guanine nucleotide–binding regulatory protein) to the enzyme adenylate cyclase. Activation of these receptors by NE or other agonists stimulates this enzyme, which increases cellular concentrations of the second messenger, cyclic adenosine monophosphate (cAMP). This increase in cAMP amplifies the receptor signal by activating a protein kinase, which in turn phosphorylates a variety of intracellular enzymes. The activity of the phosphorylated enzymes is thought to be responsible for all the responses to β-adrenergic receptor activation, including excitatory effects

> Activation of β-adrenergic receptors increases cellular cAMP.

on the heart, increased metabolic activity, and relaxation of smooth muscle of bronchi and some blood vessels.

In contrast, another adrenergic receptor type, α_2 (see Receptor Types in the Sympathetic System, later in this chapter), is coupled to adenylate cyclase through an inhibitory G protein. Thus, activation of α_2 receptors results in a decrease in the second messenger, cAMP.

Activation of α-adrenergic receptors either decreases cAMP (α_2) or increases the hydrolysis of phosphatidylinositol (α_1).

A different second messenger is involved in the activation of yet another adrenergic receptor type, the α_1 receptor (see Receptor Types in the Sympathetic System). Alpha$_1$ receptors are coupled (through another G protein) to a system that hydrolyzes phosphatidylinositol. The products of phosphatidylinositol breakdown serve as second messengers by releasing intracellular calcium stores. This initiates the phosphorylation of a number of regulatory enzymes, which are responsible for the cell response to α_1 activation.

Chronic exposure to agonists can decrease the number of receptors, and chronic exposure to antagonists can increase the number of receptors.

Chronic treatment with adrenergic agonists can result in a decrease in the number of neurotransmitter receptors (down-regulation). Conversely, the adaptive response to chronic treatment with antagonists is an increase in the number of receptors (up-regulation). For example, treatment with an antagonist such as the β blocker propranolol (discussed later in this chapter) may result in an adaptive increase in adrenergic receptors in a fashion analogous to the phenomenon of denervation supersensitivity. If the chronic treatment with such an antagonist is terminated (and especially if it is rapidly eliminated), activation of the now-increased number of receptors will result in an exaggerated effector cell stimulation. In the case of propranolol, this could cause life-threatening cardiac arrhythmias. As a general principle, agents that stimulate or inhibit the autonomic or central nervous system should be withdrawn from chronic use gradually in a stepwise fashion. The gradual reduction in dose and frequency of administration avoids the potentially dangerous expression of adaptive changes in the receptor systems that have occurred.

Chronic treatment with propranolol can result in an up-regulation of β-adrenergic receptors.

Rapid withdrawal from chronic treatment with propranolol can cause dangerous tachyarrhythmias.

Drugs that act on the nervous system are best withdrawn gradually.

TERMINATION OF NOREPINEPHRINE TRANSMISSION

Several mechanisms contribute to the termination of the synaptic transmission that had been initiated with the release of NE (Fig. 14–3). As with all neurotransmitters, diffusion out of the cleft away from the synapse

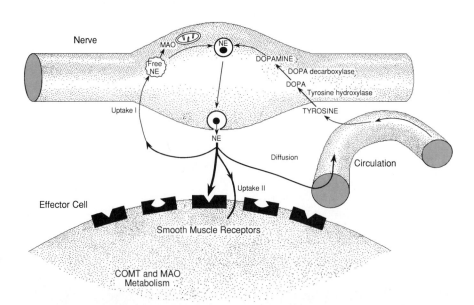

Figure 14–3

Adrenergic neuroeffector transmission; the termination of NE neurotransmission. (MAO = monoamine oxidase; COMT = catechol-O-methyl transferase.)

contributes to terminating the effects of NE. However, the main mechanism by which the effect of NE is rapidly terminated is the specific uptake of NE into the presynaptic varicosity (often referred to as reuptake or Uptake I). The NE that has been taken back up by the nerve forms the cytoplasmic pool of NE; much of this soluble NE is recycled by packaging in synaptic vesicles.

The main mechanism for terminating the action of NE is reuptake by the neuron (Uptake I).

Other tissues also take up NE and related compounds by a less specific, higher-capacity uptake mechanism, Uptake II. Most metabolism of NE and other catecholamines takes place in nonneural cells following uptake by Uptake II.

Uptake II by nonneural cells results in metabolism of NE and other catecholamines.

METABOLISM OF NOREPINEPHRINE

The catecholamines (NE, EPI, dopamine, and some synthetic analogs) are taken up (Uptake II) by many tissues of the body, metabolized, and excreted primarily as sulfated conjugates (Fig. 14–4). The mitochondria of most cells, including nerve cells, contain the catecholamine-metabolizing enzyme monoamine oxidase (MAO). The other major catecholamine-metabolizing enzyme, catechol-O-methyl transferase (COMT), is found primarily in the cytoplasm of nonneural cells (especially the liver). Other enzymes (aldehyde dehydrogenases and aldehyde reductases) occur to various extents in different organs and contribute to the formation of the final metabolic products of catecholamines. Unlike acetylcholine neurotransmission wherein enzymatic action (by acetylcholinesterase) plays the major role in ending transmission, enzymatic metabolism of NE plays no role in terminating neurotransmission. This fact is emphasized by noting that inhibitors of MAO and COMT have no effect on transmission at NE junctions, whereas inhibitors of reuptake (Uptake I), such as cocaine, potentiate the effects of NE.

MAO and COMT are the main catecholamine-metabolizing enzymes.

Enzymatic metabolism of NE plays no role in terminating neurotransmission.

The major metabolites of NE found in human plasma and urine are MHPG (3-methoxy-4-hydroxy-phenyl[ethylene]glycol, free and conjugated), VMA (vanillylmandelic acid), and NMN (normetanephrine, free and conjugated) (see Fig. 14–4). The same, or analogous, deaminated

Major NE metabolites are free and conjugated MHPG, VMA, and NMN.

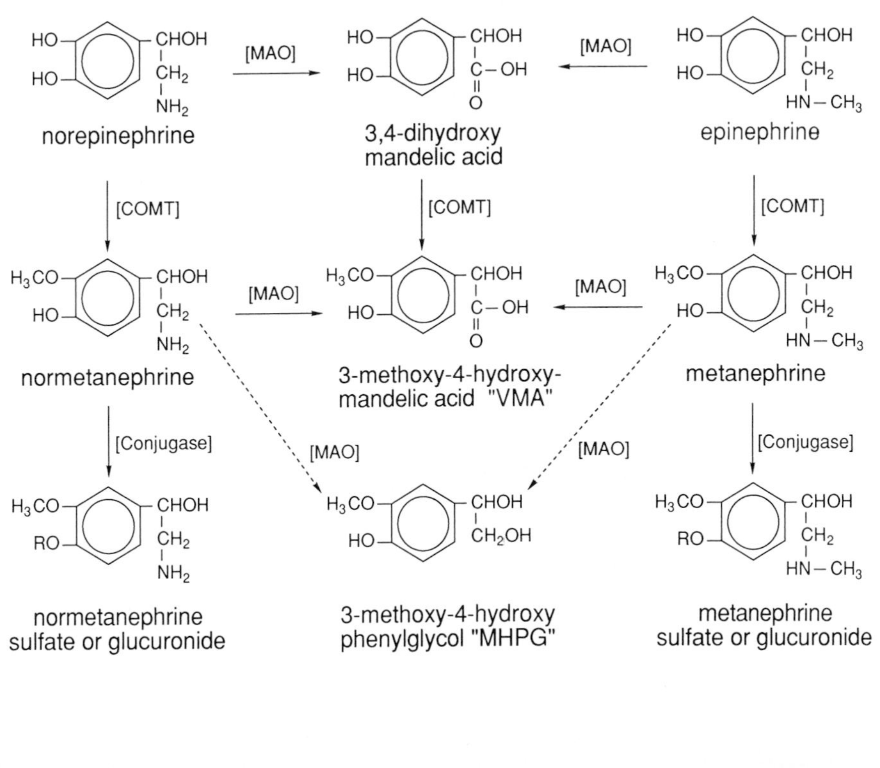

Figure 14–4

Metabolism of NE.

and methoxylated metabolites are formed from the other catecholamines.

MODIFICATION OF NOREPINEPHRINE NEUROTRANSMISSION BY DRUGS

Drugs may interact with each of the steps involved in the process of NE chemical transmission as follows:

1. Some drugs inhibit the synthesis or the packaging of NE.
2. Drugs may either block or enhance the release of NE.
3. The interaction of NE with the postsynaptic receptor may be either blocked or mimicked by drugs.
4. Some drugs prevent the termination of NE's action.

Each of the previously discussed steps in the process of NE chemical transmission can be modified by drugs, resulting in either a potentiation or an inhibition of activity at NE synapses. Some examples of drug modification are

1. Synthesis of NE is blocked by inhibiting tyrosine hydroxylase with methyltyrosine, thus inhibiting NE synaptic transmission.
2. Vesicle uptake of dopamine and NE is prevented by reserpine, depleting the nerve of transmitter and inhibiting transmission.
3. Release of NE from the nerve varicosity is enhanced by amphetamine (potentiating) and prevented by bretylium (inhibiting).
4. Receptor interaction with NE is blocked by antagonists like propranolol (inhibiting) and mimicked by agonists like isoproterenol (ISO) (potentiating).
5. Termination of NE as a transmitter by Uptake I is blocked by cocaine, thus potentiating neurotransmission.

The site of action for most adrenergic drugs in clinical use is the receptor.

Drugs are described that act through one or more of these mechanisms; however, most adrenergic drugs in clinical use exert their effects by interacting directly with adrenergic receptors.

Receptor Types in the Sympathetic System

EPI (adrenaline) stimulates some smooth muscles and inhibits others.

It has been known for nearly 100 years that the effects of an injection of EPI (adrenaline), isolated originally from adrenal glands, are similar to the effects of stimulating the sympathetic nerves. There was, however, a mystery: why did adrenaline stimulate some smooth muscles and inhibit others? As an explanation, and to explain the differences in relative activity among analogs of EPI, Ahlquist proposed in 1948 that there are two major types of adrenergic receptors:

Alpha (α) receptors—associated with most of the excitatory effects such as vasoconstriction and contraction of the uterus and spleen.
Beta (β) receptors—associated with most of the inhibitory effects such as vasodilation and relaxation of respiratory smooth muscle.

Table 14-1 RECEPTOR TYPES IN THE SYMPATHETIC (ADRENERGIC) SYSTEM

Receptor Type	Prominent Effector Organs	Response to Receptor Activation
β_1	Heart	Increased heart rate Increased force of contraction
β_2	Arterioles (and arteries in skeletal muscle)	Dilation
	Bronchial and uterine smooth muscle	Relaxation
	Several sites	Metabolic effects
α_1	Arterioles in skin, mucosa, viscera, and kidney (resistance vessels)	Constriction
	Veins	Constriction
	Uterus	Contraction
α_2	Presynaptic nerve endings	Inhibit NE release
	Postsynaptic in CNS	Decreased sympathetic tone
Dopamine	Arterioles in kidney, brain, and mesentery	Dilation

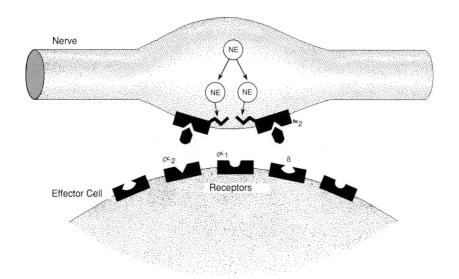

Figure 14-5

Location of α receptors; sites of NE actions.

Ahlquist also noted two important exceptions to this characterization. Namely, some α receptors mediate relaxation of gastrointestinal (GI) smooth muscle, and some β receptors mediate increases in the force and rate of contractions of the heart.

The modern view of adrenergic receptors is still based upon Ahlquist's original description, but receptor subtypes can now be defined in greater detail. A knowledge of the locations and characteristic responses of the adrenergic receptor subtypes allows one to summarize and to predict the effects of various adrenergic drugs. A classification of adrenergic receptors and their responses to activation is described here and outlined in Table 14-1.

> EPI's actions are mediated through two major types of receptors: α—associated with most excitatory effects; and β—associated with most inhibitory effects.

> Exceptions to the previous rule: α—relaxation of GI muscle; and β—stimulation of heart.

> Adrenergic drug effects can be predicted by knowing receptor locations and characteristics.

ALPHA RECEPTORS

Alpha$_1$ receptors were the originally defined "excitatory" α receptors that mediate *constriction or contraction* of smooth muscle in a number of locations including

1. *Arterioles* in skin, mucosa, viscera, and kidneys. These arterioles are numerous and small, and thus account for a large proportion of peripheral resistance.
2. *Veins* throughout the body.
3. *Uterus, spleen, male sex organ,* and *radial muscle of the iris.*

Alpha$_2$ receptors are a more recently described subtype of α receptors that are primarily located on prejunctional membranes, where they serve to regulate the release of NE (Fig. 14-5). Activation of these prejunctional receptors inhibits further release of the transmitter. Alpha$_2$ receptors can also be found postsynaptically in the CNS (see later in this chapter) and in some peripheral sites. Alpha$_2$ receptors are responsible for relaxation of GI smooth muscle, the exception to the excitatory rule for α receptors.

> Alpha$_1$ receptors mediate contractions of smooth muscle in several locations, especially blood vessels.

> Presynaptic α_2 receptors regulate NE release.

BETA RECEPTORS

Beta$_2$ receptors are the *inhibitory* β receptors that mediate *relaxation* of smooth muscle in various locations

1. Arterioles in skeletal muscle and liver (and to some degree, in various other locations).

> Beta$_2$ receptors mediate relaxation of smooth muscle in arterioles, veins, bronchi, and uterus.

2. Many veins throughout the body.
3. Bronchial muscle and uterus.

Beta$_1$ receptors are a very important exception to the generalization that β receptor activation is inhibitory to the end-organ; β_1 receptor activation results in an increase in heart rate (positive chronotropic effect) and an increase in the force of contraction of the heart (positive inotropic effect).

Beta$_1$ receptor activation increases heart rate and force of contraction (positive chronotropy and inotropy).

In addition to having activity in smooth and cardiac muscle, β receptors also subserve several metabolic effects by increasing cellular cAMP levels. For example, by interacting with β_2 receptors EPI stimulates the conversion of liver glycogen to glucose, glycogenolysis (thus elevating blood sugar, hyperglycemia). Similarly, EPI activates β_1 receptors in adipose tissue to stimulate the breakdown of triglycerides to free fatty acids, lipolysis (elevating blood fatty acids, hyperlipidemia).

Beta receptors control several metabolic functions.

Although not truly an adrenergic receptor, a receptor for another catecholamine, dopamine, is included here. There is evidence that dopamine may serve as a neurotransmitter in certain arterioles of the kidney and mesentery. Activation of dopamine receptors found in both areas results in dilation of these vessels.

Dopamine dilates arterioles in the kidney and mesentery and may be a transmitter at these sites.

As described earlier, activation of prejunctional α_2 receptors results in a feedback inhibition of further NE release, a presynaptic "autoreceptor" control mechanism. Evidence has accumulated to support an additional autonomic control mechanism: presynaptic "heteroreceptor" regulation (Fig. 14–6). In heteroreceptor regulation, prejunctional muscarinic acetylcholine receptors serve to inhibit release of NE from sympathetic varicosities, and prejunctional α-adrenergic receptors inhibit release of acetylcholine from parasympathetic varicosities. A fine control over most organ functions results from concurrent activity of both the sympathetic and parasympathetic systems. Mechanisms such as these may contribute to this autonomic control. For example, it is proposed that adrenergic drugs (or sympathetic stimulation) decrease GI activity by activating prejunctional α heteroreceptors and inhibiting acetylcholine release. (Note that the functionally dominant innervation of the gut is normally parasympathetic.)

Presynaptic "autoreceptors" control NE release.

Presynaptic "heteroreceptors" allow for subtle interactions between the sympathetic and parasympathetic systems.

Important factors that help determine the response of an organ to adrenergic drugs are the relative proportion and density of α and β recep-

Figure 14–6

Autoreceptor and heteroreceptor regulation.

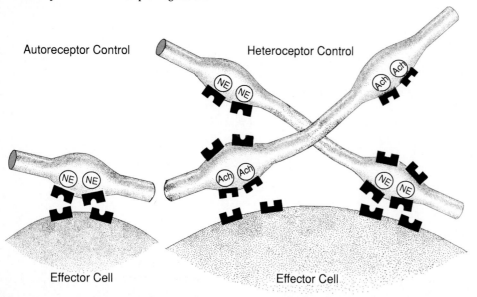

Blood Vessels in Skeletal Muscle

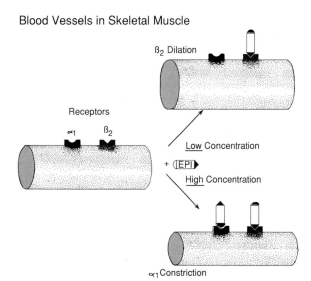

Figure 14–7

Differential receptor-related effects of low and high concentrations of epinephrine (EPI) on blood vessels in skeletal muscle.

tors in the tissue. Furthermore, receptors have different sensitivities to NE and EPI and other adrenergic drugs: NE and EPI have similar potencies at α_1 and α_2 and β_1 receptors, but EPI is much more potent than NE at β_2 receptors. The heart is generally considered to have predominantly β_1 receptors, and most blood vessels to have predominantly α_1 receptors; drug effects on these sites should, therefore, be quite predictable.

The vascular beds in skeletal muscle, on the other hand, are plentiful in both β_2 and α_1 receptors; accordingly, an agent such as EPI with activity at both receptor types is capable of producing *both* dilation *and* constriction of these vessels (Fig. 14–7). Note that the threshold of sensitivity to EPI is lower for the β_2 receptors than for the α_1 receptors. Lower (physiological) concentrations of EPI cause (β_2-mediated) vasodilation (which facilitates increased skeletal muscle perfusion during the "fight or flight" response). Only at very high concentrations of EPI (above that found *in vivo*) do the constricting effects of α_1 receptor activation become evident. This constricting effect will predominate at high levels of EPI, which can usually be produced only in a laboratory under experimental conditions.

The differences in receptor *specificity* and *sensitivity* to various adrenergic drugs can be explored by examining the chemical structures of several of the drugs in a systematic way (a structure-activity relationship [SAR] study). A number of such studies have concluded that the addition of alkyl groups to the amine substituent of catecholamines increases β activity and decreases α activity. Consider the three compounds NE, EPI, and isoproterenol (ISO), with identical catecholamine backbones (Table 14–2).

SPECIFICITY

Not only does the chemical structure of adrenergic drugs correlate with their specificity at receptor sites but structure also determines their potency at those receptors. Table 14–3 indicates the relative potencies for several of the characteristic adrenergic drugs at the α and β receptor types described earlier. For example, at β_1 receptors, ISO is more potent than EPI, which is equal to or more potent than NE, which is more potent than dopamine.

Certain drugs that have activity on the sympathetic system do so at least in part by causing the release of NE from the prejunctional membrane. Drugs that work by releasing NE are referred to as having *indirect* activity, as contrasted with those that have *direct* activity on the adrenergic receptor.

Organ responses to drugs depend largely on distribution and sensitivity of receptors.

The heart has predominantly β_1 receptors, and most blood vessels have α_1.

Skeletal muscle vascular beds have both β_2 and α_1 receptors. Low levels of EPI produce vasodilation (β_2), and very high levels produce vasoconstriction (α_1).

Chemical structure determines whether a drug will have activity at α or β receptors.

Beta specificity is increased with alkyl substitution to the amine group.

Chemical structure determines the potency of drugs at adrenergic receptors.

Direct-acting drugs have activity at the adrenergic receptor; *indirect*-acting drugs cause the release of NE.

Table 14–2 STRUCTURE-ACTIVITY RELATIONSHIP OF NOREPINEPHRINE, EPINEPHRINE, AND ISOPROTERENOL

Adrenergic Agent	Structure	Receptor Selectivity	Activity at Receptor
Norepinephrine		α	Norepinephrine (with no alkyl groups on the amine) is the most α-specific of the three compounds, with activity at α_1, α_2, and β_1 receptors; it has almost no activity at β_2 sites.
Epinephrine		$\alpha + \beta$	Epinephrine (with the addition of one methyl group on the amine) is active at all α and β receptors; the addition of the methyl group has imparted β_2 activity to this compound.
Isoproterenol		β	Isoproterenol (with the addition of an isopropyl group on the amine) is active at β_1 and β_2 receptors, with almost no activity at α sites. This most "alkyl" of the three drugs has lost all its ability to bind to α receptors.

Modified from Day M: Autonomic Pharmacology, 130. New York; Churchill Livingstone, 1979.

Hydroxyl group addition to drug structure increases direct-acting properties.

Obviously, the receptor specificity profile of indirect-acting drugs would be similar to that of NE, since it is NE that is actually stimulating the receptor. The structural features that determine the direct-acting or indirect-acting properties are the alkyl hydroxyl group and the phenyl hydroxyl group meta to the alkyl substituent (the hydroxyls shown in color on the structure of NE, shown in Table 14–4). Tyramine is a weak agonist that owes all its activity to the release of NE. The addition of one hydroxyl group (to the tyramine structure) gives rise to the partial direct-acting properties of phenylpropanolamine and of dopamine, and the addition of both hydroxyl groups results in the purely direct-acting NE.

Tyramine administration causes NE release and can produce tachyphylaxis.

The indirect-acting drugs, such as tyramine (and amphetamine and ephedrine), cause a calcium-independent release of NE that does not involve exocytosis. Facts that support this mechanism are that tyramine-induced NE release is not accompanied by the release of dopamine-β-hydroxylase (which is in the vesicles), and tachyphylaxis is observed with repeated administrations of tyramine. (*Tachyphylaxis* is the term used to describe tolerance acquired with a very short onset; tachyphylaxis is manifested by the rapid loss of effectiveness of a given dose of drug with its repeated administration.) Thus, the increase in blood pressure that results from an injection of tyramine fails to occur after the injection is repeated several times every 10–30 minutes. The soluble pool of NE that is displaced by tyramine is quite small and is rapidly depleted.

Table 14–3 AGONIST POTENCIES AT ADRENERGIC RECEPTORS

Receptor	Potency*
β_1	$ISO > EPI \geq NE > DA$
β_2	$ISO > EPI \gg NE \gg DA$
α_1	$EPI \geq NE > DA \gg ISO$
α_2	$CLO > EPI \geq NE \gg ISO$

* ISO = isoproterenol, EPI = epinephrine, NE = norepinephrine, DA = dopamine, CLO = clonidine.

Table 14-4 INDIRECT VERSUS DIRECT STRUCTURES

Adrenergic Agonist	Structure	Type of Activity
Tyramine	HO—⬡—CH₂–CH₂–NH₂	Indirect
Phenylpropanolamine (PPA)	⬡—CH–CH₂–NH₂ (OH CH₃)	Mixed, indirect, and direct
Dopamine	HO—(HO)⬡—CH₂–CH₂–NH₂	Mixed, indirect, and direct
Norepinephrine	HO—(HO)⬡—CH–CH₂–NH₂ (OH)	Direct

Modified from Day M: Autonomic Pharmacology, 129. New York; Churchill Livingstone, 1979.

Drugs that activate adrenergic receptors have important effects on the cardiovascular system. The cardiovascular changes that result are complicated by the activity of compensatory baroreceptor reflexes. These reflex responses may, in fact, be used to therapeutic advantage. For example, cases of paroxysmal atrial tachycardia may be converted with the α agonist phenylephrine. Phenylephrine stimulates vascular α_1 receptors, causing an increase in arterial blood pressure. This pressure increase elicits a baroreceptor-mediated reflex increase in vagal tone, which results in a slowing of the heart rate.

Cardiovascular Effects of Adrenergic Receptor Activation

Adrenergic drug actions may be complicated by cardiovascular reflex responses.

Figure 14-8

Results from an experimental study on the dog. (MAP = mean arterial pressure; HR = heart rate; TPR = total peripheral resistance.)

A, The potent α_1 agonist activity of NE constricts most blood vessels, increasing peripheral resistance, which results in an increase in MAP. Beta₁-receptor activation by NE causes positive chronotropy (increased HR) and positive inotropy (not shown). EPI activates β_1 receptors, increasing HR. EPI also is a potent α_1 agonist and raises MAP when given in a large dose, but note that the effect is biphasic—as the blood level of EPI declines, EPI stimulation of β_2 receptors to dilate skeletal muscle vascular beds can be seen (this effect was present throughout but was masked by α_1 vasoconstriction; see B). ISO has β_1 and β_2 activity: HR is elevated from β_1 activation, MAP is decreased from β_2-mediated dilation of vascular beds in skeletal muscle.

B, After pretreatment with an α antagonist, the responses to the same drugs were determined. All α_1-mediated vasoconstriction (increased MAP) has been prevented. The β_1 dilation of skeletal muscle vessels by EPI is now clearly revealed. Beta₁ effects on HR are not changed by α blockade.

C, After pretreatment with a β antagonist only the α-mediated vasoconstriction (increased MAP) of NE and EPI is seen.

D, Pretreatment with a combination of an α antagonist and a β antagonist blocks the actions of all three drugs.

(From Carrier O Jr: Pharmacology of the Peripheral Autonomic Nervous System, 97. Chicago: Year Book Medical, 1972.)

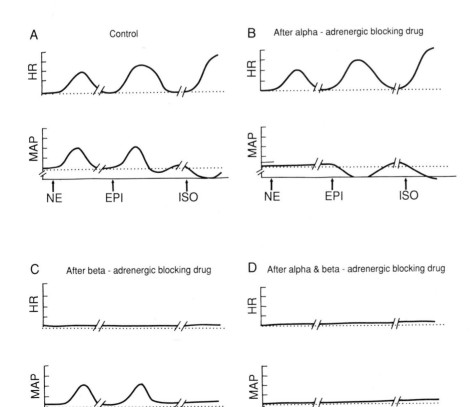

A Control

B After alpha - adrenergic blocking drug

C After beta - adrenergic blocking drug

D After alpha & beta - adrenergic blocking drug

NE EPI ISO

Time

5 Min

Figure 14-9

NE causes a dramatic α-mediated increase in TPR and BP. The β_1 effect of NE would be expected to produce an increase in HR, yet a decrease in HR is seen here. This results from baroreceptors responding to the increased BP and reflexly increasing the discharge of vagal nerves to the heart. The baroreceptor reflex effect (mediated through the vagus nerves) to lower HR overrides the direct β_1 receptor effect to raise the HR.

EPI causes a redistribution of blood flow (an effect consistent with the fight-or-flight generalization); α_1 activation results in vasoconstriction in many areas, and concurrent β_2 activation dilates vessels in the skeletal muscles. The algebraic sum of these simultaneous effects in the individual studied is a net lowering of TPR (this will vary among individuals depending on relative muscle mass and other factors). Although TPR dropped in this case, there was no decrease in BP; BP was maintained by the increase in HR and in pulse pressure (positive inotropy), both resulting from β_1 activation by EPI.

ISO increases HR by β_1 activation and lowers TPR by β_2 activation; net decreases in BP are small, as these two effects tend to oppose one another.

(Modified from Allwood MJ, Cobbold AF, Ginsburg J: Peripheral vascular effects of noradrenaline, isopropylnoradrenaline, and dopamine. Br Med Bull 19:132–136, 1963.)

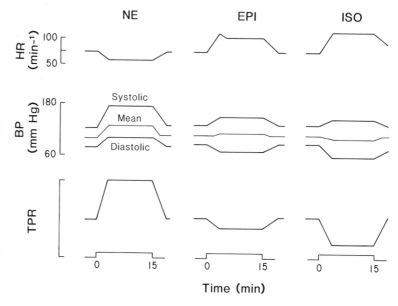

Effects of adrenergic receptor activation without baroreceptor reflexes may be examined in a laboratory preparation with the vagus nerves sectioned.

Thus, knowing the α and β receptor activities of a given drug is not sufficient to completely predict the outcome of administering the drug; baroreceptor reflexes must always be considered. However, the cardiovascular profiles of α and β receptor activation can be examined without complication by reflexes in certain laboratory preparations. Figure 14-8 presents experimental results from an anesthetized dog with the cervical vagus nerves cut (afferent and efferent) to eliminate baroreceptor reflex activity. Heart rate (HR) and mean arterial pressure (MAP) were monitored, and the dog was given intravenous (IV) injections of NE, EPI, and ISO.

In contrast, when the drugs are given in the presence of intact reflexes the resultant actions may be quite different. The responses seen in this laboratory preparation are somewhat modified by reflex action when the same drugs are administered to an intact animal. Figure 14-9 shows the heart rate (HR), blood pressure (BP), and total peripheral resistance (TPR) for a human who received IV infusions of NE, EPI, and ISO.

The baroreceptor reflex response overrides the direct effect of NE on heart rate response.

Adrenergic Agents and Their Therapeutic Uses

The three endogenous catecholamines, NE, EPI, and dopamine, activate adrenergic receptors in varying degrees (see Table 14-3). In addition to these agents, there are numerous synthetic agents that also have adrenergic agonist properties.

Many adrenergic drugs have similar properties, and clinicians may vary in their choice of drug in a given situation. For these reasons, only the model drugs used for a given therapeutic application are discussed. A more comprehensive listing of adrenergic drugs and their receptor specificities appears in Table 14-6 at the end of this chapter.

Alpha$_1$ activation causes vasoconstriction.

Beta$_1$ activation stimulates the heart.

Beta$_2$ stimulation relaxes bronchial smooth muscle.

Adrenergic agonists that mimic NE at α_1 receptors cause vasoconstriction. This property is useful in many situations in which control of blood flow is required. The agents with β_1 activity have some application in stimulating the heart. Bronchial smooth muscle is relaxed with β_2 stimulation, making drugs with this property valuable in treating asthma.

ALPHA AGONISTS

Alpha₁ Agents — Vasoconstriction

Control Hemorrhage. An agent with α_1 agonist properties, often *epineph-rine* (ADRENALIN), is used to constrict vessels in the area of superficial sur-gery. This application controls capillary bleeding and is especially useful in tooth extractions. (*Caution:* Alpha agonists should *not* be used to control bleeding in anything other than superficial surgery; deep bleeding could recur after surgical closure and drug absorption.)

Alpha₁ agonists constrict vessels to decrease local bleeding.

Contain Local Anesthetic. Alpha₁ agonists (again, usually *epinephrine*) are sometimes injected along with local anesthetics to cause localized vasocon-striction. The decreased blood flow in the area slows the absorption of the anesthetic and localizes the effect of the anesthetic. This gives more effec-tive anesthesia in the area of surgery, and it minimizes systemic toxicity from the anesthetic. (*Caution:* Special care must be taken to avoid injection into a vessel; a bolus of epinephrine could be life-threatening.)

Alpha₁ agonists constrict vessels, which prevents the spread of local anesthetics.

Nasal Decongestant. Alpha agonists are applied locally or taken orally to constrict the swollen vessels in edematous tissue in order to relieve the symptoms of mucosal congestion in the common cold, hay fever, and other allergic rhinitis. Both indirect-acting agents (which act by causing NE re-lease), such as *phenylpropanolamine,* and direct-acting agents, such as *phenylephrine* (NEOSYNEPHRINE), are used in many over-the-counter nasal decongestant products. (*Caution:* Repeated application of these agents often results in a "rebound" after-congestion that is possibly more severe than the original rhinitis.)

Alpha₁-mediated constriction of swollen vessels relieves nasal congestion.

Allergic Shock (Anaphylaxis). *Epinephrine* is the drug of choice in treating the medical emergency of anaphylactic shock. The α_1 properties of epi-nephrine will relieve the swelling of edematous mucosa, glottis, and facial tissue. In addition, the β_2 activity of epinephrine will relax the constricted bronchial smooth muscles. Both receptor-activating properties of epineph-rine contribute to reversing the life-threatening respiratory crisis of allergic shock. (*Caution:* Epinephrine is also a potent β_1 agonist; care must be used to avoid excessive cardiac stimulation.)

EPI is the drug of choice in treating anaphylactic shock; α_1 activity relieves swelling, and β_2 activity relaxes bronchioles.

Hypotension. In some hypotensive situations (e.g., during spinal anesthe-sia, following pheochromocytoma surgery, and in certain cases of shock), α agonists (or dopamine [INTROPIN]) are used for their pressor action. They are administered by IV infusion to raise blood pressure until the hypoten-sive crisis has passed or until other long-term measures are taken. (*Cautions:* Care should be taken to frequently change the site of administration of the IV drip; localized ischemia may cause tissue necrosis. Ischemia may occur in the extremities or in some organs with prolonged administration of a pressor agent. When blood pressure is supported by administration of a pressor agent, withdrawal of the agent should be done cautiously and slowly to avoid the precipitous recurrence of hypotension.)

Some hypotensive conditions are treated with pressor agents with α agonist activity.

Care must be taken with IV administration of α agonists; ischemia can result.

Shock. Shock is a cardiovascular syndrome distinguished by inadequate perfusion of tissue. Several insults to the body can bring about shock: hypovolemia (usually due to hemorrhage), cardiac insufficiency, or venous pooling (e.g., that which can occur with septicemia or some drug over-doses). Usually characterized by hypotension, clouding and loss of con-sciousness, and metabolic acidosis, the ischemia of shock may progress to cause extensive organ damage and death.

Compensatory autonomic responses result in high blood levels of adrenal catecholamines during shock.

Because of the obvious hypotension, sympathomimetic vasopressor drugs have often been employed in the past in the treatment of various types of shock. However, the wisdom of this approach is doubtful. The response of the autonomic nervous system to this stressful condition is a compensatory sympathetic discharge, resulting in high circulating levels of the adrenal catecholamines, NE and EPI. Thus, the addition of more vasoconstrictors to the system is of little benefit. Rather, much evidence indicates that in many situations treatment with a vasodilator (including α blockers; see later in this chapter) may be more rational.

The wisdom of administering vasoconstrictors during shock is doubtful.

Both fluids and dopamine are often administered in treating several types of shock.

Any pharmacological intervention in shock should be considered only after intravascular fluid volume has been replaced and the causative problem has been addressed. One catecholamine that currently is widely used to treat various forms of shock is *dopamine* (INTROPIN). Dopamine does have some α vasoconstricting and β cardiac-stimulating properties, but its value in shock stems from its ability to improve perfusion of the kidneys, brain, and intestines. Renal, cerebral, and mesenteric vascular beds are rich in dopamine receptors, and these vessels respond to dopamine by dilating (even in the presence of high circulating levels of NE).

Ergot Alkaloids

Ergot alkaloids are naturally occurring or semisynthetic derivatives of lysergic acid (Table 14–5). The source for these powerful and unusual compounds is the ergot fungus that can infect rye and other grain grasses. The fungus contains 30–40 lysergic acid derivatives, many of them pharmacologically active. The classification of these agents is complex because some of them are either agonists or antagonists (or have mixed actions) at adrenergic, dopaminergic, or serotonergic receptors. However, since most of the clinically important actions of the ergot alkaloids are blocked by the α antagonist phentolamine, these agents can be classed as α agonists.

Ergot alkaloids can be considered as α agonists because of their clinically relevant actions.

Ergot toxicity can result in profound vasoconstriction and CNS disturbances.

The ergot alkaloids, primarily by α receptor activation, cause very strong contraction of smooth muscles, including vascular smooth muscle, resulting in dramatic vasoconstriction. Throughout history, there have been a number of mass poisonings resulting from the consumption of bread baked from ergot-infected rye. The resulting condition is characterized by a profound vasoconstriction in the extremities, which can result in necrosis (thus the name St. Anthony's fire, as the limbs appear to have been burned in a fire). This *ergotism* is also distinguished by significant CNS effects: confusion, depression, delirium, and hallucinations (note that lysergic acid diethylamide [LSD] is an ergot derivative) (see Table 14–5). In fact, some investigators have suggested that the bizarre behavior of the Salem witches may have resulted from their eating bread made from ergot-infected rye (see also Chapter 27).

The ergot alkaloids have limited clinical application, being used primarily for their ability to contract vascular and uterine smooth muscle.

Ergonovine is used to control postpartum bleeding.

Postpartum Bleeding. This is routinely controlled or reduced by the administration of *ergonovine* (ERGOTRATE), which produces both vasoconstriction and a firm and sustained uterine contraction.

Migraine attacks can be treated with ergotamine, whereas methysergide is used in the prophylaxis of migraine.

Migraine Headaches. These can often be effectively aborted or relieved with *ergotamine* (ERGOMAR). One of the probable sources of migraine pain is the dilation of cranial vessels by an unknown mechanism (possibly involving the neurotransmitter serotonin). Ergotamine relieves migraine attacks presumably as the result of vasoconstriction; however, it is not usually effective in preventing attacks. Another ergot derivative and a serotonin

Table 14-5 STRUCTURE OF ERGOT ALKALOIDS

$$O{=}C{-}R$$

	R =
Lysergic acid	—OH
Lysergic acid diethylamide (LSD)	—N(CH₂CH₃)₂
Ergonovine	—NH—CHCH₂OH (with CH₃)
Ergotamine	

antagonist, *methysergide* (SANSERT), is useful in the prophylaxis of migraine (see Chapter 29).

(*Caution:* Ergotamine and ergonovine are potent vasoconstrictors; overdosage can produce ischemia profound enough to result in gangrene.)

Hyperprolactinemia. High serum levels of prolactin are effectively reduced in most patients by treatment with *bromocriptine* (PARLODEL). Bromocriptine is a dopamine (D2) receptor agonist, and as such it inhibits the release of prolactin from the pituitary.

Bromocriptine is effective in reducing elevated prolactin levels.

Alpha₂ Agents — Central Control of Blood Pressure

Studies on central blood pressure control mechanisms suggest that the nucleus tractus solitarius exerts an inhibitory effect on sympathetic outflow from the medulla. The receptors on the solitary tract nuclei are of the α_2-adrenergic subtype. Thus, activation of these postsynaptic receptors with selective α_2 agonists results in a reduced sympathetic outflow from the CNS and a lowering of blood pressure. Two centrally acting α_2-adrenergic agonists that are effective in lowering the blood pressure of hypertensive patients are *clonidine* (CATAPRES) and *methyldopa* (ALDOMET); the

Activation of α_2 receptors in the solitary tract inhibits central sympathetic outflow and lowers blood pressure.

Clonidine and methyldopa lower blood pressure by activating central α_2 receptors.

Methyldopa is enzymatically converted to α-methylnorepinephrine, a unique agonist for α_2 receptors.

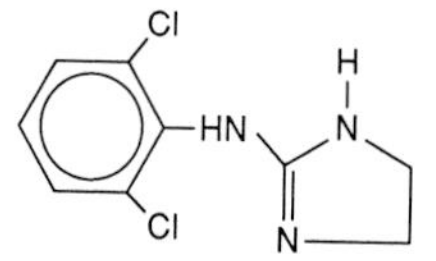

Clonidine

Methyldopa and clonidine produce less orthostatic hypotension than many other antihypertensive drugs.

Clonidine is useful in preventing the symptoms of opiate withdrawal.

activity of methyldopa is due to its enzymatic conversion to α-methylnorepinephrine.

Alphamethyldopa was originally thought to inhibit the enzyme dopa-decarboxylase in the biosynthetic pathway for NE (see Fig. 14–2). It does inhibit the decarboxylation of dopa *in vitro*, and it does lower blood pressure. However, it was learned that to be efficacious, methyldopa must serve as a *substrate* for dopa-decarboxylase, rather than as an inhibitor. Enzymatic modification of methyldopa parallels that of endogenous dopa, resulting in the production of the NE analog, α-methylnorepinephrine (Fig. 14–10). Once discovered, α-methylnorepinephrine was thought to be a "false transmitter"; that is, methyldopa-treated sympathetic nerve endings would be "shooting blanks" rather than releasing the authentic and active transmitter, NE. This hypothesis proved to be incorrect, and it is now accepted that α-methylnorepinephrine is a unique agonist for an α_2 subclass of adrenergic receptors found in the midbrain neural systems involved in the control of blood pressure. Originally designed to be a nasal decongestant, *clonidine* (CATAPRES) was also found to be a potent α_2 agonist (with no need for enzyme modification) and to lower blood pressure through this central mechanism.

Both methyldopa and clonidine are widely used and well tolerated in the treatment of hypertension. Peripheral sympathetic reflexes are little affected by these drugs, so orthostatic hypotension is not pronounced. The most common side effects of both drugs are sedation, dizziness, and dry mouth.

An unexpected relationship between clonidine and opiates was discovered as the result of a serendipitous clinical observation in a hypertensive heroin addict. Namely, clonidine prevents many of the symptoms of withdrawal from chronic opioid use. Withdrawal from chronic opioid use increases adrenergic activity in the locus ceruleus and in the peripheral sympathetic system. This "hypersympathetic state" can be ameliorated by treating with either an opioid or clonidine. Clonidine is currently a part of the pharmacological regimen used in some narcotic treatment programs. Analogously, clonidine is also used by some to ameliorate the alcohol withdrawal syndrome.

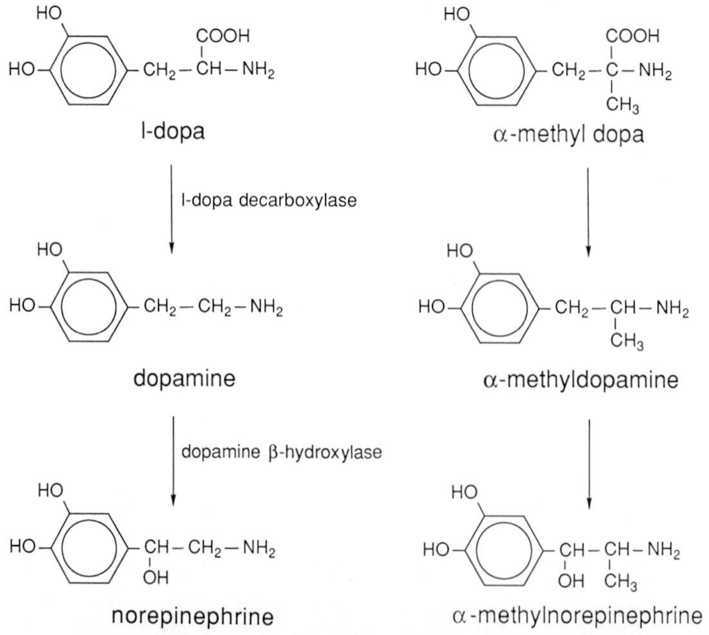

Figure 14–10

The parallel between the relationship of norepinephrine to levodopa with the relationship of α-methylnorepinephrine to α-methyl dopa.

(*Caution:* The sudden withdrawal from chronic treatment with clonidine has been reported to result in a life-threatening hypertensive crisis due, presumably, to a sudden increase in sympathetic activity in an up-regulated receptor system.)

> Sudden withdrawal from long-term clonidine treatment can produce dangerous hypertension.

BETA AGONISTS

Beta₁ Agents — Cardiac Stimulation

Stimulation of β_1-adrenergic receptors increases both heart rate and force of contraction. In cases of bradycardia, heart block, congestive heart failure, or cardiac arrest, *isoproterenol* (ISUPREL) or the β_1-selective agent *dobutamine* (DOBUTREX) can be used as cardiac stimulants.

> Agents with β_1 agonist properties can be used to stimulate the heart in cases of bradycardia or heart block.

Beta₂ Agents — Bronchial Relaxation

Stimulation of β_2 receptors causes relaxation of bronchial smooth muscle, thus decreasing airway resistance. This effect is taken advantage of in treating bronchial asthma. Both *epinephrine* (ADRENALIN) and *isoproterenol* (ISUPREL) are used in personal metered-dose inhalers to relieve an asthmatic attack. A severe asthmatic attack or the medical emergency status asthmaticus usually requires subcutaneous injections of epinephrine or isoproterenol.

> Beta₂ agonists relax bronchial muscle and are valuable in treating asthma.

Epinephrine and isoproterenol are rapid-acting and effective, but they have several disadvantages. Owing to rapid tissue uptake and metabolism, their duration of action is very short and they are not effective when administered orally. Both are active at β_1 as well as β_2 receptors; thus they have significant cardiac stimulation side effects.

> As well as β_2 activity, EPI and ISO have potentially dangerous β_1 cardiac-stimulant activity.

The need for drugs to manage asthma chronically and the stated disadvantages of epinephrine and isoproterenol fueled the search for orally active, β_2-selective agents. Useful β_2-selective drugs have been developed: *terbutaline* (BRETHINE) and *albuterol* (VENTOLIN) are effective and widely used, both in oral preparations and in metered-dose inhalers (Chapter 62).

> Terbutaline and albuterol are β_2-selective and effective orally in the treatment of asthma.

MISCELLANEOUS USES OF ADRENERGIC AGONISTS

Ophthalmic

Epinephrine is used to lower intraocular pressure in some patients with wide angle glaucoma. The vasoconstricting effect of topically applied epinephrine decreases the production of aqueous humor by the ciliary processes. The α activity of epinephrine also causes dilation of the pupil. This mydriatic property facilitates eye examinations and is useful in ophthalmic surgery (see Chapter 8).

> EPI decreases aqueous humor production and is occasionally used to treat glaucoma.

Central Nervous System

Many adrenergic agents cross the blood-brain barrier and have the potential to cause CNS stimulation, which includes increased wakefulness, nervousness, irritability, excitation, appetite suppression, and often euphoria. These effects are not seen with clinically useful doses of EPI, NE, or ISO. The CNS-stimulating effects are a prominent aspect of the actions of the amphetamines (indirect-acting adrenergic agonists). Tolerance develops to the stimulant properties of these drugs, and drug dependence can occur, notably with the amphetamines.

> Adrenergic agonists that cross into the brain can cause CNS stimulation.

Narcolepsy. *Dextroamphetamine* (DEXEDRINE) and other stimulants are used to prevent daytime sleepiness in patients with narcolepsy. A careful sched-

Dextroamphetamine and methylphenidate are stimulants that are used to treat narcolepsy.

Stimulants are used to increase the attention span in hyperactive children; the consequences of such chronic use are not well established.

ule of timing and dose must be adjusted for each patient to allow effective nighttime sleep.

Attention-Deficit Hyperactivity Disorder. Hyperkinesis—a syndrome consisting of inattentiveness, easy distractibility, impulsive behavior, and often hyperactivity—is seen most often as a developmental disorder of children. The amphetamines have a paradoxical, calming effect on this condition; the mechanisms underlying such apparently paradoxical effects are unknown. *Dextroamphetamine* and other stimulants (notably, *methylphenidate* [RITALIN]) appear to be quite effective in many of these children: attention span is increased, impulsiveness is decreased, and classroom behavior is improved. However, this is an area of much controversy in terms of how severe the disorder needs to be to warrant medication, as well as of the consequences of chronic administration over years.

Weight Loss. The anorexic central action of many adrenergic agonists has become an enormous commercial, if not medical, success. Drugs can be used, at the least, as temporary adjuncts to a weight loss program for *some* patients. They should be used only under close supervision because the many hazards of their use include dependence and cardiac arrhythmias, especially after taking excessive doses. Obviously, losing weight requires caloric restriction. Changes in eating habits, adoption of a sensible exercise regimen, perhaps counseling, and other lifestyle changes are frequently required for successful weight loss. Although *amphetamines* were prescribed as weight loss aids for many years, they are no longer recommended for this use; their adverse effects usually outweigh their limited benefit. In the late 1970s *phenylpropanolamine* (available over the counter, frequently in combination with caffeine) was reluctantly accepted for use in weight control. At best, any weight loss resulting from phenylpropanolamine use is temporary and modest in magnitude. (*Caution:* There is a considerable risk of developing dependence on amphetamines. The high abuse potential of many of these drugs warrants them a Schedule II rating under the Controlled Substances Act.) Although phenylpropanolamine is not a scheduled substance, the use of this agent as a diet aid has been implicated in incidents of hypertension, stroke, cardiac arrhythmias, renal failure, and possibly death. However, these dramatic effects are likely to have been the result of taking doses in excess of those recommended or due to the combination with caffeine.

Amphetamines have a high abuse potential.

Consumption of large doses of phenylpropanolamine can have life-threatening consequences.

In short, present evidence suggests that weight loss is facilitated by drugs in selected subgroups of obese patients. Judicious selection of dose, agent, and regimen can be useful and can avoid excessive CNS stimulation or cardiovascular side effects. Some agents, such as *fenfluramine* (PONDIMIN), produce little or no CNS stimulation or euphoria, yet retain their anorexic and weight loss effects (listed in Chapter 64 under Drug-Food Interactions).

ADVERSE EFFECTS OF ADRENERGIC AGONISTS

Side effects of adrenergic agonists may include tachycardia (β_1), hypertension (α_1), localized ischemia at infusion site (α_1), and CNS stimulation.

- *Tachyarrhythmias,* palpitations, and even ventricular fibrillation are possible adverse effects of agents with β_1 activity.
- *Hypertension* is a potential side effect of any agent with α_1 activity.
- *Localized ischemia* can occur at the infusion site of α_1 agonists. If the site of an IV infusion is not changed periodically, localized vasoconstriction can result in necrosis. As a related caution, great care must be taken to avoid *extravasation* of these drugs.

Infusions of α_1 agonists must be discontinued gradually to avoid precipitous hypotension.

- *Precipitous hypotension* can occur if a patient is suddenly withdrawn from an infusion of an α_1 agonist. Such infusions must be discontinued gradually to allow receptor and reflex regulation mechanisms to readjust.

■ *CNS stimulation* in the form of nervousness, anxiety, insomnia, and drug dependence can result from the use of adrenergic agonists that cross the blood-brain barrier (the amphetamines are notable in this respect).

The major therapeutic impetus to the use of adrenergic blocking drugs is to lower blood pressure in hypertensive patients by decreasing sympathetic influence on the vasculature. This can be accomplished by blocking the α_1-adrenergic receptors that mediate vasoconstriction, by blocking β_1-mediated renin release, by blocking peripheral sympathetic neuron activity, or by altering CNS mechanisms and decreasing centrally mediated sympathetic outflow (see Chapter 8). Another important application for adrenergic blockade is to decrease sympathetic stimulation of the heart in patients with certain cardiac diseases.

Adrenergic Blocking Drugs and Their Therapeutic Use

The primary interest in drugs that decrease sympathetic activity (by several mechanisms) is for treating hypertension.

BETA BLOCKERS

The β blockers are competitive antagonists for NE and EPI receptor sites in the heart (β_1), the bronchioles (β_2), and the blood vessels in skeletal muscle (β_2). The four most important β blockers are propranolol (shown here), metoprolol, atenolol, and timolol (see Chapter 33 for the last three). Propranolol (INDERAL) and timolol (TIMOPTIC, BLOCADREN) are nonselective antagonists, with β_1- and β_2-antagonist properties. The use of such agents with β_2-antagonist activity increases airway resistance and runs the risk of precipitating an asthmatic attack in patients with a history of asthma or bronchitis. This consideration has stimulated the search for β blockers that are selective for β_1-adrenergic receptors. Two agents that are relatively more β_1-selective are metoprolol (LOPRESSOR) and atenolol (TENORMIN).

Propranolol is a competitive antagonist for NE at β_1 (heart) and β_2 (bronchioles and some blood vessels) receptors.

Propranolol

Beta$_1$-selective antagonists, like metoprolol and atenolol, have been developed to avoid the increased airway resistance caused by β_2 blockade.

Hypertension

Beta blockers have proved very effective in lowering the blood pressure in individuals with hypertension. The logic behind the use of β antagonists in lowering blood pressure is not obvious, for good reason; the mechanism for this effect is unknown. Suggested mechanisms responsible for the lowering of blood pressure produced by β antagonists include

1. Decreased cardiac output — This effect is seen soon after administration of β blocker, but the decrease in blood pressure develops only slowly thereafter.
2. A CNS effect that decreases central sympathetic output.
3. Presynaptic β receptor inhibition — analogous to the previously described presynaptic autoinhibitory α receptors. Some have proposed presynaptic β receptors, activation of which would enhance NE release. A β antagonist would block these receptors, thus decreasing NE release.
4. Inhibition of renin release — Renin is released by activating β_1 receptors on the juxtaglomerular apparatus; this effect can be blocked by a β_1 antagonist. Further, β blockers are nearly always effective in reducing high-renin hypertension.

Propranolol (INDERAL), in addition to being nonselective for β_1 and β_2 receptors, displays a remarkable degree of variation in bioavailability, both between individuals and within the same individual (possibly owing to wide differences in plasma protein binding and metabolism). Metoprolol (LOPRESSOR) and atenolol (TENORMIN) are longer-acting and more predictable in producing therapeutic plasma levels than propranolol. They also have the advantage of being more β_1-selective, making them safer to use in patients with a history of asthma or bronchitis. Atenolol is the least lipid-

Beta blockers are used widely to treat hypertension, but the mechanism of their salutary effect is not clear.

Beta$_1$ blockers decrease renin release, and β blockers usually reduce high-renin hypertension.

Propranolol exhibits a wide range in bioavailability.

Compared with propranolol, atenolol is safer to use with asthmatic patients, has fewer CNS side effects, and produces more predictable plasma levels.

Beta blocker therapy should be discontinued gradually to avoid dramatic cardiac stimulation (from up-regulated receptors).

soluble of the β blockers; consequently it does not readily cross the blood-brain barrier and has fewer CNS side effects than the other agents. The clinical application of β blockers in the management of hypertension is covered in Chapter 35. (*Caution:* Beta blockers can cause dramatic bradycardia, hypotension, and bronchial constriction. The sudden cessation of β blocker treatment can precipitate ventricular tachycardia, myocardial infarction, unstable angina, and sudden death.)

Cardiac Arrhythmias and Angina Pectoris

Beta blockers decrease cardiac responses to sympathetic stimulation, cardiac work, and oxygen demand; thus they may be useful in treating angina pectoris and tachyarrhythmias.

Beta antagonists attenuate the cardiac responses to sympathetic stimulation: they decrease heart rate and contractility, cardiac output, and myocardial oxygen demand (see Fig. 14–8). These effects are valuable in treating angina pectoris and supraventricular and ventricular tachyarrhythmias. The ensuing decrease in cardiac work and oxygen demand make β blocker therapy effective in reducing the incidence of reinfarction and death after myocardial infarction. For the clinical application of β blockers in managing these cardiac diseases, see Chapters 33–36. (See Caution for previous section of Hypertension.)

Other Uses

Timolol decreases intraocular pressure without producing miosis or altering accommodation.

Glaucoma. Topical application of β blockers such as *timolol* (TIMOPTIC) decreases the production of aqueous humor by the ciliary body. The lowering of intraocular pressure that results brings relief in most types of glaucoma. Unlike pilocarpine, β blockers do not cause miosis or spasm of accommodation; thus they are especially valuable in treating younger patients who possess active accommodation.

Propranolol is effective for prophylaxis of migraine attacks by an uncertain mechanism.

Migraine Headaches. When used chronically, *propranolol* (INDERAL) produces a marked reduction in the number of attacks in approximately one third to one half of individuals with migraine. Such β blocker therapy is useful for prophylaxis of migraine attacks, but it is not usually effective in the acute treatment of headache, although it can be in some patients. The mechanism for the preventive effect is not known, but the β_2 activity of propranolol may block dilation of extracranial arteries and thus prevent the pain associated with the expansion of these vessels.

For some performing artists, the anxiety cycle of stage fright can be broken with β blockers.

Stage Fright. The anxiety of stage fright ("anticipational anxiety") may be relieved by β blockers. Controlled studies, as well as anecdotal reports from performing artists and public speakers, indicate that these agents may be quite effective in individuals whose performance is degraded by excessive tremor, anxiety, or palpitations. In part, the effectiveness of these agents may be due to the dampening of the anxiety cycle of sensing palpitations or tremor and thus becoming even more anxious, which causes more palpitations, etc. (possibly related is the fact that the tremor of the disease of essential tremor is reduced by propranolol as well as by ethanol [Chapter 24]).

ALPHA BLOCKERS

Phenoxybenzamine forms a covalent bond with α receptors, but the other α blockers are competitive antagonists.

The α blockers are reversible, competitive antagonists for NE receptor sites, primarily in vascular smooth muscle. However, phenoxybenzamine (DIBENZYLINE) is unusual in that it forms a covalent bond with the α receptor; it is an alkylating agent with a nitrogen mustard–like structure (thus producing long-lasting effects). The older α antagonists phentolamine (REGITINE) and phenoxybenzamine (DIBENZYLINE) are nonselective, with affinity

Phentolamine

Phenoxybenzamine

Prazosin

for both α_1 and α_2 receptors. The newer agent prazosin (MINIPRESS) is selective for α_1 receptors. Alpha blockers decrease sympathetically mediated vasoconstriction (see Fig. 14–8). Since these drugs are antagonists, they owe their pharmacological activity to blocking the action of the agonists NE and EPI. Thus, the degree of vasodilation produced by α blockers is dependent on the level of adrenergic tone of the vascular beds. The level of sympathetic activity will vary among and within vascular beds and will also vary with physiological state (e.g., exercise, stress).

Prazosin selectively blocks α_1 receptors.

Alpha blockers decrease sympathetically mediated vasoconstriction (thus lowering blood pressure).

The extent of vasodilation produced by α blockers depends on the degree of sympathetic tone to the vascular beds.

Hypertension

Because α blockers can produce a marked degree of vasodilation, they would seem a logical choice of drug to lower blood pressure in the treatment of hypertension and to treat other hemodynamic problems. Unfortunately, the nonspecific α blocker agents produce a profound orthostatic (postural) hypotension and reflex tachycardia. These adverse effects are severe enough to limit the clinical utility of these α blockers. The major exception to this limitation is the newer, α_1 selective agent prazosin (MINIPRESS). Prazosin does produce some degree of orthostatic hypotension, but this effect decreases with repeated administration. Prazosin also produces considerably less tachycardia than the nonselective agents; it has thus become a useful antihypertensive medication. The clinical application of prazosin and other drugs used to treat hypertension is covered in Chapter 35.

The nonspecific α blockers are not useful in treating hypertension because the side effects they produce are too severe.

Alpha$_1$-selective antagonists (e.g., prazosin) produce acceptably mild side effects and are useful in treating hypertension.

Although it is unclear why prazosin treatment produces relatively milder side effects than the non–selective α blockers, possible mechanisms have been suggested. One such mechanism is depicted in Figure 14–11. Nonselective α antagonists (phentolamine and phenoxybenza-

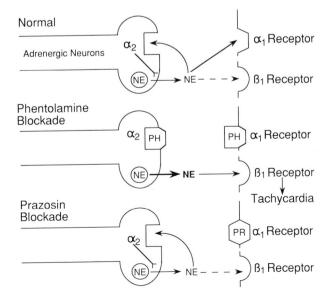

Figure 14–11

Action of prazosin.

Nonselective α antagonists increase NE release (producing side effects) by blocking presynaptic α_2-mediated feedback inhibition.

Prazosin has negligible activity at presynaptic α_2 receptors; thus it should not interfere with negative feedback mechanisms.

Blockade of a presynaptic α_1 receptor–mediated inhibition of acetylcholine release may also contribute to the low incidence of tachycardia in prazosin therapy.

Blood vessels that are seriously damaged by atherosclerosis do not respond to vasodilators; α blockers may worsen existing ischemia.

Alpha blockers are useful in correcting vasospastic conditions like Raynaud's disease and the sequelae of frostbite.

A combination of α and β blockers is useful to protect against the huge releases of catecholamines from adrenal tumors.

In some cases of late shock, α blockers are used to relax constricted postcapillary vessels.

Labetalol is a combination of isomers with α_1 and nonselective β blocking activity.

mine) not only block the (desired) postjunctional α_1 receptors; they also block the prejunctional α_2 receptors. This latter effect would reduce the negative feedback inhibition of NE release. The resulting *increased* NE release from sympathetic neurons in the heart would activate β_1 receptors and produce tachycardia. Since prazosin has negligible activity at α_2 receptors, it will produce only the intended postjunctional α_1 blockade, and not enhance NE release.

An additional possibility for the lack of significant tachycardia after prazosin administration involves heteroreceptor regulatory mechanisms (see Fig. 14–6). There is evidence that presynaptic α_1 receptors exert control on the release of acetylcholine nerve endings in the heart. The selective antagonism of prazosin would interfere with this α_1-adrenoceptor inhibition of acetylcholine release. The combination of increased acetylcholine release and decreased NE release (see preceding paragraph) may explain the low incidence of tachycardia with prazosin therapy.

Peripheral Vascular Disease

Most cases of vascular disease, including multi-infarct dementia, involve chronic occlusive atherosclerosis. The vessels in the ischemic areas of these patients are coated with plaque, damaged, and no longer resilient. Such vessels do not respond to vasodilator therapy. Introduction of an α blocker will cause a "stealing" of blood from already poorly perfused areas to other parts of the body with healthy, compliant vessels, which do respond to vasodilators. Thus, although the use of α blockers and other vasodilators to treat peripheral vascular disease is widely promoted, the wisdom of such therapy is questionable.

Nevertheless, there are some instances of peripheral ischemia that result from vasospasm; such conditions can often be improved with α blockers. The vigorous vasoconstriction of the extremities resulting from exposure to the cold in Raynaud's disease is relieved by phenoxybenzamine or prazosin. Likewise, the sequelae of frostbite and intermittent claudication are effectively treated with α blockers.

Other Uses

A pheochromocytoma may release large amounts of EPI and NE into the blood stream, especially when it is manipulated during surgery. This can, of course, result in dramatic changes in heart rate and blood pressure. Thus, before and during surgery to remove such a tumor, patients are protected from the cardiovascular effects of catecholamines by treatment with a combination of α and β blockers.

Likewise, during shock compensatory mechanisms may release large quantities of adrenal catecholamines into the blood stream, producing a prominent vasoconstriction. Such constriction in postcapillary resistance vessels results in the concentration of blood. Concentrated, viscous blood exacerbates the already inadequate perfusion characteristic of shock. In some cases, α blockers and other vasodilators have been shown to reverse this vasoconstriction and improve the survival rate from shock.

ALPHA AND BETA BLOCKERS

Labetalol (NORMODYNE) is unique in having both α (α_1-selective) and β (nonselective β_1 and β_2) blocking activity. Strictly speaking, however, labetalol can be viewed as a mixture of drugs: it has two asymmetric carbons, resulting in four optical isomers, and it is given as a racemic mixture of all four. Two of the isomers are inactive, one is a potent α blocker, and one is a potent β blocker.

Labetalol lowers total peripheral resistance without producing tachycardia and has thus proved useful in treating hypertension. An oral preparation is given to treat essential hypertension, and labetalol is administered intravenously to treat hypertensive emergencies. (*Caution:* All the precautions and contraindications relating to the use of α blockers *and* β blockers apply to the use of labetalol.)

Labetalol

The β blocker property of labetalol allows it to lower peripheral resistance (α₁ block) without producing tachycardia.

NEURON-BLOCKING DRUGS

In addition to the actions of α- and β-adrenergic receptor antagonists considered earlier, there are several other mechanisms by which drugs may decrease the effects of sympathetic activity. Included among these mechanisms is the depression of the output of NE from peripheral sympathetic neurons; drugs with this action are referred to as *neuron-blocking drugs.* As with the receptor antagonists, the primary clinical interest in these neuron-blocking drugs is for treating the prevalent condition of essential hypertension.

Several steps in the process of neurotransmission by NE are susceptible to interference by drugs.

Neuron-blocking drugs decrease sympathetic activity and are useful in treating hypertension.

Synthesis of Norepinephrine

The rate-limiting step in the enzymatic synthesis of NE is the conversion of tyrosine to levodopa by tyrosine hydroxylase (see Fig. 14–2). Thus, an inhibitor of this enzyme should markedly decrease the synthesis of neuronal NE and lower adrenergic nerve activity. The tyrosine analog α-methyltyrosine (DEMSER) effectively inhibits tyrosine hydroxylase and lowers the urinary output of NE metabolites in humans by 70%. However, this drug produces such severe side effects (pronounced sedation, diarrhea, anxiety, and tremors) that it is not useful in the management of essential hypertension. Alphamethyltyrosine is occasionally used in the management of pheochromocytoma, in those patients who are hypersensitive to or unresponsive to combined α and β blockers (see earlier).

Inhibition of the rate-limiting enzyme (tyrosine hydroxylase) in NE biosynthesis has proved to be a disappointing approach to treating hypertension. A considerable research effort was expended to produce inhibitors of the next enzyme in the NE biosynthetic pathway, dopa-decarboxylase. The agent that emerged from this work was α-methyldopa. Alphamethyldopa does effectively lower blood pressure in many hypertensive patients, but the mechanism underlying this effect eventually was proved to be unrelated to inhibition of dopa-decarboxylase (see previous section on α₂ agonists).

Alphamethyltyrosine inhibits tyrosine hydroxylase and decreases NE synthesis; its side effects are severe.

Packaging of Norepinephrine

The alkaloid *reserpine* is transported into adrenergic neurons, where it associates with the synaptic vesicle membrane and prevents the packaging of both dopamine (for conversion to NE) and cytoplasmic NE into synaptic vesicles (Fig. 14–12). This leads to a long-lasting and nearly complete depletion of neuronal NE and dopamine, both in the peripheral sympathetic system and in the CNS. This depletion can be demonstrated *in vitro* with reserpine-treated preparations (e.g., the guinea pig vas deferens), in which electrical stimulation results in the release of dopamine-β-hydroxylase but not NE (i.e., releasing the contents of "empty" synaptic vesicles).

Reserpine depletes nerve endings of NE by blocking the uptake of dopamine and NE into synaptic vesicles.

Figure 14–12

Action of reserpine.

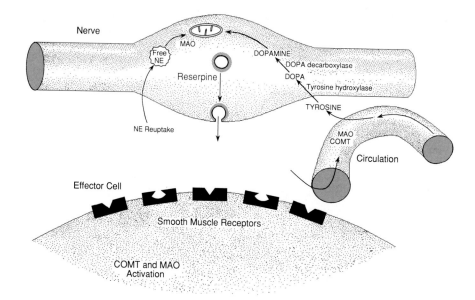

Reserpine lowers blood pressure, but at the expense of serious side effects: orthostatic hypotension, GI distress, and profound psychological depression.

With reserpine treatment, a lowering of blood pressure does ensue, along with several major side effects. As with many sympatholytic agents, reserpine produces orthostatic hypotension. The peripheral NE depletion caused by reserpine also results in an up-regulation of postjunctional adrenergic receptors, producing a supersensitivity to sympathetic agonists that is similar to denervation supersensitivity. The depletion of NE in the CNS can lead to depression severe enough to occasionally end in suicide. Extreme GI discomfort (diarrhea and abdominal cramps) also occurs as parasympathetic tone is unopposed by sympathetic activity following the "chemical sympathectomy" produced by reserpine. Although reserpine is far from an innocuous drug, it still finds some limited use as a last-resort drug in treating hypertension (for a clinical perspective, see Chapter 35). (*Caution:* Note the severe side effects of this drug. Because of the supersensitivity produced by reserpine, patients must not use sympathomimetics; even the use of some over-the-counter cold preparations may precipitate a life-threatening hypertensive or cardiac crisis. Use of reserpine must be avoided by all who have a history of depression. In addition, there is some evidence that reserpine use may be associated with an increased prevalence of breast cancer in women.)

After reserpine administration even an over-the-counter cold medicine could be dangerous.

Release of Norepinephrine

The neuronal release of NE is blocked by bretylium or guanethidine.

The two drugs *bretylium* (BRETYLOL) and *guanethidine* (ISMELIN) decrease adrenergic nerve activity by blocking neuronal NE release (see Chapter 33). In the same fashion as for reserpine, bretylium and guanethidine are taken into the adrenergic neuron by the specific amine uptake pump used for NE reuptake (Uptake I). As these drugs are transported into the neuron they displace cytoplasmic NE and cause its release, producing a transient sympathomimetic effect. Following the brief period of increased adrenergic activity, all three drugs produce a prolonged decrease in adrenergic activity. Bretylium and guanethidine, like reserpine, produce the side effects of severe orthostatic hypotension and supersensitivity to sympathomimetic drugs.

Bretylium and guanethidine produce dramatic postural hypotension and supersensitivity to sympathomimetics.

Despite the similarities between guanethidine and bretylium, there are some differences in their mechanisms and their applications. They both appear to block the process of release of NE from the neuronal membrane

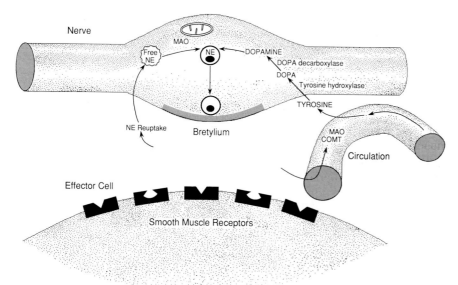

Figure 14 – 13

Action of bretylium.

(Figs. 14 – 13 and 14 – 14). However, guanethidine causes depletion of neuronal NE, whereas bretylium does not. Some researchers consider guanethidine to be a "false transmitter," because it is packaged in synaptic vesicles and, in certain experimental conditions, can be released by nerve stimulation.

The use of guanethidine is reserved for patients with severe hypertension. Bretylium is no longer used to treat hypertension; rather, it is currently approved as an antiarrhythmic agent, limited to use in emergency situations. The antiarrhythmic action of bretylium appears to be unrelated to its adrenergic neuron-blocking property. Through unknown mechanisms bretylium increases cardiac action potential duration and effective refractory period (see Chapter 33). (*Caution:* As noted earlier for reserpine, guanethidine and bretylium can produce severe orthostatic hypotension and a potentially dangerous supersensitivity to sympathomimetics. Unlike reserpine, however, these drugs do not cause CNS side effects because they fail to cross the blood-brain barrier.)

Guanethidine displaces NE in synaptic vesicles and is released upon nerve stimulation as a "false transmitter."

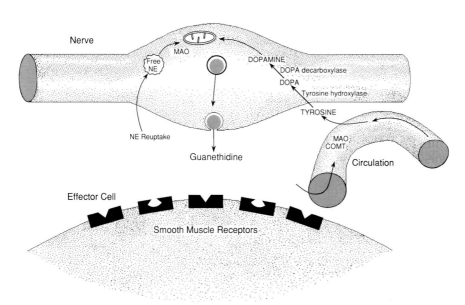

Figure 14 – 14

Action of guanethidine.

Table 14-6 ADRENERGIC DRUGS

Agents	Receptor	Therapeutically Useful Property
Alpha Agonists		
Epinephrine	Nonselective	Vasoconstriction (α_1)—prevent bleeding or hypotension
Norepinephrine	Nonselective	Vasoconstriction (α_1)—control hypotension
Dopamine	Indirect	Vasoconstriction (α_1)—control hypotension
	Dopamine	Vasodilatation—of certain areas (e.g., kidneys) during shock
Phenylpropanolamine	Indirect	Vasoconstriction (α_1)—nasal decongestant
		Anorexia (CNS)—component of weight-loss program
Pseudoephedrine	Nonselective	Vasoconstriction—nasal decongestant
Phenylephrine	α_1-selective	Vasoconstriction—treat hypotension, nasal decongestant
Methoxamine	α_1-selective	Vasoconstriction—treat hypotension
Metaraminol	α_1-selective	Vasoconstriction—treat hypotension
Mephentermine	α_1-selective	Vasoconstriction—treat hypotension
Ergotamine	α_1-selective	Vasoconstriction—treat migraine headache
Ergonovine	α_1-selective	Vasoconstriction—treat postpartum bleeding
Methyldopa	α_2-selective	Decrease sympathetic output (CNS)—treat hypertension
Clonidine	α_2-selective	Decrease sympathetic output (CNS)—treat hypertension
Guanfacine	α_2-selective	Decrease sympathetic output (CNS)—treat hypertension
Guanabenz	α_2-selective	Decrease sympathetic output (CNS)—treat hypertension
Beta Agonists		
Epinephrine	Nonselective	Bronchial relaxation (β_2)—treat asthma and anaphylactic shock
		Cardiac stimulation (β_1)—treat depressed contractility
Isoproterenol	Nonselective	Bronchial relaxation (β_2)—treat asthma
		Cardiac stimulation (β_1)—treat depressed contractility
Ethylnorepinephrine	Nonselective	Bronchial relaxation (β_2)—treat asthma
		Local vasoconstriction (α_1)—treat asthma
Dobutamine	β_1-selective	Cardiac stimulation—treat depressed contractility
Terbutaline	β_2-selective	Bronchial relaxation—treat asthma
Albuterol	β_2-selective	Bronchial relaxation—treat asthma
Pirbuterol	β_2-selective	Bronchial relaxation—treat asthma
Bitolterol	β_2-selective	Bronchial relaxation—treat asthma
Ritodrine	β_2-selective	Uterine relaxation—treat premature labor
Miscellaneous Agonists		
Dopamine	Dopamine	Vasodilatation—of certain areas (e.g., kidneys) during shock
Bromocriptine	Dopamine	Inhibit prolactin release—treat hyperprolactinemia
Phenylpropanolamine	Indirect	Anorexia (CNS)—component of weight-loss program
Pemoline	Indirect	CNS stimulation—treat attention-deficit hyperactivity
Amphetamine	Indirect	CNS stimulation—treat narcolepsy and hyperactivity
Methylphenidate	Indirect	CNS stimulation—treat narcolepsy and hyperactivity
Fenfluramine	Indirect	Anorexia (CNS)—component of weight-loss program
Alpha Antagonists		
Phenoxybenzamine	Nonselective	Vasodilatation—treat vasospasm of Raynaud's disease and frostbite; protect against pheochromocytoma
Phentolamine	Nonselective	Vasodilatation—treat vasospasm of Raynaud's disease and frostbite; protect against pheochromocytoma
Prazosin	α_1-selective	Vasodilatation—treat hypertension
Terazosin	α_1-selective	Vasodilatation—treat hypertension
Beta Antagonists		
Propranolol	Nonselective	Inhibit renin release(?)—treat hypertension
		Decrease cardiac output—treat angina and arrhythmia
Timolol	Nonselective	Decrease cardiac output—prophylaxis of myocardial infarction
		Decrease aqueous humor production—treat glaucoma
Nadolol	Nonselective	Inhibit renin release(?)—treat hypertension
		Decrease cardiac output—treat angina
Pindolol	Nonselective	(?)—treat hypertension
Metoprolol	β_1-selective	Inhibit renin release(?)—treat hypertension
		Decrease cardiac output—treat angina and arrhythmia
Acebutolol	β_1-selective	Inhibit renin release(?)—treat hypertension
		Decrease cardiac rate—treat tachyarrhythmia
Atenolol	β_1-selective	Inhibit renin release(?)—treat hypertension
Esmolol	β_1-selective	Decrease cardiac rate—treat tachyarrhythmia
Labetalol	β_1, β_2, and α_1	Lower peripheral resistance—treat hypertension
Neuron-Blocking Drugs		
Alphamethyltyrosine	NE synthesis	Decrease NE—protect against pheochromocytoma
Reserpine	NE packaging	Deplete NE—treat hypertension
Guanethidine	NE release	Prevent NE release—treat hypertension
Bretylium	NE release	Block NE release—antiarrhythmic

ADVERSE EFFECTS OF ADRENERGIC BLOCKERS

- *Hypotension,* in particular *orthostatic* (postural) *hypotension,* is a potential side effect of any agent with α antagonist or neuron-blocking activity.
- *Nasal congestion* is a complication of α antagonist use.
- *Inhibition of ejaculation* can also result from the use of agents with α antagonist or neuron-blocking activity.
- *Bradycardia* is a likely side effect when using agents with β blocking properties.
- *Bronchoconstriction* (precipitation of an asthmatic attack) can result from using agents with β antagonist properties.
- *Sedation* is a possible consequence of administration of any of these agents (e.g., propranolol) that cross the blood-brain barrier.
- *Severe CNS depression* is uniquely associated with the use of reserpine.

References

Abramowicz M: Phenylpropanolamine for weight reduction. Med Lett Drugs Ther 26:55–56, 1984.

Cooper JR, Bloom FE, Roth RH: The Biochemical Basis of Neuropharmacology. 5th ed. New York: Oxford University Press, 1986.

Day MD: Autonomic Pharmacology: Experimental and Clinical Aspects. New York: Churchill Livingstone, 1979.

DiStefano PS, Brown OM: Biochemical correlates of morphine withdrawal. 2. Effects of Clonidine. J Pharmacol Exp Ther 233:339–344, 1985.

Gilman AG, Goodman LS, Rall TW, Murad F: Goodman and Gilman's The Pharmacological Basis of Therapeutics. 7th ed. New York: Macmillan, 1985.

Kopin IJ: Catecholamine metabolism: Basic aspects and clinical significance. Pharmacol Rev 37:333–364, 1985.

Laduron PM: Presynaptic heteroreceptors in regulation of neuronal transmission. Biochem Pharmacol 34:467–470, 1985.

McGratten PA, Brown JH, Brown OM: Parasympathetic effects on *in vivo* rat heart can be regulated though an α_1-adrenergic receptor. Circ Res 60:465–471, 1987.

Minneman KP: α_1-adrenergic receptor subtypes, inositol phosphates, and sources of cell Ca^{2+}. Pharmacol Rev 40:87–119, 1988.

Rangno RE: Stopping beta blockers in patients with angina. Rational Drug Ther 15(9):1–4, 1981.

Weil WH, Shubin H, Carlson R: Treatment of circulatory shock, use of sympathomimetic and related vasoactive agents. JAMA 231:1280–1286, 1975.

Drugs Acting on the Sensory and Central Nervous Systems

Receptor Signal Transduction Mechanisms

15

Suzanne G. Laychock

The pharmacology of receptors began with the conceptualization that different receptor molecules were responsible for the myriad responses of living cells to chemically diverse extracellular substances. Later studies described quantitatively the interaction of specific ligands with protein receptors and provided the basis for the general classification schemes of the major receptor classes currently in use. The development of potent receptor agonists and antagonists paved the way for the analysis of structure-activity relationships that form the cornerstone for much of today's experimental and clinical pharmacology. The cellular characterization of receptors progressed as the subcellular structure and integration mechanisms of cells were defined through advanced technologies in histology and biochemistry. A major advance in cellular pharmacology was the localization of receptors to plasma membranes and intracellular compartments. Later, the biochemical purification and reconstitution of receptors and their subunits defined their chemical reality.

> Receptors are localized to plasma membranes and intracellular compartments.

Because stimulatory ligands often do not possess direct intracellular activity, second messengers generated in response to receptor-ligand binding translate the biophysical membrane response to an intracellular one. The identification of second messengers heralded in the era of cellular transduction mechanisms and biochemical amplification. A composite model for receptors today includes the concept of biophysically unique receptor units responding dynamically to ligand interactions through exquisitely modulated cell membrane topographical rearrangements and interactions or through intracellular traffic patterns that integrate a number of different biophysical and biochemical processes (Fig. 15–1). In addition, receptor stimulation by ligand binding often results in a pleiotropic response characterized by more than a single cellular response mechanism. There are also distinct cell signals translating the ligand response of identical receptors in different cell types, which conveys the unique nature of characteristic cellular responses in various tissues.

> Second messengers translate the biophysical membrane response to an intracellular one.

> Pleiotropic responses are characterized by more than a single cellular response mechanism or second messenger.

Receptor responses are determined by the chemistry of the ligand molecule. Most neurotransmitters, hormones, and local chemical mediators that do not enter the blood stream are water-soluble (hydrophilic). Hydrophilic molecules do not pass directly through the plasma membrane lipid bilayer of a target cell; instead, the molecules bind to specific receptor proteins within the plasma membrane and initiate specific transduction responses within the cell.

Hydrophilic Ligand Receptor Mechanisms

Figure 15-1

A model for cellular receptors and pleiotropic responses. Biophysically unique receptor units (R) in the plasma membrane respond to specific ligands (L) through direct interactions with ion channels or G proteins. G proteins modulate the activity of enzymes, ion channels, and transport processes and mediate the formation of second messengers. Receptors may also cluster and be internalized to endocytic vesicles that modify the ligand or the receptor, or both. Internalized ligand may act on intracellular effectors while the receptor is recycled to the plasma membrane.

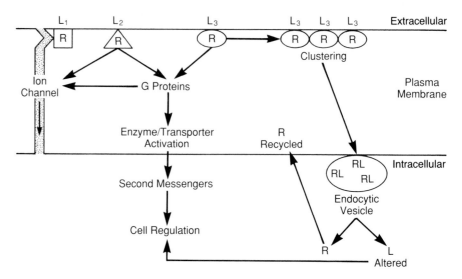

Hydrophilic molecules are water-soluble and require receptors in the plasma membrane to transduce a signal across the lipid boundary.

Receptor binding may initiate effector mechanisms in the plasma membrane or promote the internalization of the receptor-ligand complex to initiate cellular responses.

Cell-surface protein receptors can be categorized broadly as (1) those receptors that upon complex formation with ligand remain within the plasma membrane domain, and there behave as transducers initiating one or a number of enzyme or ion channel effector mechanisms; or (2) those receptors that upon complex formation leave the physical domain of the plasma membrane. The latter type may initiate effector responses within the plane of the membrane prior to exit into the cytoplasm. Alternatively, the receptor-ligand complex may travel intracellularly, become structurally transformed, and initiate unique cellular responses. Whatever the mechanism of effector activation, the movement of receptors into the cytoplasm (internalization) effectively reduces the concentration of surface receptors and decreases the sensitivity of cells to subsequent ligand exposure (desensitization or down-regulation).

ION CHANNELS/PUMPS

Voltage-gated Ca^{2+} channels allow large amounts of Ca^{2+} to enter the cell down a concentration gradient.

Many receptors regulate gated ion channels in the plasma membrane to modulate the cellular levels of Ca^{2+}, K^+, and Na^+. A small change in ion concentration in electrically excitable cells, such as neurons, muscle cells, and certain endocrine cells, alters the membrane potential and activates the voltage-sensitive channels to generate an action potential. The action potential amplifies the initial receptor response by opening voltage-gated Ca^{2+} channels that allow large amounts of Ca^{2+} to enter the cell down a concentration gradient. Ca^{2+} is a ubiquitous second messenger that initiates many cellular responses, including enzyme activation and the secretion of hormones and neurotransmitters.

Receptors mediating responses to the inhibitory neurotransmitters glycine and gamma-aminobutyric acid (GABA) elicit an increase in the chloride conductance of the neuronal membrane (see also Chapter 20). A chemically gated anion-selective transmembrane channel is formed upon interaction of the ligand with the receptor glycoprotein (Fig. 15-2A). The water-filled channel allows ions to diffuse across the membrane. The nicotinic cholinergic-receptor ion channel mediating the passage of sodium and potassium ions across membranes is also an integral part of the receptor-protein complex. The nicotinic acetylcholine (ACh)-receptor is a well-characterized chemically gated channel (see Chapter 9). The central axis of the channel is surrounded by a ring-like formation of membrane-spanning

Chemically gated channels are an integral part of the receptor-protein complex.

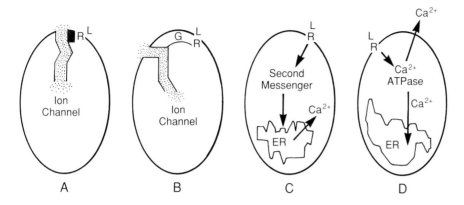

Figure 15-2

Different ways in which receptors (R) regulate ion levels in cells. Ligand (L) binding the receptor: *(A)* opens an ion channel that is linked to the receptor; *(B)* opens an ion channel in response to the receptor complexing with a G protein; *(C)* leads to the production of a second messenger, which releases Ca^{2+} from intracellular stores; *(D)* activates an ATPase, which pumps ions such as Ca^{2+} out of the cell or into sequestered pools within the cell. (ER = endoplasmic reticulum.)

subunits that dictate ion selectivity and conductance. Different ligand-regulated channels appear to have a similar subunit structure.

Other types of receptors interact with guanine nucleotide binding regulatory proteins (G proteins) in the membrane. The family of G proteins mediate many different transduction signals for receptors and are activated by the binding of guanosine triphosphate (GTP). Specific G proteins mediate conformational changes in ion channel proteins that allow ions, such as Ca^{2+} or K^+, to flow down a concentration gradient (Fig. 15-2*B*). For example, the muscarinic cholinergic receptor interacts with a G protein that modulates the activity of Ca^{2+} channels. In addition, receptors can regulate the mobilization of intracellular stores of Ca^{2+} through the generation of second messengers, including cyclic adenosine monophosphate (AMP) and inositol 1,4,5-trisphosphate (Fig. 15-2*C*).

Intracellular stores of Ca^{2+} are mobilized through the generation of second messengers.

Ion concentrations in cells are also regulated by adenosine triphosphate (ATP)-dependent pumping mechanisms (Fig. 15-2*D*). Ca^{2+}-ATPase and Na^+-K^+-ATPase are activated in receptor-stimulated cells and serve to lower or maintain intracellular ion levels. Thus, a Ca^{2+}-driven second messenger response of cells may be terminated by the activation of a Ca^{2+}-ATPase. Ca^{2+} is removed against an electrochemical gradient to the cell exterior or sequestered into pools within intracellular membrane–limited organelles such as the endoplasmic reticulum (Fig. 15-2*D*). Mitochondria also take up Ca^{2+} from the cytosol, whereas Na^+-driven antiports in the plasma membrane act to expel Ca^{2+} from the cell by ion exchange. Phosphates and Ca^{2+}-binding proteins also buffer and reduce the free intracellular Ca^{2+} concentration of cells. The net result is that the concentration of free Ca^{2+} ions in the cytosol (approximately 10^{-7} M) is a thousandfold lower than the extracellular Ca^{2+} concentration (approximately 10^{-3} M) in resting cells.

ADENYLATE CYCLASE/CYCLIC ADENOSINE MONOPHOSPHATE

Cyclic AMP (adenosine 3':5'-cyclic monophosphate) is a ubiquitous second messenger synthesized from ATP by the enzyme adenylate cyclase. Many hormones, neurotransmitters, and pharmacological agents, acting through distinct receptors, stimulate membrane-bound adenylate cyclase. However, the receptor is a distinct entity from the transduction component identified as a stimulatory G protein (G_s). A schematic representation of receptor-stimulated adenylate cyclase activation is provided (Fig. 15-3). Ligand binding of the receptor induces a change in conformation and movement of the receptor within the lipid bilayer of the membrane to

Ligand-receptor complex interacts with a G protein to promote the exchange of GDP for bound GTP, thus activating the G protein for interaction with adenylate cyclase.

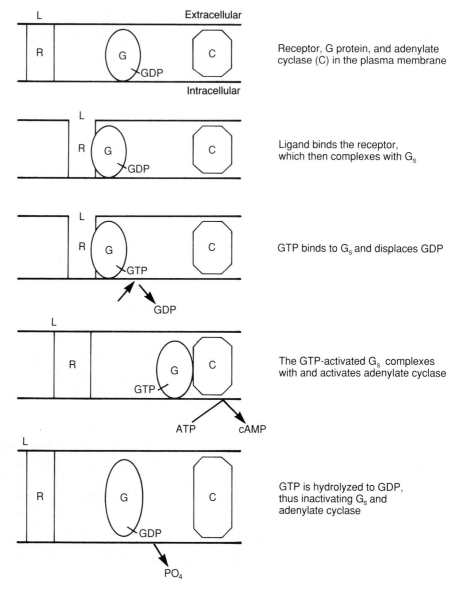

Figure 15–3

Receptor-stimulated adenylate cyclase. Receptor (R), G protein (G) bound to GDP, and adenylate cyclase (C) reside in the membrane. When a molecule of ligand (L) binds a receptor, the ligand-receptor complexes with a G protein. The GDP then exchanges for a molecule of GTP on the G protein. The G protein with GTP changes conformation, loses affinity for the receptor, and forms an activating complex with adenylate cyclase. Adenylate cyclase catalyzes the conversion of ATP to the second messenger cyclic AMP. The response is terminated upon hydrolysis of GTP to GDP.

G proteins are heterotrimers characterized by three unequal peptide subunits — α, β, γ.

interact with G_s and form a ligand-receptor–G_s monomer complex. The complexed G_s changes conformation and is activated upon exchange of a molecule of guanosine diphosphate (GDP) for GTP. The associated receptor moiety dissociates from the complex upon GTP binding, and the affinity of the receptor for agonists is reduced.

The family of G proteins that interacts with many diverse receptors in membranes are heterotrimers characterized by three peptide subunits (α, β, and γ) which dissociate upon activation. The α subunit has a high-affinity binding site for guanine nucleotides. The G_s-GTP complex orients within the plane of the membrane, interacts with adenylate cyclase, and catalyzes the enzymatic conversion of ATP to cyclic AMP. Many molecules of cyclic AMP are produced for every G_s-adenylate cyclase complex formed, resulting in amplification of the original receptor signal. The adenylate cyclase response is terminated upon deactivation of G_s by GTP hydrolase activity intrinsic to the α subunit. GTP is converted to GDP, and the α, β, and γ subunit oligomer is reconstituted. The use of nonhydrolyzable analogs of GTP, such as guanylimidodiphosphate (Gpp(NH)p) or guanosine-5'-(3-o-thio) triphosphate (GTP-gamma-S), induces prolonged activation of the G

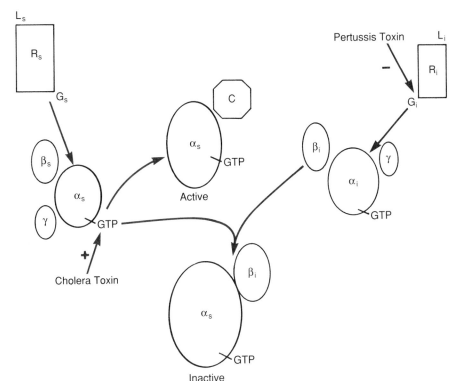

Figure 15-4

G proteins and cellular regulation. Stimulatory or inhibitory ligands (L_s or L_i) bind specific receptors and interact with stimulatory or inhibitory G proteins (G_s or G_i), respectively. The G_s and G_i dissociate into three peptide subunits, α, β, and γ. α_s bound by GTP activates adenylate cyclase (C). Cholera toxin inhibits GTP hydrolysis and prolongs activation (+) by α_s. The β_i subunit can interact with α_s and form an inactive complex. Alpha$_i$ may also inhibit the α_s response. Pertussis toxin inhibits (−) the G_i response.

protein and adenylate cyclase. In addition, the α subunit of G_s and certain other G proteins are substrates for cholera toxin, which ADP-ribosylates the subunit, thus inhibiting the GTPase and causing persistent activation of G_s and adenylate cyclase or other associated enzymes.

In contrast to G_s, there is an inhibitory G protein (G_i) that interacts with G_s-adenylate cyclase to inhibit enzyme activity. Specific receptors, including the α_2 adrenoceptor, interact with G_i to induce GTP binding and subunit dissociation similarly to that observed for G_s (Fig. 15-4). In contrast to signal transduction by G_s, however, the β subunit of G_i possesses marked inhibitory activity against adenylate cyclase and may complex with the α subunit of G_s to impede association of the stimulatory α subunit with adenylate cyclase. The α subunit of G_i probably also possesses inhibitory activity against G_s. Another bacterial toxin, pertussis toxin, ADP-ribosylates the α subunit of G_i and certain other G proteins, except the G_s type, blocking the ability of these proteins to interact with receptors. Hence, pertussis toxin contributes indirectly to enhance cyclic AMP production through the removal of inhibitory control mechanisms.

The production of cyclic AMP is not sufficient to complete the cellular transduction mechanism initiated by receptor stimulation. Cyclic AMP must react with and activate an intracellular cyclic AMP–dependent protein kinase. A great variety of proteins serve as substrates for cyclic AMP–dependent protein kinase, a number matched only by the great diversity of physiological functions attributed to adenylate cyclase activation. Thus, the activity of protein kinase amplifies the response of cyclic AMP production, because for every protein kinase activated by a molecule of cyclic AMP, many proteins are phosphorylated. Termination of the action of cyclic AMP includes not only the dephosphorylation of a phosphorylated substrate by a protein phosphatase, but also the metabolism of cyclic AMP to inactive 5'-AMP catalyzed by the enzyme phosphodiesterase.

Another cyclic nucleotide, guanosine 3':5'-cyclic monophosphate (cy-

Inhibition of GTP hydrolysis results in persistent G protein activation and responses.

Inhibitory G protein α and β subunits antagonize the activity of other G proteins.

Protein phosphatases and phosphodiesterase terminate cell activation by cyclic AMP.

Guanylate cyclase is the receptor for atrial natriuretic peptide, and cyclic GMP is a putative second messenger.

clic GMP), is a putative second messenger in many cells, including vascular smooth muscle cells. Guanylate cyclase, which synthesizes cyclic GMP from GTP, exists in both soluble and particulate forms in the cell. The receptor for atrial natriuretic peptide has been characterized as the membrane-bound form of guanylate cyclase. Cyclic GMP also requires a specific protein kinase as an effector, although in retinal cells cyclic GMP directly affects ion channel activity. Cyclic GMP-modulated events in cells include the regulation of Ca^{2+} levels and metabolism with associated effects on cell division and tumor growth. Termination of the cyclic GMP response occurs by phosphatase inactivation of phosphorylated substrates and by a cyclic GMP specific phosphodiesterase.

LIPIDS/PHOSPHOLIPIDS

The stimulation of many types of receptors results in dynamic changes in the composition of the membrane lipid bilayer. The enzymes primarily responsible for the rapid synthesis and turnover of membrane phospholipids are the phospholipid hydrolases (phospholipases). Although the *de novo* synthesis of lipids, base exchange, and other aspects of lipid biosynthesis may be stimulated also, they will not be discussed here because the involvement of receptors/second messengers in the processes is indirect.

Phospholipases respond to receptor stimulation and generate second messengers.

Phospholipases, including phospholipase C (which cleaves the polar base group from the phospholipid molecule) and phospholipase A_2 (which hydrolyzes the fatty acid from the 2C position of phospholipids) (Fig. 15–5) respond to receptor stimulation and generate second messengers. The other phospholipases, A_1 and D, which hydrolyze the fatty acid from the 1C position or the base group at the 3C phosphate bond, respectively, play less prominent roles in receptor regulation of eukaryotic cells. Phospholipase A_2 is stimulated in response to many different receptors, probably through changes in Ca^{2+} availability. In some cells, receptor stimulation of phospholipase A_2 is modulated by a G protein(s). Phospholipase A_2 liberates unsaturated fatty acids, and particularly arachidonic acid, which are primarily (1) metabolized as fuel for the cell; (2) converted to the eicosanoid group compounds (prostaglandins, thromboxanes, or leukotrienes); or (3) incorporated into membrane phospholipids by the actions of acyl-CoA acyltransferase (Fig. 15–6). The content of unsaturated fatty acids in membrane phospholipids modulates membrane fluidity and membrane fusion events.

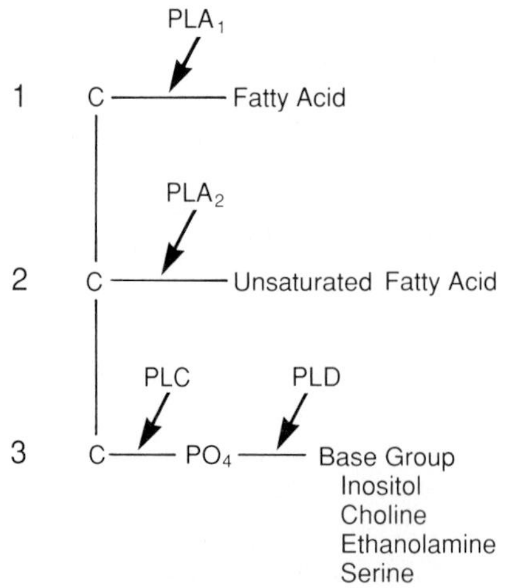

Phospholipase A_2 promotes the synthesis of prostaglandins that modulate smooth muscle contractility, secretion, and membrane permeability.

Figure 15–5

Phospholipase hydrolysis of phospholipids. Phospholipase A_1 (PLA$_1$) hydrolyzes the fatty acid from 1C; phospholipase A_2 (PLA$_2$) hydrolyzes the unsaturated fatty acid from 2C; phospholipase C (PLC) hydrolyzes the phosphate bond at 3C; phospholipase D (PLD) hydrolyzes the base group from the phosphate bond. The base groups of common phospholipids are listed.

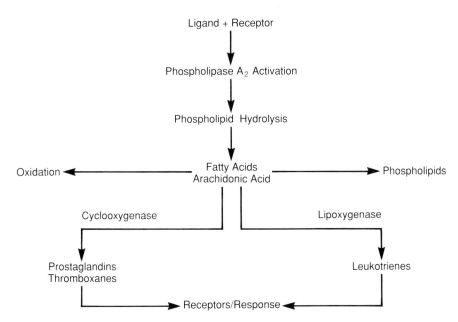

Figure 15-6

Phospholipase A_2 activation and cellular regulation. Ligand binds to a receptor that stimulates phospholipase A_2. Phospholipase A_2 hydrolyzes phospholipids and liberates arachidonic acid or other unsaturated fatty acids. Fatty acids can be oxidized for energy or incorporated into phospholipids in cell membranes. In addition, arachidonic acid can be metabolized by cyclooxygenase to prostaglandins and thromboxanes, or by lipoxygenase to leukotrienes, including hydroperoxyeicosatetraenoic acids. Each eicosanoid product has second-messenger potential and can interact at intracellular sites or with plasma membrane receptors.

Prostaglandins (E_2, F_2, D_2, and prostacyclin among others) and thromboxanes (A_2 and B_2) are cyclooxygenase-derived arachidonic acid metabolites (Fig. 15-6). The leukotrienes (LTB_4 among others) are lipoxygenase-derived arachidonic acid metabolites (Fig. 15-6). These eicosanoids serve as second messengers with the potential to act intracellularly or bind to membrane receptors on the parent cell or on neighboring cells to act as local hormones. Prostaglandins are a class of ubiquitous mediators that modulate diverse cell responses in either a positive or negative manner. They exert effects on smooth muscle contractility (with marked effects on uterine and vascular smooth muscle especially), secretory responses (platelet and endocrine systems), and membrane permeability. The transduction mechanisms affected most commonly by prostaglandins are Ca^{2+} entry and mobilization, protein kinase C, and cyclic AMP (Table 15-1). Prostaglandin receptors on cells can interact with G proteins and affect adenylate cyclase activity. Receptors for leukotrienes are present also on certain cell types, including polymorphonuclear leukocytes and bronchiolar smooth muscle cells. However, the leukotrienes appear to be less ubiquitous than the prostaglandins (see also Chapter 28).

Prostaglandin transduction mechanisms include Ca^{2+} entry and mobilization and changes in protein kinase C and adenylate cyclase activity.

Table 15-1 PROSTAGLANDIN EFFECTS ON TRANSDUCTION MECHANISMS		
Eicosanoid	**Effects**	**Cell Type**
Stimulatory		
PGE_1	Increased Ca^{2+} entry	Fibroblasts
	Increased Ca^{2+} mobilization	Uterine tissue
	Activated adenylate cyclase (G_s)	Platelets, fibroblasts, others
Inhibitory		
PGE_2	Suppressed glucose oxidation	Blastocysts, pancreatic islets
$PGF_{2\alpha}$		
PGE_2	Suppression of inositol phosphate pathway activity	Neutrophils, pancreatic islets T lymphocytes
	Inhibited Ca^{2+} influx	
	Down-regulation of receptors	
PGE_1	Inhibits adenylate cyclase (G_i)	Acid-secreting cells
PGE_2	Inhibits protein kinase C	Platelets

Figure 15-7

The second messengers inositol 1,4,5-tris-phosphate and diacylglycerol. A ligand-stimulated receptor initiates phospholipase C activation through a transducing G protein. Phospholipase C hydrolyzes phosphatidylinositol 4,5-bisphosphate (PIP_2) formed as a result of the sequential phosphorylation of phosphatidylinositol (PI). PIP_2 hydrolysis results in the formation of two second messengers, inositol 1,4,5-trisphosphate ($InsP_3$) and diacylglycerol. $InsP_3$ interacts with intracellular receptors and releases intracellular stores of Ca^{2+}. Diacylglycerol activates protein kinase C. (ER = endoplasmic reticulum; PIP = phosphatidylinositol 4-phosphate.)

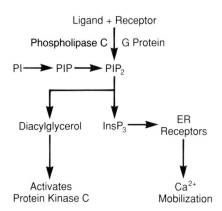

Phosphoinositide-specific phospholipase C generates diacylglycerol and inositol 1,4,5,-trisphosphate second messengers.

Inositol 1,4,5,-trisphosphate mobilizes Ca^{2+} from intracellular stores in the endoplasmic reticulum.

Diacylglycerol remains within the plasma membrane and activates protein kinase C.

Phospholipase C responds also to receptor stimulation, probably through a G protein mediator. The primary receptors responsible for phospholipase C activation are the muscarinic cholinergic receptor, the α_1 adrenoceptor, and certain peptide receptors. Inositol phospholipids and phosphatidylcholine are the major substrates for phospholipase C activity in cells. Phosphatidylinositol is unique in that it is phosphorylated by specific kinases in the membrane to produce polyphosphoinositides. Ligand-receptor stimulation activates a specific phospholipase C (phosphoinositidase), which rapidly hydrolyzes phosphatidylinositol 4,5-bisphosphate to the second messengers inositol 1,4,5-trisphosphate and diacylglycerol (Fig. 15-7). Other inositol phosphates are produced also; however, their role in cell activity has not been established.

Inositol 1,4,5-trisphosphate ($InsP_3$) is a Ca^{2+}-mobilizing second messenger that increases intracellular Ca^{2+} concentrations. $InsP_3$ enters the cytoplasm and interacts with an intracellular receptor on the endoplasmic reticulum, triggering the release of Ca^{2+} from sequestered stores within the cell (Fig. 15-7). The rapid increase in intracellular Ca^{2+} concentrations amplifies the stimulus response through the activation of many different Ca^{2+}-dependent cellular processes.

Diacylglycerol, the other second messenger generated in response to phospholipase C activation, remains within the membrane and interacts with a specific protein kinase C that phosphorylates serine and threonine residues of proteins. The combined stimulatory action of diglyceride and Ca^{2+} on protein kinase C results in augmented enzyme phosphorylation activity. The subspecies of protein kinase C within the enzyme family possess individual enzymological and histological characteristics and probably play specific roles in cell function in response to receptor stimulation in different cell types. Among the varied responses of cells to protein kinase C activation are increased secretory activity of endocrine and exocrine cells, neurons, mast cells, and platelets; alterations in glucose transport and metabolism in adipocytes and hepatocytes; and changes in gap junction activity in epidermal cells. Protein kinase C probably affects gene activation and transcription also. A class of tumor promoter, the phorbol esters, mimics the effects of diacylglycerol and activates protein kinase C.

RECEPTOR INTERNALIZATION

Certain receptors, including those for insulin, β-adrenergic agonists, and growth factors, become internalized subsequent to ligand binding. Following ligand binding, these types of receptors localize often to a portion of the plasma membrane known as a *coated pit* (an area of the plasma membrane

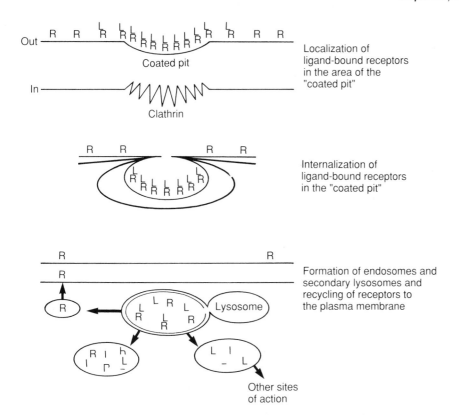

Localization of
ligand-bound receptors
in the area of the
"coated pit"

Internalization of
ligand-bound receptors
in the "coated pit"

Formation of endosomes and
secondary lysosomes and
recycling of receptors to
the plasma membrane

Other sites
of action

Figure 15–8

Receptor internalization. Ligand-bound receptors localize within the plane of the membrane to "coated pits," regions of the plasma membrane with an electron-dense cytoplasmic clathrin lining. The coated pit areas endocytose to form endosomes or receptosomes. Fusion with lysosomes promotes the degradation/alteration of ligand, which may then act within the cell at specific effector sites. Receptors may be degraded or returned to the plasma membrane for recycling.

lined on the cytoplasmic face with the protein clathrin) (Fig. 15–8). The area of the coated pit is internalized then by the process of endocytosis, and the ligand-receptor complex is found in intracellular endosomes or receptosomes. In many instances the ligand is delivered to lysosomes where it is altered/degraded by proteolysis while the receptor is recycled to the plasma membrane. The Golgi apparatus appears to play a role in ligand-receptor sorting following endocytosis. Some growth factor receptors are degraded in the lysosome with the ligand and do not recycle; the insulin receptor is either recycled or degraded. Endosomal packaging and metabolism of ligands may aid in their intracellular translocation to active sites, such as the nucleus. Peptide fragments formed in lysosomes may possess unique stimulatory properties also. Ultimately, however, the receptor number on the surface of stimulated cells diminishes as internalization progresses. This results in the phenomenon of down-regulation or desensitization with an associated loss of ligand binding and sensitivity of the cells to stimuli.

Some receptors are phosphorylated in response to ligand binding. Receptors to epidermal and platelet-derived growth factors, insulin and somatomedin C, possess intrinsic tyrosine-specific protein kinase activity that on ligand binding autophosphorylates the receptor. The significance of this event for cellular transduction responses is not fully understood. In the case of the β-adrenoceptor, however, desensitization is accompanied by receptor phosphorylation, which seems to affect receptor cycling. Initially, the receptor is uncoupled from adenylate cyclase and lost from the surface of the cell to another membrane environment from which it can be recycled following removal of the agonist (Fig. 15–9). In this desensitization process, a cyclic AMP–dependent protein kinase A and β-adrenergic receptor kinase have been postulated to phosphorylate the liganded β-adrenergic receptor and promote uncoupling from G_s with subsequent internalization of the receptor. Once internalized, the recovery of the β-ad-

Certain receptor-ligand complexes cluster in the plasma membrane and become internalized by endocytosis.

Internalized receptor may either be degraded in lysosomes or be recycled back to the plasma membrane.

Intrinsic protein kinase activity autophosphorylates ligand-bound receptors.

Figure 15-9

Model of the beta-adrenergic receptor internalization. The receptor (R) binds a stimulatory ligand (L) and interacts with a G protein (G_s) and adenylate cyclase. A beta-adrenergic receptor kinase (βARK), and cyclic AMP-dependent protein kinase A (PKA), phosphorylate the receptor, inducing internalization of the phosphorylated receptor. A phosphatase removes the phosphate from the receptor, and the receptor recycles to the plasma membrane. (C = adenylate cyclase.)

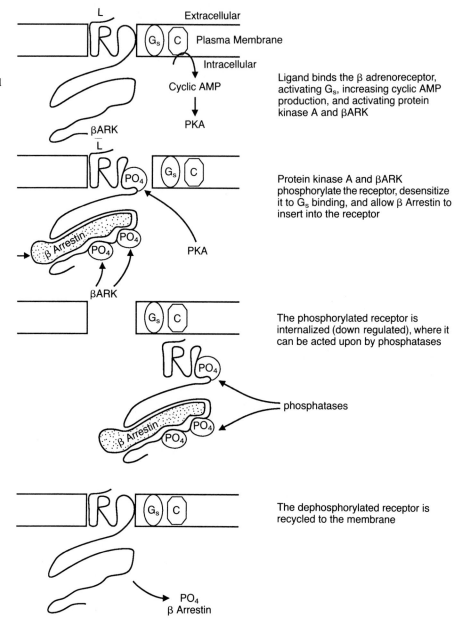

Ligand binds the β adrenoreceptor, activating G_s, increasing cyclic AMP production, and activating protein kinase A and βARK

Protein kinase A and βARK phosphorylate the receptor, desensitize it to G_s binding, and allow β Arrestin to insert into the receptor

The phosphorylated receptor is internalized (down regulated), where it can be acted upon by phosphatases

The dephosphorylated receptor is recycled to the membrane

renergic receptor and cell sensitivity is achieved through phosphatase dephosphorylation of the receptor and return of the receptor to the cell surface.

Hydrophobic Ligand Receptor Mechanisms

In contrast to hydrophilic ligands, hydrophobic molecules, such as steroid and thyroid hormones, pass through the plasma membrane of cells to interact with specific receptor proteins in the cytoplasm or nucleus to initiate cellular response processes. Steroid hormones dissociate from plasma-binding proteins and cross the plasma membrane to enter target cells. Steroid hormone receptors are tissue-specific binding proteins found in low concentrations in the cytoplasm of target cells. When steroid receptors are occupied by ligand they change conformation and become activated with enhanced affinity for nuclear interphase chromatin (Fig. 15-10). The activated hormone-receptor complex accumulates in the nu-

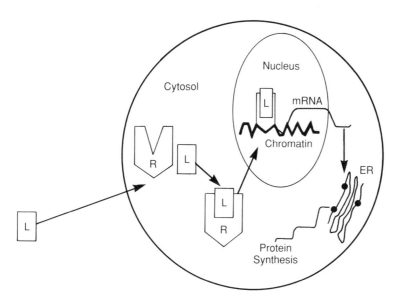

Figure 15 – 10

Model of steroid-receptor activation. The hydrophobic steroid molecule enters the cell and binds to a receptor in the cytoplasm. The hormone-receptor complex enters the nucleus, binds to chromatin, and initiates RNA transcription. The RNA leaves the nucleus to translate protein synthesis and transduce cellular responses. (ER = endoplasmic reticulum; mRNA = messenger RNA.)

cleus bound to chromosomal DNA containing acceptor sites for the complex. The estrogen receptor may deviate from the model for other steroid hormone receptors, because it has been localized to the nuclear fraction in the presence or absence of bound estrogen.

The high-affinity interaction of the steroid-hormone receptor complex with nuclear chromatin results within 30 minutes in DNA transcription and the synthesis of a high molecular weight precursor to messenger RNA. The early activation of nuclear RNA polymerase by steroids results apparently from an increase in the number of initiation sites. How DNA recognizes steroid receptors and responds through the expression of different genes is not known presently. However, polymerase activation patterns may differ in tissues based upon whether steroids induce tissue growth (polymerase I and II activation with rRNA and mRNA synthesis enhanced), as in the long-acting estrogenic response of the uterus, or more transient responses (polymerase II activation and new mRNA synthesis) such as the hypothalamic response to estrogen. When the intervening sequence (intron) RNA is removed, the mature mRNA relocates to the cytoplasm where it attaches to ribosomes and codes for the synthesis of cell-specific proteins mediating the hormonal response. A reduction of the steroid hormone response occurs as cytoplasmic receptor concentration is depleted due to the continued migration of receptor-hormone complex to the nucleus. In addition, fine-tuning of the steroidal response is achieved through the synthesis of certain proteins that either turn off responding genes or turn on secondary response genes, thereby amplifying the initial steroid stimulus.

The receptors for thyroid hormone are also in the nucleus, whether or not hormone is present, associated with the chromatin. Thyroid hormones enter cells and travel to the nucleus; 3,5,3′-triiodothyronine (T_3) rather than thyroxine (T_4) is the predominant ligand possessing physiological activity. Specific mRNAs are under thyroid hormone control, and their translation results in the synthesis of cell proteins. Thyroid hormone may also have some extranuclear sites of action at the plasma membrane or another subcellular organelle. Whether these events are receptor mediated is debated.

Thus, the orchestration of cellular events in response to receptor stimulation is discrete and varied. Responses are discrete in the specialized proteins that must interact with each other in a specialized order for a signal to be

Steroid and thyroid hormones pass through the plasma membrane and interact with specific receptor proteins in the cytoplasm or nucleus.

The early activation of nuclear RNA polymerase by steroid receptors results from an increase in the number of initiation sites.

mRNA relocation to the cytoplasm codes for the synthesis of cell-specific proteins mediating the hormonal response.

Thyroid hormone receptors are in the nucleus associated with chromatin.

Summary

transduced into the cell. However, the wide diversity among tissues having cellular responses characteristic of their unique natures dictates an almost infinite variety of second messenger systems and their interactions that are responsible for eliciting a vast array of physiological responses.

References

Berridge MJ: Inositol trisphosphate, calcium, lithium, and cell signaling. JAMA 262:1834–1841, 1989.

Gilman AG: G proteins and regulation of adenylyl cyclase. JAMA 262:1819–1825, 1989.

Poste G, Crooke ST (eds): Mechanisms of Receptor Regulation. New York: Plenum Press, 1985.

Strange PG: The structure and mechanism of neurotransmitter receptors. Biochem J 249:309–318, 1988.

General Anesthesia and General Anesthetics

16

Cedric M. Smith

The idea of a state of reversible suspension of awareness and pain that permitted surgery on the living body is as old as Genesis, "And God caused a deep sleep to fall on Adam . . . ", and alterations in consciousness have been produced and discussed throughout the ages. Alcoholic intoxication to the point of stupor and coma was and is commonplace in many societies. Casual social experimentation with a variety of intoxicants, including alcohol, nitrous oxide, and ether, as well as opiates, occurred in the 1800s. Sir Humphrey Davy, one of the prominent scientists exploring the properties of nitrous oxide, suggested in the early part of the nineteenth century that it might prove useful in medicine. Crawford W. Long, a rural practitioner in Georgia who had witnessed the effects of ether during "ether frolics," was the first to use ether for surgery to incise a boil. Most of the observations and suggestions for treatments to reduce the pain and suffering of surgery, which even included animal experiments with carbon dioxide, essentially went unpublicized and unnoticed.

The first explicit attempt at what was to be called *anesthesia,* the use of nitrous oxide for surgery, was deemed unsuccessful even though it had clearly been effective in preventing the pain of tooth extractions. Thus, it was not until October, 1846, four years after Crawford Long had used it to incise a boil that medical student and sometime dentist, William T.G. Morton, convincingly demonstrated to a small skeptical medical audience that inhalation of the pungent vapors from a secret substance, later revealed to be ether, could produce such a profound sleep that the surgical removal of a tumor of the jaw was accomplished without pain or struggling.

Although perhaps the most celebrated event in medical history, memorialized with the "ether dome" at Massachusetts General Hospital, the magic of anesthesia was born amid controversy. Each of the principals involved directly or indirectly sought to claim credit and reap financial benefits. In the years following the discovery of ether a large variety of agents were tested and within a few years chloroform and nitrous oxide were added to the list of practical agents. During the mid-1900s with the development of accurate and reliable gas machines, a number of gases (notably cyclopropane and ethylene) were introduced. Although quite effective, their use was associated with rare, but catastrophic, explosions and fires.

It was not until nearly 100 years after the demonstration of the effects of ether that nonflammable fluorinated derivatives—halothane, enflurane, isoflurane, and others—had been studied sufficiently for their introduction into clinical medicine. In spite of the passage of many years and extensive investigations, the two agents first discovered, ether and nitrous oxide, remain in some use. Nitrous oxide continues to be extensively employed and ether continues to serve as the type agent against which other anesthetics are compared. Although slow in onset and recovery, and relatively unpleasant to receive or administer, ether is still probably the safest, from the standpoint of the patient, of all general anesthetics.

For the modern use of the words *anesthesia* and *anesthetics* we are indebted to Oliver Wendell Holmes, who is perhaps most well known (and frequently misquoted) for his denunciation of the medicines and their use in his time:

> Throw out opium, which the Creator himself seems to prescribe, for we often see the scarlet poppy growing in the cornfields, as if it were foreseen that wherever there is hunger to be fed there must also be pain to be soothed; throw out a few specifics which our art did not discover, and is hardly needed to apply; throw out wine, which as a food, and vapors which produce the miracle of anesthesia, and I firmly believe that if the whole *materia medica, as now used,* could be sunk to the bottom of the sea, it would be all the better for mankind—and all the worse for the fishes.

OW HOLMES: ADDRESS TO THE MASSACHUSETTS MEDICAL SOCIETY, MAY 30, 1860

Note that he did not "throw out" opium, wine, and the vapors that "produce the miracle of anesthesia" and a few "specifics" for the betterment of mankind.

Definition

Anesthesia is the unique condition of reversible unconsciousness and absence of response to otherwise painful stimuli. This is the condition produced by certain chemical substances that have been called anesthetics.

The condition of anesthesia is characterized basically by four reversible actions: unconsciousness (or unawareness), analgesia, immobility permitting surgical procedures, and, upon recovery, amnesia. In addition, anesthesia has come to encompass a wider scope. Literally, anesthesia means loss of feeling or sensation. At one extreme, it can be viewed as a neural phenomenon reflecting specific changes in the neuronal systems of the brain and peripheral nervous system; at the other extreme, it is a unique behavioral state of nonresponsiveness to many stimuli that would otherwise produce excitation or flight. By context, anesthesia refers also to the medical specialty and the practice of anesthesiology.

Because the state of anesthesia is one in which the individual has lost the ability to respond to and remember major changes in sensory inputs, it renders the individual helpless; thus, it requires continuous, minute-by-minute care by others.

Essential to understanding anesthesia is the recognition of its reversibility. It is critical that there should be no sustained or significant impairment of cardiovascular or respiratory functions, especially those supplying the brain and other vital organs with adequate blood, nutrients, and gases.

Although intoxication by alcohol and other substances had been known since the dawn of human history, the utility of such conditions in forms that were controllable and readily reversible was not generally recognized until after the introduction of ether. Most of the major anesthetic agents in current use (Table 16–1) have been introduced into medicine only recently. Their development and practical use in anesthetic practice became feasible only with the invention of sophisticated techniques and the machinery for handling and delivery of the anesthetic gases. Essential to the development of modern anesthesia and surgery were instruments for measuring the effects of anesthesia; ways to measure precisely the amounts and delivery of gases and the anesthetic agent; knowledge and the scientific investigation of the optimal methods for the delivery of anesthetics; and adjunct medications that make the anesthetic and surgical procedures

Table 16-1 GENERAL ANESTHETICS CURRENTLY IN USE

Administered by Inhalation	Boiling Point (°C)	Minimal Anesthetic Concentration (MAC)	Water/Gas Partition Coefficient	Oil/Gas Partition Coefficient
Nitrous oxide — N_2O	Gas	101%*	0.39	1.3
Halothane (Fluothane) ($CF_3CHBrCl$)	50	0.77%	0.63	197.0
Enflurane (Ethrane) (CHF_2—O—CF_2—CHFCl)	57	1.68%	0.78	96.5
Isoflurane (Forane) (CHF_2—O—$CHClCF_3$)	48	1.15%	0.54	90.8

* MAC not reached alone with concentrations that cannot safely exceed 80% with the remaining 20% devoted to oxygen. However, larger amounts can be achieved using hyperbaric chambers, and under such conditions nitrous oxide can produce the defined minimal anesthesia required for the MAC.

Administered Intravenously

Barbiturates
   Thiopental (Pentothal)
   Methohexital (Brevital)
Benzodiazepines
   Diazepam (Valium)
   Midazolam (Versed)
Propofol (Diprivan)
Ketamine (Ketalar)

feasible. The advances in anesthesia and anesthetic techniques have paralleled the remarkable progress in surgical techniques and improvements in pre- and postoperative care.

Explanations of the actions of anesthetics ultimately require defining the relationships among their molecular actions on single nerve cells, their actions on synaptic transmissions, and the ultimate changes in functions and behavior of the whole individual. It is the functional interactions among the various intervening levels of neural organizations that constitute the explanatory power of theories and explanations of anesthesia.

It is implied frequently that because the agents are termed *general anesthetics* they act generally on nervous tissue. Although this has partial validity, it is in no way an accurate reflection of the actual situation. General anesthetics produce a state affecting overall body function, but in anesthetic concentrations they do not produce detectable generalized effects on all nerves or all nerve cell membranes. Thus, the state of anesthesia is directly and specifically a selective state in which certain functions, such as those of the respiratory and cardiovascular systems, remain functionally adequate while the systems of memory, sensation, and volitional movement are depressed. Only in lethal concentrations of anesthetics is there a generalized effect of these agents on the majority of membranes of central neurons. Thus, explanations of anesthesia involve the description of the selectivity and the spectrum of actions of each of the anesthetic agents. It is recognized that such a description is a tall task because it does, in fact, pose major questions of physiology and psychology and even philosophy, inasmuch as the agents affect consciousness, memory, pain, anxiety, and volition. The explanation of anesthesia, of necessity, involves an understanding of the neuronal and the molecular bases of these biological functions.

Mechanisms of Action of Anesthetics

General anesthetics have effects on general body functions of volition and cognition, but general anesthetics do not act generally.

DOSE- AND CONCENTRATION-DEPENDENT EFFECTS

Every general anesthesia can be viewed as a unique determination of the relationship between concentration (dose) of the anesthetic and the response of that individual.

General anesthesia and the process by which it is observed are analogous to a concentration or dose-response study in a single individual inasmuch as the inhalation of the anesthetic gas mixture exposes the relevant portions of the brain to progressively increasing concentrations over time. Because only a finite amount can be taken up by blood within a given respiratory cycle, each breath results in the incorporation of a certain amount of anesthetic into the blood stream, which is then distributed to tissues such as the brain. The rates at which the uptakes and the increases in brain concentration occur vary with the concentration in the inhaled mixture, the physical properties of the agent, and the blood flow through the lungs and to the brain. In any event, the concentration in blood and in the tissues rises progressively with continuing inhalation of the anesthetic mixture, until eventually a relatively steady state, with little net uptake or excretion, is obtained. Theoretically at least, the steady state is characterized by equal partial pressures in all tissue compartments of the body and in the alveolar gas.

Steady state of an anesthetic is defined as no net change in concentrations of the anesthetic agent in tissues over time.

At any given time following the beginning of such inhalation, the condition of the individual can be assessed and correlated with the level of the anesthetic in the blood and, more importantly, correlated with the concentration of the anesthetic in the nervous tissue. For many of the general anesthetics this is a relatively simple relationship, because the anesthetic agent does not bind strongly to any of the tissues and is distributed predictably according to the physical properties of the agent (largely its solubilities in various tissues) and the biological systems with which it interacts. Thus, the anesthetic effects can be related to the concentration of the anesthetic in a tissue and, therefore, describes a dose- or concentration-related relationship. Not only is it possible to measure the intensity of anesthetic effects; there are qualitatively different actions associated with different levels of anesthesia. In the usual anesthetic situation, both time and amount of anesthetic vary concurrently; the longer after the anesthetic is introduced, the higher is its level in tissues. It is also customary to speak of the level of anesthesia as *light* or *deep,* light being that degree of anesthesia that is associated with low concentrations of anesthetics, especially in relation to the onset of anesthesia. Deep levels of anesthesia refer to the effects of high concentrations of anesthetic in the tissues usually only reached after many minutes of breathing the anesthetic agent.

STAGES AND PLANES OF ANESTHESIA

Although outmoded clinically, the use of *stages* and *planes* of anesthesia to describe the levels and progression of anesthesia produced by diethyl ether proved to be conceptually and practically useful. These stages and planes, with planes dividing the different stages into substages, were introduced by Guedel largely as a teaching tool for training anesthesiologists and technicians at the time of World War I (Guedel, 1937). It is not important for medical students to know specifically what the definitions of stages and planes of anesthesia are with ether, because both the stages and planes are obsolete *per se* and diethyl ether is an obsolete anesthetic agent. Yet the concepts of stages and planes still have significant utility in teaching; many teachers, the author included, reintroduced them in their teaching after abandoning them, because it appeared that students' understanding of anesthesia was enhanced by having them as a background for the consideration of the other anesthetic agents. This description of the stages and planes of anesthesia is included strictly for reference and to illustrate that such explicit descriptions, as exemplified by the stages and planes of ether anesthesia, have the potential to characterize the anesthetic syndrome produced by any specific anesthetic.

The introduction of a 5–10% concentration of ether *gas* into the inspired gas mixture causes irritation of mucous membranes, and a common response is breath-holding, both voluntary as well as involuntary. Eventually, the individual takes a breath and inhales the gas mixture; over some minutes of continued breathing, the individual experiences changes in subjective feelings similar to intoxication by alcohol, with lightheadedness; some euphoria; and characteristically, the development of analgesia for otherwise painful skin incisions. If sufficient levels of ether in the brain are achieved with continued breathing, the individual experiences sleepiness and, eventually, loss of consciousness. This loss of consciousness, in the classic description, marks the transition from Stage I to Stage II of ether anesthesia; thus, low levels of ether, Stage I, are characterized by analgesia, loss of consciousness, and upon wakening, amnesia for at least a portion of the time during and immediately prior to the apparent loss of consciousness.

With continued inhalation of ether there supervenes a period of heightened reflex responses and involuntary movements and actions that may include vomiting, thrashing about, fluctuating respiration and blood pressure, fighting, and struggling. This is Stage II of ether anesthesia and has been referred to as the Stage of Delirium or the Stage of Excitement. The individual is amnesic for the entire event. The usual management of Stage II is to minimize the excitation and to move as quickly and smoothly as possible from that stage of anesthesia to the next stage, which is referred to as Stage III, or Surgical Anesthesia.

Stage III, Surgical Anesthesia, with ether is marked by the onset of almost automatically regular respiration with full deep inspiration and expiration. During surgical anesthesia, with the increasing concentrations of ether in the blood and brain, there occurs a progressive depression and modification of a variety of autonomic functions as well as reflex responses, including movement of the eyes; muscle tone of the extremities and of the abdomen; and changes in the reflex responses to skin stimulation, to traction of the mesentery, and to stimulation of the bronchi. Within the stage of surgical anesthesia a series of planes are defined, each of which is characterized by the presence or absence of specific reflexes. These planes serve as a guide to what surgical procedures could be done effectively and what would be the predictable reflex consequences.

The stages and planes of ether anesthesia were reproducible and readily learned.

The onset of the terminal stage of ether anesthesia, Stage IV, is denoted by the cessation of respiration due to the anesthetic (i.e., not due to hyperventilation or other changes in respiratory drive) in the face of an adequate cardiovascular function in terms of blood pressure, heart rate, and general cardiovascular status. Although cardiac output has been shown to be reduced significantly in Stage IV, blood pressure remains at normal levels, and cardiac function in Stage IV of ether anesthesia is adequate to maintain blood pressure and life. With maintenance of adequate artificial respiration, recovery can be readily reinitiated following complete respiratory arrest. Such recovery after respiratory arrest due to ether can be dramatically produced simply by discontinuing the ether and respiring the individual with oxygen for a few breaths; spontaneous respiration usually appears within a minute.

Modes and Sites of Action of General Anesthetics

The condition of anesthesia may well be the consequence of more than one mechanism of action.

Numerous neural sites are acted on in anesthesia by anesthetics.

How is it that simple chemical substances can be inhaled, not be metabolized, not be bound to tissue, and excreted quantitatively through pulmonary expiration, yet can affect the brain in such a profound and selective fashion? The fact of ready reversibility, and the absence of metabolism or any obvious tissue binding, gave rise to what can be called "general theories of general anesthesia"; it was thought that the agents acted nonspecifically and generalized to produce a change in the physicochemical processes of nerve membranes.

It is probable that anesthetics produce the analgesia and amnesia that permit surgery by more than one ultimate molecular mechanism. The minimal requisites for prevention of excessive suffering in surgery and anesthesia include an appropriate change in consciousness and decreases in reflex responses that permit the surgeon to carry out the desired procedures.

The potential sites of anesthetic actions can be viewed along a number of different dimensions and at different levels of neural integration, including:

- molecular and submolecular: interactions between anesthetic and subcellular components such as membranes, receptors, receptor systems, intracellular messengers, mitochondria, or various enzymes
- cellular: actions of anesthetics on neurons and neuronal nervous tissue elements, e.g., on membrane potential and ionic fluxes
- intercellular and synaptic: influence of anesthetic on excitatory and inhibitory neuronal interactions
- functional neural networks: anesthetic effects on systems such as those involved in sleep, in analgesia, in memory, in consciousness, and in the production of organized nervous activity, such as that measured by the electroencephalogram (EEG)

(The functional state characteristic of anesthesia and a condition that permits operations can be produced by a number of different agents and also by the lack of oxygen; hypoxia rapidly produces unconsciousness. Unfortunately, hypoxia is difficult to control and has a large number of extremely detrimental effects on human functioning and as such is rarely employed purposely. Cerebral concussion by a blow can also produce a state of unconsciousness and amnesia that would permit surgical procedures, but the inability to control the intensity, plus the likelihood of permanent damage, is such that it is not practical.

Prior to the discovery of anesthetic agents such as ether, surgical procedures were commonly undertaken in individuals who had received large amounts of an alcoholic beverage. Indeed, ethyl alcohol (ethanol) can produce a condition of amnesia, unconsciousness or obtunded consciousness, and an appreciable analgesia (the latter due in part to the release of endorphins), but it has a narrow margin of safety and large doses are poorly reversible. In addition, it was known early in the history of the development of anesthesia that carbon dioxide itself in high concentrations not only could produce a seizure-like behavior in animals, it also could produce an anesthetic state during which surgery could be performed. Also, certain steroids are among the agents that are known to produce conditions similar to anesthesia; the most well-studied steroids are structurally related to progesterone. One such steroid anesthetic has been on the market for a number of years, although it has never found wide clinical use.)

Table 16–2 presents an overview of the various neural sites and mechanisms possibly responsible for anesthesia. Note that different categories within the table are not mutually exclusive and, in fact, an anesthetic could both produce changes on nerve membranes and have selective effects on the cerebral cortex.

It is noteworthy that although the table is extensive, it is not complete; many of the potential sites for anesthesia have yet to be examined experimentally, and all the potential mechanisms have yet to be examined for each of the various sites. In fact, relatively few neuronal systems, synaptic systems, or neuronal sites in the nervous system have been assessed explicitly and quantitatively for the effects of anesthetic agents. Furthermore, although it is stated frequently that the anesthetics act by virtue of their

---

Table 16–2 SITES AND MECHANISMS OF ACTION OF GENERAL ANESTHETICS

(A partial integration of actions across systems)

I. Neuronal systems selectively influenced by general anesthetics (by function):
 Consciousness
   —Cerebral cortex
   —Reticular and other ascending activating systems
   —EEGs reveal at least two classes of anesthetics: one exemplified by halothane (chloroform and trichloroethylene), and another that includes nitrous oxide, diethyl ether, and cyclopropane
 Memory/amnesia
   —Cerebral cortex, hippocampus, amygdala
 Analgesia/pain perception
   —Descending pain modulating systems, midbrain periaqueductal gray matter, spinal cord dosal horn gray matter (endorphin release after nitrous oxide, ethanol)
II. Neuronal systems functionally impaired by higher concentrations of most general anesthetics:
 Respiration
   —Respiratory centers; carotid chemoreceptors by halothane, enflurane
 Blood pressure
   —Hypothalamic center control of cardiovascular system by way of autonomic outflow
 Skeletal muscle movement and tone
   —Cerebellum, midbrain, basal ganglia, cerebral cortical systems involved in initiation of movement, spinal cord
III. Synaptic processes potentially affected by general anesthetics:
   —Transmitter synthesis
   —Transmitter release—halothane (cerebral cortex)
   —Transmitter metabolism
   —Postsynaptic effects:
     Augmentation of inhibition
     Augmented or prolonged presynaptic inhibition (benzodiazepines, barbiturates, ethanol, ether)
     Augmented endorphin release (nitrous oxide and possibly ether, but not halothane)
     Augmented GABA-induced inhibition
   —Depression of transmitter-induced postsynaptic excitation (All inhalation anesthetics in high concentrations as well as barbituates, ethanol)
   —Alteration of neurotransmitter receptor proteins (demonstrated to date with an acetylcholine receptor); anesthetics cause desensitization of the receptor and accelerated closing of the ion channels associated with the receptor (other receptor systems and proteins are likely to be affected by anesthetics)
IV. Direct effects on neurons:
 Depression of membrane excitability, decrease in sodium conductance, possibly the consequence of increased membrane thickness/volume, increased fluidity of membranes
   —Hyperpolarization of small fibers in the cerebral cortex
   —Intracellular components: mitochondria oxidative systems depressed (hypoxia produces unconsciousness, hypoxia and anesthetics are additive or synergistic in actions); calcium-mediated mitochondrial functions are depressed by anesthetics
   —General anesthetics are localized selectively to lipids and hydrophobic regions of proteins; anesthetic potencies are correlated with lipid solubility as well as hyperpolarization of small fibers
V. Outline of differential actions of various general anesthetics:
   —Markedly different chemical structures and physical properties, some actions appear to be *receptor-mediated*, whereas for others the receptors not readily identified
   —Different EEGs with different agents
   —Different margins of safety and spectra of neural actions
   —Differential sensitivities of various synaptic and neural systems to different agents
   —Differential genetically determined sensitivities among agents
   —Genetic influences occur as demonstrated in mice, *Drosophila*, and nematodes

presence in the nervous system, there have been no systematic measurements of the actual concentrations of different anesthetics in the various parts of the brain. (This is in striking contrast to the studies of many other drugs in which it is standard procedure to investigate the concentrations in particular tissues and to express the overt effects in relation to such concentrations. This is a pertinent area of investigation for anesthetics but it has not, for the most part, been addressed.)

A useful way of examining the effects of the anesthetics is to ask, "What are the major effects observed and what are the neuronal sites and systems that are associated with the functional deficit or change in function induced by the anesthetic agent?"

With respect to *consciousness*, the loss of consciousness is obviously a cerebral cortical function influenced by a variety of neuronal activating systems. The most extensively studied and understood is that of the activating system originating in the midbrain reticular system whose anterior elaboration innervates the entire cerebral cortex. Activation of this reticular system is associated with awakening and an alerting shift toward low-voltage, high-frequency activity in the EEG. It has been well established that anesthetic agents, such as barbiturates and ether, selectively depress the activation of the cerebral cortex induced by sensory stimulation or by stimulation of the reticular activating system; this depression of the activating response occurs after amounts of anesthetics that produce directly only small alterations in cerebral cortical functions. This anesthetic-induced depression of the reticular system is correlated temporally with the depression of consciousness and the induction of sleep.

With respect to *memory* and *amnesia*, it is probable that the anesthetic agents act on the cerebral cortex, on the hippocampus, and on the amygdala, systems known to be involved in memory.

Another cardinal sign of anesthesia is the production of *analgesia*, the depression of the response to pain, its perception, and the reflex consequences induced by nociceptive stimulation (nociceptive refers to pain-producing). The analgesia probably results from actions at a number of different sites. With certain anesthetic agents — nitrous oxide, ethanol, and probably ether — there is a modulation in pain responses involving endorphin release that probably originates from, among other areas, the midbrain periaqueductal gray matter. It is also plausible that the analgesia is the consequence of direct effects of the anesthetic on the midbrain and hypothalamus as well as the cerebral cortex.

The electrical activity of the cerebral cortex, as recorded with an EEG, provides direct information about the effects of anesthetic agents. Not only does the qualitative and quantitative nature of the electrocortical effects reflect different levels of anesthesia, they vary with the anesthetic agent and with the individual's unique encephalographic pattern.

> EEG patterns reflect not only the state of consciousness but also the patterns of sensory input and effects of drug actions; they are as individually unique as fingerprints.

It has been shown, nevertheless, that the electroencephalographic changes during anesthesia do allow the categorization of the anesthetics into at least two major classes. One of these groups is exemplified by halothane anesthesia, which is associated with a rather quiet EEG with an absence of high-voltage, fast activity, leaving only rather low-voltage slow waves. Patterns similar to those observed after halothane are obtained also with methoxyflurane, chloroform, and trichlorethylene.

Another group, exemplified by ether, cyclopropane, and nitrous oxide, produce an active EEG consisting of fast activity that decreases during anesthesia to be replaced by relatively high-voltage slow waves. These differences in the EEG among anesthetic agents are not intrinsically of much import, but the fact that they vary with level of anesthesia and are unique for different agents clearly demonstrates that different general anesthetics have distinguishing neuronal actions. The different EEGs reflect different patterns of electrical activity in the cortex and in the neuronal input to the cortex; therefore, they, at least in part, must have different sites or mechanisms of action.

Not only do the anesthetics have different effects on large populations of neurons, they also have been shown to have different direct effects on the individual neurons themselves (see Table 16–2).

SYNAPTIC SYSTEMS AS A SITE OF ACTION

The functioning of the nervous system intrinsically involves the synaptic connections between neurons. Anesthetic agents act to disrupt selectively such synaptic transmission. Both neuron cell bodies and axons tend to be less influenced by the anesthetics than are synapses. Moreover, it has been a general observation that the more complicated and complex the synaptic and neuronal arrangement, the more susceptible the system is to disruption by anesthesia. For example, thought processes, muscular coordination, and alertness appear to be more sensitive to anesthetics than are simple reflexes or respiration.

Although it is feasible to determine the effects of anesthetics on the various neurotransmitter systems, most of these have received little research attention. In general, in concentrations required for clinical anesthesia, anesthetics do not alter the biochemical synthesis of most of the different neurotransmitters. On the other hand, the release of neurotransmitters can be reduced by anesthetics; at least one of the anesthetic agents, halothane, does reduce the transmitter released with a given stimulus as measured in one neuronal system in the cerebral cortex. Whether it has such an effect on transmitter metabolism or on the termination of action of other transmitters remain open questions (see Table 16–2).

In contrast to presynaptic systems, the postsynaptic actions of anesthetics have been studied in a number of preparations. One of the more important synaptic effects of anesthetics so far discovered is the augmentation of a specific type of inhibition between neurons — presynaptic inhibition. This augmentation of presynaptic inhibition has been demonstrated for a number of agents, including benzodiazepines, barbiturates, ethanol, and ether. Receiving greatest attention has been the gamma-aminobutyric acid (GABA)–mediated presynaptic inhibition that is potentiated by all of these anesthetic agents. Not only are anesthetic agents such as benzodiazepines and barbiturates known to affect GABA-mediated presynaptic inhibitory systems, they have been elegantly shown to directly affect different parts of the GABA-receptor complex, all with the end result of augmented presynaptic inhibition.

> Augmentation of inhibitory neuronal systems is a likely primary mechanism of anesthesia; effects on GABA-receptor systems are probably involved.

Only more recently have the effects of inhalation anesthetics (halothane, isoflurane, enflurane) on GABA-receptor systems been investigated with the finding that concentrations that are associated with surgical anesthesia markedly potentiate neuronal membrane currents produced by GABA. Although the effects on such currents are complex, it was suggested that the primary action of these inhalation anesthetics is to potentiate the GABA-receptor channel response (to GABA) (Nakahiro et al, 1989).

These effects of anesthetics on GABA systems are consistent with the observations of anesthetic-induced increases in inhibitory synaptic potentials observed in the hippocampus, spinal cord, and other neural sites.

Another example of a postsynaptic effect is the release of endogenous endorphins that can explain at least a part of the analgesia produced by nitrous oxide (and perhaps anesthetics such as ether as well as ethanol) even in concentrations insufficient to cause loss of consciousness.

The postsynaptic excitation produced by neurotransmitters is depressed by anesthetics, but this usually requires higher concentrations than for presynaptic action. Whether such postsynaptic effects occur with the concentrations obtained in surgical anesthesia remains uncertain. It seems unlikely that postsynaptic depression is the primary mechanism of action or site of action *of the anesthetic actions* of anesthetics; however, it probably contributes to the widespread neuronal effects of exposure to lethal concentrations. (The acetylcholine [ACh] postsynaptic system has been studied as a model system in recent years; anesthetics have at least two different effects on this postsynaptic receptor system and the receptor protein for ACh. First, they cause an increase in the receptor desensitization process, with desensitization consisting of a decreased affinity of the receptor for its agonist, such as ACh, upon exposure to the agonist. This desensitization is marked by an acceleration of closing of the ACh-activated ion channels associated with the receptor. Each of the various receptor systems is connected with one or more ion channels, and the receptor's function is to modulate the ion channel permeability and its affinity for an agonist and antagonist. Thus, the anesthetics decrease the responsiveness of the isolated ACh receptor by increasing its desensitization and by altering the ion channel associated with that receptor system. It is likely that in the future other receptor systems will be found that can be influenced by anesthetic agents.)

A comprehensive account of anesthesia can be developed only when it is possible to carry out systematic comparative analyses of the sensitivities of the various neuroreceptor systems to anesthetics with reference to the sites that are most selectively affected by the anesthetic agents, and with reference to the nature of these effects on the receptor systems and associated ion channels. Although it is known that the anesthetics have effects on synaptic systems in concentrations obtained clinically, it is not possible to explain the correlation of the effects of the anesthetics on these systems to the altered functions, such as loss of consciousness or pain perception. Present experimentation serves to establish the feasibility of eventually achieving that requisite knowledge.

NERVE MEMBRANE ACTIONS

Neuronal membranes have received most of the attention as possible cellular and subcellular sites of action of anesthetics, because it has been an underlying assumption that the mechanisms of anesthesia must entail a decrease in the electrical activity of at least certain neurons, such as those associated with cortical excitability, consciousness, sleep, and responses to nociceptive stimulation. It has been assumed, and shown in a few instances, that the decrease in neuronal membrane excitability and action potential generation is associated with a decrease in sodium conductance. Also, much attention has been given to the observation that anesthetics applied to isolated membrane preparations produce an increase in membrane thickness or volume, associated with an increased fluidity of the membranes. The theory of anesthetic action involving an increased membrane fluidity implies a decrease in the orderliness of the membrane molecular structure associated both with an increased fluidity and an increased volume. These changes in membrane structure and function by anesthetics may reflect also the same process that results in specific alterations in membrane ionic conductances.

An important effect of general anesthetics is increased membrane potential in small fibers, i.e., hyperpolarization (Fig. 16–1). Although the

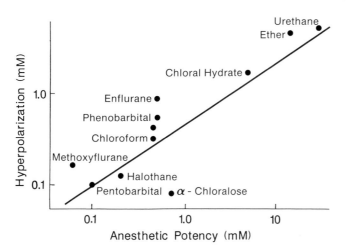

Figure 16–1

Hyperpolarization of spinal motor neurons by general anesthetics. Minimal effective hyperpolarizing concentration (mM) of the anesthetic (ordinate) plotted against the anesthetic potency of the agent (expressed as mM). (Redrawn from Nicoll RA, Madison DV: General anesthetics hyperpolarize neurons in the vertebrate central nervous system. Science 217:1055–1057, 1982. Copyright 1982 by the AAAS.)

cortical neuronal systems have received little research attention because of the technical difficulties of such experiments, such an increase in membrane potential would have profound effects if it occurred over the entire cortex. Such a hyperpolarization change in small fibers may well have been overlooked in the past because of the focus on larger cell bodies that are more accessible for recording. Yet, cerebral cortex function depends on the interaction among millions of small fibers in the neuropile of the cerebral cortex. Thus, such hyperpolarization of cortical nerve branches by anesthetics could explain their actions on cerebral cortical functions.

AN INTRACELLULAR SITE OF ACTION

With respect to intracellular components of neurons, it has long been noted that anesthetics depress mitochondrial oxidation. An analogy with hypoxia is a particularly obvious one. Hypoxia produces unconsciousness, and hypoxia and anesthetics are at least additive in their anesthetic effects. So mitochondria are another plausible site of action of anesthetics. It is known also that calcium is a critical component for mitochondrial function, as well as for the function of many intracellular systems; anesthetics are known to depress some calcium-mediated processes, and the calcium channel blocking agent, verapamil, potentiates anesthesia.

ANESTHESIA IN RELATION TO SOLUBILITY IN LIPIDS

In general, general anesthetics are distributed preferentially to lipids and hydrophobic regions of proteins because of their high lipid solubilities. Anesthetic potency has been long known to be correlated almost directly with lipid solubility (Fig. 16–2). Whether this correlation with lipid solubility, i.e., the partition between oil and water, of anesthetics has any explanatory power as a mechanism of anesthesia still remains to be established. Simply the fact that the anesthetic is present in the lipid phase really only describes its distribution; it does not provide any direct information about the functional significance. On the other hand, it can be theorized that the presence of the anesthetic in the lipid phase or in the hydrophobic regions of membrane proteins will modify the structure and function of those molecular systems. This oil solubility of anesthetics can be correlated also with the membrane-disorganizing effect described earlier. Thus, it is conceivable that the anesthetic is, in fact, dissolved in lipids, hydrophobic regions of proteins, or both, which results in increased disorganization in

Can the correlation of solubility in lipids and anesthetic potency be an explanation of anesthesia?

Figure 16–2

Concentrations of inhalation anesthetics required to produce anesthesia are inversely correlated with their solubilities in lipids. The lower the concentration required, the more potent the agent; thus, the potency of anesthetics is directly correlated with their solubilities in lipids. (Adapted from Strichartz G, Krieger N: Neurobiology of Anesthesia—Supplement to the Grass Calendar for 1988. Quincy, MA: Grass Instrument Co, 1988; and Miller KW: The nature of the site of general anesthesia. Int Rev Neurobiol 27:1–61, 1985, based on data summarized by Janoff and colleagues, on the aqueous concentrations required to abolish the righting reflex in tadpoles plotted against the lipid/aqueous partition coefficient. [Janoff AS, Pringle MJ, Miller KW: Correlation of general anesthetic potency with solubility in membranes. Biochim Biophys Acta 649:125–128, 1981].)

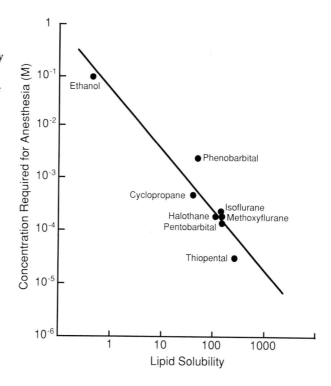

membranes. Although this lipid solubility and the disorganizing effect on membranes may be a molecular basis of anesthetic action, by themselves they fail to provide insight as to origin of the selectivity of action of anesthetic agents that is a hallmark of anesthesia.

Although the correlation between oil solubility and anesthetic potency is true generally, there are two reservations. First, these correlations are approximate ones in terms of how anesthesia potency is actually measured. The measurement of the minimal anesthetic concentration (MAC) (see Table 16–1) is time-dependent, because it is measured conventionally by administering a constant concentration for only 15 minutes. Thus, for those agents with a high solubility in water the kinetics are such that the actual measurement *in vivo* of the MAC is confounded by time. Therefore, the relative oil and water solubilities of the agents in relation to MAC are not fully independent. Secondly, the examination of the points on a graph relating to oil solubility and potency (see Figure 16–2) illustrates that although there is a strong correlation, this is by no means a sharply quantitative one-to-one correlation; there are significant deviations with some substances from an ideal relationship. It is necessary to be aware of this correlation; however, by itself it is insufficient as an explanation for the mechanism of anesthesia.

Organ System Effects of Anesthetics

RESPIRATION

A number of neuronal systems including the *respiratory system* are impaired functionally by higher concentrations of most of the general anesthetics; both rate and depth of respiration are depressed along with a reduction in the reflex responsiveness of the respiratory center to increases in carbon dioxide level and decreases in oxygen tension. Halothane is unique among the anesthetics in that its respiratory depressant effects are due not only to depression of central respiratory centers but also to its effects on the carotid body chemoreceptors. (It and other drugs with effects on sensory receptor systems are discussed in Chapter 26.) This direct depression of carotid chemoreceptors by halothane results in decreased responsiveness of these receptor systems to hypoxia and hypercapnia. It is also one of the mechanisms by which halothane, in moderate concentrations, produces its characteristic depression of respiration, consisting usually of a marked decrease in depth accompanied by an increase in rate.

Among the multiple sites of action of general anesthetics are peripheral chemoreceptors.

All general anesthetics have a small safety margin. A major hazard in any anesthesia (with the possible exception of nitrous oxide given alone) is respiratory and cardiovascular depression that, if not alleviated and reversed quickly, can be fatal. Such ultimately fatal effects may well be due in the end to a generalized effect on many different neuronal elements and many different tissue elements that have in common excitable membranes (e.g., the depression of the rhythmic neuronal activity associated with respiration or depression of the responses of skeletal muscle and autonomic nerves as well as depression of cardiac function). Widespread depression by general anesthetics of any one of the systems just mentioned is life-threatening.

All general anesthetics are potentially lethal.

CARDIOVASCULAR SYSTEM

Cardiovascular functions are influenced by anesthetic agents; a useful generalization is that there is depression of cardiovascular function occurring to some degree during every general anesthesia. Nevertheless, the primary clinical question in anesthesia is the degree of depression of cardiorespiratory functions relative to the operative procedure and the physiological needs of the particular patient. The decreases in cardiac function are due in part to direct effects on the heart such as occur with halothane. They are due also to a decrease in baroreceptor and other cardiovascular reflexes that result from both peripheral and central effects of the anesthetic agents. Depression of the reflexes associated with cardiovascular function is part of the syndrome of general anesthesia. The end result of these actions is a physiological system that can meet basal functional needs while under general anesthesia but whose ability to respond to changes in demand is severely limited.

SKELETAL MUSCLE FUNCTION (OTHER THAN RESPIRATORY)

Skeletal muscle movement and tone are depressed in anesthesia. Movement is limited generally to small movements or none at all, although reflex movements can occur, for example, to sudden otherwise painful stimuli or to muscle stretch. Thus, the initiation of muscle movement is depressed, although not necessarily abolished. The *control* of muscle movement is more markedly depressed than is movement itself, and the cerebellar and spinal cord regulation are reduced significantly. Of particular interest in anesthesia is the degree to which the responses to muscle stretch and the sustained muscle tone are retained. The anesthetic agents differ in the degree to which they produce muscle relaxation relative to depression of other nervous functions. Muscle relaxation is essential for certain surgical procedures, such as an exploratory laparotomy. The extensive use of neuromuscular blocking agents has reduced the need to select the anesthetic agents on the basis of their ability to produce skeletal relaxation. At the present time, the degree of relaxation produced by the anesthetic agents is not critically important inasmuch as whatever relaxation is needed can be provided by the administration of neuromuscular blocking agents.

Genetic and Other Factors Influencing Anesthesia

The susceptibility to, and character of, anesthesia are under a variety of genetic influences. These influences are currently being explored in various model systems. Among *Drosophila* mutants that are used extensively for genetic studies are some that exhibit sensitivity to one anesthetic while they are unaffected by other anesthetics. Such results are not consistent with the concept of a general, uniform molecular mechanism responsible for anesthesia. Rather, it appears that the anesthetic state as defined earlier can possibly result from more than one molecular mechanism or site of action. This idea of more than one mechanism and site of action for anesthesia is consistent with the striking differences of the spectrum of other actions of general anesthetics and the fact that the condition can be produced in reality by a wide variety of diverse molecules ranging from nitrogen under pressure; to nitrous oxide, diethyl ether, carbon dioxide, and ethanol; to a variety of halogenated hydrocarbons, barbiturates, some opioids, benzodiazepines, and even ketamine.

Anesthetic actions are also under a wide variety of other influences, most of which have not received much attention. One of the more prominent ones is the condition of pregnancy. Pregnant women are more susceptible not only to general anesthesia but to local anesthesia than are nonpregnant individuals. In part, the differences in the pregnant individual may be due to the known anesthetic effects of certain steroids, such as progesterone.

Anesthesia is influenced by, among other factors, genetics, pregnancy, anxiety, stress, metabolic rate, and other drugs.

Conditions of stress and anxiety have complex interactions with anesthesia. Undoubtedly anxiety not only alters the susceptibility to agents that produce unconsciousness but clearly modifies pain reflexes and the responses of pain systems. Certain kinds of stress, alone, tend to produce an analgesic state. On the other hand, anxiety by itself tends to decrease the pain threshold and, thus, increase the amount of an analgesic drug required to alleviate a given level of pain.

Other influences on anesthetic needs include increased requirements in the presence of elevated body temperature and a high basal metabolic rate. On the other hand, older patients usually require less anesthetic.

Drug Interactions

Essentially all of the drugs that produce central nervous system (CNS) depression, including anesthetics, are at least additive in their effects with other agents, e.g., opioids, barbiturates, and benzodiazepines. Amphetamines and related compounds, conversely, tend to increase the amount of the anesthetic required for anesthesia. When certain substances are taken chronically, such as alcohol, the anesthetic requirements depend on the level of tolerance and on the time and amount of the last dose. If the last dose was relatively recent there will be an addition with the anesthetic; if a somewhat longer time has elapsed there may be either tolerance to the anesthetic or even antagonism due to increased neuronal excitability resulting from a withdrawal syndrome. Analogous, but of opposite sign, changes appear with chronic administration of amphetamines or cocaine. Administered together with an anesthetic, amphetamines increase the anesthetic requirement, whereas during withdrawal from chronic amphetamine use the individual may be more sensitive to anesthetics.

Onset and Distribution of Inhalational Agents

A diagram of a closed system for administration of inhalational anesthetics is presented in Figure 16–3. Components include a source of the gas and a method of vaporization. The agents are inhaled in the form of gases, not

Circle System

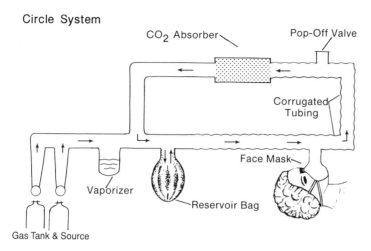

Figure 16-3

A simplified sketch of a closed, "circle" anesthetic system showing the essential components and direction of flow of gases: source, vaporizer for volatile agents, reservoir or rebreathing bag, face mask (or endotracheal tube), and carbon dioxide absorber. Anesthetics and other gases are supplied as gases, and the flow rate of supply equals that stored or metabolized in the body plus that exhaled. The excess, if any, escapes from the pop-off valve or from any loose hosing connection. As the anesthetic and oxygen are administered, they displace the gases present in the body. The displaced nitrogen, especially, then tends to accumulate in the reservoir bag. Thus, it is essential that the bag be emptied and refilled with freshly prepared inhalation mixture a number of times early during the anesthesia administration.

aerosols. Accurate and steadily reliable flow meters are essential, because the concentrations have to be regulated to less than a tenth of 1% in the inhaled gas mixture. Upon initiation of the flow of gases, oxygen and the anesthetic fill the bag and the system, which consists of conductive rubber tubing and noncorrosive connectors. In the closed system shown in Figure 16-3, the patient inhales from the bag and exhales through a carbon dioxide absorber back into the bag. Thus, little of the anesthetic mixture is allowed to escape. It is obvious that the inhaled mixture has to include at least 20% oxygen and preferably more; the maximal anesthetic gas concentration can only be 80%.

The factors that regulate the rates of onset and recovery of anesthesia are presented in Table 16-3. Note that only two of these factors are under, at least potentially, the control of the anesthetist: the composition of the inhaled mixture and the respiratory exchange.

The anesthetic mixture (oxygen and anesthetic) displaces the nitrogen normally present in air and dissolved in body tissues. With continued respiration of the anesthetic the nitrogen concentration in the rebreathing bag rises, diluting the anesthetic mixture. Thus, the anesthetic mixture must be replaced and refreshed periodically, especially during the first few minutes after the introduction of the anesthetic.

Practical matters include ensuring that the anesthetic mixture does not

The anesthesia machinery and its management are as critical to the quality of anesthesia as is the drug.

Table 16-3 FACTORS REGULATING THE RATES OF ONSET AND RECOVERY OF ANESTHESIA

Factors Regulating Rate of Onset of Anesthesia and Differences Among Agents

I. *Respiration* rate, depth, respiratory minute volume probably most important quantitatively
II. *Alveolar membrane-blood translocation* — rapid relative to other processes, in absence of lung pathology
III. *Cardiac output* and functional perfusion of brain and tissue (essential consideration but variations among usual patients and agents are not large)
IV. *Concentration (i.e., partial pressure) of anesthetic* in the inspired mixture
V. *Solubility in blood and tissues* (i.e., solubility in water as measured as blood : gas partition coefficient) — the more soluble in tissues the slower the rate of rise of alveolar blood concentration at any given inhaled concentration

Factors Regulating the Rate of Recovery from Anesthesia

I. All factors involved in *rate of onset* plus the following
II. Solubility in adipose tissues
III. Circulatory perfusion of tissues, especially adipose for potent, highly lipid soluble agents

interact with the soda lime in the carbon dioxide absorber or with the material in the hoses and mask. For example, some anesthetics such as halothane are absorbed extensively by rubber tubing.

In studies of the kinetics of anesthesia, the concept of equilibrium has been important (see Figs. 16–4 and 16–5). In this instance equilibrium refers to the condition in which there is no *net* movement of a gas such as an anesthetic in or out of tissues, blood, or the inhaled mixture. The kinetics of onset and recovery from anesthetics have been studied extensively and mathematically modeled usually *using the following artificially fixed conditions: the composition and concentrations in the inhaled mixture are kept constant; the prime variables measured are the concentrations at the end of inspiration at the time at which there is a steady state between concentration in blood and alveolar gas concentration, i.e., that the partial pressures of the gases in the pulmonary capillaries and within the alveolus are equal,* **expressed as a percent of the concentration achieved at equilibrium;** *variables are analyzed relative to time after the introduction of the specific inhaled mixture.* Comparisons of these kinetics among agents are made as well as correlations of these with other properties, for example, the solubilities of the anesthetics in body tissues.

For all agents the alveolar capillary concentration rises within minutes as the individual inspires the gas mixture containing the anesthetic gas (Fig. 16–4). But after a few minutes with active respiration and competent

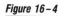

Actual concentrations, rate of changes in concentration, effect, and equilibrium are each *different* variables.

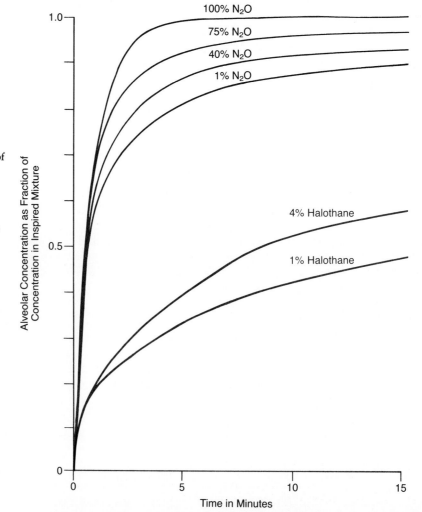

Figure 16–4

The effect of increasing the concentration of an anesthetic in the inspired mixtures (theoretical simulation). Y axis: Alveolar concentration as a *fraction of the concentration in the inspired mixture.* For example, a value of 1.0 is obtained when the partial pressure of anesthetic in blood returning to the alveolus is equal to that in the anesthetic being inspired. For the initial few minutes the *rate* of rise of anesthetic concentration in the alveolus is similar for both agents and different concentrations; this fast increase in concentration reflects primarily the rate at which the anesthetic reaches all the alveolar space. Over time, the differences relating to absolute concentration become apparent.

After 15 minutes of inhalation, the alveolar concentration of halothane, as a correlate of its great solubility in tissues, reaches a level less than half its concentration in the inspired mixture; so long as anesthetic is supplied and adequate respiratory and cardiac functions are maintained, its alveolar concentration will continue to increase gradually over hours until it finally reaches equilibrium with the inspired mixture. (Data from Eger EI: Anesthetic Uptake and Action. Baltimore: Williams & Wilkins, 1974.)

cardiovascular function, significant differences among agents appear with respect to *the rate at which the alveolar capillary concentration approaches the concentration it will obtain at equilibrium.* This final rate at which the alveolar air, in equilibrium with pulmonary capillary blood, reaches equilibrium with the inspired mixture is correlated inversely with the solubility of the gas in tissues (tissues are mostly composed of water). For example, equilibrium with nitrous oxide with a low solubility in tissues (see Table 16–1) is approached quite rapidly, whereas with the more soluble agents the rate at which equilibrium is established is slower. These differences in rate of approach to equilibrium, in relation to tissue solubility, are primarily due to the tremendous tissue reservoir for soluble agents (a large volume of distribution compartment), whereas the capacity of the blood and the cardiovascular system to carry the anesthetic to the tissues is inherently limited.

Because the brain is well perfused by arterial blood and anesthetics readily diffuse into brain tissue, the concentration of an anesthetic gas in the brain closely parallels its arterial concentration. (Theoretically, agents with different solubilities in tissues could be selected for study and example; this is not practical because the only anesthetic with a low blood and tissue solubility [tissue solubility parallels solubility in water] is nitrous oxide. However, this agent has the severe limitation of low potency largely precluding its use for studies of other variables. There are no potent agents in current use that have low tissue solubility comparable to nitrous oxide.)

In spite of the analytical utility of studying kinetics in terms of equilibrium, equilibrium is not actually obtained in practice. Differences among agents with respect to rates of equilibrium between inspired concentration and tissues are of little practical significance because, with the exception of nitrous oxide that is relatively insoluble in tissues and has a rapid rate of equilibrium, the rates of onset of anesthesia can be as rapid as respiration and circulation permit. The use of high concentrations of the potent anesthetics such as halothane in the initiation of anesthesia (higher concentration than needed for maintenance of anesthesia or "over pressure") can more than offset any undesired slowness in the establishment of *equilibrium* (between inhaled gas and tissues), because the critical aspect for anesthesia is the actual *concentration of an anesthetic agent at the neural sites of anesthetic action.* Concentrations in the brain adequate for anesthesia can be achieved within a minute or so of inhalation of any of the inhalation anesthetics if they are given in appropriate concentrations.

Anesthesia involves the minute-by-minute to hour-by-hour adjustments based on the patient's condition. Those agents with high tissue solubilities, in any event, require adjustment of the inhaled mixture as the anesthesia continues. Except for nitrous oxide, all of the inhalation anesthetics in current use are potent and highly soluble in lipids as well as in water and tissues (see Table 16–1 and Fig. 16–2).

The kinetics of anesthetic and other gases are influenced not only by simple respiratory exchange and relative solubilities and related partial pressures but by other factors as well. With the uptake of large volumes of anesthetic, usually nitrous oxide, remaining alveolar gases are concentrated; this *concentration effect* is such that the higher the inspired concentration the more rapid is the relative rise in alveolar concentration. In addition, the *second gas effect* is a phenomenon in which the uptake of large volumes of a first or primary gas (usually nitrous oxide) accelerates the rate of rise of alveolar concentration of a second gas given concomitantly (Eger, 1985). These two effects, the concentration effect and the second gas effect, are important during the first 5–10 minutes of induction.

Distinguish among lipids, lipid phase, body lipids, and adipose tissues.

Figure 16–5

Time course of changes in gas tension in various tissues with the inspiration of nitrous oxide. The gas tension is expressed as a percentage of that in the inspired mixture; 100% would signify equal gas tensions in the tissues and in the inspired mixture, i.e., equilibrium. Note that the concentrations in tissues that have ample blood supply (exemplified by brain, heart, and kidney) are almost the same as in the lung and blood. On the other hand, the tensions in muscle and fat, tissues with much more limited blood flow, lag behind the changes in tensions in blood by minutes to hours. (Modified from Cowles AL, Borgstedt HH, Gillies AJ: Uptake and distribution of inhalation anesthetic agents in clinical practice. Anes Analg 47:404–414, 1968.)

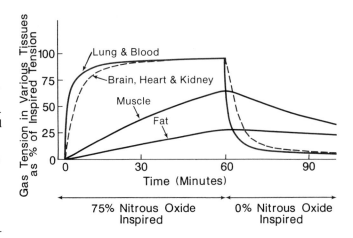

The slow uptakes and release of anesthetics by adipose tissues are due primarily to the low vascular perfusion of adipose tissue.

As anesthesia proceeds, the concentrations of anesthetics in poorly perfused tissues tend to rise slowly. Thus, adipose tissues, which can constitute 20% to 80% of body weight, generally have poor circulation and accumulate anesthetic agents over time; the longer the anesthetic is administered, the greater is the concentration in body lipids. Moreover, the more that is dissolved in lipids, the slower is the overall recovery from the anesthetic (Fig. 16–5). Thus, the more fat-soluble the anesthetic, the fatter the patient, and the longer the anesthesia, the more prolonged is the elimination of the anesthetic and the recovery. For example, halothane's solubility in fat is some 200 times its solubility in water; and the proportion present in fat (at equilibrium) would be more than 95% of the total anesthetic present in the entire body.

Present and Future Practice of Anesthesia and Surgery

For decades general anesthesia commonly was a major life event that took place exclusively in a general hospital, where the individual was in the hospital for one or more days prior to the surgery and was retained in the hospital for days following. This stereotype is out of date. At the present time there are a wide variety of procedures and techniques that permit surgical interventions. Only few of these fit under the category of general anesthesia. Many different kinds of procedures that have been carried out in the past using general anesthesia are currently undertaken using other techniques, such as mixed anesthesia with barbiturates. So-called conscious sedation procedures using a benzodiazepine in combination with local anesthesia or short-lasting opiates are now routine for minor surgery such as tooth extractions or endoscopy. These amnesia, tranquilization, analgesia, and sedation procedures now far outnumber those that employ the more classic general anesthesia using a general anesthetic agent in combination with the two to ten additional drugs commonly used as adjuncts. Thus, there is a range of drug-induced facilitation of surgical procedures that extends from no anesthesia to mild analgesia, antianxiety medication, opioid analgesia, opioid/local anesthesia, amnesic/sedation medication, to small or large amounts of a general anesthetic.

Specific Anesthetics

The agents discussed in this section start with those that are gases at standard temperature and atmospheric pressure, followed by the volatile liquids. In each section the agents currently in use are presented first, followed by substances that are currently clinically obsolete but that have had extensive use in the past.

GAS INHALATION ANESTHETICS

Nitrous Oxide

Actions. Nitrous oxide is available as a medical gas in tanks under pressure. It is nonflammable (but supports combustion in the same way as oxygen) and essentially odorless; it lacks any irritating qualities. The major drawback of nitrous oxide is its lack of potency. By itself in most individuals it can produce intoxication, analgesia, and amnesia. But it does not produce, given alone with at least 20% oxygen, either complete unconsciousness or surgical anesthesia (see Table 16–1).

Nitrous oxide is administered using a gas machine with the concentration monitored by the use of accurately calibrated flow meters, in combination with at least 20% oxygen in the inhalation mixture.

In view of the critical need to maintain a high level of oxygen as well as nitrous oxide, rebreathing is limited. Scavenging any nitrous oxide released into the operating room atmosphere is of critical importance; this has taken on added interest with the recent recognition of the toxic effects to operating room personnel exposed chronically to low levels of nitrous oxide.

The subjective effects of nitrous oxide alone are usually reported as pleasant with euphoria and a sense of well-being frequently accompanied by fantasies. Emotional liability is present and may be manifested, for example, by uncontrollable laughing ("laughing gas") or crying. The subjective effects are described commonly as similar to intoxication with ethyl alcohol.

Analgesia can be observed with inhaled concentrations as low as 20%; larger concentrations produce profound analgesia, an analgesia that is potentially equivalent in intensity to that obtainable with large doses of morphine.

In addition to analgesia, nitrous oxide produces a marked amnesia for the events taking place while exposed to the agent. This amnesia is frequently not explicitly recognized by the subject, but is obviously a desirable aspect of nitrous oxide when it is used for either its analgesic or anesthetic effects.

Because of the limited potency of nitrous oxide it is almost always combined with other CNS depressants: anesthetics, sedatives, opioids, or antianxiety agents, e.g., thiopental, morphine, or diazepam.

Kinetics and Time Course of Action. The effects of nitrous oxide are extremely rapid in onset, within a few circulation times, and there is an equally rapid rate of recovery. In correlation with its low solubility in blood and tissues, equilibrium between the concentration in the inhaled mixture and the concentration in body tissues is reached within a few minutes (see Fig. 16–5).

Organ System Effects. By itself in concentrations up to 80% in the inhaled mixture, nitrous oxide has only slight effects on the cardiovascular system, respiration, or skeletal muscle tone. When combined with other agents, such as thiopental, nitrous oxide can contribute to the respiratory depression.

Toxicities and Side Effects of Nitrous Oxide. Acute toxicity of nitrous oxide is of relevance almost exclusively as a hazard of inadvertent exposure or of nonmedical self-administration. The subjective effects, as noted earlier, may be quite enjoyable or reinforcing to repeated use. The major *acute* hazards of such exposure as an anesthetic or in its nonmedical use consist of altered judgment, confusion or loss of consciousness, decrease of pain perception, and minor to profound amnesia. When self-administered the confusion, impaired judgment, plus possible concomitant hypoxia, have resulted in tragic accidental deaths; death is commonly due to suffocation associated with rebreathing from a plastic or paper bag to the point of unconsciousness (see Chapter 67). Homemade nitrous oxide presents the additional hazard of the probable presence of the highly toxic contaminants, nitrogen dioxide and nitrogen oxide.

Chronic Toxicity. Chronic toxicity associated with repeated exposure in the operating room setting or repeated nonmedical use consists of bone marrow suppression, blood dyscrasias, peripheral neuropathy, increased rate of spontaneous abortion, deficits in cell-mediated immunity, and inactivation of methionine synthetase. The inactivation of methionine synthetase is associated with impaired folate uptake, and recovery requires folic acid. Chronic exposure to nitrous oxide results in inactivation of vitamin B_{12} and clinical signs of cobalamin deficiency.

OBSOLETE GAS ANESTHETICS

Cyclopropane

Cyclopropane is an explosive, odorless, flammable, potent anesthetic that had wide popularity in recent decades; its extensive use declined abruptly after the introduction of and sufficient experience with halothane. Cyclopropane produces a rapid anesthesia with smooth onset and a rapid recovery with some analgesia prior to the onset of unconsciousness. The signs of anesthesia are similar to those with ether but with less dramatic and marked changes over the range of clinically used concentrations. Nevertheless, delirium could appear with cyclopropane. The major reason for the discontinuation of interest in cyclopropane is its flammability and explosiveness.

Ethylene

Ethylene is only of historical interest. It is a potent, rapidly reversible, unpleasant-smelling anesthetic that frequently produces nausea and vomiting. Its most restricting properties are its flammability and explosiveness.

VOLATILE ANESTHETICS

Halothane (FLUOTHANE)

Actions. For many years halothane was the most widely used general inhalation anesthetic; more common at present is isoflurane (FORANE) discussed later. Halothane is considered in detail because of extensive knowledge about its effects; isoflurane and other agents are then introduced and compared with halothane.

Halothane is liquid, nonflammable, nonirritating, with a distinct odor. Halothane is a potent agent with an MAC of less than 1% (0.75%). In contrast to ether and cyclopropane, the anesthesia produced by halothane is not marked by obvious signs or stages. There is a time- and concentration-dependent depression of reflex responses, depression of respiration, and of blood pressure. In distinction from nitrous oxide and ether, it produces little or no analgesia until unconsciousness supervenes.

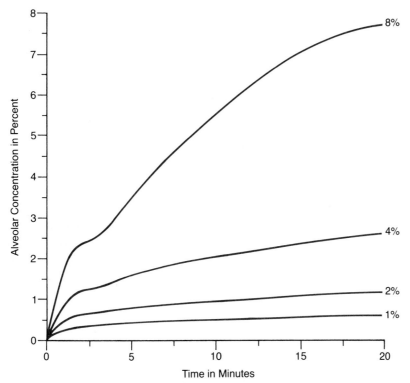

It is supplemented frequently with nitrous oxide, opiates, and muscle relaxants.

Kinetics. Because the MAC of halothane is less than 1%, large concentrations *can* be used during induction because oxygenation can be more than adequate with concentrations of oxygen exceeding 95% (Fig. 16–6).

Induction and anesthesia can be smooth and uneventful although somewhat slow. Recovery is due largely to exhalation of the anesthetic gases; 80% or more is excreted through the lungs. The remainder, some 15% or more, is destroyed by metabolism by the liver microsomal mixed-function oxidase system. Chloride and bromide ions are removed from the halothane with the production of fluoride ions and the ultimate excretion by way of the urine of fluorine-containing compounds, mostly trifluoroacetic acid and trifluoroethanol. The possibility of microsomal enzyme induction is present with repeated exposure.

Organ System Effects

Respiration. The respiration with halothane is shallow and rapid; the degree of respiratory depression is related to both the concentration and the rate of increase in concentration. During anesthesia the respiration becomes progressively more and more shallow. Because respiration may be inadequate it is frequently assisted; this poses the possibility that there will be a significant overdosing, because the signs of anesthesia associated with respiration are removed. In addition, the respiratory and chemoreceptor reflexes are markedly obtunded by halothane. This is due to both peripheral and central actions of the agent.

Circulation. With halothane anesthesia there is a progressive decrease in blood pressure due to a depression of cardiac contractility and a decrease in peripheral resistance. This depression of blood pressure is related both to the concentration of the anesthetic in the body as well as the rate at which it has been introduced. The faster the induction, the more profound and the more rapid is the drop in blood pressure. In addition to the direct effects on cardiac output, halothane has a number of effects on the cardiac rhythm. Bradycardia is common and due both to effects on autonomic function and to direct actions on the heart. The appearance of nodal rhythm is common, as well as the sensitization of the myocardium to the arrhythmic effects of epinephrine. The arrhythmias are usually not a problem in otherwise healthy individuals but may become so in the presence of those with cardiac disease or with electrolyte abnormalities.

Halothane depresses uterine tone. The production of skeletal muscle relaxation also occurs with halothane but is usually insufficient for major abdominal surgery and, thus, it is commonly supplemented with skeletal muscle relaxants. Halothane does sensitize the neuromuscular junction to competitive neuromuscular blocking agents.

A rare but serious abnormality of skeletal muscle function has been associated with the use of halogenated inhalation anesthetics, including halothane and enflurane. This syndrome is termed *malignant hyperpyrexia* and is characterized by a rapid rise in body temperature and an increase in oxygen consumption and carbon dioxide production. It appears to be due to a change in calcium uptake into skeletal muscle in genetically susceptible individuals. What the exact roles of halothane or succinylcholine are in the production of this malignant hyperthermia are not established (see Chapters 13 and 24).

Liver. There is little evidence that halothane directly produces liver damage. However, *hepatitis* has been reported in approximately one in 3000 to 7000 halothane anesthesias; the liver damage is not explainable on the basis of viral infections or known hepatotoxic drugs. Repeated exposures to halothane are associated with an increased likelihood of the occurrence of this hepatitis, and it is generally concluded that either it is a hypersensitivity reaction or is due to toxic metabolic products. Nevertheless, the most common causes of hepatitis in the postoperative period are viral infections and exposure to known hepatotoxic agents.

Isoflurane (FORANE)

Actions. Isoflurane, 1-chloro-2,2,2-trifluoroethyl difluoromethyl ether, is currently the most extensively used inhalation anesthetic. Isoflurane is a potent agent with a pungent smell. The pungent quality may make induction slow when it is given alone; however, anesthesia is commonly induced using intravenous barbiturate. The agent appears to have many of the desirable features of halothane and enflurane.

Organ System Effects. With respect to respiration, isoflurane depresses respiration progressively as the concentration in the inhaled mixture is increased. Respiration is somewhat more depressed than with comparable concentrations of the other agents; thus, it is commonly assisted or controlled.

With respect to the cardiovascular effects, isoflurane is similar qualitatively to halothane or enflurane; however, the hypotension is less marked and the cardiac reserve appears to be greater in comparison to other anesthetic effects. It does not sensitize the heart to epinephrine. Also, in contrast to enflurane, isoflurane does not produce seizure-like activity in the EEG.

Isoflurane, like enflurane, potentiates the neuromuscular blocking effects of skeletal muscle relaxants. These muscle relaxant activities are due to central effects as well as effects on the neuromuscular junction.

Uterine muscle is relaxed by isoflurane.

Enflurane (ETHRANE)

Actions. Enflurane is 2-chloro-1, 1, 2-trifluoroethyl difluoromethyl ether, a colorless, nonflammable liquid with a sweet odor. The anesthesia produced by enflurane is similar to that of halothane; however, the anesthesia itself is a mixture of CNS depression and seizure activity. The seizure activity is seen most prominently in the examination of the EEG, and actual seizures have been reported in rare instances. Enflurane is a relatively potent agent with an MAC of 1.68%, and modest increases above this amount permit a fairly smooth and rapid introduction of anesthesia, for example, using a 4% mixture of enflurane in 96% oxygen. As with halothane, anesthesia can be induced using a barbiturate to produce unconsciousness, after which the anesthetic gas mixture is introduced.

Organ System Effects. As with halothane, enflurane anesthesia is accompanied by a gradual decrease in both respiration and blood pressure. The depression of blood pressure is due, in part, to depression of myocardial contractility. Reportedly, there is a lesser likelihood of arrhythmias to occur with enflurane than with halothane. With regard to respiration, the respiratory depth decreases as the concentration of enflurane is increased; the reflex respiratory responses to both hypoxia and hypercarbia are depressed equal to or to a greater extent than after halothane. However, the increase in rate of respiration is less than with halothane.

Skeletal muscle relaxation does occur with enflurane and is somewhat greater than that produced by halothane. It potentiates the effects of competitive skeletal muscle relaxants similarly to halothane.

Liver damage has occurred during and after anesthesia with enflurane, but its mechanism remains obscure. Obviously, it should be avoided if the individual patient had exhibited liver damage following a previous exposure to that agent.

Kinetics and Time Course. The onset and recovery from enflurane is satisfactorily rapid. The bulk of the anesthetic is excreted unchanged in the expired gas. Only some 2–5% is metabolized by the liver.

OBSOLETE VOLATILE ANESTHETICS

Diethyl Ether

Ether has a pungent characteristic odor that is irritating to the nose, throat, and respiratory tract. It is flammable and explosive in concentrations used in anesthesia. The onset and induction with ether are slow and prolonged owing to the combination of its relatively low volatility, its modest potency, as well as its marked irritation of the respiratory tract. This irritation on the initial exposure leads to both voluntary and involuntary breath-holding. The actions of ether have already been described earlier in the section on stages and planes of anesthesia as exemplified by ether.

Methoxyflurane (PENTHRANE)

Methoxyflurane is the most potent of available inhalation anesthetics, but it is little used. Its low vapor pressure precludes inhaling an inspired concentration greater than 3%. Moreover, an appreciable amount of the methoxyflurane is absorbed in rubber tubing. It has been utilized for analgesia during labor and delivery. The patient is provided with a special inhaler that delivers the anesthetic as it limits the amount that can be obtained.

Methoxyflurane is metabolized extensively. It also has a definite potential for producing kidney damage after prolonged exposure. Possible kidney damage, its high water solubility, and associated slow tissue uptake and reversal have led to its infrequent clinical use.

(Methoxyflurane's actions reveal that the tissue [or blood]: gas partition coefficient has little to do with the actual rate of onset and the recovery from the anesthetics in current use. Although methoxyflurane has a high partition coefficient of 12, almost ten times that of isoflurane, induction of anesthesia can be accomplished in a relatively short time; concentrations of 2–3% in the inspired mixture are sufficient to produce anesthesia within minutes because they are extremely potent with a MAC of less than 0.16%. In fact, the administration of the same concentration of methoxyflurane as isoflurane would be expected to produce a similar rate of onset of anesthesia.)

Intravenous Induction, Analgesia, Sedation

Propofol

INDUCTION

Thiobarbiturates

Rapidly acting, short-duration-of-action barbiturates (thiopental, methohexital) have been used extensively for induction of sleep and anesthesia and as a component of "conscious sedation" (see later in this chapter and Chapter 20). Intravenous injection resulting in sleep and some amnesia is usually followed by an inhalation anesthetic or other agents. The rapid onset of sedation and sleep is the direct result of the rapid translocation of the agent from blood to brain. The short duration of a given dose is due to the redistribution of the agent from well-perfused tissues, such as brain, to tissues that are less well perfused, especially adipose tissue. The overall duration of these thiobarbiturates is determined by their distribution to fat and, eventually, their metabolism in the liver.

The barbiturates have all the expected effects of a general anesthetic agent—including respiratory depression, cardiovascular depression after large doses, and ultimately death if given in excess. These depressant effects are at least additive with any other drug with CNS depressant actions.

Propofol (DIPRIVAN) is a new agent of unique structure (2,6 diisopropylphenol). It is marketed as an emulsion for intravenous administration for induction and maintenance of anesthesia. It has the advantages of a very rapid onset after infusion or bolus injections (similar to thiobarbiturates) plus a very short recovery period of 8 minutes or less. The plasma levels after a bolus injection reveal two phases: a rapid phase with a half-life of 1.8–8.3 minutes and a slower phase with a half-life of 34–64 minutes. These two phases are analogous to similar phases of the thiobarbiturates and reflect a similar movement into highly perfused tissues, followed by redistribution to less well perfused tissues. Its disadvantages include large variety of adverse reactions, including hypotension, movements such as twitching, myoclonus, seizures, nausea, and vomiting. Note that this is a new agent with a relatively limited experience of use.

CONSCIOUS SEDATION

The term *conscious sedation* has become widely used to describe drug-induced states that permit short-lasting surgical interventions and endoscopic procedures. The essential feature is a sedated, calm patient with analgesia and amnesia. Although calm and relaxed, patients under conscious sedation techniques retain the ability to respond to simple questions and commands.

Diazepam

An opioid, such as meperidine or morphine, given in combination with diazepam—both usually given intravenously—can result in a patient who is calm, analgesic, and subsequently amnesic for most events over the next hour or so, yet who has an adequate blood pressure and respiration and who can be oriented to person, place, or time. Such combinations enjoy a relatively large safety margin and at the same time are adequate for a variety of painful or discomforting procedures or surgery; however, there are potential risks of excessive respiratory or cardiovascular depression.

Typically, diazepam is given slowly over minutes starting with a selected dose with added smaller increments given to achieve the desired end-point of a patient who is comfortable but who also has the ability to respond to simple direct commands and questions, such as "open your eyes," "lift your arm," or questions of person and place. Most important is a decrease in anxiety level so that patients are cooperative and unperturbed by the events around them. If left alone, patients usually tend to go to sleep, a sleep from which they can be readily awakened. Speech tends to be slurred and nystagmus is usually prominent, at least during the initial phases.

In addition, such amounts of diazepam usually produce marked amnesia that is only partially appreciated by the patient. The amnesia is characterized by a patchy recollection of only a small portion of the events that transpired during the drug action; bizarre dreams or sexual fantasies have been reported by some patients receiving either diazepam or midazolam (Chapter 20). To a baseline state produced by the benzodiazepine are then added other agents, depending on the nature of the procedure being performed. Among the agents employed commonly are meperidine (DEMEROL), given intravenously and resulting in analgesia; however, it carries the hazard of respiratory depression, which is augmented by the benzodiazepine. Also commonly employed is a small amount of an intravenous barbiturate that will tend to produce even more profound depression and overt sleep at least for a short period of time. In addition to the antianxiety and analgesic medications, local anesthetics are used for procedures in which appreciable pain is anticipated, such as tooth extractions or dental restorations.

As in all anesthesias, the drugs employed and the doses are largely adjusted on the basis of the patient's responses to the procedures undertaken. Conscious sedation techniques such as the ones just described have found wide popularity and great utility for a wide variety of procedures, including many different kinds of endoscopy, vascular catheterizations, and most minor surgical procedures. The great attraction of conscious sedation is the fact that the patients are not fully unconscious. Although they do not require the intensity of monitoring as in general anesthesia, continuous monitoring of respiration and blood pressure is necessary. Because patients may not be receiving oxygen inhalation, covert unrecognized levels of hypoxia may result. Monitoring of oxygen level is important.

Appropriately managed, recovery from conscious sedation is rapid and smooth. Amnesia is present for most of the events that transpire; nausea, vomiting, and other postoperative events common with general anesthetics are rare. In fact, in skillful hands the recovery is so uneventful as to be deceptive. It is absolutely necessary to be quite rigid in ensuring that day surgery patients (outpatients) have somebody else present to take them home for eventual recovery. Some patients appear for such procedures without having arranged for transportation and assistance. All patients postoperatively are at serious risk for a wide variety of accidents; it is essential that there is appropriate postoperative monitoring.

It is emphasized that although patients receiving benzodiazepines are largely amnesic they may appear to be conscious, awake, and hearing what is being told, yet unable to recall events subsequently. Thus, any kind of direction must be given to the patient days in advance of the drug administration. Not only do all of the directions need to be written down, the instructions have to be provided to the responsible third party.

Midazolam (VERSED)

The other benzodiazepine that has received attention for use for conscious sedation is midazolam. Although it has many of the same properties as diazepam and is less irritating on intravenous administration, difficulty has been encountered with its use. In fact, the most recent package insert has been corrected with a warning statement: "When used for conscious sedation, dosage must be individualized and titrated. Versed should *not* be administered by rapid or single bolus intravenous administration. Individual response will vary with age, physical status and concomitant medications but may also vary independent of these factors. (See WARNINGS concerning cardiac/respiratory arrest.)"

The major problems encountered with midazolam appear to be related to two factors. First, some individuals administering it have not appreciated the fact that there is a significant lag of many minutes between the time the drug is administered and the full appearance of its effects on the CNS. This lag appears to be related largely to the slowness of the translocation of the drug from blood to brain. Second, midazolam appears to have a significant respiratory depressant effect and this, coupled with the occasional excessive dose, has resulted in serious respiratory depression or cardiac arrest. In addition, the other drugs used commonly with conscious sedation as described earlier have distinct respiratory depressant effects, for example, the opioids or barbiturates. The respiratory depressant effects of all these agents are at least additive and may even be synergistic with midazolam. As noted earlier, serious degrees of hypoxia can occur in the absence of any overt manifestations, and cyanosis is notably unreliable.

Thus, conscious sedation using midazolam appears to be more difficult to manage than has been the case with diazepam. The result has been a number of cases of serious cardiorespiratory adverse events, including respiratory depression or cardiac arrest and death. The doses of midazolam needed for different patients varies widely; a given dose cannot be specified in advance. This unpredictability in terms of dosage, coupled with the long latency of effects, makes it a difficult agent to utilize on a routine basis.

In addition, as might be anticipated, intravenous doses of midazolam should be decreased for elderly and debilitated patients. Its sedative effect is magnified by opioid analgesics, by secobarbital, and by alcohol. Midazolam, expectedly, decreases the minimal anesthetic concentration required for general anesthesia by inhalation anesthetics.

Clinical tests of recovery from conscious sedation do not provide a valid prediction of a patient's ability to operate machinery or an automobile; at least a day or so should elapse before driving is permitted. As with all anesthetic agents and all kinds of anesthesia, including local anesthesia, the provision of devices and staff for immediate monitoring, detection, and correction of any cardiorespiratory adverse events, including oxygen levels, should be routine; equipment and personnel prepared for resuscitation should be available with no more than 2–5 seconds delay. *The patient must be monitored at all times directly by one person whose primary task is the patient's monitoring. This should include regular routine measurements of respiration, oxygen level, and cardiovascular function. Arrangements for emergency back-up by anesthesiology services should be established prior to implementation of any procedures involving conscious sedation, as well as any other kind of anesthesia.*

Dissociative Anesthesia

Surgical invasions of the body are now possible under a variety of drugs as well as other influences such as hypnosis. The catatonic state that can be produced by some drugs is a candidate for use in anesthesia and to permit surgery. One such drug, ketamine, has achieved an accepted status; its use is limited to patients with high cardiorespiratory risk factors.

Ketamine (KETALAR)

The unique form of anesthesia produced by ketamine was discovered only recently. After intravenous administration, the individual, although not asleep, fails to respond appropriately to the environment. Moreover, there are no responses to painful stimuli and there is subsequent amnesia. Yet, cardiac and respiratory behaviors and functions are maintained without significant change (except usually the patients exhibit some tachycardia). Thus, there is a state of catalepsy, maintained posture or positions, and no purposeful movement, all with an apparent lack of response to external stimuli. Muscle tone is sustained and the only movements that occur are small and nonpurposeful. The eyes frequently remain open and appear to stare or to move with slow nystagmoid movements but without significant awareness. The term *dissociative* refers to the fact that there is a disassociation between the individual's response and the environment—a functional dissociation of the thalamocortical and limbic systems.

The subjective state is reportedly sometimes pleasant and sometimes unpleasant. Bizarre dreams and hallucinations may occur, and these may be remembered by the patient as unpleasant. Approximately 12% of patients will have an "emergence reaction" consisting of dream-like states, hallucinations, delirium, confusion, or irrational behavior.

The state produced by ketamine is quite similar to that produced by a chemically close relative, phencyclidine (PCP), a drug used under the trade name SERNYLAN in veterinary medicine to produce an anesthetic state. PCP has been widely used nonmedically and is discussed further in the chapters on substance abuse (Chapter 67) and drug-induced psychiatric symptoms (Chapter 27).

Ketamine is used for high-risk patients for whom any general anesthetic of the more conventional type would be expected to compromise respiratory or cardiovascular function. Under such circumstances, anesthesia with ketamine can be carried out with ease. When given intravenously, the onset is within 1 minute with a duration of 5–10 minutes, although the half-life for the effects of ketamine is some 3 hours. Anesthesia can be maintained by repeated injections. There are no known antagonists.

The mechanism(s) of action of ketamine and PCP are being researched actively; it appears probable that at least certain classes of serotonin receptors are essential for the production of its effects; some investigators believe that the sigma opioid receptor class is also involved in PCP actions.

Opioids in Anesthesia

Morphine and meperidine have been long used in association with anesthesia — preoperatively, postoperatively, as well as during anesthesia — to obtain increased analgesia (rather than increasing the general anesthetic). In recent years, opioids have found much wider and varied use. With the availability of fentanyl (SUBLIMAZE), a rapid-acting, short-lasting (and potent) opioid agonist, a new era of techniques for anesthesia was initiated. With such agents, patients can be rapidly and easily sedated and are markedly analgesic without appreciable cardiovascular risk. Although respiration can be depressed by the drug, such depression is of little consequence because the patients in whom they are used can be readily respired artificially.

FENTANYL (SUBLIMAZE), ALFENTANIL (ALFENTA), AND SUFENTANIL (SUFENTA)

Fentanyl, alfentanyl, and sufentanyl have almost immediate onset after intravenous injection. The degree of analgesia or anesthesia is dose-related, and they can be used for: induction and as the primary anesthetic in patients in whom tracheal intubation and mechanical ventilation are required; as an adjunct for analgesia with other anesthetics (such as nitrous oxide and barbiturate); and with continuous infusion for anesthesia maintenance.

As opioid agonists they can be expected to produce all of the effects of such opioids. In addition to respiratory depression, tachycardia, rigidity of muscles of chest, hypotension, and cardiac arrhythmias have been reported. Histamine release is not marked, although itching is a side effect. Moreover, these agents can be antagonized by naloxone.

These are potent agents with each differing from the other in terms of potency. The technique of use determines the dose and regimen of administration. For example, sufentanil is five to ten times as potent as fentanyl, depending on use. A Dosage Range Chart is included in the package insert, and it should be consulted and read in its entirety *prior* to the anesthesia.

All opioid agonists with rapid onset of action have great abuse liability.

Anesthetic Accidents

Fortunately, serious life-threatening reactions to anesthetics and anesthesia are rare. However, when they do occur they can be truly tragic with consequences not only to the affected patient but also to the family, physician, and institution. Such adverse events are referred to as anesthetic mishaps, accidents, or pitfalls, but actually these are euphemisms for any serious adverse event occurring during or around anesthesia, or the recovery. Retrospective studies of accidents that have occurred around anesthesias, and that have been attributed in some way or another to the anesthesia, reveal that more than 50% of all anesthetic accidents are preventable. In the opinion of the peers that have evaluated the circumstances of such accidents, the majority (70–90%) of such "accidents" were the consequence of, or complicated by, errors that a competent practitioner would not have made. Thus, most anesthetic accidents are really not accidents at all; they are anesthetic tragedies based on simple ignorance of facts that

Most anesthetic tragedies associated with anesthetics are due to preventable failure of the anesthetist to know what should have been known or to exercise reasonable judgment.

should have been known or errors in judgment that the well-trained physician (or professional anesthetist) should not have made.

These conclusions are heartening in the sense that they indicate the source of the already infrequent problems and the means for their solutions. It is also apparent from such studies that the information needed for the safe use of anesthetic agents has been, or at least can be, obtained by research. The agents and their effects are sufficiently predictable and safe for the benefit-risk evaluations of most individuals; moreover well-designed studies can establish the potential for untoward effects.

Because of the nature of modern anesthesia and surgery, surgical procedures involve the administration of numerous drugs—before the procedure, during the anesthesia and surgery, and in the recovery period. Awareness of all of the agents involved, as well as the disease state and operative procedure, is important inasmuch as there are interactions, in terms of effects as well as pharmacokinetics. To illustrate, the following provides a scheme and minimal examples of the agents that could be used in a patient, arranged according to the time course:

Drug Combinations and Interactions in Anesthesia

Modern anesthesia is accomplished using many drugs and many sophisticated techniques.

The night before:
    Hypnotic—a benzodiazepine to reduce anxiety and promote sleep
    Nothing to eat or drink after a given time, e.g., midnight
The day of surgery:
    Preanesthetic medications
        Analgesic—opioid
        Antianxiety—a benzodiazepine
        Anticholinergic—atropine or scopolamine
    Establish IV lines and start IV fluids
    Induction of anesthesia
        Thiopental, intravenous
        Opioid
        Primary anesthesia, e.g., isoflurane
        Diazepam or midazolam, IV
        Neuromuscular blockade
    Maintenance of anesthesia (during anesthesia and surgery)
        Maintenance anesthetic—the above or additional agent, e.g., halothane, enflurane, or isoflurane
        Opioid—morphine, fentanyl, alfentanil, sufentanil
        Neuromuscular blocking agent(s)—succinylcholine, pancuronium, atracurium, or tubocurarine
        Anticholinergic drug
        Cardiovascular drugs—hypotension-producing or blood pressure–elevating or antiarrhythmic agent
    Termination of anesthesia and recovery
        Turn off the slowly reversible anesthetic agent, such as halothane
        Antagonist for opioid(s)—naloxone
        Antagonist for tubocurarine—neostigmine (usually with an anticholinergic agent such as atropine)
    Postoperative period
        Antinauseant
        Analgesic
        Cough induction or antitussive
        Antianxiety or hypnotic
        Antibiotic
        IV fluids

References

Eger EI II (ed): Nitrous Oxide/N_2O. New York: Elsevier, 1985.

Firestone LL, Miller JC, Miller KW: Tables of physical and pharmacological properties of anesthetics (Appendix). *In* Roth SH, Miller KW (eds): Molecular and Cellular Mechanisms of Anesthetics. New York and London: Plenum Medical Book Company, 1986.

Guedel AE: Inhalation Anesthesia, A Fundamental Guide. New York: MacMillan, 1937.

Marais ML, Maher MW, Wetchler BV, et al: Reduced demands on recovery room resources with propofol (Diprivan) compared to thiopental-isoflurane. Anesthesiol Rev 16:29–39, 1989.

Miller KW: The nature of the site of general anesthesia. Int Rev Neurobiol 27:1–61, 1985.

Miller KW, Roth S: Molecular and Cellular Mechanisms of Anesthetics. New York and London: Plenum Medical Book Company, 1986.

Miller KW, Roth S: The Nature of the Site of General Anesthesia, 1–61. Orlando, Florida: Academic Press, 1985.

Miller RD: Anesthesia. 2nd ed. New York: Churchill Livingstone, 1986.

Nakahiro M, Yeh JZ, Brunner E, Narahashi T: General anesthetics modulate GABA receptor channel complex in rat dorsal root ganglion neurons. FASEB J 3:1850–1854, 1989.

Nicoll RA, Madison DV: General anesthetics hyperpolarize neurons in the vertebrate nervous system. Science 717:1055–1057, 1982.

Papper EM, Kitz RJ: Uptake and Distribution of Anesthetic Agents. New York: McGraw-Hill, 1963.

Prys-Roberts C, Hug CC Jr: Pharmacokinetics of Anaesthesia. Boston: Blackwell Scientific Publications, 1984.

Roizen MF: Anesthesiology. JAMA 263:2625–2627, 1990.

Sedensky MM, Morgan PG, Meneely PM: A gene that changes anesthetic sensitivity in *C. elegans* works via neurons. Anesthesiology 71:A637, 1989.

Stoelting RK: Pharmacology and Physiology in Anesthetic Practice. Philadelphia: JB Lippincott, 1987.

Local Anesthesia and Local Anesthetics

17

Cedric M. Smith

By definition, local anesthetics are agents that act to produce a loss of sensation from a local area of the body. The demonstration by a Viennese junior intern Carl Koller in 1884 of anesthesia of the conjunctiva and cornea after instillation of a 2% solution of cocaine in the conjunctival sac prompted its almost immediate acceptance (Liljestrand, 1967). The primary medical use of local anesthetics then as well as now is the prevention and alleviation of pain by their application to sensory nerve fiber trunks or endings. The ultimate mechanism of this reduction in pain perception is the interruption of the conduction of propagated action potentials along certain sensory nerves. This depression of the conduction along nerves is commonly referred to as conduction anesthesia, or *block,* or *nerve block* meaning a decrease in the perception of pain that results from the application of the agent to nerve endings or along the nerve fiber. The effective and safe use of local anesthetics requires not only that the drugs block conduction in some nerves but that such action be readily and fully reversible and without major systemic toxic effects.

Lidocaine (XYLOCAINE) and procaine (NOVOCAINE and others) are considered the prototype agents in the drug class of local anesthetics not only because they have had extensive clinical use, but more importantly because of the extensive research and knowledge about their mechanisms of action. Although cocaine was the first drug discovered to produce local anesthesia, it has a relatively minor place in therapeutic use today. For a discussion of its systemic effects refer to Chapter 67 on substance abuse.

Although the alteration of pain perception is the usual goal of the clinical use of local anesthetics, the analogous depression of the excitation of other excitable membranes, such as those of cells in the central nervous system (CNS), heart, or muscle, is commonly considered to be a *local anesthetic effect.* The mechanisms underlying the depression of excitability and conduction produced by local anesthetics and drugs claimed to possess local anesthetic effects are similar whichever excitable tissue has been exposed to the drug.

The prime objective of the clinical use of local anesthetics is a reduction of the sensory input to the CNS, thereby reducing both the perception of, and the reflex responses to, sensory nervous input that is ultimately perceived as pain. (Mechanisms of pain are discussed in Chapters 18 and 28.)

Reversible block of the conduction along nerve fibers can be produced not only by the application of local anesthetics, but by ischemia, cold, and direct physical compression of the nerve. For example, ethyl chloride has

Definition

Local anesthetics act by depressing the excitability of excitable tissues.

Lidocaine

Procaine

The objective of local anesthesia is to decrease or abolish pain.

Pain will be prevented by decreasing the number or frequency of action potentials in nociceptive nerves.

been used clinically, especially in sports medicine, as a topical spray on the skin to cause intense cold by evaporation, which results in localized numbness. Although these techniques have limited use, the most clinically useful agent for producing local anesthesia is a local anesthetic, administered by a clinician trained in effective methods of administration.

Anesthesia and surgical techniques for ambulatory procedures have been well developed over many years, and recently these advances have been implemented with the widespread practice of ambulatory surgery using regional block or local anesthesia, frequently in combination with sedative, analgesic, or antianxiety medications. For example, the specialized clinics that treat only inguinal hernias now send patients home the day after surgical repair done with regional block anesthesia, no matter how complex the repair (Baue, 1986).

Sites and Mechanisms of Action

ACTIONS

Lidocaine and procaine and their analogs act on the membranes of nerves and other electrically excitable cells. The following are the important characteristic actions of local anesthetics; these are illustrated in Figures 17–1 to 17–4:

- The threshold for initiation of a nerve action potential is elevated. That is, with exposure to the anesthetic a greater change in the membrane potential is required to initiate an action potential, yet the resting membrane potential is *not* appreciably altered by the anesthetic. (The threshold of a nerve can be operationally defined as the membrane potential that will result in an action potential when the membrane is depolarized from its resting potential within a given time.)

Figure 17–1

Action potential and associated changes in permeability of the nerve membrane to sodium and potassium ions. The ordinate of top recording shows the nerve membrane potential recorded intracellularly, and the ordinate of the bottom recording gives the associated ion conductances. The effects of a local anesthetic are shown in color—a decrease in the rate of rise and in the size of the action potential in association with a corresponding decrease in sodium permeability. (Local anesthetics have only small effects directly on potassium conductances.) (This figure is a general illustration based ultimately on the pioneering work of Hodgkin and Huxley [1952] relating the membrane electrical properties and ionic permeabilities.) Membrane potential is recorded as the difference in potential between the intracellular electrode and the external service expressed in millivolts (mV). (E_{Na} = sodium equilibrium potential—the membrane potential at which there would be no net influx or efflux of sodium ions; E_K = potassium equilibrium potential.) Conductance is expressed as gNa = sodium conductance; gK = potassium conductance.

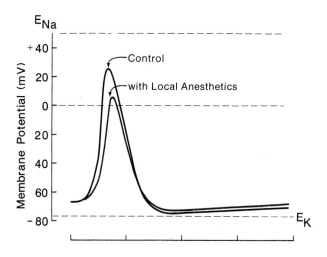

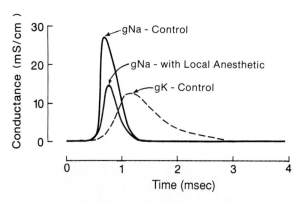

■ The conduction of action potentials along certain nerve fibers in the area exposed to the anesthetic is impaired or blocked. The direct consequence of such impaired conduction is a *decrease in the discharge frequency* along a given individual sensory nerve ranging in intensity from a partial block

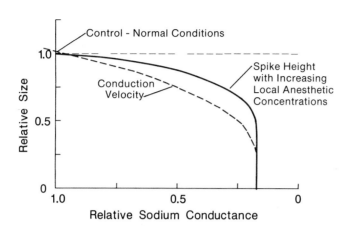

Figure 17–2

Relation of nerve conduction velocity and action potential spike height to maximal sodium conductance. With a decrease in sodium conductance, as might be produced by a local anesthetic, both the spike height and the conduction velocity fall. Finally, as the conductance decreases to about one sixth of the normal sodium conductance (the normal is shown as 1.0 at the origin on this graph), impulse conduction fails; i.e., there is a safety factor of 6. (This example is plotted from a computer simulation of data pertaining to frog nerve of 20 μm diameter at 20° C. Replotted from Ritchie JM: An overview of the mechanisms of local anesthetic action past, present, future. *In* Roth SH, Miller KW [eds]: Molecular and Cellular Mechanisms of Anesthetics, 196. New York: Plenum, 1984.)

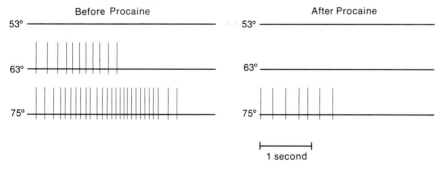

Figure 17–3

Electrical responses of a single afferent nociceptive ("pain") fiber from the tooth pulp induced by application of hot water to the crown of the tooth. The greater the temperature, the greater the frequency and the longer the repetitive discharge of action potentials. Each upward spike is a propagated action potential. Note that at rest at temperatures of 53° C (and below), there are no action potentials. After the application of procaine to the pulp (in this preparation through the circulation), the threshold for activation is increased and the discharge frequency decreased or abolished. (The rationale for studying the tooth pulp is that stimulation of the afferent nerves from tooth pulp gives rise almost exclusively to sensations of pain.)

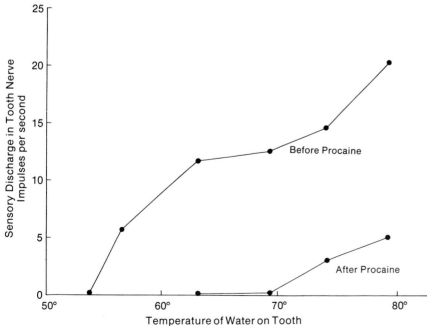

Figure 17–4

The impulse frequencies from a tooth pulp afferent nerve taken from data obtained as described in Figure 17–3 as a function of the temperature of the water applied to the tooth. After procaine, the responses to the lower temperatures are abolished and the responses to the higher temperatures markedly decreased.

of some of the propagated potentials to a total block of conduction through the exposed area (see Figs. 17–1, 17–3, and 17–4). A second result is a *decrease in the total number of fibers activated* by a given sensory stimulus. Both of these effects decrease the occurrence and the intensity of the perception and reflex responses to a given sensory input.

■ In many clinical situations in which anesthetics are used, for example, their application to a nerve trunk containing hundreds of nerves sheathed by connective tissues, only some fibers are exposed to concentrations of the anesthetic sufficient to produce complete blockade. Thus, it is more accurate to describe and to think of local anesthetic action as the *obtunding or decreasing of nociceptive input*, rather than an absolute block. Patients may not perceive low intensities of stimulation as painful, yet more powerful stimulation may produce pain; this demonstrates that local anesthesia may be relative and limited, rather than an absolute block of sensory input (Fig. 17–5).

Local anesthetic actions are relatively more pronounced on tonically repetitively discharging nerves — "frequency and use dependence."

■ The probability of a block of nerve conduction is greater in repetitively discharging nerve fibers. The intensity of the local anesthetic action is dependent on the frequency and the amount of use a given fiber has experienced—the more rapidly and the more recently that fiber has been conducting impulses, the greater the likelihood of conduction block by local anesthetic. Thus, local anesthetics exhibit what is called *frequency and use dependence*.

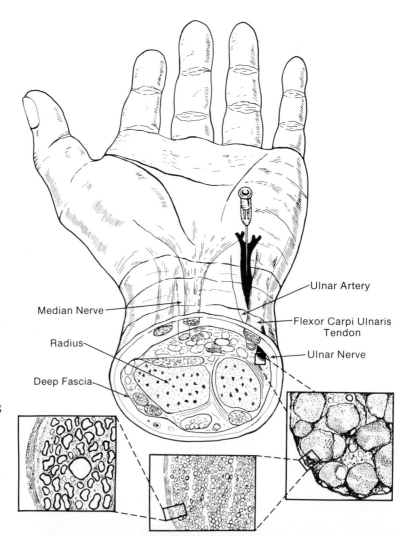

Figure 17–5

Example of the technique and landmarks for an ulnar nerve block illustrating the nerve encased in connective tissue, the close proximity of vessels, and the relatively long diffusion distance from local anesthetic applied external to the nerve sheath. The rectangular, successive enlargements are included to emphasize further the complex diffusion paths and, consequently, the delay in onset of anesthesia and the varying local anesthetic concentrations to which different nerve fibers and bundles may be exposed. (Adapted and expanded from Cousins MJ, Bridenbaugh PO [eds]: Neural Blockade in Clinical Anesthesia and Management of Pain. 2nd ed. Philadelphia: JB Lippincott, 1988; and Scott DB: Techniques of Regional Anesthesia. Norwalk, CT: Appleton & Lange/Mediglobe, 1989.)

Median Nerve

Radius

Deep Fascia

Ulnar Artery

Flexor Carpi Ulnaris Tendon

Ulnar Nerve

■ Local anesthetics are sometimes applied to sensory nerve endings, for example, with subdermal *infiltration* or by *topical* application. When nerve endings are so exposed the site of action of the local anesthetic is usually the site of origin of the repetitively generated action potentials. This site in myelinated nerves is the first node of Ranvier. The frequency of the sensory nerve discharge is proportional to the localized generator potential of the sensory ending, and the first node serves to convert the graded, local sensory generator potential to action potentials. In so doing, the nodal membrane serves as the pacemaker governing the frequency of discharge of that sensory nerve. (In nonmyelinated fibers, a site functionally analogous to the first node serves to convert the local generator potential to impulse initiation.) The end effects of procaine application on afferent nerve endings in the tooth pulp are illustrated in Figures 17–3 and 17–4.

■ There is a differential sensitivity to local anesthetics among nerve fibers. For example, pain and temperature sensations tend to be more susceptible to depression after local anesthetic application than tactile or limb movement sensations. Also, sensory systems appear in general to be more affected than motor systems. Historically, it was discovered in the early experiments that in frog sciatic nerves and in a limited number of other nerves the smaller, more slowly conducting fibers were the most susceptible to local anesthetics. However, recent investigations among a wide variety of nerves has led to the conclusion that it is not possible to generalize about nerve size and the likelihood of block by a local anesthetic.

> Smaller nerve fibers are commonly, but not always, more susceptible to local anesthesia.

■ Because pain may be prevented with block of only some of the nerves to an area, it is important to understand that patients may experience diminution of pain, yet at the same time continue to be aware of surgical procedures, of being touched, or of movement of tissues.

SITES OF ACTION

The primary site of action of local anesthetics is the cell membrane of excitable cells, such as the nerve membrane. Moreover, the site of action has been localized to be near the internal surface of the membrane, as opposed to the external surface. (Some anesthetics may have effects on the outer portion of the membrane in addition.)

> A primary site of action of local anesthetics is the inner portion of the membrane sodium channel.

MECHANISM OF ACTION

The singularly most important aspect of the actions of local anesthetics is the reduction of the transient increase in sodium permeability associated with the rising, i.e., depolarization, phase of the action potential. This reduction in sodium permeability is due to the drug's effects on the voltage-sensitive membrane channels for sodium (see Figs. 17–1 and 17–2; see also Fig. 33–3); a high density of such channels is located at the nodes of Ranvier. This action to reduce the increased sodium permeability associated with the action potential has been shown experimentally to be competitive between sodium and the local anesthetic, such as procaine. The sodium ion channels can exist dynamically in four conformational states — resting, closed, open, and inactivated. During the refractory period the channels move from the inactivated to the resting state. Membrane depolarization results in the transition from the resting to the closed state, and then to the open conformation associated with the action potential. Although the receptor for local anesthetics is not the channel itself, its binding results in an inhibition of the channel's permeability to sodium, as already described. Moreover, the binding of the local anesthetics to the receptors is a function of both the specific agent and the conformational state of the channel. In general, most local anesthetics are bound more avidly to the receptors of activated or inactivated channels than to those of resting channels. But there is a complex interrelationship in that some local anesthetics bind with higher affinity to the receptors of open channels, others to those of inactivated states, and some bind most strongly to the receptors of closed channels (see Fig. 33–3).

After repolarization, the return of the receptors and the ion channels to the active state is slow, accounting for the accumulation, with repetitive nerve activity, of channels that cannot be activated to increase sodium permeability. This accumulation with repetitive depolarizations of channels that cannot be activated can account for the *use dependence* exhibited by local anesthetics. (The increased local anesthetic binding that occurs with repetitive depolarizations, designated *phasic block*, could represent either greater accessibility of the local anesthetic to more channels or increased binding affinity [Butterworth and Strichartz, 1990].)

The interactions of local anesthetics with sodium channels are consistent with their electrophysiological actions: to decrease the rate of rise of the action potential; to increase the threshold; and to decrease the size of the action potential (see Fig. 17–1). The conduction of the impulse along a nerve consists of the sequential production of action potentials along a nerve with the action potential at each spot on the nerve membrane giving rise to currents that depolarize the next segment of the nerve. Local anesthetics decrease the action potential currents as well as increase the threshold; thus, the safety margin for propagated conduction is decreased. Eventually, no conduction occurs through the area exposed to the anesthetic, and conduction is then truly blocked in that fiber.

Local anesthetics are amines with pKas in the range of 8–9 (see Fig. 17–6). Thus, they can exist in solution as either the charged (cationic) or uncharged species depending on the pH in the immediate vicinity. The active form of most local anesthetics at the site of action is the ionized, cationic form favored by acid pH. In contrast, the un-ionized form diffuses more rapidly to the site of action; diffusion is thus favored by an alkaline pH. (Exceptions to these generalizations are to be found with benzocaine, which lacks the secondary or tertiary amine of other local anesthetics, as well as with some potent experimental local anesthetics containing a cationic quaternary moiety.)

The kinetics of the actions of local anesthetics are covered in the next sections, but note that the strength of the anesthetic-receptor binding varies appreciably among agents. Some, such as lidocaine and procaine, appear to be relatively weakly bound and their actions are rapidly reversible. Others, such as bupivacaine (MARCAINE), are much more tenaciously attached and are slowly reversible. These differences in binding to the receptor account in part for the different durations of action of the agents when used for infiltration or nerve block (see Table 17–1).

Local anesthetics have little or no effect on the resting membrane potential and no effect on the sodium pump or other active transport systems (in concentrations producing local anesthesia). Moreover, they have only minimal effects on the generator potentials integral to the function of sensory endings; it follows that the site of action upon topical application or infiltration around nerve endings must be the site of the generation of the action potential, e.g., the first node of Ranvier in myelinated fibers.

Although an understanding of the effects of local anesthetics on sodium permeability constitutes an adequate basis for their use, their phar-

Local anesthetic action is *not* associated with changes in resting membrane potential, Na$^+$-K$^+$ ATPase, sodium pump, or active membrane transport systems.

macological actions also include complex interactions with the permeabilities and membrane effects of both calcium and potassium. Also, the ionic permeability of glia is modified by local anesthetics, and thus they can influence neuronal function indirectly.

Both arrhythmias and seizures involve abnormal or excessive excitability of excitable membranes. A number of the therapeutic agents that are useful in these conditions are known to have actions on cardiac membranes that are the same or quite similar to those of local anesthetics. For example, the Class I type antiarrhythmics, such as quinidine, lidocaine, and procainamide, decrease the voltage and frequency-dependent sodium permeability and raise the threshold for initiation and repetitive discharge of action potentials. With respect to anticonvulsants, intravenous lidocaine has been used effectively in interrupting status epilepticus, and phenytoin and carbamazepine exhibit marked frequency-dependent depression of sodium permeability; these agents thus act to decrease the interneuronal spread of repetitive activity that constitutes a seizure (Catterall, 1987; Chapters 23 and 33).

The rate of onset, duration, and intensity of action are all directly or indirectly related to not only the concentration of the drug and the amount, but also the site of application and the operative procedure. Specifically, the primary factors governing the time course of local anesthetic action are as follows:

- the total volume injected/applied
- concentration
- site of application
- which relevant nerves are exposed
- potency of the local anesthetic
- rate of diffusion from the site of application to the sites of action
- diffusion to sites of loss
- diffusion away from the sites of action such as into blood vessels
- local metabolic breakdown of the agent

     All these factors are interrelated.

RATE OF ONSET

For most procedures and agents the rate of onset of local *anesthesia* is largely a function of the rate of diffusion from site where the agent is applied or injected; for example, when applied topically on skin or injected in the proximity of a regional nerve, the agent must diffuse through the tissues to reach the nerve fibers mediating the sensation of pain. Such diffusion is relatively slow, and the time of onset of effects depends on the distance as well as concentration of the agent. Typically, the onset of topical or nerve block anesthesia with lidocaine may require 5 minutes or longer. Because pain induced prior to the onset of the maximal anesthesia predictably increases patient anxiety and the pain experienced (see Chapter 18 and Fig. 17–4), it is crucial to the avoidance of pain and anxiety that sufficient time be allowed for diffusion to take place.

     Diffusion is favored by an alkaline pH for all agents currently in use for injection because the un-ionized form diffuses more readily through various tissue membranes than the ionized form. It has been stated frequently that the reason local anesthesia is more difficult to produce in inflamed tissues is because such tissues tend to be more acidic than normal.

Local Anesthetic Actions of Drugs Used to Treat Cardiac Arrhythmias and Seizures

Local anesthetics potentially have local anesthetic actions on any excitable cell—all kinds of muscle, nerve, or cardiac cells.

Time Course of Action

Most local anesthetics are weak bases.

The un-ionized form diffuses more rapidly.

The ionized form of the local anesthetic is the active form *at the membrane site of action.*

DURATION OF ANESTHESIA

The duration of nerve block is determined by the rate of diffusion away from the sites of action, *not* local metabolism.

The duration of local anesthesia is largely based on the duration of exposure of the nerve to adequate blocking concentrations of the anesthetic. The major loss of the agent is by diffusion away from the injection site and from the nerve. For all practical purposes, it can be assumed that little or no metabolism takes place at the site of action. Thus, diffusion and absorption into the circulation, followed by widespread distribution and dilution, account for the diminution of effects of the local anesthetics over time.

Absorption of the anesthetic into the circulation accounts for the extensive use of vasoconstrictors, such as epinephrine in a 1 : 200,000 dilution or phenylephrine in the anesthetic solution, in order to extend the effective duration of the agent's action. (All of the local anesthetics either cause local vasodilation or have no effect on local circulation, except for cocaine, which causes vasoconstriction.) Such added vasoconstrictors are absorbed eventually and may lead to systemic effects on the nervous and cardiovascular systems, such as cardiac arrhythmias. Thus, it is important to keep the total amount of the vasoconstrictor administered as low as possible.

METABOLISM

Metabolism plays essentially no role in determining the *duration of the local actions* of local anesthetics. The simple esters are metabolized rapidly by hydrolysis catalyzed by plasma cholinesterase (e.g., procaine). The metabolism of the amides, such as lidocaine, involves enzymes of the hepatic endoplasmic reticulum. For example, lidocaine is metabolized initially by N-dealkylation followed by hydrolysis. Other factors regulating the duration of the systemic existence of the agent in the body include protein binding in the case of lidocaine, as well as tissue binding at the application site and in the lung.

Systemic Actions

Systemic toxicity is determined by the amount absorbed relative to the amount metabolized.

After absorption or intravascular administration, local anesthetics may have effects on essentially any cell possessing an electrically excitable membrane, such as nervous elements centrally and peripherally, as well as all kinds of muscle—smooth, striated, and cardiac. Except for their use as antiarrhythmics, most of these systemic effects are important as potential toxic actions rather than of therapeutic significance.

In general, the systemic effects of local anesthetics are dependent on both the total amount given (i.e., dose) and concentration, as well as on the site of administration and techniques used. In short, the actions of local anesthetics are consistent with general pharmacological principles.

CENTRAL NERVOUS SYSTEM

Anxiety, tremor, drowsiness, jerks, and seizures may be signs of CNS toxicity.

Circulating local anesthetics may cause stimulation of the CNS as manifested by nervousness, tremor, restlessness, and anxiety; this excitation may culminate in clonic seizures. Quite a large variety of symptoms have been reported. All local anesthetics appear to have the potential to produce dose-dependent CNS excitation, although drowsiness is also a common clinical complaint.

Seizures and excitation may be followed by coma and respiratory depression. Other than supportive and protective treatment, diazepam may be given intravenously to stop or prevent seizures.

Cocaine is renowned for its subjective effects of euphoria, feelings of energy, and mental alertness, and it is extremely habit-forming. The habit-forming and dependence properties of this and related substances are discussed further in the chapter on substance abuse (Chapter 67).

PERIPHERAL NERVOUS SYSTEM

When administered systemically, such as by intravenous injection, local anesthetics can depress the ongoing activity of a number of nerves, including peripheral sensory nerves. The site of action on the sensory nerves of such effects is probably the fine terminal branches or the site of impulse generation. Actions on sensory nerves would be expected to be dependent in part on the blood supply as well as on the safety factor for conduction along the sensory axon. (As noted earlier, the safety factor for conduction is lower in smaller nerves; in myelinated fibers it is 6 or more in terms of sodium permeability, as can be deduced from Fig. 17–2.) Although this peripheral action of agents with local anesthetic activity has been demonstrated repeatedly, depression of sensory input has not been utilized therapeutically except for cough suppression (see Chapter 26).

Sensory nerves can be depressed by circulating local anesthetics.

The skeletal nerve-muscle junction and ganglia are both susceptible to reduction of transmission by local anesthetics; these actions may be evidenced after toxic overdoses. Most apparent may be neuromuscular blockade, which is manifested as weakness or paralysis of respiration. Local anesthetic depression of neuromuscular transmission is at least additive with neuromuscular and ganglion-blocking agents.

Local anesthetics can induce neuromuscular block.

The effects of local anesthetics on smooth muscle are complex because the local anesthetics act at least potentially not only on the muscle directly, but on local reflexes and the autonomic innervation. For example, spinal anesthesia results in increased gastrointestinal (GI) tone, whereas uterine contractions during childbirth are rarely affected by epidural or regional anesthesia.

CARDIOVASCULAR SYSTEM

The use of local anesthetics and agents that have properties similar to local anesthetics are covered in the chapter on antiarrhythmic agents (Chapter 33). In summary, the local anesthetics have dose- and concentration-related, predictable effects on the heart, consisting of decreased excitability, slowed conduction, and decreased force of contraction. They may cause a variety of cardiac arrhythmias also, including arrest or ventricular fibrillation.

Cardiac antiarrhythmic agents possess local anesthetic properties.

Toxicity

LOCAL

The occurrence of hypersensitivity reactions to procaine is well documented in both dental patients as well as in dental professionals. The most frequent reaction is local tissue edema that can be at least partially relieved by systemic antihistamines. In contrast to procaine, local allergic reactions to the amide anesthetics, such as lidocaine, are rare but can occur. However, anesthetic solutions contain other agents in addition to the local anesthetic. A common preservative is methylparaben, a substance whose structure is quite similar to that of procaine and to which some individuals may exhibit an allergic reaction.

Allergy to local anesthetics can be local or systemic.

Local side effects of practical import are more often those related to technique and location of application, such as neurologic complications due to damage of nerve fibers by the needle, or by compression such as occurs with injection of the local anesthetic solution directly into the tightly closed fascial sheath of the nerve bundle (see Fig. 17–5). In addition, there are appreciable potential complications of the injection itself, for example, a pneumothorax that may be associated with the attempt to perform an intercostal nerve block.

Allergy can occur to the anesthetic, the solvent, or vehicles.

SYSTEMIC ABSORPTION

It is reasonable to assume that all local anesthetics are absorbed and have systemic actions.

All anesthesias are accompanied by some systemic absorption of the agent into the vascular system. If the amount absorbed is sufficient, the systemic actions will become apparent. These include cardiac irregularities or arrest, hypotension, and CNS excitation ranging from tremor to overt seizures. However, drowsiness or coma may occur instead of CNS excitation.

The distinction among these possibilities may be difficult when faced with an emergency or in the face of the sudden onset shortly after application or injection of an anesthetic. The possible causes of collapse or unresponsiveness following local anesthetic injection range from the usually transient neurogenic hypotension of fainting, to cardiac arrest, to seizures or coma. In the absence of an electrocardiogram (ECG) or electroencephalogram (EEG), collapse with or without jerking movements may signify cardiac arrest, mandating immediate cardiopulmonary resuscitation. Because such serious toxicity can occur with almost any local anesthetic procedure, adequate means for resuscitation should always be available for *immediate* use, preferably including an assistant, a running intravenous infusion, and resuscitative drugs and equipment.

The means and ability to carry out immediate CPR are essential to every local anesthetic procedure.

Systemic toxic reactions can result from the injection of excessive doses or amounts of local anesthetic solutions (see Table 17–1 for illustration of concentrations and total amounts that are commonly used), accidental intravenous injections, abnormal rates of absorption or metabolism, or allergic reactions.

Anaphylactoid shock has been reported to occur after administration of local anesthetics, but in view of the possibility of systemic absorption and actions on the cardiovascular and CNS, it is usually not possible to differentiate direct systemic actions from anaphylaxic shock that is based on a hypersensitivity mechanism. Treatment in either instance is essentially symptomatic and resuscitative.

Although it is common practice while injecting a local anesthetic to attempt to withdraw the syringe plunger to check if the needle is in a blood vessel, the technique is of only limited value. The failure to obtain blood upon withdrawing the plunger is *no* guarantee that a vessel has not been entered or impaled. The vessel could have been ruptured or the walls could collapse on the needle lumen when suction is applied. On the other hand, if blood appears in the syringe, it is obvious that the needle is in or has ruptured a vessel. In fact, in view of the extensive blood supply to most tissues, including peripheral nerves, it is likely that the puncture or rupture of blood vessels occurs with most regional or infiltration local anesthesias.

Clinical Uses

Rational therapeutic use consists of matching the properties of the anesthetic with the goal and technique of the procedure.

The clinical uses of local anesthetics fall into three basic categories: *therapeutic* to control acute postoperative or post-traumatic pain and to permit surgical or other painful procedures; *diagnostic* to determine site and cause of pain; and *prognostic* to predict effects of nerve section or damage. In addition, the clinical uses of these agents can be considered separately according to the site of application and the procedure to be carried out, such as topical to skin or mucous membranes, infiltration, peripheral nerve block, epidural, and spinal anesthesia.

INFILTRATION AND NERVE BLOCK

Because the anesthetics are used in a wide variety of sites and conditions, their rational clinical use requires knowledge and skill in the specific procedures as well as intimate knowledge of the pharmacology of the specific local anesthetics. A large number of agents are available, and their application consists of meshing their individual properties with the planned procedure. The agents vary with respect to potency, speed of onset, diffusibility, duration of action, and relative toxicity. The potential for systemic toxicity approximately parallels potency as expressed as the concentration and amount required for infiltration or nerve block. These relationships are illustrated in Table 17–1. The major facts to be gleaned from the table are as follows:

- local anesthetics differ in terms of latency, penetrance, and duration
- the prototypic agents include procaine, which has a moderate speed of onset, moderate potency and diffusibility, and short duration of action
- lidocaine is twice as potent as procaine, is more rapid in onset, and has a moderate duration of action

Anesthetics differ in potency, latency, penetrance, and duration of action.

Table 17–1   CLINICAL CHARACTERISTICS AND CONCENTRATIONS OF SELECTED LOCAL ANESTHETICS

Low Potency, Short Duration

	Procaine (NOVOCAINE)	2-Chloroprocaine (NESACAINE)	Lidocaine (XYLOCAINE)
CHARACTERISTIC			
Latency (speed of onset)	Moderate	Fast	Fast
Penetrance (diffusibility)	Moderate	Marked	Marked
Duration	Short	Very short	Moderate
CONCENTRATION			
Optimal concentrations (%)			
Infiltration	0.5	0.5	0.25
Spinal nerve and plexus block	1.5–2	1.0–2	0.5–1.0
Maximal amount (mg/kg)	12	15	6

Intermediate

	Mepivacaine (CARBOCAINE)	Prilocaine (CITANEST)
CHARACTERISTIC		
Latency (speed of onset)	Moderate	Moderate
Penetrance (diffusibility)	Moderate	Moderate
Duration	Moderate	Moderate
CONCENTRATION		
Optimal concentrations (%)		
Infiltration	0.25	0.25
Spinal nerve and plexus block	0.5–1.0	0.5–1.0
Maximal amount (mg/kg)	6	6

Potent, Long Duration

	Tetracaine (PONTOCAINE)	Bupivacaine (MARCAINE, SENSORCAINE)	Etidocaine (DURANEST)
CHARACTERISTIC			
Latency (speed of onset)	Very slow	Fast	Very fast
Penetrance (diffusibility)	Poor	Moderate	Moderate
Duration	Long	Long	Long
CONCENTRATION			
Optimal concentrations (%)			
Infiltration	0.05	0.05	0.1
Spinal nerve and plexus block	0.1–0.2	0.25–0.5	0.5–1.0
Maximal amount (mg/kg)	2	2	2

■ in contrast to the above agents, bupivacaine and etidocaine are more potent, longer lasting, and more toxic

A short duration of action is consistent with rapid diffusion of the anesthetic away from the nerve or into the circulation or its rapid metabolism.

The differences among agents in the various properties are the rational basis for selection of lidocaine or procaine for many infiltration or peripheral nerve block procedures. For other procedures, different agents might be preferred. For example, the specialized technique of *intravenous regional anesthesia* frequently employs bupivacaine because of its longer duration of action.

TOPICAL TO SKIN OR MUCOUS MEMBRANES

Topically effective anesthesia requires agents that penetrate and remain in the skin.

Most of the local anesthetics on the market are water-soluble and poorly soluble in oil; most are also poorly absorbed through the skin. An exception to this general rule are agents used for topical anesthesia. One of the most widely used drugs for topical anesthesia is benzocaine, which is both oil-soluble and permeates the skin. Hence, benzocaine is available in ointments and creams for topical application on intact skin to relieve pain or itch associated with such conditions as skin rashes and sunburn.

For application to mucous membranes, cocaine, lidocaine, and a number of other agents have been found to be effective (such as tetracaine [CETACAINE] and proparacaine [ALCAINE, OPHTHAINE]). For both skin and mucous membranes, only the most superficial layers are exposed to effective concentrations of the anesthetic agent.

EPIDURAL AND SPINAL APPLICATIONS

The anesthetist's skill, knowledge, and judgment are the major factors determining the effectiveness and the safety of local and spinal anesthesia.

These routes of administration are widely used and involve extensive knowledge, training, and experience in the medical specialty of anesthesiology. The principal mechanism of action of the agents remains the same. The unique, specialized administrations in terms of different procedures, sites, patient preparation, concentrations, selection of vehicles, amounts and rates of administration, and other aspects of management require special training and experience far beyond the scope of basic pharmacology. (A newly developed technique uses opioids injected intrathecally to produce analgesia limited to the distribution of the agent. This type of pain relief is discussed in Chapter 18.)

References (See Also References for Chapter 33)

Baue AE: General surgery. JAMA 256:2066–2068, 1986.

Bonica JJ: Local anesthesia and regional blocks. *In* Wall PD, Melzack R (eds): Textbook of Pain, 541–557. New York: Churchill Livingstone, 1984.

Butterworth JF IV, Strichartz GR: Molecular mechanisms of local anesthesia: A review. Anesthesiology 72:711–734, 1990.

Catterall WA: Common modes of drug action on Na+ channels: Local anesthetics, antiarrhythmics and anticonvulsants. Trends Pharmacol Sci 8:57–65, 1987.

Cousins MJ, Bridenbaugh PO (eds): Neural Blockade in Clinical Anesthesia and Management of Pain. 2nd ed. Philadelphia: JB Lippincott, 1988.

Covino BG: Pharmacology of local anesthetic agents. Rational Drug Ther 21:1–9, 1987.

Hodgkin AL, Huxley AF: A quantitative description of membrane current and its application to conduction and excitation in nerve. J Physiol 117:500–544, 1952.

Hille B: Ion channels of excitable membranes. Sunderland, MA: Sinauer Associates, 1984.

Liljestrand G: Carl Koller and the Development of Local Anesthesia. Acta Physiol Scand (Suppl) 299:2–30, 1967.

Ritchie JM: An overview of the mechanisms of local anesthetic action past, present, future. *In* Roth SH, Miller KW (eds): Molecular and Cellular Mechanisms of Anesthetics, 191–201. New York: Plenum, 1984.

Savarese JJ, Covino BG: Basic and Clinical Pharmacology of Local Anesthetic Drugs. *In* Miller RD (ed): Anesthesia. 2nd ed, 985–1014. New York: Churchill Livingstone, 1986.

Scott DB: Techniques of Regional Anesthesia. Norwalk, CT: Appleton & Lange/Mediglobe, 1989.

Strichartz GR (ed): Local Anesthetics. Vol 81 of Handbook of Experimental Pharmacology. Berlin: Springer-Verlag, 1986.

Strichartz GR, Wang GK: The kinetic basis for phasic local anesthetic blockade of neuronal sodium channels. *In* Strichartz GR (ed): Local Anesthetics, 217–226. Vol 81 of Handbook of Experimental Pharmacology. Berlin: Springer-Verlag, 1986.

Wall PD, Melzack R (eds): Textbook of Pain. New York: Churchill Livingstone, 1984.

18

Opioid Analgesics—Agonists and Antagonists

Cedric M. Smith

One of the two prime objectives of medicine is the alleviation of suffering. Thus, the drugs that relieve pain and suffering are a major, perhaps the major, subject in all of pharmacology. The hallmark and standard of all medicines used to relieve suffering and pain are the opiates, specifically morphine. Not only is morphine *the* standard, it remains today after centuries of use an extremely valuable and useful therapeutic agent to prevent or relieve moderate to severe pain of whatever cause.

Morphine is the major active ingredient in an ancient medicinal plant, the opium poppy. In addition, it has served as the parent substance for a host of synthetic compounds, some of which share some or all of morphine's actions (opioid agonists), whereas some are complete or partial antagonists (opioid antagonists).

The study of the receptors to morphine has led only recently to the remarkable discovery that within the body and the nervous system are a number of naturally occurring substances that bind to the morphine receptors to produce morphine-like effects. These naturally occurring substances—endorphins, enkephalins, and dynorphin—are discussed briefly. However, because the theme of this chapter is the drug therapy that can result in the prevention or relief of pain, the nature of pain and its measurement is addressed initially.

A note about words and language is in order. Strictly speaking, *opiate* refers to a substance derived from opium and possessing opium-like (i.e., morphine-like) actions. *Opioid* refers to a compound with morphine-like effects or that binds to an opiate receptor. Until the last few years the opioid agonists with morphine properties were referred to as *narcotics* or *narcotic analgesics;* it is still acceptable to refer to them as narcotic analgesics in the context of their medical use as analgesics. The word narcotics has at least three different meanings: first, it refers in old popular literature to any agent that can induce *narcosis,* a state of drugged sleep; second, narcotics can refer in the legal system to whatever the laws, in that jurisdiction and time, define as narcotics (these frequently have included not only opiates but many substances that do not have morphine-like effects); and third, it can refer to narcotic analgesics, which usually means opiates and opioids with morphine-like actions.

The effective and rational use of analgesics to alleviate pain derives directly from three related knowledge bases: one, the knowledge of their acute and chronic actions and the mechanisms of these analgesic actions; two, the relationships between these actions and their potentially serious side effects; and three, the pharmacokinetics of these effects in the context of the variability of their actions in different individuals and disease conditions.

Opium contains morphine, codeine, papaverine, and thebaine.

The pharmacological activity of opium is due to its content of morphine.

The terms opioids and narcotic analgesics refer to drugs that have actions similar to those of morphine.

Narcotics can mean opioids, drugs producing narcosis, or what the *narcotics* laws list as narcotics.

In order to relieve pain or to assess drug effects on pain, pain itself needs to be examined. Pain varies with respect to (1) the stimuli, conditions, and sites of pain; (2) the subjective perception of pain as well as the objective responses to pain stimuli (nociception); and (3) the emotional, psychological, and behavioral counterparts of the perception of pain.

Stimuli and *conditions* causing pain are quite varied and depend in part on the specific tissue, the nature of the stimulus (e.g., heat, cold, cutting, stretching, ischemia), the duration of the painful stimulus, as well as the intensity of the stimulation. For example, depending on the tissue, pain may be associated with incising the skin, stretching of tissues such as muscle or omentum, hypoxia of contracting skeletal muscle, immobility of extremities, distension (of bowel, bladder, and so forth), inflammation, or neuralgia. In short, the nature and intensity of the pain experienced vary with the number and types of nerves excited, the tissues involved, the excitability and conduction through central nervous system (CNS) pathways, the amount of concurrent stress and anxiety, as well as the levels of the endogenous endorphin and neurotransmitters. In general, the stimuli that are perceived as painful have the potential to cause damage to tissues.

Nociception is a *subjective* phenomenon that can vary along the dimensions of intensity or severity, character (sharp, dull, boring, aching, burning, vise-like), duration, frequency, recurrence, pattern, and location(s). The *objective* counterparts of pain perception include changes in heart rate, blood pressure, respiration, vasoconstriction, pallor, sweating, restlessness, withdrawal, and avoidance.

The *emotional* and *psychological* components of pain are inexorably intertwined with the perceptual and reflex components. Among the more important in relation to treatment is the *meaning* of pain to the individual. Pain perception and reactions are heavily based on expectations and learned responses, some of which are culturally conditioned. A particularly important factor influencing severe, chronic pain is its significance to the patient as actual or potential loss, with an attendant loss of personal control and autonomy. Not only is pain experienced, it is commonly accompanied by strong reactions of anger, anguish, fear, sadness, anxiety, depression, or frustration. These reactions need to be assessed on their own merits, but many are mutually interactive with pain. For example, anxiety and depression aggravate and potentiate all kinds of pain; providing patients with greater control over their lives and medication, or relieving their anxiety, can result in marked decreases in perceived pain.

Thus, the experience or expectation of pain may be associated with a variety of pain-related behaviors that can have major influences over choice of medication, the route of administration, and the regimen. For example, pain medication needs of those stoic patients who deny all but life-threatening pain are different from the needs of those who seek medications of all kinds for even the most minor of injuries.

Assessment and Measurement of Pain

Pain consists of stimuli and conditions, perceptions, feelings, complex reflexes, emotions, and personal and social behaviors.

Matching the drug with the pain, the person, and the disease

Principles in the Prevention and Alleviation of Pain

The analgesic drugs are used clinically in the context of all the factors involved in pain. Rational therapy seeks to address each of the factors mentioned earlier to

- remove the cause (treat the etiology)
- antagonize the mechanisms of pain and suffering
- relieve anxiety
- relieve depression
- increase sense of personal control
- promote positive suggestions of well-being
- reduce sensory input that aggravates the pain

- provide as effective and complete pain relief as possible as early as possible
- prevent anxiety, fear, and learned responses that may augment perceived pain and pain-related behaviors.

Many drug classes have effects and uses in the alleviation of pain.

Drugs used in the prevention and treatment of pain include not only the opioid analgesics as such but local anesthetics, general anesthetics, and the nonsteroidal anti-inflammatory drugs (aspirin, acetaminophen, ibuprofen, and the many others). Pain can be markedly influenced also by a variety of so-called adjunctive agents including, but not limited to, caffeine, amphetamines, α_2 adrenergic agonists, tricyclic antidepressants, carbamazepine, phenytoin, and hydroxyzine.

Classification of Opioids, Opiates, and Narcotic Analgesics

Agonists, antagonists, mixed agonist/antagonists

Multiple opioid receptors: more than 12 different classes

Prior to discussing the actions and uses of the type of agent, morphine, and related compounds, it is useful to provide a frame of reference for all the compounds in this class according to receptor action and specificity. The multiple opioid receptors were the first receptors in the brain to be identified and characterized, and the first clues of their existence were provided by the study of the selective agonists and by the availability of opioid antagonists. Five major classes of molecular opioid receptors have been defined. Three of these general classes (there are many subclasses) are designated mu (μ), kappa (κ), and sigma (σ). Theoretically, any agent could bind to each of these classes of receptors and act as either an agonist or antagonist, or it could have mixed properties.

Table 18–1 shows the specific receptor classes pertinent to most of the clinically used opioid analgesics. Nevertheless, the specificity (as deter-

Table 18-1 CLASSIFICATION OF OPIOIDS, OPIATES, AND NARCOTIC ANALGESICS*

Compound	Major Receptor Types†		
	μ	κ	σ
AGONIST			
Morphine (and codeine, oxycodone, meperidine, hydromorphone, and the like)	<u>Ag</u>	Ag	
MIXED AGONISTS/ANTAGONISTS			
Buprenorphine (Buprenex)	<u>pAg/Ant</u>		
Pentazocine (Talwin-Nx)	Ant	<u>Ag</u>	Ag
Nalbuphine (Nubain)	Ant	<u>Ag</u>	
Butorphanol (Stadol)	(Ant)	<u>Ag</u>	
ANTAGONISTS			
Naloxone (Narcan)	<u>Ant</u>	<u>Ant</u>	
Nalorphine (Nalline)	<u>Ant</u>	pAg	Ag

* *Analgesia is due to agonist activity at certain μ or certain κ receptors, or both.* Note also that drugs binding to the same class of receptors may have different relative affinities for such receptors. The receptor action for which the compound is used clinically is underlined. (In this simplified table, areas were left blank because either the information is not available or the results are not particularly pertinent.)

A *partial agonist* is a substance that binds only to limited degree (i.e., has limited efficacy) to a population of receptors; for example, a drug that can bind to a receptor in two ways, one of which is agonistic and the other not. The apparent end effect of such an agent would be a function of the relative affinities for the two ways of binding. An example is buprenorphine at μ receptors.

A *mixed agonist/antagonist* results when the agent is a partial agonist alone but is antagonistic to a strong agonist, such as in the example given for partial agonist. (The same end result of apparent mixed agonism-antagonism could occur when the opioid agent acts on one subgroup of receptors as an agonist and on another subgroup as an antagonist.)

† Ag = opioid agonist; pAg = partial agonist; Ant = antagonist.

mined by the specificities of agonists and antagonists in relation to their pharmacological actions and receptor topography) varies both with the species and with the neural locations.

The primary source of morphine is opium obtained from the opium poppy, and the pharmacological effects of opium, such as smoked opium, are due to its content of morphine. Thus an *opiate* is a substance that produces the effects of opium, i.e., morphine; an *opioid* is a substance not derived directly from opium but possessing the same properties. In modern usage opioid and opiate tend to be employed interchangeably.

In addition to morphine, opium contains a number of alkaloids (nitrogen-containing bases derived from plants) including the therapeutically useful codeine and two not therapeutically significant agents, papaverine and thebaine.

Actions of Opioids as Typified by Morphine

Alkaloids — nitrogen-containing bases derived from plants

CENTRAL NERVOUS SYSTEM EFFECTS OF MORPHINE

The primary uses of morphine derive from its dose-related effects on the CNS to cause analgesia, sedation, mental clouding, and euphoria. It also depresses respiration and the cough reflex, and causes constipation, pupillary constriction, nausea, vomiting, and antidiuretic hormone release. (All of these effects are dose-related and occur after all the usual routes of administration — intramuscular, subcutaneous, intravenous, or oral.)

Relief of pain — analgesia — is produced by μ and κ opioid receptor agonists.

Analgesia

The analgesia following administration of morphine is characterized by a sense of relief and well-being accompanying the decrease in pain — its perception and the reflex responses to the pain stimulus. The decrease in responses to pain applies to almost all kinds and intensities of pain; the depression of nociceptive (i.e., pain) reflexes occurs even in the body below the level of a complete spinal cord section.

"Morphine! God's own medicine" — Sir William Osler

Not only is there an increase, after morphine, in the sensory threshold for pain, the relief from suffering may exceed that of pain reduction. This has given rise to the partially accurate statement that morphine decreases the painfulness without a fully corresponding change in the level of perceived pain. After receiving morphine for pain, patients may describe the effects according to the cliché: "I have just as much pain, but it doesn't hurt as bad."

Although there is relief of pain and a change in nociception, morphine has no effects on other sensory modalities. (There may be reduced visual acuity because of pupillary constriction, but not because of any direct effect on the visual system.) Yet, the relief of pain can be dangerous.

A major side effect of all analgesics is the abolition of symptoms and reflexes *absolutely essential* to diagnosis, e.g., giving morphine or any analgesic for abdominal pain in the face of an unrecognized appendicitis has tragic consequences.

Doses of analgesics which suppress the dysphoric sensations connected with the functions of the protective system do not influence sensory perceptions like touch, taste, vision and hearing and their mental assimilation. In this respect, analgesics contrast with general anesthetics. The invaluable relief given by the analgesics rests on their ability to suppress the protective system with its dysphoric sensations and anxiety. *When using analgesics we have to keep in mind that they inactivate this protective system which serves the useful purpose of warning against injury. Therefore the use of analgesics should be permitted, or indeed ordered, only when the warning has been heeded or the functions of the system have lost their meaning* (italics added). (Schaumann O: Some new aspects of action of morphine-like analgesics. Br Med J 2:1091, 1956.)

Morphine frequently produces dysphoria.

Closely associated with the relief of pain is morphine's effects of relieving anxiety, worry, and tension. In this respect alone morphine has a

Opioids relieve all kinds of pain, worry, and anxiety.

dramatic, acute effect to relieve anxiety and to induce a feeling of relaxation and tranquility, including the relief of painful memories and frustrations. For some individuals at least, morphine and other opioids produce an elevation of mood, an outright euphoria. Characteristic of this mood elevation is an increase of feelings of well-being, increased energy, and increased effectiveness. Nevertheless, for most people in the absence of pain, the effects of an opiate are most often perceived as mildly unpleasant, dysphoric, with anxiety or irritability.

Morphine affects higher cortical functions; there may be difficulty in concentrating or maintaining a train of thought. In the absence of external stimulation, morphine induces sedation in the sense of drowsiness and may induce a dream-filled sleep. With moderate analgesic doses the patient may sleep but can be readily aroused. With larger doses coma or a state of unconsciousness or anesthesia results.

Characteristically, morphine causes a decrease in libido, a decrease in sexual drive, and a decrease in sexual performance.

In spite of all these neuronal actions morphine has neither selective muscle relaxant effects nor antiepileptic/antiseizure effects. If anything, the threshold for seizures is lowered after opioids.

Depression of Respiration

Depression of respiration is a serious, predictable, dose-related side effect of all morphine and opioid agonists.

After morphine, or any of the opioids, the rate and depth of respiration are both decreased; the respiratory minute volume declines correspondingly. This depression of respiration is largely due to a decrease in the responsiveness to CO_2; this depression is synergic with sleep. With suppression of the carbon dioxide drive to respiration, hypoxia, by way of the carotid chemoreceptors, may be the only major drive for respiration. Under such a condition a *sudden* increase in oxygen in the inspired air may result in cessation of respiration, resulting in further acidosis and CNS depression.

The opioid-induced respiratory depression is the major serious dose-related, predictable side effect of opioids. All opioids produce this dose-dependent depression of respiration and it occurs with the doses used clinically for analgesia. Analgesic doses (doses that produce equivalent degrees of analgesia) of all opioids produce approximately equivalent degrees of respiratory depression (the only exception may be large doses of codeine). The acute toxicity of all opioids is related primarily to their depression of respiration, an effect that can be fatal.

The increased CO_2 level consequent to decreased respiration results in an increase in cerebrospinal fluid pressure.

Depression of the Cough Reflex

Independent of the effects on respiration, morphine and many of the opioids decrease or abolish the cough reflex. Depending on the patient's condition, a decreased cough reflex could be either a desirable relief of coughing or an undesirable effect when it is helpful for the patient to cough actively, for example, after inhalation anesthesia. Cough suppression is mediated by unique opiate receptors that are not stereospecific (in contrast to most of the other receptor systems; see dextromethorphan, later in this chapter).

Constriction of the Pupil

A characteristic effect of morphine and many, but not all, opioids is constriction of the pupil. This constriction is the consequence of central effects on the oculomotor (Edinger-Westphal) nucleus; morphine has little direct effect on pupillary muscles. Although this constriction occurs with most doses of morphine, it is not diagnostic of opioids. Moreover, with asphyxia resulting from morphine overdose there may be pupillary dilation.

Nausea and Vomiting

Morphine induces nausea, and even vomiting in some patients, due to its stimulation of the chemoreceptor trigger zone in the medulla. With large doses, the converse, a decrease in vomiting, occurs because of morphine's depression of the vomiting center.

Expect that opioids will produce nausea or vomiting.

Endocrine Effects

Morphine has a complex group of effects on the endocrine system including the depression of the release of a number of hormones, including antidiuretic hormone, adrenocorticotropic hormone (ACTH), prolactin, growth hormone, and gonadotrophic hormones.

SITES AND MECHANISMS OF ANALGESIC ACTION OF MORPHINE AND OPIOIDS

Sites

Morphine has actions at a number of sites along the pain-analgesic pathways in the CNS. It has spinal, midbrain, thalamic, and cortical sites of action. Nociceptive spinal reflexes are depressed by morphine by way of the actions in the dorsal horn (substantia gelatinosa). (Spinal intrathecal or epidural injections of morphine and other opioids can produce relief of pain, and this route has therapeutic utility in certain patients with severe chronic pain.)

Morphine has multiple central and peripheral sites of action. Opioid receptors are widely distributed in brain and peripheral tissues.

When administered systemically morphine acts in the midbrain (periaqueductal gray matter) as well as by modulating the functions of the spinal, limbic, hypothalamic, and prefrontal cortical areas. Thus, it has multiple sites of action, each of which has been demonstrated to play a role in opioids' analgesic effects. Nevertheless, the analgesic actions of opioids are limited to their effects in the CNS; they do not act outside the brain on the nociceptive pain pathways, in contrast with the nonsteroidal anti-inflammatory analgesics (Chapter 28). (Studies since 1988 have found that opioid receptors may indeed exist in peripheral tissues, and that alleviation of pain by opioids might involve peripheral as well as central actions.)

Mechanisms—Opioid Receptors

Morphine binds as an agonist stereospecifically to specific receptors that have unique distributions in the nervous system, including (but not limited to) the sites enumerated earlier. These receptors and the binding have been characterized by studies of a large number of chemical analogs, on receptors from various neural sites, and by histochemical mapping. Thus, the receptors and receptor systems can be described by

- neuronal location
- correlation of chemical structure with pharmacological effects
- kinetics of binding
- interactions among ligands
- influences of other factors possibly associated with the receptor systems such as ions (Ca^{2+}, Na^+) and various neuroamines

The μ opioid receptor possesses at least 11 reactive sites; four of these are *nuclear* and 6 are secondary or *satellite* sites.

An example of the complexity and some of the mechanisms underlying the remarkable specificity of different opioid compounds to the different receptor systems is presented in Figure 18–1. This figure shows a minimal topography necessary to account for much of the structure activity relationships among a series of opioid derivatives. The entire receptor system is most likely a part of the nerve membrane and contains binding sites for the major moieties on morphine such as nitrogen and its substituents, the hydroxyl groups, the planar benzene ring, and the large bulky constituents. Not only can the binding sites be identified, their approximate size and shape can be deduced from study of the molecular structures that bind to specific sites as compared with those in which the orientation or the size of the important groups precludes effective attachment.

The steric theory of opioid receptors has several components. It assumes that opioid receptors have *nuclear sites* that are responsible for initiating the pharmacologic action of the drug. In addition to these nuclear sites are *secondary sites* that play two roles: they determine the affinity of the drug for the receptor, and they define or limit the orientation of the drug on the receptor. Differences in the configuration of these two components may result in several effects on drug-receptor interactions. Changes in the molecular groups that bind to either the nuclear or the secondary sites will result in a change in activity. (*Allomorphism* is a term proposed to describe a change in the position of the active moieties of the nuclear part of the receptor, whereas *allosterism* is a change in the positions of the satellite [secondary] sites. Changes in either can result in changes in affinity or orienting properties of the receptor for a drug. In addition, the term *allotaxia* has been coined to refer to the property whereby a drug can occupy the receptor in several orientations or positions [Martin, 1988].)

Figure 18–1

A topographic model of one version of a hypothetical opioid receptor and the morphine molecule ligand. The reactive binding sites are shown as shaded areas.

Top, The model of the receptor and morphine molecules are shown separately, including a conventional chemical drawing of the morphine molecule.

The topography of the receptor was established using a general opioid ligand based on extensive data on the relationships between chemical structure and opioid activity. The reactive sites and associated bond energies are included in the original presentation of this model (Martin, 1983). This adaptation depicts the receptor embedded in a neuronal membrane, but data for its cellular and membrane location are lacking.

Bottom, The hypothetical relationship between the molecule and the various binding sites. The viewer is asked to envision the hydrogens and the electron clouds surrounding the basic structure. The oxygen moieties are shown as solid colored spheres; the nitrogen is in shaded color at the right side of the figure. (Adapted from Martin WR: Pharmacology of opioids. Pharmacol Rev 35(4):283–323, 1983, © by American Society for Pharmacology and Experimental Therapeutics.)

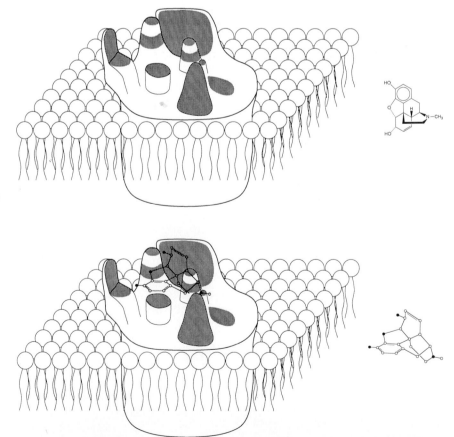

Future research will undoubtedly define the protein and peptide sequences of isolated opioid receptors and permit the reconstruction of the complete receptor including detailed definition of its pre- and postsynaptic locations on neuronal membranes.

Receptor-Mediated Mechanisms of Opioid Action

Although receptor research has been remarkably successful in defining receptor structures, locations, and drug specificities, the mechanisms that are set in motion by agonist-receptor binding involved in analgesia are as yet not well defined. Presumably, opioids act to modify ionic permeabilities such as K^+ conductance of nerve membranes, which in turn results in hyperpolarization and depression of excitability in the neuronal system. But to date how this is accomplished has not been established. The end results of such actions include alterations in some portions in most, if not all, of the central cholinergic, adrenergic, serotonergic, and dopaminergic neurotransmitter systems.

Each reactive binding site on a receptor binds with a unique energy and a unique capacity for agonism and antagonism.

It is also likely that opioids act by way of modifications of calcium uptake and binding in nerve endings. Electrophysiologically some of the systems affected by opioids exhibit decreased cell discharge, membrane hyperpolarization, augmentation of hyperpolarization produced by repetitive neuronal firing, decreases in neuronal afterdischarges, and decreases in temporal summation. In any event, the most relevant action is the ultimate effect of blocking the transmission of nociceptive information in ascending neuronal projections.

Reviewing these many actions serves to emphasize that the nociceptive systems utilize a number of neurotransmitters: substance P, enkephalins, and serotonin are involved at the spinal cord level; serotonergic, adrenergic, cholinergic, and dopaminergic systems are involved in the medulla and midbrain pain pathways and reticular activating system, as well as in the periaqueductal gray. Adrenergic agents, such as amphetamine and dopamine, tend to reduce pain, whereas cholinergic and serotonergic agents tend to exacerbate it.

Nociceptive neuronal systems involve a variety of neurotransmitters.

Depending on how many distinctions one wants to make, there are from 5 to more than 12 molecularly distinct classes of opioid receptors. For the purposes of understanding current agents used in therapy it is sufficient to identify 4 major classes of opioid receptors whose binding characteristics can be readily correlated with their pharmacological spectra of action. One of these, the cough suppressant receptor, is not stereospecific and is usually not considered among the *stereospecific opioid receptors*. Three of the most therapeutically relevant stereospecific receptors, as shown in Table 18–1, are the μ, κ, and σ receptors. The stereospecificity applies both to compounds that are agonists (morphine-like) and to antagonists (such as naloxone). There are compounds with pure agonist action at specific sites, e.g., morphine, and compounds with almost pure antagonist actions, e.g., naloxone. In addition, many compounds with mixed agonist/antagonist properties are known and some of these have found clinical utility, e.g., pentazocine.

The analgesic effects of morphine and the related opioids are the consequence of its binding to μ and to κ receptors; moreover, only a proportion of these μ and κ receptors, which are localized at a relatively few specific sites, are actually involved in eliciting analgesia. In addition, μ receptors are involved in the respiratory depression, pupillary constriction, and the changes in feeling states of increased self-image, energy, and effectiveness produced by opioid agonists. Not only do the opioids act on specific receptors, but different neurons differ in their complement of the various receptor subtypes, and not all nociceptive systems contain opioid

Analgesic effects of opioids are mediated through agonistic actions of μ and κ receptors.

Only some of the μ and κ receptors are involved in pain and analgesia.

All actions of opioids involve specific constellations of opioid receptors.

receptors. (A δ class of receptors selectively binds enkephalins and may also be involved in opioid analgesia.)

(The σ receptor has relatively little relevance to therapeutics at present inasmuch as it mediates the perceptual, psychotomimetic, and increased irritability effects of certain experimental compounds, and may possibly be involved in the actions of phencyclidine [see Chapters 16, 26, and 67]. Some of the agonist-antagonists [pentazocine, butorphanol] bind to sigma receptors and have psychomimetic effects in large doses.)

Binding to κ receptors, in addition to producing analgesia, is also responsible in part for feelings of sedation and personal ineffectiveness produced by opioids.

The characterization and discovery of the multiple opioid receptors are major accomplishments of recent research. Current active advances in the treatment of pain, the prevention of fatal poisoning, and the understanding of drug dependence are direct results of a long search for safe, nonaddicting substitutes for opiates. The evidence for the different receptors came from observations made in prison patients (at the U.S. Public Health Service's Addiction Research Center in Lexington, Kentucky) who were participating in studies on the safety and abuse potentiality of new analgesics. These studies were part of well-integrated efforts — chemical, analytical, animal experiments, human volunteers, and patients — involving the pharmaceutical industry, laboratories at the National Institutes of Health, and experimental studies in animals in academic departments of pharmacology and medicine (Martin, 1988). As this chapter and Chapter 67 attest, these goals have been partially, albeit not fully, achieved with the availability of potent analgesics with improved safety margins and lesser abuse liabilities.

MORPHINE-RELATED COMPOUNDS USED AS COUGH SUPPRESSANTS

Dextromethorphan

The lack of stereospecificity in the cough suppressant effects was revealed by the discovery and introduction of dextromethorphan (ROMILAR and many others) — the dextroisomer of a synthetic opioid. Dextromethorphan is an effective cough suppressant essentially devoid of any of the analgesic, respiratory depressant or euphorigenic effects of opioid agonists. Dextromethorphan is now widely available in over-the-counter cough and cold remedies; it has largely replaced codeine as a cough suppressant medication.

OPIOID PEPTIDES

The discovery and characterization of opioid receptors led directly to searches for endogenous ligands for these receptors. These searches were rewarded with the discovery of a number of peptides that bind to opiate receptors and that have morphine-like effects. The availability of the remarkably selective and specific antagonist, naloxone, made the research feasible. The following is a short list of known endogenous compounds:

- leucine-enkephalin (H-Tyr-Gly-Gly-Phe-Leu-OH)
- methionine-enkephalin (H-Tyr-Gly-Gly-Phe-Met-OH)
- beta-endorphin
- dynorphins

Beta-endorphin is the sequence 61–91 in the amino acid sequence in the polypeptide known as β lipotropin (of previously unknown function). Note that leucine-enkephalin is identical to met-enkephalin except for the replacement of Met by Leu. Dynorphin is a 17-amino acid peptide containing the leucine-enkephalin sequence. These peptides are not synthesized directly, but rather are the products of the cleavage of larger precursor polypeptides. Their local application to parts of the brain results in effects similar to those of opiates, and the actions are blocked by antagonists. Although a large number of derivatives have been studied, none has yet been found to have clinical utility. But the search is not over. A number of as yet unidentified opioid peptides have been detected in brain extracts, and an opiate receptor ligand (binding agent) different from known endorphins has been reported in cerebrospinal fluid. (Not only are there opioid peptides in brain, but morphine and codeine can be synthesized by mammalian tissues.)

The functions of these endogenous peptides with opiate actions remain an area of intense research. In general it appears that they are not elaborated or active as analgesics in the normal state. This is consistent with the fact that the administration of opioid antagonists does not result in pain or other effects opposite to the opioids, as would be expected if they antagonized existing opioids in the brain.

> Opioid antagonists do not produce pain.

On the other hand, these endogenous opioid systems appear to be involved in the modulation of the responses to pain and nociceptive input by way of the extensive neural systems that modulate pain perception and responses. Sustained pain and certain types of stress are associated with the release of endogenous opioids. Consistent with such pain-induced release is the observation that naloxone administration can increase the intensity of pain experienced by noxious stimulation.

Thus, the endorphins/enkephalins and related substances probably have specific functions in specific neural systems but not directly as neurotransmitters. Evidence suggests that they *may* be involved as *modulators* of the presynaptic mechanisms involved in neurotransmitter synthesis/release in nociceptive pathways, including the descending modulation of nociceptive pathways.

> The intensity of pain is modified by anxiety, depression, expectation, prior experiences, and levels of a variety of neurotransmitters.

In addition to pain systems, the endorphins are involved in central systems of appetitive drives (e.g., food, water, sex), memory, mood states, mental processes, and traumatic nervous system damage. In experimental animals naloxone dramatically increases the recovery of neurons damaged by trauma such as spinal cord compression. Other tissues, such as the placenta, are being found to contain endorphin-like peptides and their macromolecular precursors.

In recent years not only have morphine-like peptides been discovered, a wide variety of other peptides have been identified as being involved in the regulation of organ function and behavior. Some examples of these peptides are the octapeptide involved in the control of food intake; pentagastrin; somatostatin; and thyrotropin releasing factor (TRF), luteinizing hormone releasing factor, (LRF), and follicle-stimulating hormone (FSH).

EFFECTS OF MORPHINE ON OTHER SYSTEMS

Smooth Muscle

Intestine. Many opioids share with opium and morphine the property of causing constipation and a decrease of propulsive activity in the small and large intestines. This constipative effect has been known and utilized since antiquity. The decrease in motility and propulsion is the consequence of nonpainful, sustained contraction of the smooth muscles of the gut.

> Endogenous opioids and opioid receptors are present in the gastrointestinal wall, nerves and plexuses, and muscles.

This constipating effect of opioids is a common, and sometimes distressing, side effect of all of the opioid agonists. Diarrhea is characterized by persistent propulsion, and morphine, even in doses below those needed for analgesia, provides effective temporary symptomatic relief of diarrhea.

The mechanism of the constipating action of opioids is complex but it is

> Constipating and antidiarrheal actions are not necessarily identical.

Antidiarrheal effects of opioids are due to actions on the intestine and on the CNS.

Opioid antidiarrheal effects are due to decrease in propulsion and increased net water absorption from the gut.

The name LOMOTIL provides no clue that this product contains atropine as well as the opioid diphenoxylate.

known to be due to both central and peripheral actions: actions in the CNS to increase vagal innervation of the bowel, and local actions directly on smooth muscle and on cholinergic neuroeffector transmission. At least a significant portion of the constipative, smooth muscle contractions can be antagonized by atropine, indicating that the opioid actions involve activation of cholinergic systems. (Both central and peripheral opiate receptors are involved in coordinated smooth muscle activity, as evidenced by the fact that naloxone, in experimental investigations, has been shown to increase intestinal motility.) The antidiarrheal actions are due not only to changes in motility but to an enhancement of net water and electrolyte absorption in both large and small bowel. This antisecretory action of opioids is stereospecific and blocked by naloxone.

Antidiarrheal Preparations. The time-honored antidiarrheal preparation of paregoric (paregoric is a tincture of opium containing benzoic acid, camphor, and anise oil) is still available as an over-the-counter drug; its active ingredient is morphine.

Newer antidiarrheal agents that act selectively on opioid receptors include diphenoxylate (LOMOTIL is the trade name preparation that includes also atropine) and loperamide (IMODIUM). Loperamide as IMODIUM is now also available over-the-counter. The fact that LOMOTIL contains atropine is not commonly appreciated and has contributed to anticholinergic toxicity, especially in the elderly.

Biliary Tract, Bronchi, Ureter, Urinary Bladder. Opioids increase biliary tract tone and pressure and can produce biliary colic. Morphine and other opioids can cause bronchoconstriction or contraction of the ureters. For most patients these effects do not cause symptoms, but in the face of disease, such as cholelithiasis or bronchial asthma, the benefits and need for the analgesic effects have to be weighed against the risk of aggravating pre-existing conditions. For example, although opioids do cause contraction of the ureter, they are commonly administered, in spite of this action, to relieve the excruciating pain that may be caused by kidney stones.

In addition, morphine causes an increase in the tone of the detrusor muscle and urinary bladder as well as the vesical sphincter, all of which may lead to urinary retention or difficulty in urination.

All of these effects on smooth muscles can occur with doses equal to or sometimes less than those needed for analgesia. Thus, they all may be present as side effects when using opioids as analgesics.

Histamine Release

Morphine and many opioid agonists, such as heroin, cause peripheral vasodilation and itching. These effects are mediated at least in part by the release of histamine.

Cardiovascular Effects

In doses used to produce analgesia, morphine and opioid agonists have little influence on the cardiovascular system. A flush of the skin is not uncommon and a minor degree of orthostatic hypotension consistent with moderate peripheral vasodilation can be detected. This peripheral vasodilation is due partly to histamine release.

TIME COURSE OF MORPHINE ACTIONS

After intramuscular or subcutaneous administration the onset of action of morphine is prompt, yet the peak of analgesia may be delayed for 30 or 40 minutes. This delay appears to be in part related to the penetration to brain sites, because a similar time course for the appearance of peak analgesia is observed upon intravenous administration. Agents with greater lipid solubilities have a somewhat more rapid onset of action.

All narcotic analgesics are weak bases, moderately ionized at pH 7. Morphine is effective after oral administration, but the degree of first-pass effect differs appreciably among patients so that the dose and frequency of oral administration must be adjusted on an individual basis.

Morphine is metabolized to two glucuronides, at the hydroxyl groups at positions 6 and 3 of the structure. The 6 glucuronide has, to the surprise of many, been found not only to have morphine-like effects but it appears to be many times as potent as morphine. In relation to the relevant kinetics, after intramuscular injection the active agent is primarily morphine. After single oral doses both morphine and the 6 glucuronide are present in active levels. With chronic oral administration the 6 glucuronide accumulates to a greater degree than does morphine; thus, the glucuronide metabolite plays an increasingly significant role with chronic administration (see Fig. 18–3).

The glucuronide metabolites are excreted by the kidney along with some free morphine; 90% of administered morphine can be accounted for in urinary excretion products over 24 hours. (As discussed later, tolerance to an opioid is not due to alterations in metabolism.)

Not only are the metabolism and excretion of morphine and its active metabolite important to morphine, they are also important to codeine and heroin, two agents whose actions are due, at least in part, to their conversion *in vivo* to morphine.

The duration of action of morphine and metabolite is directly related to blood (i.e., brain) levels; the analgesic effects are greater with higher blood levels and the relief of pain decreases in parallel with the decline in blood (i.e., brain) levels. Thus, there is no absolute or discretely definable *duration of action;* rather, in the face of continuing pain system activity, the administration of morphine or other agonists such as meperidine results in a maximal pain relief within an hour followed by a gradual increase in pain over a period of 2–6 hours (Figs. 18–2 and 18–3). *Thus, the time course of the relief of pain depends on the dose and the blood level achieved, the severity of the pain, and the individual patient's threshold for pain and its relief (see Fig. 18–4).*

The time course of the *relief* from pain *in that individual patient* is the prime concern. Average duration of action statements provide only a rough guess of what can be expected.

The magnitude of pain relief is dependent on severity of pain, the individuals' sensitivities to pain and to the opioid, and the level of the opioid at the opioid receptors.

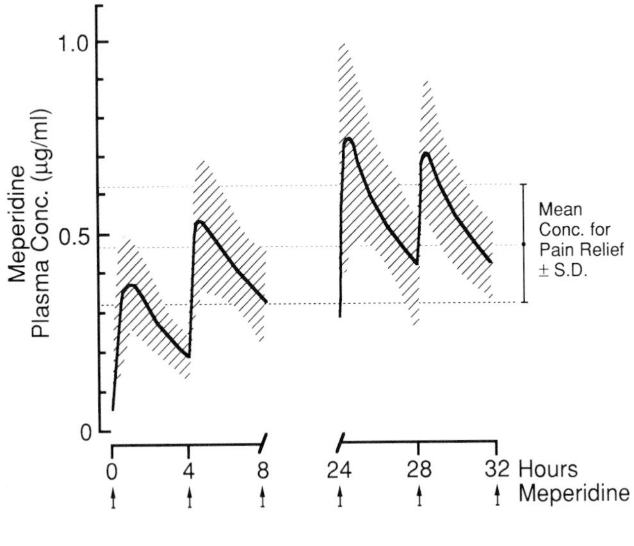

Figure 18–2

Practical aspects of blood levels—The importance of regular dosing and cumulation was explicitly examined in patients receiving meperidine (Demerol) postoperatively, every 4 hours. The intensity of the pain experienced by patients postoperatively was measured at the same time as a blood sample was taken to measure the meperidine level.

The mean blood level of meperidine associated with pain relief (the minimal analgesic level) is plotted on the graph as the *horizontal dotted line* at ~0.48 µg/ml, with the ±1 standard deviation shown by the *horizontal dotted lines.*

The *heavy solid lines* indicate the actual mean blood levels obtained after the first, second, and last two doses; the *shaded areas* depict the standard deviation. Note the apparent absence of tolerance and the cumulation of levels into the analgesic, pain-relieving blood level range. (From Austin KL, Stapleton JV, Mather LE: Relationship between blood meperidine concentrations and analgesic response: A preliminary report. Anesthesiology 53:460–466, 1980.)

Figure 18-3

Plasma concentrations (mean + SEM) of
morphine, morphine-6-glucuronide
(M-6-G), and morphine-3-glucuronide
(M-3-G). *A,* After intravenous administration of morphine, and *B,* after oral
administration of morphine. Note the
logarithmic scale for the plasma concentrations. (From Osborne R, Joel S, Trew D,
Slevin R: Morphine and metabolite
behavior after different routes of morphine
administration: Demonstration of the
importance of the active metabolite
morphine-6-glucuronide. Clin Pharmacol
Ther 47:12–19, 1990.)

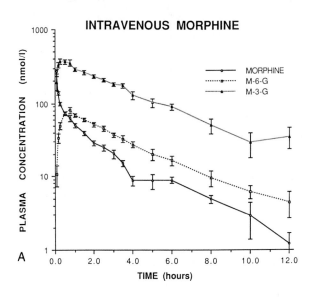

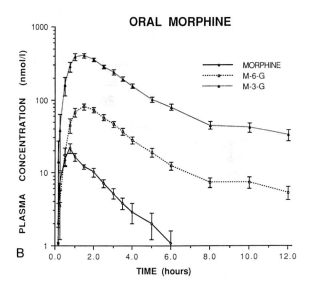

TOLERANCE

With repeated administration of opioids there develops a tolerance to the
effects of the agent. (By tolerance it is meant that a larger dose is needed to
produce a given effect, or that a given dose produces quantitatively less
effect). In general, this tolerance to opioids is limited to the so-called de-

pressant effects of analgesia, respiratory depression, antianxiety effects, and drowsiness. Even though individuals may be relatively tolerant to the respiratory depressant actions, sufficiently large doses can produce respiratory depression and possibly death. In contrast, little tolerance develops to the constipation or pupillary constriction produced by opioids.

The development of tolerance is dependent on dose, the repetition rate, and regularity. The maximum degree of tolerance with opioids can be large such that doses 10–20 times the initial dose can be tolerated.

The mechanism of functional tolerance and physical dependence involves the opioid and neurotransmitter system described earlier. In addition, the *N*-methyl-D-aspartate (NMDA) type of glutamate receptors and calcium channels are also known to be involved, because blockade of these receptor systems reduces development of tolerance and dependence with chronic opioid administration.

Although marked tolerance can be observed in those dependent on opioids, in the clinical use of analgesics for pain relief, the development of tolerance is rarely a problem. Tolerance development is almost never a problem during the 1–3 days of opioid analgesic use commonly needed postoperatively or following trauma (see Fig. 18–2). Even when opioids are used for the management of chronic pain, for example, for those terminal cancer patients who have pain, the tolerance that develops can be readily managed by dosage adjustment. Patients vary markedly in their sensitivities (Fig. 18–4).

Cross tolerance occurs among all opioid agonists.

With repeated administration of opioids both habituation and dependence can develop (see Chapter 67). Presumably the development of the habit of repeatedly taking a drug is related to a drug's potential to produce desirable subjective states such as euphoria or the relief of anxiety or some other feeling state. Physical dependence occurs also after chronic adminis-

Although marked tolerance can be observed with chronic opioid administration, tolerance is *not* of significance in the 1–3 days required for the treatment of acute pain or postoperatively.

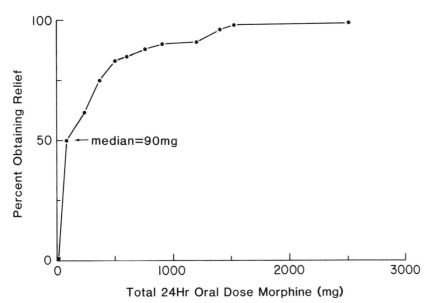

Figure 18–4

Variability among cancer patients with chronic pain with respect to the amount of morphine required for relief of pain. All the patients were receiving doses of morphine sufficient to relieve their pain. The cumulative frequency expressed as percent of patients is plotted against the total 24-hour oral intake of morphine. Note that the median daily dose, the dose that half of the patients were receiving, is relatively low, only 90 mg, whereas some patients required many times that dose level in order to obtain satisfactory analgesia. (Data from McQuay HJ, Caroll D, Faura CC, et al: Oral morphine in cancer pain: Influences on morphine and metabolite concentration. Clin Pharmacol Ther 48:236–244, 1990.)

tration of progressively larger amounts, so that upon discontinuation of such administration a characteristic withdrawal, or abstinence, sickness appears. Amounts required to induce such physical dependence can exceed, for example, 60 mg/day of morphine or its equivalent (analgesic doses of morphine are 6–10 mg, commonly given every 4–6 hours).

(The signs and symptoms of the abstinence syndrome are as follows: autonomic—sweating, vomiting, diarrhea, abdominal cramps, runny nose, shivering, goose flesh, increased heart rate and blood pressure, increased body temperature, mydriasis; CNS—sleeplessness, restless sleep [yen], irritability, tremor, joint and muscle pains, anorexia, yawning, dehydration, ketosis, weight loss, hypophoria. The peak severity occurs some 36–72 hours after the last dose and the symptoms gradually wane over a period of 2–5 weeks. This withdrawal is not life-threatening to an otherwise healthy individual and can be alleviated by any narcotic analgesic of the opiate-opioid class [see Chapter 67]. A protracted abstinence syndrome of months in duration has also been identified.)

SIDE EFFECTS OF MORPHINE AND OPIOIDS

The major side effects are the dose-related predictable effects just described. Allergic reactions do occur; however, the claim of patients that they are allergic to one or another of the opioids needs to be assessed accurately. These claims can range from outright allergic reactions, to precipitation of bronchial asthma, to the occurrence of predictable opioid effects such as nausea, vomiting, or constipation.

ACUTE POISONING

Acute poisoning with morphine and other opioids occurs with overdoses relative to the person's sensitivity, accidentally due to misjudgment in clinical settings, and to overdosing by addicts, as well as in suicide attempts. Among fatal drug poisonings, the narcotic analgesics are among the most commonly encountered, exceeding even alcohol. The signs and symptoms of poisoning are predictable on the basis of a knowledge of the pharmacology of the drug; it includes characteristically coma, pin-point pupils, and respiratory depression. With severe respiratory depression, there is also impairment of cardiovascular function. Nevertheless, although respiratory depression with pin-point pupils is highly suggestive of opioid intoxication, barbiturate poisoning can present similarly. Conversely, with sustained hypoxia morphine intoxication can result in pupillary dilation.

The treatment of suspected opioid overdose consists of the support of respiration and the cardiovascular functions plus the administration of the definitive antagonist, naloxone. This naloxone administration will probably have to be repeated, inasmuch as naloxone has a shorter duration of action than morphine or any other opioids that might have caused the poisoning.

CLINICAL USES

Morphine remains a mainstay in the treatment (and prevention) of moderate to severe pain and the situations and factors associated with such pain. Among the common situations and uses are

The medication of choice for severe pain is morphine—or a morphine-like opioid—in doses sufficient to relieve the pain, given often enough to maintain analgesia.

1. preoperatively to relieve anxiety, produce analgesia, and reduce amount of anesthetic required, and postoperatively to produce some degree of analgesia;

2. to treat severe pain, e.g., pain of fracture, large tissue trauma, a

stone in a hollow viscus such as ureteral stone, or metastatic carcinoma of bone;

3. postoperatively to relieve pain and discomfort in the immediate postoperative period. In the absence of complications, postoperative pain requiring opioid medication usually lasts no more than 1–2 days.

The important principles of use of morphine as well as all opioid analgesics address the classic questions of "who, what, where, when, how much." The following are all firmly established by medical research as well as by legal precedent. Failure to adhere to these can have tragic consequences because the opioid drugs have great potential for harm as well as benefit.

- The selection of the drug, dose, route, and regimen should be based on the pain being experienced and anticipated; that is, the drug therapy needs to correspond to the pain syndrome.
- The opioid or any analgesic should be administered only *after the diagnosis,* even a preliminary diagnosis, because the analgesic can mask the pain that is required for an accurate diagnosis.
- In severe acute pain, doses should be adequate to effect relief of the pain, and then repeated frequently enough to maintain pain relief. Pain intensities, the degree of suffering, and individual sensitivity to the opioids vary markedly among different patients. Moreover, adequate pain management requires the regular administration of doses in order to obtain the requisite accumulation (see Fig. 18–2). (It is now well established that p.r.n. [*pro re nata,* as needed] orders and prescriptions for management of severe pain are inappropriate and should be avoided. Rather, a specific repetition rate should be prescribed and then modified on the basis of the patient's actual responses.) The established best prevention for the development of the *chronic pain syndrome* is the appropriate and adequate treatment of acute pain (see Fig. 18–4).
- Automated intravenous delivery systems are now available that permit intermittent self-administration of opioids. This technique has been found useful for relief of pain associated with surgery, sickle cell crises, and cancer. By avoiding the potentially wide swings in blood levels associated with infrequent intramuscular administration, patient-controlled analgesia (PCA) can provide more constant and uniform analgesia. In addition, it provides the patient a sense of control and, more often than not, results in less analgesic drug use than the more conventional intramuscular injections. The potential addictive aspects of opioid infusions have been negligible. Typical opioid side effects can occur, and operator errors can potentially result in continuous or excessive doses.
- The major caution when selecting doses is to be certain that excessive CNS depression and depression of respiratory gas exchange are avoided. Special caution is in order when used with other CNS depressants or in the presence of emphysema, bronchial asthma, or any other limitation of respiratory gas exchange.

A number of different opioids are available for clinical use (Table 18–2). Meperidine is considered next because it has been one of the most frequently ordered opioids for moderate to severe pain, and for pre- and postoperative pain. It is a synthetic congener with a simpler structure than morphine. Nevertheless, it has, with a few exceptions, all of the major properties described earlier for morphine. In short, meperidine is approximately one sixth as potent as morphine, and in sufficient doses it can produce equivalent degrees of analgesia. In equianalgesic doses, meperidine is somewhat shorter acting, less constipating, and without pupillary constriction or cough suppressant activity.

Individualize dosage and schedule. Assess and evaluate (directly or indirectly) patient's response to pain treatments and medication; for example, assess patient at time of expected peak of action.

Acute appendicitis and other causes of acute surgical abdominal emergencies still occur and still cause death or protracted morbidity.

Matching pain, disease, drug, and regimen

The patient is the authority regarding his or her pain. Patient control of opioid dose and frequency is usually more effective, more efficient, and less likely to result in abuse than arbitrary intermittent p.r.n. medication.

Meperidine (DEMEROL, PETHIDINE)

Meperidine (DEMEROL) itself is neither safer nor more effective than morphine.

Table 18-2   SELECTED OPIOID ANALGESICS LISTED FROM LONGEST TO SHORTEST DURATION OF ACTION*

Morphine-like	Trade Name	Duration of Action (Hours)	Analgesic Doses (mg) IM	Oral	Used IV
Methadone	Dolophine	≥4–6	10	20	—
Levorphanol	Levo-Dromoran	≥4–6	10	20	—
Codeine		4–5	130	120	—
Hydromorphone	Dilaudid	4–5	1.5	7.5	—
Oxymorphone	Numorphan	4–5	1	6	—
Morphine		**4–5**	**10**	**60**	**+**
Meperidine		2–4	75–100	300	+
		IV			
Fentanyl	Sublimaze	<1 hour	0.1	NA	+
Sufentanil	Sufenta	<1 hour	NA	NA	+
Alfentanil	Alfenta	<1 hour	NA	NA	+
Marketed As Combinations					
Oxycodone	Percodan, with aspirin		NA	30	
	Percocet, with acetaminophen				
Hydrocodone	Hycodan, with homatropine methylbromide		NA	10	

* *Notes:* NA = not applicable.
    Lower doses used for cough suppression (e.g., 10–20 mg for codeine).
    Not antitussive—meperidine, oxymorphone.
    Less constipation—meperidine, hydromorphone.

PHARMACOLOGICAL EFFECTS

Analgesia

The maximum level of analgesia obtainable with meperidine is equivalent to that obtained with morphine. Meperidine is less potent; 80–100 mg intramuscularly produces analgesia equivalent to that obtained with 10 mg of morphine sulfate.

Behavior and Subjective State

Meperidine produces an affective state similar to that of morphine with feelings of calmness and well-being. Anxiety is relieved and a dreamy drowsiness is common. Large doses result in progressive depression of awareness and cognition, and finally coma. In toxic doses, CNS excitation occurs also with tremor, muscle twitches, and even seizures. (This excitation is due at least in part to a metabolite of meperidine, normeperidine, as described later.)

Respiration

In equianalgesic doses, acute doses of meperidine produce equivalent degrees of respiratory depression. Thus, the acute margin of safety is the same as with morphine.

Cough Reflex

In analgesic doses meperidine does not suppress cough or produce pupillary constriction.

In contrast to morphine and codeine, meperidine does *not* depress the cough reflex. The absence of effects on the cough reflex is neither intrinsically medically beneficial nor harmful. An active cough reflex is frequently desirable postoperatively after inhalation general anesthesia when coughing and deep vigorous respiration help prevent atelectasis.

Pupil

In analgesic doses, meperidine does not produce pupillary constriction. (After toxic doses there is some pupillary constriction, but this is not remarkable.)

Smooth Muscle

Meperidine is spasmogenic on gastrointestinal, ureteral, and biliary smooth muscle, but these effects are somewhat less than those obtained with morphine. The clinical significance of this difference from morphine has long been a matter of dispute.

SIDE EFFECTS

The side effects of meperidine are similar to those of morphine and include respiratory depression, mental clouding, dizziness, sweating, nausea, vomiting, dysphoria, and urinary retention. Large doses or chronic administration may give rise to seizures (discussed in following paragraphs).

TIME COURSE OF ACTION

Meperidine, on average, has a shorter duration of action than morphine— approximately 2–4 hours. In severe pain such as in sickle cell crises, only 1–2 hours of pain relief might be obtained in some patients. Figure 18–2 illustrates the effects that can be predicted with meperidine. The mean blood level of meperidine associated with at least minimal pain relief did not change over a 32-hour period with repeated administration of meperidine (100 mg intramuscularly) every 4 hours. Thus, *there was no tolerance to the analgesic effects of meperidine even when given regularly on a 4-hour schedule.*

Meperidine, on average, has a slightly shorter duration of action than morphine. But individual differences are far more important in determining actual duration of pain relief.

From these investigations it can be concluded that

1. Essentially no tolerance to the analgesic effects of meperidine develops during the immediate postoperative period (2–4 days).
2. The blood levels of meperidine in most of the patients after the first dose did not even achieve a minimal analgesic level, but an analgesic level was achieved with the accumulation occurring with the second and later doses. Thus, better pain relief is obtained when the meperidine is given on a regular basis rather than on the erratic basis of a p.r.n. order.
3. Individuals differ markedly with respect to the blood levels obtained after given doses, as well as with respect to the levels needed to produce a relief of pain. Hence, there is a large variation in the dose needed to obtain relief of pain; there is also a large individual variability in time course and half-lives with meperidine (and other opioids); for example, meperidine could well have been given on a shorter schedule, e.g., 3 hours, in many patients.

Meperidine is metabolized in the liver to normeperidine. Normeperidine is not only twice as toxic as meperidine, but it has a longer half-life. As might be expected, with chronic administration of meperidine, normeperidine can accumulate. In addition, meperidine metabolism is subject to induction; for example, chronic phenobarbital administration is associated with increased normeperidine levels. As a consequence, *meperidine should not be used chronically,* and it should be avoided in patients who have been receiving phenobarbital or any other drug likely to cause hepatic drug-metabolizing systems to be increased.

Meperidine should not be administered chronically, and beware of drug interactions, such as with phenobarbital.

Without doubt the repeated administration of meperidine is associated with habit formation, tolerance, and physical dependence with withdrawal upon discontinuation. (That is, meperidine [DEMEROL] is an addicting substance. See Chapter 67.)

Methadone (DOLOPHINE and generics)

ACTIONS

Methadone is a synthetic agent with effects similar to those of morphine, but it has a slower onset and longer duration of action and is said to be more predictable on oral administration. The analgesia obtained is equivalent to that of morphine with equivalent risk of respiratory depression relative to analgesic effects. (Chemical structures of many opioids are included in Chapter 67.)

SIDE EFFECTS

The side effects and risks of methadone are similar to those of morphine.

Chronic use of methadone results in tolerance and dependence. The withdrawal syndrome may be months in duration.

CLINICAL USES

There are three established uses of methadone: as an analgesic, for treatment of the acute withdrawal syndrome after stopping any chronic administered opioid, and for long-term management of opioid dependence (methadone maintenance, see Chapter 67).

As an analgesic, methadone is suited especially for oral administration and when a longer-acting agent than morphine is desired. The use of the shorter-acting morphine or meperidine permits ready dosage and frequency adjustments but frequent dosing. On the other hand, methadone need not be administered as frequently, but dosage adjustment in the event of excessive sedation or inadequate pain relief may be more difficult.

Codeine

ACTIONS

The effects of codeine are basically similar to those of morphine. By tradition, codeine has been used mostly for oral administration in relatively low doses for either cough suppression (antitussive) or for relief of mild to moderate pain. For example, low doses of codeine are combined frequently with aspirin or other nonsteroidal anti-inflammatory compounds for the management of moderate pain when the nonsteroidal agent is not adequate, such as in the management of pain following dental procedures, or postoperative pain that does not require the usual parenteral doses of morphine. Actually, if a sufficient dose is administered codeine has the potential of producing analgesia equivalent to that produced by morphine. In fact, the activity of codeine is due in part to its metabolism to morphine.

SIDE EFFECTS

The side effects of codeine are essentially those described for morphine. When administered in the usual oral doses (30 or 60 mg), the most common complaint is constipation. Some patients are aware of vague peculiar or unpleasant feelings, although some find the feelings pleasant and desirable; codeine, even orally, has a potential of being habit-forming.

Codeine and alcohol are the intoxicants involved in the abuse of cough

Codeine's side effect of constipation is a predictable opioid action.

syrup. The abuse potential is considered to be low, probably a reflection of the fact that the preponderance of prescriptions are for oral administration of relatively low doses.

CLINICAL USES

Codeine is a relatively frequently used analgesic, commonly combined with nonopioid analgesics. Such combinations are, in principle, rational inasmuch as the combination provides more pain relief than either one alone, and the use of low doses of each reduces the potential toxic effects of both.

Codeine is available in parenteral form and can be used for the management of mild to severe pain.

ACTIONS

Fentanyl is a potent opioid agonist of relatively recent origin, available only for intravenous or intramuscular administration. It has rapid onset and short duration of action; both are shorter than morphine or meperidine. (A dose of 100 μg is approximately equivalent in analgesic activity to 10 mg of morphine or 75 mg of meperidine.) The rapid onset is consistent with its much greater lipid solubility than that of morphine.

The major actions are similar to those of morphine. It is used for its sedative and analgesic effects almost exclusively in the context of anesthesia and operative procedures as a principal anesthetic agent or as an analgesic in combination with other agents (see Chapter 16).

SIDE EFFECTS

Fentanyl produces dose-related depression of respiration ranging from decreased sensitivity to CO_2 to outright apnea. Some depression of respiration can persist longer than effective analgesia and is manifested by shallow, slow respiration. The respiratory depression appears 5–15 minutes after intravenous injections and can persist for up to 4 hours after a single dose.

In view of the potent, rapidly occurring actions of fentanyl, it should be given only by those trained in its use and when the opioid antagonist naloxone, resuscitative equipment, and staff are immediately available.

Fentanyl may cause skeletal muscle rigidity, which can be especially troublesome when this involves respiratory and trunk muscles. The muscle activity can be so marked that it can interfere with the induction of anesthesia.

Fentanyl is associated with few direct effects on cardiac function except for the production of moderate bradycardia.

Histamine release is rarely a problem.

CHRONIC TOXICITY

Although fentanyl is not chronically administered therapeutically, repeated self-administration results in a morphine-type dependence; the availability of the drug presents a significant risk for abuse by anesthesia professionals.

COMPOUNDS RELATED TO FENTANYL

Sufentanil (SUFENTA) is similar in actions and therapeutic uses to fentanyl, yet it is even more potent, up to 10 times more than fentanyl. Using doses

A number of effective opioid agonists are available—most are effective, but none has significant advantages over morphine, codeine, methadone, and the mixed agonist/antagonists.

Analgesics from different pharmacological classes are, in general, at least additive of their effects.

Fentanyl (SUBLIMAZE)

Opioids with rapid onset and relatively short durations of action include fentanyl, sufentanil, alfentanil, and heroin.

such as 8 μg/kg intravenously, it produces profound analgesia almost immediately. It has a distribution time of a few minutes and an elimination half-life of approximately 2–3 hours. More than 90% is bound to plasma proteins.

Sufentanil is employed as the sole analgesic, as an anesthetic, or in combination with other anesthetics. Like fentanyl, it can produce muscular rigidity. Also, like other opioids, it can depress respiration, but this is usually not of major concern because patients receiving sufentanil commonly receive a neuromuscular blocking agent also before and at the same time. Obviously, it is essential that respiration must be maintained, assisted or supported at all times.

The respiratory depression produced by sufentanil or fentanyl can be reversed by naloxone; the duration of action of naloxone may be shorter than that of sufentanil, necessitating continuous postoperative monitoring and possibly repeat doses of naloxone.

There are insufficient data on safety of sufentanil during pregnancy or in labor and delivery to support its use in these conditions.

Sufentanil, like fentanyl, is a Schedule II controlled drug substance that can produce dependence of the morphine type.

ALFENTANIL (ALFENTA)

Alfentanil is, like the others in this group, a potent opioid, but it is distinguished by a rapid onset and an even shorter duration of action than that of sufentanil. The rapid action and short duration of action allow it to be used not only by intravenous injection but also by intravenous infusion. (Even though the time required for recovery, recurrence of pain, and adequate respiration vary markedly according to blood level, individual patient, and the procedure, as a generalization alfentanil is shorter-acting than sufentanil, which is of significantly shorter duration of action than fentanyl, which in turn is much shorter acting than morphine. If recovery from morphine might require approximately 2 hours, fentanyl would require 1 hour, and sufentanil and alfentanil 20 minutes or less.) The level of analgesia or "anesthesia" with alfentanil can be regulated by close observation of the patient or by blood levels. Thus, it is currently enjoying wide use (1) as an analgesic adjunct in the maintenance of anesthesia with other agents such as barbiture/nitrous oxide/oxygen and (2) as a primary anesthetic for induction of anesthesia for general surgery.

These fentanyl derivatives have found widespread use in anesthesia, especially for cardiac surgery. But they have a number of disadvantages or unwanted side effects. In addition to the anticipated respiratory depression, amnesia is not always complete, episodes of hypertension or bradycardia occur, and muscle rigidity is common.

Propoxyphene (DARVON)

ACTIONS

Propoxyphene has been extensively used as an analgesic for mild to moderate pain in conditions for which low dose oral codeine has been traditionally prescribed. It is commonly administered in combination with aspirin or caffeine (or both) or acetaminophen. Although the claim is made that the combinations are more effective in relieving mild pain than aspirin or acetaminophen alone, the magnitude of analgesia produced by propoxyphene alone is probably small. Unlike codeine, propoxyphene is not antitussive. Its rather limited analgesic efficacy in the face of significant potential toxicity makes the benefit-risk ratio so small that its use has doubtful justification.

Avoid and discourage the use of propoxyphene (DARVON) because it has significant toxicity, is not very effective as an analgesic, and has appreciable abuse liability.

TOXICITY

Propoxyphene has long been viewed erroneously by the public and many physicians as being useful for relatively mild pain and devoid of serious side effects. On the contrary, its acute and chronic potential toxicity places it in doubtful status as even a prescribed drug. In acute overdoses it can be rapidly fatal. Its toxic effects are additive or more than additive with other CNS depressants such as alcohol or muscle relaxants. The CNS depression produced by propoxyphene is complicated by convulsions that are difficult to treat. It is second only to barbiturates as a prescription drug associated with drug fatalities, many of which are suicides or accidental overdoses.

The treatment of acute overdosage centers on the maintenance of an adequate airway, assisted or artificial respiration, followed by the administration of naloxone (0.4–2 mg) intravenously, and repeated every 2–3 minutes until an adequate respiratory response is obtained or a total of 10 mg is given.

Not only is acute toxicity a potential problem, the chronic ingestion of propoxyphene can result in drug dependence with habituation, tolerance, and physical dependence.

Thus, the inclusion of propoxyphene (DARVON and combination preparations DARVOCET, DARVON-N with A.S.A.) in this textbook is justified largely on the basis of continuing misuse by dentists and physicians when equally or more effective, less hazardous, and frequently less expensive medications are available.

In addition, patients need to be educated regarding the facts about the drug as described in the package insert and patient information brochures. They need to be made aware especially of the potential interactions and the potential for abuse. Although the potential for abuse (or *abuse* liability) of codeine or of propoxyphene is less than that of parenteral morphine or meperidine, it remains a significant liability that deserves attention and prevention.

Heroin

Heroin is the diacetyl derivative of morphine; the sale and manufacture of heroin have been illegal since the 1930s.

The effects of heroin given intramuscularly are indistinguishable from those of morphine given by the same route. It is an effective opioid (narcotic) analgesic when administered in clinical situations.

Upon intravenous injection heroin has a rapid onset of effects, both objectively and subjectively; this onset is much more rapid than after an equianalgesic dose of morphine, owing probably to its more rapid entry into the brain (see Chapter 67).

Heroin is metabolized extensively to morphine, and most of its pharmacological effects are due to morphine as well as to the heroin itself.

There are many other opioid agonists that could be used clinically; none of these possesses major advantages over those covered here.

Mixed Opioid Agonist/Antagonists

PENTAZOCINE (TALWIN, TALWIN-NX, TALWIN COMPOUND WITH ASPIRIN)

Actions

Investigation of the subjective effects of the first known morphine antagonist, the *N*-allyl derivative (nalorphine, NALLINE), revealed that it had analgesic effects. The substance produced unpleasant subjective effects also that precluded further consideration as an analgesic. Nevertheless, that observation established that a compound could be, at the same time, both an analgesic and an antagonist, and was thought unlikely to be abused. This observation set the stage for the discovery decades later of therapeutically useful agents that were *mixed agonist/antagonists.* The first of these widely marketed as an analgesic was pentazocine.

The analgesia produced by pentazocine has been shown to be due in large part to its agonistic actions at the κ class of opioid receptors.

Pentazocine produces analgesia and drowsiness similar to that produced by morphine with 30 mg of pentazocine, equivalent to 10 mg morphine, or equivalent to 80–100 mg of meperidine. Its time course of action of 3 hours is similar to that of morphine.

Pentazocine and the other mixed agonist/antagonists produce respiratory depression, which on a single acute dose is equivalent to that produced by an equianalgesic dose of morphine. The cardiovascular effects are similar to those of morphine. It has no antidiuretic effect. The gastrointestinal effects are not prominent, and they have not been studied extensively.

Toxicity and Side Effects

Pentazocine can produce respiratory depression and some sedation, and some patients may experience hallucinations, confusion, or disorientation. Seizures have occurred after administration of pentazocine in patients susceptible to seizures.

Chronic administration results in tolerance and in dependence. Its oral use has low abuse liability, but with injection a small number of cases of abuse (frequently medical professionals) have occurred. Pentazocine became a drug of abuse; it was used intravenously in combination with the antihistaminics tripelennamine (PYRIBENZAMINE) or diphenhydramine (BENADRYL). This abuse led to the development of a unique oral preparation, TALWIN-NX, consisting of pentazocine combined with naloxone. In the event the combination is injected intravenously, the naloxone effectively antagonizes the opioid effects of the pentazocine. On the other hand, when the combination is ingested the naloxone is rapidly metabolized, leaving the pentazocine alone to produce its desired analgesic effects.

One of the toxic consequences of repeated parenteral injections of pentazocine is the unsightly and nearly irreversible induration of connective tissues in the skin.

Opioid Antagonism

All opioids have the potential for serious allergic or hypersensitivity reactions in patients sensitive to any one agent. (It may be difficult to distinguish allergic reactions from the dose-related predictable effects of opioids.)

Pentazocine, and potentially all the mixed agonist/antagonists, can antagonize the actions of opioid agonists such as morphine. Obviously, it should be avoided in anyone who has received an opioid recently or those dependent on any opioid.

NALBUPHINE (NUBAIN)

The κ receptor is involved in the analgesia produced by pentazocine, nalbuphine, and butorphanol.

Nalbuphine is an effective analgesic with approximately the same potency and duration of effect as morphine. The analgesia is the consequence of κ agonism.

Nalbuphine, as well as butorphanol, has proportionately less respiratory depressant effect after large doses than does morphine. Consequently, for possible chronic use or when high doses are used, these agents may have a wider margin of safety and may represent a useful alternative to morphine.

BUTORPHANOL (STADOL)

Butorphanol is a more potent κ agonist with a usual analgesic dose of 2–4 mg intramuscularly. Its duration of action and side effects are similar to those of morphine but with less respiratory depression following large doses or overdoses.

BUPRENORPHINE (BUPRENEX)

Buprenorphine is a unique opioid; it is long acting and quite potent. A dose of 0.3 mg intramuscularly has analgesic effects equivalent to 10 mg of morphine. Peak effects occur in approximately 1 hour, and the analgesic action can be sustained for up to 6 hours. Not only is it effective parenterally but it is also well absorbed upon sublingual administration.

The actions of buprenorphine are the consequence of its tight binding to the μ opioid receptor.

Buprenorphine is a potent, long-lasting μ partial agonist that also has some antagonistic actions.

Some individuals will probably develop dependence on each of these mixed agonists/antagonists, but the data to date suggest that they are all less likely to produce physical dependence than morphine. The physical dependence in buprenorphine-maintained patients is of a low order of intensity and long duration. Upon detoxification, the patients exhibit only mild signs of acute abstinence and discomfort.

NALOXONE (NARCAN)

Naloxone is the prototype drug and the antagonist drug of choice at the present time. It antagonizes opioid-induced euphoria, analgesia, drowsiness, and respiratory depression. It appears to be less effective against the stimulant actions, such as pupillary constriction and smooth muscle contraction. It is selectively effective against these effects induced by any of the narcotic analgesics. (Naloxone, as a selective and specific antagonist at the μ receptor, has been employed extensively as a tool in investigating whether or not opioids are involved in a particular toxic state or physiological function.)

Of major importance clinically is the pharmacokinetics of naloxone. It is appreciably shorter acting than most opioids; therefore, it must be given repeatedly in most instances in which it is used to manage toxic overdoses of opioids.

In individuals tolerant because of chronic use of narcotic analgesics, naloxone evokes an acute, severe withdrawal syndrome.

Prior to the introduction of naloxone, nalorphine (NALLINE, N-allyl normorphine) and levallorphan were available for use as antagonists. They are both mixed agonist/antagonists that, when given after narcotics, reverse the opiate syndrome; however, given alone they produce respiratory depression, cough suppression, miosis, and analgesia. Because many individuals experience unpleasant reactions, such as feelings of unreality, dreams, hallucinations, sweating, nausea, or groggy sensations after these drugs, they have not been used except as antagonists; they are now clinically obsolete.

Longer-acting antagonists have been tested for the treatment of addiction, i.e., secondary prevention of relapse to heroin use. Such agents include naltrexone, longer acting than naloxone, and cyclazocine, which is longer acting than naltrexone. Although these are effective antagonists, addict-patients have not generally liked or stayed on these antagonists chronically.

Narcotic Antagonists

The impressive advancements in knowledge of the opioid receptors and endogenous opioids were only possible with the availability of the selective, reversible opioid antagonist naloxone.

Naloxone's antagonism of intoxication by opioids is almost always of shorter duration than the opioid's actions.

The Future

To date, no new therapeutic drug has resulted from the breathtaking advances in knowledge of pain, analgesia, and addiction. For example, the endorphin structures primarily confirm the structural conclusions from studies of thousands of morphine-like substances. Current limitations on use of the endorphins depend as much as anything on the practical concerns for predictable absorption and appropriate durations of action. Nevertheless, there is already significantly improved use of these agents, and new advances are likely. Preliminary evidence is that given intravenously, the endorphins can relieve narcotic withdrawal symptoms without producing euphoria. There is good evidence that certain opioid peptides can enter the CNS after their intravenous administration.

References

Akil H, Watson SJ: Neuropeptides in Brain and Pituitary: Overview. *In* Meltzer HY (ed): Psychopharmacology: The Third Generation of Progress, 367. New York: Raven Press, 1987.

Austin KL, Stapleton JV, Mather LE: Relationship between blood meperidine concentrations and analgesic response: A preliminary report. Anesthesiology 53:460–466, 1980.

Burks TF: Actions of drugs on gastrointestinal motility. *In* Johnson LR (ed): Physiology of the Gastrointestinal Tract, 2nd ed, 723–743. New York: Raven Press, 1987.

Duggan AW, North RA: Electrophysiology of opioids. Pharmacol Rev 35:219–281, 1984.

Gebhart GF: Opioid analgesics and antagonists. *In* Neidle EA, Yagiela JA (eds): Pharmacology and Therapeutics for Dentistry, 3rd ed, 276–292. St. Louis: CV Mosby Co., 1989.

Jaffe JH, Martin WR: Opioid analgesics and antagonists. *In* Gilman AG, Rall TW, Nies AS, Taylor P (eds): Goodman and Gilman's The Pharmacological Basis of Therapeutics, 8th ed, 485–521. New York: Pergamon Press plc, 1990.

Kromer W: Endogenous and exogenous opioids in the control of gastrointestinal motility and secretion. Pharmacol Rev 40:121–162, 1988.

Leslie FM: Methods used for the study of opioid receptors. Pharmacol Rev 39:197–249, 1987.

Martin WR: Clinical evidence for different narcotic receptors and relevance for the clinician. Ann Emerg Med 15:1026–1029, 1986.

Martin WR: The evolution of concepts of opioid receptors. *In* Pasternak GW (ed): The Opiate Receptors, 3–22. Clifton, NJ: The Humana Press, 1988.

Martin WR: Pharmacology of opioids. Pharmacol Rev 35:283–323, 1983.

McQuay HJ, Caroll D, Faura CC, et al: Oral morphine in cancer pain: Influences on morphine and metabolite concentration. Clin Pharmacol Ther 48:236–244, 1990.

Meltzer HY (ed): Psychopharmacology: The Third Generation of Progress. New York: Raven Press, 1987.

Osborne R, Joel S, Trew D, Slevin R: Morphine and metabolite behavior after different routes of morphine administration: Demonstration of the importance of the active metabolite morphine-6-glucuronide. Clin Pharmacol Ther 47:12–19, 1990.

Pasternak GW: Opioid receptors. *In* Meltzer HY (ed): Psychopharmacology: The Third Generation of Progress, 281. New York: Raven Press, 1987.

Twycross RG, McQuay HF: Opioids. *In* Wall PD, Melzack R (eds): Textbook of Pain, 686. New York: Churchill Livingstone, 1989.

Wall PD, Melzack R (eds): Textbook of Pain. 2nd ed. New York: Churchill Livingstone, 1989.

Yaksh TL, Aimone LD: The central pharmacology of pain transmission. *In* Wall PD, Melzack R (eds): Textbook of Pain, 2nd ed, 181. New York: Churchill Livingstone, 1989.

19

Alcohols

Peter K. Gessner

Chemically, the term *alcohol* identifies compounds with aliphatic hydroxy groups. The three simplest alcohols, methanol, ethanol, and ethylene glycol, all tend to be abused. Ethanol is imbibed by the majority of the population who enjoy its inebriating effects. A minority do so excessively; the consequences of this constitute a major public health and social problem. Methanol and ethylene glycol have some inebriating effects, but they are also profoundly toxic. Their consumption, even in small quantities, precipitates a life-threatening medical emergency. Much of the methanol that reaches the retail market is sold mixed with ethanol. The toxicity of such mixtures is determined largely by their relative content of methanol and ethanol.

CH_3OH Methanol
CH_3CH_2OH Ethanol
CH_2OH Ethylene glycol
$|$
CH_2OH

Ethanol is inebriating.
Methanol and ethylene glycol are poisons.

Beverage alcohol is formed when yeast is forced to oxidize sugars anaerobically. This process continues until either all the sugar is used up or the ethanol concentration reaches 12–14%. That is the concentration of ethanol in table wine. The ethanol concentration in beers, which are made from brews containing initially less sugar, is usually only 4–5%. Spirits, or liquor, are usually marketed as 80–100 proof, that is 40–50% ethanol (proof = ethanol concentration × 2). To obtain ethanol this concentrated it is necessary to distill it off. Some wines (sherry, vermouth, etc.) are fortified, using distilled alcohol, to an ethanol content of 18%. When quantitating ethanol consumption clinically, it is usual to report it in multiples of 15-g quantities of pure ethanol, one such "drink" being approximately equivalent, therefore, to a 1-oz shot of 100-proof liquor, a 4-oz glass of table wine, or a 12-oz bottle of beer.

    In scientific writing, *in vivo* ethanol levels are most often reported in milligrams per deciliter (mg/dl). The earlier notation for this measure was milligrams percent (mg%). Alternatively, a unit of concentration, millimoles (mM), is used, in which a 1-mM ethanol solution contains 4.6 mg/dl. Yet another notation, and one that survives in the popular media and the courts, is as weight per volume percent blood ethanol content. Thus the 0.1% blood alcohol level, which in many jurisdictions is considered presumptive evidence of driving while intoxicated, is equivalent to a blood ethanol concentration of 100 mg/dl.

Ethanol

ABSORPTION, DISTRIBUTION, AND ELIMINATION

Ethanol is absorbed primarily in the small intestine. Although there is some absorption from the stomach, it is much slower than that from the intestine.

251

Accordingly, the presence of food in the stomach, by slowing the rate of gastric emptying, will delay the absorption, and the resulting peak plasma alcohol levels will be lower. At high concentrations (50 proof or better) ethanol itself inhibits gastric motility, delays gastric emptying, and results in a "bottling-up" phenomenon. The absorption of ethanol in the intestine is complete, and the rate is proportional to its concentration.

Ethanol partitions as body water.

The *in vivo* distribution of ethanol is governed by its partitioning between water and fat as 30/1. Accordingly, at equilibrium, its distribution is much the same as that of body water. Since fat constitutes a higher proportion of the body weight in women than in men, the resultant volume of distribution of ethanol in women is 0.6 l/kg while that in men is 0.7 l/kg. Accordingly, absorption of a given quantity of ethanol will result in a higher blood ethanol level in women than in men of equal weight. This differential is further enhanced by the fact that whereas the average man weighs 70 kg, the average woman weighs only 55 kg.

Ethanol is excreted in breath, urine, and sweat. In each instance, the amount cleared from the body by these means is small, but the concentration of ethanol in these excreta is proportional to that in blood and can be utilized for a noninvasive assessment of blood ethanol levels.

Ethanol is eliminated at a constant rate.

At moderate to high blood ethanol concentrations, the metabolic elimination of ethanol occurs by apparent first-order kinetics, that is at a constant rate rather than at a rate that is proportional to its concentration, as is the case for most other drugs. On average, the body clears about ⅔ of a "drink"/hour. Hepatic metabolism constitutes the major route of ethanol elimination. Ethanol is oxidized first to acetaldehyde, then to acetate, and eventually to carbon dioxide. In hepatic homogenates, three enzymes — alcohol dehydrogenase, the microsomal ethanol-oxidizing system (MEOS), and catalase — all can mediate the oxidation of ethanol to acetaldehyde. *In vivo* in humans, however, only aldehyde dehydrogenase is considered to play a significant role, although ethanol consumption does induce the MEOS levels.

ACUTE EFFECTS ON THE NERVOUS SYSTEM

On the basis of the similarities in withdrawal symptoms and pharmacological effects on the central nervous system (CNS), ethanol is classified as a CNS depressant of the same type as the barbiturates and the sedative-hypnotics.

Progressive and monophasic CNS depression

Ethanol induces a depression of the CNS that leads to a progressive and monophasic impairment of cerebellar and cognitive function. A good test of cerebellar function is the ability to stand steadily with one foot directly in front of the other and one's eyes closed. As blood ethanol levels increase, a progressive deterioration of standing steadiness is observed (Fig. 19–1). The effects of a given blood ethanol level are somewhat smaller in moderate drinkers and markedly smaller in heavy drinkers than those observed in abstainers, clear-cut evidence of tolerance. Arithmetic subtraction proficiency is a good test of cognitive function. It also progressively deteriorates as blood ethanol levels rise; here too tolerance among moderate and heavy drinkers is evident. In tests of driving ability, significant impairment of function is observed at blood ethanol levels of 35 mg/dl. Under laboratory conditions, significant effects of ethanol on brain function can be shown at substantially lower levels still. Thus, the ability of subjects to detect a flickering in a light source is impaired at blood ethanol levels as low as 13 mg/dl. Additionally, ethanol induces a progressive impairment of judgment: in tests of standing steadiness, such as that illus-

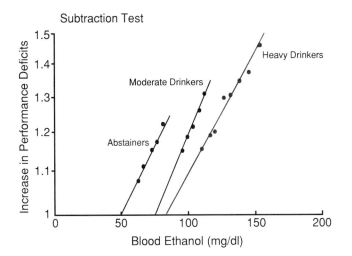

Subtraction Test

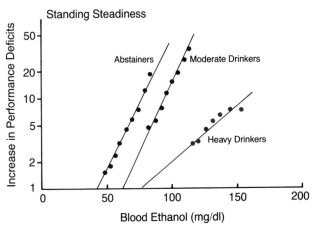

Standing Steadiness

Effect of blood ethanol levels on cerebellar and cognitive function. (Redrawn from Goldberg L: Quantitative studies on alcohol tolerance in man. Acta Physiol Scand 5:S16, 1943.)

Figure 19–1

trated in Figure 19–1, subjects with raised blood ethanol levels assert that their performance is improved even in the presence of patently obvious objective evidence to the contrary, that is, even when they are visibly swaying, losing their balance, or falling.

An important consequence of the impairment in coordination and judgment brought about by ethanol is the increased probability of involvement in a vehicular accident. In excess of 50% of fatal automobile accidents involve at least one intoxicated driver. In this regard, the ability of ethanol to impair muscle proprioception, and hence a body sense of acceleration, is important. It results in the driver being much more dependent on responses to visual stimuli and thus more reactive. The probability of being involved in a vehicular accident rises in an exponential manner with blood alcohol levels (Fig. 19–2). Moreover, for special at-risk groups, such as those people under age 18 or over age 75, even blood levels of 25 mg/dl are correlated with a fourfold and eightfold higher incidence, respectively, of involvement in accidents. As might be expected, alcoholic intoxication is also found to be a concomitant of a quarter or more of pedestrian highway deaths, serious injuries in the home, and private plane crashes.

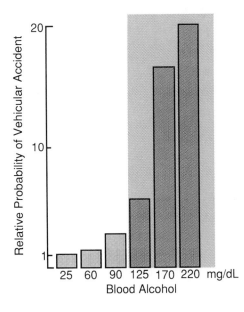

Figure 19–2

Relationship between probability of vehicular accident and blood ethanol level.

Action at GABA receptors

Identification of the mechanism mediating ethanol's pharmacological effects on the CNS has been difficult because of alcohol's many neurochemical actions. There is a degree of consensus, however, that many of the CNS effects of ethanol are due to its augmentation of the chloride flux induced by gamma-aminobutyric acid (GABA) at its GABA$_A$ receptors. GABA functions as an inhibitory neurotransmitter in the CNS, where it is present in significant concentrations (only trace amounts of it are found in the peripheral nervous system). GABA-ergic neurons are, for the most part, short interneurons. The postsynaptic GABA receptor is an oligomeric one that incorporates a chloride ion channel. GABA increases the chloride ion flux through this channel, and this causes hyperpolarization of the target neuron and postsynaptic inhibition. The augmentation of the GABA-induced chloride flux brought about by ethanol occurs by an allosteric action of ethanol, that is, by an action at a site other than the GABA recognition site on the receptor. The GABA receptor is a very complex structure with separate allosteric sites for benzodiazepines, pentobarbital and other barbiturates, and picrotoxin. One of these sites, the benzodiazepine one, can exist in two interconvertible transitional states: one state favors benzodiazepine anxiolytic-type ligands, the other favors anxiogenic ligands of the β-carboline type. Ethanol recognition appears to occur at yet another and separate site, although one that may in some way be interconnected with the benzodiazepine site (see also Chapter 20).

The sites and mechanisms of ethanol and other alcohols have been studied in a number of systems. In addition to GABA receptors, the sites and mechanisms of alcohol action may turn out to involve binding or modification of the binding properties of NMDA (N-methyl D-aspartate) and nicotinic ACh receptors, ATPases, cyclic GMP, and central prostaglandin systems. In addition, ethanol has been shown to produce vasoconstriction of cerebral vessels, alterations in the calcium release and neurotransmitter-secretion coupling, and altered release of endogenous anxiogenic substances. In large concentrations, concentrations that would be lethal *in vivo*, ethanol has widespread effects on neuronal membrane fluidity and excitability (discussed further in Chapter 16).

Positional alcohol nystagmus

Ethanol has a number of other acute centrally mediated effects. It affects the organs of balance, causing a biphasic positional alcohol nystagmus (PAN), whereby the eyes of a supine subject with the head turned to one side beat initially, as blood ethanol levels rise, to that side. Later, while blood ethanol levels are falling, the direction of the beating is reversed. These phenomena, which tend to be accompanied in the ambulatory individual by nausea and vomiting, are a consequence of a more rapid equilibration of ethanol in the semicircular canals of the inner ear with the cupula than with the endolymph. As a result, since the density of ethanol is only 0.79, the specific density of the cupula becomes initially lower, and later higher, than that of the endolymph. This causes the inner ear, an organ normally sensitive only to the effects of acceleration, to also become sensitive to the effects of gravity, thereby suggesting motion when none is occurring.

Ethanol causes cutaneous and mucosal vasodilation. This results in a sensation of warmth but also in an overall increase in the rate of heat loss and a lowering of central core temperature. In cold winter environments this has been known to result in fatal hypothermia. Ethanol also causes a stimulation of gastric secretion, which results in increased appetite and enhanced peristalsis. The effect is a central one that is abolished by vagotomy. Finally, consumption of ethanol leads to diuresis through inhibition of antidiuretic hormone secretion.

ACUTE EFFECTS ON INTERPERSONAL BEHAVIOR

In our society, alcohol consumption is strongly correlated with aggressive and destructive behavior. It is commonly, but erroneously assumed, therefore, that such behavior is purely a manifestation of a pharmacological effect of ethanol. The assumption frequently takes the form of the assertion that such behavior is generated by the lower brain centers being released from higher brain controls. However, consumption of ethanol *per se* (that is, in subjects ignorant of the fact that they are consuming it) does not increase the aggressive behavior of social drinkers, even when their blood ethanol levels rise to 100 mg/dl. On the other hand, such individuals exhibit significantly more aggressive behavior if they believe that they have consumed alcohol, even if the belief is an incorrect one. A consequence of this is that by excusing behavior that would be otherwise unacceptable, on the basis that it is ethanol-induced, heavy drinking is rewarded.

To determine whether observed behaviors are due to the pharmacological action of ethanol or to expectancies that subjects bring to the situation, it is necessary to perform studies in which some subjects are purposefully deceived regarding the presence or absence of ethanol in beverage they are given to drink. Specifically, in such "balanced placebo studies" the object is to deceive some of the subjects to believe they are imbibing an alcoholic beverage while, in fact, they are drinking an alcohol-free concoction and *vice versa*, and to compare the effects in these groups with the effects observed in subjects informed correctly. It is found that subjects who are told they are receiving alcohol tend to behave more aggressively than those who are told they are receiving placebo (tonic water), regardless of what they actually received, even with ethanol doses sufficient to raise the blood ethanol level to 100 mg/dl (Fig. 19–3). In contrast, a belief on the part of these same subjects that they have consumed ethanol has no effect whatever on the length of time it takes for them to respond to a stimulus (response latency), whereas ethanol unambiguously increases it.

Ethanol is popularly perceived as generally having stress-relieving properties. Experimentally, it has been found that ethanol ingestion results in decreased cardiovascular responses in some stressful situations (e.g., anticipating having to give a short speech on the topic "what I like and dislike about my body and physical appearance") in those individuals

Alcohol expectancy effects

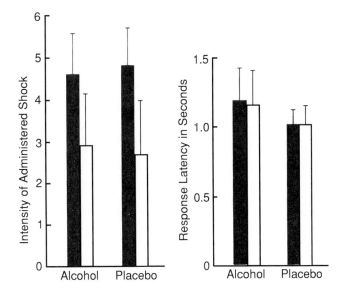

Figure 19–3

Effect of experimental conditions on aggressive behavior and response latency. Subjects were made to believe that they were consuming a beverage containing ethanol *(color bars)* or an alcohol-free beverage *(white bars).* The nature of the beverage they actually consumed is indicated under the bars. (Data from Lang AR, Goeckner DJ, Adesso VJ, Marlatt GA: Effects of alcohol on aggression in male social drinkers. J Abnorm Psychol 84:508–518, 1975.)

likely to have a marked cardiovascular reaction to such stress (Type A individuals) but not in Type B individuals, whose response is less marked. In men, ethanol ingestion also reduces, in a dose-dependent fashion, the cardiovascular response to the stress of having to make a favorable impression on an unresponsive person of the opposite sex during a 5-minute interaction. So also, however, does expectancy. In women placed in a similar contingency, moderate doses of ethanol have the opposite effect.

HEPATIC METABOLISM AND EFFECTS

Hepatic metabolism

The oxidation of ethanol to acetaldehyde occurs in the liver and is catalyzed by a zinc-containing cytosolic enzyme, alcohol dehydrogenase. In the process oxidized nicotinamide-adenine dinucleotide (NAD^+), a cofactor, is reduced to nicotinamide-adenine dinucleotide (NADH) (Fig. 19–4). The amount of NAD^+ in the cytosol is rapidly reduced and becomes the factor limiting the rate of ethanol metabolism. Regeneration of the NAD^+ from NADH can occur by the reduction of various substrates, for instance, of pyruvate to lactate. Measurement of the pyruvate/lactate ratio in hepatic vein blood during ethanol metabolism gives a measure of the redox state of the cytosolic compartment of the hepatocyte: it is found to decrease 6.5-fold. Oxaloacetate is another cytoplasmic substrate that, in the process of being reduced to malate by malic dehydrogenase, regenerates NAD^+ from NADH. Its cytoplasmic levels too are low, but malic dehydrogenase (unlike lactic dehydrogenase) is also a mitochondrial enzyme, and malate can readily cross into the mitochondrion (NADH cannot). Reoxidation of the malate to oxaloacetate in the mitochondrion occurs at the expense of the reduction of mitochondrial NAD^+. In this manner, reducing equivalents are shuttled from the cytoplasm to the mitochondrion. In the mitochondrion, the NADH is reoxidized to NAD^+ by the action of the respiratory electron transport system found there.

Effect on redox state of liver

It is possible to measure the redox state in the mitochondrial compartment by measuring the hepatic vein ratio of β-hydroxybutyrate/acetoacetate. During ethanol metabolism this ratio is decreased threefold. This is an

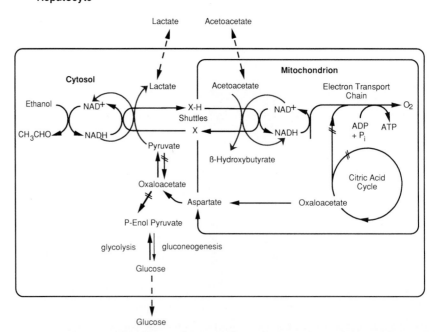

Figure 19–4

Metabolic scheme for events related to ethanol metabolism in the hepatocyte. Reactions inhibited or blocked during ethanol metabolism are shown crossed by double lines.

indication that the respiratory electron transport train is not regenerating NAD^+ as fast as it is utilized. This is so because the rate of operation of this system is independent of the NADH concentration; it is controlled instead by the ratio of adenosine diphosphate (ADP) and inorganic phosphate to adenosine triphosphate (ATP). Since ethanol metabolism has acutely no effect on the utilization of ATP, this ratio remains constant and, as a consequence, so does the rate of ethanol oxidation.

Chronically, high doses of ethanol are found to bring about, over a period of about 48 hours, an increased rate of cellular utilization of ATP and thereby a higher rate of operation of the respiratory electron transport chain. This is brought about by an increase in the activity of the membrane-bound Na^+/K^+ adenosine triphosphatase (ATPase), which suggests that ethanol renders the cell membrane more leaky to these ions. The higher rate of operation of the electron transport chain results in higher oxygen utilization by the hepatocyte and, incidentally, in a higher rate of ethanol metabolism.

A faster rate of oxygen utilization by the hepatocyte causes the oxygen to be extracted more efficiently as the blood percolates through the liver lobule to the centrolobular vein. Ethanol is, however, also a central respiratory depressant. Consequently, a heavy chronic drinker who imbibes enough ethanol to bring about the enhancement in the rate of hepatic oxygen extraction can subsequently again imbibe enough to significantly depress the respiratory rate. The combination of these two circumstances can cause the oxygen tension in the blood reaching the centrolobular vein to be so low that anoxia and necrosis of hepatocytes in the centrolobular region ensue.

Effect on hepatic oxygen utilization

During ethanol metabolism gluconeogenesis is blocked because gluconeogenesis involves formation of enol phosphopyruvate from pyruvate by oxaloacetate, and during ethanol metabolism, the pyruvate is removed by reduction to lactate. The citric acid cycle is also inhibited by the scarcity of NADH (ethanol oxidation provides all the energy needed by the cell). Fatty acid utilization by the liver is inhibited as well. The latter involves, as a first step, β-oxidation, a process that requires reoxidation of cofactors by the electron transport chain. Since β-oxidation is in competition for reducing equivalents with the NADH produced by the oxidation of ethanol, it is also blocked. Heavy ethanol consumption, accordingly, is correlated with fatty acid infiltration of the liver. The condition is reversible.

TOLERANCE, PHYSICAL DEPENDENCE, AND ALCOHOLISM

Although, as indicated previously, both functional and metabolic tolerance develop to ethanol, the functional tolerance is quantitatively more important. Whereas tolerance develops even when only small amounts of ethanol are used, physical dependence does not, unless the amount used is elevated above that initially necessary to induce significant pharmacological effects. Consumption of ethanol in quantities insufficient to induce physical dependence is nonetheless considered abuse if, because of the pharmacological effects of the ethanol, the user experiences significant problems, whether medical, legal, occupational, or economic. Drinking behaviors can therefore be divided into four types: abstinence, social or non-problem drinking, problem drinking, and ethanol dependence or alcohol addiction. This represents a behavioral progression, and although the vast majority of individuals who imbibe alcoholic beverages do not become addicted to ethanol, this is the progression followed by those who do.

Those who become addicted to alcohol progress from social drinking, through problem drinking, to ethanol dependence.

Assessment of drinking is an integral part of any medical history.

Loss of control, although a common complaint, is not an established phenomenon.

The term *alcoholism,* as used generally in this country, encompasses both alcohol addiction and problem drinking. Also in this country, the notion that alcoholism is a disease has assumed the form of a credo. Whatever label is attached to alcoholism, when alcohol abusers require medical attention they should receive it. An important example of such attention is the recognition and diagnosis of problem drinking and alcohol dependence in patients by their physicians. Confronting patients with the medical conclusion that their drinking has assumed proportions dangerous to their health and well-being is a first and crucial step in the treatment of the condition. Some of the diagnostic characteristics held to suggest a diagnosis of alcoholism are the occurrence of tremor, having a drink first thing in the morning, the occurrence of memory lapses (or alcoholic "blackouts," whereby individuals remember nothing of a period of time during which, although they were under the influence of ethanol, their function was not severely impaired), missing meals because of drinking, continuous drinking for periods of 12 hours or more, and the assertion that they incurred a "loss of control." The latter construct is invoked by subjects who state that they were determined to have no more than 1 or 2 drinks, but having started to imbibe they were unable to stop. Although the assertion is a common one, repeated efforts to duplicate this phenomenon under controlled laboratory conditions have been uniformly unsuccessful. What has been found, however, is that individuals with a diagnosis of alcoholism, told they are drinking an alcoholic beverage, will drink more of it and behave in a more inebriated manner than if told that they are drinking tonic water, regardless of whether the beverage actually contains ethanol. This finding suggests something akin to a conditioned response.

The basis of the Temperance Movement in the U.S., the efforts of which culminated in the 1919–1933 Prohibition Amendment, was the belief that ethanol, imbibed in any quantity, possessed a behavioral toxicity that necessarily predestined the drinker to become a hopeless drunkard. That position has become discredited. It is nonetheless true, however, that when it is consumed in large amounts, ethanol possesses a behavioral toxicity. Thus, in adult males the imbibing of 6 or more drinks per day is correlated over time with an escalation of consumption; chronic consumption of approximately 10 or more drinks per day necessarily leads to the development of ethanol dependence.

Alcoholism is very much a familial condition. Research with twins and adoptees in Scandinavia indicates that there is a genetic component, although only one eighth of the overall prevalence of alcoholism can be attributed to it with certainty. (Although the genetic contributions to alcohol actions and alcohol dependence are difficult to define quantitatively in human populations, the actions of ethanol in experimental animals are under genetic control[s]. Among these actions and interactions are the intensity and nature of ethanol's acute behavioral effects, taste sensitivity and palatability of alcoholic beverages, reinforcing or aversive effects of ethanol, the magnitude of tolerance on chronic administration, enzyme systems involved in metabolism of ethanol, the nature and severity of physical dependence, and the susceptibility to neurologic damage. The evidence supports the possibility that each of these aspects is regulated by different genes.)

Research in France and Scandinavia has revealed that the frequency distribution of the amount consumed is unimodal and log-normally distributed. One conclusion that can be drawn from this distribution is that those suffering from alcoholism, although they may consume the bulk of the alcohol, do not form a separate population. Additionally, it is found that, although the mean of this distribution is determined by the overall per capita consumption of the population, its standard deviation is independent of per capita consumption, remaining virtually constant as per capita consumption changes. From this it follows that, free will notwithstanding, the number of individuals who report, for instance, 10 or more drinks per day is a function of the overall per capita consumption. It also suggests that, in the aggregate, how much ethanol a person consumes is strongly affected by the consumption of that individual's drinking friends and acquaintances. At the same time, because ethanol is in market terms an elastic commodity its per capita consumption decreases as its price increases. Since alcoholic beverages are easy to make, however, too high a price leads to illicit manufacture and marketing.

Individual alcohol consumption is primarily environmentally determined; the genetic components are small.

THE ACUTE WITHDRAWAL SYNDROME

In those physically dependent on ethanol, the early symptoms of the withdrawal syndrome are observed within hours of the cessation or significant reduction of alcohol consumption. Also, if the level of physical dependence is high, marked symptoms and signs of the withdrawal may be evident while the subject's blood ethanol levels are sufficiently high to cause intoxication in a nontolerant subject. A characteristic gross tremor is the most prevalent sign, and it can become extreme. Severe weakness, effusive perspiration, hyperreflexia, insomnia, anorexia, nausea, retching, vomiting, and diarrhea are other early signs. More serious symptoms are an elevation of blood pressure, hallucinations (during which the patient tends to retain insight), and grand mal–type seizures. If mild, the syndrome responds to general supportive therapy, which includes reality orientation. If the syndrome is more severe, pharmacological therapy is indicated. This consists of the administration of increasing amounts of an appropriate CNS depressant until tolerance is exceeded, and thereafter its gradual withdrawal. If such therapy is instituted in the first 2 days of withdrawal, the condition usually responds well to it.

Untreated, the symptoms and signs peak, as a rule, after 48 hours, and an improvement in the patient's condition then ensues. In a fraction of the patients who are dependent on high levels of ethanol (in excess of 390 g of ethanol or 26 drinks/day) and who do not receive pharmacological treatment during the first 2 days of withdrawal, a secondary condition called *delirium tremens* develops. Untreated, it has a mortality rate of as much as 30%, and even in those receiving expert care, a mortality rate of 3–7% persists. The condition is characterized by overactivity of the autonomic nervous system, with tachycardia, dilated pupils, excessive sweating, and fever of noninfectious origin. The gross delirium that develops is characterized by a loss of insight, and an inability to identify people and to interpret properly what is seen, heard, or perceived by other sensory means.

The acute alcohol withdrawal syndrome, if severe and untreated, is frequently followed by delirium tremens, which has a substantial mortality.

THERAPY OF THE WITHDRAWAL SYNDROME

Because of the tendency of patients in withdrawal to hallucinate, an effort is made to keep the patients in contact with reality by checking on them at 30-minute intervals, and engaging them in conversation with emphasis on where and who they are and what is happening at the time. It has been found that the presence of windows and good lighting are helpful. Attention has to be given also to keeping the patient hydrated; administration of thiamine is essential. For many individuals in mild withdrawal such treatment may be sufficient, and some advocate the routine adoption of this

The acute alcohol withdrawal syndrome can be terminated by titration of patient with a CNS depressant until sedation is observed.

approach, relying on frequent checks of the cardiovascular system's status and body temperature to detect the development of more severe withdrawal, which would necessitate the patient's transfer to a hospital setting. Others maintain that the severe withdrawal that will develop in some, if this approach is used, is difficult to manage, and that pharmacological therapy of the withdrawal at this stage assures a much better uniform outcome. The basis of the pharmacological approach is stepwise reintoxication of the patient with a relatively short-acting depressant until signs of mild CNS depression are evident. This is followed by a gradual lowering of the maintenance dose to zero over a 10-day period. Drugs that have been successfully used to this end include paraldehyde, chlordiazepoxide, and more recently oxazepam. Although diazepam has perhaps been the most widely used, the dependence potential of this drug leads to concern regarding its use in individuals prone to substance abuse.

Although a number of drugs will control the adrenergic concomitants of the alcohol withdrawal syndrome, they do so without controlling the process that leads to the more severe manifestations of the withdrawal. Accordingly, their use tends to render problematical the monitoring and appropriate timely treatment of the withdrawal. Among these agents are the phenothiazines, which actually lower seizure threshold, propranolol, and most recently clonidine. Also, phenytoin and other anticonvulsants are not effective in preventing the seizures of alcohol withdrawal and should not be used in the absence of a history of epilepsy.

HANGOVER

In the majority, but not all individuals, acute ingestion of 5 or more alcoholic drinks is followed some hours later by a discomforting set of postintoxication symptoms collectively referred to as a *hangover*. The symptoms start soon after blood alcohol levels begin to decline and peak before ethanol is completely cleared from the blood. The intensity of the symptoms is related to the quantity of alcoholic beverage consumed and they are seldom reported following consumption of fewer than 5 drinks. The symptoms are significantly worse following consumption of beverages high in congener content, such as bourbon, than ones free of them, such as vodka. Thirst, the most common hangover symptom, is likely the result of the diuresis induced by ethanol. Headache is the next most common symptom; its etiology is not known. One cluster of symptoms—namely, giddiness, nausea, and vomiting—is probably due to the vestibular effects of ethanol discussed earlier. Finally, a second cluster consisting of tremor, disturbances of thermoregulation (sweating, hot flashes, cold chills, and so on), and nervousness is common to both hangover and mild or early alcohol withdrawal syndrome.

TOXICITY

Acute intoxication with large amounts of ethanol results in emesis, unconsciousness, and surgical anesthesia. The combination can be fatal because of the aspiration of vomitus and consequent obstruction or pneumonia. High blood ethanol levels induce hypotension through a direct action on peripheral blood vessels. This hypotension is unresponsive to norepinephrine and can result in cardiovascular shock, a frequent cause of death in ethanol overdose. If the cardiovascular shock is counteracted, renal failure is a frequent sequela of ethanol poisoning. It occurs because, during cardiovascular shock, the blood flow to the kidneys is shut down and renal ischemia results. Although ethanol causes a depression of the brainstem respiratory center, respiratory arrest is not the usual cause of death.

Ethanol, consumed chronically in large quantities (the amount imbibed by alcoholics can be 150–600 g or 10–40 drinks/day), is a systemic poison. The toxic sequelae involve so many organ systems that it has been said that to know ethanol toxicity is to know medicine. The most important among these sequelae are those on the CNS, the induction of liver cirrhosis and pancreatitis, the hypertensive and teratogenic effects, and the ability to cause damage to skeletal and cardiac muscle.

> Consumed chronically in large quantities, ethanol is a systemic poison.

Even relatively modest chronic consumption of ethanol (75 g or 5 drinks/day or more) results in intellectual and memory impairment that is correlated with an enlargement of cerebral ventricles. Given the fixed size of the cranium, this phenomenon is usually taken as evidence of cerebral atrophy. With abstinence, there follows a partial reversal of both the cognitive deficit and the ventricular enlargement, at least in some patients but not all.

Thiamine deficiency, caused in part by the heavy drinker's diet being vitamin-deficient and partly by ethanol's inhibition of thiamine absorption, is known to be the cause of Wernicke's encephalopathy. The symptoms of this condition include paralysis of ocular and facial muscles, nystagmus, loss of appetite, vomiting, and disorientation. The condition is readily reversible upon administration of thiamine, and since the latter is not toxic, thiamine is routinely administered parenterally at the beginning of detoxification. Thiamine deficiency is also thought to be responsible for Korsakoff's psychosis. The chief characteristic of this *irreversible* condition is an inability to convert short-term to long-term memory. This results in a compensatory tendency of the subject to confabulate. Peripheral neuralgias, from which alcoholics commonly suffer, have also been attributed to the thiamine avitaminosis. Additionally, alcoholics are prone to develop cerebellar degeneration. This manifests itself initially as a loss of proprioception in the lower extremities and progresses to the point that individuals cannot walk or even get up unaided. The varied chronic neurologic effects of alcohol are likely to be due to the combination of the direct neurotoxic effects of ethanol plus the nutritional derangements.

> Thiamine deficiency is a common finding in heavy drinkers; it can lead to Wernicke's encephalopathy and probably to Korsakoff's psychosis.

Ethanol is a human teratogen. It increases the incidences of spontaneous abortions, low–birth-weight babies (although only if the mother also smokes), and congenital abnormalities. When the latter are present in an aggregate and extreme form, the condition is termed the *fetal alcohol syndrome*. This consists of a triad of facial dysmorphology, prenatal and postnatal growth deficiencies, and CNS involvement, which includes mild to moderate mental retardation. The facial dysmorphology involves the eyes, which have short palpebral fissures (i.e., small eyeballs); the nose, which is short and upturned and lacks a bridge; and the mouth, which has a hypoplastic upper lip with a thinned upper vermilion and a diminished to absent philtrum. The CNS involvement can include microcephaly, hypotonia, irritability in infancy, and hyperactivity in childhood. The syndrome was first described among Washington State residents, mostly Pacific Coast Native Americans, and a large proportion of reported cases have been from that area. How prevalent the syndrome is in other venues or how large an intake of ethanol it is correlated with is not clear, but a woman who drinks heavily during pregnancy places her unborn child at substantial risk. Moreover, whereas both ethanol abuse and cigarette smoking each separately increases the risk of growth retardation, when these are done conjointly that risk is multiplied.

Although liver cirrhosis can have a number of etiologies, mortality from this condition is very closely correlated with ethanol consumption

Figure 19–5

Incidence of yearly liver cirrhosis mortality as a function of per capita ethanol consumption in discrete geographical locations in Ontario, Canada. (From Schmidt W, Popham RE: Alcohol Problems and Their Prevention: A Public Health Perspective. Toronto: Addiction Research Foundation, 1977.)

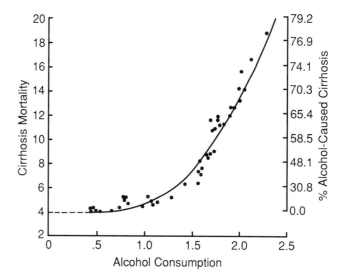

Chronic high ethanol consumption is the primary cause of liver cirrhosis.

Cardiomyopathy, hypertension, myopathy, and pancreatitis are all pathologies associated with excessive ethanol consumption.

(Fig. 19–5); so much so that its incidence has been used as an index of alcoholism. As evident from the figure, in the absence of ethanol consumption liver cirrhosis mortality is quite low, but it rises rapidly once that consumption reaches a certain level. The condition is characterized by the hepatic deposition of fibrous tissue (a healing process) as a consequence of focal necrosis. Such fibrous tissue, however, impedes hepatic blood flow. The liver is supplied with blood through the hepatic artery and the portal vein. Resistance to blood flow results in the development of portal hypertension. This leads to transudation of fluid into the peritoneal cavity, which becomes filled and distended (ascites). Additionally, portal hypertension causes the development of varicose veins in the esophagus, which is supplied with blood through the portal system. Internal hemorrhages from such esophageal varices are frequently the cause of death in alcoholism. In individuals with liver cirrhosis, the inability of the liver to remove toxic metabolic products from the blood leads to hepatic coma, another frequent cause of death in alcoholism. Additionally, hepatomas are a complication in as many as one fifth of the patients with alcoholic liver cirrhosis. Clearly, the prognosis of individuals with alcoholic liver cirrhosis is guarded at best, but it is particularly poor in those unable to cease their ethanol consumption (Fig. 19–6).

Liver cirrhosis is not the only organic pathology that is quantitatively correlated with the amount of ethanol consumed. As shown in Figure 19–7, this is generically true of other nonhepatic alcohol-related conditions. In particular, the severity of both myopathy and cardiomyopathy is a function of the lifetime ethanol consumption. Myopathy occurs in individuals with a lifetime ethanol consumption of 13 mg/kg (equivalent to 12 drinks/day/70 kg man for 20 years). It is functionally evident as proximal muscle weakness and atrophy; such patients have elevated serum creatinine levels. Electron microscopic examination of biopsies shows nonspecific but definite ultrastructural changes. Cardiomyopathy results in a lowering of the ejection fraction and an increased left ventricular mass. Electron microscopic analysis of biopsy specimens reveals increased endometrial thickness, interstitial fibrosis, and loss of myofibrils. An abnormally low ejection fraction has been found in some 43% of individuals with a daily ethanol consumption of 243 g/70 kg man for 16 years.

Pancreatitis is yet another condition induced by heavy ethanol consumption. Compared with idiopathic pancreatitis, alcoholic pancreatitis

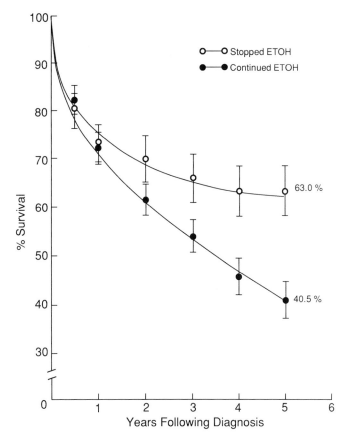

Figure 19-6

Percentage survival following diagnosis of alcoholic liver cirrhosis as a function of time and abstinence from ethanol. (From Powell WJ Jr, Klatskin G: Duration of survival in patients with Laennec's cirrhosis. Influence of alcohol withdrawal, and possible effects of recent changes in general management of the disease. Am J Med 44:406–420, 1968.)

has a higher incidence of severe pain, pancreatic calcification, overt diabetes, and a higher death rate (26%) in the 5 years following initial diagnosis. With abstinence, the severe pain either partially or completely disappears within a year in 90% of such patients, but it persists in about half of those who continue to drink.

Chronic heavy ethanol consumption (in excess of 4–6 drinks/day on average) results in a significant increase in the incidence of hypertension, although moderate drinkers have hypertension rates no different from abstainers. Acutely, ethanol increases both systolic and diastolic pressure, as well as pulse rate, although it has only slight effects on blood catecholamine levels.

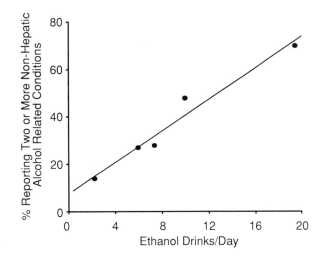

Figure 19-7

Percentage of alcoholics reporting two or more medical conditions (anemia, weakness in limbs, numbness of legs, dizziness, loss of balance, or fractures) in the previous 6 months as a function of their mean daily alcohol consumption. (Data from Polich JM, Armor DJ, Braiker HB: The Course of Alcoholism: Four Years After Treatment, Tables 3.23 and 3.24. Santa Monica, CA: Rand Corp, 1980.)

Finally, heavy ethanol consumption has an immunosuppressant effect on circulating T lymphocyte counts and results in nonspecific B lymphocyte activation. These effects on cell-mediated immunity may contribute to the high incidence of tuberculosis and other infections among alcoholics.

THERAPY OF ALCOHOLISM

Since the primary problem in alcoholism is the imbibing of immodest amounts of ethanol, preventing ethanol ingestion is an obvious therapeutic strategy. The discovery that following administration of disulfiram (ANTABUSE) in a dose that produces no evident pharmacological effect of its own, ingestion of ethanol results in a distinctly unpleasant reaction, now termed the *disulfiram-ethanol reaction* (DER), suggested this drug could be used therapeutically in the treatment of alcoholism. Within minutes of the ingestion of ethanol, subjects pretreated with disulfiram experience a sensation of facial heat that is accompanied by flushing, a rise of several degrees in facial skin temperature, conjunctival injection, and an odor of acetaldehyde on the breath. Soon they experience palpitations, a throbbing in the neck, and a rather disturbing dyspnea (Fig. 19–8). For some, pallor, profuse perspiration, nausea, and vomiting follow. These phenomena are accompanied by an increase in respiration, a tachycardia, and drops in both diastolic and systolic pressure. At one time, when very large doses of disulfiram (1000 mg/day or more) were used, the reaction was sufficiently severe to result in cardiovascular collapse, and a number of fatalities occurred.

In current clinical practice, disulfiram is prescribed in a daily dosage of 250–500 mg/kg and the nature of the DER is explained to the patients, but patients are neither challenged with ethanol nor encouraged to do so on their own. Nonetheless, many patients given disulfiram do deliberately, if carefully, test whether the reaction occurs.

The primary action of disulfiram is the inhibition of the low K_m hepatic aldehyde dehydrogenase isozyme that is responsible for the metabolism of the acetaldehyde formed during ethanol metabolism. If this enzyme is blocked, the acetaldehyde formed accumulates. The intensity of the DER correlates closely with the blood level of acetaldehyde. The main effect of acetaldehyde on the cardiovascular system is to lower peripheral resis-

Individuals treated with disulfiram experience an aversive reaction within minutes of ingesting ethanol.

Disulfiram inhibits acetaldehyde dehydrogenase, causing accumulation of acetaldehyde during ethanol metabolism.

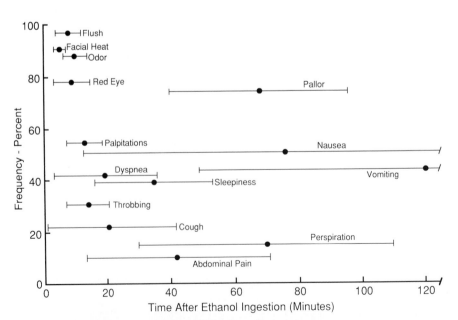

Figure 19–8

Incidence and mean onset time (*solid circle*) of symptoms and signs of the disulfiram-ethanol reaction. *Horizontal bar* represents ± 1 standard deviation of onset time. (Data from Hine CH, Burbridge TN, Macklin EA, et al: Some aspects of the human pharmacology of tetraethyl thiuram disulphide (Antabuse)–alcohol reactions. J Clin Invest 31:317–325, 1952; Raby K. Investigations on the disulfiram-alcohol reaction: Clinical observations. Quart J Stud Alc 14:545–556, 1953.)

tance. In the normal person this results in sympathetic stimulation and a compensatory increase in the force of myocardial contraction. As a result, while diastolic pressure drops, systolic pressure does not change appreciably. However, disulfiram has a second effect: it inhibits dopamine-β-hydroxylase, the enzyme responsible for transforming dopamine to norepinephrine. With the synthesis of norepinephrine blocked, the cardiac stores of norepinephrine are depleted and there is little to release when the sympathetic nerves are reflexly stimulated. Accordingly, a drop in systolic pressure is also seen (Fig. 19–9). It is this, if severe, that can lead to cardiovascular collapse. DERs that call for medical intervention are very rare at present. Should one occur, however, the treatment of choice is administration of the alcohol dehydrogenase inhibitor 4-methylpyrazole. It abrogates the reaction by inhibiting the metabolism of ethanol to acetaldehyde.

Disulfiram is a very effective drug—taken daily it results in total abstinence in the vast majority of patients. Like all effective drugs, it will not work if it is not taken. If a period of a month during a course of treatment of alcoholism is considered, a clear correlation is observed between the number of disulfiram-free days and the number of drinking days (Fig. 19–10). If no disulfiram is taken at all, drinking occurs on about half the days. If compliance is assured, disulfiram therapy is very effective indeed, both in terms of virtually eliminating drinking and in very substantially reducing the number of days lost from work, days institutionalized, and other indices of alcohol-induced life disruption. In the North American context, however, the compliance of most alcoholics with disulfiram therapy, when left to their own devices, is very poor.

Disulfiram therapy, if followed, assures abstinence and is a very effective treatment of alcoholism.

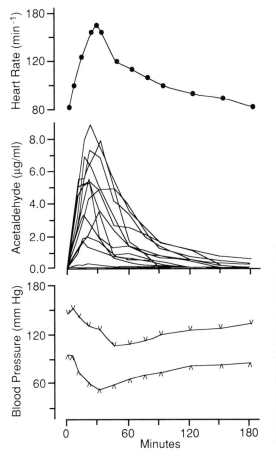

Figure 19–9

Time course of blood acetaldehyde levels and cardiovascular changes during the course of the disulfiram-ethanol reaction. Patients were administered 400 mg disulfiram daily for 3–6 days and were challenged with a 13.2-g dose of ethanol at zero time. (Data from Beyeler C, Fisch HU, Preisig R: The disulfiram-alcohol reaction: Factors determining and potential tests predicting severity. Alcoholism (NY) 9:118–124, 1985; Beyeler C, Fisch HU, Preisig R: Kardiovaskuläre und metabolische Veränderungen während der Antabus-Alkohol-Reaktion: Grundlagen zur Erfassung des Schweregrades. Schweiz Med Wochenschr 117:52–60, 1987.)

Figure 19-10

Correlation between the mean number of days on which disulfiram was not taken (disulfiram-free days) and the mean number of drinking days per 30-day months in groups of alcoholics being treated for alcoholism. (Data from Azrin NH, Sisson RW, Meyers R, Godley M: Alcoholism treatment by disulfiram and community reinforcement therapy. J Behav Ther Exp Psychiatry 13:105–112, 1982.)

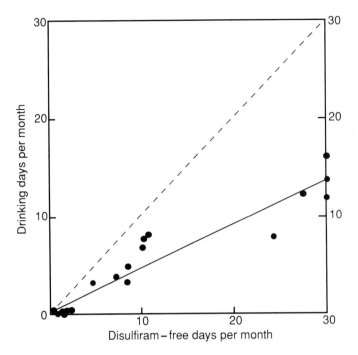

Disulfiram is almost totally insoluble in water and is therefore administered orally. By itself it does not inhibit the low K_m aldehyde dehydrogenase *in vitro*. It must act through a metabolite. Chemically disulfiram is the disulfide of dithiocarb, and it is reduced to the latter *in vivo*. Dithiocarb is in turn hydrolyzed to diethylamine, which is excreted in urine, and carbon disulfide, which is excreted in breath. It is therefore possible to ascertain objectively the patient's compliance with disulfiram therapy. It tends to be very low indeed unless, in designing the therapy, appropriate environmental contingencies are incorporated. If patients can be persuaded to involve their spouses and ask them to help maintain compliance by witnessing the ingestion of the disulfiram, preferably in a liquid suspension, therapy is usually very successful. Alternatively, high levels of therapeutic success are attained if patients agree to enter into a contract with the clinic whereby access to the treatment or a financial deposit is forfeited if tests fail to confirm compliance, or if the daily ingestion of disulfiram (supervised by a plant nurse or a probation officer) is made a condition of continued employment (or parole).

For many years total lifelong abstinence was considered the only appropriate goal of alcoholism therapy; an accepted dictum was that, in becoming alcoholic, individuals irreversibly lost the ability to control their drinking. Then, in a large follow-up study of patients who had received abstinence-oriented therapy, the Rand Corporation found that a significant proportion of the subjects had apparently returned to stable moderate ethanol consumption (Fig. 19–11). These findings were treated as highly controversial by the alcoholism treatment community, which felt the publicity surrounding the findings might lead abstinent alcoholics to try drinking, a situation likened to giving a loaded gun to a child. For the same reason there was strong opposition to any effort to teach alcohol abusers how to drink in a controlled fashion. Since then it has become apparent that, whatever the treatment goals are, some of those treated embrace long-term abstinence whereas others return successfully to relatively stable moderate drinking. This is also true of those in the community who recover without treatment (Fig. 19–12). From the Rand study it is apparent that the controlled drinking outcome is much more frequently observed in those whose alcohol consumption at the time of entry into therapy was not very high.

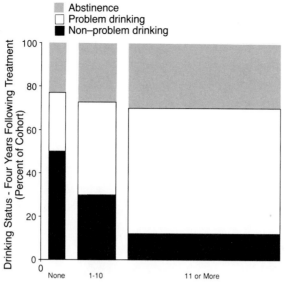

Figure 19-11

Long-term outcome of abstinence-oriented treatment of alcoholism as a function of the severity of the alcohol dependence at entry into treatment. *Entry status:* The treatment population (n = 508) was divided into three cohorts depending on the incidence of alcohol-dependence symptoms (continuous drinking for 12 or more hours, missing meals because of drinking, memory lapses—blackouts, loss of control, drinking first thing in the morning, having "the shakes"—severe tremor) experienced in the 30 days preceding entry into treatment. The relative size of the three cohorts is given by the width of the respective columns. (Among those who reported no dependence symptoms many sought treatment because of other adverse consequences.) *Outcome status:* The individuals in each cohort were classified at 4 years following entry into treatment according to whether their drinking behavior corresponded to abstinence—no consumption of ethanol in the last 6 months *(color)*; problem drinking— consumption of ethanol resulting in either dependence symptoms during the preceding 30 days or adverse consequences in the previous 6 months *(white)*; or non-problem drinking—consumption of ethanol without any dependence symptoms or adverse consequences in the stated periods *(black)*. At entry into treatment, the average ethanol consumption of individuals in the none, 1-10, and ≥11 dependency symptom-cohorts was 7, 14, and 23 drinks per day, respectively. At 4 years, the average ethanol consumption by the individuals in the problem and non-problem drinking groups was 13.5 and 5 drinks per day, respectively. (Data from Polich JM, Armor DJ, and Braiker HB: The Course of Alcoholism: Four Years after Treatment, Tables 3.27 and 3.28. Santa Monica, CA: Rand Corp, 1980.)

Conversely, many individuals with moderate alcohol problems find the goal of lifelong abstinence, and the necessary restructuring of their whole social life, unacceptable and fail to remain in treatment. At the same time, there is evidence that individuals who have been dependent on ethanol find learning to drink in a controlled fashion very difficult. Accordingly, the emerging treatment paradigm appears to favor lifelong abstinence as a goal for those who have progressed to alcohol dependence, and achievement of stable moderate drinking a goal for those who have not progressed beyond problem drinking (Fig. 19-13).

Heavy chronic consumption of ethanol induces an impairment of memory and cognitive function. At the same time, a great deal of learning is required to remain abstinent and even more to achieve stable moderate drinking. Accordingly, it is not surprising that one of the best predictors of treatment outcome is the degree of cognitive impairment patients present

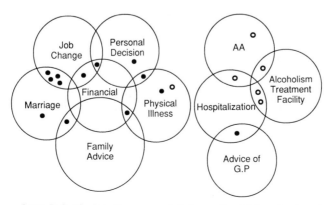

Figure 19-12

Previously alcoholic individuals *(small closed circles)* and the reasons they gave *(large open circles)* for ceasing to abuse alcohol. Subsample of 3600 individuals chosen at random from those on the electoral register; mean duration of the recovery: 6.5 years, range 1-25 years. *Open circles:* individuals who had become abstinent; *closed circles:* individuals who had become moderate drinkers (mean consumption 2.5 drinks/day, range 0-5 drinks/day). Individuals positioned at the intersection of more than one circle gave more than one reason for ceasing alcohol

abuse. Individuals in the group of circles on the right received professional help; those in the group on the left recovered without seeking or receiving such help. (Data from Saunders WM, Kershaw PW: Spontaneous remission from alcohol—A community study. Br J Addict 74:251-265, 1979.)

Figure 19–13

Progression of drinking behaviors and the range of advocated treatment goals.

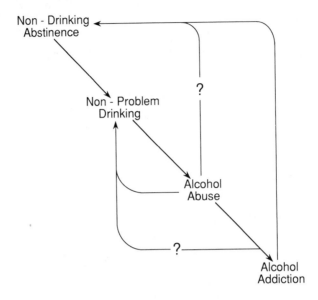

upon entry into therapy: the greater the impairment the less likely the success of therapy. With abstinence there is a partial reversal of such impairment. Accordingly, an initial period of abstinence is therapeutically desirable, whatever the long-term treatment goals. As an interim treatment goal, temporary abstinence is acceptable even to individuals who are desirous of eventually returning to controlled drinking. Disulfiram can be used to achieve such interim abstinence.

Methanol

Produced when wood is heated in the absence of air (hence, wood spirits), methanol is widely used as antifreeze and windshield-washing fluid. It is also used, frequently in mixtures with ethanol, as a solvent for shellacs, varnishes, and paints or as an adulterant to make ethanol unfit for consumption.

METABOLISM AND EXCRETION

Methanol is oxidized to formaldehyde and formic acid; both are toxic.

Methanol is eliminated by oxidation to formaldehyde and formic acid. The first step in this process is mediated by alcohol dehydrogenase, a reaction for which ethanol is an effective competitive inhibitor, completely blocking methanol oxidation at blood levels of 100–200 mg/dl. Another effective inhibitor of alcohol dehydrogenase is 4-methylpyrazole. The oxidation of formaldehyde, by formic acid, to carbon dioxide is a rather limited capacity pathway in humans. The alternate route of elimination is excretion in the expired air. As much as 30% of the dose can be eliminated in this fashion.

A major pathway of methanol elimination is excretion in expired air; if its metabolism is blocked, more will be eliminated in this manner.

TOXIC EFFECTS

Consumption of methanol is followed by mild and transient CNS intoxication and the development, with a characteristic delay of several hours, of headache, clammy skin, nausea, and vomiting. Blurring of vision is a characteristic toxic effect of formaldehyde. Untreated, it progresses to irreversible blindness. It can be reversed in its early stages by hemodialysis. However, if all the methanol is not cleared from the blood by this means, once hemodialysis is stopped more formaldehyde will be formed and vision impairment will return. Patients also experience severe lower abdominal pain, which is due to the development of formate acidosis and is relieved by infusion of 5% bicarbonate.

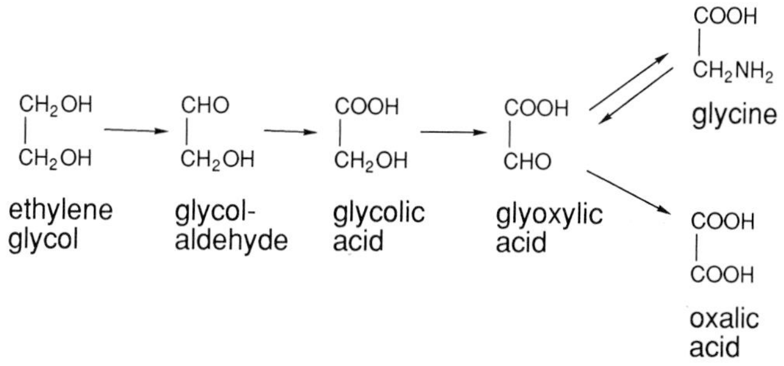

$$\underset{\text{ethylene glycol}}{\overset{\text{CH}_2\text{OH}}{\underset{\text{CH}_2\text{OH}}{|}}} \rightarrow \underset{\text{glycol-aldehyde}}{\overset{\text{CHO}}{\underset{\text{CH}_2\text{OH}}{|}}} \rightarrow \underset{\text{glycolic acid}}{\overset{\text{COOH}}{\underset{\text{CH}_2\text{OH}}{|}}} \rightarrow \underset{\text{glyoxylic acid}}{\overset{\text{COOH}}{\underset{\text{CHO}}{|}}}$$

$$\underset{\text{glycine}}{\overset{\text{COOH}}{\underset{\text{CH}_2\text{NH}_2}{|}}}$$

$$\underset{\text{oxalic acid}}{\overset{\text{COOH}}{\underset{\text{COOH}}{|}}}$$

Figure 19-14

Scheme of the biotransformation reactions involving ethylene glycol metabolism.

The course of the intoxication is frequently insidious, since symptoms although delayed for many hours develop rapidly once they begin to appear. The delay can be in part a consequence of the ethanol content of material ingested because the oxidation of methanol to its toxic metabolites is impeded as long as significant body burdens of ethanol persist. Additionally, the delay encompasses a period of compensated metabolic acidosis. Once the respiratory and metabolic compensating mechanisms are exhausted, blood pH falls rapidly.

TREATMENT OF INTOXICATION

Three approaches need to be utilized for the successful treatment of this condition. First, either ethanol or, if it is available, 4-methylpyrazole should be administered to inhibit the metabolism of methanol to formaldehyde. Second, the acidosis, if present, should be corrected by infusion of bicarbonate. Third, if blurring of vision indicates significant blood levels of formaldehyde, hemodialysis should be instituted.

METABOLISM, INTOXICATION, AND TREATMENT

Ethylene Glycol

Ethylene glycol, a compound frequently used as a permanent antifreeze in car radiators, is first metabolized to glycolaldehyde by the action of alcohol dehydrogenase. Its further metabolism is to glycolic acid and glyoxylic acid (Fig. 19–14). The latter is metabolized by a limited-capacity pathway to glycine. When that pathway is saturated and the levels of glyoxylic acid rise, significant formation of oxalic acid occurs. As oxalate levels rise, formation of crystals of calcium oxalate, a very sparingly soluble compound, occurs. Deposition of these crystals in renal tubular cells causes their necrosis and renal failure. Following larger doses of ethylene glycol, calcium oxalate deposition in other tissues, notably in cerebral capillaries, can also occur.

Ethylene glycol can be metabolized to oxalic acid; calcium oxalate crystals form in the kidneys and elsewhere because of the low solubility of this salt.

The intoxication, which occurs without a smell of alcohol on the breath, can present with nausea, vomiting, and hematemesis. Proteinuria and presence of calcium oxalate crystals in the urine, tachycardia, and coma are further presenting signs. As in methanol intoxication, the therapy should include three approaches: First, inhibition of the metabolism of ethylene glycol by administration of either ethanol or 4-methylpyrazole; second, correction of the acidosis by infusion of bicarbonate; and third, hemodialysis for the removal of glycolic aldehyde, glycolic acid, and glyoxylic acid.

General References

Blane HT, Leonard KE (eds): Psychological Theories of Drinking and Alcoholism. New York: Guilford, 1987.

Brewer C: Supervised disulfiram in alcoholism. Br J Hosp Med 35:116–119, 1986.

Chan AWK, Welte JW, Whitney RB: Identification of alcoholism in young adults by blood chemistries. Alcohol 4:175–179, 1987.

Deitrich RA, Dunwiddie TV, Harris RA, Erwin VG: Mechanism of action of ethanol: Initial central nervous system actions. Pharmacol Rev 41:489–537, 1989.

Gessner PK: Drug therapy of the alcohol withdrawal syndrome. *In* Majchrowicz E, Nobles EP (eds): Biochemistry and Pharmacology of Ethanol. Vol 2, 375–435. New York: Plenum, 1979.

Gessner PK, Gessner T: Disulfiram and Its Metabolite, Dithiocarb: Pharmacology and Status in the Therapy of Alcoholism, HIV Infections, and Heavy Metal Intoxication. London: Chapman & Hall (in press).

Harris RA, Allan AM: Alcohol intoxication: Ion channels and genetics. FASEB J 3:1689–1695, 1989.

Jacobsen D, Hewlett TP, Webb R, et al: Ethylene glycol intoxication: Evaluation of kinetics and crystalluria. Am J Med 84:145–152, 1988.

Johlin FC, Fortman CS, Nghiem DD, Tephly TR: Studies on the role of folic and folate dependent enzyme in human methanol poisoning. Pharmacol 31:557–561, 1987.

Lieber CS: Biochemical and molecular basis of alcohol-induced injury to liver and other tissues. New Engl J Med 319:1639–1650, 1988.

McLelland AT, Woody GE, O'Brien CP: Development of psychiatric illness in drug abusers: Possible role of drug preference. New Engl J Med 301:1310–1314, 1979.

Orrego H, Blake JE, Blendis LM, et al: Long-term treatment of alcoholic liver disease with propylthiouracil. New Engl J Med 317:1421–1427, 1987.

Peele S: The Meaning of Addiction: Compulsive Experience and Its Interpretation. Lexington, MA: Lexington Books, 1985.

Wilkinson PK: Pharmacokinetics of ethanol: A review. Alcoholism (Baltimore) 4:6–21, 1980.

Antianxiety Drugs

20

Cedric M. Smith

This chapter addresses the agents used in the treatment and prevention of anxiety, anxiety syndromes, and panic disorders. The focus is on the benzodiazepines and buspirone. The older, largely obsolete sedative/hypnotic barbiturates and related compounds are described briefly because they are still on the market and used occasionally.

Drugs used in the therapy of disorders of feelings, thoughts, and behaviors are now usually classified according to their uses in the therapy of identified diseases or conditions, such as epilepsy, anxiety and anxiety disorders, depression, panic attacks, or sleep disorders (e.g., insomnia). In contrast, in the past it was usual to classify and discuss these agents either according to their chemical class—for example, the barbiturates or benzodiazepines—or according to their general pharmacological effects, such as sedatives, hypnotics, or central nervous system (CNS) depressants.

The discovery of the antianxiety and calming effects of a newly synthesized novel class of compounds, the benzodiazepines, in the late 1950s signaled the beginning of a new era of more effective and safe treatment of a variety of anxiety states as well as epilepsy and sleep disorders. In addition to their use in anxiety, the benzodiazepines have extensive clinical application in anesthesia procedures and as muscle relaxants. The discovery of the properties of benzodiazepines was initiated by innovative organic chemists who provided the novel benzodiazepine, chlordiazepoxide, to experienced pharmacologists. It was observed that this compound and other congeners produced a unique calming action in laboratory animals. When following up on this observation, it was established that these compounds had unique, heretofore undiscovered, mechanisms of action and a margin of safety far better than barbiturates, the then-established sedative or hypnotic agents. The efficacy, unique spectrum of action, and wide margin of safety of benzodiazepines were observed subsequently in human subjects. These observations sparked monumental research programs and have resulted in the discovery of hundreds of potentially useful compounds, new therapeutic approaches, and a variety of new receptors and receptor systems.

Although the benzodiazepines have a large margin of safety on acute administration (when comparing dosages required to reduce anxiety and promote sleep with the dosages that result in respiratory depression), they are not without adverse effects. The variability among patients in the time course of action and pharmacokinetics presents problems for effective clinical use. All the benzodiazepines are at least additive in their effects with other CNS depressants such as opioids or alcohol. In addition, with

The other drug groups discussed in this chapter are the barbiturates, buspirone, and various drugs used in the treatment of panic disorders.

The major drug classes are the benzodiazepines—the first truly selectively acting antianxiety drugs.

Benzodiazepines have unique spectra of actions—varying with the compound and with individual sensitivities.

271

chronic administration and use, all have the potential for abuse and dependence at a risk level, in terms of prevalence, similar to that of alcoholic beverages (i.e., some 5–10% of those exposed).

Major therapeutic uses of benzodiazepines: short-term treatment of anxiety disorders and insomnia; skeletal muscle relaxation; conscious sedation procedures; and epilepsy.

The current major uses of the benzodiazepines are for the relief of anxiety and as hypnotic, sleep-promoting agents. In addition, some of them have found important therapeutic niches as skeletal muscle relaxants (diazepam, see Chapter 25), as agents for anesthetic conscious sedation techniques (diazepam, midazolam, see Chapter 16), and in the treatment of seizures and seizure disorders (diazepam, clonazepam, see Chapter 23). The differential utility of a specific agent for a given patient and symptom, follows from both the unique spectra of action of different agents as well as the differences among agents in terms of their onsets and durations of action.

Treatment of Anxiety

Anxiety is both the feeling and the behaviors of the natural reaction to fear-inducing situations.

Anxiety is a complex of subjective feelings and characteristic behaviors. The subjective feelings consist of tension, apprehension, fear, worry, and difficulty with thinking or concentrating. These feelings are usually accompanied by behavioral signs and symptoms of trembling, tremors, muscle tension, restlessness, and fatigue with autonomic hyperactivity in the respiratory, cardiovascular, urinary, and gastrointestinal (GI) systems. Such signs and symptoms of anxiety can be altogether normal, appropriate, and beneficial responses to threatening or tragic situations. But anxiety can take on harmful and medically meaningful dimensions when it is inappropriate to the situation or functionally disabling. For example, intense chronically sustained anxiety or unrealistic worry about oneself or a close relative, such as a parent or child, can be truly disabling. Thus, the need for diagnosis and treatment is a function not only of the symptoms but of their intensity, duration, and the degree to which they interfere with other activities.

Excessive anxiety, anxiety out of proportion to the external situation, can be incapacitating.

Among the identified anxiety disorders are generalized anxiety disorder, panic disorder, agoraphobia, social phobia, simple phobias, post-traumatic stress syndrome, and obsessive-compulsive disorder. Anxiety is also a common concomitant of many organic diseases, such as hypoglycemia, anemia, vitamin B_{12} deficiency, hyperthyroidism, coronary heart disease, and mitral valve prolapse. Anxiety may also be a prominent symptom in patients in many of the other psychiatric diagnostic categories—those with personality disorders, mood (affective) disorders, or schizophrenia.

Anxiety syndromes can be produced by drugs and other chemical substances, as well as being endogenous or due to the situation.

It is important to recognize that anxiety symptoms are commonly produced or aggravated by a wide variety of drugs including, notably, caffeine, theophylline, ephedrine, amphetamines, cocaine, thyroid hormones, digitalis, imipramine, indomethacin, baclofen, levodopa, propranolol, as well as rebound or withdrawal from alcohol or benzodiazepine use (see Chapter 27).

The antianxiety drugs can antagonize and relieve anxiety in many of the syndromes listed earlier, as well as the anxiety of everyday life; however, their use in therapy is best limited to administration for relatively short periods of time—a few days to a month—and to those situations and conditions in which such short-term therapy is useful, such as preoperatively, for acute grief reactions that impair functioning, or for insomnia of brief duration due to worry over short-lived transient external events.

For chronic use for chronic anxiety syndromes the drugs have only limited applicability; the major long-term therapeutic goal in such syndromes is the learning and training by the patient in the avoidance of, and adaptation to, anxiety-producing thoughts and situations.

A comment on terminology is pertinent. In a general sense *sedation* refers to any of a variety of calming or nervous system depressant effects as determined subjectively by the individual or by observation of the demeanor or behavior. The terms *sedation* and *sedative* lack precise definitions or operational meanings, and at present they refer usually to the actions of the benzodiazepines to relieve anxiety or to be anxiolytic. (Traditionally, the sedative-hypnotic drugs have included a large variety of agents including the barbiturates, benzodiazepines, meprobamate, and a miscellaneous group of substances that possess actions similar to the barbiturates; of these miscellaneous agents the following are still on the market: glutethemide, methyprylon, and chloral hydrate. In addition, many drugs used primarily for other purposes have sedative or hypnotic effects; these include phenothiazines, tricylic antidepressants, diphenhydramine, and many other antihistamines, opioids, and clonidine.) In contrast, *hypnotic* agents rather specifically refer to substances that produce or promote sleep; *hypnosis,* on the other hand, is a general term used usually in reference to the phenomenon of hypnosis and hypnotic trances. Thus, in common parlance, benzodiazepines are sedative-hypnotic, antianxiety agents, some of which are used therapeutically for the temporary relief of anxiety or insomnia.

Alone benzodiazepines have a large therapeutic index.

Before discussing the actions and uses of benzodiazepines and other antianxiety agents, the following are situations and *conditions in which they are not used, are hazardous or contraindicated:*

Benzodiazepines have a number of potentially serious side effects.

- if mental alertness is required, for example, for driving or operating dangerous machinery;
- in depressive mood disorders or psychosis;
- in individuals who may have the potential to develop drug dependence (i.e., 20% of the general population and all moderate to heavy drinkers);
- with concomitant alcohol use or combined with other CNS depressants;
- in pregnant women, and possibly in all women of childbearing age;
- in the elderly, inasmuch as drug effects (acute and chronic) may be indistinguishable from or contribute to organic brain disease.

The structures of the first agents introduced therapeutically, chlordiazepoxide (LIBRIUM) and diazepam (VALIUM), illustrate the chemistry of the benzodiazepines that includes a rather unusual 7-member ring. Since their introduction, these drugs have become among the most frequently prescribed of all drugs, and a variety of related substances have been discovered and studied, some of which have been accepted as effective, relatively safe, and therapeutically useful agents. These are presented in Tables 20–1 and 20–4.

Benzodiazepines

Chlordiazepoxide (LIBRIUM)

ACTIONS AND SPECTRA OF ACTION OF BENZODIAZEPINES

Acute Effects

Benzodiazepines have many dose-related reproducible actions, almost all of which are the consequence of selective effects on the CNS. Common among them are relief of anxiety, calming, sedation, drowsiness, amnesia, and impairment of cognitive functioning. Subjectively, there may be feelings of physical and mental relaxation akin to alcohol intoxication. Some individuals report the feeling state to be pleasant and desirable, whereas others find it dysphoric. Patients appear to be relaxed and relieved of worries, sometimes talkative, somnolent, with slurred speech, muscle incoordination, and ataxia.

There may be wide individual differences in the effects of a given dose

Diazepam (VALIUM)

Desmethyldiazepam

Alprazolam (XANAX)

Flurazepam (DALMANE)

Oxazepam (SERAX)

Lorazepam (ATIVAN)

of a specific agent, actions of the specific agent, and differences in dose-related intensity and quality of effects. Among the more adverse potential effects are subjective feelings of dizziness, headache, nausea, nervousness, and cloudy mentation. Behavioral disinhibition, as manifested by increased aggressiveness and hostility, may also be observed.

Skeletal muscle relaxation is prominent with only one currently available compound, diazepam. Most of the other benzodiazepines, such as chlordiazepoxide or the active metabolite of diazepam, desmethyldiazepam, lack selective or clinically useful muscle relaxant effects. The full assessment of the spectrum of effects in humans of the more recently introduced compounds has not been investigated specifically, e.g, for their muscle relaxant or antidepressant actions. The selectivity of action of diazepam as a muscle relaxant provides strong evidence for a unique pattern of effects for each of the benzodiazepines; although the benzodiazepines now available share a number of effects, *each of them has a unique spectrum of action.*

Another distinguishing property of some benzodiazepines is their ability to alleviate symptoms of depression or of anxiety that accompanies depressive mood disorder. For example, alprazolam has antidepressant actions not detectable with diazepam; diazepam has either no effect or makes depression symptoms worse.

The amnesia produced by the benzodiazepines is characterized by its patchy character and the fact that it is generally not recognized by the patient. (Obviously patients are amnesic for events taking place while they are comatose or unconscious, but the amnesia being referred to here is that taking place while the patients are responding and interacting with their environment.) The amnesia can be retrograde where events in the past are not remembered, but most frequently it is anterograde with the events taking place following drug administration lost to recall at a later time. This amnesia has great therapeutic potential, as in the management of surgical and operative procedures, as well as great potential for harm. To illustrate, an investigation of the effects of the administration of 10 mg of diazepam preoperatively found approximately a 40% loss of memory that would have been recalled in the absence of the drug; and 40% of the individuals receiving it did not even remember the operating or recovery room.

This drug-induced amnesia is usually desirable, whereas the equivalent memory loss, unrecognized by the patient, could have devastating consequences to a business executive or to an elderly patient with pre-existing marginal memory functioning. The benzodiazepines have been widely prescribed to patients who are also undergoing psychotherapy. Obviously, any amnesia for the discussions and counseling taking place in such psychotherapeutic sessions makes the worth of such sessions doubtful.

The CNS depressant effects of the benzodiazepines, and all agents discussed in this chapter as well, are additive or synergistic with the CNS depressant actions of alcohol, barbiturates, phenothiaziness, opioids, and tricyclic antidepressants.

Depression of respiration and the appearance of a comatose state are dose-related actions of benzodiazepines, but they occur only with doses that exceed those needed for relief of anxiety or the promotion of nighttime sleep. Moreover, respiratory depression or coma requires, relative to therapeutic effects, greater doses of benzodiazepines than of barbiturates or the other antianxiety drugs. Nevertheless, although by themselves the benzodiazepines are remarkably safe substances, they all too commonly contribute to the nervous system depression following poisoning with ethanol and many other CNS depressants. For example, deaths due to alcohol and sedative drug interactions exceed 2500 per year in the United States, and such interactions are involved in more than 47,000 emergency room admissions.

Effects with Chronic Administration

Acute tolerance to the depressant effects of benzodiazepines occurs during the time course of action of a single dose. Acute tolerance means that greater effects occur while the blood levels are rising than occur at the same blood level during recovery. This acute tolerance has been observed for both subjective effects and for the motor relaxation and incoordination effects.

Tolerance to the effects of repeated dosages has been observed even with a single hypnotic dosage repeated up to weeks later. Tolerance to single daily hypnotic dosages at bedtime can be detected with most agents within 1 week or less of daily treatment. It appears that tolerance develops more rapidly to frequently repeated dosing, for example, every 4 hours, as opposed to daily. It is also said that tolerance is more likely to occur to the daytime drowsiness and sedation than to the antianxiety or antiepileptic effects; however, at least some tolerance to the antianxiety effects does occur over periods of days and weeks of administration. Moreover, high levels of tolerance can be achieved with progressive escalation of dosage and the frequency of administration. (This acquired tolerance is usually mostly functional in origin, but can be metabolic also as discussed later. As a general approximation, the degree of tolerance obtained with benzodiazepines is such that two to three times the dosage that originally produced sedation would be required in the tolerant state to produce equivalent sedation.)

Not only does tolerance develop with chronic administration, but habituation and physical dependence also occur with therapeutic and larger dosages (discussed later).

Triazolam (HALCION)

Tolerance, habitual, and physical dependence can occur with therapeutic and higher dosages.

SITES AND MECHANISMS OF ACTION OF BENZODIAZEPINES

Sites of Action

As a useful generalization and conclusion, it can be assumed that the benzodiazepines act directly on those CNS systems that mediate the functions modified by the agents. The mood and emotional effects of the benzodiazepines result, most probably, from their actions on limbic systems (amygdala and hippocampus). Spontaneous and evoked neuronal activity in these areas is decreased; the long feedback networks in these systems appear especially vulnerable, such as the loop from limbic forebrain to reticular system and back to cortex.

Mental confusion and amnesia are readily associated with benzodiazepine effects on hippocampus and cortical association areas.

The sleep-promoting properties of benzodiazepines appear to arise from the cortical effects or effects on sleep-wakefulness clocks. In contrast to barbiturates, they do not have selective effects on the reticular activating system. After receiving a dose of a benzodiazepine at bedtime, there is, on average, an increase in total sleep time, decreased sleep latency, decreased awakenings, an increase in Stage 2, and a decreased time in Stages 3 and 4.

The effects of benzodiazepines (specifically diazepam) on muscle function and motor control are due to their effects on supraspinal, reticular,

Benzodiazepines have antianxiety, amnesia, sleep-promoting, intoxicating, and atactic effects.

Some benzodiazepines produce skeletal muscle relaxation, some are useful as antiepileptic agents, and at least one has antidepressant and antipanic actions.

Sites of action include cerebral cortex, amygdala, hippocampus, sleep centers, midbrain and cerebellar motor systems.

and cerebellar systems. Although there are demonstrable spinal effects of diazepam, e.g., to increase presynaptic inhibition, these are of less importance in producing muscle relaxation than the supraspinal actions. In addition to the direct effects on motor control systems, relaxation of tense skeletal muscles is one of the consequences of the supraspinal antianxiety effects.

In summary, benzodiazepines affect a large number of nervous system sites including hypothalamic areas involved in stress responses. Moreover, the spectra of the actions of different benzodiazepines, albeit similar, actually reveal unique differential actions. These differential actions are probably best explained on the basis of the distribution, functions, and the specificities and heterogeneity of the benzodiazepine receptor systems.

Mechanisms of Action — Benzodiazepine Receptors and Receptor Systems

The actions of benzodiazepines and the other sedative-hypnotics can be assessed at a number of levels of integration in terms of effects on behavior, neurophysiology of single neurons and networks, and receptors isolated or *in situ.*

Benzodiazepine receptors are widely distributed in the central nervous system.

Behavior. A well-established characteristic effect in humans and animals of the benzodiazepines is their decrease in the subjective and behavioral manifestations of fear and anxiety. In experimental animals this is reflected by tame and relaxed behavior with decreases in the autonomic (blood pressure, heart rate, respiratory rate, piloerection, GI motility) concomitants of fear and escape behavior. In operant behavior systems the benzodiazepines characteristically result in increases in learned behaviors that had been suppressed by the introduction of concomitant punishment. This test has been commonly used as one among many models of anxiety.

In humans, analogous behavioral changes are observed in addition to a subjective sense of relaxation and absence of tension and anxiety.

Benzodiazepine effects have been described on single neurons, neuronal discharge patterns, neuronal networks, benzodiazepine receptors, and on the processes of excitation and inhibition.

Neurophysiological Actions. At the level of single neurons, such as those in the limbic system, the *benzodiazepines depress the repetitive afterdischarges* that occur in response to single shock. This depression of repetitive activity is plausibly associated with the antiseizure and antiepileptic actions. It could also represent some of the neural equivalents of the neurophysiological components of memory.

In synaptic systems, most of which are normally repetitively active, benzodiazepines alter and depress the potentiation of synaptic transmission that occurs after a period of repetitive activity (posttetanic potentiation — PTP). This *depression of PTP* occurs with dosages that have no effect on the transmission itself of single or regular impulses. This depression of PTP is probably correlated also with the muscle relaxant and antiseizure effects.

Perhaps most studied of the neurophysiological effects of these agents is their *enhancement of presynaptic inhibition* at both spinal and supraspinal sites. Presynaptic inhibition refers to depression (inhibition) of transmission at a given synapse by activity of other nerves that have their terminations on the presynaptic nerve terminals of the given synapse. The inhibition is manifested by a decrease in transmitter output from the presynaptic terminals of the given synapse — hence a decrease, an inhibition, over the original transmission.

One of the most extensively studied of the presynaptic systems is that affecting the spinal excitatory transmission from primary afferent fibers from muscle spindles to the homonymous motor neurons. Repetitive stimulation of skin afferent fibers of the same spinal segment results in the simultaneous inhibition of the homonymous monosynaptic reflex. This inhibition is not due to effects on those motor neurons; rather, it is the consequence of effects on the afferent terminals mediating the motor neuron excitation. The inhibition is the consequence of the skin afferents exciting interneurons that, in turn, end on the presynaptic terminals of the synaptic endings causing a depression of their transmitter output. This decrease in transmitter output is the result of a decrease in the presynaptic membrane potential associated with an increase in chloride permeability; the transmitter at this synapse between an interneuron and the presynaptic terminations is gamma-aminobutyric acid (GABA). This reflex and the influence of diazepam are discussed further in Chapter 26 on muscle relaxants.

Many benzodiazepine receptors are intimately connected with GABA receptor systems and chloride channels.

Consistent with the effect of benzodiazepines to augment presynaptic inhibition is the observation that the benzodiazepines also *augment the effects of GABA* on the same synaptic system. (These observations are fully consonant with the results of studies of the effects of benzodiazepines and of GABA on isolated neuronal and receptor systems.)

At a number of supraspinal sites GABA acts postsynaptically and here, too, benzodiazepines act to augment the actions of GABA.

Biochemical and Molecular Actions. Although the benzodiazepines potentiate GABA and GABA-ergic transmission, they do not act as GABA agonists or antagonists nor do they affect GABA release, synthesis, or metabolism. Rather, they act on unique benzodiazepine receptors, many of which are closely associated with the GABA receptors and the transmembrane channel for chloride.

The benzodiazepines bind stereospecifically with receptors and with nonspecific receptors, both of which are widely distributed in the nervous system. The receptors that bind the benzodiazepines have been characterized as *heterogeneous* or *polymorphic* to summarize the fact that there is a wide variety of specificities of receptor binding with respect to neural sites, molecular specificity, affinities, agonist *versus* antagonist actions, and neuronal synaptic consequences of binding. In contrast to opioid receptors there have yet to be well-defined classes of benzodiazepine receptors, although there is support for three or more subclasses of benzodiazepine receptors in brain. (BZ-1 and BZ-2 classes have been postulated. A correlation has been found in animal studies for the BZ-1 receptors in cognition, memory, and motor function, whereas the BZ-2 receptors were more involved in sleep [Barnett et al, 1985; Ankier and Goa, 1988]).

Benzodiazepine receptors are heterogeneous, with the possibility of numerous classes and subclasses of receptors.

The consequence of this widespread, highly complex heterogeneous family of systems is that the various benzodiazepines affect many neuronal systems and that, although the spectra of their actions are similar, they are not identical—as illustrated already by the muscle relaxant actions of diazepam, which are not evident with chlordiazepoxide.

Receptors are classified on the basis of location, and allosteric coupling with other receptor systems, as well as on the specificity of their binding and interaction with other analogs.

In addition, the benzodiazepines can now be classified according to the degree to which they have "agonist" or "antagonist" effects on specific receptors. Thus, each compound can now be classified according to the characteristics of its binding to populations of isolated receptors, to populations of receptors at specific neuronal sites, and to characteristics of its binding interactions with other compounds—e.g., as agonist, antagonist, and partial agonist.

Benzodiazepines can be assessed relative to their actions as agonists, antagonists, partial agonists, and inverse agonists.

(Benzodiazepines are known to have actions other than the augmen-

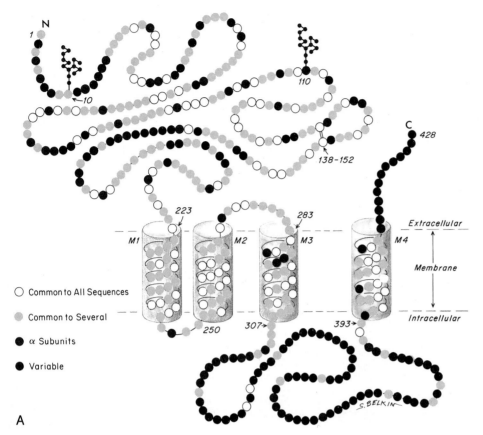

A

Figure 20-1

(A) Generic GABA_A receptor protein subunit sequence and putative topological structure. The numbering follows that of the rat α_1 sequence used by Khrestchatisky M, MacLennan AJ, Chiang MY, et al: A novel alpha-subunit in rat brain GABA_A receptors. Neuron 3:745–753, 1989. Note the NH_2 terminal (labeled N, residue 1) presumed extracellular domain, with probable sites for asparagine glycosylation (polymeric black circles at positions 10 and 110), and the cystine bridge (solid line connecting 138 and 152). Four putative membrane-spanning α-helical cylinders M1, M2, M3, and M4 are shown. The COOH-terminus (labeled C, residue 428) is again extracellular. A large intracellular cytoplasmic loop between M3 and M4 is present. The color code indicates the degree of variability within the family of rat polypeptides published to date: α_1, α_2, α_4, β_1, β_2, β_3, γ_2, and δ. Those amino acids identical in all the clones are shown in white, those identical in two or more types are gray, those identical in all α but not in β, γ, or δ are black, and those that vary between types are in color.

tation of GABA effects, including a glycine-like action and alterations in many other synaptic systems involving cholinergic, adrenergic, serotonergic, or dopaminergic neurotransmitters. However, most of such alterations appear at present not to be primary actions because many of them could have occurred secondary to effects on GABA systems.)

The causal connections between the interactions of benzodiazepines with the family of GABA receptor systems and their antianxiety and antiseizure actions are not well understood; the affected GABA systems are not directly involved in anxiety or seizures; serotonergic and other neurotransmitter systems appear to be more directly involved. Benzodiazepine receptors probably have endogenous ligand(s) that are anxiogenic: a number of possible candidates are under active scrutiny at present. Likely candidates include one or more β-carbolines found to be elevated in conditions associated with high levels of anxiety. Nevertheless, it remains possible that the endogenous ligand has actions similar to those of the benzodiazepines or that there is, in reality, no functional endogenous ligand for benzodiazepine receptors.

The study of large numbers of compounds has revealed that the binding to benzodiazepine receptors can be characterized by one of the following classes of effects:

1. Agonist—examples include diazepam and chlordiazepoxide with stereospecific binding of different affinities at different receptors.

2. Antagonist—the example is flumazenil, which has antagonistic actions and competitive binding with agonists at certain benzodiazepine receptors (discussed later).

3. "Inverse agonist"—a term describing those benzodiazepine derivatives found to bind to some benzodiazepine receptors and that are associated with increased anxiety or seizure activity, actions opposite (i.e., inverse) to the usual effects of benzodiazepines.

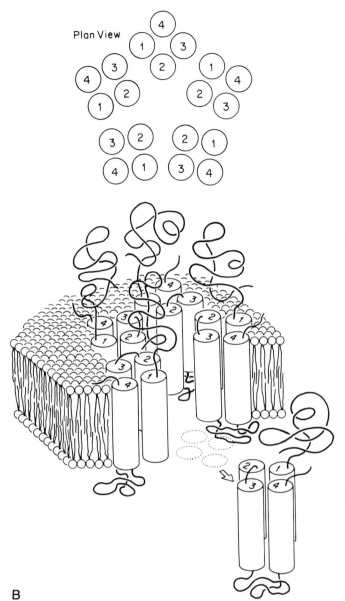

Plan View

B

Figure 20 – 1 Continued

(B) Model of the GABA$_A$ receptor-chloride channel protein complex. The ligand-gated ion channel is proposed to be a hetero-oligomer composed of five subunits of the type shown in A. Each subunit has four membrane-spanning domains (cylinders numbered 1 – 4), one or more of which contribute to the wall of the ion channel. The structure is patterned after the well-characterized nicotinic acetylcholine receptor, another member of the same gene superfamily. The naturally occurring oligomers are composed of some of the α, β, γ, and δ polypeptides, but the exact subunit composition, stoichiometry, and number of subunits are not known at this time. (From Olsen RW, Tobin AJ: Molecular biology of GABA$_A$ receptors. FASEB J 4:1469 – 1480, 1990.)

A proposed model of the benzodiazepine receptor systems can serve to summarize the complex relationships of the benzodiazepine binding site(s) with the receptor systems for GABA, the primary gating ligand for transmembrane chloride ion channels. The same receptor systems possess other binding sites for barbiturates, some convulsants, and other substances. Figure 20 – 1 illustrates a generic GABA$_A$ receptor protein sequence and possible topological structure. The GABA receptor system is a hetero-oligomeric protein consisting of several distinct polypeptide types (α, β, γ, δ). Multiple different subunits are expressed in brain with different subtypes showing regional variations consistent with the pharmacological evidence of heterogeneity. The arrangement of some of the major allosteric relationships established experimentally follows:

- The receptor is associated with and modulates the transmembrane chloride ion channel that is gated by the primary ligand, GABA; the chloride channel can exist in an open and a closed configuration. The channel is composed of a number of protein subunits.

- The GABA site on this receptor complex is associated primarily with the β subunit, whereas the α subunit contains the binding site for benzodiazepines. The γ subunit appears to be required for the benzodiazepine receptor–mediated modulatory effects.
- The benzodiazepine binding site appears to be able to modulate allosterically the affinity and availability of GABA-binding sites in either direction; it may also modulate the coupling of the GABA receptor with the chloride channel.
- More than two types of GABA receptors are present in brain, based on structural and function diversity. The binding sites probably can exist in high- and low-affinity states. The receptor complex is ultimately connected to intracellular protein kinases and cyclic adenosine monophosphate (cAMP) sites.
- Kinetic and binding studies have led to the conclusion that each channel may have two or more benzodiazepine (BZ) binding sites, each of which can bind either an agonist or an antagonist. At one site, binding with benzodiazepine agonists results in a "depressant" effect (i.e., an augmentation of GABA binding and an increase in chloride conductance), whereas binding at the other, a "convulsant" or "inverse agonist" site, results in a decrease in chloride conductance. (This is one theory to explain the fact that similar substances with similar binding characteristics can actually have opposite effects.)
- Each channel receptor system also has related but molecularly different sites that bind barbiturates (agonist) and picrotoxin (antagonist and convulsant). Binding at such sites also modifies GABA effects on chloride permeability; in high concentrations binding at these sites directly affects the chloride channel.
- The presence of GABA enhances the affinity of agonists to benzodiazepine receptors; conversely, benzodiazepine agonists enhance GABA-receptor binding.
- Barbiturates, ethanol, and other agents can enhance agonist binding to the benzodiazepine receptor.
- Benzodiazepine antagonists, such as flumazenil, primarily bind to benzodiazepine receptors and have little effect on GABA-induced chloride fluxes.
- At least three subtypes of benzodiazepine receptors exist in brain; and the subtypes have different regional distribution in brain sites, with different distributions between GABA and benzodiazepine binding and between different benzodiazepines.

The concentrations of benzodiazepine receptors are modified by prior exposure and other influences such as stress.

The receptor concentrations may be increased — up-regulation — or decreased — down-regulation.

Benzodiazepine binding is regulated and influenced by a variety of factors. The binding itself is modified by the ionic composition of the test media, by the presence of GABA, by phenytoin, and by many influences, such as the prior occurrence of seizures or the administration of benzodiazepines. Chronic administration of a benzodiazepine results in a decrease in the benzodiazepine receptor concentration (down-regulation), one factor, but not the only factor, responsible for the development of tolerance. With discontinuation of chronic benzodiazepine administration, a rapid up-regulation of the benzodiazepine receptor concentrations occurs, consistent with the appearance of the withdrawal syndrome.

What is not known is how the binding to the GABA or the benzodiazepine receptors actually produces effects on other binding sites, that is, how the allosteric actions are created molecularly. The diagrams reflect only a relationship or association, not a mechanistic model. In fact, this is a minimal model and represents only a small sample of the total information available on benzodiazepine receptors. Also largely unknown are the functional connections between this model and the neural activities in the networks involved in anxiety and sleep disorders, as well as those responsible for tolerance and physical dependence.

The benzodiazepine receptors have many homologies with the nicotinic and adrenergic receptors. Like those, the benzodiazepine actions are ultimately linked with cyclic guanosine monophosphate (cGMP) systems as well as prostaglandin systems. Although benzodiazepine effects on chloride channels and GABA systems have been investigated extensively, their actions are not strictly limited to the chloride channels because they depress sodium and potassium conductances, at least in isolated nerve preparations; such actions could be related to their anticonvulsant properties.

TIME COURSE OF ACTION

Absorption

Oral. Although the benzodiazepines are orally effective, there are significant differences among them. Diazepam, flurazepam, and desmethyldiazepam (the active metabolite formed in the stomach after administration of the prodrug clorazepate) are among the most rapidly absorbed; on the other hand, oxazepam is one of the most slowly absorbed (Table 20–1).

Intramuscular. The intramuscular (IM) route should be avoided for diazepam and chlordiazepoxide because they are absorbed poorly and erratically after IM injection. Midazolam and lorazepam are marketed for both intravenous (IV) and IM use.

Avoid IM routes of injection for diazepam and chlordiazepoxide.

Intravenous. Most of the benzodiazepines are poorly soluble in water and are not available for IV use. The agents useful for this route are diazepam and midazolam, the two agents used for conscious sedation techniques (see

Table 20–1	BENZODIAZEPINES: DURATION OF ACTION AND POTENTIAL FOR ACCUMULATION AFTER ORAL ADMINISTRATION*		
Class/Agent	**Half-life (Range — hours)**	**Onset of Action (t 1/2 — minutes)**	**Rebound Insomnia/Anxiety**
Short-Acting			
Triazolam (Halcion)	1–5	Fast 2–30	++++
Medium Duration of Action			
Lorazepam (Ativan)	8–24	Intermediate 30–55	+
Oxazepam (Serax)	3–20	Slow 45–90	+
Temazepam (Restoril) (plus active metabolite, oxazepam)	6–20	Slow 45–90	+
Alprazolam (Xanax)	6–27	Fast-Intermediate 30–45	
(and metabolite oxazepam and desmethyldiazepam)	(20–200)		
Halazepam (Paxipam)	14 (median)	Intermediate 45	
Long Duration of Action			
Agents acting directly and as desmethyldiazepam			
(nordiazepam)	30–200	Fast 15–45	
Clorazepate (Tranxene)			
Clobazam			
Prazepam			
Halazepam			
Diazepam			
Chlordiazepoxide			
Quazepam (Doral) (directly plus active metabolites)	27–53	Fast 30	
	(~70–195)		
Flurazepam (Dalmane), plus its longer-lasting	1.5	Fast 15–45	
metabolite, desalkylflurazepam	30–200		

*Note that the range of values observed from samples of given population increases as the size of sample is expanded, i.e., the likelihood of having a patient possessing a very long or very short half-life increases as the number of patients observed increases (sample size). The ranges in this table were individual values from reported relatively small samples of patients, and in actual practice even larger and smaller individual values are to be expected.

Chapter 16). Intravenously administered diazepam may be painful and is followed occasionally by phlebitis, but this route is quite useful in management of seizures, for conscious sedation techniques, and during anesthesia.

Distribution

All the benzodiazepines in use are bound 50% or more to plasma proteins. Their distribution to tissues such as brain is correlated with lipid solubility; diazepam has not only a more rapid absorption from the intestine than chlordiazepoxide, it has a higher lipid solubility and a more rapid distribution to the CNS. There is selective localization first in gray matter, followed by white matter, including even the myelin of peripheral nerves. Diazepam accumulates in fat, as do its metabolites desmethyldiazepam and oxazepam.

Metabolism and Excretion

Benzodiazepines may be prodrug, active drug, active drug plus active metabolites, or active by virtue of active metabolites.

The benzodiazepines are metabolized eventually through N-dealkylation or hydroxylation by liver microsomal systems, followed by conjugation to form inactive glucuronides that are excreted in the urine (Fig. 20–2). The durations of *action* of the different compounds are functions of three interactive processes: (1) the appearance of acute and chronic functional tolerance; (2) the kinetics of the metabolism of all of the compounds (except oxazepam and lorazepam) to active metabolites with longer durations of action than the parent compounds; (3) the metabolism to the inactive metabolites.

Many of the metabolites of benzodiazepines have longer half-lives than that of the parent compound; therefore they accumulate to a greater extent.

Not only do the compounds differ in terms of both onset and duration of action but there is also a remarkable variability among patients in the rates of onset and duration of action. In addition, and possibly related to acute tolerance, there is a wide discrepancy between observed and perceived effects of these agents and the blood (and brain) levels. Taking

Figure 20–2

All these metabolites are eventually glucuronidated and excreted as glucuronides. Essentially all are biologically active; the α-hydroxy metabolites tend to have shorter half-lives than the parent compound. All compounds in bold type are on the market, and all are biologically active except clorazepate, which is a prodrug metabolized to the active desmethyldiazepam. Nordiazepam, nordazepam, and desmethyldiazepam are different names for the same compound.

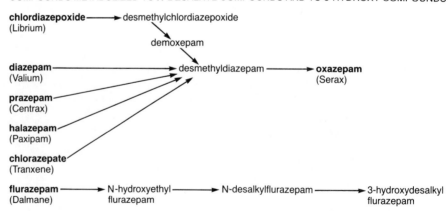

COMPOUNDS METABOLIZED TO N-DESALKYL COMPOUNDS AND TO 3-HYDROXY COMPOUNDS

COMPOUNDS METABOLIZED TO THEIR α-HYDROXY DERIVATIVES

triazolam
(Halcion)

alprazolam
(Xanax)

midazolam
(Versed)

diazepam as an example, its perceived effects are evident within a few minutes to half an hour after oral administration, and the effects appear to wane in 3–4 hours. In contrast, the peak blood level of diazepam does not occur until after 1–2 hours and the blood levels stay elevated for 6 or more hours, consistent with the pharmacokinetic half-life that ranges from *20 to 100 hours*. The usual regimen for diazepam administration is consistent with the observed effects calling for dosages every 4 hours, rather than with the blood levels and half-lives.

Not only is there marked individual variability in half-lives but also oral absorption may be quite unpredictable because of the influences of a large number of factors, including the presence of food, the type of food, and the presence of different beverages, including alcoholic. Although alcohol given alone slows diazepam metabolism, the effect of alcohol is seriously confounded by the presence of other beverage components as well as by food. Practically speaking, there are a variety of significant factors influencing oral absorption and most are actually beyond the control of the patient or prescriber, even if they were all known. In fact, the variability in time course among individuals generally tends to be even greater than the differences in the mean effects associated with such variables as gender, food, age, and weight.

As Figure 20–2 depicts, five of the benzodiazepines are metabolized to active metabolites, the desalkyl derivatives—desmethyldiazepam for chlordiazepoxide, diazepam, prazepam, and clorazepate. Desmethyldiazepam is metabolized to another potentially active metabolite, oxazepam. Except for clorazepate, which itself is inactive, all of the parent compounds are active and are the primary active species after a single dose. Corresponding desalkyl metabolites appear after flurazepam.

Because the desalkyl derivatives have half-lives ranging from approximately 30 to 200 hours in different individuals, they accumulate when given once a day or more often. It is a safe assumption that anyone receiving these compounds as often as once a day or more will be obtaining the effects of both the parent compound and any active metabolites. Moreover, the degree of accumulation obviously varies widely from individual to individual. The ranges of half-lives given in Table 20–1 are those reported in relatively small numbers of individuals taking part in rather well-controlled clinical trials. In the real world the individual differences are undoubtedly much greater.

In any event, it is vitally important to recognize the potential for extremely long durations of action of compounds whose effects appear to be relatively brief—3–4 hours. The presence of these compounds could be readily determined if blood level determinations became routine; however, in most present day practices the physician and patient must remain in the dark regarding accumulation of both the parent and the metabolite. (The long half-life of flurazepam and its metabolite is consistent with the fact that sleep duration was increased over control levels after a single bedtime dose, not only on the night it was taken but on the following night as well.)

Table 20–1 presents the major pharmacokinetic parameters for the available benzodiazepines. The compounds can be divided into three classes based on duration of action and their potential for producing rebound anxiety/insomnia. Except for the single shortest-acting substance, triazolam, all have long half-lives, from hours to up to a week.

Although all are effective upon oral administration, some are much more rapidly absorbed and have much more rapid onsets of action than others. The values for onset times are approximate and are given to illustrate the relative differences among the agents. There are appreciable individual differences in observed rates of onset.

Note the very long half-lives of most of the benzodiazepines.

Individuals differ markedly with respect to the duration of action of a given benzodiazepine.

Even more marked than the variability in onset of action is the variability in duration of action among individuals. For example, after administration of diazepam the peak plasma levels occur 1–4 hours after ingestion, and duration half-life for most people is *more than 1 day* for the parent compound and *up to 1 week* for the active metabolite desmethyldiazepam (referred to as either nordiazepam or desmethyldiazepam). But the mean durations cannot be used to define the dose and frequency regimen in the usual clinical setting, because for one person the half-life of the drug and metabolite may be approximately 1 day, whereas for another patient it may be 1 week. Thus, the amount of accumulation with repeated dosing is vastly different among individuals.

TOXIC EFFECTS

Acute

The major toxic effects are the predictable dose-related drug actions.

The major and most frequent adverse effects are the dose-related extensions of the anticipated actions of the agents, i.e., excessive depression of CNS functions. Prominent among these at relatively low doses are drowsiness, sleep, mental confusion and slow mentation, disorientation, ataxia, slurred speech, nystagmus, mild to marked amnesia (commonly not fully appreciated by the patient), and the production or aggravation of symptoms of dementia. In some individuals the benzodiazepines cause aggressive behavior, hyperactivity, delirium, and sometimes insomnia or serious depression. Larger than recommended therapeutic doses, or therapeutic doses in the presence of alcohol or other depressants can result in respiratory depression, coma, hallucinations, nightmares, confusion, delirium, amnesia, disorientation, and depression; all of these acute toxic effects may be more severe in the older patient.

Some individuals may exhibit apparently "paradoxical" hyperactivity, delirium, or hallucinations.

Therapeutic or greater doses of benzodiazepines can impair driving ability, the ability to stay awake, as well as the ability to assess one's own level of functional impairment. In these respects the benzodiazepines are driving hazards and especially so in anyone who also consumes any amount of an alcoholic beverage. These interactions and effects on driving can occur for up to 1 day following a single dose, a duration of action consistent with the long half-life of many of these agents.

When used to promote sleep, the shorter-acting agents, such as triazolam, oxazepam, and temazepam, may cause early morning awakening or rebound as well as *rebound insomnia* the following night.

The elderly are particularly susceptible to the amnesia or dementing effects of benzodiazepines.

Benzodiazepines are frequently involved in deliberate overdoses, usually associated with other CNS depressants such as alcohol. Although the margin of safety of benzodiazepines alone is large, and larger than alcohol or barbiturates, overdoses can result in serious respiratory depression. Death after overdoses is commonly the result of the combined effects of these agents plus alcohol and other compounds.

Rebound insomnia or anxiety may be a stimulus to habitual drug taking.

If detected and treated with cardiorespiratory support the outcome of poisoning by a benzodiazepine is rarely fatal. If unattended the respiration may be compromised, and aspiration of regurgitated stomach contents is a serious risk.

Allergic hypersensitivity reactions might be expected; however, there have been few reports of either skin rashes or major hypersensitivity reactions.

Local reactions, such as pain at the site of the injection, have been experienced after injection of the IV preparation of diazepam and after IM injections of lorazepam.

Toxicity with Chronic Use

The chronic use of these agents presents a number of potential toxic effects; most of these are predictable extensions of their acute actions. Noteworthy among these are the impairment of cognitive intellectual functions of thinking and memory. It is frequently not appreciated by the physician or caretaker that such symptoms in a patient may actually be manifestations of drug effects. Such dementing effects of benzodiazepines can actually impair the learning and adaptive process of ongoing psychotherapy, and in older patients these dementing actions may cause or aggravate the signs and symptoms of organic mental syndromes. The benzodiazepines are among that large list of potentially dementing agents that includes prominently the anticholinergics of all types as well as digitalis glycosides (see Chapter 27).

In addition, chronic benzodiazepine medication can result in undesirable weight gain or, in some, a weight loss (see Chapter 64).

It is possible, although presently disputed, that benzodiazepines produce birth defects; in any event they should be avoided unless absolutely necessary in all patients who are or who may become pregnant.

COMPLIANCE

Many patients will take the benzodiazepines as prescribed; the usual problems with compliance are the same as those with any other medication. Many of those who are noncompliant do not take the medication because they experience unpleasant subjective effects of slowed mentation, mental clouding, or sleepiness. In addition, many patients admit that they have discontinued taking the medication or take it as prescribed only to relieve acute effects "when I need it." At the other end of the spectrum are patients who are noncompliant because they take more than prescribed at a time, at shorter intervals, or take it along with other drugs or alcohol. Accurate data on the frequencies of these different patterns of compliance are hard to come by and subject to appreciable dispute among practitioners and investigators; nevertheless, it can be conservatively estimated that the majority are usually compliant, or discontinue the medication, whereas some 5–10% may escalate the dose occasionally or habitually.

Most patients are compliant—some do not take and some take excessive amounts.

Some individuals perceive and express a liking for the subjective effects of certain of the benzodiazepines. Although all of them have been accused of producing a sense of well-being or euphoria, this has actually been reported and studied for only a few agents. Diazepam has been most studied in this regard. In contrast, the administration of chlordiazepoxide rarely results in directly perceived subjective effects; the difference between these two compounds could well be due to the much slower rate of onset of effects of chlordiazepoxide as compared with diazepam. Although some individuals express a liking for the effects of diazepam and will take it when available, the majority of those receiving the agent do not like it. Moreover, most alcoholic and sedative drug abusers do not prefer benzodiazepines when other psychoactive substances, such as alcohol, barbiturates, or opioids, are available; but they do take them, usually in combinations, when the other agents are not available.

DRUG INTERACTIONS

As already discussed the administration of benzodiazepines is at least additive, and is usually synergistic, with other psychotropic agents. These potentially dangerous interactions can have either pharmacodynamic or pharmacokinetic origins. For example, the ingestion of alcohol along with a

Benzodiazepines are additive or synergistic with other CNS depressants including ethanol.

There are many potential interactions between benzodiazepines and other drugs.

Check an up-to-date reference for reactions for each patient.

benzodiazepine results in an acute pharmacodynamic addition or potentiation of the central effects of the two agents, plus an increase in the plasma levels of diazepam.

Other documented interactions include increased blood levels of imipramine and desipramine in patients receiving alprazolam as well as imipramine. Erythromycin administration may result in elevated blood levels of triazolam. Cimetidine coadministered with diazepam has resulted in increased half-life of both diazepam and its desmethyl derivative. These potentially important, but rather unpredictable, interactions emphasize the need to consult current, up-to-date compilations of drug interaction reports prior to prescribing any drug, especially psychoactive drugs.

TOLERANCE

Acute and chronic acquired tolerance develops to the benzodiazepines, and there is some cross tolerance among the benzodiazepines (agonists). The fact that the cross-tolerance to the acute effects, between benzodiazepines and alcohol or barbiturates, is only partial and limited in extent probably reflects the differences in the basic mechanisms of action of these different drugs.

That acute and chronic tolerance develops to the sedating, CNS-depressant actions of benzodiazepines there is no doubt. Even single hypnotic doses of flurazepam given once a day result on the initial night in marked increase in sleep time; with continued daily administration, the sleep duration gradually returns toward the baseline level, as illustrated in Figure 20-3.

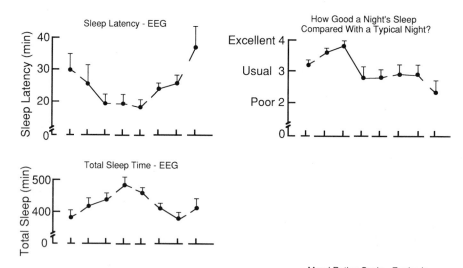

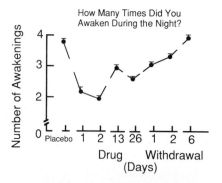

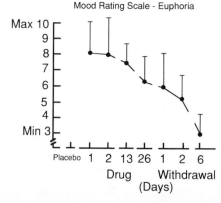

Figure 20-3

Sleep duration after nightly administration of flurazepam. Note on the first and second nights of flurazepam the decreased sleep latency, increased sleep time, decreased awakening, and better sleep. On the twenty-sixth night, total sleep time has decreased, awakenings have returned, and quality of sleep has declined. Rebound of symptoms upon withdrawal does not occur until the sixth day after flurazepam discontinuation. (Redrawn from Mendelson WB: Human Sleep—Research and Clinical Care. New York: Plenum Medical Book Co, 1987.)

Whether and to what possible degree tolerance develops to the therapeutic antianxiety, muscle relaxant, or antiseizure effects is less well established. The evidence suggests that tolerance does develop at least to the muscle relaxant and antianxiety effects, but this tolerance is relatively slow in onset and perhaps less apparent than the tolerance to the daytime drowsiness and sedation.

The mechanisms involved in the chronic acquired tolerance to the benzodiazepines include acute and chronic behavioral (functional) tolerance, down-regulation of benzodiazepine receptors, and metabolic tolerance. Tolerance appears to develop not only to the parent drug, but to the active metabolites as well. Although tolerance most likely develops with chronic administration of any of the benzodiazepines, it has not been studied definitively except with few compounds, i.e., diazepam and the agents used for insomnia.

PHYSICAL DEPENDENCE

Discontinuation of the administration of any of the benzodiazepines after regular administration for weeks or more can result in a withdrawal syndrome. The signs and symptoms of the withdrawal syndromes with the various benzodiazepines have not been studied experimentally in human beings; however, clinical case reports suggest that they are similar, but not identical, to those after chronic barbiturate or alcohol consumption. One difference apparent with diazepam withdrawal is the long latency of 5 or more days before symptoms appear. The nature and magnitude of the withdrawal illness are graded and appear to relate, at least in part, to the levels of both the parent and metabolite compounds and the duration of exposure to given levels of these (see Chapter 67). It is probable, but has yet to be firmly established, that not only the quantitative but the qualitative character of the withdrawal syndromes will be unique to the specific benzodiazepines, and especially to their psychoactive metabolites that accumulate with chronic administration of these drugs. The dependence follows pharmacological principles in that the withdrawal syndrome follows unique patterns, can vary from mild to severe, and can be precipitated by specific antagonists (such as flumazenil) as well as relieved by drugs with similar actions.

The possible dependence-producing capability of benzodiazepines has been the subject of appreciable controversy. Much of this has arisen because of the absence of explicit studies in patients and human subjects, plus the fact that the drugs are used to alleviate anxiety or insomnia while the primary withdrawal symptoms are the identical symptoms—anxiety and sleep disturbances. Thus, the potential for the appearance of withdrawal symptoms exists whenever a benzodiazepine is being discontinued or dosage reduced. Accordingly, whenever these agents are being reduced or discontinued the dosage should be tapered over weeks and months; patient understanding and cooperation are essential. Even so, it may be difficult to differentiate between the appearance of withdrawal signs that will subside eventually and a rebound increase in symptoms due to a combination of withdrawal and symptom recurrence. Nevertheless, some studies clearly establish that a withdrawal syndrome is an almost inevitable consequence of abruptly stopping even modest therapeutic doses of a benzodiazepine. Moreover, even when using a gradual tapering of the dose over weeks, more than 30% of patients were unable to achieve a drug-free state (Rickels et al, 1990; Schweizer et al, 1990). The possibility remains that some benzodiazepines (or their metabolites) may be much more likely to produce physical dependence than others.

Tolerance and physical dependence occur with therapeutic doses of benzodiazepines.

THERAPEUTIC USES AND IMPLICATIONS OF BENZODIAZEPINES

Treatment of Anxiety

Benzodiazepines may be useful for short-duration treatment of symptomatic anxiety.

The symptom of anxiety warrants treatment only when it is concluded that the patient's well-being is being threatened by anxiety and that its relief will result, in both the short and the long term, in significant improvement in the patient's ability to function. In general, only short-lasting treatment of days to a few weeks, at most, can be justified. Although temporary relief of anxiety can usually be readily obtained with benzodiazepines, sustained relief in chronic anxiety disorders is unlikely; long-term chronic administration is associated with a number of undesirable consequences. It is recommended that prescriptions for the antianxiety effects of benzodiazepines be limited to less than 1 month's supply. In the event that longer periods of use are warranted, this routine limitation will serve as an alert regarding the probable need for further diagnostic or therapeutic interventions. For example, phobic syndromes, panic, and generalized anxiety syndromes are not likely to benefit from chronic benzodiazepine administration. For some patients a trial of antidepressants, or of alprazolam, may prove to be more effective.

In the event that the anxiety appears severe and treatment is indicated, what agent would be the best choice? At present, it is suggested that flurazepam or chlordiazepoxide given once a day at bedtime might be a rational choice. This initial regimen is suggested because of the role of sleep disturbances in aggravating anxiety as well as the need to minimize self-medication and avoid overdosage.

The other agents used to treat anxiety include diazepam, alprazolam, oxazepam, lorazepam, prazepam, and chlorazepate (see Table 20–4).

Treatment of Panic Attacks and Agoraphobia

Separately identified anxiety syndromes of panic and agoraphobia are frequently treated with benzodiazepines. But the responsiveness to other agents suggests that, at least in terms of therapy, panic syndromes have a different neurochemical basis than generalized anxiety disorder. Among the drugs that have been found to be effective in some patients are imipramine, phenelzine, alprazolam, and clonazepam. In contrast, carbamazepine is not associated with a reduction of panic attacks. In the presence of obsessive-compulsive features clomipramine and fluoxetine may be more effective.

Caffeine can produce or exacerbate anxiety disorders.

Similarly to anxiety disorders, panic can be caused or aggravated by caffeine, even in rather small amounts. As with some individuals with insomnia, patients may not make the connection between their caffeine intake and their symptoms. Because the symptoms of anxiety and panic are so commonly aggravated by caffeine and other drugs, a critical initial approach to therapy is a detailed dietary evaluation and documentation of all medications, including all sources of caffeine as well as alcohol.

Relief of Symptoms of Alcohol Withdrawal

Benzodiazepines effectively reduce the acute ethanol withdrawal syndrome.

The benzodiazepines are mainstays in the management of withdrawal symptoms appearing with the discontinuation of alcohol consumption. Dosages and frequency of administration are based on the amounts required; these are usually titrated so that only minor tremulousness is present. Chlordiazepoxide and diazepam have been used more extensively for this purpose than the others, but reports of the effectiveness of oxazepam, alprazolam, chlorazepate, and lorazepam have appeared. None seems to have any particular advantages. Oxazepam might seem to be a preferred choice on the theoretical grounds that it acts directly, has no active metabolites, and is absorbed relatively slowly on oral administration (see Chapters 19 and 67).

Insomnia

All the benzodiazepines are potentially effective in promoting sleep when taken at bedtime to either facilitate falling asleep or sustain sleep throughout the night. Agents particularly advanced for the short-term treatment of insomnia are temazepam, triazolam, quazepam, and flurazepam. The sleep-promoting effects are most evident when sleep is disturbed because of acute anxiety, an observation consistent with their well-established actions. In contrast, although they are commonly ordered for acutely hospitalized patients, they are relatively ineffective in maintaining sleep that is being disturbed by external stimuli such as the lights and noise typical of a busy hospital.

Insomnia is a symptom, not a diagnosis.

When insomnia is caused by anxiety, benzodiazepines are effective for short-duration relief.

The use of any hypnotic requires assessing the nature of the sleep disorder (e.g., is it really due to anxiety in the face of caffeine consumption?) and matching the therapeutic objective with the time course and potential side effects of specific agents.

The major causes of insomnia, including drugs, are listed in Table 20–2. It should be clear that the use of a hypnotic such as a benzodiazepine is not warranted or appropriate in the face of caffeine- or drug-induced insomnia.

When patients complain of difficulty sleeping, a sleeping pill is frequently *not* indicated nor the treatment of choice.

For drugs to promote the onset of sleep in the face of time-limited anxiety, the benzodiazepines are the agents of choice. Diazepam or flurazepam at bedtime (as part of the ritual of getting ready and going to bed expecting to sleep, i.e., good sleep habits) can decrease sleep latency (time until sleep occurs), decrease awakenings during the night, and increase total sleep time. However, their long durations of action tend to produce some daytime sedation the next day (hypnotic "hangover") and to impair finer mental processes, especially in the elderly. Short-acting agents, typically triazolam (HALCION), have the same initial effects and few carry-over hangover effects the next day; however, their use can result in early morning awakening or rebound insomnia the next night.

In the event that the insomnia is due to depression, one of the most common causes of insomnia, the benzodiazepines are not likely to be effective and actually may aggravate the depression. In addition, insomnia is not common in younger age groups in the absence of disease, drugs, or alcohol, whereas it is common in older age groups. Yet, it is the older patients who are at high risk of experiencing the harmful effects of benzodiazepines.

The benzodiazepines are contraindicated in heavy alcohol drinkers and may serve to aggravate the sleep disturbances associated with acute or chronic heavy drinking.

Alternatives to benzodiazepines for the treatment of insomnia include a number of drugs that have a potential sleep-inducing property as a side effect (Table 20–3). Among the agents commonly prescribed for administration at bedtime to promote sleep is the antihistamine diphenhydramine and the more sedating antidepressants such as amitriptyline.

Over-the-counter sleep medication: diphenhydramine, an antihistamine.

Most of the currently available over-the-counter sleep aids utilize either diphenhydramine or another antihistamine, doxylamine. Although these antihistamines do produce drowsiness in many people, some individuals experience the opposite, CNS excitation and wakefulness. Each of the

Table 20–2 INSOMNIA: CAUSES AND TREATMENTS (N.B.: Differentiate transient versus chronic!)

Causes/Mechanism	Treatment
Psychophysiological (in absence of psychiatric disorder)	Relieve specific situation or condition such as environment, schedule, anxiety-inducing social factors.
Medical disorders	Diagnose and treat medical disorder such as pain, itch, bowel or bladder discomfort, cardiac failure.
Psychiatric	Endogenous depression—treat depression, follow sleep patterns, maximize hypnotic properties of antidepressant drugs.
	Depression and anxiety secondary to situation—improve sleep habits, sleep environment, exercise early in the day, counseling, antidepressants, and lastly, time-limited use of hypnotics: NO MORE than 1 week; do not increase dosage; do not provide extra medication; use with caution, if at all, in heavy snorers; follow patient after drug stopped; do not use hypnotics in elderly if at all possible but if so then 1/2 usual dosage, not every night, not chronically.
	Hypnotic drugs may be a major cause of dementia.

Drugs That Can Cause Insomnia*

This list serves as a reminder that sleep and sleep cycles involve all of the following neurotransmitter and receptor systems: serotonergic, cholinergic, endorphin, opioid, benzodiazepine, sleeping-promoting peptides, and others yet to be discovered.

Caffeine
Amphetamines
Diet pills
Theophylline
Methylphenidate
Alcohol !
Benzodiazepines/hypnotics !
ACTH
MAOI
Propranolol
Thyroid hormone
Cancer chemotherapeutic agents
Phenytoin
Alpha methyldopa
Oral contraceptives
Antihistamines—some in some people !
Digitalis glycosides

Alcohol or drug dependence/withdrawal !

*! Exclamation points follow those agents after which insomnia or sleep disturbances may appear to be paradoxical.

Table 20–3 DRUGS THAT MAY CAUSE DROWSINESS OR SLEEP

Antihistamines
Alcohol
Digitalis
Opiates
Anticholinergic agents (such as scopolamine)
Antidepressants (such as amitriptyline)
Phenothiazines
Centrally acting muscle relaxants
Anticonvulsants
Propranolol
Methysergide
Cyproheptadine

drugs listed in Table 20–3 might be conceivably prescribed, apart from other indications, yet administered to maximize the sleep-promoting property in patients with insomnia. Conversely, they might be prescribed to minimize daytime drowsiness.

Although not as universally effective as benzodiazepines, large doses (e.g., 5 gm) of L-tryptophan (the essential amino acid and precursor of serotonin) at bedtime do promote sleep. Tryptophan has been sold almost exclusively by health food stores and not as a medication. It has now been removed from the market after the connection between its consumption and *eosinophilia-myalgia syndrome* (EMS). Almost all of the more than 1321 cases of EMS reported as of February 1990 were associated with the use of supplemental L-tryptophan manufactured by five Japanese companies, and there is preliminary evidence that the syndrome is caused by a contaminant, but this has yet to be established and if so what the nature of the specific contaminant(s) responsible is (Division of Epidemiology, 1990; Centers for Disease Control, 1990).

Not only do many drugs increase or decrease sleep, some have been implicated in causing *somnambulism* (sleepwalking); these include phenothiazines, hypnotics, antidepressants, stimulants, antihistamines, and alcohol.

Anesthesia

Many of the benzodiazepines are used preoperatively; they are given frequently the night before or shortly before induction of anesthesia to relieve anxiety, cause sleepiness, and produce amnesia for the events occurring on the day of surgery. Their administration can be expected to also reduce the amount of general and local anesthetic required for a given operative procedure. (See Chapter 16 for further descriptions of diazepam and midazolam for conscious sedation.)

Benzodiazepines are used for conscious sedation techniques and for skeletal muscle relaxation.

Other Therapeutic Uses of Benzodiazepines

Lorazepam and midazolam are both rapidly acting agents that are now available for IM injection; their use is being promoted for the management of aggressive and violent patients, alone or in combination with antipsychotic agents. This use is relatively new and untested in terms of the relationship between efficacy and the intrinsic risks of excessive sedation, respiratory depression, confusion, and loss of memory.

Other therapeutic uses include diazepam as a muscle relaxant (see Chapter 25) and for the management of seizures (see Chapter 23). Alprazolam has a potential for use in depressive mood disorders, especially those associated with anxiety (see Chapter 22); it is demonstrably effective as an antidepressant, but not quite as effective in severe depression as the tricyclic antidepressants such as amitriptyline.

Dosage and Preparations

Approximate oral dosages for antianxiety or sleep promotion effects are given in Table 20–4. These should be reduced at least by half for elderly patients. In view of the large variability in individual responsiveness and half-life it is better to observe the effects of one or more small doses and then adjust dosage and frequency to match the individual patient's response.

Preparations for IV injection are now available for diazepam, midazolam, and lorazepam. Injection solutions must be prepared according to package directions and must be given into the vein; perivascular or intraarterial injections must be absolutely avoided, because these can result in severe pain, tissue damage, or outright necrosis. Parenteral administration of these agents should be carried out only in an anesthesia or recovery room setting where staff and equipment to maintain a patent airway and assistance of respiration are immediately available.

IM injection formulations of lorazepam and midazolam have been introduced. None of the other benzodiazepines are available in clinically useful formulations for IM use (e.g., diazepam is absorbed erratically after IM injection).

Benzodiazepine Antagonist(s) — Flumazenil

Benzodiazepine antagonists are under active investigation. The first agent likely to become clinically available is flumazenil. It effectively antagonizes the CNS effects of benzodiazepines, including the depression of respira-

Table 20–4 USUAL INITIAL ORAL DOSAGE FOR ANTIANXIETY OR HYPNOTIC EFFECTS*

Benzodiazepines	Dosage (mg)
Short Duration of Action	
Triazolam (Halcion)	0.5–1
Medium Duration of Action	
Lorazepam (Ativan)	1–2
Oxazepam (Serax)	15–30
Temazepam (Restoril)	10–30
Alprazolam (Xanax)	0.25–0.5
Long Duration of Action	
Chlordiazepoxide (Librium)	10–20
Diazepam (Valium)	2–5
Prazepam (Centrax)	10–20
Halazepam (Paxipam)	20–40
Clorazepate (Tranxene)	7.5–30
Flurazepam (Dalmane)	15–30
Quazepam (Doral)	7.5–15
Buspirone (BuSpar)	5–30

*Usually given at bedtime for hypnotic action or two or more times daily for antianxiety effects.

tion. It acts as a selective, competitive antagonist of benzodiazepines, and clinical reports of effective reversal of poisonings have included a number of benzodiazepines, including diazepam, lorazepam, midazolam, and temazepam. It has little, if any, ability to antagonize anesthetics or alcohol (although some reports of antagonism have appeared). It is likely to become a routinely available antidote for coma due in part or solely to a benzodiazepine. In addition, flumazenil will probably prove useful for diagnostic purposes in poisoning, in the management of cognitive disorders and in provocative diagnosis of panic disorder (Nutt et al, 1990).

Flumazenil can be administered intravenously. Its duration of action of 1–4 hours is relatively short, and thus the treatment of poisoning usually requires continuous monitoring of the patient's vital signs and the repeated administration of flumazenil. Although the short duration of action may lead to undermedication of benzodiazepine poisoning, the brief duration allows for ready adjustment of dose and frequency as well as its use for diagnosis of possible benzodiazepine accumulation or toxicity.

As might be expected, benzodiazepine antagonists, such as flumazenil, can precipitate an abstinence syndrome in individuals who have taken benzodiazepines chronically.

Flumazenil, the benzodiazepine antagonist, is likely to become a drug of choice in benzodiazepine overdoses, in the same way as naloxone is the antagonist for opioid overdose.

CONTRAINDICATIONS

Contraindications to the benzodiazepine antianxiety agents are discussed in general terms in the section on adverse effects and in the context of the therapeutic uses. Nevertheless, in view of the extensive prescribing of these agents the following list should serve for further cautions. Contraindications include the following:

- advanced age;
- pregnancy;
- alcohol or substance abuse or the potential for abuse (10–20% of the population and 50% of inpatients);
- depressive mood disorder (with possible exception of alprazolam);
- driving or operating dangerous machinery;
- the presence of other CNS depressants (except in inpatient anesthesia setting);
- narcolepsy (and narcolepsy can present with insomnia or disturbances of sleep);
- hypersensitivity to any benzodiazepine;
- caution is warranted in relation to drug interactions with cimetidine, erythromycin, or other CNS depressants;
- chronic use for longer than 1 week to 1 month, except for epilepsy. (There remains some dispute among clinicians regarding the effectiveness or benefit of long-term treatment in some patients with generalized anxiety disorder. But by routinely limiting the duration of the prescription the patient can be thoroughly re-evaluated at least during every month of continuous therapy.)

Buspirone

Buspirone (BUSPAR)

A variety of animal models of anxiety have been employed in intensive searches for new, safer, and more selective antianxiety agents. One of the results of this research is buspirone. Buspirone not only has a unique spectrum of action different from benzodiazepines and the older barbiturates, but both it and its congeners have also become effective therapeutic agents in certain classes of patients as well as useful tools for investigation of the neurochemical bases of anxiety syndromes.

PHARMACOLOGICAL ACTIONS

Buspirone relieves anxiety symptoms in humans and in many animal models of anxiety without producing significant sedation, drowsiness, or amnesia. CNS depression is not observed after buspirone even after dosages far in excess of those needed to relieve anxiety. Moreover, in its presence benzodiazepines or alcohol is no more depressant than in its absence; thus, there is neither antagonism nor synergism with other antianxiety or hypnotic agents.

Using scores reflecting all the possible anxiety symptoms, buspirone has been found to be as effective as diazepam in the treatment of generalized anxiety disorder, with either drug significantly better than the placebo controls. The subjective effects of buspirone are minimal in contrast to benzodiazepines in some people; sleepiness, mental slowing, or amnesia does not occur. Among the various anxiety symptoms, buspirone appears to be more effective against the psychological symptoms, such as worrying or difficulty in concentration, whereas diazepam seems to be better against muscle tension and insomnia. When patients currently receiving benzodiazepines are shifted to buspirone they have reportedly experienced a return of some of their anxiety symptoms. This finding, rather than just indicating lesser effectiveness of buspirone, may reflect the possibility that patients with a cluster of certain symptoms may do better on benzodiazepines and less well on buspirone, whereas others may be benefited more by buspirone.

The antianxiety efficacy of buspirone demonstrates the potential for effective new, more selective agents for the treatment of anxiety syndromes.

Adverse effects, and the effects that can be anticipated with dosage increases, have included dizziness, insomnia, nervousness, nausea, headache, myoclonic jerks, chest pain, tinnitus, and fatigue. Some of these side effects are the same as anxiety itself, and their appearance may pose a dilemma in deciding whether to increase or decrease buspirone doses. The package insert includes an extensive list of reported side effects, a few of which are serious but most are not. However, this is a relatively new agent and only greater experience will allow the definition of the actual risks and benefits.

MECHANISM(S) OF ACTION

Buspirone, unlike all previously studied antianxiety agents, does not affect the benzodiazepine/GABA/chloride channel receptor systems directly. Rather, it appears to act as an agonist in serotonin systems, specifically the serotonin-1A (or 5-HT 1A) class of receptors. Of all of the receptors to the various neurotransmitters, buspirone has its highest affinity with this serotonin receptor (the next greatest affinity was with a dopamine receptor). Serotonin receptors that bind buspirone have been localized at plausible brain sites in the limbic system, hippocampus, midbrain, thalamus, medulla-pons, striatum, hypothalamus, and cerebellum. Also, buspirone depresses the electrical activity of known serotonergic neurons in a manner consistent with a serotonin agonist. Detailed drug interaction and discrimination studies have also led to the conclusion that buspirone is a 5-HT 1A partial agonist.

Buspirone appears to act as a partial agonist at certain serotonin receptors.

TOXICITY

The dose-related and reported side effects are discussed earlier. The only treatment for gross overdose is symptomatic. The agent appears to enjoy a wide safety margin for acute effects.

Some allergic reactions have been reported, but the significance of these is not clear.

DRUG INTERACTIONS

There are no cross-reactions—additive or antagonistic with other CNS active agents including alcohol—although concomitant use of alcohol is obviously best avoided. When given together with haloperidol an increase in serum haloperidol levels was observed, but the clinical significance of this has not been established.

THERAPEUTIC USES

Buspirone is an effective antianxiety agent for the treatment of generalized anxiety disorders. In a direct comparison with benzodiazepines it appears to be, on average, just as effective over the short term; however, patient compliance with continued medication is poorer than with benzodiazepines. On the other hand, the benzodiazepines present the risks of physical dependence and withdrawal/rebound of symptoms upon discontinuation. Buspirone is *not* effective as a hypnotic to promote sleep induction, and it does not alleviate withdrawal symptoms in individuals who have recently had a benzodiazepine discontinued.

DOSAGE AND PREPARATIONS

Buspirone is available in 5- and 10-mg tablets that are usually given three times a day. In view of the unique sensitivity to some individuals it is important to start with low dosages initially.

Barbiturates

Most barbiturates are now obsolete and of historical interest only.

Barbiturates have been divided traditionally according to time course of action into long-acting, short-acting, and ultra–short-acting agents. This division is consistent also with their major therapeutic uses. Phenobarbital, a long-acting agent, has had a long history of use as a long-acting sedative and antianxiety agent, but these uses have been essentially completely supplanted by benzodiazepines and other drugs. Phenobarbital is now solely used in the treatment of epilepsy and is covered in Chapter 23.

At the other end of the spectrum are the ultra–short-acting agents, the thiobarbiturates that are used exclusively for anesthesia (discussed in Chapter 16).

The remaining short-acting barbiturates have been used therapeutically primarily as hypnotic agents. Two of the more widely prescribed were secobarbital (SECONAL) and pentobarbital (NEMBUTAL and others). These agents were effective in promoting or causing sleep. Although they and related compounds remain on the market, they have been supplanted by benzodiazepines. As used to promote sleep at bedtime the usually recommended doses of the barbiturates are effective and present by themselves little risk except sedative hangover, i.e., the drug effects persist into the next day with grogginess and difficulty in thinking and concentrating. (In children and some individuals the barbiturates have a paradoxical excitatory action.)

The acute and chronic margins of safety of barbiturates are low.

In larger doses the barbiturates produce a dose-related depression of CNS function ranging from mild sedation and mental clouding, to sleep, to coma, to coma with respiratory depression and eventually death. Their potential lethality is well demonstrated by the fact that until the last few years barbiturates were one of the most commonly employed drugs in completed suicides.

In addition, chronic consumption of doses two to four times the hypnotic dosage leads to tolerance and physical dependence; they were the agents used to establish the classification of dependence syndromes, especially the barbiturate-alcohol class. They exhibit cross-tolerance and cross-dependence with alcohol (see Chapter 67).

For occasional use for short periods of insomnia due to situational anxiety, the benzodiazepines are at least as effective in promoting useful sleep as the barbiturates and have a much greater safety margin.

The decline in use of the barbiturate hypnotics is mostly due to the availability of less toxic agents. However, the recent increase in knowledge about sleep physiology and pathology has led to distinctly different approaches to the treatment of insomnia; for example, it has been established that there are few, if any, indications for the regular chronic use of a hypnotic at bedtime to induce sleep.

Older pharmacology textbooks contain a wealth of interesting information on the barbiturates, most of which is therapeutically obsolete.

ADRENERGIC β BLOCKERS

Other agents known to modify anxiety are propranolol and other β blockers, which have been used to prevent performance anxiety or stage fright; they suppress both the peripheral autonomic and motor symptoms of anxiety and the feelings of anxiety.

ANTIDEPRESSANTS

The tricyclic antidepressants may be useful not only in the relief of insomnia but also as treatment of anxiety accompanied by depression or for panic attacks (see Chapter 22). The major limitations center on the delay in onset of effects and the possible cardiovascular effects of orthostatic hypotension or arrhythmias.

NEUROLEPTICS

Low doses of antipsychotic agents, such as haloperidol, have been used in treatment of anxiety, especially in the elderly. A major limitation in their use is the possible development of extrapyramidal syndromes or tardive dyskinesia.

MEPROBAMATE

Meprobamate (MILTOWN), which has many of the properties of the barbiturates, remains on the market but is largely of historical interest as one of the early tranquilizing drugs developed and introduced in the 1950s. It was promoted as different from phenobarbital or other barbiturates, that it produced alleviation of tension and anxiety, and that it was less hazardous than the barbiturates. However, these touted differences in therapeutic efficacy were never thoroughly established, yet the agent enjoyed extensive popularity. One reason for its good safety record was the fact that the recommended dosages that were usually prescribed were relatively small, and these produced few side effects (or drug-induced therapeutic effects either). This compound is described frequently as having skeletal muscle–relaxing effects, but there is no basis for such claims (see Chapter 25).

ANTIHISTAMINES

A common side effect of antihistamines (H_1 blocking agents) is sedation, drowsiness, and sleep. Among the most sedating of these substances is one

Miscellaneous Agents

A variety of drugs with different mechanisms of action may produce some therapeutically useful antianxiety effects.

of the first antihistamines discovered, diphenhydramine (BENADRYL and others) (see also Chapter 65). At the present time it is perhaps the most widely used medicine for sleep by prescription as well as over-the-counter. Depending on dose it increases sleep quality and duration (Kudo and Kurihara, 1990).

Hydroxyzine (VISTARIL, ATARAX, and others) is an antihistamine that has been used as an antianxiety agent. These agents have not been the subject of well-controlled clinical trials in comparison with benzodiazepines. The place of these antihistamines in the therapy of anxiety is uncertain.

References

Ankier SI, Goa KL: Quazepam: A preliminary review of its pharmacodynamic and pharmacokinetic properties and therapeutic efficacy in insomnia. Drugs 35:42–62, 1988.

Barnett A, Iorio LC, Billard W: Novel receptor specificity of selected benzodiazepines. Clin Neuropharmacol 8(Suppl 1):S8–S16, 1985.

Billard W, Crosby G, Iorio L, et al: Selective affinity of the benzodiazepines quazepam and 2-oxoquazepam for BZ1 binding site and demonstration of ^{3}H-2-oxoquazepam as a BZ1 selective radioligand. Life Sci 42:179–187, 1988.

Bloom FE: Neurotransmitters: Past, present, and future directions. FASEB J 2:32–41, 1988.

Busto U, Sellers EM, Naranjo CA, et al: Withdrawal reaction after long-term therapeutic use of benzodiazepines. N Engl J Med 315:854–859, 1986.

Centers for Disease Control: Analysis of L-tryptophan for etiology of eosinophilia-myalgia syndrome. MMWR 39:789–790, 1990. (Also printed in JAMA 264:2620, 1990).

Ciraulo DA, Sands BF, Shader RI: Critical review of liability for benzodiazepine abuse among alcoholics. Am J Psychiatry 145:1501–1506, 1988.

Division of Epidemiology, New York State Department of Health: Eosinophilia myalgia syndrome. NY State J Med 90:380–382, 1990.

Drugs for psychiatric disorders. Med Lett Drugs Ther 31:13–20, 1989.

Eison AS, Temple DL Jr: Buspirone: Review of its pharmacology and current perspectives on its mechanism of action. Am J Med 80(Suppl 3B):1–9, 1986.

Eldefrawi AT, Eldefrawi ME: Receptors for gamma-aminobutyric acid and voltage-dependent chloride channels as targets for drugs and toxicants. FASEB J 1:262–271, 1987.

Enna SJ, Mohler H: γ-aminobutyric acid (GABA) receptors and their association with benzodiazepine recognition sites. *In* Meltzer HY (ed): Psychopharmacology: The Third Generation of Progress, 265. New York: Raven Press, 1987.

Griffith JD, Jasinski DR, Casten GP, McKinney GR: Investigation of the abuse liability of buspirone in alcohol-dependent patients. Am J Med 80(Suppl 3B):30–35, 1986.

Haefely W, Martin JR, Schoch P: Novel anxiolytics that act as partial agonists at benzodiazepine receptors. Trends Pharmacol Sci 11:452–456, 1990.

Hindmarch I, Beaumont G, Brandon S, Leonard BE (eds): Benzodiazepines: Current Concepts. New York: John Wiley & Sons, 1990.

Jick H: Early pregnancy and benzodiazepines. J Clin Psychopharmacol 8:159–160, 1988.

Kenakin T: Agonists, partial agonists, antagonists, inverse agonists and agonist/antagonists? Trends Pharmacol Sci 8:423–425, 1987.

Kudo Y, Kurihara M: Clinical evaluation of diphenhydramine hydrochloride for the treatment of insomnia in psychiatric patients: A double-blind study. J Clin Pharmacol 30:1041–1048, 1990.

Lader MH: Rational use of anxiolytic drugs. Ration Drug Ther 21:1–5, 1987.

Lloyd KG, Morselli PL: Psychopharmacology of GABA-ergic drugs. *In* Meltzer HY (ed): Psychopharmacology: The Third Generation of Progress, 183. New York: Raven Press, 1987.

Mendelson WB: Human Sleep—Research and Clinical Care. New York: Plenum Medical Book Co, 1987.

Muller WE: The Benzodiazepine Receptor: Drug Acceptor Only or a Physiologically

Relevant Part of Our Central Nervous System? New York: Cambridge University Press, 1987.

Nicoll RA: The coupling of neurotransmitter receptors to ion channels in the brain. Science 241:545–551, 1988.

Nutt DJ, Glue P, Lawson C, Wilson S: Flumazenil provocation of panic attacks. Evidence for altered benzodiazepine receptor sensitivity in panic disorder. Arch Gen Psychiatry 47:917–925, 1990.

Olajide D, Lader M: A comparison of buspirone, diazepam, and placebo in patients with chronic anxiety states. J Clin Psychopharmacol 7:148–152, 1987.

Olsen RW, Tobin AJ: Molecular biology of GABA$_A$ receptors. FASEB J 4:1469–1480, 1990.

Rampe D, Triggle DJ: Benzodiazepines and calcium channel function. Trends Pharmacol Sci 7:461–464, 1986.

Rickels K, Schweizer E, Case G, Greenblatt DJ: Long-term therapeutic use of benzodiazepines. I. Effects of abrupt discontinuation. Arch Gen Psychiatry 47:899–907, 1990.

Roy-Byrne PP, Cowley DS, Greenblatt DJ, et al: Reduced benzodiazepine sensitivity in panic disorder. Arch Gen Psychiatry 47:534–538, 1990.

Schweizer E, Rickels K: Failure of buspirone to manage benzodiazepine withdrawal. Am J Psychiatry 143:1590–1592, 1986.

Schweizer E, Rickels K, Case G, Greenblatt DJ: Long-term therapeutic use of benzodiazepines. II. Effects of gradual taper. Arch Gen Psychiatry 47:908–915, 1990.

Sussman N: Treatment of anxiety with buspirone. Psychiatr Ann 17:114–120, 1987.

Uhlenhuth EH, DeWit H, Balter MB, et al: Risks and benefits of long-term benzodiazepine use. J Clin Psychopharmacol 8:161–167, 1988.

Yocca FD: Neurochemistry and neurophysiology of buspirone and gepirone: Interactions at presynaptic and postsynaptic 5-HT$_{1A}$ receptors. J Clin Psychopharmacol 10:6S–12S, 1990.

21

Antipsychotic Drugs (Neuroleptics)

Jerrold C. Winter

Chlorpromazine revolutionized the practice of psychiatry.

The introduction in the mid-1950s of chlorpromazine can truly be said to have revolutionized the practice of psychiatry. Prior to that time no regularly efficacious treatment was available for the most common psychotic disorders. Discovery of the neuroleptics made possible the release to their homes and to their communities of many thousands of patients who previously faced the prospect of lifetime institutionalization.

Unfortunately, the early hope that psychotic patients would be cured by antipsychotic drugs has not been realized; amelioration of the signs and symptoms of the disorders better characterizes the usual course of drug therapy. In addition, despite the dozens of neuroleptics marketed since chlorpromazine, none represents a quantum advance beyond that prototypical agent.

There is a tendency among students of medicine to regard psychotherapeutic drugs in general, and neuroleptics in particular, as the province of psychiatry. In fact, surveys have indicated that two thirds of all prescriptions for antidepressants and neuroleptics are written by physicians other than psychiatrists. Even those physicians who do not themselves prescribe neuroleptics will certainly encounter patients who are maintained on these drugs. It is therefore essential that all physicians have a working general knowledge of the indications, adverse effects, and drug interactions of the neuroleptics.

Indications for Use

Psychosis is the condition most often treated with neuroleptics. Although psychosis has been variously defined, the essential feature is partial or complete separation from reality. The origins of psychosis are multiple and may include factors that are not amenable to treatment with neuroleptics. For example, a number of drugs of abuse may produce acute departure from reality that may be aggravated by the use of antipsychotic drugs. Therefore, careful medical evaluation is essential prior to the initiation of neuroleptic therapy.

The most common forms of psychosis for which neuroleptics are indicated are the schizophrenic disorders. These are characterized by chronicity, impaired function, and disturbances of thinking and affect. The American Psychiatric Association's Diagnostic and Statistical Manual of Mental Disorders third edition, Revised (DSM-III-R), provides the following specific criteria for the use of neuroleptics: (1) one or more psychotic symptoms such as delusions, hallucinations, illogical thinking, or disorganized behavior; (2) deterioration from a previous level of functioning; (3) continuous signs of the illness for at least 6 months; (4) a tendency toward onset before age 45; (5) symptoms not due to affective disorders; and (6) symptoms not due to organic mental disorder or mental retardation.

Although psychosis is the primary indication for the use of neuroleptics, they are widely prescribed as well for a variety of aberrant behaviors of nonspecific origin including aggression, hostility, and self-destructive behavior. These drugs play a significant, albeit ill-defined and sometimes controversial, role in the treatment of disturbed children. Delusions and hallucinations in the demented elderly are often treated with neuroleptics, as are the manic and delusional symptoms of manic-depressive psychosis. In a nonbehavioral application, the antiemetic properties of certain of the neuroleptics are made use of to reduce nausea and vomiting associated with cancer chemotherapy. This and other minor uses of the neuroleptics are not discussed in this chapter.

Psychosis is the primary indication for the use of neuroleptics.

History and Nomenclature

Phenothiazine is a tricyclic chemical long known to have anthelmintic properties. In 1950, chlorpromazine, a simple derivative of phenothiazine, was synthesized by Paul Charpentier and his colleagues at the Rhone-Poulenc Laboratories in France (see the structures later in this chapter). Chlorpromazine was initially examined by the French surgeon Henri Laborit as a part of his studies of the role of histamine in surgical shock. Noting that the drug produced a state of calmness and indifference ("ataraxia"), Laborit suggested possible uses in psychiatry. Confirmation of that suggestion was provided by Jean Delay and Pierre Deniker in Paris in 1952. Thirty-eight psychotic patients treated with chlorpromazine by Delay and Deniker became less aggressive and agitated and suffered fewer delusions and hallucinations.

Reserpine, a drug derived from the Indian shrub *Rauwolfia serpentina*, is best known to today's students of medicine as an antihypertensive agent. However, there is also reason to regard it as the first antipsychotic drug. As a part of traditional Indian medicine, rauwolfia was used for a variety of conditions including insanity. Although reserpine's effects in mental disturbances were reported by Indian psychiatrists as early as 1931, it was work by the American psychiatrist Nathan Kline that brought reserpine to worldwide attention. Because of a range of adverse effects, including disturbances of the extrapyramidal motor system (EPMS), and questions as to its efficacy, reserpine was quickly eclipsed for psychiatric use by the phenothiazines. Among reserpine's legacies is the word *tranquilizer*, coined by F.F. Yonkman to characterize its pharmacological effects in animals.

The neuroleptic properties of reserpine

In this chapter, the terms *antipsychotic agent* and *neuroleptic* are used interchangeably. The former has the advantage of simplicity and obvious meaning, whereas the latter has the virtue of brevity. Some continue to use the word *ataractic*, but there is little to recommend it. Least desirable of all is reference to neuroleptics as tranquilizers. Distinction between major tranquilizers, the neuroleptics, and the so-called minor tranquilizers, the anxiolytics, does not help. Phenothiazines and other neuroleptics are pharmacologically and therapeutically distinct from anxiolytics such as the benzodiazepines (see Chapter 20). The implication of a continuum of therapeutic or pharmacological activity by use of a common term, *tranquilizer*, contributes to patient misunderstanding as well as to the possibility of inappropriate prescribing by physicians.

The word *tranquilizer* is too indefinite in meaning to be useful.

Efficacy

Each of the drugs illustrated is of proven efficacy in the treatment of psychosis. However, as noted earlier, none can be considered curative. In most patients, there is rapid improvement in the most florid signs of psy-

In general, antipsychotic drugs do not cure psychosis.

chosis followed by a plateau. Whatever the degree of improvement that is maintained, there seldom is doubt as to the continued presence of the disease. This is indicated either by residual impairment of function during neuroleptic treatment or by relapse upon discontinuation of treatment.

Potency

Neuroleptics available at present have similar efficacies but differ widely in potency.

As was discussed in Chapter 2, potency is defined as the quantity of a drug, usually expressed as milligrams per patient or milligrams per kilogram, required to produce a given therapeutic effect. With respect to the neuroleptics illustrated, there is a wide range of acceptable doses for any given drug and an even wider range between drugs. For example, when haloperidol was first introduced for use, dosages of a fraction of a milligram per day

Class: phenothiazine

	R_1	R_2
Subclass: aliphatic		
chlorpromazine (Thorazine)	$-(CH_2)_3-N(CH_3)_2$	$-Cl$
Subclass: piperidine		
thioridazine (Mellaril)	$-(CH_2)_2-$ [piperidine ring, N–CH₃]	$-SCH_3$
mesoridazine (Serentil)	$-(CH_2)_2-$ [piperidine ring, N–CH₃]	$-SCH_3$ with $=O$
Subclass: piperazine		
fluphenazine (Permitil, Prolixin)	$-(CH_2)_3-N$ [piperazine] $N-(CH_2)_2-OH$	$-CF_3$
perphenazine (Trilafon)	$-(CH_2)_3-N$ [piperazine] $N-(CH_2)_2-OH$	$-Cl$
trifluoperazine (Stelazine)	$-(CH_2)_3-N$ [piperazine] $N-CH_3$	$-CF_3$
prochlorperazine (Compazine)	$-(CH_2)_3-N$ [piperazine] $N-CH_3$	$-Cl$

Class: butyrophenone

haloperidol
(Haldol)

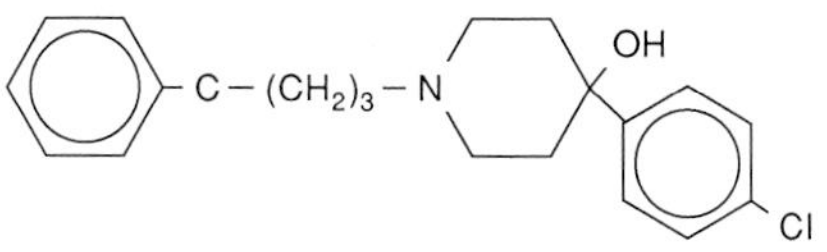

Class: dibenoxazepine

loxapine
(Loxitane)

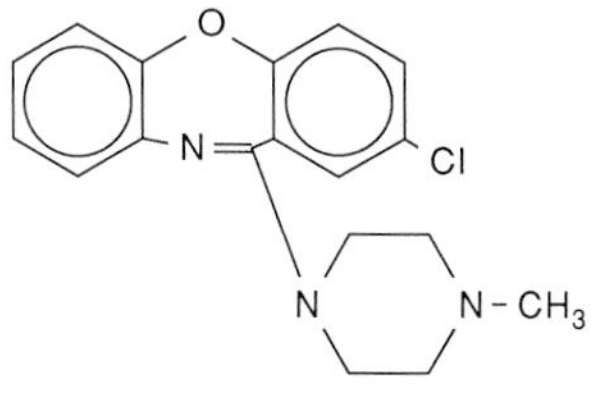

Class: dihydroindolone

molidone
(Moban)

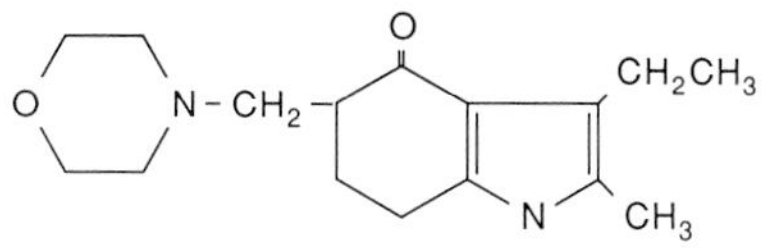

Class: thioxanthene

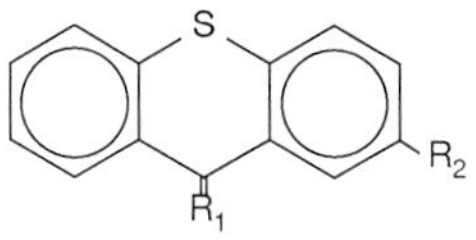

	R₁	R₂

chlorprothixene
(Taractan)

$$\overset{\parallel}{CH} - (CH_3)_2 - N(CH_3)_2$$

$- Cl$

thiothixene
(Navane)

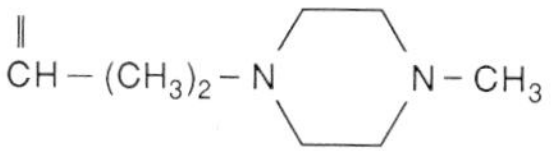

$$\overset{\parallel}{CH} - (CH_3)_2 - NN - CH_3$$

$$-SO_2 \\ \overset{|}{N(CH_3)_2}$$

were not uncommon, whereas patients have sometimes been treated with as much as 2 g/day of chlorpromazine. A portion of this high degree of variation both within and between neuroleptics is no doubt due to characteristics inherent to each drug. In addition, however, this variability is a reflection of the fact that (1) antipsychotic drugs as a group have a high therapeutic index, at least with respect to lethal effects, (2) antipsychotic drugs rarely produce completely satisfactory therapeutic results, and (3) individual patients appear to differ widely in their sensitivity to these drugs.

As is true for other classes of drugs, neuroleptics are sometimes classified on the basis of their relative potencies. For example, within the phenothiazine family of antipsychotics, the typical dose of a piperazine-type drug such as trifluoperazine is significantly less than that of chlorpromazine, an aliphatic, or of thioridazine, a piperidine. Thus, trifluoperazine is a *high-potency phenothiazine*. Although it is true that certain adverse effects are correlated with potency, the pattern of correlation is not consistent; trifluoperazine is, for example, less likely to produce sedation than is chlorpromazine but more likely to cause disturbances of the EPMS. Potency *per se* is for the phenothiazines, as for most other drugs, of little importance in the selection of the most appropriate therapeutic agent.

Mechanism of Action

The precise pharmacological mechanisms by which neuroleptics exert their beneficial effects are unknown. The explanation for this state of ignorance is simple: the etiology of the major psychotic disorders, including schizophrenia, is unknown. However, consideration of the pharmacological properties of the drugs may provide some clues.

The 12 neuroleptics available for use at present in the United States represent five distinct chemical classes. The largest group is the phenothiazines, currently represented by 7 drugs. There are two thioxanthenes, and each of the remaining three chemical classes has but a single representative. Despite their variety of chemical structures, the antipsychotic drugs share certain effects, particularly with respect to the neurotransmitter dopamine.

It was noted earlier that reserpine sometimes causes disturbances of the extrapyramidal motor system, a peculiar effect not previously produced by any pharmacological agent. However, similar effects soon were observed following treatment with chlorpromazine and, subsequently, with every other neuroleptic. A portion of the syndrome produced by neuroleptics closely resembles Parkinson's disease, a disorder caused by loss of dopaminergic neurons in the substantia nigra and their axonal projections to the striatum. It is now thought likely that neuroleptic-induced extrapyramidal disturbance is due to antagonism of striatal dopamine function.

Antagonism of dopamine by neuroleptics causes functional disturbance of the EPMS.

There is little reason to believe that activity in the EPMS is related to psychosis. However, with the discovery of other aspects of dopamine function, the notion that dopaminergic antagonism is responsible for the therapeutic effects of antipsychotics became more plausible. In particular, the rhinencephalon or limbic lobe was found to receive projections from dopaminergic neurons of the mesencephalon. The limbic system, composed of the limbic lobe and associated areas of the thalamus, epithalamus, and hypothalamus, has long been associated with emotional functions.

The dopamine hypothesis of schizophrenia

The dopamine hypothesis of schizophrenia states that hyperactivity in dopaminergic systems causes the signs and symptoms characteristic of the disease. Primary support for the hypothesis comes from the observation that all clinically effective antipsychotic drugs block one or another aspect of dopaminergic function. Further evidence is provided by the fact that chronic treatment with amphetamine, a drug believed to interact with dopaminergic systems, causes a syndrome that closely resembles paranoid schizophrenia.

Adverse Effects

The fact that there are no consistent, generally agreed upon differences in efficacy among the 12 neuroleptics illustrated in this chapter has led to major emphasis being placed upon their relative adverse effects. With reference to the whole spectrum of these possible effects, significant differences between individual agents do exist. Therapeutic advantage may sometimes be gained by taking these differences into consideration. For example, the elderly are particularly prone to orthostatic (postural) hypotension, dizziness, and life-threatening falls. In the elderly one may wish to choose a neuroleptic with minimal hypotensive activity even if the drug has a rather high incidence of another unwanted action. In the sections that follow, the adverse effects of neuroleptics are discussed first in general terms and then with respect to individual agents.

The antagonism of dopaminergic activity by neuroleptics has already been noted. In addition, there is clinically significant interaction of these drugs with a number of other chemical messengers. Of particular importance are functions mediated by acetylcholine and by norepinephrine. Although it is sometimes useful to group together those adverse effects that are related to one chemical transmitter or another, the present scheme of classification is according to organ system.

CENTRAL NERVOUS SYSTEM

Sedation

In general, neuroleptics depress activity in the central nervous system (CNS). The resulting drowsiness and sedation are sometimes useful in agitated and assaultive patients but more often are regarded as undesired properties. This is especially true during maintenance therapy. There appears to be no relationship between the degree of sedation produced and the actual antipsychotic effects. Although multiple mechanisms are probably involved, activity of neuroleptics at histaminergic and cholinergic receptors in the CNS seems a likely factor.

Antipsychotic drugs differ significantly in their sedative properties.

Neuroleptics are unlike ethanol and the barbiturates in that their depressant effects are not accompanied by disinhibition of behavior akin to drunkenness. Nonetheless, driving and other psychomotor skills may be impaired. Although effects on respiration are usually modest, particular caution must be exercised in treatment of patients with respiratory infections or chronic respiratory disorders.

The depressant effects of antipsychotic drugs are at least additive with those of ethanol, barbiturates, opiates, and other depressants of CNS activity. Although it is difficult to prove that antipsychotic drugs truly potentiate the effects of these agents, it should be assumed to occur and appropriate adjustments in dosage should be made when neuroleptics are combined with such drugs.

Sedation is most often associated with chlorpromazine and the piperidine phenothiazines, but its occurrence should be anticipated with all the neuroleptics. Potentiation of the effects of depressant drugs is not peculiar to a particular class of antipsychotic drug.

Seizures

Neuroleptics decrease the convulsive threshold and may precipitate seizures in persons with pre-existing CNS pathology. This effect is best documented with respect to chlorpromazine but should be anticipated with all neuroleptics. Potentiation of the depressant effects of barbiturates does not extend to their anticonvulsant properties. For this reason, doses of barbiturates and other antiepileptic agents should not be reduced routinely on initiation of antipsychotic drug therapy. Furthermore, neuroleptics are contraindicated in the treatment of conditions such as ethanol and barbiturate withdrawal in which there is an increased probability of seizures.

Antipsychotic drugs may increase the probability of seizures.

Hypotension

The effects of antipsychotic drugs on blood pressure appear to result from a combination of depression of activity in medullary cardiovascular centers and blockade of peripheral adrenergic receptors. Changes in resting blood pressure usually are minimal, but significant postural (orthostatic) hypotension may occur. Dizziness and transient loss of consciousness may result. Particular caution must be exercised in the use of these drugs in the elderly and in those with pre-existing impairment of the cerebrovascular circulation.

Epinephrine reversal

In the periphery, neuroleptics appear to be selectively active at α-adrenergic receptors, and epinephrine reversal may occur. This is a phenomenon in which doses of epinephrine that usually produce pressor effects result in hypotension owing to unopposed stimulation of β-adrenergic receptors. The pressor agent of choice in neuroleptic-induced hypotension is levarterenol (norepinephrine). Although antipsychotic drugs in general have higher affinities for the α_1-adrenergic receptor compared with the α_2 subtype, antagonism of the antihypertensive effects of α_2 agonists such as clonidine has been reported.

The available clinical data do not permit precise comparison of neuroleptics with respect to their hypotensive properties. However, it generally is assumed that hypotension is less likely to occur following the use of piperazine-type phenothiazines and nonphenothiazine neuroleptics. The claim that molindone is without clinically significant hypotensive effects remains to be established. For any given agent, the risk of hypotension is increased by parenteral administration.

Temperature Regulation

An early use of chlorpromazine was to facilitate the lowering of body temperature prior to cardiac surgery. However, it is now recognized that neuroleptics are not specific hypothermic agents but instead serve to loosen in general the homeostatic mechanisms that normally maintain body temperature. Thus, patients maintained on neuroleptics may become hyperthermic when exposed to high environmental temperatures, and several deaths have been reported. Although disordered temperature regulation is thought to be mediated by neuroleptic blockade of muscarinic acetylcholine receptors in the hypothalamus, any tendency toward hyperthermia may be further enhanced by peripheral cholinergic blockade that results in decreased sweating.

Antiemetic Properties

Clinical advantage is sometimes taken of the antiemetic properties of neuroleptics.

Nausea and vomiting are profoundly influenced by dopamine-sensitive receptors of a medullary center called the *chemoreceptor trigger zone* (CRT). The antiemetic properties of neuroleptics are believed to arise from dopaminergic blockade in the CRT. Thus, neuroleptics, especially chlorpromazine and prochlorperazine, often are used to control nausea and emesis in a variety of disease states as well as that associated with cancer chemotherapeutic agents. However, the antiemetic effects of neuroleptics may obscure the diagnosis and treatment of conditions characterized by nausea and vomiting. These include intestinal obstruction, brain tumor, and Reye's syndrome as well as a variety of drug intoxications.

Extrapyramidal Motor System

Neuroleptics are believed to act as antagonists of dopaminergic components of the EPMS. The functional consequences of neuroleptic-induced disturbance of the EPMS may be divided into four distinct syndromes: dystonia, akathisia, parkinsonian syndrome, and tardive dyskinesia. The first three occur soon after initiation of neuroleptic therapy and usually are amenable to treatment. In contrast, tardive dyskinesia may first appear only after years of neuroleptic use and may then be irreversible.

Dystonia

These effects may appear shortly after initiation of neuroleptic therapy and are often referred to as *acute dystonic reactions.* Dystonias are particularly common following parenteral administration. Hypertonicity of the muscles of the neck and back may progress to torticollis and opisthotonos, respectively. Difficulty in swallowing and spasms of the muscles of the jaw, tongue, and eyes may occur.

Dystonia/akathisia/Parkinson-like syndrome(s)

At the first appearance of dystonia, administration of the neuroleptic should be stopped and the patient reassured as to the essentially benign nature of the condition. Especially severe cases may require the parenteral administration of an anticholinergic antiparkinsonian agent or diphenhydramine.

Akathisia

The literal meaning of this term is "without sitting." It refers particularly to motor restlessness and a desire on the part of the patient to be in constant motion. An anxiety-like subjective state may also be present. Because of the distinctly unpleasant nature of neuroleptic-induced akathisia in normal subjects, it is reasonable to conclude that this syndrome may contribute to noncompliance by some patients. Reduction of dosage may be of value.

Parkinsonian Syndrome (Pseudoparkinsonism)

As is implied by its name, this condition closely resembles idiopathic Parkinson's disease. It is characterized by an unchanging facial expression, drooling, tremors, disturbances in posture and gait, and rigidity, especially of the upper limbs. Akinesia, a state of decreased motor activity, is often a major sign of the parkinsonian syndrome. Anticholinergic antiparkinsonian drugs are of value in treating the neuroleptic-induced condition. In contrast with true Parkinson's disease, therapy with levodopa has been found to be ineffective and, in some instances, to worsen the syndrome.

It is generally assumed that among the phenothiazines, extrapyramidal disturbances are least likely following the piperidines and most likely with the piperazines; chlorpromazine and the thioxanthenes are intermediate. There is, however, a tradeoff in that the piperidines tend to be most troublesome in terms of anticholinergic effects and disturbances of cardiac rhythm. Among the nonphenothiazines, a full spectrum of tendencies to produce extrapyramidal disturbances is seen. Haloperidol is most likely to produce extrapyramidal disturbances; more limited experience suggests that loxapine is intermediate in frequency of these effects, whereas molindone is relatively inactive.

Anticholinergic properties may protect against dysfunction of the EPMS.

A drug that deserves special mention with respect to neuroleptic-induced extrapyramidal disturbances is clozapine. Clinical trials of the drug conducted in the early 1970s demonstrated antipsychotic efficacy and a very low incidence of EPMS disturbance. However, reports of agranulocytosis caused clozapine to be withheld from the U.S. market until 1989. The decision to approve the drug was based on evidence that clozapine may be effective in some schizophrenics resistant to other neuroleptics and on the provision of a surveillance program to detect agranulocytosis. Current estimates of incidence of clozapine-induced agranulocytosis range from

1.1 to 1.5%, with nearly all cases arising within the first 5 months of treatment.

Tardive Dyskinesia

As is implied by its name, tardive dyskinesia has a delayed onset, sometimes becoming apparent only after years of treatment. Among the more prominent signs of tardive dyskinesia are involuntary movements of the tongue, face, mouth, and jaw. However, essentially all aspects of EPMS dysfunction have now been recognized as possible tardive effects. Thus, tardive dystonia, parkinsonism, and akathisia have been reported.

Tardive dyskinesia may be irreversible.

Tardive dyskinesia differs in a number of respects from the EPMS disturbances that appear in the first several weeks to months of neuroleptic therapy. Most important is the apparent irreversibility of the condition. It responds poorly if at all to antiparkinsonian agents and may worsen rather than improve with discontinuation of neuroleptic treatment. Whereas the early-onset extrapyramidal disturbances are thought to be due to the direct effects of dopaminergic blockade in the striatum, tardive dyskinesia has many of the features of a supersensitivity phenomenon.

No consensus exists regarding treatment of tardive dyskinesia. The hypothesis that a low tendency to produce acute extrapyramidal disturbance is correlated with fewer tardive effects is unproved, and all neuroleptics are suspect. It is hoped that clozapine will prove to be an exception to this rule. Principles of prevention include the use of the lowest possible doses of antipsychotic drugs for the shortest periods of time consistent with a therapeutic effect. Regular assessment of the continued efficacy of neuroleptics is essential. At the first signs of tardive dyskinesia, neuroleptic therapy should, if possible, be stopped.

Neuroleptic Malignant Syndrome

Neuroleptic malignant syndrome

An unusual and sometimes fatal reaction to antipsychotic drugs that combines features of disordered temperature regulation and extrapyramidal reactions is called the *neuroleptic malignant syndrome* (NMS). Since the syndrome was first described in 1960, fewer than 200 cases have been reported in the world literature. Concern is not with numbers but with the fact that about 10% of patients with NMS die. The hallmarks of NMS are hyperthermia and rigidity, presumably of extrapyramidal origin. In addition, delirium and increased blood pressure often occur. The most common laboratory finding is an elevated level of creatine phosphokinase.

Treatment of NMS is uncertain but should include termination of all neuroleptics and use of general supportive measures including body cooling and rehydration as needed. A variety of drugs with activity on dopaminergic systems have been tried. Among those claimed to have some beneficial effects are bromocriptine, amantadine, levodopa, and the anticholinergic antiparkinsonian agents. However, no consensus has emerged as to the efficacy of these agents. Attempts to control rigidity have most often employed benzodiazepines or dantrolene. The latter drug has been found to be of value in treating malignant hyperthermia, a condition that shares several of the features of NMS. It is not possible to attribute NMS to any particular neuroleptic at this time.

CARDIOVASCULAR SYSTEM

Neuroleptic-induced tachycardia is mediated by a combination of reflex activity triggered by hypotension and a direct antimuscarinic effect on the myocardium. The clinical significance of these actions in healthy patients is uncertain. However, in those with coronary atherosclerosis, sustained tachycardia increases the probability of overt arrhythmias and myocardial infarct.

Of all the neuroleptics, the arrhythmogenic effects of thioridazine have been best documented. Even relatively modest doses may be associated with prolongation of the QT interval, decreased amplitude of the T wave, the appearance of U waves, and a widening of the QRS complex. Although it is generally assumed that neuroleptics as a group have a high therapeutic index, there is no doubt that overdose of thioridazine and possibly others can be fatal. In addition, it is suspected that sudden unexplained death in patients maintained on antipsychotic drugs may often be due to cardiac dysfunction.

Those physicians who prescribe neuroleptics must take into account possible untoward effects on the myocardium, especially by the piperidine phenothiazines and particularly in those patients with pre-existing coronary atherosclerosis or disturbances in cardiac rhythm. In addition, combination of antipsychotic drugs with sympathomimetics should be avoided. Outpatients maintained on neuroleptics should be cautioned against the concurrent use of amphetamines, cocaine, and nonprescription products such as cold remedies and aids to weight loss that contain sympathomimetic agents.

Antipsychotic drugs and sympathomimetic agents may interact adversely with respect to cardiac function.

ENDOCRINE SYSTEMS

Dopamine released by the hypothalamus passes through the hypothalamicoadenohypophyseal portal system to the pituitary where it functions to inhibit the release of prolactin. The antidopaminergic effects of neuroleptics thus account for the increase in serum prolactin that is consistently seen in patients treated with these drugs. Neuroleptic-induced hyperprolactinemia is sometimes associated with galactorrhea, menstrual changes, and gynecomastia. A theoretical hazard of elevated levels of prolactin is an increase in incidence of hormonally mediated cancers, especially cancer of the breast. However, several studies have failed to detect an increased incidence of breast cancer in patients maintained on phenothiazines.

Hyperprolactinemia

A number of other adverse effects of antipsychotic drugs may have an endocrine component. These include sexual dysfunction and undesired weight gain. Both have most often been associated with the piperidine phenothiazines. Chlorpromazine-induced fluid retention has been reported, and a number of neuroleptics cause an increase in appetite possibly through antihistaminergic or antiserotonergic effects.

MISCELLANEOUS ADVERSE EFFECTS

Peripheral Antimuscarinic Actions

The use of antipsychotic drugs is often associated with one or more signs of an atropine-like syndrome. Thus, blurred vision, exacerbation of narrow angle glaucoma, dry mouth, sinus tachycardia, constipation, urinary retention, and decreased sweating may occur.

Jaundice

Shortly after the introduction of chlorpromazine, liver dysfunction, usually in the form of cholestatic jaundice, was associated with its use. Because this is a relatively rare condition, the risk imposed by individual agents is not known with certainty. The condition usually is reversible on discontinuation of neuroleptic use. If treatment is to continue, an agent from another chemical class should be chosen. Periodic liver function tests are indicated in patients chronically treated with phenothiazines. Reversible changes in liver function tests are commonly observed with initiation of phenothiazines.

Hematological Disorders

Blood dyscrasias, including agranulocytosis, eosinophilia, leukopenia, hemolytic or aplastic anemia, thrombocytopenic purpura, and pancytopenia, are rare. However, because of the possibly fatal outcome of these disorders, patients and their families should be warned to report sore throat or other signs of infection.

Dermatological Effects

The skin is the site of several toxic effects of the neuroleptics. Earliest in onset and presumed to have an immunological basis is an urticarial reaction. With long-term treatment, unusual sensitivity to the sun and discoloration of the skin may occur. A possibly related condition is deposition of fine particulate matter in the lens and cornea of the eye. Ocular changes have most often been associated with long-term, high-dose therapy with thioridazine. Under these circumstances, regular examinations of the eye are indicated.

Tolerance and Physical Dependence

The abuse liability of neuroleptics is very low.

It is generally assumed that some measure of tolerance develops to the sedative and hypotensive effects of neuroleptics. Nonetheless, particular care must be exercised in the use of these drugs in the elderly. Physical dependence on antipsychotic drugs is seldom reported. However, a withdrawal syndrome including vomiting and movement disorders has been described. For this reason, gradual reduction in dosage following long-term treatment is prudent.

General References

Andreason NC, Flaum M, Swayze VW, et al: Positive and negative symptoms in schizophrenia. Arch Gen Psychiat 47:615–621, 1990.

Baldessarini RJ: Drugs and the treatment of psychiatric disorders. *In* Gilman AG, Rall TW, Nies AS, Taylor P (eds): Goodman and Gilman's The Pharmacological Basis of Therapeutics, New York: Pergamon Press, 1990.

Fleischhacker WW, Roth SD, Kane JM: The pharmacological treatment of neuroleptic-induced akathisia. J Clin Psychopharmacol 10:12–21, 1990.

Hollister LE, Czernansky JG: Clinical Pharmacology of Psychotherapeutic Drugs, 3rd ed. New York: Churchill Livingstone, 1990.

Jacobsen E: The early history of psychotherapeutic drugs. Psychopharmacology 89:138–144, 1986.

Roberts GW: Schizophrenia: The cellular biology of a functional psychosis. Trends Neurosci 13:207–211, 1990.

Rosenberg MR, Green M: Neuroleptic malignant syndrome. Arch Intern Med 149:1927–1931, 1989.

Antidepressants—Drugs Used in the Treatment of Mood Disorders

22

Jerome A. Roth

The major affective disorders of endogenous origin are characterized by changes in mood and behavioral states, and are generally classified into two categories, unipolar and bipolar (manic-depressive) depression. In actuality these are likely to be overly simplistic terms to describe the variety of behavioral and mood changes, but they do represent relevant clinical states that often require drug intervention. Disorders of mood can be debilitating if the magnitude of the disorder prevents one from living a normal daily existence. Under circumstances where the affective changes are severe enough to interfere significantly with an individual's interaction with society, then drug intervention may be recommended. Depression signs and symptoms occur also in response to adverse life events such as loss of a loved one, during physical illness, and as a side effect of certain drugs, including hormones and antihypertensive agents.

As with all major behavioral disorders, it is now assumed that the affective disorders of endogenous origin result from specific biochemical changes in the brain. However, it is unlikely that depression originates from only a single biochemical alteration in all patients. It is more likely that it is caused by any one of a number of neurological changes that have, as an end result, a similar alteration in behavioral state. Thus, depression is a heterogeneous disorder most likely brought about by a number of neurochemical changes in the central nervous system (CNS). Some of the theories that have been proposed for the cause of depression are presented in this chapter.

Major Unipolar Depression

Depression or melancholia is a rather common mood change that many individuals (~ 15% over a lifetime) have experienced in their lives. In most cases depression is an experience associated with some tragic or adverse life experience such as loss of a close friend or family member. This type of depression is referred to often as *reactive* depression, because it is associated with an onset produced by a specific event in one's life. Usually, this type of depression is of relatively short duration and usually is not severe enough to fully interfere with one's daily routine. The other type of depression, *endogenous* depression, is not a consequence of a specific disturbing event and appears to result spontaneously, presumably as the result of some biochemical changes in the nervous system. Although patients are assigned frequently to one of the two classes of depression, often these classifications are not useful terms in selecting alternative modes of treatment. With either class, drug intervention is warranted if (1) the intensity of the depression is severe enough to interfere with normal daily function; (2)

Unipolar depression:

1. Reactive
2. Endogenous

Factors indicating that drug intervention is required:

1. Intensity
2. Duration
3. Quality

Retarded vs. agitated unipolar depression

the duration of the depressive symptoms is in the order of weeks or months; and (3) the depression includes thoughts of suicide. Classical symptoms of depression include not only subjective mood changes but a variety of somatic and psychic changes—sleep disturbances such as insomnia, anorexia, the loss or the gain of weight, gastrointestinal (GI) disturbances, fatigue, loss of interest, feelings of guilt, diminished ability to think or concentrate, and withdrawal from interpersonal interactions and activities.

Unipolar depression can be subclassified further into two types, retarded and agitated depression, based on the nature of the behavior expressed. Retarded depression is characterized by psychomotor retardation; the subject reacts little with the environment whether it be in response to situations, people, or some other stimuli. In contrast, agitated depression is characterized by a lack of direction of the person's activity with an excess of undirected and unproductive activity such as hand-wringing, pacing, or shouting. Moreover, the intensity and the nature of expression of the depression may be different for each individual.

Depression is usually self-limited, and even if no drug is administered patients are likely to recover spontaneously. Another common feature of unipolar depression is that it is often cyclic; most individuals will experience more than one episode of depression with an episode lasting weeks or months or longer. What causes the onset of each episode is not known, but it is likely that the diurnal rhythms of hormones are involved in the etiology of this disorder. (For a small number of individuals, exposure to light is important; this has been designated Seasonal Affective Disorder [SAD].)

ETIOLOGY

Many theories have expounded upon the cause of depression; each of these has some merit as well as some limitations. Unipolar depression is probably a heterogeneous disorder resulting from a number of different biochemical changes in the brain. The theories that have withstood the test of time and are consistent with responses to therapeutic drugs are *biogenic amine* theories of depression. These theories can be divided into two themes:

Etiology of unipolar depression—biogenic amine theory:

1. Catecholamine hypothesis
2. Indoleamine hypothesis

1. catecholamine theory—depression is associated with an absolute or relative deficiency of neuronal catecholamines, particularly norepinephrine, at functionally important adrenergic receptor sites in the brain.

2. indoleamine theory—depression is associated with an absolute or relative deficiency of indoleamines, specifically 5-hydroxytryptamine (5-HT), at functionally important receptor sites in the brain.

These biogenic amine hypotheses for depression are based on the following observations:

1. Drugs such as reserpine that deplete norepinephrine from the storage granules cause depression. Similarly, drugs that prevent synthesis of 5-HT have been shown to prevent the actions of antidepressant drugs.

2. Drugs that increase the levels of norepinephrine or 5-HT in the brain have been shown to have a mood-elevating effect and are used in the treatment of depression. These include the stimulants such as amphetamine that promote the release of norepinephrine from the storage vesicles, tricyclic antidepressant drugs that inhibit the neuronal reuptake (Uptake I) of either norepinephrine or 5-HT, and monoamine oxidase (MAO) inhibitors that prevent the breakdown of norepinephrine and 5-HT, resulting in increased levels of these neurotransmitters in the CNS.

Although the biochemical actions of drugs effective for relieving depression in a significant number of patients have been investigated extensively, the exact mechanism(s) by which these drugs alleviate depression is not well understood. This is due, in part, to the fact that all antidepressant drugs used clinically require approximately 2–3 weeks of administration before therapeutic signs are observed. Because of this delayed response to the antidepressant effects of these drugs, current theory suggests that a down-regulation of either the norepinephrine or 5-HT receptors is ultimately responsible for the therapeutic actions of these drugs. This idea of down-regulation is supported by experimental data in laboratory animals.

TREATMENT

Electroconvulsive Therapy

Although not publicized as a major method for treatment of depression, electroconvulsive therapy (ECT) is still considered to be an effective treatment for depression, especially in those depressed patients who do not respond to drug treatment. Because drug treatment takes 2–3 weeks before a therapeutic response is observed, ECT may be the treatment of choice in cases of severe depression in which attempts of suicide have occurred. It may be the preferred treatment also in cases where drug treatment is contraindicated.

Treatments for unipolar depression:

1. Electroconvulsive therapy
2. Drugs:
   Tricyclic antidepressants
   MAO inhibitors
   Second-generation antidepressants

The major disadvantage of ECT stems from the fact that patients frequently choose the drug treatment in preference of ECT because of the fears and anxieties about ECT. Accordingly, patients may view pills as an easier means of treatment even though drugs may have to be administered for prolonged periods of time and may have serious potential side effects. Another major disadvantage of ECT is that of memory loss. Most of the memory loss associated with ECT is transient; however, this treatment may cause some permanent memory loss as well. Yet, such loss of memory may be a small price to pay for improvement in severely psychotic or suicidal patients.

Drug Treatment

There are basically three classes of drugs used clinically for treatment of unipolar depression: tricyclic antidepressants; MAO inhibitors; and the so-called second-generation antidepressant drugs.

Tricyclic Antidepressant Drugs. The tricyclic antidepressant drugs are generally considered the drugs of first choice for the treatment of unipolar depression, yet they have limited efficacy in that two thirds or fewer of the depressed patients respond favorably. Table 22–1 lists the seven tricyclic antidepressants used clinically in the United States.

Tricyclic antidepressants inhibit neurol reuptake of norepinephrine or 5-HT leading to a down-regulation of their respective receptors.

The first tricyclic drug used clinically was imipramine. The structure of imipramine is similar to that of the antipsychotic phenothiazines. Imipramine was not designed originally for use in the treatment of depression but was synthesized as an analog of phenothiazine for possible use as an antipsychotic agent. However, it displayed only modest antipsychotic properties and could exacerbate schizophrenic psychosis. Surprisingly, some depressed patients improved, and clinical trials demonstrated ultimately that imipramine had a mood-elevating effect. Thus, it became one of the first so-called tricyclic antidepressant drugs. When administered to normal nondepressed individuals, the tricyclic antidepressant drugs have

Table 22–1 TRICYCLIC ANTIDEPRESSANTS

Drug	Structure	Therapeutic Dosage (mg/day)
Imipramine (Tofranil, others)	$CH_2CH_2CH_2N(CH_3)_2$	50–150 (300)*
Desipramine (Norpramin, others)	$CH_2CH_2CH_2NHCH_3$	50–300 (300)*
Amitriptyline (Elavil, others)	$CHCH_2CH_2N(CH_3)_2$	50–150 (300)*
Nortriptyline (Aventyl, others)	$CHCH_2CH_2NHCH_3$	20–100
Protriptyline (Vivactil)	$CH_2CH_2CH_2NHCH_3$	10–40
Doxepin (Sinequan)	$CHCH_2CH_2N(CH_3)_2$	40–150
Trimipramine (Surmontil)	$CH_2CHCH_2N(CH_3)_2$ / CH_3	50–150

* Recommended maximal permissible dose.

few behavioral effects other than sedation, although it has been reported that they may produce psychotic symptoms or manic behavior in some predisposed individuals.

In general, all tricyclic antidepressant drugs are equally effective in alleviating the symptoms of depression. However, they differ in their side-effect profiles. Amitriptyline and doxepin are the most sedating of the tricyclic drugs and therefore are used preferentially for treatment of agitated depression or where sedation or improved sleep is desired (see Chapter 20). Accordingly, other tricyclic antidepressant drugs listed in the table may be preferred for treatment of retarded depression.

Also available are two tricyclic antidepressant formulations in combination with other psychoactive drugs. TRIAVIL and ETRAFON are the trade names for combinations of amitriptyline plus perphenazine, designed principally for treatment of depression characterized by agitation or psychotic behavior. Another widely prescribed combination drug consists of amitriptyline combined with chlordiazepoxide (LIMBITROL), designed and promoted for the treatment of depression characterized by anxiety. Whether these combinations are any more effective than the individual drugs for treatment of these disorders is questionable.

As noted earlier, the probable mechanism of the antidepressant actions of tricyclic antidepressant drugs is through inhibition of the neuronal reuptake of either norepinephrine or 5-HT. Presumably, the increased levels of these neurotransmitters resulting from this process within the synaptic cleft result ultimately in the down-regulation (see Chapter 14) of their respective postsynaptic receptors. Because there is evidence that depression is associated with specific deficiencies of each norepinephrine or 5-HT in the brain, current research on antidepressant drugs is focusing on drugs that selectively inhibit either of these transport systems.

Time Course and Metabolism of Tricyclic Antidepressants. The two major routes for the metabolism of the tricyclic antidepressant agents are through the mixed-function oxidase enzyme system. These include hydroxylation of either or both of the aromatic rings and N-demethylation of one or both of the methyl groups associated with the side-chain amine. In both cases the end products are active pharmacologically. Accordingly, the N-demethylated products of imipramine and amitriptyline, desmethylimipramine and nortriptyline, respectively, are marketed as antidepressant agents. There is some evidence in the literature that suggests that these secondary amines, i.e., desmethylimipramine and nortriptyline, may be the functionally active forms of the parent tertiary amine drug.

Metabolism of tricyclic antidepressants through mixed-function oxidase; metabolites are pharmacologically active.

The hydroxylated aromatic rings can be conjugated by glucuronic acid or sulfate and this process ultimately inactivates the drug. The tricyclic antidepressant agents are highly lipid-soluble and tightly bound to serum proteins. Accordingly, the half-lives for the tricyclic antidepressant drugs are generally in excess of 20 hours. Although often administered in multiple daily doses, the tricyclic drugs can be given once a day, preferably at bedtime because of the sedating properties and long half-lives of the drugs.

The most common adverse effect of the tricyclic antidepressant drugs is cholinergic blockade, including dry mouth, constipation, blurred vision, and tachycardia. In general, the anticholinergic effects observed with the tricyclic antidepressant drugs are more severe than are encountered with the phenothiazine antipsychotic drugs. Tolerance to the anticholinergic effects occurs often, but in the event that the anticholinergic properties are not tolerated by the patient, the dosage of the drug can be reduced or a

Tricyclic antidepressant side effects:

1. Cholinergic blockade
2. Cardiac complications including atrial fibrillation, A-V block, and ventricular tachycardia
3. Allergic reactions
4. Potentiates pressor effects of sympathomimetics
5. Antagonism of antihypertensive effect of guanethidine
6. Hypertensive crisis in combination with MAO inhibitor

choline ester such as bethanechol can be administered along with the tricyclic drug. Amitriptyline displays the greatest anticholinergic effects, whereas desmethylimipramine displays the least.

Because of the anticholinergic side effects and because they inhibit the reuptake of catecholamines, the tricyclic drugs are contraindicated in individuals with any cardiac disease. The tricyclic antidepressant drugs may cause atrial fibrillation, A-V block, or ventricular tachycardia. In cases of mild congestive heart failure, tricyclic antidepressant drugs can be administered; however, the patients should be under careful clinical supervision for cardiac function.

Other side effects of the tricyclic antidepressant drugs include allergic reactions and a number of drug interactions. As with any other drug class, if a patient develops an allergy to any one of the tricyclic antidepressant drugs, a different class of antidepressant has to be administered. Included in drug interactions are the fact that tricyclic antidepressant drugs can potentiate the pressor effects of sympathomimetic agents, antagonize the antihypertensive effects of guanethidine by preventing its uptake into the neuron, and induce a hypertensive crisis when taken in conjunction or administered sequentially before or after an MAO inhibitor. With respect to the last point, the combination of a tricyclic antidepressant drug and an MAO inhibitor should be avoided, because it is a potentially lethal combination. The actions of the tricyclics and the MAO inhibitors potentiate each other; MAO inhibitors increase the norepinephrine stores in the nerve endings and its subsequent release upon nerve stimulation in the periphery, whereas the tricyclic drugs prevent reuptake of the released norepinephrine.

The lethality of the tricyclic antidepressant drugs is primarily the result of their effect on cardiac rhythmicity. In general, they are more toxic than the phenothiazine antipsychotic drugs, and the frequency of toxicity is greater also because they are administered to a patient population that is at risk of suicide attempts; thus, they should be dispensed with caution and in total quantities that are not likely to be lethal if taken all at once. Deaths from overdoses of the tricyclic antidepressants occur; the cause of death is most usually a cardiac arrhythmia, but respiratory failure and coma can occur also. The CNS depressant activity of the tricyclic drugs is additive with other CNS depressant agents.

The tricyclic antidepressant drugs are highly lipid-soluble compounds and remain bound to the lipid components of the body. An overdose of the tricyclic agents necessitates support of the vital functions and usually requires a prolonged period to fully eliminate the drug. Small doses (1–2 mg) of physostigmine can be administered carefully to patients who have overdosed on the tricyclics; this treatment produces a rapid recovery but for only a brief period of time because of the short duration of action of physostigmine.

MAO inhibitors are not selective inhibitors of the A and B forms of MAO.

Monoamine Oxidase Inhibitors. The MAO inhibitors were the first clinically effective drugs for the treatment of depression. The introduction in the 1950s of the MAO inhibitors for treatment of depression stemmed from the observation that isoniazid, a hydrazine derivative used for the treatment of tuberculosis, had a mood-elevating effect in these patients. At the same time these observations were being made, it was also shown that hydrazines were potent inhibitors of MAO. Numerous MAO inhibitors were synthesized by pharmaceutical companies over the next few years, but because of serious side effects associated with many of the drugs, only three are marketed currently for the treatment of depression. Although

Table 22-2 MONOAMINE OXIDASE INHIBITORS

Drug	Structure	Therapeutic Dosage (mg/day)
Phenelzine (Nardil)	$CH_2-CH_2-NH-NH_2$	45-90
Tranylcypromine (Parnate)	$CH-CH-NH_2$ / CH_2	10-30
Isocarboxazid (Marplan)	$CH_2-NH-NH-C$	10-50

these drugs are efficacious therapeutically, the potential serious side effects associated with their administration have limited their use.

The three MAO inhibitor drugs listed in Table 22-2 being used currently for the treatment of depression are all phenylethylamine derivatives. The drugs listed in the table all possess similar pharmacological activities and, therefore, the selection is based on a physician's experience with any particular agent. The three drugs are nonselective inhibitors of the two forms of MAO, Type A and Type B. As discussed in the chapter on drug metabolism, the A form of MAO is localized within the neuron and is responsible for the deamination of norepinephrine and 5-HT. Recent studies have demonstrated that it is the inhibition of the A form of MAO that imparts the antidepressant effects of these drugs.

The three drugs inhibit MAO irreversibly by covalently binding to the flavin adenine dinucleotide (FAD) cofactor. Because MAO is in excess *in vivo*, approximately 80% of the enzyme activity must be inhibited before pharmacological activity is expressed. Upon stopping an MAO inhibitor in a patient who has been receiving the drug, 10 days to 2 weeks is required for the resynthesis of new enzyme. This is an important fact, especially in cases where a patient has to be switched from an MAO inhibitor to a tricyclic antidepressant agent. As noted earlier, the combination of an MAO inhibitor and a tricyclic antidepressant drug is potentially lethal; therefore, before changing medications, a 2-week period is required to allow MAO levels to return to normal. Likewise, when shifting from a tricyclic drug to an MAO inhibitor, a 2-week period is recommended, because the tricyclics have long half-lives and remain bound in the body for extended periods of time.

The major limitation on the widespread use of the MAO inhibitors for the treatment of depression has been the potential serious side effects. The minor adverse effects of the MAO inhibitors include excessive stimulation and allergic reactions. Decreasing dosage can possibly prevent the excessive stimulation, and changing the class of antidepressant can correct these deficiencies. In contrast to what might be expected, all MAO inhibitors can produce orthostatic hypotension. In fact, the MAO inhibitor pargyline was recently introduced as an antihypertensive agent, but because of the seri-

MAO inhibitors irreversibly inhibit MAO.

Side effects of MAO inhibitors:

1. Excessive stimulation
2. Allergic reactions
3. Hypotension
4. Interaction with tricyclic antidepressants
5. Potentiate depressants such as meperidine
6. Potential hypertensive crisis with sympathomimetic amine present in food (e.g., tyramine, phenylethylamine)

ous side effects associated, it was removed from the market for this purpose. The mechanism for the hypotensive action of MAO inhibitors is not known but is presumed to be mediated centrally.

Side Effects of Monoamine Oxidase Inhibitors. The most serious side effects of the MAO inhibitors are associated with their interaction with other drugs. The consequence of the interaction of the MAO inhibitors with tricyclic antidepressant drugs has been discussed already. Another drug interaction of importance is between the MAO inhibitors and opioids such as meperidine. In the latter case, the MAO inhibitors can potentiate the action of depressants by interfering with their metabolism. However, the major reason why the MAO inhibitors are not widely used is their potential interaction with sympathomimetic amines. This interaction has led to a number of cases of lethal hypertensive crises. Any food or cold medication that contains any sympathomimetic amine is contraindicated in patients receiving MAO inhibitors. Thus, diets of patients receiving these drugs have to be monitored carefully for agents that contain tyramine, phenylethylamine, and for over-the-counter cold remedies that contain phenylephrine or similar vasoconstricting agents. For example, foods that contain tyramine, such as bananas, red wines, cheeses, and chocolate, should not be consumed by patients receiving these drugs. It is because of these dietary restrictions that this class of antidepressant agent is not widely used. In the event a severe hypertensive crisis occurs, short-acting adrenergic blocking agents can be administered.

In the future new MAO inhibitors may be introduced that reversibly inhibit the enzyme. Also, more selective inhibitors may be employed that selectively inhibit only the A form of MAO because this is the form associated with the antidepressant effects of these drugs. However, all of the new drugs under investigation that are selective Type A MAO inhibitors also produce hypertensive crises when administered in the presence of sympathomimetic amines.

Second-generation antidepressants—a structurally diverse group of agents

Second-Generation Antidepressant Drugs. The name *second-generation antidepressant inhibitors* implies that these newer drugs represent a different class of agents. Initially it was thought that some of these agents worked by a different mechanism than the two classes of drugs described earlier. However, in actuality this term is used now to describe a structurally diverse group of agents that apparently are neither tricyclic antidepressant agents nor MAO inhibitors. Yet, for many of these agents their mechanisms of action appear to be similar to those of the tricyclic drugs.

Maprotiline (LUDIOMIL). Structurally this new tetracyclic antidepressant agent is chemically similar to the tricyclic. Mechanistically and functionally, this drug is also similar to the tricyclic antidepressant agents, including the side effects associated with its use. Although this agent is therapeutically effective, it has little advantage over the tricyclic agents.

CH₂CH₂CH₂NHCH₃

Maprotiline

Amoxapine (ASENDIN). As illustrated, this compound is the N-demethylated derivative of the antipsychotic drug loxapine. Mechanistically, it blocks the neuronal reuptake of both norepinephrine and 5-HT and thus provides little additional benefit over the tricyclic antidepressant drugs. In addition, it blocks dopamine receptors and, therefore, may have the potential to cause tardive dyskinesia upon prolonged use.

Amoxapine

Trazodone (DESYREL). Trazodone represents one of the new class of drugs that apparently does not inhibit MAO or the reuptake of the catecholamine neurotransmitters in therapeutic concentrations. It is reported to have less anticholinergic action and is less cardiotoxic than any of the other antidepressant agents. In addition, it appears to produce fewer side effects than the other antidepressant agents. It is at least as sedating as amitriptyline or doxepin. However, trazodone can cause priapism, and prolonged use can lead to impotence; the mechanism of this action of trazodone is not fully understood but may involve a down-regulation of either the norepinephrine or 5-HT receptor.

Trazodone

Bupropion (WELLBUTRIN). Bupropion represents a new chemical class of antidepressants introduced with hope it would avoid the drawbacks of the tricyclics. Its antidepressant effects are equivalent to those of amitriptyline. Although it lacks the cardiac toxicity of the tricyclics, it carries the potential of causing restlessness and agitation, insomnia, and seizures. The prevalence of seizures is 0.4%, with high dosages and other predisposing factors contributing to the risk. The use of bupropion is limited by the wide variety of side effects and potentially serious drug interactions (MAO inhibitors, levodopa, drugs affecting hepatic drug metabolizing enzymes, and agents that lower seizure threshold), although fatalities from overdoses have yet to be reported.

Adequate blood concentrations are achieved within 2 hours following oral administration. The half-life ranges from 8 to 24 hours; several of the metabolites have even longer elimination half-lives.

Fluoxetine (PROZAC). Fluoxetine is a new second-generation antidepressant agent and appears to function by selectively inhibiting neuronal reuptake of 5-HT. It is a highly lipid-soluble compound and has a half-life of approximately 2–3 days. It is metabolized to the N-demethylated derivative by the mixed-function oxidase, and this metabolite is also pharmacologically active, possessing a half-life of approximately 8 days.

Fluoxetine

The most common adverse effects associated with fluoxetine are nervousness, anxiety, and insomnia. Other less common side effects include arrhythmias, migraine headaches, hypo- or hypertension, increased appetite, allergic reactions, and gastritis. An increase in the frequency of suicide attempts has been reported in a series of patients taking fluoxetine, patients who reportedly did not express suicidal behavior prior to its administration.

Bipolar Depression

Bipolar depression or manic-depressive syndrome is characterized by cyclical changes in affective state between the manic and depressive phases of behavior. Bipolar patients cycle back and forth between the two affective states, and similar to unipolar depression, require treatment when the mood changes are of sufficient magnitude to disrupt their lives or the lives of people closely associated with them. There is stronger evidence that bipolar depression, as opposed to unipolar depression, is linked genetically. The etiology for this disorder is not fully understood, but it is presumed to involve biogenic amine neurotransmitters. Scientific studies have demonstrated changes in urinary biogenic amine levels and their metabolites prior to a change in the affective state of bipolar depressed patients. Whether these changes are a consequence of some hormonal change or some other biochemical event is unknown.

LITHIUM

The major drug for treatment of bipolar depression is the element lithium. Since the late nineteenth century, lithium has had a long history of various

Li⁺ is drug of choice for treatment of bipolar depression.

medical uses. In the early part of this century, lithium was believed to be the active ingredient in many tonics and was touted as the cure-all agent for a variety of maladies. In the 1940s it was used as an effective salt substitute until reports of several deaths from lithium overdose. It was not until 1949 with the studies of John F.J. Cade in Australia that lithium was used for treatment of bipolar depression. Cade had performed a series of experiments involving the injection of urine of normal and bipolar-depressed patients into guinea pigs. The culmination of these studies was the finding that lithium prevented death of the guinea pigs injected with urine from bipolar patients; in so doing he found that lithium sedated the guinea pigs. From these findings he successfully went on to test lithium for the treatment of bipolar depression. Although the European scientific community started using lithium for bipolar depression in the 1950s, it was not until over a decade later that this drug was accepted for use in the United States for treatment of this affective disorder.

Although lithium has been used extensively for treatment of bipolar depression, the mechanism of its actions remains almost totally unknown. Recent studies have demonstrated that lithium inhibits the phosphatase responsible for the conversion of inositol monophosphates to inositol, but how or whether this inhibitory process leads to suppression of the manic behavior is still a mystery.

Lithium is used primarily to prevent the occurrence of the manic phase of bipolar depression. It is not useful for the acute manic episodes in which the more classical antipsychotic drugs or benzodiazepines are required to quell the extreme mania and to treat the psychotic symptoms. Lithium is used as maintenance therapy and appears to modulate the cycling as well as prevent the mania. Whether lithium can be used to prevent the occurrence of depressive episodes appears to depend on the patient. In those patients whose depressive episodes do not respond to ongoing lithium treatment, an appropriate antidepressant drug is administered along with the lithium during the depressive phase.

Lithium has an extremely low therapeutic index, and blood levels have to be monitored and maintained to ensure efficacy and to prevent toxicity. When a patient is treated with lithium initially, his or her blood levels are monitored carefully so that the blood levels fall within the therapeutic range. Acceptable therapeutic blood levels of lithium range between 0.8 and 1.2 mEq/L of blood. Between 1.6 and 2.0 mEq/L toxic manifestations are observed, which include GI disturbances, weakness, thirst, and hand tremors. Blood levels above 2.0 mEq/L are associated with severe toxicity, including coma, convulsions, and death. Chronic treatment with lithium that maintains plasma concentrations at the higher end of the therapeutic scale has been reported to lead to polyuria and impairment of renal function manifested by glomerular necrosis. In a few individuals lithium has been reported to cause thyroid enlargement, which may lead to the development of goiter; in such cases lithium treatment must be discontinued.

Lithium levels may vary widely in a given patient at different times. Lithium is reabsorbed in the kidney by the same system for the reabsorption of sodium. About 95% of ingested lithium is eliminated through the kidney. Thus, changes in sodium concentrations in blood are associated with altered lithium levels. During periods of excessive sodium loss in the summer due to sweating, lithium reabsorption may increase and its blood concentrations rise to toxic levels. Under these conditions sodium intake has to be adjusted to meet the loss of excreted sodium. Lithium has a long half-life of approximately 20 hours and is administered normally as lithium carbonate in multiple daily dosages or twice a day in slow-release formulations.

Li^+ has a low therapeutic index:

0.8–1.2 mEq/L blood — therapeutic range
1.6–2.0 mEq/L blood — GI toxicity
>2.0 mEq/L blood — CNS toxicity

Li^+ side effects:

1. Impairment of renal function
2. Thyroid enlargement

Na^+ intake must be maintained to prevent increased Li^+ reabsorption in the kidney.

OTHER DRUGS USED IN DISORDERS OF MOOD

In certain patients other drugs are known to produce reproducible improvement in mood. Among these are carbamazepine (TEGRETOL), which can have antidepressant and antimanic effects (discussed further in Chapter 23); thus, it is among two additional second-line drugs for depressive illness. Some patients with anxiety associated with depression respond to alprazolam; however, most benzodiazepines have no effect on, or actually aggravate, depression. Whether alprazolam has equivalent efficacy as amitriptyline in severely depressed patients is currently disputed; it is agreed that in the less severely depressed patients alprazolam has antidepressant effects.

References

Bunney WE Jr, Murphy DL, Goodwin FK: The "switch process" in manic-depressive illness. Arch Gen Psychiatry 27:295–302, 1972.

Cade JFJ: Lithium salts in the treatment of psychotic excitement. Med J Aust 2:349–352, 1949.

Coccaro EF, Siever LJ: Second generation antidepressants: A comparative review. J Clin Psychopharmacol 25:241, 1985.

Cooper JR, Bloom FE, Roth RH: The Biochemical Basis of Neuropharmacology. 3rd ed. New York: Oxford University Press, 1978.

Frommer DA, Kulig KW, Marx JA, Rumack B: Tricyclic antidepressant overdose: A review. JAMA 257:521, 1987.

Herrington RN, Lader MH: Antidepressant drugs (Chapter 1). Lithium (Chapter 2). *In* van Praag HM (ed): Handbook of Biological Psychiatry. Part V: Drug Treatment in Psychiatry—Psychotropic Drugs, 1–72. New York: Marcel Dekker, 1981.

Hollister LE: Current antidepressants. Annu Rev Pharmacol Toxicol 26:23–37, 1986.

Hollister LE, Csernansky JG: Clinical Pharmacology of Psychotherapeutic Drugs. 3rd ed. New York: Churchill Livingstone, 1990.

Kaplan HI, Sadock BJ (eds): Comprehensive Textbook of Psychiatry IV. 4th ed. Baltimore: Williams & Wilkins, 1985.

Meltzer HY (ed): Psychopharmacology—The Third Generation of Progress. New York: Raven Press, 1987.

Schildkraut JJ: The catecholamine hypothesis of affective disorders: A review of supporting evidence. Am J Psychiatry 122:508, 1965.

Sulser F: Antidepressant treatments and regulation of norepinephrine receptor-coupled adenylate cyclase systems in the brain. Adv Biochem Psychopharmacol 39:249, 1984.

Veith RC, Raskind MA, Caldwell JH, et al: Cardiovascular effects of tricylic antidepressants in depressed patients with chronic heart disease. N Engl J Med 306:954, 1982.

23

Drugs Used in the Treatment of Epilepsy

Arthur W. K. Chan

Prevalence of epilepsy is usually three to six cases per 1000 population.

The term *epilepsy* is used collectively to include a group of syndromes of central nervous system (CNS) disorders characterized by sudden, transitory, and recurring seizures involving one or more of the following systems: motor (convulsion), sensory, autonomic, or psychic. Most investigators do not include single isolated seizures in the definition of epilepsy. Abnormal and excessive discharges in the electroencephalogram (EEG) nearly always accompany the seizures. Synonyms of the term epilepsy are convulsive disorders and seizure disorders. Most estimations on the prevalence of epilepsy fall within the narrow range of between three and six cases/1000 population. However, much lower (1.5/1000) or higher (15–30/1000) prevalence figures have been reported also, the latter being documented in Africa and South America (Hauser, 1978; Schoenberg, 1985).

Because different drugs effectively prevent or modify different types of seizures, rational drug therapy requires a basic understanding of the seizure types. Although objective studies of physicians' perspectives of epilepsy are scarce, there have been concerns about the lack of interest and knowledge in doctors and medical students about epilepsy and the deleterious effect such negative attitudes could have on epileptic patients. With the proliferation of health maintenance organizations around the country, the doctors that new epileptic patients will first encounter most likely will not be neurologists. Therefore, it is important that medical students are educated about the epilepsies and antiepileptic drugs.

The International League Against Epilepsy (ILAE), through its Commission on Classification and Terminology, adopted an international classification of epileptic seizures (ICES) in 1981. This ICES is a revised version of the one recognized by the ILAE in 1969. Although there are still ongoing debates about certain terminologies in the ICES, by and large this is a useful classification, albeit somewhat lengthy for convenient clinical use. Table 23–1 presents a shortened version of the ICES that is based on clinical manifestations together with ictal and interictal EEGs.

Basic Mechanisms of Epilepsy

It would be a gross oversimplification to suggest a single mechanism or cause for epilepsy. Because of the diversity of seizure types, it is understandable that a common denominator has so far not been found; rather, there is likely to be more than one neurophysiological and biochemical mechanism for seizure disorders. Because the most prominent feature of an epileptic seizure is sustained synchronous neuronal discharges, any plausible mechanism needs to account for such a phenomenon. Some investigators have proposed that synchronous firing may require specifically timed

Table 23-1 CLASSIFICATION OF EPILEPTIC SEIZURES

Seizure Type		Features
I. Partial seizures (focal, local seizures)*	A. Simple partial seizures	Consciousness not impaired. Convulsions involving only the motor (jacksonian motor epilepsy) or sensory system (jacksonian sensory epilepsy); may also occur with autonomic or psychic symptoms, depending on the local contralateral EEG discharge in the cortical area.
	B. Complex partial seizures	Impairment of consciousness either at onset or following simple focal onset. Manifestations are varied and complex, involving confused behavior. Interictal EEG generally shows unilateral or bilateral focal discharge in the temporal or frontal region. Ictal EEG shows diffuse discharges.
	C. Partial seizures leading secondarily to generalized seizures	Progresson of A or B to generalized seizures, or from A→B→generalized seizures.
II. Generalized seizures (convulsive or nonconvulsive)*	A.1. Absence seizures	Brief (few seconds to half a minute) attack with sudden onset and termination; impairment of consciousness. Ictal EEG usually shows bilateral and synchronous 3-Hz spike-and-wave pattern but may be 2–4 Hz. Symptoms may include blank stare, eye movement, with or without jerking of the limbs or body,
	A.2. Atypical absence seizures	Slower onset and cessation than those usually seen for absence seizures. EEG more heterogenous.
	B. Myoclonic Seizures	Brief, single, mild-to-volent jerks of arms or head with brief bursts of multiple spikes in ictal or interictal EEG.
	C. Clonic seizures	Rhythmic, multiple jerks of all parts of the body, with loss of consciousness.
	D. Tonic seizures	Rigid, violent muscular contractions, fixing the limbs in some strained position. Loss of consciousness.
	E. Tonic-clonic seizures (grand mal)	Generalized tonic muscle contractions with flexion of the upper extremities and forced extension of the lower extremities, followed by rhythmic contractions of the limbs. Usually lasts several minutes. Loss of consciousness.
	F. Atonic seizures	Sudden loss of muscle tone, leading to a head drop or slumping to the ground.
III. Unclassified Seizures		Incomplete data.

* The term *status epilepticus* denotes seizures that are repeated frequently enough that recovery between attacks does not occur. Status epilepticus may be focal or generalized.

inhibitory and excitatory neuronal activity. However, the specific mechanism for sustaining the synchronous firing is still unknown. It has been suggested that most seizures begin with, and are sustained by, the synchronous firing of a relatively localized group of neurons, namely, the *seizure focus.* A reduction in inhibitory neurons in the focus may be a plausible explanation. Alternatively, the primary seizure focus may originate or be triggered by factors such as congenital defects, hypoxia at birth, local biochemical changes, neoplasm, head trauma, ischemia, or endocrine disorders. The seizure focus may remain quiescent over long periods of time, discharging only intermittently as revealed by surface EEG analysis, and may not lead to overt clinical seizures. What is not known is the exact mechanism for the transition from a dormant focus to one that can initiate the spread of synchronous electrical discharges to neighboring areas. Presumably, inhibitory pathways and mechanisms exist that prevent the spread of abnormal discharges. The notion of positive feedback loops has been proposed also, but there has been little evidence to support this idea.

Posttetanic potentiation (progressive enhancement of synaptic transmission that occurs following rapid, repetitive stimulation) may contribute to self-maintenance and spread of the excessive discharges. Physiological and biochemical factors that may also facilitate the spread of abnormal electrical activity to other parts (presumably normal) of the brain include changes in blood gas tension, blood glucose levels, plasma pH, and electrolyte composition of extracellular fluid; fatigue; sleep deprivation; drug withdrawal; nutritional deficiencies; emotional stress; and endocrine

Sustained synchronous neuronal discharges constitute a prominent feature of a seizure.

Various mechanisms of epilepsy

changes. Other less common triggering factors include hot water baths, music, reading books, brushing teeth, eating, watching TV, and doing mathematics.

Alterations in the membrane or metabolic properties of individual neurons may render the neurons pathologically hyperexcitable. Such changes may in turn affect Ca^{2+} and Na^+ conductances. The microenvironment surrounding neurons may effect neuronal discharges. Elevated extracellular potassium may be associated with seizure activity. Some findings indicate that such changes in extracellular potassium are preceded by a decrease in extracellular calcium concentration. This series of events may increase neuronal excitability by decreasing synaptically mediated inhibition and by decreasing the inhibitory influence of calcium-dependent potassium efflux. Another mechanism involves a reduced level of $Na^+ + K^+$ATPase found in the synaptosomal membrane derived from a freeze-lesion focus; this may lead to a reduced capability to reclaim lost K^+.

Biochemical lesions affecting the synthesis, storage, release, and reuptake of inhibitory amino acid neurotransmitters may be another possible mechanism for enhancing neuronal excitability. A major inhibitory neurotransmitter is γ-aminobutyric acid (GABA). Many convulsive agents are known to affect GABA metabolism. Some agents related to GABA metabolism and its receptors have been shown to possess some antiepileptic activity. Some of the antiepileptic properties of benzodiazepines may be related to the receptor complex involving both benzodiazepine and GABA receptors that are linked intimately to chloride conductance and synaptic inhibition (see Chapter 20).

Animal models of epilepsy indicate that there is at least one initiation site for seizures in the rat brain, the area tempestus, and at least two policing areas, the substantia nigra and the anterior thalamus. It remains to be determined whether the same brain regions in the human brain regulate seizure activity. Other animal models of seizure disorders also provide basic information about epilepsy. For example, the method of kindling involves inducing seizures with chronically administered repetitive low-intensity and below-threshold electrical stimuli. The relevance of kindling to human epileptogenesis has been debated, but a review (Schmutz, 1987) suggests that kindling and related processes can occur in humans as well as in animals. Another model is to generate seizure-like discharges in brain tissue slices (e.g., hippocampus) under *in vitro* conditions. One limitation is that hippocampal slices do not truly represent the brain tissue in its normal environment where it is intricately connected with other brain areas.

General Features of Antiepileptic Drug Therapy

Antiepileptic drugs suppress but do not cure seizure disorders.

The Main Objective of Using Antiepileptic Drugs Is to Suppress Seizures and Seizure Recurrence. Unfortunately, currently available drugs do not suppress seizure activity in all epileptics. The therapeutic success appears to be dependent on the type of seizure and the accompanying neurological abnormalities. Drug therapy is protracted often and, in some instances, may last several decades. Thus, compliance with therapy and chronic drug toxicity are major concerns.

Effective Management Depends Initially on an Accurate and Comprehensive Diagnosis. Underlying causes, such as hypoglycemia, tumor, and infections, require treatment. An accurate medical history is not only a *sine qua non* but may also alert physicians to possible seizure-inducing factors.

Drug Levels Should Be Checked Routinely. Because of the variability of responses to drug therapy among patients and the unpredictable nature of seizure recurrence, the monitoring of plasma antiepileptic drug levels is extremely helpful in determining compliance, kinetic drug interaction, and inadequate or excessive drug dosage.

The Drugs Are Usually Administered Orally. The intravenous route is instituted only for treatment of status epilepticus and certain neonatal and infantile seizures. Drugs such as diazepam are sometimes administered rectally to treat febrile seizures.

The Antiepileptic Drugs Are Metabolized in the Liver. Some form initial metabolites (see individual drugs later) that possess antiepileptic activities also. The unmetabolized drugs and their metabolites are excreted in the urine, usually as conjugates of glucuronic or sulfuric acid.

An Initial Therapeutic Aim Is to Use Only One Drug. When drug dosages are increased gradually, sufficient time (usually five to seven half-lives) should be allowed for serum drug level to reach plateau. If the drug fails to control seizures, another drug may be substituted as the first drug is slowly withdrawn. The use of only one drug is favored by most specialists. In refractory seizures a combination of two or more drugs may be required. However, in some cases the indiscriminant use of multiple drug therapy can be the cause of poor seizure control. With multiple drug therapy the metabolism of one drug may be altered by the intake of other drugs, and the incidence and severity of adverse effects may be higher (Schmidt and Seldon, 1982). Other risks of multiple drug therapy include exacerbation of seizures and inability to evaluate the effectiveness of individual drugs.

Precipitating or Aggravating Factors Can Affect Seizure Control by Drugs. Some examples include stressful situations, sleep deprivation, progressive neurological disease, and alcohol intake.

Sudden Withdrawal of Drugs Should Be Avoided. Seizures or status epilepticus may be triggered by the abrupt cessation of antiepileptic drugs.

Avoid sudden withdrawal of antiepileptic drugs.

Neuropsychological Impairments May Occur With Antiepileptic Drug Use. There is sufficient evidence to indicate that prolonged use of antiepileptic drugs may be associated with neuropsychological impairments, especially at high, but not necessarily toxic, serum drug levels.

The Teratogenicity of Antiepileptic Drugs Is Unknown. Well-controlled studies on the teratogenicity of antiepileptic drugs have not been performed, primarily because of the difficulty in controlling for many confounding variables. Nevertheless, the available evidence suggests that children of epileptic mothers who took antiepileptic drugs during pregnancy have an approximately two to three times higher prevalence of a variety of birth defects compared with children born to mothers of the general population. This increased risk of birth defects may be due to the antiepileptic drugs, to genetic factors, or to the occurrence of seizures. Although pregnancy *per se* appears to have little influence on seizure frequency, about 25% of pregnant epileptic patients have increases in seizure frequency, whereas 25% show decreases and 50% have no change in seizure frequency. The increases in seizures could be the result of either noncompliance or altered disposition of antiepileptic drugs. Hormonal, metabolic, respiratory, and psychological factors may play a role also. At the least, there is evidence to indicate that, of the currently available antiepileptic drugs, trimethadione is strongly teratogenic, and therefore it should not be prescribed to women who might become pregnant.

Antiepileptic drugs should not be discontinued in pregnant epileptic patients.

In spite of the potential hazards of antiepileptic drugs they should *not* be discontinued in pregnant epileptic women for whom the medication is essential for the prevention of major seizures, because abrupt discontinuation may trigger status epilepticus, which will be hazardous for both the fetus and the mother. The decision to reduce dosage to a minimum or to change to another drug should be made only on an individual basis after a careful review of the patient's history of frequency and severity of seizures. Because drug metabolism may be altered during pregnancy, the monitoring of antiepileptic drug concentration should be instituted, especially when dosage reduction is contemplated. Women with epilepsy who are planning to become pregnant need to be counseled about the risks of congenital malformations associated with antiepileptic medication during pregnancy, the possibility of injury to the fetus or infant should the mother have a seizure, the potential hazards of antiepileptic drugs in breast milk, and the risk of genetic transmission of epilepsy. The chance of an epileptic woman having a normal child is better than 90% (Dalessio, 1985).

Deficiency of folic acid and vitamin K may exist in the newborn whose mother received phenytoin, phenobarbital, or primidone. These disorders may lead to serious hemorrhage in the third trimester or during the neonatal period. This can be prevented by administration of vitamin K.

Several Classes of Antiepileptic Drugs Share Some Common Structural Features (Fig. 23–1). These (representative drugs listed in parentheses) are the hydantoins (phenytoin), barbiturates (phenobarbital), deoxybarbiturates (primidone), succinimides (ethosuximide), and oxazolidinediones (trimethadione). However, there are other drugs, such as carbamazepine, valproic acid, and diazepam (Fig. 23–2), that differ widely in their chemical

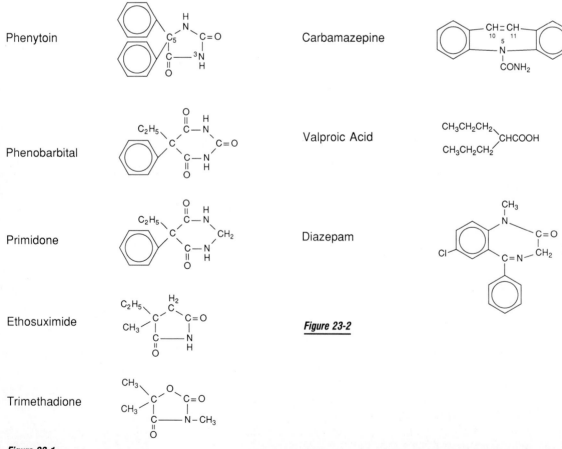

Phenytoin

Phenobarbital

Primidone

Ethosuximide

Trimethadione

Carbamazepine

Valproic Acid

Diazepam

Figure 23-2

Figure 23-1

Table 23-2   COMMONLY USED ANTIEPILEPTIC DRUGS

| Generic Name (Common Trade Name) | Adult Dosage | | | Therapeutic Blood Level | Clinical Use |
	Common Formulations	Initial	Maintenance		
Phenytoin (Dilantin)	Caps 300 mg, 100 mg; Tabs 50 mg; Susp 30 or 125 mg/5 ml; Inj 50 mg/ml	3–5 mg/kg day; For status epilepticus, 20 mg/kg up to 50 mg/min	4–6 mg/kg/day, maximum 500 mg	10–20 μg/ml	Most types of seizures except absence seizures.
Phenobarbital (Luminal and many others)	Tabs 8–100 mg; Caps 16, 65 mg; Inj 50–150 mg/ml	1–5 mg/kg/day; for status epilepticus, 10–20 mg/kg at 60 mg/min or up to 1 g IV	5 mg/kg/day	10–25 μg/ml	Generalized tonic-clonic and partial seizures. Drug of first choice for neonatal seizures. Ineffective against absence seizures.
Primidone (Mysoline)	Tabs 50, 250 mg; Susp 250 mg/5ml	100–125 mg/day	750–1000 mg/day in divided doses	5–12 μg/ml; active metabolite is phenobarbital	Useful against generalized tonic-clonic and both simple and complex partial seizures. Ineffective against absence seizures. Sometimes useful for myoclonic seizures.
Carbamazepine (Tegretol)	Tabs 100, 200 mg	400 mg/day	800–1200 mg/day	5–12 μg/ml	All types of seizures except absence seizures.
Valproic Acid (Depakene)	Caps 250 mg; Syrup 250 mg/5 ml	12–15 mg/kg/day	Up to 4 g/day	50–100 μg/ml	Absence seizures; also used for generalized and complex partial seizures in other countries.
Ethosuximide (Zarontin)	Caps 250 mg; Syrup 250 mg/5ml	250 mg/day	Incremental increase of 250 mg at 3–7 days interval, up to 40 mg/kg or 1.5 g/day	40–100 μg/ml	Drug of choice for absence seizures.
Trimethadione (Tridione)	Caps 300 mg; Tabs 150 mg; Solution 40 mg/ml	900 mg/day	Increment of 300 mg/week up to 2.4 g	700 μg/ml or more for the active metabolite, dimethadione	Absence seizures; usefulness limited by serious side effects.
Clonazepam (Clonopin)	Tabs 0.5, 1, 2 mg	Not > 1.5 mg/day	Increment of 0.5–1 mg every 3 days, not > 20 mg/day	5–70 ng/ml	Absence and myoclonic seizures.
Diazepam (Valium)	Tabs 2, 5, 10, 15 mg; Inj 5 mg/ml	5–10 mg IV repeatable up to 30 mg	—	—	Drug of choice for status epilepticus.

structures. Table 23–2 summarizes information on dosages, therapeutic blood levels, and clinical indications for the primary drugs. Detailed information on individual drugs is described in the following text.

HYDANTOINS

Phenytoin

Phenytoin was introduced as an anticonvulsant by Merritt and Putnam in 1938. It has a broad range of action against many types of seizures (see Table 23–2) but is ineffective against absence seizures. When used intravenously, phenytoin (50 mg/minute, IV) is effective also in controlling tonic-clonic status epilepticus. However, a major drawback with intravenous (IV) phenytoin is the lag time of 15–20 minutes before a reduction in seizures will occur. Therefore, some researchers suggest the simultaneous IV administration of both diazepam and phenytoin. The contraindications for the use of phenytoin in status epilepticus are severe arteriosclerotic heart disease, a history of idiosyncratic reaction to the drug, congestive heart failure, heart block, and bradycardia.

Drug Therapy

Phenytoin is used for many types of seizures except absence.

Actions and Uses. Phenytoin is a weak acid with a pKa of about 9.0. It is extremely insoluble at the pH of gastric juice and, therefore, is only poorly and slowly absorbed in the stomach. Most phenytoin absorption takes place in the small intestine; however, its solubility in the intestinal fluid is still relatively low (100 μg/ml). Therefore, a portion of an oral dose of phenytoin can remain unabsorbed and be lost in the feces. There are considerable individual differences in the absorption of phenytoin, and these differences may be complicated by the availability of different generic formulations of the drug.

Phenytoin is inexpensive and can be administered in one daily dose. A peak blood level is reached approximately 8–12 hours after dosing. There is a high degree of variability (10–34 hours) in half-life (average of 24 hours in adults) and in individual blood levels from a standard dosage of phenytoin. Consequently, it is desirable to determine blood levels frequently. In children the elimination half-life is shorter, about 5–18 hours.

Phenytoin is almost 90% bound to plasma proteins in adults. Over 95% of the drug is metabolized by the liver cytochrome oxidase system to the inactive parahydroxyphenyl derivative, which constitutes 60–70% of a single dose of the parent drug. This major metabolite is excreted in the urine as a glucuronide. Because of the dose-dependent inhibition of its own metabolism, a steady state serum concentration of phenytoin may not be reached until 4–12 weeks after the beginning of therapy. Moreover, with the usual therapeutic dosage, the enzyme system for the metabolism of phenytoin can be saturated completely. Therefore, a small increase in dose may lead to a large increase in phenytoin blood level and unexpected drug toxicity.

A small increase in dose may lead to a large increase in phenytoin blood level.

Mechanism of Action. The exact mechanism of action of phenytoin in the prevention and modification of seizures has not been established, even though a number of plausible mechanisms have been studied extensively (Levy et al, 1989; Jones and Wimbish, 1985). Phenytoin has a stabilizing effect on neuronal membranes, including those of peripheral nerves, which results in an increase in the threshold, especially evident in repetitively discharging neurons. A characteristic of phenytoin is a decrease in the spread of seizure activity in neural networks that is apparent in the absence of a major effect on the seizure focus itself. It also causes a hyperpolarization and decrease in posttetanic potentiation, presumably due to its action upon calcium and sodium conductance. It has been suggested that phenytoin could block sodium conductance by occupying calcium-binding sites on the outer nerve membrane. The reduction in calcium influx by phenytoin might in turn inhibit the release of neurotransmitters. Phenytoin has been shown to activate Na^+-K^+-ATPase in extraneuronal systems, but it has yet to be demonstrated conclusively that phenytoin stimulates active transport of sodium in a normally functioning neuron *in vivo* or *in vitro*. The binding of phenytoin to specific receptors in brain synaptosomal fractions is enhanced in the presence of chloride ions, and this may facilitate GABA-mediated chloride conductance in the postsynaptic membrane.

Drug Interactions. The concurrent administration of phenytoin with other drugs can result in either marked increases or decreases in plasma phenytoin levels, depending whether the drugs inhibit or enhance the metabolism of phenytoin and whether they displace phenytoin from protein-binding sites. Some examples of drugs that can increase plasma phenytoin levels are disulfiram, dicumarol, isoniazid, chloramphenicol methsuximide, phenobarbital, and benzodiazepines. Drugs that can lower plasma phenytoin levels include ethanol, valproic acid, phenobarbital, salicylates, carbamazepine, phenylbutazone, sulfisoxazole, and tolbutamide.

On the other hand, phenytoin, when coadministered with phenobarbital or methsuximide, can elevate the serum concentration of phenobarbital and N-desmethyl-methsuximide derived from methsuximide, probably by competitive inhibition of hydroxylation of the phenyl ring. It can lower the serum levels of the following drugs also, probably either by competing with protein-binding sites or by enzyme induction: warfarin, carbamazepine, bishydroxycoumarin, digitoxin, valproic acid, vitamin D, metyrapone, dexamethasone, thyroxine, contraceptive pill, and quinidine (Wilder and Bruni, 1981).

Other drugs may affect serum phenytoin levels and *vice versa.* Phenytoin has a stabilizing effect on neuronal membranes.

Side Effects and Toxicity. The toxic effects are dependent on the dosage as well as the route and duration of administration. Acute overdosage (phenytoin levels > 40 μg/ml) by the oral route produces toxic signs such as stupor, seizure exacerbation, nystagmus, movement disorders, ataxia, and even coma. When the drug is administered intravenously too rapidly, toxic signs such as cardiac arrhythmias (with or without hypertension) and CNS depression may occur. Arrhythmias occur more frequently in older patients and those with cardiac problems, but they can also occur in young healthy patients.

The dose-dependent side effects arising from chronic medication include gingival hyperplasia, folate deficiency, vitamin K deficiency, behavioral changes, gastrointestinal (GI) symptoms, coarsening of facial features, hirsutism, cerebellar-vestibular dysfunctions, and megaloblastic anemia. The common side effect of gingival hyperplasia can be reduced by good oral hygiene or it may require periodic gingivectomy to remove the excess tissue. This condition is associated with an increase in the number of fibroblasts and in the amount of connective tissue due to altered collagen metabolism.

Gingival hyperplasia and folate and vitamin K deficiency are some possible side effects of phenytoin.

Phenytoin may have endocrinological effects also, such as elevation of plasma cortisol levels, inhibition of release of antidiuretic hormone (ADH) in patients with inappropriate ADH secretion, minor hypocalcemia, and inhibition of insulin secretion leading to hyperglycemia and glycosuria. It may affect thyroid function also.

Idiosyncratic side effects of phenytoin include rashes (morbilliform, erythema multiforme, and Stevens-Johnson syndrome). Rare instances of systemic lupus erythematosus, hepatic necrosis, red-cell aplasia, agranulocytosis, and thrombocytopenia have been reported.

Infants born to mothers taking phenytoin, when compared with those of the general population, have a two- to threefold increase in teratogenesis, which is expressed as cleft lip, cleft palate, and congenital heart disease. A so-called fetal hydantoin syndrome has been reported also, characterized by mental retardation, craniofacial anomalies, hypoplastic fingernails, and hypertelorism. There is still uncertainty as to whether the teratogenicity is caused by phenytoin, by uncontrolled seizures during pregnancy, or by both factors. However, it is believed generally that the teratogenetic risks are lower than the risk from uncontrolled seizures during pregnancy.

Mephenytoin

Mephenytoin (MESANTOIN; 3-methyl-5,5-phenylethylhydantoin) was introduced in 1945 as an anticonvulsant. It is approved by the Federal Drug Administration (FDA) for treatment of tonic-clonic, simple partial, and complex partial seizures in patients who have been refractory to less toxic

Other hydantoins include mephenytoin and ethotoin.

antiepileptic drugs. It is not useful for, and may even exacerbate, absence seizures. Because of the toxicity of mephenytoin, it is advisable to keep the initial dosage at 50 to 100 mg/day during the first week, with increases of 50 or 100 mg at weekly intervals.

Compared with phenytoin, mephenytoin causes less gingival hyperplasia, ataxia, hirsutism, nausea, and vomiting, but it also causes a greater incidence of drowsiness, hepatitis, skin rashes, aplastic anemia, and leukopenia; at least part of these are due to the formation of the active metabolite nirvanol, which accumulates with chronic administration. Therefore, therapy with mephenytoin should be supplemented with regular physical and laboratory examinations. Patients should be alerted about prompt reporting of symptoms such as skin rash, jaundice, bleeding, and nausea. Mephenytoin and nirvanol can interact with other drugs (e.g., carbamazepine, benzodiazepines, and barbiturates) in much the same ways as phenytoin does.

Ethotoin

Ethotoin (PEGANONE; 3-ethyl-5 phenylhydantoin) is used for the treatment of tonic-clonic and complex partial seizures. Although ethotoin has a much lower incidence of side effects than phenytoin or mephenytoin, it has a lower efficacy. Therefore, it is used only occasionally as an adjunct to other antiepileptic drugs. Another disadvantage of ethotoin is that it must be given (after meals) in four to six divided dosages daily to minimize fluctuations between peak and trough plasma concentrations.

BARBITURATES

Phenobarbital

First introduced for the treatment of seizures in 1912, phenobarbital (5-ethyl-5-phenylbarbituric acid) has since become one of the most widely used antiepileptic drugs. It has a broad spectrum of activity, few serious side effects, and is relatively inexpensive. It is considered a safe drug, but there are some subtle and potentially harmful effects associated with chronic therapy. It is effective against generalized tonic-clonic as well as simple and complex partial seizures. In contrast, it is not useful for treating absence, myoclonic, and related seizures. It is effective also in treating status epilepticus by IV administration, but peak brain levels and antiepileptic activity may not be attained for 20–90 minutes. Other indications of phenobarbital include the prevention and treatment of febrile seizures, as well as alcohol- and drug-withdrawal seizures.

Actions and Uses. With a pKa of 7.3, phenobarbital is well absorbed from the GI tract, being predominantly in the un-ionized form in the stomach and to a lesser degree in the intestine. After an oral dose, peak plasma level can be reached within 2–3 hours, and the drug is 40–60% bound to plasma proteins. Unlike drugs such as phenytoin, carbamazepine, and valproic acid, phenobarbital has a relatively low affinity for proteins and phospholipids.

Phenobarbital is parahydroxylated by the mixed-function oxidase enzyme systems in the liver. This metabolite is inactive and is excreted (about 30–50% of the dose) in the urine as glucuronide or sulfate. Twenty-five to 40% of the unchanged drug is excreted in the urine, and the rate of excretion can be enhanced by alkalization of the urine. Phenobarbital can be excreted as the *N*-glucoside derivative also.

Phenobarbital has a broad spectrum of antiepileptic activity.

Compared with other antiepileptic drugs, phenobarbital has a relatively long elimination half-life, approximately 100 hours in adults and even longer in neonates. However, in children the average half-life is approximately 48 hours. Because of its lengthy half-life, phenobarbital can be administered once daily to produce relatively constant serum levels. In contrast, the long half-life can be burdensome in cases of toxic reactions or drug overdose.

Phenobarbital has a long elimination half-life.

Mechanism of Action. Although the precise mechanism of action of phenobarbital has not been established, several plausible mechanisms have been proposed. It may act by suppressing brain electrical activity and the discharges of epileptic foci, elevating the seizure threshold and inhibiting the kindling process. Other evidence suggests that phenobarbital may act by augmenting responses to GABA, suppressing glutamic acid activation, and depressing some postsynaptic potentials (see Chapter 20). High concentrations of phenobarbital may decrease transmitter release and postsynaptic excitation by blocking Ca^{2+} entry into nerve terminals.

Drug Interactions. Phenobarbital can interact with other antiepileptic drugs through its inducing effects on the liver drug-metabolizing enzymes or by competition for the same enzymes for hydroxylation. Drugs such as phenytoin, valproate, and methsuximide are known to elevate serum levels of phenobarbital, presumably by a competitive inhibition of p-hydroxylation. In the case of coadministration with valproate, the plasma concentration of phenobarbital can rise by as much as 40%. In addition, the combination of ethanol or benzodiazepines with phenobarbital is to be avoided because of possible synergistic interactions.

Serum phenobarbital levels are elevated when the drug is coadministered with valproic acid.

Side Effects and Toxicity. Sedation is the most common side effect, especially during the initiation of phenobarbital therapy; the degree of sedation is quite variable among individuals. Most patients develop tolerance to the sedative effect after several weeks, yet the sedative effect may be a limiting factor for controlling seizures in some patients. Minor overdosage causes ataxia and nystagmus, but lethal consequences can result from accidental or purposeful overdose, especially in cases where phenobarbital is combined with other drugs such as ethanol, narcotics, and benzodiazepines. Although other serious systemic side effects are infrequent, neurotoxic and seemingly paradoxical effects can occur in children, with hyperactivity, irritability, and sleeplessness the prominent symptoms; cognitive functions may be disturbed also. In the elderly, paradoxical effects may be manifested as excitement, agitation, or confusion.

Allergic reactions occur in only 1–2% of patients. Side effects such as hepatitis, bone marrow depression, and lupus erythematosus are rare. Newborns of mothers who received phenobarbital during pregnancy may show withdrawal signs, and occasionally they may have hypoprothrombinemia with hemorrhage; the latter can be treated with vitamin K administration.

Mephobarbital

Mephobarbital (MEBARAL) is the N-methyl analog of phenobarbital. The N-demethyl substitution imparts a higher lipid-solubility to mephobarbital compared to phenobarbital. About 50% of an oral dose of mephobarbital is absorbed from the GI tract. Because the primary metabolic route of mephobarbital is N-demethylation to phenobarbital, this drug has the same pharmacological properties, clinical uses, and side effects as those of phenobar-

Mephobarbital is metabolized to phenobarbital.

bital. It has not been established whether mephobarbital *per se* has any significant antiepileptic actions. About 75% of a single oral dose is converted to phenobarbital in 24 hours. Therefore, chronic administration of mephobarbital leads to accumulation of phenobarbital.

DEOXYBARBITURATES

Primidone

Primidone shares a similar chemical structure with phenytoin and phenobarbital.

Like phenobarbital, primidone (MYSOLINE; 2-desoxy-phenobarbital) is effective against tonic-clonic and partial seizures. It is used also as an adjunct to other antiepileptic drugs such as phenytoin or carbamazepine.

Actions and Uses. Primidone, being un-ionized, is readily absorbed from the GI tract after oral administration, with peak plasma levels appearing usually about 3 hours after an oral dose. It is minimally bound to plasma proteins. The elimination half-life varies, with a range of 5–18 hrs. Two active metabolites are formed from the metabolism of primidone, namely, phenobarbital and phenylethylmalonamide (PEMA). Primidone and PEMA are excreted unchanged by the kidney. Whereas the phenobarbital and PEMA serum concentrations remain relatively stable, the primidone level tends to be much more variable during the day. It is advisable to monitor at least the primidone and phenobarbital serum concentrations in patients on primidone.

Drug Interactions. Both phenytoin and carbamazepine induce the biotransformation of primidone, leading to decreased levels of primidone but increased levels of phenobarbital. Isoniazid can increase primidone serum levels (Pippenger, 1982). Other drug interactions to be expected are those involving its active metabolite, phenobarbital.

Side Effects and Toxicity. Most of the side effects of primidone are those usually seen with phenobarbital, although there is convincing evidence that primidone itself produces neurotoxicity. It is advisable to build up the primidone dosage slowly to avoid effects such as sedation, dizziness, and incoordination. Like phenobarbital, serious adverse effects are relatively rare for primidone.

SUCCINIMIDES

Ethosuximide

Ethosuximide is the drug of choice for absence seizures.

Ethosuximide (ZARONTIN; 2-ethyl-2-methylsuccinimide) is currently the drug of choice for absence seizures. Among the three marketed succinimide antiepileptic drugs, ethosuximide is the most effective against pentylenetetrazol seizures in animals. This correlates well with its clinical efficacy in humans. In contrast, the other two succinimides, methsuximide and phensuximide, have some efficacy against maximal electroshock seizures in animals (which correlates with efficacy against tonic-clonic and complex partial seizures in humans), with ethosuximide ranked the least effective. Ethosuximide has no clinical efficacy against tonic-clonic and complex partial seizures.

Actions and Uses. Ethosuximide is absorbed rapidly, with peak plasma levels occurring within several hours after oral administration. It is not appreciably bound to plasma proteins. Because of its water solubility, the drug does not accumulate in fat. About 20–25% of ethosuximide is excreted unchanged by the kidney, and about 40–50% is excreted as the inactive hydroxyethyl derivative, which is the major metabolite of ethosuximide. Several other minor hydroxylated metabolites have been identified in the urine also.

The elimination half-life of ethosuximide averages 20–60 hours in adults and is usually shorter in children (about 30 hours). However, in some children under 10 years of age, the half-life may be as long as that in adults.

Drug Interactions. Ethosuximide rarely interacts with other antiepileptic drugs. Valproic acid may or may not increase ethosuximide serum concentration. Ethosuximide may increase the lethargy and somnolence produced by barbiturates.

Side Effects and Toxicity. In general, ethosuximide is well tolerated, although minor side effects occur in 25–40% of patients. These include drowsiness, nausea, vomiting, anorexia, dizziness, lethargy, fatigue, photophobia, and abdominal pain. Tolerance to some of these effects may develop with continued treatment. Occasionally, patients may have behavioral changes, dystonic movements, hiccups, and skin rashes. Serious toxic effects are uncommon, but a small number of cases of leukopenia, pancytopenia, lupus erythematosus, Stevens-Johnson Syndrome, parkinsonian symptoms, and psychotic episodes, as well as several cases of fatal bone marrow depression, have been reported.

Methsuximide

This drug (CELONTIN; N-2-dimethyl-2-phenylsuccinimide) has been largely replaced by ethosuximide for the treatment of absence seizures. Some investigators have reported success with methsuximide as an adjunctive antiepileptic drug for complex partial seizures and complex atypical absences (Wilder and Buchanan, 1981). Methsuximide is not useful for treating tonic-clonic and simple partial seizures. The drug has a short elimination half-life of 1–2.6 hours. Its major metabolite, N-desmethylmethsuximide, possesses antiepileptic activity, and because of its relatively longer half-life (about 40 hours) it accumulates in the serum during chronic administration of methsuximide.

Unlike ethosuximide, methsuximide interacts with phenytoin or phenobarbital, causing appreciable elevations in the plasma levels of either drug. Conversely, the plasma concentration of methsuximide's metabolite N-desmethylmethsuximide is increased when methsuximide is coadministered with either phenytoin or phenobarbital. The side effects of methsuximide are similar to those reported for ethosuximide, but patients on methsuximide tend to be less likely to develop tolerance to these effects than if they are on ethosuximide.

Methusuximide can interact with phenytoin or phenobarbital.

Phensuximide

This drug (MILONTIN; N-methyl-2-phenylsuccinimide) was the first succinimide to be introduced for treating absence seizures, but it is now considered the least effective of the marketed succinimides. Like methsuximide, it has a short elimination half-life (4–8 hours), as does its major active metabolite N-desmethyl-phensuximide. This drug is seldom used because of its low efficacy and the presence of serious side effects (idiosyncratic reactions and renal toxicity).

OXAZOLIDINEDIONES

Trimethadione

Prior to the discovery of ethosuximide, trimethadione (TRIDIONE; 3,5,5-tri-methyl-2,4-oxazolidinedione) was the agent of choice against absence seizures. Because of its toxicity, it is now used only in patients whose absence seizures are not well-controlled or who do not tolerate other drugs.

Actions and Uses. When taken orally, trimethadione is absorbed rapidly, and peak plasma concentrations occur within 0.5–2 hours. It is demethyl-ated to the active metabolite dimethadione by the hepatic microsomal drug-metabolizing system, and no further metabolism of this product occurs. Thus, almost all of the administered dose of trimethadione is excreted slowly in the urine as dimethadione. This major metabolite accumulates slowly in the serum during chronic therapy with trimethadione, and because of its long elimination half-life (10–20 days), it takes over 30 days to reach steady and therapeutic serum levels of dimethadione (see Table 23–2).

Side Effects and Toxicity. Both trimethadione and dimethadione are CNS depressants; therefore, at high doses they produce sedation, ataxia, and incoordination. Tolerance to drowsiness tends to develop with continued administration of trimethadione. Another common side effect is hemeralopia, or light blindness. About 10% of patients on trimethadione have dermatologic side effects such as rash, exfoliative dermatitis, and erythema multiforme. Neutropenia can develop in about 20% of patients. More serious and fatal cases of pancytopenia have been reported. Other less common serious toxic effects are a nephrotic syndrome and a myasthenic syndrome.

There is strong evidence suggesting that trimethadione has teratogenic effects.

Paramethadione

Paramethadione (PARADIONE; 3,5-dimethyl-5-ethyl-2, 4-oxazolidinedione) is almost identical to the structure of trimethadione except for the substitution of one of the methyl groups on the 5C position by an ethyl group. Therefore, its clinical pharmacology, metabolism, dosage, indications, and toxicity are similar to those of trimethadione. There are some indications that the incidence of severe side effects may be less with paramethadione than with trimethadione. However, paramethadione appears to have less consistent efficacy against absence seizures.

VALPROIC ACID

The antiepileptic properties of valproic acid (DEPAKENE; *n*-dipropylacetic acid) were recognized serendipitously in 1960. Since then it has been used widely in Europe, but it did not gain FDA approval for the treatment of absence seizures in the United States until 1978. It is approved also as an adjunctive therapy for other types of seizures occurring in conjunction with absence seizures.

Valproic acid has a broad spectrum of antiepileptic activity. It is useful particularly for absence seizures, especially in cases where ethosuximide proves to be ineffective. It is also the drug of choice against myoclonic seizures, coexisting absence and tonic-clonic seizures, as well as atonic seizures, although the latter seizures are relatively intractable to treatment.

Dimethadione is an active metabolite of trimethadione.

Usefulness of trimethadione is limited by side effects; there are teratogenic effects.

Valproic acid has a broad spectrum of antiepileptic activity.

Other indications for valproic acid include treatment of partial seizures, febrile seizures, and primary and secondary generalized tonic-clonic seizures. Better results tend to be obtained when valproic acid is used as the only drug rather than in polydrug therapy.

Actions and Uses. When administered orally, valproic acid is absorbed rapidly, with peak blood levels occurring in 1–5 hours, depending on whether the patient is in a fasting or fed state, and whether the tablet is enteric-coated. Valproic acid is about 90% bound to plasma proteins, but the percentage of free valproic acid increases at the high range of therapeutic dosages due to saturation of protein-binding sites.

Valproic acid is metabolized by β and ω oxidations to at least five metabolites with the former being the preferred metabolic pathway in humans. None of these metabolites contribute markedly to the therapeutic effects of valproic acid. Formation of the valproic acid glucuronide and subsequent excretion represent another pathway of metabolism. The elimination half-life of valproic acid is relatively short, and it varies between 6 and 18 hours; because of this, blood levels tend to fluctuate considerably. There is wide variability and little correlation between the blood concentration and the clinical response.

Mechanism of Action. Although animal studies suggest that the antiepileptic effect of valproic acid may be mediated by way of some aspects of brain GABA metabolism, the concentrations of valproate studied were well above the therapeutic ranges seen in humans.

Drug Interactions. Interactions of valproic acid with several other antiepileptic drugs may lead to clinically important changes in blood levels of valproate and the coadministered drugs. When phenobarbital is coadministered with valproic acid, the serum level of phenobarbital may be increased by 30–50%. This is due to a decreased formation of p-hydroxyphenobarbital. However, when primidone is combined with valproic acid, no increase in the metabolically derived phenobarbital has been reported. The combination of carbamazepine and valproic acid causes reduction in plasma level and increase in the clearance of the latter drug. Conversely, valproate can decrease carbamazepine protein binding, causing higher free carbamazepine levels, especially at times of peak serum concentrations. The combination of phenytoin and valproic acid can cause a transient (during first week of coadministration) increase in the percentage of free phenytoin and decrease in total plasma phenytoin concentration because of displacement of phenytoin from protein-binding sites; there is also a transient increase in phenytoin metabolism and excretion of its hydroxylated metabolite. However, when equilibrium is achieved, free phenytoin levels generally remain unchanged. Epileptic children receiving valproic acid and antipyretic dosages of aspirin may have an increase in valproate-free fraction, presumably due to a decrease in protein binding as well as inhibition of metabolism of valproate. A pharmacodynamic interaction between valproic acid and clonazepam has been reported in children, resulting in drowsiness in some patients or absence status in others.

Valproic acid can interact with carbamazepine, phenobarbital, phenytoin, and other anticonvulsants.

Side Effects and Toxicity. The incidence of minor side effects has been reported to vary between 16 and 80%; these include nausea, diarrhea, vomiting, fatigue, and abdominal cramps, and most occur transiently during the early phase of therapy. These effects can be minimized by using enteric-coated tablets and administering the drug with or after a meal. Sedation is another common side effect and occurs in about half of the

Sedation is a common side effect of valproic acid.

patients, being more common when phenobarbital is coadministered with valproic acid. Much less common effects include ataxia, tremor, rash, alopecia, and stimulation of appetite.

Asymptomatic elevation in serum glutamic-oxaloacetic transaminase (SGOT) and serum glutamic-pyruvic transaminase (SGPT) activity occurs in 15–30% of patients during the first several months of drug treatment. A more serious and potentially fatal hepatotoxicity can occur also, with an apparent rate of 1 in 20,000 to 40,000 patients. Most but not all of these cases involved patients under 15 years of age and occurred during the first 6 months of therapy. The majority of these patients took multiple antiepileptic drugs. Among these cases of hepatic failure, two occurred in one family; this suggests a possible genetic predisposition to the toxic actions of valproate. Animal studies suggest that a toxic metabolite, 2-n-propyl-4-penetenoic acid, formed by the metabolism of valproate by isoenzymes of cytochrome P-450 that have been induced specifically by coadministration of phenobarbital or other antiepileptic drugs, may lead to valproate-induced liver injury. Other rare toxic effects that have been reported are acute hyperammonemia and pancreatitis.

Although valproic acid is teratogenic in animals, no human congenital anomalies associated specifically with this drug have been reported.

IMINOSTILBENES

Carbamazepine

Carbamazepine (TEGRETOL; 5-carbamoyl-5H-dibenz [b,f] azepine; 5H-dibenz [b,f] azepine-5-carboxamide) was introduced in 1962 for the treatment of trigeminal neuralgia. It was later approved by the FDA as an antiepileptic agent for patients 6 years of age or older. Carbamazepine is used for complex partial seizures, tonic-clonic seizures, and mixed seizures, which include complex partial, tonic-clonic, and other partial or generalized seizures. It has not been proven to be useful for absence seizures.

Carbamazepine is useful for complex partial and generalized seizures.

Actions and Uses. Absorption of carbamazepine is slow after oral administration, probably because of its poor water solubility. Taking the drug with meals can enhance its absorption, presumably owing to improved solubilization by the increase in secretions of gastric juice and bile. Peak plasma levels occur within 6–24 hours after an oral dose, but may appear earlier during long-term carbamazepine therapy. The drug is 70–80% bound to plasma proteins, and it distributes rapidly into all tissues. The initial major biotransformation product is the 10,11-epoxide, which possesses antiepileptic activity and is further metabolized to inactive products, mostly 10,11-dihydroxide. Further investigations are needed to determine the metabolic fate of carbamazepine.

Drug Interactions. Because carbamazepine can cause autoinduction of its metabolism during chronic administration, a decrease in its elimination half-life and acceleration of the metabolism of other drugs, such as warfarin and tetracycline, occur. The combination of carbamazepine with phenytoin decreases phenytoin clearance and increases plasma phenytoin concentration. However, carbamazepine does not alter the plasma concentration of phenobarbital, even though it may elevate phenobarbital levels derived from primidone. Phenobarbital and phenytoin may accelerate the metabolism of carbamazepine. The drug manufacturer suggests that carbamazepine should not be coadministered with monoamine oxidase (MAO) inhibitors, presumably on theoretical grounds. There are reports indicating that carbamazepine lowers the plasma level and increases the clearance of ethosuximide and valproic acid; it also decreases the plasma level and elimination half-life of clonazepam.

Side Effects and Toxicity. The more common side effects, which occur with dosages in the upper recommended therapeutic range, include drowsiness, headache, GI upset, diplopia, and blurred vision. With acute massive overdosage the following symptoms may occur: respiratory depression, coma, tremor, myoclonus, seizures, rigidity, hyperreflexia, hyporeflexia, dilated pupils, ophthalmoplegia, nystagmus, urinary retention, sinus tachycardia, and atrioventricular (A-V) conduction delay. Although serious hepatotoxicity is rare, fatal carbamazepine hepatitis has been reported. There may be transient elevations of hepatic enzymes also. Idiosyncratic reactions include skin rashes, exfoliative dermatitis, pruritic eruptions, lymphatic hyperplasia, aplastic anemia, thrombocytopenia, and pancytopenia. Cases of serious bone marrow depression have been reported, but recent reviews of clinical data indicate that the hematopoietic toxicity of carbamazepine is much less than originally feared. Most of the earlier reports of hematopoietic toxicity involved patients using other antiepileptic drugs together with carbamazepine. Nevertheless, it is prudent to monitor blood cell counts and plasma drug levels for patients who are on carbamazepine therapy. This drug should not be administered to patients with a history of hepatic disease or serious blood dyscrasia or with known hypersensitivity to any of the tricyclic compounds.

Carbamazepine can have serious side effects but they are not common.

Carbamazepine appears to have a low to negligible teratogenic effect, but a significant decrease in head circumference of neonates born to mothers taking carbamazepine has been reported. Such growth defects were not present in neonates born to mothers taking monotherapy of phenytoin or phenobarbital.

BENZODIAZEPINES

The benzodiazepines are used primarily as sedative-antianxiety drugs and are discussed in detail in Chapter 20. This section covers only their uses as antiepileptic drugs. Currently, the following are used as antiepileptic drugs in the United States: diazepam, clonazepam, and clorazepate dipotassium. Other benzodiazepines that have undergone some clinical trials as antiepileptic drugs include lorazepam, nitrazepam, and oxazepam. The benzodiazepines mentioned all have the 1,4-configuration. Clobazam is a benzodiazepine with the 1,5-configuration, and it possesses antiepileptic activity also.

Diazepam

Given intravenously, diazepam (VALIUM) is useful for the initial treatment of status epilepticus. It is indicated particularly when transient high serum and brain concentrations of the drug are needed to control uninterrupted and long-duration tonic-clonic status. However, repeated doses of IV diazepam are not recommended because of the risk of serious toxic effects, especially respiratory depression and hypotension; therefore, an adequate loading dose of another long-acting antiepileptic drug, e.g., phenytoin or phenobarbital, is usually administered in addition. Cardiorespiratory toxicity may occur if diazepam is administered to patients who have been taking high doses of other depressant drugs or antiepileptic medications. Diazepam is used sometimes as an adjunct to other primary antiepileptic drugs in treating infantile spasms, atypical absence, myoclonic, atonic, and photo-

Diazepam is the drug of choice for status epilepticus.

sensitive seizures. It has been used also in Europe as a prophylactic drug for febrile seizures in children.

Both of the main metabolites of diazepam, *N*-desmethyldiazepam and oxazepam, possess antiepileptic activity. Peak diazepam plasma concentrations occur in 0.5–3 hours after an oral dose, and steady state serum levels are reached after 4–10 days of chronic dosing (see Chapter 20).

Diazepam potentiates actions of other CNS depressants.

The common side effects of diazepam are drowsiness, ataxia, and fatigue; other symptoms include paradoxical excitement, agitation, blurred vision, confusion, and diplopia. Hepatotoxic and renal toxic side effects are rare. Physical dependence can occur with chronic diazepam administration, more commonly with high doses but it does occur with therapeutic doses. Thus, abrupt discontinuation of the drug may precipitate seizures, including status epilepticus. Diazepam potentiates the action of other CNS depressant drugs such as ethanol and barbiturates, and *vice versa*.

Clonazepam

Clonazepam is useful for myoclonic and atonic seizures as well as infantile spasms.

Although clonazepam (CLONOPIN; 5-(2-chlorophenyl)-1,3-dihydro-7-nitro-2H-1,4-benzodiazepin-2-one) is recognized by the FDA for use alone or as an adjunctive antiepileptic drug, it is used most often as an adjunct. It is effective in the treatment of absences (typical and atypical), infantile spasms, and myoclonic and atonic seizures. It has shown some efficacy also against simple and complex partial seizures and tonic-clonic seizures.

Clonazepam is absorbed rapidly from the GI tract and is mostly un-ionized at physiological pH. It is about 40–50% bound to plasma proteins. Its major metabolite is the 7-amino derivative, formed by reduction of the nitro group. Plasma levels after a given dose of clonazepam vary appreciably, making accurate prediction of plasma concentrations based on dosage difficult. The elimination half-life varies between 20 and 40 hours, with peak plasma concentrations occurring 1–3 hours after an oral dose.

Tolerance to the antiepileptic effect of clonazepam occurs in about 30% of patients, usually after 1–6 months of therapy. Of these, approximately one third will no longer respond to the drug at any dosage, whereas the remainder of the patients will still experience therapeutic benefits with increased dosage of the drug.

The most common side effects of clonazepam are drowsiness, ataxia, and behavioral changes. These effects may be accentuated by coadministration of barbiturates. Some patients may develop tolerance to drowsiness and ataxia during chronic drug therapy, but for some patients these side effects cannot be reduced to tolerable levels even by reduction of dosage. Children affected by behavioral changes may be hyperactive, irritable, aggressive, disobedient, and violent. Less common side effects include dizziness, hypotonia, hypersalivation, anorexia, increased appetite, nausea, skin rashes, and thrombocytopenia. Bronchial hypersecretion and hypersalivation can cause respiratory problems in children. When clonazepam is coadministered with valproic acid, there may be exacerbation of absence seizures. Paradoxically, clonazepam can also increase seizure frequency.

Clorazepate Dipotassium

Clorazepate dipotassium (TRANXENE; 7-chloro-2,3-dihydro-2,2 dihydroxo-5-phenyl-1H-1,4-benzodiazepine-3-carboxylic acid dipotassium salt) is used as an adjunctive drug for partial seizures. After oral administration, clorazepate is converted rapidly to *N*-desmethyldiazepam, which is the same as the active metabolite of diazepam. Peak plasma concentrations of *N*-desmethyldiazepam occur in 0.5–1 hour after an oral dose, with an elimination half-life of about 40 hours. Therefore, the ultimate metabolism of clorazepate dipotassium follows the same pathway as that of diazepam, but side effects occur apparently with less frequency than with diazepam.

MISCELLANEOUS ANTIEPILEPTIC DRUGS

Acetazolamide

Acetazolamide (DIAMOX; 5-acetamido-1,3, 4-thiadiazole-2-sulfonamide), a carbonic anhydrase inhibitor, is sometimes effective against absence seizures. It is sometimes useful also as an adjunct in the treatment of tonic-clonic, myoclonic, and atonic seizures, particularly in women whose seizures occur or are exacerbated at specific times in the menstrual cycle. However, its usefulness is transient often because of rapid development of tolerance. Its antiepileptic effect may be due to its inhibitory effect on brain carbonic anhydrase, which leads to an increased transneuronal chloride gradient, increased chloride current, and increased inhibition.

Acetazolamide is absorbed mainly from the upper small intestine, although some absorption takes place in the stomach. Peak plasma levels are reached 2 or 3 hours after oral administration. The drug is about 90% protein bound. Diffusion of the free drug into tissue is pH-dependent. Acetazolamide is not metabolized by the liver, but is excreted unchanged in the urine. The elimination of acetazolamide from the plasma follows an initial rapid phase with a half-life of 95 minutes, and a slower phase with a half-life of 10–15 hours.

Only about 10% of patients who receive treatment with acetazolamide suffer from side effects, usually mild, which include drowsiness, loss of appetite, paresthesia, and confusion. Hypersensitivity reactions, though possible, are not common. In animal studies, acetazolamide at high doses was teratogenic and embryocidal. Therefore, its use in pregnant epileptic women should be avoided whenever possible.

Miscellaneous antiepileptic drugs

Adrenocorticotropic Hormone

Adrenocorticotropic hormone (ACTH; corticotropin) is used as adjunctive therapy in infantile spasms and refractory seizures of infancy and childhood. For short-term therapy of infantile spasms there seems to be little difference between ACTH treatment and oral steroids or other antiepileptic drugs such as benzodiazepines and valproic acid. However, ACTH appears to have a better long-term outcome in terms of later epilepsies and developmental status.

Because ACTH is inactivated by proteolytic enzymes in the GI tract, it is ineffective when administered orally. Therefore, it is given in an intramuscular repository form, by subcutaneous injections, or by the IV route. It is metabolized rapidly with a plasma half-life of only 15 minutes.

The synthetic analogs of corticosterone and cortisol (e.g., prednisolone, prednisone, and dexamethasone) have been used in the treatment of infantile spasms and other refractory seizures of infancy and childhood.

Lidocaine

The local anesthetic lidocaine (XYLOCAINE) is useful for the treatment of refractory status epilepticus, although it is not approved by the FDA for the

Lidocaine is useful for refractory status epilepticus.

treatment of epilepsy. (For example, the recommended initial IV dose is 1–3 mg/kg given slowly. A second injection dose of 1 mg/kg can be given after 30 minutes.) High dosages of lidocaine may themselves cause convulsions; constant electrocardiogram (ECG) and blood pressure monitoring is necessary to detect possible cardiovascular complications.

Phenacemide

Introduced in 1949, phenacemide (PHENURONE; 1-(2-phenylacetyl)-urea) is now used rarely or is used as a reserved agent because of its serious toxic effects to most organ systems as well as severe behavioral effects. It is useful for refractory complex partial seizures and other severe, uncontrollable types of seizures.

Other Treatments

Surgical procedures may be useful in certain cases of refractory seizures.

Ward (Browne and Feldman, 1983) has suggested that a patient with epilepsy must meet four criteria if surgical therapy is to be considered: (1) the patient's seizures are intractable and are refractory to adequate medical therapy; (2) there must be an identifiable epileptogenic focus generating the seizures, and the focus needs to be confirmed by several lines of evidence; (3) the focus must be located in a dispensable part of the cortex so that it can be resected without causing major neurologic deficit; (4) the focus to be removed must be surgically accessible. Repeated studies have shown that, when patients were selected for surgical therapy based on the above strict criteria, good seizure control was obtained in a high percentage (60–80%) of the cases.

Other surgical procedures include cerebellar stimulation, stereotactic lesions, hemispherectomy, and commissurotomy. The technique of cerebellar stimulation in the treatment of epilepsy reportedly has fairly good success in seizure control and abolition of seizures, but more confirmations are needed. There is evidence that the surgical technique may damage the underlying cerebellum. The stereotactic technique for producing focal lesions was applied to the treatment of epilepsy over 20 years ago with limited effectiveness (20–40%). Hemispherectomy is used in patients whose epileptogenic lesion is distributed widely throughout much of one hemisphere. An essential criterion for the choice of this procedure is the lateralization of epileptogenic activity to one hemisphere. This surgical technique requires a large exposure and the removal of large areas of the cortex. Commissurotomy involves sectioning the cerebral commissures with the idea of preventing the spread of seizure discharges. Patients whose generalized seizures are medically intractable may have their seizures reduced dramatically after sectioning of the corpus callosum, anterior commissure, or the hippocampal commissure. However, the incidence of focal seizures is often unchanged by this procedure.

Need for New Drugs

There are several compelling reasons for the development of new antiepileptic drugs. Although antiepileptic drugs permit many patients to lead rewarding lives, clinical data do not support the widely held but erroneous belief that a large percentage of epileptic patients are adequately controlled by drug therapy. However, it should be noted that the major cause of poor seizure control is patient noncompliance with regularly taking their medications. Another consideration is that chronic toxicity is associated often with the prolonged administration of antiepileptic drugs. Therefore, the need for new drugs is clear, and the search for more effective and safer antiepileptic drugs continues, with nearly 20 new agents currently undergoing clinical evaluation and several new compounds with novel structures undergoing preclinical evaluation.

References

Beghi E, Mascio RD, Tognoni G: Drug treatment of epilepsy. Outlines, criticism and perspectives. Drugs 31:249–265, 1986.

Browne TR, Feldman RG (eds): Epilepsy: Diagnosis and Management. Boston: Little Brown & Company, 1983.

Dalessio DJ: Seizure disorders and pregnancy. N Engl J Med 312:559–563, 1985.

Delgado-Escueta AV, Treiman DM, Walsh GO: The epilepsies. Part 1. N Engl J Med 308:1508–1514, 1983.

Delgado-Escueta AV, Treiman DM, Walsh GO: The treatable epilepsies. Part 2. N Engl J Med 308:1576–1583, 1983.

Delgado-Escueta AV, Wasterlain CG, Treiman DM, Porter RJ (eds): Status Epilepticus. Mechanisms of Brain Damage and Treatment. Vol 34 of Advances in Neurology. New York: Raven Press, 1983.

Fariello RG: Biochemical approaches to seizure mechanisms: The GABA and glutamate systems. *In* Porter RJ, Morselli PL (eds): The Epilepsies, 1–19. Boston: Butterworths, 1985.

Hauser WA: Epidemiology of epilepsy. Adv Neurol 19:313–339, 1978.

Janz D, Dam M, Richens A, et al (eds): Epilepsy, Pregnancy, and the Child. New York: Raven Press, 1982.

Jones GL, Wimbish GH: Hydantoins. *In* Frey HH, Janz D (eds): Antiepileptic Drugs, 351–419. Vol 74 of Handbook of Experimental Pharmacology. Berlin: Springer-Verlag, 1985.

Knudsen FU, Vestermark S: Prophylactic diazepam or phenobarbitone in febrile convulsions: A prospective, controlled study. Arch Dis Child 53:660–663, 1978.

Kutt H: Interactions between anticonvulsants and other commonly prescribed drugs. Epilepsia 25(Suppl 2):5118–5131, 1984.

Lee K, Taudorf K, Hvorslev V: Prophylactic treatment with valproic acid or diazepam in children with febrile convulsions. Acta Paediatr Scand 75:593–597, 1986.

Levy RH, Dreifuss FE, Mattson RH, et al (eds): Antiepileptic Drugs. 3rd ed. New York: Raven Press, 1989.

Lombroso CT: A prospective study of infantile spasms: Clinical and therapeutic correlations. Epilepsia 24:135–158, 1983.

Marciani MG, Gotman J: Effects of drug withdrawal on location of seizure onset. Epilepsia 27:423–431, 1986.

Meldrum BS, Porter RJ (eds): New Anticonvulsant Drugs. Vol 4 of Current Problems in Epilepsy. London: John Libbey & Co, 1986.

Morselli PL, Pippenger CE, Penry JK (eds): Antiepileptic Drug Therapy in Pediatrics. New York: Raven Press, 1983.

Oxley J, Janz D, Meinardi H (eds): Chronic Toxicity of Antiepileptic Drugs. New York: Raven Press, 1983.

Pippenger CE: An overview of antiepileptic drug interactions. Epilepsia 25(Suppl 1):581–586, 1982.

Porter RJ, Morselli PL (eds): The Epilepsies. Boston: Butterworths, 1985.

Rodin EA: The Prognosis of Patients with Epilepsy. Springfield, IL: Charles C Thomas, 1968.

Schmidt D, Seldon L: Adverse Effects of Antiepileptic Drugs. New York: Raven Press, 1982.

Schmutz M: Relevance of kindling and related processes to human epileptogenesis. Prog Neuropsychopharmacol Biol Psychiatry 11:505–525, 1987.

Schoenberg BS: Epidemiology of epilepsy. *In* Porter RT, Morselli PL (eds): The Epilepsies, 94–105. Boston: Butterworths, 1985.

Trimble MR (ed): Chronic Epilepsy: Its Prognosis and Management. New York: John Wiley & Sons, 1990.

Wilder BJ, Bruni J: Seizure Disorders. A Pharmacological Approach to Treatment. New York: Raven Press, 1981.

Wilder BJ, Buchanan RA: Methsuximide for refractory complex partial seizures. Neurology 31:741–744, 1981.

Wolf P: The classification of seizures and the epilepsies. *In* Porter RT, Morselli PL (eds): The Epilepsies, 106–124. Boston: Butterworths, 1985.

24

Drugs Used in the Treatment of Parkinson's Disease and Other Movement Disorders

Linda A. Hershey

Parkinson's Disease

Parkinson's disease affects about 1% of the population over the age of 50.

Other forms of parkinsonism include vascular parkinsonism, progressive supranuclear palsy, Alzheimer's-type dementia, and drug-induced parkinsonism.

Tremor, rigidity, and bradykinesia (slowness on initiation and execution of body movements) make up the symptom complex first described by James Parkinson in 1817. Parkinson's disease, or idiopathic parkinsonism, is one of the most common forms of this symptom complex. It affects about 1% of the population over the age of 50. In addition to the classic triad of symptoms, patients with Parkinson's disease may also develop sialorrhea (drooling), dysarthria (inarticulate speech), masked facies, postural instability, gait disorder, hypotension, depression, and dementia.

Differential Diagnosis. Essential tremor is a more common cause of rhythmic, regular involuntary movements, affecting 5% of the general population. It is more likely than Parkinson's disease to be familial. Essential tremor is symmetrical and seen best with arms held in extension, whereas the parkinsonian tremor is usually asymmetrical and most apparent at rest. Essential tremor is usually faster (4–11 cps) than the tremor of Parkinson's disease (3–5 cps). Parkinsonian tremor may affect the tongue, lips, and jaw in addition to any of or all four extremities. The head or voice may be involved along with arms (but not legs) in essential tremor (Jankovic and Fahn, 1980). The pharmacological differentiation between Parkinson's and essential tremor is described in Table 24–1.

A patient whose chief complaint is stiffness should be evaluated to see whether the resistance to passive stretch is velocity- or direction-dependent (spasticity is affected by these parameters, whereas rigidity is not). Spasticity is associated with strokes, head injury, multiple sclerosis, and spinal cord diseases but not with Parkinson's disease. Vascular parkinsonism, like stroke, usually begins acutely in patients who are hypertensive or diabetic. It responds poorly to antiparkinsonian medications and may improve with time.

A patient whose chief complaint is slowness should have his or her eye movements evaluated carefully. Patients with progressive supranuclear palsy may present with rigidity and bradykinesia and respond initially to antiparkinsonian therapy. Later they develop paralysis of vertical gaze (downgaze paralysis, in particular). They have slow saccades also and irregularities of smooth pursuit. They have a "reptilian stare" because their eye-blink frequency (5–10/minute) is slower than that seen in patients with Parkinson's disease (10–15/minute). These eye movement abnormalities are not under the control of nigrostriatal neurons and thus do not respond to antiparkinsonian therapy.

Some patients with Alzheimer's-type dementia may develop bradykinesia, rigidity, and gait disorder a year or two after the cognitive disorder

Table 24-1 PHARMACOLOGICAL DIFFERENTIATION OF TREMOR

	Parkinson's Disease Rest Tremor	Essential Tremor
Drugs that relieve tremor	Amantadine Anticholinergics Levodopa Bromocriptine Pergolide	β blockers Primidone Phenobarbital Benzodiazepines Alcohol
Drugs that worsen tremor	Physostigmine Phenothiazines Butyrophenones Metaclopramide Reserpine MPTP	Epinephrine Terbutaline Theophylline Lithium Divalproex Tricyclics

becomes apparent (this differs from Parkinson's disease, in which dementia follows the onset of motor signs by several years). Other disorders that can mimic Parkinson's disease include Shy-Drager syndrome, olivopontocerebellar atrophy, carbon monoxide poisoning, and pugilism.

However, the most common cause of parkinsonism is drugs. Antipsychotic agents and metoclopramide can cause parkinsonian signs by blockade of central dopamine receptors (see Chapter 21). Reserpine can cause these signs by depleting nerve endings of dopamine. A byproduct in the synthesis of meperidine, 1-methyl-4-phenyl-1,2,5,6-tetrahydropyridine (MPTP), can kill dopamine neurons and produce a clinical and pathological condition nearly identical to that of Parkinson's disease. MPTP-induced parkinsonism has been recognized in young people who are intravenous drug abusers (Davis et al, 1979) and replicated in primate animal models.

> Dopamine-blocking agents are the most common cause of parkinsonism.

Clinical Stages. Parkinson's disease patients with unilateral signs (usually tremor and rigidity) have Stage I disease, according to the staging system of Hoehn and Yahr (1967). Bilateral symptoms and signs, in the absence of gait or balance problems, constitute Stage II disease. Once patients develop unsteadiness of gait or begin falling, they have Stage III Parkinson's. Stage IV patients require assistance with ambulation (a cane, walker, or another person), whereas Stage V patients are either wheelchair-bound or bed-bound.

Pathology. In Parkinson's disease, there is selective degeneration of dopamine-containing neurons in the substantia nigra and hypothalamus in addition to loss of norepinephrine-containing neurons in the locus ceruleus. There are no ischemic changes or signs of inflammation. The cause for this selective death of neurons is still unknown. The selective vulnerability of pigmented brainstem nuclei (substantia nigra and locus ceruleus) to MPTP appears to be related to the affinity of MPP$^+$ for neuromelanin (D'Amato et al, 1987). To become neurotoxic, MPTP must be converted to 1-methyl-4-phenylpyridinium (MPP$^+$) by the B isozyme of monoamine oxidase (MAO-B).

> Degeneration of substantia nigra neurons is the cause of dopamine deficiency in Parkinson's disease.

ANTICHOLINERGIC AGENTS

History. Belladonna alkaloids were used in the treatment of parkinsonism over 100 years ago. They were intended initially to relieve the sialorrhea of parkinsonism, but they were partially effective also in managing tremor. Synthetic analogs of these alkaloids were developed in an effort to find drugs with fewer adverse effects (see also Chapter 11).

Table 24-2 SYNTHETIC BELLADONNA ALKALOIDS

Generic Name	Brand Name	Dosage Forms	Daily Dosage*
Trihexiphenidyl	Artane	Tabs (2, 5 mg) Caps (5 mg)	Start: 2 mg bid Max: 5 mg qid
Benztropine	Cogentin	Tabs (0.5, 1, 2 mg) Ampule (2 mg)	Start: 0.5 mg bid Max: 2 mg qid
Ethopropazine	Parsidol	Tabs (50, 100 mg)	Start: 50 mg bid Max: 200 mg qid
Diphenhydramine	Benadryl	Caps (25, 50 mg)	Start: 25 mg bid Max: 50 mg qid

* bid = twice a day; qid = four times a day.

Chemistry. Trihexyphenidyl (ARTANE) is the prototype of the synthetic belladonna alkaloids. Table 24-2 lists dosage forms and daily dosage ranges. Benztropine (COGENTIN) was synthesized in an effort to combine the beneficial effects of an antihistamine (diphenhydramine) with those of a belladonna alkaloid (atropine). One phenothiazine with weak dopamine-blocking effects but potent anticholinergic activity is ethopropazine (PARSIDOL). If one drug in this class is not effective or causes adverse drug effects, another should be tried.

Mechanism of Action. The involvement of central cholinergic mechanisms in Parkinson's disease was inferred by the observation that a centrally acting cholinesterase (ChE) inhibitor, physostigmine, worsens signs of the disease, whereas peripherally acting ChE inhibitors have no effect. Centrally acting anticholinergic agents are able to reverse physostigmine's action (Duvoisin, 1967).

Anticholinergic agents counteract the relative excess of striatal cholinergic activity in Parkinson's disease.

Organ Pharmacology. These observations fit well with evidence that the striatum (caudate and putamen) contains the highest concentration of acetylcholine (ACh) in the brain. The striatum also contains high activities of enzymes involved in ACh synthesis and degradation. As Parkinson's disease progresses, there is less inhibitory (dopaminergic) input to the striatum from the substantia nigra. This results in excessive central cholinergic activity that can be controlled to some extent with anticholinergic agents.

Adverse Effects. Central side effects of anticholinergic agents include confusion, hallucinations, and impairment of memory. Lethargy and depression are seen less commonly. Demented patients are more vulnerable to these central adverse effects of anticholinergic agents than are those without cognitive impairment. Peripheral side effects of these agents, such as dry mouth and constipation, must be tolerated usually in order to achieve an antiparkinsonian effect. Patients should be advised to stop the drug if they experience urinary retention or blurred vision. A lower dose can be resumed once the possibility of prostatic hypertrophy or glaucoma has been excluded.

Therapeutic Uses. Anticholinergic agents are sometimes effective in treating mild tremor and rigidity in early Parkinson's disease, but their most effective use is in the treatment of drug-induced parkinsonism and dystonia. In Parkinson's disease, they are more effective when used in combination with levodopa than when used alone. Use of anticholinergic agents is not advised in patients known to have dementia, benign prostatic hypertrophy, or glaucoma.

Drug Interactions. Anticholinergic agents delay gastric emptying and thus interfere with the absorption of levodopa or neuroleptics, drugs known to be absorbed in the duodenum and destroyed in the stomach (Rivera-Calimlim, 1976). Anticholinergic drugs also have additive adverse effects with other agents, such as tricyclic antidepressants, antihistamines, and antispasmodics.

Preparations and Dosages. Table 24–2 outlines the dosage forms of currently marketed anticholinergic agents in addition to the daily dosage ranges used in the treatment of Parkinson's disease. Much higher doses of these drugs are required for the treatment of the idiopathic dystonias (20–30 mg/day). Early-onset Parkinson's disease patients (onset between 20 and 40 years) commonly experience painful dystonia even before antiparkinson therapy is initiated. They may respond favorably to high doses of anticholinergic agents.

Summary. As monotherapy, anticholinergic agents are more effective in the treatment of drug-induced parkinsonism and dystonia than they are in the treatment of Parkinson's disease. The exception to this rule is the patient with early-onset Parkinson's disease, whose dystonia may be the most striking clinical feature. In most Parkinson's disease patients, anticholinergic agents are more effective when used in combination with levodopa than when used alone.

Anticholinergic agents are most effective in treating drug-induced parkinsonism and the dystonia seen in early-onset Parkinson's disease.

AMANTADINE

History. Amantadine was developed initially as an antiviral agent. In 1968, a woman with Parkinson's disease was being treated with amantadine for protection against the influenza virus when she noticed marked improvement in her parkinsonian symptoms. This led to clinical trials in Parkinson's disease patients (Schwab et al, 1969).

Chemistry and Mechanism of Action. Amantadine is a 10-carbon-cage amine that is soluble in water. Its primary mechanism of action is the enhancement of dopamine release, but it is also a weak dopamine agonist and a blocker of dopamine and norepinephrine reuptake.

Amantadine works primarily to enhance the release of central dopamine.

Adverse Effects. Few patients experience serious side effects from amantadine. Some are unable to tolerate ankle edema or livido reticularis (a mottled reddish-purple pattern on the legs). Amantadine rarely causes dizziness, nausea, abdominal pain, confusion, hallucinations, or headache. These symptoms diminish with dosage reduction and disappear with discontinuation.

Therapeutic Uses. Amantadine is useful in treating Parkinson's disease patients early in their disease course (Fahn and Isgreen, 1975). Patients with Stage III–IV disease may develop tolerance to its therapeutic effect over weeks to months. However, as many as 40% experience significant improvement lasting a year or more (Butzer et al, 1975). Patients who do not respond well to amantadine alone may notice a synergistic effect with the addition of carbidopa/levodopa. Use of amantadine in epileptic patients is not advised, because excessive dosages or drug interactions may precipitate seizures. Use in acute renal failure is contraindicated also, because this drug depends on renal clearance.

Amantadine is most useful in the early stages of Parkinson's disease.

Drug Interactions. The synergistic interaction of amantadine with levodopa may be exploited for the benefit of patients who lose (or never had) therapeutic benefit with amantadine alone (Fahn and Isgreen, 1975). Patients with tremor alone may benefit from the synergistic action of amantadine with an anticholinergic agent.

Preparations and Dosages. Amantadine is available in a liquid form (50 mg/5 mL) as well as in tablet form (100 mg). The usual starting dose is 200 mg/day in two divided doses, and the usual maintenance dose is 300 mg/day. Early-onset Parkinson's disease patients may be able to tolerate 400 mg/day. Frail elderly patients with Parkinson's or Alzheimer's disease may benefit from small doses of the liquid formulation (50–100 mg/day in two to four doses).

Summary. Amantadine is an excellent first-line drug in managing Parkinson's disease patients early in the course of their disease. When the disease has progressed to the extent that therapeutic benefit is lost, amantadine can be used as an adjunct to carbidopa/levodopa. The liquid form of amantadine is useful in treating the rigidity of frail elderly patients with Parkinson's or Alzheimer's disease.

LEVODOPA

History. Birkmayer and Hornykiewicz (1962) were the first to demonstrate the effectiveness of intravenous (IV) levodopa in Parkinson's disease patients. In addition, they showed that neither dopamine nor 5-hydroxytryptamine (5-HT) (a precursor to serotonin) was effective. In the same year, Barbeau demonstrated the benefit of oral levodopa in reducing parkinsonian rigidity and akinesia. Five years later, Cotzias and coworkers (1967) reported sustained effectiveness with higher daily doses of oral levodopa than those used in earlier clinical trials. All these early investigators noted that reduction of tremor required much higher doses of levodopa than did reduction of the signs of rigidity or bradykinesia.

Chemistry. Levodopa is an aromatic amino acid that is produced naturally by tyrosine hydroxylase as the product of the rate-limiting step of catecholamine synthesis. It is the immediate precursor to dopamine and, unlike dopamine, is capable of crossing the blood-brain barrier. The dopamine reuptake system in striatal neurons is able to transport levodopa into dopamine-synthesizing neurons.

Levodopa

Levodopa stimulates dopamine synthesis in central nigrostriatal pathways.

Mechanism of Action. Levodopa stimulates dopamine synthesis in the remaining healthy neurons in Parkinson's disease patients and at least partially corrects central dopamine deficiency. In order to reduce peripheral side effects and maximize the amount of levodopa delivered to the central nervous system (CNS), levodopa is almost always given in combination with an inhibitor of the peripheral amino acid decarboxylase (carbidopa or benserazide). Oral carbidopa has been shown to double the bioavailability of orally administered levodopa (Nutt et al, 1985).

Organ Pharmacology. Parkinson's disease patients are known to have reduced spinal fluid concentrations of homovanillic acid (HVA), a metabolite of dopamine. The fact that HVA concentrations in spinal fluid increase with levodopa therapy provides evidence that this drug enhances the central synthesis of dopamine. Autopsy data also show higher concentrations of dopamine and HVA in the caudate nuclei of levodopa-treated patients, compared to similar brain regions of untreated Parkinson's disease patients.

Acute Adverse Effects. The most common acute side effects of levodopa are nausea, vomiting, anorexia, and "dizziness" due to orthostatic hypotension. These symptoms can be prevented by preloading the patient with 75 mg/day of carbidopa (available to physicians through the manufacturer). Because carbidopa does not cross the blood-brain barrier, there is still a risk of central side effects acutely (dyskinesias, confusion, hallucinations, nightmares). For these reasons, low doses of carbidopa/levodopa are prescribed initially (50/200 mg/day in two divided doses). Central adverse effects can be overcome by simply lowering the total daily dose of carbidopa/levodopa.

Carbidopa reduces the peripheral adverse effects of levodopa, but not the central adverse effects.

Chronic Adverse Effects. Prior to the introduction of levodopa, certain motor fluctuations, such as freezing episodes, could cause a patient to become suddenly immobile. Conversely, a patient could experience "kinesia paradoxica," or sudden mobility, triggered by a startle reflex (a call of "fire," for example).

Today when a patient becomes increasingly immobile about 2–3 hours after his dose of carbidopa/levodopa, it is most likely due to the *wearing-off effect,* a sign of reduced storage capacity for dopamine in degenerating neurons (Spencer and Wooten, 1984; Fabbrini et al, 1987).

The excessive mobility ("on") that patients develop within minutes to hours of taking a dose of carbidopa/levodopa is referred to as *peak-dose dyskinesia.* These choreiform movements coincide with peak concentrations of levodopa in plasma. Patients are most functional when they are "on." When "on" and "off" episodes occur with no particular relationship to the timing of the carbidopa/levodopa dose, the patient is said to be experiencing the *"on-off"phenomenon.* Postsynaptic, as well as presynaptic, changes are thought to be involved in this chronic adverse effect (Fabbrini et al, 1987).

Therapeutic Uses. Most authors recommend starting carbidopa/levodopa when the patient is functionally disabled and unresponsive to less potent antiparkinsonian drugs (Fahn and Bressman, 1984). The rationale for this is to avoid as many of the long-term complications of levodopa as possible, especially because the drug's effectiveness seems to wear off after 3–4 years. Some start the drug whenever parkinsonian symptoms become a nuisance (Markham and Diamond, 1981). Others advise saving levodopa for patients with balance and gait problems.

Carbidopa/levodopa is recommended for Parkinson's disease patients who are either functionally disabled or unresponsive to less potent drugs.

Contraindications. Although levodopa is quite effective in treating the symptoms and signs of idiopathic Parkinson's disease, it is less helpful in treating other forms of parkinsonism. The rigidity of progressive supranuclear palsy and Alzheimer's disease may respond to low doses of carbidopa/levodopa, but these patients are more vulnerable than nondemented patients to drug-induced confusion and hallucinations. Schizophrenic patients should not be treated with carbidopa/levodopa for drug-induced parkinsonism, because they are also more vulnerable to the drug's neurotoxic effects.

Drug Interactions. There is a significant dietary interaction with levodopa, because it competes with amino acids for its absorption into the gut and across the blood-brain barrier (Nutt et al, 1984). In order to reduce the likelihood of adverse gastrointestinal (GI) side effects, patients are advised initially to take carbidopa/levodopa with meals. Later in the course of therapy (after the development of tolerance to acute side effects), patients are usually encouraged to take the drug on an empty stomach in order to

Table 24-3 LEVODOPA AND DOPAMINE AGONISTS			
Generic Name	**Brand Name**	**Dosage Forms**	**Daily Dosage***
Levodopa	Larodopa	Tabs (100 mg, 250 mg, 500 mg)	Start: 100 mg bid Max: 2000 mg qid
Carbidopa/levodopa	Sinemet	Tabs (25/100, 10/100, 25/250)	Start: 25/100 bid Max: 50/500 qid
Benserazide/levodopa	Madopar	Caps (125/250)	Start: 125/250 qd Max: 250/500 qid
Bromocriptine	Parlodel	Tabs (2.5 mg) Caps (5 mg)	Start: 1.25 mg qhs Max: 10 mg qid
Pergolide	Permax	Tabs (0.05 mg, 0.25 mg, 1 mg)	Start: 0.05 mg qhs Max: 1 mg qid

* bid = twice a day; qid = four times a day; qd = every day; qhs = at bedtime.

Patients who are losing the therapeutic effect of carbidopa/levodopa are advised to reduce the amount of protein in their diets.

Motor fluctuations can be avoided if low dosages of carbidopa/levodopa are used in combination with dopamine agonist or deprenyl.

speed absorption and maximize bioavailability. Patients who seem to be losing the therapeutic effect of levodopa are advised to minimize protein in their morning and noon meals in order to maximize bioavailability of levodopa during daytime hours.

Preparations and Dosages. The most appropriate carbidopa/levodopa preparation for initial therapy is the 25/100 formulation (Table 24-3). This allows for enough carbidopa to block the peripheral decarboxylase (usually 75-100 mg/day is required). A low dosage (50/200/day in two divided doses) should be used for the first few days to avoid orthostatic hypotension and nausea. A maintenance dosage of 75/300/day may be effective for a year or more in many Stage III Parkinson's disease patients. Adjunctive therapy with amantadine, bromocriptine, pergolide, or deprenyl may prolong the safe use of low-dose carbidopa/levodopa.

Some advanced Parkinson's disease patients require up to 2000 mg/day of levodopa (the 25/250 formulation can be given in four to eight divided doses per day). Once "on-off" develops, the dosages should be reduced and given more frequently (the 10/100 formulation can be given every 2 hours in eight or ten divided doses per day). The patient should understand that the goal of therapy is to restore function, not to erase every sign and symptom of the disease. Patients should not be permitted to take "as needed" dosages, because that practice may lead to peak-dose dyskinesia.

Summary. The carbidopa/levodopa preparations available today remain the most effective therapy for Parkinson's disease patients who are functionally disabled (Stages III-V). Because motor fluctuations are such a common adverse effect of long-term carbidopa/levodopa use, newer sustained-release preparations are under investigation. Other studies are focusing on finding the optimal combination of adjunctive therapies to minimize long-term adverse effects and maximize long-term benefits from carbidopa/levodopa.

BROMOCRIPTINE

History. Bromocriptine, an ergot derivative that acts as a dopamine agonist, was developed initially as a drug to treat hyperprolactinemia and its associated signs of amenorrhea and galactorrhea (Parkes, 1979). The dosage that suppresses prolactin is one tenth of that which improves the symptoms of Parkinson's disease. Bromocriptine also reduces plasma levels of growth hormone in patients with acromegaly through a direct inhibitory effect on the pituitary.

Chemistry and Mechanism of Action. This chemically complex ergot derivative (2-bromo-alpha-ergocryptine) must be extracted from fungi because it cannot be synthesized easily. Bromocriptine works as a D2 agonist and a D1 antagonist. There are two types of striatal dopamine receptors: the D1 receptor that stimulates adenyl cyclase and depolarizes (excites) the postsynaptic neuron, and the D2 receptor that inhibits adenyl cyclase and hyperpolarizes (inhibits) the postsynaptic neuron. The D2 receptor is located both pre- and postsynaptically. Dopamine acts as both a D1 and D2 agonist. The increased efficacy of bromocriptine when given in combination with carbidopa/levodopa is most likely due to the ability of dopamine (acting at D1 sites) to put the D2 site into its high-affinity state (Clark and White, 1987).

Bromocriptine is more effective when used in combination with carbidopa/levodopa than when used alone.

Organ Pharmacology. Coadministration of bromocriptine with carbidopa/levodopa is an appropriate treatment for Parkinson's disease patients who have developed diminished responsiveness to, or peak-dose dyskinesias from, levodopa. Agonist therapy is particularly helpful when there are fewer neurons available to synthesize dopamine. Dyskinesias are thought to be mediated through D1 receptors. This explains why dyskinesias are reduced when bromocriptine is added and the dose of carbidopa/levodopa reduced.

Adverse Effects. Patients should be warned about the *first-dose phenomenon* (collapse due to orthostatic hypotension) that is seen in 1% of subjects given a single bromocriptine dose of 1.25 mg (one half of a 2.5-mg tablet). Hypotension results from relaxation of smooth muscle in the splanchnic and renal circulations as well as central sympathetic inhibition (Parkes, 1979).

Other adverse effects of bromocriptine include nausea and vomiting. Raynaud's phenomena may occur with the hands turning purple or blue when immersed in cold water or exposed to cold air. Livedo reticularis is a purplish discoloration that gives the legs a mottled appearance. Hallucinations may result from hydrolysis of the lysergic acid fragment from the bromocriptine molecule or from agonist action at D2 receptors. Hallucinations can be avoided usually by gradually dropping the dose of carbidopa/levodopa while increasing the bromocriptine dose.

Therapeutic Uses. Bromocriptine was recommended originally for advanced Parkinson's disease patients who had become less responsive to carbidopa/levodopa or who had developed response fluctuations. Recent studies have suggested combining bromocriptine with carbidopa/levodopa early in an effort to prevent the development of motor fluctuations (Rinne, 1985). Monotherapy with bromocriptine is not recommended because it is less effective, more costly, and more toxic (nausea and vomiting) than monotherapy with carbidopa/levodopa.

Relative contraindications for bromocriptine include patients with dementia, because they are more likely to experience hallucinations and confusion. Patients with peripheral vascular disease and ischemic heart disease are more likely to develop adverse vascular effects.

Drug Interactions. The synergistic value of using bromocriptine in combination with carbidopa/levodopa was discussed earlier. Amantadine, which enhances the release of dopamine presynaptically, also acts in synergy with bromocriptine. In fact, the three drugs can be used in combination with one another, provided the adverse effects of each are monitored carefully (Parkes, 1979).

Preparations and Dosages. Bromocriptine tablets of 2.5 mg and capsules of 5 mg are currently available (see Table 24–3). Patients are advised to take half of the 2.5-mg tablet at bedtime for the first week in order to prevent orthostatic hypotension. Dosage increases should be made no more rapidly than 2.5 mg/week in order to avoid adverse effects. The optimal maintenance dose, when given in combination with carbidopa/levodopa, is about 10–20 mg/day (Hoehn and Elton, 1985).

Summary. Bromocriptine, a D2-selective agonist, is most useful as adjunctive therapy for Parkinson's disease patients who have reduced effects or who have developed peak-dose dyskinesias from carbidopa/levodopa. Bromocriptine also prevents motor fluctuations if it is used as an adjunct to carbidopa/levodopa early in the course of the disease.

PERGOLIDE

History. Pergolide is marketed as adjunctive therapy for use in the management of advanced Parkinson's disease when there is loss of therapeutic benefit from or dyskinesias caused by carbidopa/levodopa.

Chemistry and Mechanism of Action. Pergolide mesylate is an ergoline derivative that is primarily a D2 agonist, but it has some weak D1-activating properties also. It is 10–100 times more potent than bromocriptine on a milligram per milligram basis. Like bromocriptine, it inhibits the secretion of prolactin in humans.

Involuntary movements are less common with bromocriptine and pergolide because of their selective blockade of D2 receptors.

Adverse Effects. In early clinical trials, more orthostatic hypotension was seen in groups that received pergolide in addition to carbidopa/levodopa than in those treated with carbidopa/levodopa alone. Tolerance to this side effect usually develops over the first 3–4 weeks of therapy. Tolerance is less likely to develop to the visual hallucinations or daytime sedation that is seen in some patients. Reduction in the dose of carbidopa/levodopa is recommended when these adverse effects appear, although discontinuation of the pergolide is sometimes necessary (Ahlskog and Muenter, 1988a). Involuntary movements are uncommon with pergolide because of its D2 selectivity. Nausea, nasal congestion, anxiety, ankle swelling, and an erythematous rash have been reported also with pergolide.

Pergolide and bromocriptine are similar to each other in both their therapeutic and toxic effects.

Therapeutic Uses. The effectiveness of pergolide as an adjunct to carbidopa/levodopa has been shown to be comparable to that of bromocriptine in a crossover study of Parkinson's disease patients with a wide range of baseline disabilities (LeWitt et al, 1983). It is particularly effective as an adjunct in Parkinson's disease patients who are experiencing motor fluctuations or declining levodopa efficacy (Jankovic, 1986; Ahlskog and Muenter, 1988b).

Drug Interactions. The synergistic interaction between pergolide and carbidopa/levodopa is evident in the studies described earlier. In one of these, the addition of pergolide permitted a 46% reduction, on average, in the daily dose of carbidopa/levodopa (Jankovic, 1986). In another, the addition of pergolide allowed for a reduction in the carbidopa/levodopa dosing frequency from a median of 7.5 doses/day to 5.0 doses/day (Ahlskog and Muenter, 1988b). Dopamine antagonists such as neuroleptics or metoclopramide should not be administered concurrently with pergolide, because they will diminish the drug's effectiveness.

Preparations and Dosages. If the patient has not been treated previously with bromocriptine, then the 0.05-mg preparation of pergolide should be given at a dosage of one tablet at bedtime for the first few days (see Table 24–3). The dosage can be increased by 0.1-mg increments every 3 days over the first 2 weeks of therapy. The 0.25-mg and 1.0-mg formulations can be used for subsequent dosage adjustments as a stable daily dose of 1–5 mg is reached. If the patient has been treated previously with bromocriptine, then either a gradual or an abrupt substitution can take place using the 1 : 10 ratio as a guideline (1 mg of pergolide for every 10 mg of bromocriptine).

Summary. Pergolide, like bromocriptine, is effective as an adjunct to carbidopa/levodopa in the treatment of advanced stages of Parkinson's disease. Future studies are needed to determine whether it might be useful early in the disease to prevent progression or the development of motor fluctuations.

DEPRENYL

History. Deprenyl (selegiline) was shown originally in an animal model of parkinsonism to prevent MPTP-induced destruction of neurons in the substantia nigra. In a retrospective study, Parkinson's disease patients who took deprenyl and levodopa in combination lived longer than patients who took levodopa alone (Birkmayer et al, 1985). These data have provided the impetus for several larger prospective clinical trials.

Chemistry and Mechanism of Action. Deprenyl, or phenylisopropyl-N-methylpropynylamine, is a Type B-selective MAO inhibitor that slows the catabolism of dopamine and reduces the formation of oxygen radicals. It is rapidly absorbed from the GI tract and readily crosses the blood-brain barrier. Deprenyl is metabolized to L-amphetamine and L-methamphetamine. Ongoing studies are examining whether the effects of deprenyl are symptomatic (by increasing synaptic availability of dopamine), protective (by reducing formation of oxygen radicals), or both. Several studies have suggested that oxidatively mediated mechanisms contribute to the degeneration of pigmented neurons in the substantia nigra of patients with Parkinson's disease (Parkinson Study Group, 1989a).

> Deprenyl slows the catabolism of dopamine and reduces the formation of oxygen radicals.

Adverse Effects. At the recommended dosage of 5 mg twice a day, deprenyl does not cause the same side effects as nonselective MAO inhibitors (especially hypertension after ingestion of tyramine-containing foods and beverages). At daily dosages higher than this, however, deprenyl begins to lose its MAO-B selectivity. If taken in combination with carbidopa/levodopa, deprenyl can exacerbate or precipitate dopaminergic adverse effects such as chorea, confusion, or hallucinations. These side effects can be eliminated by reducing the dose of carbidopa/levodopa by 10–30%. Insomnia, nausea, and dry mouth are other common complaints.

Therapeutic Uses. Deprenyl ameliorates the wearing-off effect for 1–2 years in about 50% of advanced Parkinson's disease patients, whereas it benefits fewer patients who experience either random fluctuations (on-off)

In untreated Parkinson's disease patients, deprenyl delays the need for carbidopa/levodopa by about 1 year.

or decreased benefit from carbidopa/levodopa (Elizan et al, 1989). In early, untreated Parkinson's disease patients, deprenyl has been shown in a double-blind study to delay the need for carbidopa/levodopa by about a year and to prolong the duration of full-time employment (Parkinson Study Group, 1989b).

Drug Interaction. The synergistic interaction between deprenyl and carbidopa/levodopa has been used for therapeutic benefit in patients with advanced disease who are experiencing the wearing-off effect. Ongoing studies will determine its effectiveness in slowing the progression of disease in early levodopa-treated Parkinson's disease patients. Deprenyl is contraindicated for use with meperidine; caution is warranted for any opioid.

Preparations and Dosages. The only preparation of deprenyl currently available is the 5-mg tablet formulation (ELDEPRYL). This is administered twice daily with breakfast and lunch (to minimize both insomnia and nausea). Reduced dosages (5 mg/day) are beneficial to some patients.

Summary. Deprenyl (selegiline) is useful for a few years in augmenting the effectiveness of carbidopa/levodopa in Parkinson's disease patients who are experiencing the wearing-off phenomenon. It is effective also in early, untreated Parkinson's disease patients in that it delays the onset of significant disability and maintains the patient's ability to continue full-time employment.

Essential Tremor

Essential tremor affects about 5% of the general population, whereas Parkinson's disease affects less than 1%. Essential tremor is seen in all age groups, although the frequency of tremor falls and the amplitude rises with age (Jankovic and Fahn, 1980). The frequency of this postural tremor is usually faster (4–11 cps) than that of the parkinsonian rest tremor (3–6 cps). In addition to the postural tremor, the head may shake with a yes or a no motion and the voice may be affected also (vocal tremor). Essential tremor is referred to as *familial tremor* when a positive family history is elicited. Essential tremor is uniquely abolished by alcohol.

Differential Diagnosis. Other tremors that are rapid, symmetrical, and postural are those caused by drugs (β agonists, theophylline, amphetamines, lithium, tricyclic antidepressants, neuroleptics, adrenocorticosteroids, and divalproex). Syndromes that can produce a postural tremor include hyperthyroidism, hypoglycemia, pheochromocytoma, and chronic anxiety disorders. Situational anxiety and fatigue can cause tremor as well.

PROPRANOLOL

Propranolol reduces tremor amplitude in 50–70% of patients with essential tremor.

History. Propranolol was the first β blocker to be used in the treatment of essential tremor (Dupont et al, 1973; Winkler and Young, 1974). Although it may not abolish essential tremor, propranolol can reduce tremor amplitude in 50–70% of patients so affected.

Mechanism of Action. Peripheral adrenergic mechanisms are intact in essential tremor. Infusion of intra-arterial isoproterenol increases the amplitude of essential tremor, and this increase (not the underlying tremor) can be blocked by intra-arterial propranolol. In contrast, chronic oral propranolol is capable of reducing the amplitude of the underlying tremor. These findings suggest that propranolol has a sensory or central action in the treatment of essential tremor (Young et al, 1975).

Adverse Effects. Because propranolol can induce bronchospasm, it is contraindicated in patients with chronic obstructive lung disease or asthma. A selective β_1 antagonist, such as metoprolol, is preferable for these patients. Propranolol is contraindicated also in patients with brittle diabetes, because it may mask the symptoms of hypoglycemia (tremor, tachycardia, and diaphoresis). It can lower blood pressure, so it should be used cautiously, or not at all, in patients whose blood pressure is lower than normal.

Therapeutic Uses. Propranolol is useful in the treatment of not only essential tremor, but also drug-induced postural tremors such as those unmasked by tricyclic antidepressants or lithium. Lower doses than those used in essential tremor are usually effective in the treatment of drug-induced tremors. Essential tremor patients who are not compliant with taking three or four doses of propranolol each day should take nadolol, a β blocker with a 24-hour half-life that can be given once daily (Koller, 1983).

Drug Interactions. Because propranolol can depress cardiac output and reduce hepatic blood flow, it can decrease the clearance (and cause toxicity) of drugs that are metabolized by the liver (e.g., lidocaine, cimetidine, theophylline).

Preparations and Dosages. Propranolol is usually started at low doses (10 mg three times a day) in normotensive individuals in order to avoid hypotension. If this dose is well tolerated, the therapeutic range (120–320 mg/day) can be reached within 1–2 weeks, provided the increments are made gradually. Nadolol may be started at 40 mg/day in a single daily dose, and the therapeutic range (120–240 mg/day) can be approached within 1–2 weeks.

Summary. Although propranolol reduces the amplitude of essential tremor in 50–70% of patients, it does not usually abolish the tremor completely. Combination with primidone is now recommended for optimal therapeutic management of essential tremor. Nadolol is effective in treating essential tremor and is more convenient because of its once-daily dosing.

PRIMIDONE

History. In 1981, O'Brien and colleagues noted that a patient with both epilepsy and essential tremor experienced reduction in tremor amplitude while being treated with the anticonvulsant primidone. They treated 20 other essential tremor patients and found a good clinical response in 12 (six could not tolerate the drug's adverse effects).

Primidone produces more acute toxicity than does propranolol, but is slightly more effective in treating essential tremor.

Chemistry and Mechanism of Action. Primidone, whose half-life is 10 hours, is converted to two active metabolites: phenylethylmalonamide (PEMA) with a half-life of 24–48 hours, and phenobarbital with a half-life of 50–120 hours. PEMA is not effective in reducing the amplitude of essential tremor. It is unlikely that phenobarbital adds to the benefit of primidone, because maximal benefit can be seen within the first seven hours after a single dose before plasma phenobarbital concentrations are measurable. The mechanism for primidone's antitremor action is unknown (Koller and Royse, 1986).

Adverse Effects. Vertigo, nausea, and unsteadiness are early adverse effects of primidone that are often dose-limiting. Patients should be warned that they may experience a flu-like syndrome (headache, nasal congestion, and nausea), but this is usually short-lived. Some authors have noted that essential tremor patients tolerate primidone less well than do seizure patients (O'Brien et al, 1981). Nevertheless, Koller and Royse (1986) found only 12% of essential tremor patients to be intolerant of primidone, provided the doses were built up gradually.

Therapeutic Uses. Treatment of essential tremor can be started with either primidone or propranolol. Lower doses of both medications can be used to maximize therapeutic benefit and minimize adverse effects.

Drug Interactions. The synergistic interaction between primidone and propranolol may be exploited for patients who gain only partial benefit from propranolol alone.

Preparations and Dosages. Primidone is available in 50-mg and 250-mg tablets. The usual starting dosage is 50 mg at bedtime. The dosage may be increased slowly to 250 mg at bedtime. Further increases are unlikely to provide more therapeutic benefit for essential tremor.

Summary. Some clinicians now use primidone as a first-line drug in the treatment of essential tremor. Although a small percentage cannot tolerate its adverse effects, the majority find it to be more effective than propranolol in the reduction of tremor amplitude. Use of the two drugs in combination is more advantageous than either drug used alone.

Huntington's Disease

This autosomal dominant disorder is characterized early on by chorea (jerky, unpredictable involuntary movements) and psychiatric disturbances (personality change, psychosis, or depression). Later in the course of the disease, patients develop progressive intellectual impairment (dementia), gait disorder, and slurred speech (dysarthria). The symptoms initially appear in the fourth or fifth decade of life in most patients. Juvenile-onset cases (before the age of 20) are often not recognized, because the primary clinical symptoms (seizures, dystonia, and rigidity) are so different from those seen in adults. Senile-onset cases (over the age of 60) are difficult to recognize as well, because symptoms are mild, dementia is rare, and progression is slow.

Differential Diagnosis. A careful drug history should be taken from patients suspected of having Huntington's disease, because drug-induced chorea (tardive dyskinesia or levodopa-induced dyskinesia) is common and may appear to be clinically similar (Jankovic, 1981). The acute onset of hemichorea should suggest a lacunar infarction of the basal ganglia. Young adults with chorea should be screened for Wilson's disease, systemic lupus erythematosus, thyrotoxicosis, and hypoparathyroidism. In children, the possibilities of Sydenham's chorea or chorioathetoid cerebral palsy should be considered. Senile chorea is a more benign syndrome than Huntington's, because the chorea is unaccompanied by dementia, psychiatric disturbance, or family history.

There is a relative excess of nigrostriatal dopamine in Huntington's disease.

Pathology. There is preservation of the dopaminergic pathway of the nigrostriatal system in Huntington's disease in spite of widespread destruction of other striatal neurons (Martin, 1984). Concentrations of several neurotransmitters are decreased: gamma-aminobutyric acid (GABA), ACh, substance P, and enkephalins, whereas dopamine concentrations are either normal or elevated. The most striking abnormality on imaging studies or on gross examination of the brain is severe caudate atrophy, even though cortical atrophy is usually present in addition.

HALOPERIDOL

History. Haloperidol was administered to psychotic inpatients originally, mostly schizophrenics, who had been refractory to phenothiazine therapy (Ayd, 1972). Its use in Huntington's disease began with the treatment of the associated psychosis, but it was later found to ameliorate the chorea as well. It is now the drug used most commonly to treat this condition.

Haloperidol improves both the psychosis and the chorea of Huntington's disease.

Chemistry. Haloperidol is a butyrophenone with a chemical structure completely different from that of the phenothiazines. It is absorbed rapidly and almost completely with a plasma half-life of 12–20 hours. Although there seems to be a therapeutic range of plasma concentrations required for the treatment of acute psychoses (10–40 ng/mL), lower concentrations are effective in the treatment of movement disorders (Rivera-Calimlim and Hershey, 1984).

Mechanisms of Action. Central dopamine receptor blockade is the mechanism by which haloperidol is thought to work in treating both the psychosis and the chorea of Huntington's disease. Both of these signs are thought to be caused by a relative excess of central dopamine.

Adverse Effects. The most common adverse effects of haloperidol are motoric; acute dystonia is seen within days of initiating therapy, drug-induced parkinsonism within weeks, and tardive dyskinesia within months to years. Tardive dyskinesia can be minimized by using the lowest dose that is still effective in controlling psychosis and chorea.

Therapeutic Uses. Whereas extremity chorea may respond to haloperidol, the gait disorder of Huntington's disease does not (Koller and Trimble, 1985). Psychosis, anxiety, agitation, and hostility are the most common psychiatric disturbances seen in Huntington's disease. All respond well to haloperidol. Nevertheless, the drug does not change the long-term course of the disease.

Preparation and Dosages. Haloperidol is available in 0.5-mg, 1-mg, 2-mg, and 5-mg tablets and as a colorless and tasteless solution containing 2 mg/mL. It is available also in ampules of 5 mg (1 mL) for intramuscular (IM) and IV injection. Doses of 1–4 mg/day in two divided doses are used to initiate therapy. Doses in excess of 10–20 mg/day are rarely required. Ironically, less drug is usually needed as the disease progresses, because the chorea lessens in severity over time.

Summary. Haloperidol is probably the most commonly used neuroleptic in patients with Huntington's disease. It is an excellent antipsychotic agent and also can reduce chorea to some extent. It is not effective in treating the gait disorder of Huntington's disease. Patients on long-term therapy with haloperidol should be examined at each visit for the presence of tardive dyskinesia, because this movement disorder is reversible in its early stages.

Malignant Hyperthermia

Rigidity in the masseter, pterygoid, and temporalis muscles (trismus) is often the first sign of malignant hyperthermia. Fever is not necessarily present early on, but tachycardia, tachypnea, and flushing are usually

The clinical presentation of neuroleptic malignant syndrome is similar to that of malignant hyperthermia.

quick to follow the onset of rigidity. Later signs include fever, excessive bleeding (consumption coagulopathy), heart failure, metabolic acidosis, myoglobinuria, and renal failure. Most patients with malignant hyperthermia are recognized in the operating room, but others do not show signs of the fully developed syndrome until they arrive in the recovery room. Virtually all inhalation anesthetics can produce malignant hyperthermia (for example, halothane) as can skeletal muscle relaxants (succinylcholine). Mortality rates were once 60–70%, but these are now closer to 10–30% (Britt, 1974; Britt, 1979).

Differential Diagnosis. Neuroleptic malignant syndrome bears many similarities to malignant hyperthermia. Fever, rigidity, tachycardia, and myoglobinuria can be seen in both conditions (Kurlan et al, 1984). Two important differences include drug exposure histories (neuroleptic malignant syndrome is usually seen in acutely psychotic patients who are being treated with accelerating dosages of neuroleptic agents) and family histories (the propensity to malignant hyperthermia is a dominantly inherited trait). Serum creatine phosphokinase is elevated in both disorders (a syndrome similar to the neuroleptic malignant syndrome has been reported in the absence of neuroleptics [Parsa et al, 1990]).

Heat stroke patients are usually hypotonic, not rigid. They are hypotensive, not hypertensive. Otherwise, they are similar to patients with malignant hyperthermia in that they are febrile, have elevated creatine phosphokinase levels, and may develop myoglobinuric renal failure and consumption coagulopathy. Lethal catatonia seen in schizophrenia usually involves severe rigidity without hyperthermia, tachycardia, tachypnea, or elevated enzyme levels.

Pathology. Excessive cytoplasmic calcium accumulation can be induced by certain anesthetic agents in muscle biopsy tissue removed from patients who have experienced malignant hyperthermia. Ryan and associates (1974) showed reduced adenosinetriphosphatase (ATPase) activity in biopsy material obtained at the time a patient was symptomatic. In this tissue there was also reduced calcium uptake into the sarcoplasmic reticulum. When the same patient underwent a second surgical procedure under ketamine, an anesthetic agent not associated with malignant hyperthermia, the muscle ATPase activity and calcium uptake were normal.

Malignant hyperthermia is caused by drug-induced interference with calcium reuptake into the sarcoplasmic reticulum.

Summary. Malignant hyperthermia is a rare, but potentially lethal, condition that is due to drug-induced interference with calcium uptake into the sarcoplasmic reticulum. Without the relaxation that calcium uptake normally provides for the excitation-contraction coupling process, a hypermetabolic state develops that is manifested by rigidity, fever, hypertension, tachycardia, and tachypnea. The propensity for developing this condition is inherited as an autosomal dominant trait.

DANTROLENE

History. Dantrolene was developed originally as a muscle relaxant to treat the spasticity associated with stroke, multiple sclerosis, or cord injury (Dykes, 1975). Development of the porcine model for malignant hyperthermia allowed dantrolene to be tested as a therapeutic and prophylactic agent (Gronert et al, 1976). Oral dantrolene was shown later to prevent malignant hyperthermia in humans, and the intravenous form proved effective for treating the fully developed syndrome (Gronert, 1980).

Chemistry and Mechanism of Action. Dantrolene is a hydantoin derivative that is unique among muscle relaxant drugs in that it acts directly on skeletal muscle. It has no effect on neuromuscular transmission or electrical properties of muscle membranes. Instead, it decreases the rate of calcium release from the sarcoplasmic reticulum, so that less calcium is available to activate the contractile apparatus (Hainaut and Desmedt, 1974) (see Chapter 25).

By decreasing the rate of calcium release from the sarcoplasmic reticulum, dantrolene can prevent signs and symptoms of malignant hypothermia.

Adverse Effects. Potentially fatal hepatitis, pleural effusion, pericarditis, and pericardial effusion have been reported on rare occasions with chronic oral dantrolene (Utili et al, 1977; Petusevsky et al, 1979). The most common adverse effects seen with acute dosing are weakness, nausea, dizziness, and drowsiness.

Therapeutic Uses. Because oral dosing of dantrolene results in peak plasma concentrations at about 4 hours, most authors recommend confining prophylactic therapy to 24 hours preoperatively. When malignant hyperthermia develops unexpectedly, all inhalation anesthetic agents and succinylcholine must be discontinued, the acidosis treated, and dantrolene injected intravenously (Hall, 1980).

Preparations and Dosages. The 25-mg tablet preparation of dantrolene is used for prevention of malignant hyperthermia in high-risk patients. Twenty-four hours in advance of the surgery, 5 mg/kg is given in three to four divided doses. To treat the fully developed syndrome, small IV aliquots of 1 mg/kg should be given at 5–10 minute intervals until the symptoms resolve. Most patients respond to a total dose of 2–3 mg/kg, although up to 10 mg/kg has been used in the porcine model without serious adverse effects (Hall, 1980).

Summary. Whereas malignant hyperthermia once carried a mortality rate of 60–70%, it is now lethal in only 10–30% of patients. This is due in large part to a better understanding of its pathophysiology, better management of the acidosis, and prophylactic or therapeutic use of dantrolene.

General References

Ahlskog JE, Muenter MD: Pergolide: Long-term use in Parkinson's disease. Mayo Clin Proc 63:979–987, 1988a.

Ahlskog JE, Muenter MD: Treatment of Parkinson's disease with pergolide: A double-blind study. Mayo Clin Proc 63:969–978, 1988b.

Ayd FJ: Haloperidol: Fifteen years of clinical experience. Dis Nerv Syst 33:459–469, 1972.

Barbeau A: The pathogenesis of Parkinson's disease. Can Med Assoc J 87:802–807, 1962.

Birkmayer W, Hornykiewicz O: The L-dopa effect on Parkinson syndrome in man. Arch Psychiatr Nervenkr 203:560–574, 1962.

Birkmayer W, Knoll J, Reiderer P, et al: Increased life expectancy resulting from addition of L-deprenyl to Madopar treatment in Parkinson's disease: A long-term study. J Neural Transm 64:113–127, 1985.

Britt BA: Malignant hyperthermia: A pharmacogenetic disease of skeletal and cardiac muscle. N Engl J Med 290:1140–1142, 1974.

Britt BA: Malignant hyperthermia. Int Anesthesiol Clin 17:1–182, 1979.

Butzer JF, Silver DE, Sahs AL: Amantadine in Parkinson's disease. Neurology 25:603–606, 1975.

Clark D, White FJ: D1 dopamine receptor—The search for a function: A critical evaluation of the D1/D2 dopamine receptor classification and its functional implications. Synapse 1:347–388, 1987.

Cotzias GC, VanWoert MH, Schiffer LM: Aromatic amino acids and modification of parkinsonism. N Engl J Med 276:374–378, 1967.

D'Amato RJ, Alexander GM, Schwartzman RJ, et al: Evidence for neuromelanin involvement in MPTP-induced neurotoxicity. Nature 327:324–326, 1987.

Davis GC, Williams AC, Markey SP, et al: Chronic parkinsonism secondary to intravenous injection of meperidine analogues. Psychiatry Res 1:249–254, 1979.

Dupont E, Hansen JJ, Dalby MA: Treatment of benign essential tremor with propranolol. Acta Neurol Scand 49:75–84, 1973.

Duvoisin RC: Cholinergic-anticholinergic antagonism in parkinsonism. Arch Neurol 17:124–136, 1967.

Dykes MHM: Evaluation of a muscle relaxant: Dantrolene sodium (Dantrium). JAMA 231:862–864, 1975.

Elizan TS, Yahr MD, Moros DA, et al: Selegiline as an adjunct to conventional levodopa therapy in Parkinson's disease: Experience with this type B monoamine oxidase inhibitor in 200 patients. Arch Neurol 46:1280–1283, 1989.

Fabbrini G, Juncos J, Mouradian MM, et al: Levodopa pharmacokinetic mechanisms and motor fluctuations in Parkinson's disease. Ann Neurol 21:370–376, 1987.

Fahn S, Bressman SB: Should levodopa therapy be started early or late? Evidence against early treatment. Can J Neurol Sci 11:200–206, 1984.

Fahn S, Isgreen WP: Long-term evaluation of amantadine and levodopa combination in parkinsonism by double-blind crossover analyses. Neurology 25:695–700, 1975.

Gronert GA: Human malignant hyperthermia: Awake episodes and correction by dantrolene. Anesth Analg (Paris) 59:377–378, 1980.

Gronert GA, Milde JH, Theye RA: Dantrolene in porcine malignant hyperthermia. Anesthesiology 44:488–495, 1976.

Hainaut K, Desmedt JE: Effect of dantrolene sodium on calcium movements in single muscle. Nature 252:728–730, 1974.

Hall GM: Dantrolene and the treatment of malignant hyperthermia. Br J Anaesth 52:847–849, 1980.

Hoehn MM, Elton RL: Low dosages of bromocriptine added to levodopa in Parkinson's disease. Neurology 35:199–206, 1985.

Hoehn MM, Yahr MD: Parkinsonism: Onset, progression and mortality. Neurology 17:427–442, 1967.

Jankovic J: Drug-induced and other orofacial-cervical dyskinesias. Ann Intern Med 94:788–793, 1981.

Jankovic J: Pergolide: Short-term and long-term experience in Parkinson's disease. *In* Fahn S, Marsdon CD, Jenner P, Teychenne P (eds): Recent Developments in Parkinson's Disease, 339–345. New York: Raven Press, 1986.

Jankovic J, Fahn S: Physiologic and pathologic tremors. Ann Intern Med 93:460–465, 1980.

Klawans HL, Weiner WJ: Parkinsonism. *In* Nausieda PA, Goetz CG (eds): Textbook of Clinical Neuropharmacology, 1–35. New York: Raven Press, 1981.

Koller WC: Nadolol in essential tremor. Neurology 33:1076–1077, 1983.

Koller WC, Royse VL: Efficacy of primidone in essential tremor. Neurology 36:121–124, 1986.

Koller WC, Trimble J: The gait abnormality of Huntington's disease. Neurology 35:1450–1454, 1985.

Kurlan R, Hamill R, Shoulson I: Neuroleptic malignant syndrome. Clin Neuropharmacol 7:109–120, 1984.

LeWitt PA, Ward CD, Larsen TA, et al: Comparison of pergolide and bromocriptine therapy in parkinsonism. Neurology 33:1009–1014, 1983.

Markham CH, Diamond SG: Evidence to support early levodopa therapy in Parkinson's disease. Neurology 31:125–131, 1981.

Martin JB: Huntington's disease: New approaches to an old problem. Neurology 34:1059–1072, 1984.

Nutt JG, Woodward WR, Anderson JL: The effect of carbidopa on the pharmocokinetics of intravenously administered levodopa. Ann Neurol 18:537–543, 1985.

Nutt JG, Woodward WR, Hammerstad JP, et al: The "on-off" phenomenon in Parkinson's disease: Relation to levodopa absorption and transport. N Engl J Med 310:483–488, 1984.

O'Brien MD, Upton AR, Toseland PA: Benign familial tremor treated with primidone. Br Med J 282:178–180, 1981.

Parkes D: Bromocriptine. N Engl J Med 301:873–878, 1979.

Parkinson Study Group: DATATOP: A multicenter clinical trial in early Parkinson's disease. Arch Neurol 46:1052–1060, 1989a.

Parkinson Study Group: Effect of deprenyl on the progression of disability in early Parkinson's disease. N Engl J Med 321:1364–1371, 1989b.

Parsa MA, Rohr T, Ramirez LF, Meltzer HY: Neuroleptic malignant syndrome without neuroleptics. J Clin Psychopharmacol 10:437–438, 1990.

Petusevsky ML, Faling LJ, Rocklin RE, et al: Pleuropericardial reaction to treatment with dantrolene. JAMA 242:2772–2774, 1979.

Rinne UK: Combined bromocriptine-levodopa therapy early in Parkinson's disease. Neurology 35:1196–1198, 1985.

Rivera-Calimlim L: Impaired absorption of chlorpromazine in rats given trihexyphenidyl. Br J Pharmacol 56:301–305, 1976.

Rivera-Calimlim L, Hershey L: Neuroleptic concentrations and clinical response. Annu Rev Pharmacol Toxicol 24:361–386, 1984.

Ryan JF, Donlon JV, Malt RA, et al: Cardiopulmonary bypass in the treatment of malignant hyperthermia. N Engl J Med 290:1121–1122, 1974.

Schwab RS, England AC, Poskanzer DC, Young RR: Amantadine in the treatment of Parkinson's disease. JAMA 208:1168–1170, 1969.

Spencer SE, Wooten GF: Altered pharmacokinetics of L-dopa metabolism in rat striatum deprived of dopaminergic innervation. Neurology 34:1105–1108, 1984.

Utili R, Boitnott JK, Zimmerman HJ: Dantrolene-associated hepatic injury: Incidence and character. Gastroenterology 72:610–616, 1977.

Winkler GF, Young RD: Efficacy of chronic propranolol therapy in action tremors of the familial, senile, or essential varieties. N Engl J Med 290:984–988, 1974.

Young RR, Growdon JH, Shahani BT: Beta-adrenergic mechanisms in action tremor. N Engl J Med 293:950–953, 1975.

25

Skeletal Muscle Relaxants

Cedric M. Smith

Relaxation of skeletal muscle can be achieved by drug actions at many different sites.

Skeletal muscle hyperactivity is an end result of a variety of pathophysiological mechanisms.

Drugs that act at the neuromuscular junction can cause muscle relaxation; they can also cause muscle paralysis, including respiratory failure.

Drugs Acting Directly on Skeletal Muscle — Intracellular in Muscle Fibers

Dantrolene is unique with its intracellular site of action.

Clinically, spasticity is characterized by exaggerated stretch reflexes.

Drugs covered in this chapter are commonly included in the category of *centrally acting muscle relaxants,* which refers to a heterogenous group of drugs used to produce muscle relaxation, excepting the neuromuscular blocking agents such as tubocurarine used in anesthesia. The skeletal muscle relaxants have their primary clinical and therapeutic uses in the treatment of muscle spasm and immobility associated with strains, sprains, and injuries of the back and, to a lesser degree, injuries to the neck. They have been used also for the treatment of a variety of clinical conditions that have in common only the presence of skeletal muscle hyperactivity, for example, the muscle spasms that can occur in multiple sclerosis.

These drugs are a heterogenous group not only in terms of their chemistry and sites of actions but also in terms of their mechanisms of action as well as their clinical uses. Some of them are discussed in other sections of the book, for example, diazepam (VALIUM) in the antianxiety chapter (Chapter 20). General pharmacology and organ system pharmacology of such agents are not repeated in this chapter; the reader is referred to those chapters in which the drugs are discussed in greater detail.

The agents are discussed in order of their sites of action, starting in the ultimate periphery, the skeletal muscle itself, and ending with the agents that have actions at the cortical and midbrain levels in the central nervous system (CNS). Drugs used strictly in the treatment of Parkinson's disease that may have rigidity as one of its components as well as tremor, and drugs used in the treatment of tremors of central origin, are covered in Chapter 24.

DANTROLENE

Dantrolene (DANTRIUM) is a unique drug in terms of its effects and site of action. Dantrolene's action is restricted to the intracellular space inside skeletal muscle fibers; specifically, it interrupts the sarcoplasmic excitation-contraction coupling responsible for muscle contraction. This intracellular action in skeletal muscle is associated with a reduction of the release of calcium ions that initiate muscle contraction.

Dantrolene has found its greatest utility in the treatment of spasms and spasticity associated with cerebral palsy and of the spasticity and mass-reflex movements that can occur in paraplegic and hemiplegic patients. However, although it produces relaxation, in larger doses and in certain muscles it can produce muscle weakness — an extension of its therapeutic effect.

Muscle spasm and spasticity is only one of the reasons why individuals with cerebral palsy have disordered, uncoordinated muscle function. To the degree that the excessive activity of muscle spasticity impairs normal muscle coordination and strength, its relaxation is therapeutically beneficial. However, in muscle groups in which the major functional defect is primarily an inadequate coordination, relaxation and weakness frequently further impair functional capabilities. The major problem in cerebral palsy is most often a defect in the coordination of muscle activity rather than excessive tone or muscle spasticity. Although reducing spasticity may be useful therapeutically and functionally when that is impairing movement, there are limits to the numbers of individuals for whom it is helpful and to the magnitude of beneficial effects that can be achieved by any muscle relaxant.

Although dantrolene can be used in other syndromes such as low back spasm, it is not commonly used for that purpose. A unique use of dantrolene is in the management of the malignant neuroleptic syndrome and in the syndrome of malignant hyperthermia. These syndromes are described briefly in Chapter 24 where the antipsychotic drugs are covered, the agents that have been associated most closely with the malignant neuroleptic syndrome. The major objectives of the use of muscle relaxants in these conditions is the rapid reduction in the excessive muscle activity, resulting in decreased hyperthermia and avoidance of the damage to muscle that can result in myoglobinemia, myoglobinuria, and possible kidney damage.

Adverse Reactions

The most frequent reactions to dantrolene are drowsiness, dizziness, and weakness. It can also result in a wide variety of side effects, including insomnia, gastrointestinal (GI) disturbances, mental confusion, myalgia, and abnormal hair growth. The major limitation to the chronic use of dantrolene is the possible occurrence of severe liver toxicity or pleural effusion. Both these serious side effects warrant close monitoring of all patients receiving this drug. The individuals at higher risk of such side effects are those with pre-existing liver damage, females, and patients over 35 years of age; it also appears that long-term use increases the risk.

DANTROLENE

In addition to having effects on extrafusal muscle fibers responsible for developing muscle contractions, shortening, and force, dantrolene's effect on muscle intrafusal fibers results in a relaxation of these fibers and thus a decrease in the activity from muscle spindles. Muscle spindles are a major source of afferent input from skeletal muscle. Each muscle spindle has at least one primary ending or one or more afferent endings wrapped around a complex of eight to twelve intrafusal muscle fibers; all of the intrafusal fibers serve to regulate the sensitivity of the stretch receptors. At the risk of oversimplification, the primary endings sense *rate* of stretch of the muscle, whereas the secondary endings are much more exclusively involved in sensing only the *static length* of the muscle. Thus the primary and secondary endings are each under selective regulation by the contractions of intrafusal muscle fibers; the individual intrafusal fibers are specialized so that some of them primarily regulate the sensitivity to the dynamic rate of change of length, whereas others are more involved in regulating the static length sensitivity of the muscle spindle afferents.

Rigidity, clinically, is characterized by sustained, abnormally increased, skeletal muscle activity.

The malignant neuroleptic syndrome and malignant hyperthermia are both marked by excessive muscle activity, muscle damage, and hyperthermia.

The major limitation to the use of dantrolene is its potential to produce severe liver toxicity.

Drugs Acting on the Sensory Systems of Muscle — Influence on Muscle Spindle Afferents and Intrafusal Fibers

Skeletal muscle activity integrally involves the coordinated activity of afferent input with efferent output.

Skeletal muscle afferent systems also receive ongoing efferent regulation through the fusimotor system.

Muscle activity involves potentially every neuron in the brain.

The actions of drugs on sensory systems of muscle are also discussed in Chapter 26.

Relaxants With Multiple Sites of Action Including Muscle Afferents

The so-called centrally acting muscle relaxants have multiple potential sites of action in the nervous and muscle systems.

Some centrally acting drugs fail to exert clinically useful muscle relaxant effects — for example, morphine and opioids, meprobamate, most barbiturates, and most benzodiazepines other than diazepam.

Phenytoin depresses the generation and propagation of repetitive action potentials in sensory nerves, cardiac arrhythmias, and neuralgias — in addition to epilepsy.

Agents Acting on Skeletal Muscle Membrane

Myotonia congenita — Thomsen's disease

The muscle spindle system as well as the tendon organs are complex components of the even more complex motor control system; they are involved in spinal regulation of motor control as well as midbrain and cerebellar coordination of muscle activity, both postural tone as well as movements. In addition, the spindle afferents project to the cerebral cortex; however, the function of these extensive cortical projections is not well understood. For this chapter it is sufficient to note that the muscle spindle system is intricately involved in maintenance of muscle tone, the occurrence of muscle spasm and muscle rigidity, and disturbances of muscle coordination. (Agents that excite muscle spindle afferent endings do not play a role as muscle relaxants; these are discussed in Chapter 26 on sensory actions of drugs.)

METHOCARBAMOL

Mephenesin was the first compound with selective muscle relaxant actions that did not act directly on muscle. It is obsolete therapeutically because of its short duration of action. Another drug of the same chemical class and with many of the same actions is methocarbamol (ROBAXIN). Mephenesin, and probably methocarbamol, depress muscle spindle afferent activity, presumably by a direct effect on the muscle spindle ending; this effect occurs with doses that are associated with muscle relaxation. These and related compounds have spinal cord sites of action and are discussed further later.

PHENYTOIN

Phenytoin (DILANTIN), the well-known antiepileptic drug, has been shown experimentally and in clinical studies to have a relaxing effect, especially when it is combined with chlorpromazine. Phenytoin's action is to decrease the excitability of the sensory ending of muscle spindles to stretch; this effect has been found to occur in experimental preparations of rigidity in concentrations consistent with those obtained clinically.

QUININE

The old drug quinine (QUINAMM), which has a long time-honored use as an antipyretic, analgesic and antimalarial drug, remains in medicine for its unique ability to stabilize the muscle membrane against repetitive activity. It is used in two specific disease conditions. One is myotonia congenita (Thomsen's disease), a congenital condition in which there are repetitive action potentials generated in the muscle fibers following a single or brief excitation/contraction. In this condition, there appears to be a failure in the ability to relax a previously contracted muscle. Another condition of repetitive muscle activity is the nocturnal muscle cramp, which can be particularly distressing in the elderly. Quinine is effective in these disease states because it decreases the repetitive generation of action potentials along membranes and especially along the membranes of skeletal muscle fibers.

Site and Mechanism of Action

A muscle contraction is initiated by an action potential that travels down the axon from the motor neuron to the neuromuscular junction, and the release of the neurotransmitter followed by the generation of a single propagated action potential along the muscle fiber. In myotonia a single action potential generated from the neuromuscular junction along the muscle membrane is associated not with just a single potential but with a burst of repetitive action potentials that results in a short-lasting tetanus; with many muscle fibers these repetitive action potentials give rise to a muscle cramp. This repetitive activity occurs not only in a single motor unit in single muscle fibers but in a number of muscle fibers at approximately the same time. The action of quinine is quite similar to the action and mechanism of action of its optical isomer quinidine, consisting of an antiarrhythmic effect on the heart. The mechanism of action of quinine is similar to that of quinidine in three ways: a membrane-stabilizing action, interference with the voltage-dependent sodium permeability, and increased threshold for action-potential generation (see Chapter 33).

Quinine, optical isomer of quinidine

Side Effects

For the most part the side effects of quinine are similar to those of quinidine. These side effects have received the time-honored name of *cinchonism*, which derives from the fact that quinine is obtained from the bark of the cinchona tree. These side effects consist of disturbances of hearing and vision, including tinnitus, deafness, vertigo, blurred vision, photophobia, and even retinal ischemia. Disturbances of GI function are common and include nausea, vomiting, or diarrhea; somewhat less common side effects consist of rashes, pruritus, angioedema, and hypersensitivity. The side effects of quinine, like quinidine, can include cardiac irregularities also. The chronic use of quinine has been associated with headaches and fever. (Quinine is also mentioned as an example of a drug that affects sensory systems in Chapter 26.)

Cinchonism — the syndrome of quinine toxicity

CALCIUM/CALCIUM CHANNEL-BLOCKING AGENTS

The intravenous administration of calcium salts in the form of calcium gluconate has been used in the past for the treatment of muscle cramps. But this therapy has been largely discontinued. There are also clinical reports of the effectiveness of verapamil, the calcium channel–blocking agent, for the treatment of muscle cramps (discussed in greater detail in Chapter 31).

Muscle cramps may be a side effect of calcium channel blockers, yet these agents are sometimes used to treat muscle cramps.

METHOCARBAMOL

Methocarbamol (ROBAXIN) is the prime agent of this class that remains in the clinical armamentarium. Methocarbamol and mephenesin were shown in the early 1950s to have selective effects on spinal cord reflexes that were mediated over multineuronal pathways, as compared with its effects on the monosynaptic reflex. When the mono- and polysynaptic reflexes of a given segment of the spinal cord were tested with barbiturate or with ether anesthesia, the two types of reflexes were depressed to approximately equivalent degrees; a 50% depression of the monosynaptic reflex would be accompanied by approximately 50% depression of the polysynaptic reflex. In contrast, mephenesin and methocarbamol selectively depressed the polysynaptic spinal reflexes to a greater degree than the monosynaptic. This simple observation led to the categorization of a class of agents that were assumed to act as muscle relaxants by blocking interneurons in multisynaptic reflex chains.

Other agents frequently included in this category of interneuron blocking agents, and presumed to act in a similar fashion, are chlorzoxazone (PARAFLEX), metaxalone (SKELAXIN), and carisoprodol (SOMA). As a mat-

Drugs Acting Solely or in Part on Spinal Cord Reflexes

What are the therapeutic objectives of using a muscle relaxant? Relief of pain, of anxiety, of incoordination, limitation of movement, of muscle spasm. . . . Which??

ter of fact, however, these agents are not selective in their effects on inter-neurons, and in larger concentrations actually depress motor neurons as well. Their actions on interneurons are not the sole site or mechanism of their muscle relaxant actions. They also depress reflexes that impinge on fusimotor neurons (those neurons that innervate intrafusal muscle fibers) and thereby depress muscle spindle afferent activity indirectly. In addition, these agents have a number of other actions that are plausibly associated with their clinical utility as muscle relaxants in cases of spasticity and rigidity, such as depression of repetitive activation of neurons and depression of posttetanic potentiation, as tested with spinal monosynaptic reflexes.

DIAZEPAM

Diazepam (VALIUM) is unique among the benzodiazepines in having a selective effect to produce muscle relaxation in doses equal to or below those that cause a reduction in anxiety or sleep. The muscle relaxant activity of diazepam is in part related to its action at the spinal cord level where it augments presynaptic inhibition; diazepam increases the gamma-amino-butyric acid (GABA)–mediated actions presynaptically on the excitatory boutons on the motor neuron. In fact, it was the demonstration of the site of this action that helped define the unique action of the benzodiazepines, first on presynaptic inhibition and second on GABA-mediated inhibition. (The site and mechanism of action of diazepam is discussed in the chapter dealing extensively with benzodiazepines, Chapter 20.)

The major limitations in the therapeutic use of most of the muscle relaxant drugs including diazepam are the dose-related side effects of sedation, drowsiness, and muscle incoordination; sufficient doses of the agents result in ataxia or sleep.

BACLOFEN

Baclofen (LIORESAL) has unique actions at the spinal, and probably supra-spinal, levels to reduce the excitatory synaptic influences on the motor neuron and other neurons in the descending excitatory pathway to skeletal muscle. Baclofen reduces the release as well as the efficacy of the excitatory amino acid transmitters. In this connection it probably acts to block the release and action of both aspartate and glutamate at least at the spinal cord level. Interestingly, the drug is a structural analog of GABA, and it was synthesized originally with the idea that it would interact with the GABA system. It acts, at least in part, as an agonist on GABA β receptors at spinal and supraspinal sites in the substantia nigra (Turski et al, 1990). Thus, it decreases the reflex excitation of the motor neuron as well as the influence of descending excitation inasmuch as these depend upon an adequate level of excitability of the motor neuron in order to evoke muscle contraction or sustained muscle activity.

Baclofen has found its greatest use in muscle spasm associated with neurological disease, such as multiple sclerosis and spinal cord injury.

The side effects of baclofen, in addition to the predictable weakness and fatigue, include nausea, GI disturbances, confusion, headache, insomnia, urinary frequency, and mania. A variety of neurological symptoms following baclofen have been reported, but it may be difficult to interpret whether they are due to the drug, the underlying disease, or the combination.

CYCLOBENZAPRINE

Cyclobenzaprine (FLEXERIL) is a close chemical relative of amitriptyline. Somewhat unexpectedly it was found to produce relaxation of experimentally produced rigidities and, subsequently, the muscle spasms in human disease conditions. Cyclobenzaprine appears to have a unique profile of action. Its site of action is in the midbrain and at the spinal level, resulting in a depression of repetitive motor neuron activity. It produces a selective depression of the experimental rigidity following spinal cord ischemic damage with a wider margin of safety than most other relaxants. In addition, in larger doses cyclobenzaprine has sedative and sleep-inducing activity and has a side effect profile quite similar to amitriptyline. Evidence to date suggests, nevertheless, that cyclobenzaprine is much more effective as a muscle relaxant than is amitriptyline or any other tricyclic antidepressant. (The complexity of clinical low back syndromes and drug actions can be illustrated by the fact that psychiatric depression itself predisposes individuals to low back syndromes. Depression also augments and aggravates pain. In addition, the tricyclic antidepressants have a limited analgesic effect and are used in the management of a variety of chronic pain conditions.)

> Cyclobenzaprine has a side effect profile similar to tricyclic antidepressants.

In addition to causing drowsiness, cyclobenzaprine has the same side effects as amitriptyline, including the cardiac and atropine-like effects. It has all of the characteristic effects of anticholinergic agents, including drowsiness and mental confusion, as well as the peripheral autonomic effects of dry mouth, paralysis of accommodation, and changes in GI function.

> In treating low back pain/spasm due to muscle and tendon strain, learn to use a few drugs well.

As might be anticipated, the muscle relaxant drugs already mentioned act not only at the spinal level but also at the supraspinal level. To the degree that they have been investigated, most have actions at supraspinal, midbrain, or higher levels that may be more important quantitatively than their actions at the spinal cord level. This general conclusion is not based on extensive research of all available agents; those that have been examined and found to have midbrain and supraspinal actions are diazepam, methocarbamol, orphenadrine, cyclobenzaprine, baclofen, phenytoin, and chlorpromazine.

Drugs and Drug Action at Supraspinal and Cerebellar Levels

> The specific sites of the supraspinal actions of muscle relaxants have not been elucidated.

ORPHENADRINE

Orphenadrine (NORFLEX) has some clinical efficacy as an adjunct to rest and physical therapy in the relief of painful musculoskeletal disorders. It produces relaxation of skeletal muscle hyperactivity, notably that associated with strains and sprains of the low back muscles, ligaments, and tendons.

Orphenadrine has been shown to act supraspinally to decrease experimental rigidity in part by decreasing the excitation of fusimotor neurons and the fusimotor outflow to muscle spindles and, thereby, depressing stretch reflexes.

The side effects of orphenadrine are associated with its anticholinergic action — dry mouth, tachycardia, urinary retention, blurred vision, mental confusion, drowsiness, constipation, or hallucinations.

CHLORPROMAZINE

Chlorpromazine (THORAZINE) has been long known to depress the fusimotor system at some site(s) between the cerebellum and midbrain to the spinal cord level. In conditions in which there is hyperactivity of fusimotor neurons, chlorpromazine depresses fusimotor neuron outflow and thereby depresses muscle spindle sensitivity and the associated stretch reflexes.

The combination of phenytoin with chlorpromazine has been found to be effective in reducing muscle spasm and spasticity. It appears that the muscle spindle activity is effectively suppressed by combining an agent that acts directly on the afferent ending with an agent (chlorpromazine) that decreases fusimotor outflow. (The possibility of using other agents, such as methocarbamol or cyclobenzaprine in combination with phenytoin or other spindle afferent depressants, has not been explored; there are few data by which one could predict what such a combination might accomplish. It is theoretically possible that the combination would be appreciably more effective and less toxic than any single agent.)

Comments on Sites and Mechanisms of Action

In the treatment of low back syndromes, the muscle relaxant drugs are solely *adjuncts* to physical therapy, rest, nonsteroidal anti-inflammatory agents, and other therapy.

Table 25–1 summarizes various sites of action of the different drugs mentioned. The muscle spasm and spasticity, such as that associated with acute strains or repeated strains of the lower back, are made worse by anxiety or depression. In addition, poor posture and generally inadequate muscle tone are primary risk factors.

The recovery from an acute low-back insult requires the individual to avoid further strain and stress and to limit motion until the inflammation and reflex hyperactivity resolves. Thus, *bed rest, the use of nonsteroidal anti-inflammatory agents, and application of physical therapy interventions are essential components of the overall management of an acute back strain.* Drugs are appropriately viewed as adjuncts of the overall management of the disease condition, and not as the primary or definitive therapy. Overall, any drug that promotes bed rest or restful sleep will tend to be beneficial for acute back strains, and any drug that tends to improve the level of anxiety or depression will also be potentially beneficial. The complexity of back injuries and their reflex consequences has made it difficult to ascertain the specific sites of drug action. It is generally accepted that the drugs presented in this chapter have some limited efficacy and when used appropriately as adjuncts do provide some benefit. Nevertheless, their effects are not profound, and other influences may be equally or more important than the drug therapy itself.

Table 25–1   PRIMARY SITES OF ACTION OF SKELETAL MUSCLE RELAXANTS

Drug or Class:	Muscle	Muscle Membrane	Neuro-muscular Junction	Muscle Spindle Afferent	Muscle Spindle Fusimotor	Spinal Cord: Presynaptic	Motor Neuron	Inter-neurons	Mid-brain	Basal Ganglia	Cortex (Antianxiety, Sedation)
Dantrolene	+										
Quinine		+									
Phenytoin				+							
Chlorpromazine					+						+
Tubocurarine/ succinylcholine (and related)			+		+						
Methocarbamol				+	+	+	(+)	+	+		+
Diazepam					+	+			+	S.N.	+
Baclofen						+	+			S.N.	
Cyclobenzaprine									+		+
Antiparkinsonian Agents											
Amantadine										+	
Biperiden, trihexyphenidyl (and related)										+	

S.N. = substantia nigra

When utilizing drugs as muscle relaxants, the objectives of therapy need to be addressed at the outset — whether this be muscle spasm and its reduction, improved muscle coordination, or the modification of pain. These objectives need to take into account the many factors that can influence the syndromes or their persistence, such as anxiety and depression.

The therapeutic management of many patients with low back and other syndromes in which muscle spasm is a feature remains far from satisfactory. Drugs are not uniquely useful, in part because the primary objectives of treatment are other than on muscle spasm. For example, for many conditions the major goals of therapy may be to increase range of motion or to abolish pain, whereas these so-called relaxant drugs in fact may have little effect on mobility or pain as such. Moreover, only a limited number of clinical trials have been carried out; head-to-head comparisons of the different drugs for relaxant effects have not been done.

Some clinicians suggest that the drug against which they would compare other drugs would be cyclobenzaprine, whereas others would select diazepam or an adequate dose of one of the nonsteroidal anti-inflammatory drugs. These differences in clinical opinion reflect the fact that these agents may be effective but only to a limited degree. A useful strategy would be to use a given agent and increase the dose until benefit or side effects occur. If no useful effect is obtained and the condition persists, an alternate drug could be tried using a similar approach.

In addition to the low-back syndromes, there are a number of conditions that are associated characteristically with skeletal muscle hyperactivity in which drug therapy may be beneficial. These include the hand-shoulder syndrome, the temporomandibular joint syndrome, stiff neck or wry neck, stiff man syndrome, black widow spider bites, nocturnal muscle cramps, the neck pain associated with the use of new eyeglasses, as well as the muscle spasms that accompany arthritis, spinal cord injury, and multiple sclerosis.

Comments on Therapeutic Uses of Muscle Relaxants

Skeletal muscle relaxant drugs are a diverse group of agents used to treat a diverse group of clinical syndromes.

References

Barnes CD, Fung SJ, Gintautas J: Brainstem noradrenergic system depression by cyclobenzaprine. Neuropharmacology 19:221–224, 1980.

Basmajian JV: Acute back pain and spasm. A controlled multicenter trial of combined analgesic and antispasm agents. Spine 14:438–439, 1989.

Bennett RM, Gatter RA, Campbell SM, et al: A comparison of cyclobenzaprine and placebo in the management of fibrositis. A double-blind controlled study. Arthritis Rheum 31:1535–1542, 1988.

Borenstein DG, Wiesel, SW: Low Back Pain: Medical Diagnosis and Comprehensive Management. Philadelphia: WB Saunders Co, 1989.

Brooks VB: The Neural Basis of Motor Control. New York: Oxford University Press, 1986.

Cohan SL, Raines A, Panagakos J, Armitage P: Phenytoin and chlorpromazine in the treatment of spasticity. Arch Neurol 37:360–364, 1980.

Davidoff RA: Antispasticity drugs: Mechanisms of action. Ann Neurol 17:107–115, 1985.

Delwaide PJ: Electrophysiological analysis of the mode of action of muscle relaxants in spasticity. Ann Neurol 17:90–95, 1985.

Eldred E, Yellin H, Desantis M, Smith CM: Supplement to bibliography on muscle receptors: Their morphology, pathology, physiology and pharmacology. Exp Neurol 55(Part 2):1–118, 1977.

Hershey LA: Newer muscle-relaxant drugs. In Yetiv JS, Bianchine JR (eds): Recent Advances in Clinical Therapeutics II: Psychopharmacology, Neuropharmacology, and Gastrointestinal Therapeutics, 113–125. San Diego: Grune & Stratton, 1983.

Kirkaldy-Willis WH (ed): Managing Low Back Pain. 2nd ed. New York: Churchill Livingstone, 1988.

Martyn J, Goldhill DR, Goudsouzian NG: Clinical pharmacology of muscle relaxants in patients with burns. J Clin Pharmacol 26:680–685, 1986.

Nauta WJH, Feirtag M: Fundamental Neuroanatomy. New York: WH Freeman & Company, 1986.

Raines A: Centrally acting muscle relaxants. *In* Pradhan SN, Maickel RP, Dutta SN (eds): Pharmacology in Medicine: Principles and Practice, 184–188. Bethesda, MD: SP Press International, 1986.

Raines A, Mahany TM, Baizer L, et al: Description and analysis of the myotonolytic effects of phenytoin in the decerebrate cat: Implications for potential utility of phenytoin in spastic disorders. J Pharmacol 232:283–294, 1985.

Share NN, McFarlane CS: Cyclobenzaprine: A novel centrally acting skeletal muscle relaxant. Neuropharmacology 14:675–684, 1975.

Smith CM: The pharmacology of sedative/hypnotics, alcohol, and anesthetics: Sites and mechanisms of action. *In* Martin WR (ed): Drug Addiction I, 413–587. Vol 45/1 of Handbook of Experimental Pharmacology. Heidelberg: Springer-Verlag, 1977.

Turski L, Klockgether T, Schwarz M, et al: Substantia nigra — A site of action of muscle relaxant drugs. Ann Neurol 28:341–348, 1990.

Ward A, Chaffman MO, Sorkin EM: Dantrolene: A review of its pharmacodynamic and pharmacokinetic properties and therapeutic use in malignant hyperthermia, the neuroleptic malignant syndrome and an update of its use in muscle spasticity. Drugs 32:130–168, 1986.

Ward NG: Tricyclic antidepressants for chronic low-back pain. Mechanisms of action and predictors of response. Spine 11:661–665, 1986.

Sensory Pharmacology

Cedric M. Smith

26

Sensory pharmacology is the study of actions of drugs on neuronal sensory receptors resulting in an increase, decrease, or modification of afferent nerve activity. *Sensory* here means (1) *afferent* to the central nervous system (CNS) and (2) *afferent* to local nervous reflexes such as in the axon reflex and intrinsic nerve circuits of the gastrointestinal (GI) tract. Thus, in analogy with other drug classifications, drugs that have effects on sensory and afferent systems are appropriately termed *sensory* or *afferent* drugs.

An important reason for examining the drugs that alter sensory afferent systems is the fact that most drugs alter sensory systems either directly or indirectly. In doing so, they have the potential to affect many organ systems, inasmuch as most body functions are under nervous control and are thus *potentially* alterable by drugs that alter the afferent limb of nervous reflexes.

The knowledge of drug effects on sensory systems has three primary applications: *therapeutic use; detection of side effects;* and *tools for research.*

It is easy to understand that drugs can alter sensory input from the major exteroceptors, such as ringing in the ears after aspirin, itching with histamine, or warmth with pepper. By contrast it is difficult to appreciate that most of the afferent nerve activity is *not* perceived directly. For example, color and taste are usually perceived, but muscle stretch, intestinal tone, or oxygen tension in blood is not. Essentially all of the visceral (interoceptive) afferent traffic is *not* consciously perceived or remembered (such as changes in neuroendocrine, cardiac, kidney, and respiratory functions). Nevertheless, altered functions consequent to such drug-induced effects on the sensory system may well be perceived. For example, alteration in the length detectors in skeletal muscle produces discoordination. Although the change in muscle length is not experienced directly in such a situation, discoordination is perceived as the mismatch between what one wishes to accomplish and what is accomplished with muscle activation.

Another example is the drop in blood pressure induced by excitation of baroreceptors (which is not perceived), resulting in fainting and falling that is perceived; stimulation of carotid chemoreceptors is not perceived, but hyperventilation and air hunger might be.

The autonomic, unconscious alterations of sensory input that can be produced by drugs can only be appreciated in the context of attention and awareness in which the change in afferent input occurs. As the old proverb goes: "We can look, but not see. See, but not perceive. Perceive, but not think. Think, but not act." More often than not, organisms respond to a change in sensory input yet frequently do not perceive the stimulus; commonly we perceive and become aware of *only* the responses after the fact.

Drugs can have actions on afferent nerve endings and on local nervous reflexes.

Changes in Afferent Input and Conscious Awareness, Perception

Many drugs can alter sensory systems, either directly or indirectly.

Almost all of the visceral (interoceptive) afferent traffic is *not* perceived consciously.

The qualitative and quantitative changes in reflexes or the more indirect responses can be predicted only with difficulty, because the actions are functions of a great number of factors. These include route of drug administration, dosage, drug distribution, the degree of excitation or depression of sensory ending, the numbers and type of sensory endings affected, the anatomical distribution of these endings, and finally, their ultimate destinations in the CNS.

A number of examples of sensory drug actions are presented in Tables 26–1 to 26–3. Before considering certain classes in detail, it may be helpful to consider the factors that are implicitly involved in a description and analysis of such actions.

Analyses and Principles of Sensory Drug Actions

The primary questions that need to be asked in any consideration of afferent drugs (i.e., drugs acting on afferent systems) are the following (see Tables 26–1 and 26–2):

1. Specificity of—
   Site(s) of action, which sensory endings at which locations
   Mechanisms of action
   Reflexes or perceptual consequences
   Chemical structure and drug action
   Drug localization and differential distribution
2. Spectrum of—
   Effects of individual agents on various endings and on other organ systems (see Table 26–2)
3. Varieties of actions producible by afferent drugs
4. Rationale of understanding and classification—
   Levels of integration—molecule, localization, end-organ, reflex, and adaptive nervous functions (see Table 26–3)

Table 26–1 THERAPEUTIC AND POTENTIAL USES OF DRUGS AFFECTING AFFERENT INPUT

A. Therapeutic Action	Some Examples
Depression of sensation, analgesia	Local anesthetics, ethylchloride spray Salicylates, NSAIDs, bradykinin and substance P antagonists, counterirritants, capsaicin, methyl salicylate
Anti-inflammatory	NSAIDs, capsaicin, substance P antagonists, heat, cold
Local vasodilation, counterirritation	Capsaicin, methyl salicylate
Muscle relaxation	Phenytoin, mephenesin, carbamazepine
Decreased muscle tremor	(e.g., a sensory site of action of propranolol in reducing essential tremor is conceivable)
Antitussive	Benzonatate (Tessalon), menthol, camphor
Relief of dyspnea	Morphine insufflation
Nausea, vomiting	Apomorphine, ipecac, lithium (many drugs as side effect)
Modification of intestinal motility	Irritant laxatives, alcohol
Decreased blood pressure	Veratrum alkaloids, calcium channel blockers
Sensitization of warm receptor	Capsaicin, methyl salicylate
Sensitization/stimulation of cold receptors	Menthol, eugenol
Abolition of triggers of neuralgic attacks	Carbamazepine, phenytoin
Respiratory stimulation	Nicotine, choline esters, carbon dioxide, cyanide, doxapram
Antiemetic, antivertigo	(Possible sensory effects of phenothiazines, nabilone, diphenidol, scopolamine)

SITES OF DRUG ACTION ON AFFERENT SYSTEMS

It follows that drugs that affect physiological and biochemical processes at the same time also alter certain afferent systems, either directly or indirectly. Moreover, either one or several afferent systems *may be the site of the main action of a drug or may be a site of origin of side effects.*

Drug effects on a sensory system may arise from drug actions on sites in the sensory ending itself, on the sensory end organ, on the surrounding and supporting structures that are frequently involved in the transduction process, and on the impulse conducting sensory nerve or its afferent terminals in the CNS. Furthermore, drugs may act on the efferent regulation that many sensory organs possess (e.g., the γ-fusimotor system to the muscle spindles), or on the efferent outflow to the tissue in which the sensory ending is located (e.g., effects on temperature receptors that might be brought about by changes in skin blood flow).

Certain drugs can produce dramatic alterations in sensory activity that are not perceived even though they have afferent projections to the cerebral cortex. Among the most well-known are succinylcholine and decamethonium, which cause marked excitation of muscle spindle stretch receptors. Likewise, ethanol has stimulant effects on skeletal muscle afferents that are not, as far as is known, perceived.

Sensory ending, location, excitation or depression, perceptual and reflex consequences

SPECIFICITY AND SPECTRUM OF ACTION

The rationales for classification of drugs with sensory effects involve consideration of various levels of integration, spanning from the molecular

Table 26-1 THERAPEUTIC AND POTENTIAL USES OF DRUGS AFFECTING AFFERENT INPUT Continued

B. Potential or Other Action

Antiepileptic for the reflex epilepsies	
Altered odors, tastes, sound, and heat (more aversive or less aversive)	Sodium lauryl sulfate in toothpaste makes orange juice more bitter, less sweet
Alteration of appetite or consumption of foods, such as increasing sweetness, food flavors, or conversely, conditioned food aversion	Sweeteners, salt substitutes, glutamic acid, food and beverages mixtures, lithium
Antieating	
Antismoking	
Antidrinking	
Modification of *trophic* influences of sensory nerves	
Drugs as conditioned stimuli—drugs as discriminative stimuli, and possibly as one basis of placebo responses to drugs or other chemicals	Nicotine, alcohol, beverages, hallucinogens, opioids, amphetamines, sedative/hypnotics, psychotropic drugs, disulfiram-alcohol reaction
Anesthetic states	Possibly dissociative conditions or new anesthetics
Anti-itch	
Production of itch, pain, unpleasant sensations	Itch powder, tear gases
Detection of toxic levels	Yellow vision with digitalis, diuretics
Use of drugs for esthetic purposes to enhance or modify senses and perception	Perfumes, food seasonings and flavor additives, cannibinols, LSD
Diagnosis of panic disorder	Caffeine taste test (DeMet et al, 1989)

Table 26-2   DRUG CLASSES HAVING POTENTIAL FOR EFFECTS ON MANY SENSORY SYSTEMS

Drug Classes	Unique Site or Effect
Local anesthetics (on systemic administration) e.g., lidocaine, tocainide, encainide, amiodarone	
Quinine and quinidine	Tinnitus, peripheral neuropathy, blurred vision
Nonsteroidal anti-inflammatory drugs Aspirin Indomethacin Naproxen Butazolidin	Tinnitus, peripheral neuropathy, blurred vision
Agents that alter calcium or calcium permeability Nifedipine Copper- or vitamin-deficient state Penicillamine Etidronate	
Cholinergic agonists Nicotine, acetylcholine, succinylcholine	Skin, polymodal C nociceptive fibers, carotid body muscle spindles
Histamine	C nociceptive, pain, itch
Lithium	
Drugs altering Na+, K+ levels Diuretics, thiazides	Xanthopsia, vertigo, headache, paresthesias
Reserpine	Deafness, dizziness, headaches, pruritus
Tricyclic antidepressants	Numbness, tingling, paresthesias, neuropathy, tinnitus
Retinoids	Numerous side effects on visual, auditory, and muscle as well as other major systems—CNS, GI, cardiovascular, neural

characteristics of the drug, to the localization and distribution of the agent, the specificity and spectrum of the action on specific end organs, the reflex connections of the sensory systems, and finally to the role of these sensory systems in adaptive nervous functions.

Specificity of action can be assessed in a number of ways. It may relate to the site(s) of action, that is, the location and type of nerve endings affected; it may refer to location and function in terms of reflex consequences; or it may refer to mechanism of action of the agent on the endings under consideration. For example, does a drug increase or decrease the frequency of afferent discharges? What are the reflex changes or changes in perception such as muscle relaxation, bitter taste, or sensation of pain resulting from afferent drug action? What are the structure-relationships

From sights, sounds, and smells to palsy, paresthesia, and pain

Table 26-3 / A FRAME OF REFERENCE FOR CLASSIFICATION OF NEURAL RESPONSES TO DRUG EFFECTS ON AFFERENT SYSTEMS

Connectivity	Examples
Tight and narrow	Knee jerk; muscle tone; cardiovascular reflexes; esthesia—hypoalgesia, analgesia, hyperalgesia, local anesthesia
Tight and broad—nonspecific or generalized	Flexor response to pain; depression of monosynaptic reflex with massive afferent excitation; tear gas immobility
Loose and narrow—effect readily influenced by other sensory input or changes in CNS functions	Special senses
Loose and general/complex	Learned and conditioned responses such as drugs as conditioned stimuli; complex behavior that is a function of drug state; some placebo responses

among compounds exerting actions on a given end organ? Is drug specificity the result of differential distribution of the agent or of route of administration?

A characterization of afferent drugs also includes a delineation of the spectrum of their actions, described by the dose-response relationships for various different sensory endings, and for effects on other organ systems. For example, certain drugs act on reflex systems that are *tightly connected*, that is, a change in afferent input is regularly associated with a specific consequence; examples include the knee jerk reflex to a tendon tap and the widespread vasoconstriction reflex in response to a drop of pressure in the carotid sinus. The reflex consequences of activation of specific afferents in such tightly connected systems are confined to rather narrow anatomical connections; in addition, they can be readily predicted (see Table 26–3).

In contrast, in other afferent systems the consequences of activation do not result in obligatory or tightly connected responses. For example, the end effects of the stimulation of the special senses such as taste or smell of pungent materials, such as pepper, are often defined only by previous experience, context, and expectations. In such a loose and complex system, drug influence could well involve conditioning or the drugs could serve as *conditioned stimuli*. Some types of placebo effects of drugs belong in this category.

Between the two extremes of the *tight-narrow* and the *loose-complex* systems is the possibility of a tight but rather *widespread, generalized* system, such as the flexor withdrawal response to painful stimuli and a kind of loose, yet rather narrow, system in which certain of the senses, such as taste and olfaction, induce only limited, simple reflex responses.

Specific Drug Actions on Sensory Receptors

Drug effects on sensory systems are discussed in relation to *selective effects* on given receptors, including those of the special senses, and by defining the effects and *side effects of individual drugs*.

SENSORY EFFECTS AS SIDE EFFECTS

Some drugs and drug classes have prominent or widespread effects on many sensory systems. As would be expected, all drugs that are local anesthetics or have local anesthetic properties, such as cardiac antiarrhythmics, can produce a variety of sensory disturbances, among which are paresthesias, numbness, vertigo, dizziness, visual disturbances, abnormal taste or smell, and tinnitus (Table 26–4; see also Table 26–2).

Most drugs have side effects; many side effects consist of sensory disturbances of GI function, vision, taste, smell, and pain.

The knowledge about side effects of drugs derives largely from reports from patients, many of whom are receiving multiple drugs. For some drugs, the sensory side effect may occur so frequently that the majority of individuals receiving the drug will experience the effect. For others, the sensory effects may reproducibly appear only with large doses or in only a small percentage of patients. In addition, for drugs commonly used clinically together, such as diuretics and digitalis, it may be difficult to ascertain which drug is responsible for a given side effect, for example, the yellow vision reported relatively frequently with digitalis and with thiazide diuretics.

The haphazard way in which the data on side effects have been collected over the years, plus the varied terms used to describe such side effects, makes it difficult to draw precise comparisons among agents or to

Table 26-4 EXAMPLES OF SIDE EFFECTS ATTRIBUTABLE TO ACTIONS OF DRUGS ON SENSORY SYSTEMS*

Alterations In	Drug
Vision and Hearing	
Color vision (usually yellow)	Digitalis, pheniramine, thiazide diuretics
Vision	
Acuity	Toxic amblyopia with nicotine, nicotinic acid
Blurred vision	Anticholinergic, atropinic compounds, phenothiazines, tricyclic antidepressants, urinary antispasmodics, enalapril, ranitidine, guanabenz, diphenidol, digoxin, nadolol, many others
Audition	
Tinnitus	Aspirin, quinine, quinidine, ibuprofen, naproxen
Hearing loss	Streptomycin, amikacin, kanamycin, chloroquine, erythromycin, tocainide, quinine, NSAIDs, naproxen, ketoprofen, indomethacin, bumetanide, ethacrynic acid, reserpine, erythromycin, antihistaminics, antiarrhythmic drugs, tricyclic antidepressants, phenothiazines, allopurinol, cholestyramine, and reported for many others
Skeletal Muscle Systems	
Ataxia, incoordination	Phenytoin, ethanol
Muscle pain postoperatively	Succinylcholine
Tremor	Lithium, phenothiazines, nicotine
Gastrointestinal System	
Nausea and vomiting	Lithium, aspirin, morphine, opioids, alcohol, digitalis, antibiotics, levodopa, NSAIDs, ergotamine, metronidazole, triazolam, guanadrel, baclofen, meclofenamate, methocarbamol, antineoplastic agents, yohimbine
Taste (or Smell)	
Reduced	
	Amebicides and anthelmintics (metronidazole, others)
	Anesthetics, local (benzocaine, procaine, cocaine, tetracaine, encainide)
	Anticholesteremic (clofibrate)
	Anticoagulants (phenindione)
	Antihistamines (chlorpheniramine)
	Antimicrobial agents (amphomycin, ampicillin, cefamandole, griseofulvin, ethambutol, lincomycin, sulfasalazine, streptomycin, tetracyclines, tyrothricin)
	Antiproliferative, including immunosuppressive agents (doxorubicin and methotrexate, azathioprine, carmustine, vincristine)
	Antirheumatic, analgesic-antipyretic, anti-inflammatory agents (allopurinol, colchicine, gold, levamisole, D-penicillamine, phenylbutazone, 5-thiopyridoxine)
	Antiseptics (hexetidine)
	Antithyroid agents (carbimazole, methimazole, methylthiouracil, propylthiouracil, thiouracil)
	Diuretics and antihypertensive agents (captopril, diazoxide, ethacrynic acid, acetazolamide)
	Hypoglycemic drugs (glipizide, phenformin and derivatives)
	Muscle relaxants and drugs for treatment of Parkinson's disease (baclofen, chlormezanone, levodopa, cyclobenzaprine)
	Opioids (codeine, hydromorphone, morphine)
	Psychopharmacologic, including antiepileptic drugs (carbamazepine, lithium carbonate, phenytoin, trifluoperazine)
	Autonomic drugs (amphetamines, phenmetrazine/phenbutrazate, anticholinergic)
	Vasodilators (oxyfedrine, bamifylline)
Altered	Captopril, griseofulvin, histidine, lithium, benzonatate, trialkyl tin, phytonadione, diethylpropion, fenfluramine, pentoxifylline, phentermine, amoxapine, perphenazine, tricyclic antidepressants, mazindol, sodium lauryl sulfate (toothpaste)
Bitter	Carbamazepine, levodopa, phenylbutazone, organophosphate insecticides
Metallic	Allopurinol, ethambutol, gold preparations, metronidazole, methocarbamol, lithium
Pain	
Headache	Numerous substances including aspirin, NSAIDs, vasodilators, sulfonamides, clonidine, buprenorphine, aminoglutethimide, benzodiazepines, cephalosporin antibiotics, ranitidine, piroxicam, antihistamines, terfenadine, guanadrel, antiarrhythmics, digoxin, lithium, amiloride, tricyclic antidepressants, baclofen, famotine, enalapril, butorphanol, meclofenamate, nifedipine, verapamil, diltiazem, maprotiline, mexiletine, acebutolol, naltrexone
Paresthesias	
	Many drugs, including verapamil, probucol, buspirone, tocainide, amiodarone, nadolol, pindolol, guanadrel, cephalosporins, dronabinol, phenytoin, ergotamine

Adapted and expanded from Schiffman SS: Taste and smell in disease. N Engl J Med 308:1275–1279, 1337–1343, 1983.
* Partial list grouped roughly by class.

ascertain the actual probability of a given drug or drugs causing a certain sensory side effect. The Interactions and Side Effects Index to the Physicians' Desk Reference [PDR] allows an initial access through the book (or a CD-ROM disc) to the side effects of drugs, at least as they are tabulated in the Federal Drug Administration [FDA]–approved package inserts included in the PDR. Grossly underrepresented in these lists are older drugs, notably such agents as aspirin or digoxin.)

Side effects listed as frequent (e.g., greater than 3–5% of a population) can be assumed to be associated with the drug, to err on the cautious side. Sensory side effects reported at lower frequencies could well be due to the drug, but might also be due to other causes. Although sensory disturbance side effects may be due to a specific drug, they could also be due to the disease itself. In the case of antihypertensive drugs such as guanadrel or methyldopa, both the drugs and the hypertension itself can cause headaches and paresthesias; either could be the result of drug effects or symptoms of hypertension. In the absence of good placebo-controlled studies, a distinction between the two possible causes is impossible to make.

In addition to the special chemical sense of taste and smell, only a few chemoreceptive sensory systems have received much research attention. Among these few are the carotid and aortic bodies, the baroceptors, stretch receptors of skeletal muscle, and vagal afferents from the GI tract. (Major reviews on this subject are cited in the reference list.)

The sensory side effects of drugs can be problems for any group of patients, but they are of major significance to the elderly. With aging there is frequently a deterioration in sensory function, as well as the taking of many drugs. The consequence of both of these results in aggravation of the very functions critical to the maintenance of healthy elders—awareness of their environment and active participation. Flavor enhancement can improve the nutritional status of the elderly (Schiffman et al, 1990). Among the common drug side effects are alterations of vision, hearing, taste, or smell. Decreased visual acuity and blurred vision may be of endogenous origin, but they are frequently contributed to by many drugs—perhaps most commonly by the many drugs with anticholinergic actions.

Tinnitus and hearing loss are frequent with aspirin, nonsteroidal anti-inflammatory drugs (NSAIDs), a wide variety of antibiotics, and psychotropic drugs. A change in hearing acuity in a patient mandates a major review of all medications received over past weeks and months.

Patients frequently complain of alterations in taste and smell of foods. Such symptoms usually have an identifiable organic cause and are an indication for the review of medications in a search for a possible culprit. Drug effects include reduction or altered or specific tastes, most commonly bitter or metallic tastes (see Table 26–4).

The vast majority of the population have headaches at one time or another. Yet drugs are a frequently overlooked cause of such headaches. Moreover, some of the most frequent causes are agents that are used commonly to treat headaches, such as aspirin and the NSAIDs. The number of possible perpetrators is extensive, as the partial list in Table 26–4 illustrates.

Patients are most often truthful, and their reports deserve to be accepted in the search for possible causes. Unfortunately, all too often the causes of such symptoms are the very drugs prescribed to alleviate disease and distress. As indicated in Table 26–4, one of the following symptoms *could be* caused by any of hundreds of drugs:

anorexia	paresthesias, tingling
nausea (e.g., 1000 entries in the PDR)	pruritus
vomiting (almost 900 entries)	numbness
diarrhea (500–600 entries)	dizziness
constipation	blurred vision
abdominal pain or cramps	double vision
headache	

> The majority of patients suffer one or more iatrogenic diseases during hospitalization; drugs are a major cause of iatrogenic disease.

Therefore, each of such symptoms *deserves an explicit consideration and inquiry regarding the possibility that a drug may be responsible.*

THERAPEUTIC USES OF DRUGS ACTING ON SENSORY RECEPTORS

A compilation of the therapeutic uses of drugs acting on sensory receptors is presented in Table 26–1. Those that illustrate the therapeutic applications best are listed first. The local anesthetics by their very nature act to modify sensory input. Usually they are given locally so that they act directly on the endings or the nerve axon, but systemic administration also has had limited use.

> The site of action of a major class of analgesics, the NSAIDs, is the afferent nerve ending.

The salicylates and NSAIDs act specifically on peripheral afferent receptor systems to decrease nociceptive nerve activity and receptor sensitivity, as well as to antagonize the process of inflammation (see Chapter 28). This class of agents illustrates, perhaps better than any other, the potential for drug actions at specific sensory targets. Among other therapeutic drugs acting on sensory endings are phenytoin and muscle relaxants used to modify afferent activity from skeletal muscle; benzonatate (TESSALON), an antitussive used as a moderately useful cough remedy, and ipecac and apomorphine, used for emesis.

Topical Drugs for Relief in Joints, Muscles, and Associated Soft Tissue — "Counterirritants"

The uses of the locally applied or injected local anesthetics and steroids are described briefly under those drugs (Chapters 17 and 43).

Counterirritant is one of those classifications that is not well defined; unfortunately, it implies a probably incorrect mechanism of action. The agents do produce some of the signs of inflammation and irritation, but the "irritating" properties of these agents are an insufficient and incomplete characterization. This group includes a rather wide variety of substances that have in common only the fact that they produce irritation. They are applied topically to the skin as creams or ointments for the symptomatic relief of muscle stiffness and soreness following (1) bruises, extensive muscle use, or exposure to cold; (2) tendinitis or bursitis associated with specific repeated movements; and (3) the pain and muscle stiffness frequently accompanying rheumatoid arthritis and osteoarthritis. An FDA advisory review panel has recognized the agents and classes shown in Table 26–5 as being "safe and effective."

> Counterirritant drugs cause signs of irritation, but how they act to relieve pain and muscle spasm is probably through local and segmental reflexes.

Except for capsaicin, the active ingredient from the red pepper *Capsicum*, the mechanism by which these so-called counterirritants act has not been established, although a number of plausible mechanisms have been advanced: reflex vasodilation of underlying muscles, distraction, placebo effects, and presynaptic inhibition.

Table 26–5   COUNTERIRRITANTS

Group	Characteristics (Actions)	Active Ingredients
A	Erythema, irritation	Mustard (allyl isothiocyanate), methyl salicylate, turpentine oil
B	Cooling followed by warmth	Menthol, camphor
	Warmth	Eucalyptus oil
C	Erythema, vasodilation	Histamine, methyl nicotinate
D	Irritation, sensation of warmth, erythema, and pain with large concentrations	Capsaicin, Capsicum, Capsicum oleoresin

Methyl Salicylate. In sufficient concentrations the compounds in Groups A and D (see Table 26–5) produce reddening and erythema of the skin. The most widely used of all of these agents is methyl salicylate (oil of wintergreen). When applied to intact skin methyl salicylate, like most of the agents in this class, produces a sense of warmth and skin reddening. It is widely available in numerous creams by itself or in a variety of combination with other agents; for example, BENGAY preparations consist of methyl salicylate (15–29%) and menthol (7–16%) in a variety of bases. It is used for the topical treatment of muscle and joint pain. (Oil of wintergreen is also used in low concentrations for its pleasant taste and aroma. But it is extremely toxic; as little as 4 ml of methyl salicylate has been fatal in children. However, as a topical ointment it has had a long and safe marketing history.)

Mustard oil (allyl isothiocyanate) and turpentine not only cause irritation and erythema, but they have the potential to produce blisters, vesication, urticaria, and tissue damage.

Capsaicin. Capsaicin is the active ingredient in hot pepper; as most people who have had direct experience with hot pepper know, capsaicin is not only hot to the taste, it is hot to the skin and augments the intensity of any warm stimulus (temperature or infrared radiation). It has a remarkable specificity and potency. The threshold concentration for its perception in the taste of foods is of the order of less than 1 part per million. Beyond its fascinating history and variety of its uses as a food flavoring, it has found widespread therapeutic use, and recently it has taken on major importance as a tool for unraveling the neurophysiology of a variety of neural and sensory systems. Tolerance develops to the taste, heat, and pain induced by oral or topical capsaicin.

Acute Topical Effects. Capsaicin selectively stimulates certain primary afferent neurons at their sensory endings, sometimes along their axons as well as at their terminations. When applied to the intact skin or mucous membranes in low concentrations it may not have detectable effect, except that upon exposing the skin to a mild heat source, a sense of warmth localized to the area of the capsaicin application results. After higher concentrations, the agent alone produces the characteristic sensation of warmth and heat; in large concentrations it causes heat and pain. Thus, capsaicin results in a local warming effect coupled with a decrease in the pain threshold to heat sufficient to produce spontaneous burning pain. These sensations can be abolished rapidly by cooling the skin surface (Fig. 26–1). These effects are, in the lowest concentrations, specific for afferents mediating heat; capsaicin appears to be without appreciable effects on cold receptors. Nevertheless, there can be increased responses to stimulation by other modalities such as mechanoreception, i.e., mechanical hyperalgesia.

Electrophysiological studies reveal that capsaicin selectively excites afferents responding to nociceptive chemical stimuli, the so-called polymodal C fiber nociceptors. These endings are assumed to possess at least two membrane conductance systems, one of which is a transducer to heat and others transduce mechanical and other chemical stimuli. This conception implies that chemicals such as capsaicin act proximally to the sensory receptor–nerve activity mechanisms. (Alternatively, the cross-modality perceptual responses that have been observed could take origin from two different afferent receptors and nerves that converge on a second-order sensory neuron.)

The major therapeutic use of capsaicin is in over-the-counter topical ointments and creams used to facilitate relief of pain and muscle spasm in

Figure 26-1

The dependence of threshold for heat pain (ordinate) on capsaicin concentration and time. Capsaicin was applied at the indicated concentrations (abscissa) to a linear array of skin patches on the anterior aspect of the forearm. The heat threshold was determined at 4 hours (*circles*), 11 hours (*squares*), and 21 hours (*triangles*) following application. (From Culp WJ, Ochoa J, Cline M, Dotson R: Heat and mechanical analgesia induced by capsaicin—Cross modality threshold in human c-nociceptors. Brain 112:1317–1331, 1989. By permission of Oxford University Press.)

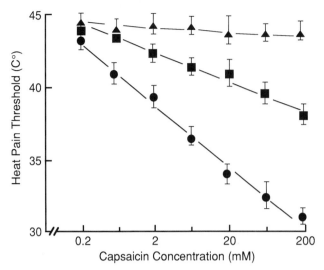

conditions of skeletal muscle aches, strains, sprains, or inflammatory states such as rheumatoid arthritis. In addition, it sometimes relieves postherpetic neuralgia, local stump pain, and in some otherwise refractory painful diabetic neuropathy. (Examples of many preparations available are AXSAIN, containing 0.075% capsaicin in a cream base; ZOSTRIX, with 0.025% capsaicin in a cream base; HEET, which contains oleoresin *Capsicum*, 0.4%; camphor, 3.6%; methyl salicylate, 15%; alcohol, 70%; and SLOAN's, which contains turpentine oil, 46.7%; pine oil, 6.74%; camphor, 3.35%; methyl salicylate, 2.66%; *Capsicum* oleoresin, 0.62%; kerosene, 39.8%.)

The symptomatic relief following application of capsaicin is commonly accompanied by a feeling of warmth and erythema at the site of application. Although capsaicin can produce profound stimulation of warm receptors of skin or of mucous membranes, it produces almost no evidence of tissue damage or destruction. Thus, although it activates one of the systems critically involved in inflammation, it cannot be considered as an inflammatory substance.

Mechanism of Action. One of the prime actions of capsaicin, after local as well as systemic adminstration, is to cause the depletion of the peptide, substance P, from certain sensory neurons. Substance P, an undecapeptide, is thought be a neurotransmitter or neuromodulator involved in afferent C fibers. In general, the major capsaicin-sensitive neurons are probably the polymodal nociceptive receptors with free nerve endings. (But this may not be absolutely or exclusively true. It is probable that some sensory neurons containing substance P are not sensitive to capsaicin; and there may be primary afferents altered by capsaicin that do not contain substance P. Not only is substance P important, a number of other neuropeptides can probably be affected by capsaicin.)

Systemic and Chronic Effects. The interest in the specificity of action of capsaicin derives from the observation that the sustained excitation of the sensitive sensory neurons by capsaicin is followed by a sustained refractoriness, a refractoriness *not* limited to only capsaicin but that extends to a wide variety of apparently chemically unrelated irritants and excitants as well. This refractoriness is associated with the depletion of substance P.

Not only is depletion of substance P found upon local or topical application of capsaicin, depletion occurs after systemic administration. Even more intriguing, when capsaicin is administered to neonatal rats, it results in degeneration and *permanent loss* of the majority of afferent C fibers. These observations were the initial starting points to extensive research endeavors that continue to the present time (Buck and Burks, 1986). To date none of the fascinating projects have realized improvements in therapy. However, there remains great potential for the application of capsaicin or analogs in new types of management of troublesome chronic pain syndromes as well as the elucidation of the pathophysiological roles mediated by peptides and local nerve activity.

Caution. Cautions that apply to all these agents are that they are only to be used externally; some of them can be extremely toxic if ingested. In addition, some individuals are known to be especially sensitive; sensitization can also occur.

Drug Effects on Sensory Receptors of Skeletal Muscle

In contrast to fibers that mediate pain, the large, rapidly conducting afferent fibers from the muscle spindles can be dissected from the largely parallel fiber bundles in dorsal roots entering the spinal cord. Each skeletal muscle spindle is a complex organ with usually two or more afferent endings and four to twelve intrafusal muscle fibers on and around which the sensory endings terminate (or from which the activity takes origin, depending on the point of view). The sensory endings function physiologically to signal muscle length in response to stretch or the contraction of the long polar portions of the intrafusal muscle fibers.

Some so-called centrally acting muscle relaxants (methocarbamol, phenytoin, chlorpromazine, dantrolene) actually act on or through the peripheral sensory systems.

Some drugs such as succinylcholine can produce truly dramatic excitation of the muscle spindle afferents. Because one of the reflex consequences of this excitation is an excitation of motor neurons innervating the same muscle, the muscle spindle afferent stimulation is one of the causes of the fasciculations, twitches, and exaggerated stretch reflexes that are observed immediately following the intravenous injection of succinylcholine (see Chapter 13).

A variety of quaternary nitrogen compounds as well as nicotine also produce muscle spindle afferent excitation. This excitation is due conceivably to direct effects on the sensory endings, but it is more likely due to contraction and contracture of the specialized intrafusal muscle fibers. The pharmacology of these endings is illustrative of many sensory systems, because they have unique cholinergic structure-activity-relationships for stimulation (agonism) as well as for antagonism. In general, the more nicotinic (as opposed to muscarinic) the cholinergic agents are, the more potent they are, the more excitation they produce, and the more selectively they act on primary endings. There are differential sensitivities of the primary and secondary endings, as indicated by marked effects of both nicotine and succinylcholine on the primary endings but only moderate effects on the secondary endings. The specificity of the receptors on the sensory receptor is evident not only from the actions of cholinergic agonists, but it is apparent also with the selective block of most agents by tubocurarine but not by the antimuscarinic agent atropine.

A few agents other than cholinergic drugs are known to excite these same receptors, including ethanol in blood concentrations associated with ataxia, as well as capsaicin and high potassium levels. (A stimulatory effect of potassium at most sensory endings would be anticipated in view of the membrane depolarization it would be expected to produce.)

The excitatory action of cholinergic agents is also selective for muscle spindle afferents, in that tendon organs in the same muscle are not excited even though they have large afferent fibers of the same size and conduction velocity as many spindle afferents.

In contrast to these excitants, a number of agents are known to depress the spindle afferent response to stretch. As might be expected, local anesthetics lead this list. The therapeutic muscle relaxant effects of mephenesin and phenytoin are attributable, at least in part, to their depressant effects on the spindle afferents; the side effect of ataxia is also consistent with muscle afferent actions. Benzonatate, a drug used therapeutically because of its cough suppressant action, depresses muscle spindle afferent activity analogous with its depressant, "local anesthetic" effect on receptors in the lung and bronchi.

In addition to spindles and tendon organs, there are other muscle afferents with afferent nerve fibers in the Group III and IV categories. In contrast to the muscle spindles, almost nothing is known of the actions of drugs on their receptors except that bradykinin is probably an excitant, a fact consistent with the function of kinins to mediate muscle pain. Anti-inflammatory agents are likely also to be depressants of these small afferents, but this has yet to be demonstrated experimentally. (Local application of cholinergic agents such as nicotine and acetylcholine excites a number of other sensory endings such as those in skin, mucous membranes, and tongue. The cholinergic agents that excite these endings have a unique spectrum of action at each site; each site also exhibits unique structure-activity relationships to excitants and to their antagonists.)

Future investigations will undoubtedly explore the many possibilities for selective drug actions on all kinds of sensory systems, as outlined in Table 26–1.

General References

Akoev GN, Alekseev NP, Krylov BV: Mechanoreceptors: Their Functional Organization. Berlin, Heidelberg: Springer-Verlag, 1988.

Aronson JK, Ford AR: The use of colour vision measurement in the diagnosis of digoxin toxicity. Q J Med (New Series XLIX) 195:273–282, 1980.

Berstein JE, Korman NJ, Bickers DR, et al: Topical capsaicin treatment of chronic post-herpetic neuralgia. J Am Acad Dermatol 21:265–270, 1989.

Buck SH, Burks TF: The neuropharmacology of capsaicin: Review of some recent observations. Pharmacol Rev 38:179–226, 1986.

Cagan RH: Neural Mechanisms in Taste. Boca Raton, FL: CRC Press, 1989.

Culp WJ, Ochoa J, Cline M, Dotson R: Heat and mechanical hyperalgesia induced by capsaicin—cross modality threshold modulation in human C-nociceptors. Brain 112:1317–1331, 1989.

DeMet E, Stein MK, Tran C, et al: Caffeine taste test for panic disorder: Adenosine receptor supersensitivity. Psychiatry Res 30:231–242, 1989.

Eldred E, Yellin H, DeSantis M, Smith CM: Supplement to bibliography on muscle receptors: Their morphology, pathology, physiology and pharmacology. Exper Neurol 55(Part 2):1–118, 1977.

Feldman EG (dir), Davidson DE (ed): Handbook of Nonprescription Drugs, 8th ed. Washington, DC: American Pharmaceutical Association, The National Professional Society of Pharmacists, 1986.

Green BG: Capsaicin sensitization and desensitization on the tongue produced by brief exposures to a low concentration. Neurosci Lett 170:173–178, 1989.

Green BG, Mason JR, Kare MR: Chemical Senses, vol 2. Irritation. New York: Marcel Dekker, 1990.

Hartung M, Leah J, Zimmerman M: The excitation of cutaneous nerve endings in a neuroma by capsaicin. Brain Res 499:363–366, 1989.

Hu H, Fine J, Epstein P, et al.: Tear gas—harassing agent or toxic chemical weapon? JAMA 262:660–663, 1989.

Karrer T, Bartoshuk L: Oral capsaicin desensitization and its effect on taste. Chem Senses 15:597, 1990.

Lammers JWJ, Minette P, McCusker MT, et al: Capsaicin-induced bronchodilation in mild asthmatic subjects—possible role of nonadrenergic inhibitory system. J Appl Physiol 67:856–861, 1989.

Lembeck F: Columbus, capsicum and capsaicin: Past, present and future. Acta Physiol Hung 69:265–273, 1987.

Mattes RD, Cowart BJ, Schiavo MA, et al: Dietary evaluation of patients with smell and/or taste disorders. Am J Clin Nutr 51:233–240, 1990.

Rayner HC, Atkins RC, Westerman RA: Relief of local stump pain by capsaicin cream. Lancet 2:1276–1277, 1989.

Ross DR, Varipapa RJ: Treatment of painful diabetic neuropathy with topical capsaicin. N Engl J Med 321:474–475, 1989.

Schiffman SS: Taste and smell in disease. N Engl J Med 308:1275–1279, 1337–1343, 1983.

Schiffman SS, Frey AE, Warwick ZS: Nutritional assessment of elderly persons eating flavor-enhanced foods. Chem Senses 15:633, 1990.

Smith CM: The effects of drugs on afferent nervous systems. *In* Burger A (ed): Chemical Constitution and Pharmacodynamic Action. Vol 1. Drugs Affecting the Peripheral Nervous System. New York: Marcel Dekker, 1967.

Smith CM: Variety of Effects Resulting From Drug Action on Sensory Receptors. Vol 4 of Pharmacology and the Future of Man. Basel: S. Karger, 1973.

Taché Y, Wingate D: Brain-Gut Interactions. Boca Raton, FL: CRC Press, 1990.

27

Drug-Induced Psychiatric Symptoms

Katherine R. Bonson
Jerrold C. Winter
Cedric M. Smith

Many drugs can cause psychiatric symptoms.

Many drugs can produce effects on the central nervous system (CNS), including those drugs that are primarily used for their peripheral effects. Medically, agents that rely on a central action for therapeutic benefit are prescribed most often by psychiatrists in an attempt to alleviate mental disturbances. However, in obvious contrast to this practice, millions of people self-medicate with street drugs that are centrally reinforcing. It is important to remember that the noticeable effects of a drug are dependent on the dose and on the biological state of the person taking the compound. Thus, a relative increase in the dose of any drug may produce extremes in central nervous stimulation or depression. This explains why it is not uncommon for various psychiatric symptoms to develop in people taking a variety of available drugs, whether they be prescribed, over the counter, or illicit. A physician aware of this fact will be able to distinguish judiciously whether such symptoms as delirium, hallucination, anxiety, or aggression are of endogenous origin or the product of a substance a patient has consumed or administered.

Delirium and Hallucination

Delirium is marked by clouded consciousness.

A clear distinction can be made between delirium and hallucination. The essential feature of delirium is a clouded state of consciousness, i.e., a reduction in the clarity of awareness of the environment. This is manifested by a difficulty in sustaining attention to either external or internal stimuli because of sensory misperception or disordered stream of thought. In addition, disturbances of sleep-wakefulness and psychomotor activity are commonly present.

> A 42-year-old man was brought to the emergency room by police after he was found apparently intoxicated, wandering the streets dressed only from the waist up. On admission, the patient was extremely agitated and was disoriented to time, place and person. [Goldfrank et al, 1982]

Agitation and disorientation are characteristic of delirious patients; these patients often do not know where they are or what day it is. In the previous case study, the man had suffered a delirium after a woman had secretly put scopolamine, an anticholinergic drug, into his drink.

Hallucination is different from delirium in that people who are hallucinating have a false sensory perception that occurs in the absence of relevant or adequate stimuli. Although the hallucination may have a compelling sense of reality, people may be able to identify that it is in fact not a real occurrence.

> My eyelashes grew to infinity and like golden threads wound around little wiry spindles that spun by themselves with dazzling speed. About me were rivers, many torrents of gems of all colors, with endlessly changing floral patterns that I can only compare with kaleidoscopic patterns. . . . One of the guests addressed me in Italian, which the drug in its omnipotence changed into Spanish. The questions and answers were almost reasonable and touched upon such important subjects as literature or the theatre. [Gautier, 1865]

The visual hallucinations described by the French poet Gautier occurred to him following ingestion of hashish. Such vivid hallucinations are possible without the loss of a clear sensorium or confusion about who one is or where one lives. However, the effect of a drug is influenced not only by the chemical itself but by the mind/brain upon which it is acting. The frame of mind and situation a person is in when taking a drug is commonly referred to as the effect of *set* and *setting*. For example, when ministers were given a hallucinogen in a church on Good Friday, there was a preponderance of religious hallucinations among them. Conversely, when convicts with hostile personalities were administered the same drug while in prison, they tended to become very violent. The complexity of the brain accounts for the vast differences in behavior and thought among individuals that can result from a single agent.

Clinical lore has it that drug-induced hallucinations tend to be visual, whereas those that result from schizophrenia are generally auditory. This conclusion is not based on strong evidence, however, so it is not a good basis for an accurate diagnosis of the source of a hallucination. In addition, hallucinations and delirium may present together and should be noted as distinct conditions.

It is useful to distinguish "true" hallucinogenic substances from agents that can produce hallucinations as a side effect. The classic example of a true hallucinogen is lysergic acid diethylamide (LSD), which produces profound behavioral manifestations including sensory distortions and hallucination. Table 27–1 is an outline of true hallucinogens. These can be contrasted with other drugs that induce hallucinations secondarily to their main effect, or that occur only upon chronic administration or on abrupt withdrawal after chronic exposure.

LSD is capable of causing its intense effects at the minute dose of 50 μg or greater. It was discovered serendipitously by Albert Hofmann, a Swiss medicinal chemist who was working in the field of obstetric pharmacology. In 1938 he developed a series of compounds from ergot alkaloids that enhanced the strength of uterine contractions during labor. While testing these chemicals in 1943, Hofmann began to notice peculiar sensations. He left the laboratory, experiencing a fantastic bicycle trip home before he was able to lie down. During the ensuing hours Hofmann hallucinated colors and moving patterns and felt that his ego had left his body. He surmised upon recovery that he had absorbed one of the compounds through his skin while at the laboratory bench. Hofmann then went back to the laboratory and proceeded to systematically ingest the drugs in the series he had

---

A hallucination is a false sensory perception.

Table 27–1 TRUE HALLUCINOGENS: SOME DRUGS WHOSE PRIMARY KNOWN EFFECT IS THE PRODUCTION OF HALLUCINATIONS

I. Indoles
  A. N,N-dimethyltryptamine (DMT)
  B. (4-phosphoryloxy-DMT) psilocybin (phosphorylated psilocin; *Psilocybe mexicana* Heim)
  C. Lysergic acid diethylamide (LSD)
II. Phenethylamines
  A. Mescaline (3,4,5-trimethoxyphenylethylamine; *Lophophora williamsii*; peyote)
  B. DOM (2,5-dimethoxy-4-methylamphetamine)
III. Tetrahydrocannabinols

Hallucination and delirium do not always appear together.

A hallucination is a uniquely individual experience.

Indole and Phenethylamine Hallucinogens

Drugs that produce hallucinations as a primary action can be distinguished from those for which hallucinatory effects are secondary.

The discovery of lysergic acid diethylamide (LSD)

been working with. One of them was LSD, and Hofmann's personal experiments opened a long and colorful history for this hallucinogen. (The initials for lysergic acid diethylamide are *LSD* rather than *LAD* because the German word for *acid* is *Sauer*.)

Hallucinogens with an indole ring in their structure

LSD is one of many hallucinogens that contain an indole ring in its chemical structure. This ring structure was not developed in a laboratory; this ring is found naturally in the form of dimethyltryptamine in many Central and South American plants. People in these regions have used hallucinogenic plants for thousands of years, often in conjunction with religious ceremonies, because of the drugs' intense effects. Another drug with dimethyltryptamine as its base is the 4-phosphoryloxy derivative, psilocybin, a compound found in hallucinogenic mushrooms. The mechanism of action of these drugs in the brain is thought to be very similar, especially at serotonin receptors.

Mescaline is a phenethylamine hallucinogen.

In addition to indole compounds, hallucinogens are also derived from phenethylamines. Mescaline, the active agent in the peyote cactus, is a phenethylamine with methoxy substitutions at three positions. Mescaline has been used for centuries by native people throughout the Americas in peyote cults. These cults have even incorporated the side effects of nausea and vomiting into the ceremony as a cleansing ritual. Mescaline is the only hallucinogen that has been legal in the United States for religious purposes—but only if one belongs to the Native American Church.

Ring-substituted amphetamines are hallucinogenic.

When the basic phenethylamine structure is substituted at the α position with a methyl group, it becomes amphetamine. There are many hallucinogenic derivatives of amphetamine, including DOM (2,5-dimethoxy-4-methamphetamine, also known at one time as STP). The presence of the α-methyl group delays deamination in the body, giving compounds a longer half-life and therefore more time to act in the brain. This class of hallucinogens tends to produce a more "speed-like" effect than indolamines in connection with their amphetamine structure. Another phenethylamine popular "on the street" is MDMA (methylenedioxymethamphetamine, "ecstasy"). MDMA is one of a variety of psychoactive substances that have been tested for their potential as disorienting chemical weapons. There is currently some scientific concern that MDMA may be a neurotoxin in serotonergic systems.

Indoleamine and phenethylamine hallucinogens both act through the serotonergic system of the brain.

Generally, indoleamines and phenethylamines produce strikingly similar perceptual and subjective effects despite their structural differences. Pharmacological research with both classes of hallucinogens suggest that these drugs act at a specific subtype of serotonergic receptor (5-HT_2) in the brain, with possible interaction at dopamine sites. The neurochemical model of schizophrenia proposes similar receptor stimulation, based on initial studies of hallucinogens in humans that showed effects thought to resemble psychosis. In fact, the term *psychotomimetic* was coined by the French psychiatrist J. J. Moreau de Tours in the nineteenth century as a classification for drugs that produce hallucinations. Although this term is a rather simplistic reduction of the symptoms of both schizophrenia and hallucinogen intoxication, it does illustrate how basic research in pharmacology lends itself directly to medical theories of the origin and pathophysiology of mental disorders.

Symptoms of hallucinogen intoxication can be physical, somatic, and psychic.

The typical hallucinogenic experience can be understood by its physical, somatic, and psychic effects. Sympathetic stimulation characterizes the physical signs, e.g., pupillary dilation, tremor, increased pulse rate, and increased deep tendon reflexes. These effects are joined by somatic symptoms that may include nausea, loss of appetite, dizziness, paresthesia, blurred vision, weakness, or drowsiness. After several hours, such psychic effects as decreased concentration, difficulty in communication, depersonalization, mystical interpretations of events, and changes in mood may predominate. Anxiety in response to the effects of the drug may augment the physical response, particularly if one has been given the drug unwittingly or if the effects are more intense than was expected. This may be especially true as uncontrollable visual and thought distortions develop.

The duration of a hallucinogenic "trip" with LSD may last up to 8–12 hours, depending on the dose and the individual. The appearance of anxiety that may bring the user of a hallucinogen to the attention of a physician tends to occur after the peak of the drug's hallucinatory effects. For LSD, the peak occurs after about one half-life, or 3–4 hours. The period following the peak is especially susceptible to negative responses because users may expect they will not be under the influence of the drug once the hallucinations subside. Knowledge of the usual time course for the effects of a chemical among the drug-using community has meant that the panic that may occur from hallucinogen ingestion is now often dealt with effectively at home rather than in an emergency room.

The effects of LSD may persist for 8–12 hours.

Although campaigns against the nonmedical use of LSD and related drugs during the 1960s and 1970s stressed its hazards, much of the evidence was anecdotal. Accidents have happened in reaction to panic states, feelings of persecution, and delusional misjudgment, but fatalities from such events have been the result of behavioral manifestations of the drug, not direct toxic effects. Believing that one can fly or leap tall buildings can lead to such behavior with tragic consequences, yet there is no evidence that anyone has ever died from any physical toxicity produced by hallucinogens.

Life-threatening effects of LSD are *not* the result of its direct physical/organic toxicity.

Likewise, the claim that LSD causes chromosome damage has not been borne out by teratogenic and mutagenic studies. Nevertheless, the principle still stands that women intending to become pregnant or are already pregnant should avoid all drugs if possible. This is especially true for LSD because it is derived from compounds that induce uterine contractions.

Another fear that was promoted when LSD was first being used extensively was the possibility that the psychic effects would continue beyond the time the drug was acting on the brain. Before this concern in modern times, even Albert Hofmann reported that during his second exposure to LSD, "I was overcome by a fear that I was going out of my mind." The term for the reappearance of the hallucinogenic experience in the absence of retaking the drug is a *flashback*. As a phenomenon, flashbacks are actually rather uncommon. When they do present, either as prolonged disorientation or as hallucinations, they can be interpreted as indicating that an individual has a predisposition to psychiatric instability. It is also possible, however, that as with any overwhelming emotional experience, fragments of time spent while on a hallucinogen could be persistently remembered and that these memories could be an alternate explanation of flashbacks.

A flashback is a rare phenomenon.

In any case, it is impossible to predict with accuracy who will have an adverse reaction to a hallucinogen. Should a "bad trip" occur, treatment is generally supportive, e.g., creating a calm environment and reassuring the person she or he is not going crazy. Although chlorpromazine and other antipsychotics have been used to antagonize adverse effects of a hallucinogen, an antianxiety agent such as a benzodiazepine may be preferable if pharmacological treatment is to be used at all.

In contrast to the recreational use of hallucinogens and their potential negative effects, hallucinogenic substances have also been explored for their use in clinical psychotherapy. A variety of circumstances have been proposed in which LSD could be a useful adjunct in therapy because of its

LSD has not been found to be an efficacious adjunct to psychotherapy.

ability to produce emotional lability and openness. These include the management of dying patients, rehabilitation of convicts, counseling people with difficult emotional issues, and treatment of alcoholism. An obscure indole hallucinogen called ibogaine has been receiving attention for its use in Dutch efforts to break drug addiction. However, despite their theoretical attractiveness, none of the hallucinogens has ever been shown to have clinical efficacy in any psychological situation.

Hallucinogens remain classified as Schedule I drugs, a category of illegal drugs that indicates high abuse potential without accepted medical use; heroin and marijuana are other examples. The scheduling system of drugs in the U.S. proceeds through four other categories for drugs of varying abuse potential that are medically accepted. Hence, drugs found on the street are not always Schedule I; cocaine and opium are Schedule II drugs because they are used clinically despite their risk of abuse. A further discussion of the scheduling system can be found in Chapter 66. Tetrahydrocannabinol (THC), the active ingredient in marijuana, is now being made available as a Schedule II drug for use in lessening the nausea resulting from cancer chemotherapy. It has also been experimentally tested for use in reducing intraocular pressure in glaucoma. As with indole and phenethylamine hallucinogens, there are no reports of directly fatal effects due to marijuana; it should be kept in mind that adequate doses of THC can be hallucinogenic.

Tetrahydrocannabinol (THC), the active ingredient in marijuana, is now legally available for certain medical uses.

Nonhallucinogenic Drugs that Induce Hallucinations

Hallucinations can occur as a side effect of drugs not usually classified as hallucinogenic.

Many drugs can produce hallucinations as a secondary effect. Often these agents have also been classified as *psychotomimetic*, but as with the true hallucinogens the behavioral changes do not faithfully replicate clinical psychosis. Drugs that cause hallucination as a side effect often produce delirium as an additional component of the intoxication. This is especially true of the first category of drugs to be discussed, the anticholinergics.

ANTICHOLINERGICS

Atropine and scopolamine can cause CNS disturbances.

Antagonists of the neurotransmitter acetylcholine are found in many members of the plant family *Solanaceae*, which includes deadly nightshade, jimsonweed, and the eyes of the common potato. It is the alkaloids atropine (hyoscyamine), scopolamine (hyoscine), and a number of related substances in these plants that act on the nervous system centrally and peripherally.

Varieties of the genus *Datura* contain these alkaloids in their leaves, flowers, stems, and seeds. *Datura stramonium* (the common jimsonweed or thorn apple) can be smoked or brewed as a tea. Its effects are described in this account.

Delirium, dilated pupils, and dry mucous membranes characterize anticholinergic intoxication.

A 16-year-old girl was admitted with a six-hour history of bizarre behavior. She was seen by the casualty officer, a neurosurgeon, and by a psychiatrist before the possibility of poisoning was considered on the clinical presentation of an acute psychosis with disorientation. She was agitated, talking incoherently and plucking at the bed clothes. The skin and mucous membranes were dry, the pulse was 100/min. and the bladder was slightly distended. The pupils were dilated and reacted sluggishly to light, rotary nystagmus was present, and the tendon reflexes were hyperactive with flexor plantar responses. Her agitation was controlled with diazepam and within 24 hours of admission she was rational and admitted eating two Surama cigarettes. She described vivid frightening hallucinations of dead babies in a satanic black mass. [Ballantyne et al, 1976]

The clues that these symptoms were not the result of indole or phenethylamine hallucinogens are the classic signs of dry mucous membranes and distended bladder typical of parasympathetic blockade.

Another case illustrates why it is important to consider anticholinergic intoxication when delirium and hallucinations are presenting behavior.

Recently we were asked to see a 71-year-old woman admitted for evaluation of her long-standing problem of dizziness. Although she exhibited normal behavior on admission, within 24 hours she became psychotic, displayed agitation and paranoid behavior and complained of visual hallucinations. Her transfer medications were listed as propranolol hydrochloride, 40 mg twice daily; isosorbide dinitrate, 10 mg four times daily; digoxin, 0.125 mg four times daily; furosemide, 40 mg four times daily; and meclizine hydrochloride, 15 mg/day.

The patient was not clinically hypoxic and on physical examination her condition was essentially normal except for a tachycardia of 100 beats per minute, a BP of 220/111 mmHg, widely dilated pupils, and aberrant behavior that did not seem to be altered by the intramuscular administration of 2 mg of haloperidol.

Although not listed on her transfer medications, the patient finally admitted on further questioning to have had "some medicine stuck behind my ear three days ago." A Transderm-V disk (containing scopolamine) was removed and physostigmine salicylate, 1 mg intramuscularly, was administered with complete resolution of her psychotic features, tachycardia and cycloplegia within three hours. [Osterholm and Camoriano, 1982. Copyright 1982, American Medical Association.]

Older people tend to be more sensitive to the behavioral effects of drugs, as seen in this case with a scopolamine patch, so dosages should be monitored. Table 27–2 provides a guide to screening procedures recommended when prescribing to elderly patients. Clinicians should remember

Over-the-counter medicines may be an unrecognized cause of psychiatric symptoms.

Table 27–2   ROUTINE SCREENING PROCEDURES RECOMMENDED FOR ELDERLY PATIENTS IN WHOM USE OF PSYCHOTROPIC DRUGS IS BEING CONSIDERED

History

Is a medical illness causing the "psychiatric" symptoms?
Is a drug the patient is currently taking causing the psychiatric symptoms?
Has the patient had these or other psychiatric symptoms in the past? If so, what was the diagnosis and what medication, if any, was therapeutically effective? What side effects, if any, developed?

Physical Examination

Is there evidence of neurologic, renal, hepatic, or other medical disease that would further increase the elderly patient's risk for side effects?

Mental Status

Is there a psychiatric illness of recent onset?
Is there evidence of dementia or delirium?

Laboratory Studies

Is there evidence of decreased hepatic synthesizing function (e.g., decreased serum albumin) or decreased renal function (e.g., decreased creatinine clearance)?

Drug Interactions

What adverse drug interactions might develop if the psychotropic drug was added to medications the patient is currently taking?

From Thompson TL III, Moran MG, Nies AG: Psychotropic drug use in the elderly. Reprinted, by permission of the New England Journal of Medicine 308:134–138, 1983.

Many common medications have anticholinergic actions.

that medications as diverse as over-the-counter allergy remedies (antihistamines), phenothiazine-type antipsychotics, and tricyclic antidepressants produce anticholinergic effects; frequently overlooked as a source of anticholinergic toxicity are bladder and urinary antispasmodics. The wide spectrum of such anticholinergic effects have been summarized.

Signs of extreme parasympathetic blockade are present with anticholinergic toxicity.

Confusion and incoordination may develop as CNS effects.

The symptoms and signs of toxicity develop promptly after ingestion of the drug. The mouth becomes dry and burns, swallowing and talking become difficult or impossible, and there is marked thirst. The vision is blurred and photophobia is prominent; the pupils are dilated. The skin is hot, dry and flushed. The body temperature tends to rise. The pulse is weak and rapid. Palpitations may occur and the blood pressure is elevated. Urinary urgency and difficulty in micturition occurs especially in older men. The behavior and mental symptoms may suggest an acute organic psychosis. Memory is disturbed, orientation is faulty, hallucinations (especially visual) are common, the sensorium is clouded and mania and delirium are not unusual.

The patient may be restless, excited and confused, and exhibit muscular incoordination. Gait and speech are disturbed. The diagnosis of an acute schizophrenic episode or alcoholic delirium has been mistakenly made. [Weiner, 1980, p. 127]

These symptoms have given rise to various mnemonics such as the following:

- Dry as a bone (blockade of salivation and sweating)
- Blind as a bat (mydriasis and paralysis of accommodation)
- Hot as a hen (hyperthermia and peripheral vasodilation)
- Red as a beet (no sweat and peripheral vasodilatation)
- Mad as a hatter (delirious; reference from insanity seen in hat makers in nineteenth-century England who were chronically exposed to mercury)

Anticholinergic poisoning can be antagonized by physostigmine; physostigmine has a short duration of action and a narrow margin of safety.

The treatment for anticholinergic overdose is as for atropine poisoning. This includes gastric lavage, control of body temperature, and maintenance of urine flow. Because anticholinergics act as competitive antagonists at acetylcholine receptors, their effects may be overcome by the careful use of physostigmine. If sedation is required, a barbiturate or benzodiazepine may be given.

PHENCYCLIDINE

Phencyclidine, known also as PCP or "angel dust," was developed in the 1950s as a potential anesthetic-analgesic. Its chemical structure as an arylcyclohexylamine resembles that of ketamine, an anesthetic used in humans. Both agents can cause marked delirium and hallucinations. Phencyclidine (under the trade name SERNYL) was removed from the market in the 1960s because these effects were frequent and pronounced upon recovery from the anesthesia. It is very easy and inexpensive to synthesize, however, which helped to make it a popularly available street drug in the 1970s.

Although PCP has some euphorigenic effects, it also can produce delirium and unpleasant hallucinations.

PCP is generally termed a *dissociative* anesthetic (see Chapter 16 concerning anesthetics). It has been shown to inhibit the reuptake of dopamine, serotonin, and norepinephrine and may act at an opioid receptor. Evidence also suggests that PCP acts at excitatory amino acid receptors, specifically the N-methyl-D-aspartate (NMDA) receptor. The common features are shown in these case reports:

PCP has effects on many neurochemical systems.

A 22-year-old male was traveling at approximately 5 mph at 4:15 p.m. on a busy highway. He was pulled over by police who described the subject as sitting behind the wheel, staring straight ahead, clenching and unclenching his fists and foaming at the mouth. There was no response to questions. The attending physician described the patient as non-responsive to verbal commands, eyes open but unable to follow moving objects and nonresponsive to painful stimuli. [Clardy et al, 1979]

Unresponsiveness to environmental stimuli is typical with PCP intoxication.

A 29-year-old man . . . became floridly psychotic after . . . having smoked a marijuana cigarette laced with [PCP]. He suffered from auditory hallucinations that told how his hands had offended him, and commanded punishment by biting both his arms. It is possible the phencyclidine serves as the trigger in the development of a long-lasting psychosis. [Grove, 1989]

In addition to these bizarre effects, PCP symptoms include changes in body image, feelings of inebriation, hypertension, negativism or hostility, coma or stupor without respiratory depression (Luby et al, 1959). The lethal dose of 20–100 mg is associated with convulsions, hypotension, and cardiac arrhythmias. There is no specific antagonist, so treatment of PCP intoxification is symptomatic. General care appropriate for possible hypertension, coma, or violence should be provided, and stimuli should be minimized. Acidification of urine increases PCP excretion but may increase the risk of renal failure. If convulsions develop, they may be treated with diazepam.

Convulsions may occur with a lethal dose of PCP.

STIMULANTS

Stimulants of the CNS include such drugs as amphetamine, cocaine, and methylphenidate. Although many stimulants share a structure that resembles amphetamine, this is not always the case. Hence, although there are many pharmacological similarities among the various compounds, each stimulant also has effects that are unique.

Psychosis can result from chronic stimulant use.

Chronic use of relatively low levels of a stimulant, as well as large acute doses, can result in a syndrome resembling psychosis. This was first noted in individuals who were using amphetamines for their anorexic effects as appetite suppressants (Connell, 1958), although related behavior has been seen in people using cocaine. Agitation and paranoia are characteristic, and these may be accompanied by tactile hallucinations of bugs crawling underneath the skin. This syndrome is often seen in people who take stimulants to maintain adequate work performance.

Agitation and paranoia are prominent with stimulant overdose.

A 27-year-old truck driver shot his boss in the back of the head because he thought the boss was trying to release a poison gas into the back seat of the car in which he was riding. "I thought they had gassed me. My boss kept reaching down beside him and pulling on something. I rolled the window down to let the gas out. I got nauseated and passed out due to the gas. I then got up on my elbow and shot my boss, who was driving." Over the previous 20 hours, in order to make a nonstop 1,600 mile trip, Mr. A had ingested 180 mg of amphetamine; he had not slept for 48 hours. [Ellingwood, 1970]

Acute high-dose intoxication has been encountered from what has been called the *cocaine body-packer syndrome.* This results from the rupture of condoms filled with cocaine that had been swallowed to smuggle co-

Smuggling cocaine in body cavities presents serious risk of poisoning.

Cocaine can cause death from cardiac arrhythmias.

caine through customs at border checks. It is clear that cocaine can be lethal. The causes of death appear to include fatal cardiac arrhythmias and cerebrovascular accidents as well as uncontrollable seizures. The following case report is condensed from Jonsson and colleagues (1983).

> A 44-year-old man was admitted after having been arrested for suspicion of cocaine smuggling. He admitted to having hidden 14 rubber condoms filled with cocaine in his rectum before departure from a South American country.
>
> Initially, the patient appeared well. On the day of admission the patient was given oral laxatives and subsequently passed 11 rubber condoms, each containing approximately 20 g of a white powder substance identified as cocaine on toxicologic study. The patient remained asymptomatic that day. In an attempt to induce elimination of the remaining balloons, a tap-water enema was given the next morning. An hour later, agitation, diaphoresis and tachycardia suddenly developed in the patient, followed by a generalized seizure, after which he was apneic with a rapid feeble pulse and hypotension (systolic blood pressure of 90 mmHg).

"Crack" and "ice" pose major hazards from overdoses.

With the rising popularity of smokable forms of cocaine ("crack") and amphetamines ("ice"), the possibility of overdose from stimulants increases because users often administer these drugs repeatedly within a short period of time.

Experimental evidence shows that all stimulants acutely block the reuptake of the monoamine neurotransmitters, and some also cause the release of these chemicals. With prolonged use, there is depletion of neurotransmitters and compensatory up-regulation of receptor numbers, making the systems more sensitive. Treatment of stimulant intoxication with antipsychotics has been suggested, based on neurochemical changes in the brain, but it is preferable to give clinical support and protection. Acidification of the urine is theoretically of value but has not been practically useful in increasing stimulant elimination.

SELECTED THERAPEUTIC AGENTS

The following are but a few examples of other drugs that can produce mental disturbances when given in sufficient quantity or to a sensitive person. A more extensive list of agents that cause psychiatric symptoms is found in Table 27–3; this list can serve as a checklist when a patient presents with psychiatric symptoms.

Behavioral toxicity is common with digitalis; especially vulnerable are older patients.

Digitalis glycosides are one of the very common but frequently overlooked causes of peculiar behavior in elderly adults. The ability of digitalis to induce clouded perception was recognized in 1874 by Duroziez who called it *délire digitalique.* This case history is but one from hundreds in the literature.

> A 56-year-old white male . . . [had] an aortic valve replacement. He was discharged 24 days after the operation feeling well, apyrexial, with no evidence of cardiac failure, and mentally normal. Therapy at the time of discharge was digoxin, furosemide, potassium, and coumarin. Two weeks after returning home he became progressively more confused and disoriented, particularly at night, with hallucinations typical of . . . a toxic delirious state. He was restless, paranoid and extremely agitated and there was marked intellectual deterioration. He was readmitted. In view of the absence of congestive cardiac failure, his digoxin and diuretic were stopped. . . . Within 24–48

Table 27–3   PSYCHIATRIC SYMPTOMS PRODUCED BY DRUGS, AND A PARTIAL LIST OF THE DRUGS (Similar drugs are grouped together)

Delirium: Ranging From Mild Confusion and Disorientation to Frank Delirium

Anticholinergic, including anticholinergic and possibly related
 Antiasthmatic preparations
 Urinary tract antispasmodics
 Atropine, scopolamine, belladonna alkaloids
 Antiparkinsonian
 Antihistaminics
 Phenothiazines
 Trazodone
 Tricyclic antidepressants
Digitalis glycosides
Quinidine
Barbiturates
Sedative/hypnotics
Anticonvulsants
 Phenytoin
Diuretics
Chlorambucil
Amphotericin B
Cisplatin
Cephalosporins
Chloroquine
Chloramphenicol
Cycloserine

Gentamicin
Trimethoprim-sulfamethoxazole
Tobramycin
Atenolol
Cimetidine
Ranitidine
Disulfiram
Indomethacin
Naproxen
Salicylates (chronic)
Levodopa
Methyldopa
Pentazocine
Propoxyphene
Lidocaine
Tocainide
Metrizamide
Niridazole
Podophyllin
Acyclovir
Aminocaproic acid
Asparaginase
Captopril
Folate deficiency

Depression

Corticosteroids
Naproxen
Ibuprofen
Indomethacin
Digitalis glycosides
Thiazide diuretics
Ethionamide
Phenacetin
Timolol
Levodopa
Methyldopa
Amitriptyline
Disulfiram
Pentazocine
Meperidine

Phenylephrine
Reserpine, rescinnamine
Vinblastine
Thyroid hormone deficiency
Benzodiazepines
 Diazepam
 Alprazolam
Bromides
Asparaginase
Cimetidine
Prazosin
Trichlormethiazide
Folate deficiency
Baclofen
Oral contraceptives

Hallucinations

Anticholinergic (see Delirium list)
Levodopa
Amantadine
Ergotamine
Corticosteroids
Opioids
 Methadone
 Meperidine
 Propoxyphene
 Pentazocine
Benzodiazepines
 Triazolam
 Diazepam
 Clonazepam
Isocarboxazid
Diphenidol
Albuterol
Digitalis glycosides
Quinidine
Dapsone
Gentamicin
Ibuprofen
Indomethacin
Salicylates (chronic)
Thiabendazole

Methysergide
Niridazole
Oxymetazoline
Vincristine
Trazodone
Thiabendazole
Bromocriptine
Acyclovir
Anticonvulsants
 Ethosuccimide
 Phenytoin
 Primidone
Tocainide
Procaine
Antidepressants
Caffeine
Pseudoephedrine, phenylephrine
Chloroquine
Chloramphenicol
Tobramycin
Cimetidine
Cyclosporine
Cycloserine
Prazosin

Table continued on following page

Table 27-3   PSYCHIATRIC SYMPTOMS PRODUCED BY DRUGS, AND A PARTIAL LIST OF THE DRUGS (Similar drugs are grouped together) (Continued)

Schizophrenia-like Symptoms

Bromocriptine	Reserpine
Amphetamines	Barbiturates
Cocaine	Sedative/hypnotics
Phencyclidine	Acyclovir
Baclofen	Diuretics
Anticholinergic agents	Potassium deficiency
Corticosteroids	

Paranoia (Plus Many More Under Delirium)

Propranolol	Baclofen
Phenylephrine	Cimetidine
Albuterol	Cycloserine
NSAIDs	Clonazepam
Ibuprofen	Isoniazid
Indomethacin	Methyldopa
Salicylates (chronic)	Procainamide
Sulindac	Lidocaine
Naproxen	

hours his agitation and confusion lessened and he developed insight into his abnormal behavior. . . . After one week he had returned to complete normality. [Sagel and Matisonn, 1972]

Propranolol has been repeatedly linked to behavioral changes as a result of withdrawal as illustrated by this case.

Abrupt discontinuation of many drugs, for example propranolol, can result in withdrawal symptoms that present as behavioral disturbances.

A 52-year-old man with no previous history of psychiatric illness was admitted to our inpatient service for evaluation of acute mental status changes. Four days earlier, he had become confused and disoriented. He refused to speak to anyone and began to stare blankly into space. He began to mutter to himself about "going to jail, going to jump in the river." His family described apparent paranoid ideation; the patient talked to them about "someone coming to burn my house down," and despite their reassurances, he was convinced that he would no longer be able to live with them.

The patient's family reported that he had been taking 80 mg/day of propranolol for many weeks until a few days before the change in his behavior, when he abruptly discontinued the medication after "running out of pills."

Upon admission, the patient reported seeing bugs crawling over him and the examining physician. His mood was suspicious, hostile and perplexed. Physical examination was remarkable for mildly elevated blood pressure (144/100). The neurology consultation team . . . did not feel that CT scan findings could account for the patient's acute symptomatology.

The patient's mental status began to improve dramatically approximately 12 hours after restarting the propranolol. By the tenth hospital day, the patient was completely back to his baseline. [Golden et al, 1989]

The initial signs of a drug toxicity may be changes in behavior.

Quinidine is representative of a large group of agents that are infrequently associated with psychiatric disturbances. Nonetheless, in isolated instances, behavioral changes may be the first sign of toxicity:

A 72-year-old woman was hospitalized because of severe memory loss and chronic confusional state of several years' duration. She could not perform household tasks, cope with small amounts of money, remember a shopping list, find her way about indoors or along familiar streets or recall events.

Since suffering acute myocardial infarction 14 years previously, the patient had regularly taken 400 mg of quinidine sulfate and 50 mg of hydrochlorothiazide daily. The results of all laboratory studies—including urinalysis, lipid profile, thyroid profile, blood serologic test, skull x-ray, brain scan, cerebrospinal fluid exam, medial supraorbital telethermometry, serum vitamin B12 and magnesium levels and a computerized axial tomographic brain scan—were all normal. The EEG showed a mild and diffuse slowing. On admission the serum sodium level was 125 mEq/liter and the potassium level was 3.3 mEq/liter. Diuretic medication was discontinued on admission . . . and by the fourth day the serum sodium had risen to normal (138 mEq/liter) without any improvement in her mentation.

The patient remained severely confused and disoriented and had vivid nocturnal hallucinations. After the patient had been hospitalized for two weeks without evidencing any improvement, it was elected to discontinue the quinidine. The following day she was greatly improved; within 48 hours she was well oriented for time and place. [Gilbert, 1977. Copyright 1977, American Medical Association.]

Antihistamines can produce a variety of behavioral disturbances in different individuals. In some they cause drowsiness, in others stimulation, and in others very bizarre effects.

A 3-year-old girl received two 5 ml doses of Actifed (pseudoephedrine and tripolidine) during the night. The following day she suddenly developed episodes of uncontrollable terror, complaining of seeing spiders and insects. On examination she was intermittently pushing and brushing away invisible objects and also hitting out and stamping. The episodes continued intermittently for three days. [Sankey et al, 1984]

To what extent the pseudoephedrine or the combination contributed to this response is not known.

Medications that produce orthostatic hypotension in therapeutic doses may also be the cause of any of the following behavioral symptoms: dizziness, confusion, visual difficulties, impotence, or fatigability (Lipsitz, 1989).

A variety of drugs can produce, precipitate, or aggravate anxiety (Table 27-4). As discussed in Chapter 20 on antianxiety agents, the symptom of anxiety is an almost universal affective and physiological response to threatened or real danger, or the anxiety may consist of unrealistic fears in the absence of apparent stimuli. It is a common component of such psychiatric syndromes as schizophrenia, paranoia, depression, mania, and many personality disorders. The diagnostic work-up of an individual with symptoms of anxiety mandates that all potential sources of the anxiety be explored, including any drugs the person may be taking. Central nervous system stimulants in particular should be assessed in detail, especially the daily levels of caffeine because its use is so pervasive.

Table 27-4 DRUGS THAT INDUCE ANXIETY, PANIC, AND CENTRAL NERVOUS SYSTEM STIMULATION

Caffeine
Theophylline (cf. interactions with the numerous drugs that can alter theophylline pharmacokinetics)
Cocaine
Amphetamines
    Amphetamine (formerly Benzedrine; now in Biphetamine with dextroamphetamine)
    Dextroamphetamine (Dexedrine and others)
    Ephedrine (common ingredient in cold remedies)
Methylphenidate (Ritalin)
Other appetite suppressants
    Diethylproprion
    Phenylpropanolamine (PPA)
    Fenfluramine

Lidocaine
Procaine
2-chloroprocaine
Tocainide

Lactate intravenous infusion (experimental induction of anxiety)
CO_2 (by rebreathing, respiratory insufficiency, or drug-induced, such as with opioids or benzodiazepines)
Verapamil (increased depression and anxiety scores)
Camphor
Tricyclic antidepressants (jitteriness may be prominent; anxiety upon abrupt discontinuation)
Antipsychotics (phenothiazines, haloperidol)
Mianserin (panic anxiety increased *after discontinuation*)
Benzodiazepines (acute withdrawal after chronic use and acute paradoxical reactions)
Beta carbolines
Fluoxetine (acute vs. withdrawal effect)

People taking antihistamines can develop psychotic ideation.

Drug-Induced Anxiety

Anxiety is a common symptom resulting from the use of many kinds of drugs.

The source of anxiety may not be readily apparent.

CAFFEINE

The effects of caffeine are dependent on a person's sensitivity and rate of metabolism.

It is widely recognized that there are marked differences in the amounts of caffeine different individuals consume, the corresponding blood levels of caffeine obtained, and the magnitudes of the effects experienced. Some of the obvious factors involved are age, acquired functional and metabolic tolerance, differences in rates of metabolism, and physical dependence. Caffeine predictably produces increased alertness, decreased sleep and sleepiness, insomnia, and increased ability to work out mathematical and cognitive problems. At low doses there is usually an increased sense of well-being and mental capacity. With larger doses irritability may develop into what is commonly called *coffee nerves.* Physiological tremor is increased, and reflexes are hyperactive; there is also a modest bronchodilating effect.

Large doses of caffeine can cause marked CNS stimulation.

An ambitious 37-year-old Army lieutenant colonel was referred from a medical clinic to a psychiatric outpatient facility because of a two-year history of "chronic anxiety." The symptoms, which occurred almost daily, included dizziness, tremulousness, apprehension about job performance, "butterflies in the stomach," restlessness, frequent episodes of "diarrhea," and persistent difficulty in both falling and remaining asleep.

Determination of caffeine intake is an integral part of every adequate medical history.

Three complete medical workups had been negative. . . . In reply to questioning from the psychiatrist, he described consuming at least 8–14 cups of coffee a day . . . he also frequently drank hot cocoa before bedtime . . . and his soft drink preference was exclusively colas (3–4 a day). Total caffeine intake thus approximated 1,200 mg a day.

He was initially unwilling to limit his intake of coffee, cocoa and colas. When symptoms persisted, however, he voluntarily reduced his daily intake of caffeine and four weeks after his initial visit, he reported distinct improvement of his long-standing tremulousness, loose stools and insomnia. [Greden, 1974]

Physical exhaustion can happen with prolonged caffeine ingestion.

In the absence of a decrease in caffeine intake, sleep will eventually occur from exhaustion in spite of large doses that may have kept a person awake for up to 24 hours. Overt seizures, however, have occurred only with massive overdoses in some people.

Although not well studied, older individuals appear to have an increased sensitivity to the sleep-disturbing effects of caffeine. Probably the major source of individual differences is related to the remarkable extremes in the rates of caffeine metabolism. For some the half-life is only 2 hours, whereas others may show a half-life for caffeine of greater than 15 hours. The longer half-lives are consistent with some individual's observation that even a cup of coffee at noon or early afternoon may result in difficulty in falling asleep at night. On a population basis, the more rapid metabolizers are those who are the heaviest consumers; the slower metabolizers tend to consume much less.

An individual's rate of caffeine metabolism determines the duration of caffeine's effects.

Caffeine is present in numerous common foods and over-the-counter medicines.

The sources of caffeine are numerous, yet their intake is all too often not determined or recognized in medical diagnostic assessments. Besides the familiar sources of coffee, cola drinks, and teas, caffeine is found in over-the-counter preparations for pain, colds, asthma, and menstrual symptoms. Diet aids, sleep prevention aids, and noncola soft drinks also may contain significant amounts of caffeine. Caffeine is a primary ingredient in the mail-order "look-alike drugs" sold as energizers, stimulants, "cocaine-like" drugs, and enhancers of sexual prowess. Table 27–5 lists the caffeine content of some of the many sources of this substance.

Table 27-5 CAFFEINE CONTENT OF CERTAIN BEVERAGES AND DRUGS

Source	Approximate amount of caffeine per unit (5 oz cup or tablet)
Beverages	
Brewed coffee	80–150 mg
Instant coffee	85–100 mg
Decaffeinated coffee	2–4 mg
Tea (bag or leaf)	30–75 mg
Cocoa	5–40 mg
Cola drinks	35–60 mg*
Nonprescription (OTC) Drugs	
Analgesics	
Anacin, Bromo-Seltzer, Cope, Empirin compound	32 mg
Excedrin	60 mg
Stimulants	
No Doz	100 mg
Vivarin	200 mg
Caffedrine	250 mg
Many cold preparations	32 mg

From Oakley R: Drugs, Society and Human Behavior, 196. St Louis: CV Mosby Co, 1978.
*12 oz.

Although caffeine is demonstrably a common cause of anxiety or other disturbances, its effects are often not fully appreciated by the individual outside of the fact that routine coffee drinkers know they need the beverage to get started in the morning. Even patients with extreme insomnia frequently deny that coffee or another caffeinated beverage plays a role in their troubles with sleeping. At least some of the failure to make a connection between caffeine and one's symptoms derives from the fact that as a young adult the person may not have experienced any disruption of mood or sleep from caffeine consumption. The apparent change in sensitivity is possibly related to changes in sleep physiology with age as well as the fact that young adults are often sleep-deprived.

Sensitivity to caffeine may change over a person's life.

Assessing the impact of caffeine on a person is complicated by the fact that its chronic consumption results not only in tolerance but in physical dependence. The omission of the usual 1–4 cups of coffee in the morning in a regular user results in mental sluggishness, feelings of depression, plus an inability to think, write, or carry out cognitive procedures in a coherent manner. A dull, generalized headache and increased irritability appear late in the morning or early afternoon. These symptoms are promptly relieved by ingestion of caffeine, indicating that this is a withdrawal syndrome from a substance the person was physically dependent on. An interesting aspect of caffeine is the occurrence of increased irritability and anxiety both as acute effects and as symptoms of withdrawal.

Chronic caffeine consumption results in tolerance and physical dependence.

Caffeine augments and aggravates conditions of anxiety, depression, panic, and mania. In recognition of this, many psychiatric and substance-abuse treatment centers avoid serving any caffeine-containing beverages.

Caffeine can interfere with the treatment of behavioral disorders.

Chemically, caffeine is classified as a methylated xanthine. Another compound in this category is theophylline, which has similar excitatory actions on the CNS as caffeine yet is not as potent. Theophylline is found in various teas and is also used extensively in the clinical treatment of cardio-respiratory disease. Methylxanthines are antagonists of the sedative actions of adenosine. It is thought that the CNS excitation produced by methylxanthines are the consequence of their blockade of adenosine receptors (see Chapter 62).

Methylxanthines block the sedative effects of adenosine.

OTHER ANXIETY-INDUCING DRUGS

Stimulants are not the only drugs that cause anxiety.

As was previously discussed, cocaine and amphetamine-like drugs may cause anxious behavior and irritability; this can be true even when psychotic-like symptoms are not present. Other drugs that have been known to produce anxiety are shown in Table 27–4. The anxiety is a predictable effect for many of them, such as the local anesthetics, camphor, and the endogenously occurring β carbolines (see Chapter 20). For a number of others, such as antipsychotics, antidepressants, and benzodiazepines, the appearance of anxiety is a unique individual effect, making this possibility an easy one to overlook in management of patients with psychiatric or chronic medical disease. The source of anxiety in patients with a chronic disease may be difficult to determine because it can also be associated with postural hypotension, hypokalemia, or CO_2 retention.

Anxiety may be precipitated by withdrawal from medicines.

In addition to being an acute drug effect, anxiety is an extremely common component of the withdrawal syndrome for many agents, including benzodiazepines, antidepressants, and alcohol. Except for alcohol, withdrawal syndromes may be delayed for over a week after discontinuation of a drug, so the connection between the anxiety and the discontinuation of one or more drugs is infrequently appreciated. Moreover, withdrawal need not be absolute for anxiety to appear; a reduction in dose or an increase in drug metabolism might be sufficient to evoke such withdrawal symptoms.

Drugs That Induce Aggression

Human aggression can be thought of as being either appropriate or inappropriate. For example, when people are under physical threat or attack, aggressive self-defense is considered to be a rational response. Organized sporting events are also situations in which violent behavior is often socially acceptable. On the other hand, when hostility is unprovoked, excessive, or directed at an inappropriate target it is deemed to be of concern to society. Hence, the aggression that is produced as a side effect of certain drugs should be understood to indicate inappropriate behavior.

Inappropriate aggression may result from the use of certain drugs.

ANABOLIC STEROIDS

Anabolic steroids may affect the CNS.

During the 1980s, anabolic steroids have been brought to the public eye as one class of agents that can produce a broad spectrum of psychological derangements, including aggression. These effects were first utilized by German soldiers during World War II but are experienced today by modern athletes who take these agents primarily to build up muscle strength and dimensions.

Testosterone is the base structure of anabolic steroids.

Anabolic steroids are chemically derived from the male sex hormone, testosterone. They were developed as drugs that would produce more anabolism than testosterone yet with a lesser degree of androgenizing effects. Anabolic steroids are used clinically in male hypogonadism and hereditary angioneurotic edema, but it is their nonmedical use by athletic persons that has drawn attention to their negative side effects. A football player who had been taking massive doses of anabolic steroids reported:

Violence and irrationality can develop with chronic anabolic steroid use.

> My aggression level was so high that I got into an argument and went to my locker, put my hand through the metal mesh and ripped the door off its hinges. Then I went back to [my room] and took a baseball bat and demolished my refrigerator, smashed it to pieces and then ripped the phone off the wall. My nerves were on edge like they'd never been before. At practice one day I got into a fight with a line-

backer. . . . I threw him down . . . and smashed his eye. As he got up, bleeding and humiliated, I felt sympathy for him. But then the steroids kicked in and I said to myself, "All right! You're a tough guy!" [Chaikin and Telander, 1988]

This behavior is widely recognized by illicit users and is referred to as *'roid rage.* Anabolic steroid abuse is not restricted to professional athletes; studies indicate that up to 7% of high-school students may be using the drugs. In addition to aggression, a psychotic-like syndrome has also been described in response to anabolic steroids that can include auditory hallucinations, paranoid delusions, and manic episodes. Immediate discontinuation of the drug is called for should psychiatric symptoms occur, and violent behavior can be treated with restraint or antipsychotics.

> Symptoms of psychosis may be present after long-term administration of anabolic steroids.

CORTICOSTEROIDS

People taking corticosteroids frequently report behavioral changes that may include aggression as well as more severe psychotic symptoms.

> Another potential source of aggression are corticosteroids.

The accused had a congenital malformation of his maxilla for which an operation was necessary. He was given dexamethasone 8 mg daily for three days from the day before his operation and 4 mg on the fourth day.

During the days [following the operation] he experienced rapid fluctuations of mood, expressed suicidal ideas and attempted to jump from a car. . . . Eleven days after the operation . . . he rammed his head forcibly against a wall and attacked his fiancee with . . . a knife. After arrest he struggled violently with the police and repeatedly attempted to commit suicide. He responded to neuroleptics and his psychotic symptoms remitted within 3 days. [D'Orban, 1989]

Conclusions

These case reports and tables demonstrate that it is not possible for anyone to remember all the potential behavioral effects of all drugs. What is feasible is, first, to remember those agents that are the most common or most striking offenders and, second, to establish one's own principles and rules to follow in evaluating and assessing every patient who presents with a psychiatric symptom.

Without doubt, drugs can produce, frequently unbeknownst to the individual or others, delirium, dementia, psychosis, anxiety, hallucinations, aggression, paranoia, or disturbance of sleep/wakefulness. These effects of drugs can occur with usual therapeutic doses and blood levels as well as with overdoses; the effects can be acute or chronic.

Moreover, as emphasized in Chapter 67, in the absence of specific analysis, the identity of a street drug is never known. This is true no matter what name the drug was sold under (e.g., phencyclidine is often claimed to be THC). In addition, irrational and sometimes dangerous combinations of drugs may be present. Consequently, treatment must be guided primarily by the symptoms exhibited by the patient and not by possibly incorrect assumptions or claims about the specific drug in question. Toxicological analyses may be helpful, but efficient and effective identification of an unknown compound may depend on accurate speculation of what class the drug falls into. In preparation for meeting psychiatric emergencies it is more important to develop a good working knowledge of quickly available resource material than to try the impossible task of remembering every possible action of a drug.

> Keep in mind those drugs most often associated with behavioral changes.

> Rely on presenting symptoms in determining treatment, not what the person was supposed to have taken.

> Consultation of reference materials is frequently essential for accurate diagnosis and effective treatment of psychiatric symptoms.

Nevertheless, an up-to-date drug history that includes all of the prescription, over-the-counter, and street drugs is essential for every patient that exhibits unusual behavior.

In the management and treatment of any psychiatric or behavioral condition, every effort should be made to discontinue and avoid all drugs during the period of initial evaluation. Periodic assessments (which may include drug holidays from prescribed medication) may be recommended thereafter.

References

Abed RT, Clark PJ: Acute psychotic episode caused by the abuse of phensedyl. Br J Psychiatry 151:868, 1987.

Abramowicz M, Aaron H (eds): Drugs that cause psychiatric symptoms. Med Lett Drugs Ther 28:81–86, 1986.

Ackerman WE, Phero JC, Juneja MM: Panic disorder following 2-chloroprocaine. (Letter.) Am J Psychiatry 146:940–941, 1989.

Ballantyne A, Lippiette P, Park J: Herbal cigarettes for kicks. Brit Med J 2:1539–1540, 1976.

Brahams D: Benzodiazepines and sexual fantasies. Lancet 335(8682):157, 1990.

Braunig P, Bleistein J, Rao ML: Suicidality and corticosteroid-induced psychosis. Biol Psychiatry 26:209–210, 1989.

Cape RDT: Drugs and confusional states. *In* Crooks J, Stevenson IH (eds): Drugs and the Elderly, Chapter 25. Baltimore: University Park Press, 1979.

Chaiken T, Telander R: The nightmare of steroids. Sports Illustrated Oct 24, 1988, 82–102.

Clardy DO, Cravey RH, MacDonald BJ, et al: Phencyclidine-intoxicated driver. J Anal Toxicol 3:238–241, 1979.

Connell PH: Amphetamine Psychosis. London: Oxford University Press, 1958.

Coodley EL: Drug metabolism in the aged. Rational Drug Ther 17(12):1–6, 1983.

Cummings JL: Organic psychoses, delusional disorders and secondary mania. Psychiatr Clin North Am 9:293–311, 1986.

Denicoff KD, Joffe RT, Lakshmanan MC, et al: Neuropsychiatric manifestations of altered thyroid state. Am J Psychiatry 147:94–99, 1990.

Derlet RW: Cocaine intoxication. Postgrad Med 86:245–253, 1989.

D'Orban PT: Steroid-induced psychosis. Lancet 2(8664):694, 1989.

Drug Interactions and Side Effects Index. Oradell, NJ: Medical Economics Company, 1988. Keyed to PDR 42nd ed 1988.

Dundee JW: Do fantasies occur with intravenous benzodiazepines? SAAD Digest 6:173–176, 1986.

Ellingwood EH: Assault and homicide associated with amphetamine abuse. Am J Psychiatry 127:1170–1175, 1970.

Fisch RZ, Lahad A: Adverse psychiatric reaction to ketoconazole. Am J Psychiatry 146:939–940, 1989.

Fox AW: More on rhabdomyolysis associated with cocaine intoxication. N Engl J Med 321:1271, 1989.

Fuller MA, Sajatovic M: Neurotoxicity resulting from a combination of lithium and loxapine. J Clin Psychiatry 50:187, 1989.

Gardner EE, Hall RC: Psychiatric symptoms produced by over-the-counter drugs. Psychosomatics 23:186–190, 1982.

Gautier. *Cited in* Moreau JJ: Hashish and Mental Illness, 12. 1845. Reprint, edited by Peters H, Nahas GG, translated by Barnett GJ. New York: Raven Press, 1973.

Gilbert GJ: Quinidine dementia. JAMA 237:2093–2094, 1977.

Golden RN: Diethylpropion, bupropion, and psychoses. Br J Psychiatry 153:265–266, 1988.

Golden RN, Hoffman J, Falk D, et al: Psychoses associated with propranolol withdrawal. Biol Psychiatry 25:351–354, 1989.

Goldfrank L, Flomenbaum N, Lewin N: Anticholinergic poisoning. J Toxicol Clin Toxicol 19:17–25, 1982.

Greden JF: Anxiety of caffeinism; A diagnostic dilemma. Am J Psychiatry 131:1089–1092, 1974.

Grove VE Jr: Phencyclidine (angel dust) invades Texas. Texas Med 75:64–65, 1979.

Jonsson S, O'Meara M, Young JB: Acute cocaine poisoning—Importance of treating seizures and acidosis. Am J Med 75:1061–1064, 1983.

Larson EW, Richelson E: Organic causes of mania. Mayo Clin Proc 63:906–912, 1988.

Ling MHM, Perry PJ, Tsuang MT: Side effects of corticosteroid therapy. Arch Gen Psychiatry 38:471–477, 1981.

Lipowski ZJ: Delirium (acute confusional states). JAMA 258:1789–1792, 1987.

Lipsitz LA: Orthostatic hypotension in the elderly. N Engl J Med 321:952–957, 1989.

Luby ED, Cohen BD, Rosenbaum et al: Study of a new schizophrenomimetic drug—Sernyl. AMA Arch Neurol Psychiatry 81:363–369, 1959.

Mego DM, Omori DJM, Hanley JF: Transdermal scopolamine as a cause of transient psychosis in two elderly patients. South Med J 81:394–395, 1988.

Negrete JC: Cannabis and schizophrenia. Br J Addict 84:349–351, 1989.

Oakley R: Drugs, Society and Human Behavior. St. Louis: CV Mosby Co, 1978.

Osterholm RK, Camoriano JK: Transdermal scopolamine psychosis. JAMA 247:3081, 1982.

Ostfeld AM, Machne X, Unna KR: The effects of atropine on the electroencephalogram and behavior in man. J Pharmacol Exp Ther 128:265–272, 1960.

Pope HG, Katz DL: Affective and psychotic symptoms associated with anabolic steroid use. Am J Psychiatry 145:487–490, 1988.

Safer DJ, Allen RP: The central effects of scopolamine in man. Biol Psychiatry 3:347–355, 1971.

Sagel J, Matisonn R: Neuropsychiatric disturbances as the initial manifestation of digitalis toxicity. S Afr Med J 46:512–514, 1972.

Sankey RJ, Nunn AJ, Sills JA: Visual hallucinations in children receiving decongestants. Br Med J 288:1369, 1984.

Sherer MA: Intravenous cocaine: Psychiatric effects, biological mechanisms. Biol Psychiatry 24:865–885, 1988.

Sherer MA, Kumor KM, Cone EJ, Jaffee JH: Suspiciousness induced by four-hour intravenous infusions of cocaine. Arch Gen Psychiatry 45:673–677, 1988.

Stafford P: Psychedelics Encyclopedia. Los Angeles: JP Tarcher, 1983.

Stramonium poisoning. JAMA 262:687, 1989.

Thompson TL III, Moran MG, Nies AS: Psychotropic drug use in the elderly. N Engl J Med 308:134–138, 1983.

Verghese C: Quinine psychosis. Br J Psychiatry 153:575–576, 1988.

Wagner SL, Gallant JD: Organophosphate intoxication from over-the-counter insecticides. Ann Emerg Med 18:802, 1989.

Weiner N: Atropine, scopolamine and related anti-muscarinic drugs. *In* Goodman AG, Goodman LS, Gilman A (eds): Goodman and Gilman's The Pharmacological Basis of Therapeutics. 6th ed, 127. New York: Macmillan Publishing Co., 1980.

Wood KA, Harris MJ, Morreale A, Rizos AL: Drug-induced psychosis and depression in the elderly. Psychiatr Clin North Am 11: 167–193, 1988.

Wright HH, Cole EA, Batey SR, Hanna K: Phencyclidine-induced psychosis: Eight-year follow-up of ten cases. South Med J 81:565–567, 1988.

Zisking AA: Transdermal scopolamine-induced psychosis. Postgrad Med 84:73–76, 1988.

Autocoids and Anti-Inflammatory Drugs

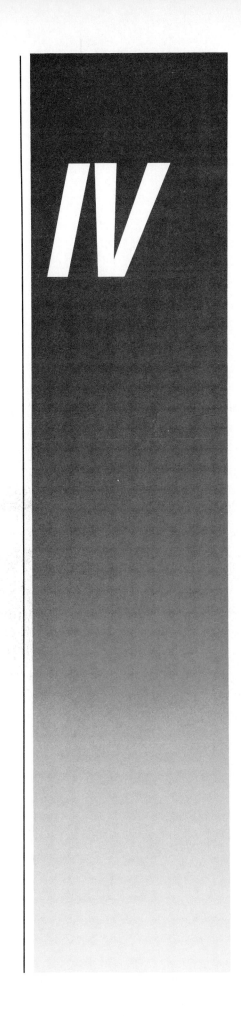

Inflammation and Nonsteroidal Anti-Inflammatory Drugs

28

James B. Lee
Shigehiro Katayama

Inflammation is a fundamental pathophysiological response designed to eliminate any noxious stimulus introduced into the host. Such noxious stimuli include radiant, chemical, physical, infectious, and immune provocations. The inflammatory reaction is readily divided into an acute and chronic response. The acute reaction, described by Celsus in the first century AD, is characterized by redness, heat, swelling, and pain (*rubor, calor, tumor,* and *dolor*) with an accompanying loss of function. It should be remembered that the pain response may be characterized by hyperalgesia or itching, both of which are submaximal expressions of the pain phenomenon.

The acute reaction is optimally observed in the skin where provocative stimuli, such as caustic chemicals, burns and wounds, infections and allergens, elicit all four classic components of the inflammatory response. The chronic reaction is characterized by persistent pain, swelling, and cellular proliferation with an accompanying chronic and often major loss of function such as that observed in rheumatoid arthritis. In this instance, redness and heat may be conspicuously absent. The two most important classes of pharmacological agents that inhibit the acute or chronic inflammatory response are (1) the nonsteroidal anti-inflammatory drugs (NSAIDs, typically carboxylic or enolic organic acids), the prototype of which is aspirin, and (2) the adrenal glucocorticosteroid hormones (SAIDs), the prototype being hydrocortisone (cortisol).

The mechanisms of acute and chronic inflammatory reactions are complex, vary from tissue to tissue, and are dependent on the etiological agent. Common mechanisms include chemotactic stimuli, phagocytosis, and lysozomal enzyme release as well as activation of the clotting, fibrinolytic, kinin, and complement pathways. Many of the chemical mediators identified so far are listed in Table 28–1. Histamine release appears to occur early in the initial stages of inflammation. Bradykinin, a nonapeptide, is formed from α_2-globulins by the release of proteases from polymorphonuclear leukocytes after they migrate to an area of inflammation. Lipases activate many arachidonic acid byproducts such as prostaglandins (PGs), thromboxanes (TXs), or leukotrienes (LTs). Platelet-activating factors and oxygen-free radicals also are released as chemical mediators of inflammation. The initial steps in these reactions involve a number of different cell types and cellular interactions. Most of these chemical mediators appear to have similar effects in that they dilate capillaries in the area of inflammation, increase capillary permeability causing greater transudation, and heighten leukocyte intracapillary adhesiveness and diapedesis into the

Inflammation

Acute and chronic inflammation is inhibited by nonsteroidal anti-inflammatory agents (NSAIDs) and glucocorticoids (SAIDs).

Mechanisms of inflammation include chemical mediators such as histamine, kinins, prostaglandins (PGs), leukotrienes (LTs), and interleukin.

401

Table 28–1 CHEMICAL MEDIATORS OF ACUTE INFLAMMATION

Vasoactive amines: histamine, serotonin
Kallikrein and kinins: bradykinin
Hageman, other clotting factors: thrombin
Fibrinolytic system: plasmin
Complement components
Eosinophile, platelet activators
Products from arachidonic acid
   Nonenzymatically
      Oxidation products of arachidonate
   Through cyclooxygenase
      Endoperoxides (PGG_2, PGH_2)
      Thromboxanes (TXA_2)
      Prostaglandins (PGE_2, PGI_2)
   Through lipoxygenase
      Hydroperoxy acids
      Hydroxy acids
      Leukotrienes
Oxygen-derived products
Lysozomal constituents (neutral protease)

PGs exert their acute anti-inflammatory effects in concert with histamine, serotonin, and kinins.

interstitium where active phagocytosis occurs. It has been disclosed that blood monocytes and tissue macrophages are primary sources of many cytokines. One of the cytokines is the polypeptide hormone termed *interleukin-1,* which not only has a potent effect on the inflammatory response but also enhances the immune response by supporting B lymphocyte proliferation and antibody production as well as T lymphocyte production of lymphokines.

ACUTE INFLAMMATION

The contribution of the various known chemical mediators to the acute inflammatory response is obscure. This is principally the result of inability to isolate the activities of one agent from another or to exclude complex interactions among all the agents. Thus, the resultant exudative potpourri containing a host of chemical inflammatory mediators has been labeled appropriately as a pharmacological "soup."

However, certain facts have emerged in the past 30 years that have led to general acceptance that the PGs and LTs may play central roles in the acute inflammatory response. In the first place, certain PGs such as PGE_1, PGE_2, and PGI_2 are capable of inducing or augmenting all four classic signs of infection. Whereas histamine and serotonin are believed to mediate the initial phase of inflammation (1 – 1½ hours), and kinins the second phase (1½ – 2 hours), PGs probably exert their proinflammatory effects in the late phases of inflammation (2½ – 6 hours). It must be emphasized that although PGs elicit all four classic signs of inflammation, the intensity and duration of PG-induced heat, redness, edema, and pain are conditioned by the presence of the many other chemical mediators outlined earlier. Thus, the marked capillary permeability and plasma exudation elicited by bradykinin and histamine are only minimally observed by administration of PGE_2 alone. However, the exudation effects of bradykinin and histamine are potentiated by PGE_2, probably the result of the latter's vasodilatory activity. The time sequence and the interdependence of the various mediators in the acute inflammatory response has been reviewed extensively by Zurier (1982).

CHRONIC INFLAMMATION

In general, acute inflammatory reactions are characterized by localized exudative effects in the target organ, such as skin and lungs, whereas chronic inflammatory reactions are systemic in nature and characterized by marked painful cellular proliferative processes without redness and heat. Such a process is exemplified by the synovial articular pannus formation of rheumatoid arthritis. The role of chemotactic factors promoting migratory and local cellular proliferation is unknown. Although the classic PGs and TXs do not appear to be involved importantly in the chemotactic migration of leukocytes to sites of inflammation, it has been demonstrated clearly that one of the products of the arachidonic acid cascade, LT B_4, is extremely chemotactic and may be importantly involved in the chronic as well as the acute inflammatory response. This is discussed more fully in the section on formation of LTs.

Although the loss of function in chronic inflammatory disease may not directly result from PGs, it is important to note that PGE_2 may contribute to other pathological processes such as induction of bone resorption observed in rheumatoid arthritis. This is derived from the potent calcium-mobilizing action of PGE_2 synthesized from synovial membrane, which may be responsible for periarticular bone demineralization and resultant disability in rheumatoid arthritis. The contributions of arachidonic acid products to the inflammatory process are summarized in Table 28–2.

One manifestation of subacute or chronic inflammation is the presence of fever often observed with systemic viral or bacterial infections. In this instance, PGs may be extremely important etiological agents because they produce fever when infused intravenously (IV) in humans. Moreover, pyrogen-induced fever is associated with a release of PGE_2 and $PGF_{2\alpha}$ in the cerebral ventricles, with both fever and PG release being inhibited by PG synthesis inhibition. Because such pyrogens are believed to be released by bacterial endotoxins during infectious processes, it is widely held that hyperthermia may be directly the result of hypothalamic release of PGs occasioned by endotoxin entrance into the central nervous system (CNS).

In all the aforementioned inflammatory phenomena, the therapeutic efficacy of aspirin and glucocorticoid treatment had long been appreciated by clinicians years before the cited chemical mediators had been delineated and cellular mechanisms outlined. These two therapeutic modalities are discussed, however, in light of the advances in our fundamental understanding of biochemical and pathophysiological pathways underlying their actions as well as their interactions with other noninflammatory pharmacological agents.

As mentioned previously, anti-inflammatory agents may be classified as either steroidal (SAIDs) or nonsteroidal (NSAIDs). NSAIDs may be subdivided further into either prostaglandin synthetase inhibitors (PSIs) or nonprostaglandin synthetase inhibitors (non-PSIs). Through convention, the generic term NSAID has come to refer to newer specific prostaglandin synthetase inhibitors exclusive of aspirin. This has led to conceptual confusion because the NSAID aspirin is, in fact, a PG synthetase inhibitor. In addition, there are many important anti-inflammatory compounds that are NSAIDs but that do not act by inhibition of PG synthetase, as illustrated in Table 28–3. It is evident that the PSIs are represented by carboxylic or enolic acid compounds, whereas the non-PSIs are a heterogeneous chemically unrelated group of compounds, classified according to their effects on various symptoms or diseases (e.g., the analgesic-antipyretic para-aminophenols, antirheumatoid arthritis agents, and antigout preparations). Therefore, this chapter refers to NSAIDs as either PSIs (including aspirin) or non-PSIs, according to the classification shown in Table 28–3. The PSIs (including aspirin) are examined first and then the non-PSIs (para-aminophenols and the antirheumatoid agents, gold and levamisole). Evaluation

---

Table 28–2 FUNCTIONS OF ARACHIDONIC ACID PRODUCTS IN INFLAMMATION

PGE_1, PGE_2, PGI_2
  Fever and local heat
  Vasodilation
  Vasopermeability synergism with bradykinin and histamine
  Hyperalgesia synergism with bradykinin and histamine
Thromboxane A_2
  Platelet aggregation
Leukotriene B_4
  Chemotaxis

Nonsteroidal Anti-Inflammatory Drugs

NSAIDs are either PG synthesis inhibitors (PSIs) or non–PG synthesis inhibitors (non-PSIs).

Table 28–3 MAJOR CLASSES OF NONSTEROIDAL ANTI-INFLAMMATORY DRUGS (NSAIDs)

Prostaglandin Synthetase Inhibitors (PSIs)		Nonprostaglandin Synthetase Inhibitors (non-PSIs)		
Carboxylic Acids	*Enolic Acids*	*Para-Aminophenols*	*Antirheumatoid Arthritis Agents*	*Antigout Agents*
Salicylic	Oxicams	Phenacetin	Gold	Colchicine
Acetic	Pyrazolones	Acetaminophen	Immunosuppressives	Allopurinol
Proprionic			Penicillamine	Uricosuric
Fenamic			Levamisole	Probenecid
			Antimalarial	Sulfinpyrazone
			Chloroquine	
			Hydroxychloroquine	

of steroidal anti-inflammatory agents and other antirheumatoid (immuno-suppressives, antimalarials, penicillamine) and antigout non-PSIs are considered elsewhere in this text (see Chapters 30, 57, and 59).

PROSTAGLANDIN SYNTHETASE INHIBITORS

Because nonsteroidal analgesics and antipyretics are perhaps the most widely prescribed over-the-counter medications used in medicine today, it is extremely important for the physician to thoroughly understand the mechanism of their action, their interactions with other drugs, and their potent and at times serious side effects. Because of widespread and often imprudent usage, serious and at times fatal sequelae have only too frequently been the result of failure to appreciate these actions of aspirin-like drugs. Because, with the exception of the para-aminophenols, all such analgesic-antipyretic preparations exhibit the property of PG synthesis inhibition, the biosynthesis of PGs (as well as LTs) is outlined in detail before the pharmacological properties of these fascinating agents are discussed specifically.

Arachidonic Acid Cascade

Noxious inflammatory stimuli lead to PG production through activation of membrane phospholipase A_2.

FORMATION OF PROSTAGLANDINS AND THROMBOXANES

As previously mentioned, arachidonic acid and its metabolite byproducts (the arachidonic acid cascade) are important mediators of fever and inflammation. The rate-limiting step in the formation of the metabolites of arachidonic acid seems to be the initial step, namely, the calcium-dependent release of free arachidonic acid from the cell membrane phospholipid pool. Noxious proinflammatory agents disrupt the cell membrane, leading to activation of phospholipase A_2 and resultant degradation of the cell membrane phospholipid layer into arachidonic acid and diacyl glycerol moieties. Although this reaction, mediated through phospholipase A_2, is predominant in most tissues and cells including leukocytes, phospholipase C may play another role in arachidonic acid release through liberating a diglyceride, which is then hydrolyzed by another lipase to yield arachidonic acid. Details of the mechanism of release of arachidonate esterified to the glycerol moiety of phospholipids are beyond the scope of this discussion. It is important to note, however, that a major action of the anti-inflammatory glucocorticoids appears to be a decrease in arachidonic acid release from phospholipids by corticosteroid inhibition of phospholipases A_2 or C. The biosynthesis of PGs and TXs is illustrated in Figure 28–1.

Following the release of arachidonic acid, three enzymes are involved in the subsequent sequence of events leading to the formation of the prostaglandins. In the first biosynthetic pathway, PG cyclooxygenase catalyzes the initial step, yielding two PG endoperoxides: PGG_2 and PGH_2. This reaction has been shown to be inhibited by aspirin, indomethacin, and other PSIs. These intermediates are labile and can be converted into stable PGs such as PGE_2, PGD_2, and $PGF_{2\alpha}$.* In addition, unstable PGG_2 and PGH_2 can be metabolized to TXA_2 by TX synthetase and to PGI_2 by prostacyclin synthetase. These labile compounds are converted rapidly to stable but biologically inactive TXB_2 and 6-keto-$PGF_{1\alpha}$, respectively.

---

* The PGs are composed of a basic 20-carbon fatty acid containing a cyclopentane ring, the so-called hypothetical prostanoic acid. The carbons are numbered 1–20 from the carboxyl to the terminal methyl group. The designations of PGE_1, PGE_2, and PGE_3 refer only to the number of double bonds in the aliphatic side chains. The PGE_2 class is the most abundant, naturally occurring group. For PG_1 the precursor is 8,11,14-eicosatrienoic acid (dihomo-γ-linolenic acid), and for PG_2 the precursor is 5,8,11,14-eicosatetraenoic acid (arachidonic acid). PG_3 is formed from 5,8,11,14,17-eicosapentaenoic acid.

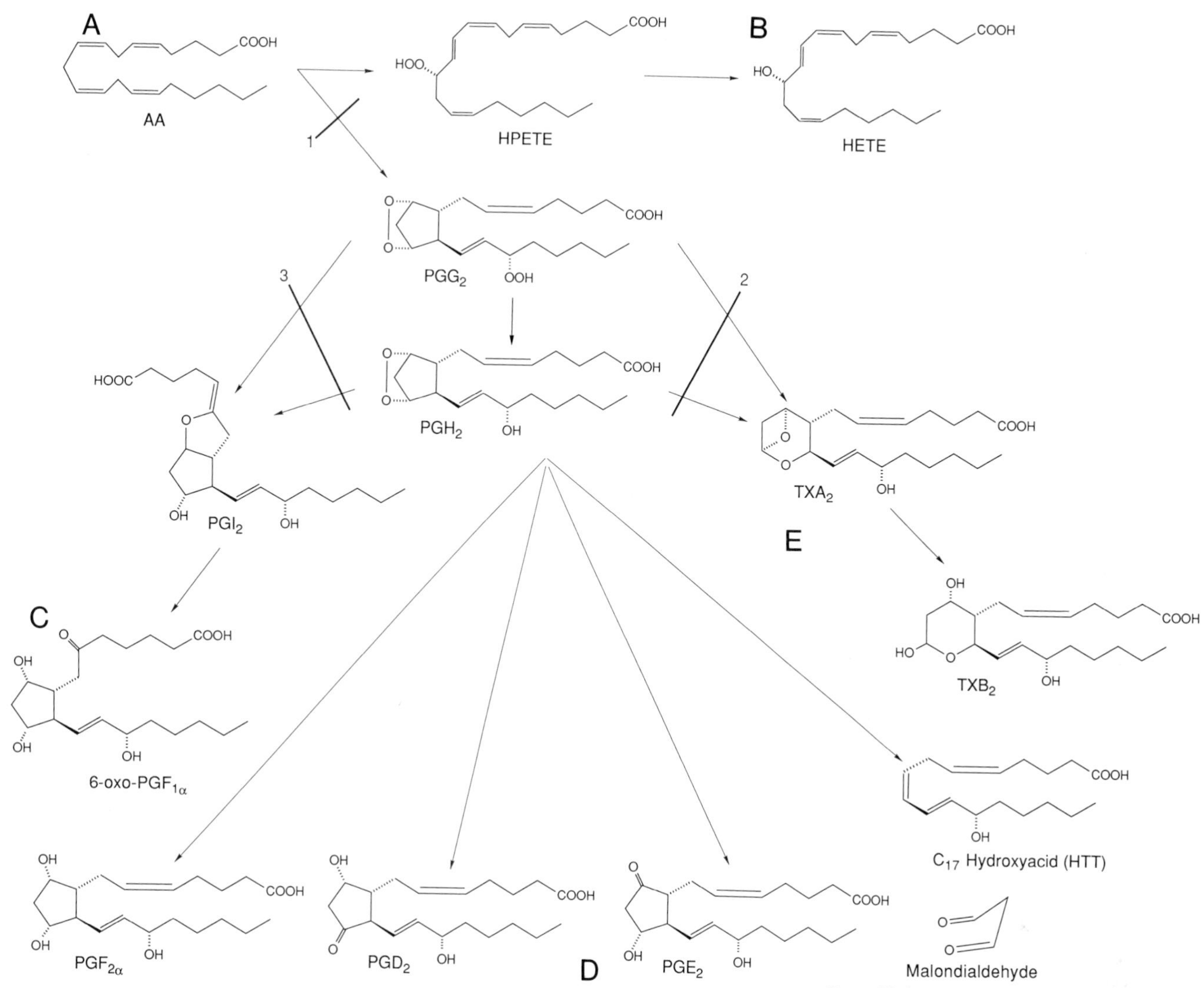

Figure 28-1

Metabolic pathways of PG synthesis from arachidonic acid (AA). Sites at which cyclooxygenase inhibitors (aspirin-like drugs —PSIs), thromboxane synthetase inhibitors (imidazole and 1-methyl imidazole), and prostacyclin (PGI₂) synthetase inhibitors (15-hydroperoxyarachidonic acid and 13-hydroperoxylinoleic acid) act are indicated by the numerals 1, 2, and 3, respectively. (HETE = 12-hydroxy-eicosatetraenoic acid; HPETE = 12-hydroperoxyeicosatetraenoic acid; TXA₂ = thromboxane A₂; TXB₂ = thromboxane B₂.) (From Moncada S, Vane JR: Unstable metabolites of arachidonic acid and their role in haemostasis and thrombosis. Br Med Bull 34:129–135, 1975.)

Arachidonic acid is converted to PGs and TXs by PG synthetase.

The relative amounts of compound formed depend on the tissue or cell being studied. When platelets are activated by collagen, subendothelial tissue, thrombin, adenosine diphosphate, epinephrine, antigen-antibody complexes, bacteria or virus, unstable TXA_2 production predominates. TXA_2 and PG endoperoxides induce a rapid and irreversible aggregation of platelets. They also contract vascular smooth muscle cells. However, in many other cells and tissues, synthesis of PGs predominates. For example, vascular endothelial cells form PGI_2, which has a potent vasodilating and antiaggregatory action as in the case of PGE_2. Neutrophils as well as monocytes or macrophages produce PGE_2, whereas PGD_2 is formed in mast cells and basophils. In kidneys, collecting duct and renointerstitial cells make PGE_2, PGA_2 and $PGF_{2\alpha}$; renovasculature endothelium synthesizes PGI_2, whereas glomerular mesangial endothelium forms PGE_2 and $PGF_{2\alpha}$. As mentioned before, PGE_2 and PGI_2 produce or augment vasodilation and enhance bradykinin- or serotonin-induced pain, resulting in redness, swelling, and pain in the inflammatory processes. As also mentioned, PGs such as PGE_2 and PGI_2 have been shown to increase during pyrogen-induced fever. In fact, PGE_2 administered into the hypothalamus increases, whereas PGD_2 decreases, body temperature, indicating a possible role of PGs in the regulation of systemic body temperature.

FORMATION OF LEUKOTRIENES

In the second pathway of arachidonic acid metabolism, 5-lipoxygenase forms a series of products named *leukotrienes* (LTs), as illustrated in Figure 28–2. Their designation was chosen because they were discovered in leu-

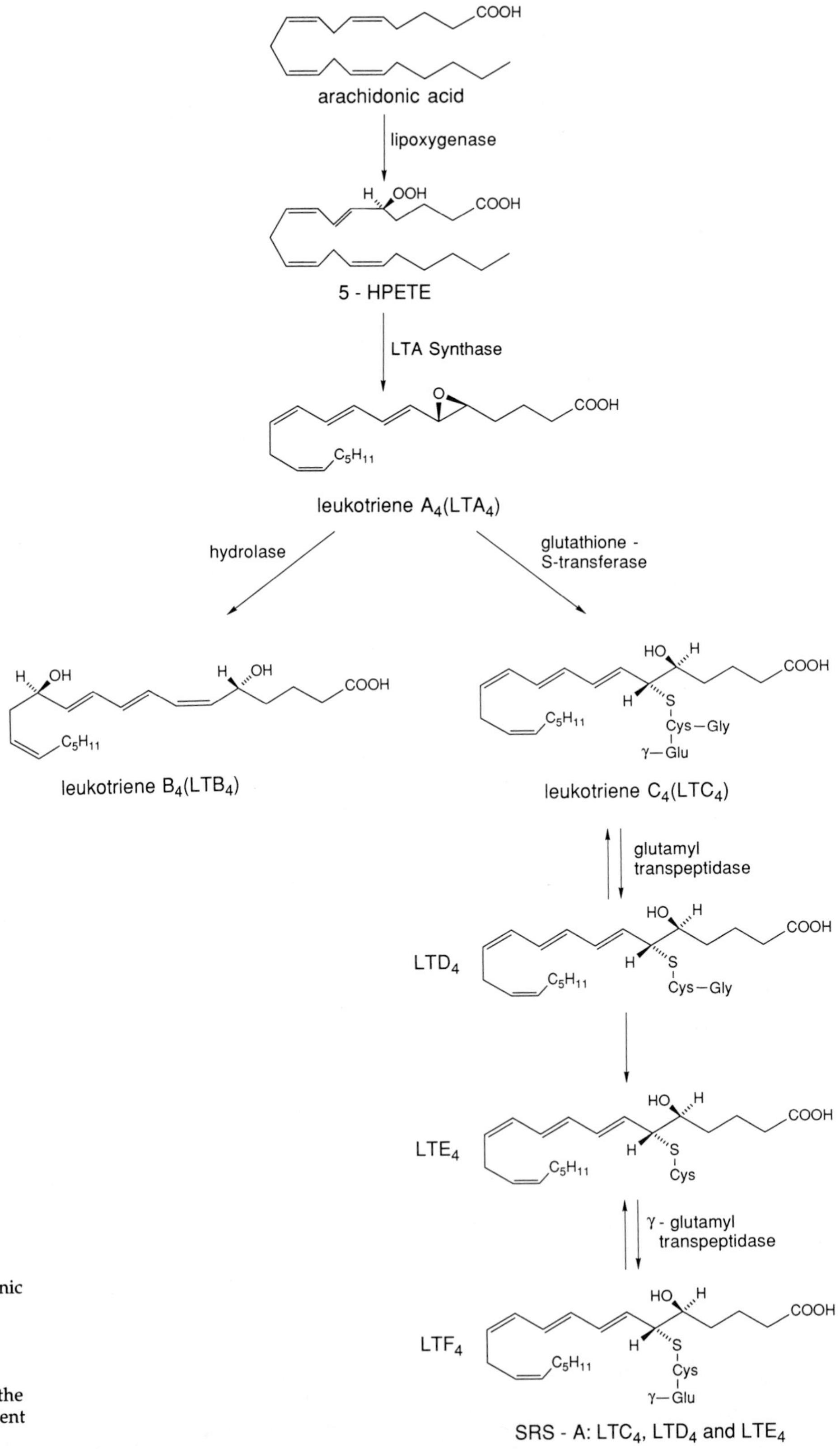

Figure 28-2

Formation of leukotrienes from arachidonic acid by way of 5-lipoxygenase pathway. (From Samuelsson B: Leukotrienes: Mediators of immediate hypersensitivity reaction and inflammation. Science 220:568–575, 1983. Copyright 1983 by the American Association for the Advancement of Science.)

kocytes and because the common structural feature is a conjugated triene. Various members of the group have been designated alphabetically, and a subscript denotes the number of double bonds. 5-hydroperoxyeicosate-traenoic acid (5-HPETE) may be enzymatically dehydrated to LTA_4 (5[S]-trans-oxido-7,9-trans-11,14-cis-eicosatetraenoic acid). Subsequent enzymatic hydrolysis of LTA_4 results in LTB_4 (5[S]-12[R]-dihydroxy-6cis-8,10-trans-14-cis-eicosatetraenoic acid). In addition to hydrolysis of LTA_4 to LTB_4, LTA_4 also interacts with a sulfhydryl compound in which addition of glutathione (Glu-Cys-Gly) by glutathione-S-transferase produces LTC_4 (5[S]-hydroxy-6[S]-glutathionyl-7,9-trans-11,14-cis-eicosate-traenoic acid). LTD_4 can be converted then from LTC_4 through elimination of glutamyl residue by a γ-glutamyl transpeptidase. The remaining peptide bond in LTD_4 is hydrolyzed to give LTE_4 by a dipeptidase.

Arachidonic acid is converted to a variety of LTs by 5-lipoxygenase.

PGs, TX, and some monohydroxy derivatives of arachidonic acid (hydroxyeicosatetraenoic acids) have been reported to have some minor chemotactic effects on polymorphonuclear leukocytes. However, LTB_4 is by far the most active substance among arachidonic acid metabolites. LTB_4 is not only chemotactic for neutrophils and eosinophils but also for monocytic macrophages. Polymorphonuclear leukocytes only survive for hours in the inflammatory area, whereas monocytes may remain for weeks, finally being transformed to fibroblasts and initiating the reconstitution and repair of inflammatory insults such as wounds. Furthermore, monocytes can present antigens to cells capable of producing antibodies and can synthesize all the members of the arachidonic acid cascade. Lastly, monocytes are capable also of forming the cytokine interleukin, interferon, complements, and proteases that are capable of tissue disruption. It is important to remember that such prolonged actions of LTB_4 on cellular proliferation renders such compounds a more prominent role in subacute and chronic inflammation, whereas the cyclooxygenase system products, i.e., PGs, modulate the acute inflammation.

LTB_4 is a major chemical mediator of chronic inflammation.

LTC_4, LTD_4, LTE_4, and their 11-trans-isomers do not have any effects on chemotaxis, enzyme release, or leukocyte aggregation. However, they do possess potent biological activities, which were formerly attributed to slow-reacting substance released from sensitized lungs treated with a specific antigen. Therefore, these LTs may be important mediators in asthma and other acute hypersensitivity reactions. Contraction of guinea pig ileum and other smooth muscle by the LTs exhibits a slow onset and relaxation, which is the basis of the original designation as slow-reacting substance, distinguishing these substances from histamine, bradykinin, and $PGF_{2\alpha}$. LTC_4 and LTD_4 are approximately 200-fold and 20,000-fold more potent than histamine in promoting small airway contraction. In addition, these LTs cause rapid arteriolar contraction and promote plasma leakage in postcapillary venules. They also slow the rate of mucous clearance from the airway of the patients with asthma after the inhalation of antigen and increase the amount of mucous glycoprotein synthesis in the human airway.

LTC_4 and LTD_4 have no effect on chemotaxis but have marked bronchiolar constrictive properties and may be important in bronchial asthma.

Pharmacological Properties of Major Classes of Prostaglandin Synthetase Inhibitors

The major mechanism whereby PSIs exert their therapeutic and toxic effects has been hypothesized to be through their ability to inhibit PG synthesis. These drugs block the cyclooxygenase pathway, nonselectively inhibiting the synthesis of PGs. Therefore, the anti-inflammatory effects of these drugs are in general related to inhibition of PG and TX synthesis. The experimental data so far do not support a specific effect on the lipooxygenase pathway.

The second property shared by the PSIs is their chemical relationship

Table 28–4 MAJOR PROSTAGLANDIN SYNTHETASE INHIBITORS

	Carboxylic Acids			Enolic Acids	
Salicylic Acids and Esters	*Acetic Acids*	*Proprionic Acids*	*Fenamic Acids*	*Pyrazolones*	*Oxicams*
Aspirin	Indomethacin	Ibuprofen	Mefenamic	Phenylbutazone	Piroxicam
Diflunisal	Sulindac	Naproxen	Meclofenamic*		
Salicylates	Tolmetin	Fenoprofen	Flufenamic†		
Sodium	Diclofenac	Ketoprofen			
Calcium†		Flurbiprofen			
Choline†					
Choline magnesium*					
Magnesium*					
Salicyl*					

* Not available in Japan.
† Not available in the United States.

in being weak organic acids. Major classes of PSIs are shown in Table 28–4. Certain of these compounds are not universally available and are not discussed further. Usual dose for anti-inflammatory therapy as well as their plasma half-lives are provided in Table 28–5. Specific characteristics for

Table 28–5 PLASMA HALF-LIFE USUAL, ANTIRHEUMATOID ARTHRITIS (RA) DOSAGE, AND COST OF PROSTAGLANDIN SYNTHESIS INHIBITORS

PSI	Plasma Half-Life (hours)	Daily RA Dosage (mg)*	Tablet Strength (mg)	Cost 100 Tablets (dollars)	Monthly Cost per Mean RA Dosage (dollars)†
Carboxylic Acids					
Salicylates					
Aspirin, generic	9–16‡	3000–5000	325	1.19	4
Diflunisal (Dolobid)	8–12	500–1000	250	77.96	70
Acetic Acids					
Indomethacin (Indocin)	4–5	75–150	25	48.49 (G. 15.85)§	72 (G. 21)§
Sulindac (Clinoril)	16	300–400	150	86.12	51
Tolmetin (Tolectin)	1–2	600–1800	200	43.63	78
Diclofenac (Voltaren)	2	150–200	50	77.61	81
Propionic Acids					
Ibuprofen (Motrin, Rufen)‖	2	1200–3200	400	17.25 (G. 11.20)§	28 (G. 19)§
Naproxen (Naprosyn, Anaprox)	13	500–1000	250	61.87	55
Fenoprofen (Nalfon)	2–4	1200–2400	200	40.77	110
Ketoprofen (Orudis)	2–4	150–300	50	71.17	46
Flurbiprofen (Ansaid)	3–9	200–300	100	99.06	74
Fenamic Acids					
Mefenamic acid (Ponstel)	2–4	—¶	250	69.26	—
Meclofenamate (Meclomen)	2–4	200–400	50	56.09	101
Enolic Acids					
Oxicams					
Piroxicam (Feldene)	50	20	10	113.46	68
Pyrazolones					
Phenylbutazone (Butazolidin)	84	—**	100	53.01	—

* Daily RA dosage in divided doses three to four times per day, except diclofenac (two to three times per day); diflunisal, sulindac, and naproxen (two times per day); and piroxicam (one time per day).
† Monthly cost rounded off to the nearest dollar.
‡ At low daily dosages (<3000 mg), plasma half-life for salicylate is 2–4 hours.
§ G. = generic.
‖ Available as over-the-counter preparations in 200 mg tablets (Advil, Nuprin, Medipren).
¶ Therapeutically useful for analgesia and dysmennorrhea but not for RA.
** Not indicated for RA.

individual PSIs are discussed initially, followed by an evaluation of some of the major adverse side effects commonly observed with almost all of the PSIs.

Because acetylsalicylic acid (aspirin) has been used empirically for years for its analgesic and antipyretic properties, antedating all anti-inflammatory agents except quinine, it is the prototype with which all other NSAIDs are compared. Although the introduction of phenylbutazone in 1952 was the first more potent aspirin-like drug to be introduced since aspirin itself was first marketed in 1915, its serious and frequent side effects precluded its wide acceptance and, in particular, its use for investigational purposes. In contrast, indomethacin, in use since 1965, represents the prototype of the newer class of more potent NSAIDs that have appeared in the last 25 years. Because aspirin and indomethacin are classic PG cyclooxygenase inhibitors and have been studied more extensively than other agents, a more detailed description of the effects and side effects of these two anti-inflammatory drugs are presented.

Aspirin and indomethacin are the classic prototype PG cyclooxygenase inhibitors.

At this point, it should be emphasized that *all* the anti-inflammatory drugs discussed provide only symptomatic relief in chronic inflammatory disorders such as rheumatoid arthritis. They do *not* alter the chronic course of the disease, including pannus formation with bone destruction, joint malformation, and loss of function.

SALICYLATES

Historical Aspects. One of the earliest analgesic-antipyretics was quinine derived from the bark of the cinchona tree. It had been recognized for years that the bark of the willow tree had similar bitter-tasting properties and also produced relief of pain and fever. This prompted Reverend Edmund Stone in 1763 to write a letter to the president of the Royal Society in England outlining his experience in successfully treating "agues" with a powdered extract of the willow tree bark. The active ingredient of the bark was shown to be salicylic acid derived from salicin isolated in 1829 by Leroux. Acetylsalicylic acid (aspirin) was discovered as a byproduct of coal tar by a German chemist Charles Gerhardt in 1853 and later prepared by another German chemist, Hoffman. The therapeutic effectiveness of acetylsalicylic acid as an anti-inflammatory–analgesic–antipyretic was described by Heinrich Dreser in 1899, who helped popularize its usage under the name *aspirin*. Aspirin is believed to be derived from the German word for acetylsalicylic acid *acetylspirsaure* (from *spirea,* a plant from which salicyclic acid had been prepared for years, and *saure* the German word for acid).

The historical aspects of aspirin

Since the introduction of aspirin, it has become the cheapest and most common of all household remedies, being used for the relief of every conceivable imaginary or real ache or pain known to humankind since the 1900s. Although it has specific important medical indications, its over-the-counter availability, low cost, and the erroneous belief by the laity that except for "gastric upset" it is essentially without side effects has led to its indiscriminate, unsupervised, and at times hazardous usage. The host of newer, more potent, aspirin-like prostaglandin synthesis inhibitors that have appeared since the mid-1960s with almost identical therapeutic and toxic properties has led to extreme pharmaceutical marketing competition and media exploitation. Although scarcely mentioned in television marketing commercials, significant serious morbidity and mortality events may result from professionally unsupervised aspirin and aspirin-like drug usage. This chapter concentrates on the indications, contraindications, toxic effects, and drug interactions of the PSIs to provide the student, physician, pharmacist, and nurse with the fundamental therapeutic principles underlying these classic effective anti-inflammatory agents. It is hoped

Although viewed as benign, aspirin and other PSIs may have serious side effects.

COOH
OH

Salicylic acid

COOH
O—C—CH₃
‖
O

Acetylsalicylic acid (aspirin)

COONa
OH

Sodium salicylate

COOCH₃
OH

Methyl salicylate

Salicylates are absorbed in the stomach, transported bound to albumin, and metabolized by the liver.

in this way to better ensure their more prudent usage and thereby minimize the occurrence of serious and at times fatal outcomes that are the consequence of excessive and ill-advised usage.

Chemistry, Metabolism, and Excretion. Salicylic acid, the parent derivative closely related to benzoic acid, is believed to be the active component of the salicylates. Acetylsalicylic acid, sodium salicylate, and salicylic acid are all absorbed as the nonionized gastric-irritating acid by the acid pH of the gastric juice. Alkalization of gastric hydrochloride (HCl) promotes absorption in the buffered salt conformation (e.g., sodium salicylate) with resultant reduction in gastric irritation. Absorption of salicylates occurs rapidly in the stomach and upper small intestines, although in the alkaline media of the latter, absorption is slower and less predictable. Thus, peak salicylate levels from rapid gastric absorption (1–3 hours) may be slightly blunted and delayed by alkalization of stomach contents and use of buffered or enteric-coated aspirin preparations. However, generally this does not alter clinical effectiveness of these preparations and may significantly reduce gastric irritation.

Following absorption, the salicylates are transported bound to albumin (90%) and as such compete with and displace a host of similarly transported naturally ocurring compounds (e.g., hormones like thyroxine and steroids) and drugs (e.g., penicillin, warfarin, and barbiturates). The salicylates have two major acetylating properties that are integral to their biochemical effects: the acetylation of plasma albumin by reacting with lysine, and the irreversible acetylation (and consequent inactivation) of PG cyclooxygenase. The salicylates are distributed throughout the body by pH-dependent passive diffusion.

The metabolic pathways of aspirin follow first and zero-order kinetics. The majority (80%) of salicylate is converted to water-soluble conjugates (salicyluric acid and salicyl-phenyl-glucuronide) by hepatic glycine conjugation that are excreted in the urine together with smaller amounts (5%) of free salicylic acid and gentisic acid. At low doses, first-order kinetics are followed, but at higher anti-inflammatory doses, zero-order kinetics occur, the result of saturation of hepatic conjugating systems. This results in an increase in half-life to 9–16 hours at high doses compared with a half-life of 3–4 hours at low doses. The renal elimination of salicylates is markedly enhanced by urinary alkalization, which promotes ionization of salicylic acid to salicylate anion, diminishing back diffusion that occurs with unionized salicylic acid. Alkalization has no effect on water-soluble salicylate glucuronide excretion.

Pharmacological Actions and Therapeutic Indications. The major anti-inflammatory analgesic and antipyretic effects of aspirin and other PSIs that are the result of PG synthesis inhibition have been discussed at length and need not be repeated here. Obviously, these pharmacological properties are central to the beneficial effects of aspirin and PSI in a wide variety of inflammatory disorders, including rheumatic fever, rheumatoid arthritis, osteoarthritis, ankylosing spondilitis, headache, fever, myalgias, and dysmenorrhea to name a few.

A more recent application of low aspirin administration has been proposed to be its potential for prevention of cardiovascular catastrophes (e.g., coronary thrombosis and cerebrovascular accident) by virtue of its preferential inhibitory action on platelet TXA_2, leading to a prolongation in the bleeding time. In normal hemostasis vascular injury like trauma, plaque formation sets into motion a train of events leading to clot formation and re-epithelialization of vascular endothelium. It is believed that adenosine diphosphate (ADP)–mediated activation of platelet phospholipase A_2 initiates this process, which in turn generates two platelet aggregating pathways, PG-TXA$_2$ and platelet activating factor (Paf-acether). In the PG pathway, PGG$_2$ and PGH$_2$ result in TXA$_2$ formation that in turn results in vasoconstriction and platelet aggregation. PGH$_2$, either from endothelial or from platelet arachidonate, yields results in production of vasodilating and platelet inhibitory PGI$_2$. In the Paf-acether pathway, Paf-acether derived from liberation of platelet arachidonate also results in platelet aggregation.

It is believed that aspirin at low dose prolongs the bleeding time by inhibiting platelet TXA$_2$ and Paf-acether production to a greater extent than vascular PGI$_2$ synthesis and for the lifetime of the platelet (i.e., 7–8 days). The net result is a preponderance of antiplatelet aggregating PGI$_2$ and a prolonged bleeding time. It is premature to state at this writing whether daily low-dose aspirin administration (81–325 mg/day) to patients with postmyocardial infarction or stroke or patients with incipient tendencies to these phenomena (e.g., higher risk subjects with abnormal plasma lipids, smokers, and positive family histories) will benefit from aspirin treatment. However, current data support the beneficial effects of such aspirin treatment, and widespread clinical trials and therapeutic recommendations for this aspirin indication are underway. It is an obvious corollary that aspirin should be avoided in patients with hypoprothrombinemia (e.g., hepatic disease), oral anticoagulant therapy (aspirin also displaces anticoagulants as warfarin from plasma-binding sites), hemophilia, and other bleeding diatheses, and in patients undergoing surgery where its usage could be hazardous.

> Aspirin may be useful in prevention of coronary thrombosis by inhibiting platelet TXA$_2$ and prolonging bleeding time.

Two additional more recent cardiovascular uses for aspirin and other PSIs have been shown to be enhancing closure of patent ductus arteriosus in the newborn and in Bartter's syndrome. Because experience in treatment of these disorders has been more extensive with more potent PSIs, these therapeutic indications are discussed in the section dealing with indomethacin.

Salicylic acid and its derivatives have two additional properties that have led to their topical use as counterirritants. These compounds are absorbed by the skin and are highly irritating, at times producing keratolysis. These pharmacological properties have led to the use of salicylic acid (often in combination with benzoic acid) as keratolytic agents in the treatment of warts, corns, and other localized hyperkeratotic skin disorders. Methyl salicylate, more commonly known as oil of wintergreen, has found a therapeutic niche as a counterirritant when applied to the skin adjacent to muscles that have become inflamed due to physical exercise; it is used also for viral infections, as well as a topical adjunctive therapy over sites of arthralgias (e.g., rheumatoid arthritis, see Chapter 59). Classic PSI side effects may occur from excessive skin absorption but are rare.

> Salicylic acid acts as a counterirritant.

Additional pharmacological effects of aspirin include action on the CNS (stimulation of the respiratory center at high dose leading to hyperventilation followed by respiratory depression at toxic doses), renal effects, and gastrointestinal (GI) effects (which are discussed later on in this chapter). Among the clinically relevant renal effects of aspirin is its uricosuric action at very high doses, which has been employed in the past for the treatment of gout but is no longer indicated for treatment of this disorder. Pharmacological effects of aspirin also include endocrine-metabolic effects (uncoupling of oxidative phosphorylation, hyperglycemia, stimulation of adrenal steroidogenesis, and decreased thyroxine turnover) and the pathophysiological state of dysmenorrhea. (The latter topic, concerned with the ameliorative effects of PG inhibition on painful premenstrual abdominal cramping in women, is discussed subsequently in the discussion on proprionic acid PSIs.)

Aspirin displaces many drugs bound to plasma protein.

Drug Interactions. Aspirin displaces a number of drugs from plasma protein-binding sites including the other anti-inflammatory PSIs, such as the acetic and proprionic acid derivatives, warfarin, methotrexate, tolbutamide, propamide, phenytoin, and probenecid. Aspirin also antagonizes the effect of diuretic therapy such as spironolactone and, by its competitive actions on the organic renal transport system, increases penicillin G concentration and decreases the uricosuric effect of sulfinpyrazone and probenecid. The anti-inflammatory effects of aspirin are affected little by other drugs, although its GI side effects such as gastritis and bleeding are increased by concomitant use of alcohol. Because the hemorrhagic effects of aspirin are accentuated by its platelet-inhibiting properties and by displacement of the anticoagulant warfarin from plasma proteins, the combination of alcohol and aspirin ingestion in patients on anticoagulant therapy can be lethal.

Availability and Dosage. *Aspirin* and *sodium salicylate* are available in 325 and 650 mg tablets (pediatric aspirin as 81 mg tablets and adult aspirin preparations as 975 mg are also available). The route of administration is always oral. Timed-release, enteric-coated, buffered preparations and suppositories are marketed. However, therapeutic levels may be blunted or delayed with timed-release and enteric-coated preparations that, however, have a definite place for use in patients prone to gastric irritation and peptic ulceration (e.g., the elderly and patients with poor food intake). The buffering capacity of buffered aspirin is often inadequate to neutralize gastric HCl and, even when effective, may enhance renal salicylate elimination by alkalization of the urine, leading to lower therapeutic levels. Rectal administration by suppository is used rarely because of unpredictable absorption and mucosal irritation.

Dosage regimens for aspirin

The analgesic and antipyretic dosage for adults ranges from 325 to 975 mg (usual dose, 650 mg) four times per day after meals and with bedtime milk or snack. Self-medication should not exceed 4–5 days before physician consultation; all high fevers in infants and young children demand immediate physician evaluation because life-threatening dehydration may occur rapidly. The usual pediatric dosage of aspirin is 60–75 mg/kg/day. Such dose schedules produce blood salicylate levels usually less than 30 mg/dl and are not associated with signs of *salicylism* (see later in chapter). The dosage regimen for more severe and chronic inflammatory disorders, such as rheumatic fever and rheumatoid arthritis, is more rigorous and prolonged (see Table 28–5).

Salicylates are also available as salicyl, choline, magnesium, and combined choline-magnesium compounds. Salicylsalicylic (salsalate) is a dimer of salicylic acid that is insoluble in acidic gastric fluids but is partially hydrolyzed to two molecules of salicyclic acid in the alkaline milieu of the small intestine. Its half-life in plasma is 14–18 hours, and twice-daily dosage yields satisfactory blood levels. Although the amount of salicylic acid available from salsalate is 15% of acetylsalicylic acid (aspirin) on a molar basis, its attenuated side effects in production of GI irritation and peptic ulceration make it a desirable choice in patients with rheumatic disorders who are prone to such GI disorders. The recommended dosage for rheumatoid arthritis or osteoarthritis is 3000 mg/day given in divided doses.

Diflunisal is a diflurophenyl derivative of salicylic acid that, however, is not metabolized to salicylic acid. It is more potent than aspirin in its anti-inflammatory and analgesic actions; moreover, its prolonged half-life (see Table 28–5) allows for twice-daily dosing. Unlike aspirin, diflunisal is devoid of significant antipyretic activity. Diflunisal appears in the milk of

Diflunisal

lactating women and in general possesses all side effects common to the PSIs, although reportedly to a lesser degree. For instance, diflunisal appears to produce less GI and auditory symptoms than aspirin and, therefore, has found acceptance as a long-acting analgesic for the relief of musculoskeletal pain, including that of osteoarthritis. It has been employed also in the treatment of rheumatoid arthritis. Diflunisal is available in 250 and 500 mg tablets, with total recommended daily dose of 500–1000 mg given in divided doses every 8–12 hours, not to exceed 1500 mg (see Table 28–5).

Toxic Reactions to Salicylates. Adverse reactions shared by all PSIs, including aspirin, are discussed separately. However, there are certain toxic effects following aspirin overdose or sensitivity that are relatively specific for salicylates. Because these may be serious and life-threatening, they are discussed in detail in this section.

Salicylism is the aggregate term applied to a well-described syndrome resulting from aspirin (and other salicylate) overdose. It is a common cause of accidental poisoning in children and has been responsible for numerous fatalities; some estimates of the incidence of morbidity due to salicylism range into the tens of thousands annually. The advent of child-proof safety caps for bottles of baby aspirin (81 mg each) has almost certainly decreased the occurrence of childhood salicylism; nevertheless, pleasant-tasting, colorful preparations should be stored in inaccessible locked cabinets.

The overdose of aspirin that has resulted in fatalities is extremely variable, depending on the patient's size, rate of absorption, and so forth. In general, mild to moderate toxicity is observed with doses between 150 and 250 mg/kg body weight, and severe to lethal toxicity in doses above 250 mg/kg body weight. However, severe intoxication has occurred at the lower ingestion doses and survival at doses far above the higher ingestion amounts. Methyl salicylate (oil of wintergreen) is particularly toxic in low doses; fatalities have been reported following ingestion of a single teaspoon (approximately 5 g). Mild salicylate toxicity is associated usually with plasma salicylate levels of 40–70 mg/dl; moderate toxicity is 70–150 mg/dl; and severe to lethal toxicity is above 150 mg/dl.

Early symptoms of salicylate intoxication include tinnitus, decreased auditory acuity, headache, sweating, nausea, and vomiting. Hyperventilation is almost always present, attributable to a direct stimulating effect of salicylates on the CNS respiratory centers and from CO_2 generated by aspirin's uncoupling of oxidative phosphorylation. This results in an initial respiratory alkalosis that is compensated within 3 days by enhanced renal sodium and potassium bicarbonate excretion. Compensated respiratory alkalosis (normal blood pH, normal or low pCO_2, and low serum bicarbonate) coupled with the aforementioned symptoms is the usual presentation of salicylism in adults and is treated by measures outlined later.

Salicylism in children represents a more ominous picture because a toxic aspirin dose produces profound CNS effects, including respiratory depression, marked hyperthermia, vomiting, diarrhea and sweating, all of which combine to produce superimposed respiratory and metabolic acidosis, ultimately leading to convulsions, coma, and death. The metabolic acidosis is the result of organic acid accumulation (salicylates and their derivatives, lactic and acetoacetic acids, sulphuric and phosphoric acids), in the face of already depleted buffer stores from renal bicarbonate loss, that occurs as a compensation for the initial phases of respiratory alkalosis.

The initial treatment of salicylism includes removing unabsorbed gastric salicylate by intubation or induction of vomiting (ipecac) as well as immediate IV therapy for correction of hypovolemia, dehydration, and

The pathophysiology and treatment of salicylism

acid-base abnormalities. Appropriate IV solutions of glucose and electrolytes are dictated by interpretation of laboratory data and invariably include sodium bicarbonate to replenish depleted stores and promote urinary alkalization to enhance renal salicylate excretion. Immediate initial treatment of hyperpyrexia by environmental cooling (e.g., alcohol sponges, tepid water) is indicated.

In all serious and potentially lethal cases of salicylism, immediate intubation for respiratory support through mechanical assistance under the supervision of an anesthesiologist is imperative. In these cases, salicylate removal by peritoneal or hemodialysis should be undertaken without delay. No attempt should be made to await the tenuous outcome accompanying standard nondialytic therapeutic maneuvers.

Aspirin hypersensitivity occurs in a small number of patients (0.3%), particularly those with asthma and nasal polyps. Although observed primarily with aspirin, hypersensitivity has also been reported in this susceptible population with many other PSIs, which should be avoided in such individuals. Manifestations of hypersensitivity include vasomotor rhinitis, urticaria, bronchial wheezing, and angioneurotic edema including full-blown lethal anaphylactic reactions with laryngeal edema, generalized edema, vasomotor collapse, and shock. The immune mechanism for such reactions is unclear. Currently, it is believed that PSI inhibition in these individuals may lead to suppression of anti-immune PGs with a rare and inappropriate persistence of bronchoconstricting $PGF_{2\alpha}$ and LTs. Such reactions constitute a true medical emergency with immediate treatment directed to relief of airway obstruction, oxygen, and parenteral administration of epinephrine and corticosteroids. Patients with this alarming hypersensitivity to aspirin should be advised to strictly avoid aspirin and all other PSIs that, in this instance, become life-threatening.

Reye's syndrome is a potentially fatal encephalopathy associated with fatty hepatic degeneration and dysfunction in children in association with influenza epidemics and with the varicella virus. Although evidence has been presented that aspirin may precipitate or accentuate this disorder, there is no unequivocal proof that this association is valid. Nevertheless, it would appear prudent to abstain from the use of aspirin in children for the symptomatic treatment of influenza and varicella.

ACETIC ACIDS

Indomethacin

Historical Aspects. Indomethacin was introduced in 1965 in a search for more potent aspirin-like anti-inflammatory agents. It is of historical interest that the research and development of indomethacin leading to its clinical availability occurred concomitantly and independently with the isolation and identification of PGEs and PGFs from seminal vesicles by Bergstrom and associates in 1962 and 1963; at the same time there was an independent discovery of sustained vasodepressor activity in the renal medulla by Lee and colleagues (1962, 1963), who isolated and identified the responsible lipids as prostaglandins PGA_2, PGE_2, and $PGF_{2\alpha}$. Thus, although both aspirin and indomethacin were utilized clinically in the 1960s for their anti-inflammatory properties, their mechanism of action and renal and extrarenal side effects were completely unknown until they were demonstrated to be potent inhibitors of PG synthetase in 1971 by Smith and Willis and Ferreira and coworkers.

In this connection, it is important to note the extensive contributions of the Upjohn Company in making PGE_1 (biosynthesized from arachidonic

Indomethacin

Historical aspects of the discovery of PGs and the PSIs

acid by sheep seminal vesicles) available to investigators throughout the world, enabling the discovery of the incredibly diverse and potent biological activities of the PGs in virtually every cell, tissue, and organ system in the mammalian hierarchy. In similar fashion, the contributions of Merck, Sharpe and Dohme in providing indomethacin for investigational use and initiating basic research on the PG synthetase inhibitory actions of indomethacin provided the impetus that ultimately led to a much more precise delineation of the role of PGs in biology and medicine. As a result, the effects and side effects of aspirin and indomethacin in reproduction, blood pressure and sodium and water homeostasis, the GI tract, the cardiovascular-hemostatic system, and the immune-inflammatory response are now believed to be, in large part, the result of PG synthesis inhibition. The body of knowledge gained in these early experiments with aspirin and indomethacin provides a standard against which all actions of subsequently discovered PSIs have been compared.

Chemistry, Metabolism, and Excretion. Indomethacin is a methylated derivative of indole, which is insoluble in water. Indomethacin is absorbed efficiently and rapidly from the GI tract, including the rectal mucosa when given by suppository. Once absorbed, indomethacin is almost entirely bound to plasma proteins, reaching a peak plasma concentration of 1 μg/ml 2 hours after ingestion of a 25 mg capsule. Indomethacin undergoes significant enterohepatic circulation following linear pharmacokinetics with a plasma half-life averaging 4–5 hours, although variable extensions to 12–13 hours have been reported. Indomethacin is metabolized by hepatic microsomal enzymes into free and conjugated desmethyl and desbenzoyl metabolites. It is excreted in urine (60%) and in bile (30% in feces) as the unchanged compound and metabolites.

Pharmacological Actions and Therapeutic Indications. Indomethacin has all the classic anti-inflammatory–analgesic–antipyretic actions of aspirin but is 20–30 times more potent, comparable in this regard to phenylbutazone. It is important to note, however, that not all the effects of indomethacin can be attributed to PG synthesis inhibition. Thus, indomethacin decreases production of renin by the juxtaglomerular cells of the kidney cortex, which may result in important blood pressure and salt and water effects independent of the prostaglandins. Similarly, indomethacin may affect cyclic adenosine monophosphate (AMP) functions by virtue of its inhibitory effect on phosphodiesterase.

The clinical indications for indomethacin include symptomatic relief in osteoarthritis, ankylosing spondylitis, and rheumatoid arthritis (e.g., alleviation of morning stiffness, increased mobility, increased grip strength), including relief of acute exacerbations with reduction in joint swelling and tenderness. Indomethacin is extremely useful in the treatment of acute gouty arthritis, acute bursitis, and acute tendinitis.

Unique indications for PG synthesis inhibition with indomethacin (and other PSIs) exist in Bartter's syndrome and patent ductus arteriosus in the newborn. Bartter's syndrome is characterized by hyperplasia of the renal juxtaglomerular apparatus, hyperreninemia, hyperaldosteronism, hypokalemic alkalosis, and normal blood pressure associated with an elevated excretion of PGs. Indomethacin provides dramatic reversal of these abnormalities, which are probably related to increased PG production. Because the hypokalemia is only partially reversed, it has been postulated that a primary deficit in renal tubular potassium chloride transport underlies this disorder and that overproduction of renal PGs is not the primary cause but rather a secondary compensatory mechanism to the related hy-

Indomethacin has unique clinical usefulness in Bartter's syndrome and closure of patent ductus arteriosus.

povolemia. Nevertheless, indomethacin treatment remains a mainstay of treatment for this disorder.

Intrauterine maintenance of a patent ductus arteriosus is dependent on oxygen tension, gestational age, and PGs. Patent ductus arteriosus in the newborn in the past was corrected by surgical closure, but because patency of this vascular channel is PG-dependent, medical treatment with PSIs such as indomethacin has led to a success rate of 60–90%, thus obviating the need for surgical intervention in many instances. The usual dose is 0.2 mg/kg orally every 12–24 hours to a cumulative maximum of 0.6 mg/kg. Because the plasma half-life of indomethacin in the infant is three to four times that of the adult (20 hours), and because renal blood flow in the infant is PG-dependent, urine flow usually decreases during standard treatment of patent ductus with indomethacin. Although this renal effect is reversible and well tolerated in normal infants, acute renal failure may be precipitated in infants with renal disease. In addition to renal failure, indomethacin is also contraindicated in infants with bleeding diatheses and GI disease (e.g., thrombocytopenia, hyperbilirubinemia, enterocolitis).

Absolute contraindications to indomethacin include pregnancy, especially in the last trimester, when indomethacin-induced premature closure of the ductus may occur; hypersensitivity reactions to indomethacin, aspirin, and other PSIs; bleeding abnormalities; and when predisposition to precipitation of indomethacin's serious side effects may occur. Not only is indomethacin one of the most potent PSIs, its side effects are prominent. Although these side effects can be attributed largely to PG synthesis inhibition, certain reactions appear to be independent of indomethacin's effects on PG synthesis. In this context, it must be remembered that *all* the PSIs share the same potentially fatal side effects. Despite claims that one or another of the PSIs may have a lower incidence of a particular side reaction, it is imperative for the physician to treat all PSIs with the same caution and respect when the potential for serious and life-threatening events is common to all such drugs.

One of the most common and disturbing effects is drowsiness and (paradoxically) headache, which can occur in over half the patients under treatment. As with other side effects, indomethacin-induced drowsiness and headache are most commonly encountered in daily doses of 100 mg or more. These symptoms are readily reversed by omitting or lowering the dose of indomethacin. Additional predominant (and more serious) side effects include those of the GI tract (dyspepsia, nausea and vomiting, abdominal pain, flatulence, diarrhea, and peptic ulceration with and without hemorrhage) and the renal system (interstitial nephritis, papillary necrosis, and acute renal failure). These are discussed in detail subsequently (see Side Effects Common to Prostaglandin Synthetase Inhibitors).

Availability and Dosage. Indomethacin is available in 25 and 50 mg capsules, 75 mg sustained-release (SR) capsules, and a suspension (25 mg/5 ml), all for oral use. The drug is also available as 50 mg suppositories and as an IV preparation (1 mg indomethacin/vial to be reconstituted with 1–2 ml saline solution or distilled water).

The initial dosage is usually 25 mg orally three times per day with daily increments of 25–50 mg at weekly intervals up to a daily maximal dose of 150–200 mg as dictated by therapeutic response or side effects. Seventy five mg sustained-release capsules one to two times per day may be substituted for 25–50 mg capsules three times per day. It is often advantageous to give a large proportion of the daily dosage (up to 75 mg) at bedtime with milk to relieve morning stiffness and pain. The use of indomethacin suppositories should be minimized to avoid rectal irritation and bleeding. Similar dose regimens may be used for acute exacerbations of rheumatoid

Contraindications and side effects of indomethacin

arthritis, osteoarthritis, ankylosing spondylitis, or acute gouty arthritis. In the latter condition, an initial daily total of 150 mg in divided doses is recommended.

Initial IV dose to infants with patent ductus arteriosus is 0.2 mg/kg with subsequent doses of 0.1, 0.2, or 0.25 mg/kg (depending on age) given at 12–24 hour intervals for a total of three doses. If the ductus reopens, a second 3-day course separated by 12–24 hour intervals may be given. Severe oliguria may occur, and urinary output must be monitored and further doses withheld until renal function returns to normal.

Sulindac

Chemistry, Metabolism, and Excretion. Sulindac, a sulfoxide indene derivative, is chemically related to indomethacin and was developed in a search for an anti-inflammatory PSI with less side effects than indomethacin.

Sulindac is a prodrug; sulindac itself is biologically inactive. Approximately 90% of the drug is absorbed following oral administration. It is rapidly irreversibly oxidized to an inactive sulfone metabolite and reversibly reduced to a sulfide metabolite, which is believed to be the pharmacologically active form. About 95% of the prodrug and its metabolites are bound to plasma proteins, with peak plasma concentrations of the active sulfide metabolite occurring in 2 hours. Because of an extensive enterohepatic circulation, the plasma half-life of the sulfide metabolite is 16 hours, which allows for a more prolonged anti-inflammatory activity and a twice-daily dosing schedule.

Approximately 50% of administered sulindac is excreted by the kidneys in the form of free and conjugated glucuronide conjugates of sulindac and its sulfone metabolite. There is little renal excretion of the active sulfide metabolite. About 25% of administered sulindac appears in the feces as the sulfide and sulfone metabolite.

Sulindac

Pharmacological Actions and Therapeutic Indications. The pharmacological indications for sulindac are identical to those of indomethacin (rheumatoid arthritis, osteoarthritis, ankylosing spondilitis, acute gout, and bursitis and tendinitis). Unlike indomethacin, sulindac has not been utilized to any degree for pharmacological closure of patent ductus arteriosus in the newborn or in Bartter's syndrome.

Sulindac possesses all the side effects of the PSIs (discussed subsequently). However, the effects may be modified or lessened to some degree because sulindac is a prodrug with little renal excretion of the active sulfide metabolite. These GI symptoms (nausea and epigastric pain) appear to be of less magnitude and occur with a decreased incidence (approximately 20%) when compared with indomethacin (30–50%). Similarly, evidence has been presented that suggests a renal sparing effect of sulindac, particularly in patients with glomerulonephritis and cirrhosis. However, the degree of renal sparing by sulindac has proven to be controversial, particularly in hypovolemic states when renal blood flow is PG-dependent and when PSIs (including sulindac) may precipitate acute renal failure. This is discussed in detail later. More recently, there have been 23 reports following sulindac administration of a rare complication of renal lithiasis with incorporation of sulindac metabolites in the renal stones. This has not been reported with other PSIs and may be related to the unique metabolism sulindac undergoes following absorption.

Availability and Dosage. Sulindac is available in 150 and 200 mg tablets. The recommended initial dosage is 150 mg two times per day with weekly increments to a maximal dose of 400 mg as determined by therapeutic response or side effects. In acute bursitis and tendinitis and acute gouty arthritis, the recommended starting dosage is 200 mg two times per day for approximately 1 week.

Tolmetin

Chemistry, Metabolism, and Excretion. Tolmetin is a pyrrolealkanoic acid. Following oral administration, it is absorbed rapidly and completely with peak plasma levels occurring in 30–60 minutes. The half-life in plasma is approximately 1–2 hours, with a slower phase declining by 5 hours. Tolmetin is almost totally bound to plasma proteins. The drug is eliminated almost entirely by renal excretion of the unchanged drug and inactive oxidized metabolites and conjugates.

Pharmacological Actions and Therapeutic Indications. As with all PSIs, tolmetin's pharmacological actions are mediated in large part by PG synthesis inhibition. It is more potent than aspirin but less potent than indomethacin. Side effects are most frequently GI with nausea, abdominal pain, diarrhea, vomiting, and dyspepsia. CNS side effects, including headache and drowsiness, are reportedly less severe and less frequent than with indomethacin. Unlike most other PSIs, tolmetin does not displace anticoagulants, such as warfarin, from plasma protein-binding sites, although it does prolong the bleeding time, presumably due to its inhibiting effect of platelet TXA_2 and prolongation of prothrombin time.

The therapeutic indications are identical to all PSIs (rheumatoid arthritis, osteoarthritis, and ankylosing spondylitis), although usage in acute gouty arthritis and other musculoskeletal disorders is not recommended.

Availability and Dosage. Tolmetin sodium is available in 200 mg tablets, 400 mg capsules, and 600 mg tablets for oral use. The initial recommended dosage is 400 mg three times per day for a total daily dose of 1200 mg. This can be increased or decreased according to the patient's response and tolerance to a daily range between 600 and 1800 mg. Doses exceeding 1800 mg are not recommended. It is recommended that the drug be administered immediately after waking and at bedtime with milk or meals. The daily pediatric dosage (greater than 2 years) for juvenile rheumatoid arthritis is 20 mg/kg given three times per day with downward or upward adjustments to 15–30 mg/kg, not to exceed 30 mg/kg/day.

Diclofenac

Chemistry, Metabolism, and Excretion. Diclofenac is a phenylacetic PSI that was first marketed in Japan in 1974 and enjoyed wide clinical usage worldwide with the exception of the United States, where more stringent Food and Drug Administration (FDA) criteria for acceptability precluded its introduction until 1988. The chemical structure, which includes a secondary amino group and a phenyl ring with two chlorine atoms in the ortho position, was developed based on structure-activity relationships of other PSIs.

Diclofenac is absorbed completely with a high rate of first-pass hepatic metabolism, so only 50–60% reaches the systemic circulation. Peak plasma concentrations occur in 2–3 hours, with a mean terminal half-life of 2 hours (early elimination due to first-pass metabolism is more rapid). Diclofenate is almost completely bound to plasma protein. Peak plasma

Tolmetin

Diclofenac

Diclofenac: Metabolism

concentrations are less than proportional to dose, with plasma concentrations ranging from 1 to 2 μg/ml following ingestion of 25 – 50 mg. Repeated administration twice a day did not result in any drug accumulation in plasma levels; concomitant food intake may retard onset but not extent of absorption. Diclofenac is distributed throughout all bodily tissues, penetrating synovial membrane to joint fluid within 4 hours, which produces synovial fluid concentrations higher than those of plasma.

Diclofenac is metabolized extensively by the liver to at least four metabolites; the most prominent is the active 4'-hydroxy-diclofenac. Conjugates of diclofenac and its three metabolites are eliminated mainly by the kidney (50%) and to a lesser extent in the bile (20%). Little diclofenac is excreted unchanged.

Pharmacological Actions and Therapeutic Indications. As with other PSIs, diclofenac is effective as an anti-inflammatory agent in the treatment of rheumatoid arthritis, osteoarthritis, and ankylosing spondylitis. It is also effective in nonrheumatic conditions as an analgesic in dysmenorrhea, renal and biliary colic, oral surgery, and chronic musculoskeletal low back pain. It is a potent PSI, approximately equal in potency to indomethacin. Although the mechanism of action of diclofenac is by PG synthesis inhibition, it also results in a decrease in lipooxygenase products (LTs) by enhancing the uptake of arachidonic acid into triglycerides. The most important attribute of diclofenac, which differentiates it from many other PSIs, is its prolonged uptake into synovial fluid, with concentrations persisting above plasma levels for 24 hours. This fact, coupled with the short 2-hour plasma half-life of diclofenac and lack of accumulation of the free acid in patients with hepatic and renal disease, allows for one to two times daily dosing, although three times daily doses are prescribed usually. Thus, diclofenac does not require dose reduction in patients with compromised hepatic and renal function. In addition, the lower circulating plasma diclofenac levels are associated with a lower incidence and severity of the classic side effects of the PSIs. In short, the pharmacological properties of diclofenac approach the ideal, because high concentrations of active drug are present where they are needed (e.g., joint synovial fluid) and in low concentrations where they produce side effects (e.g., plasma and nonsynovial organs and tissues).

The clinical experience with diclofenac worldwide (with the exception of the United States) is vast, where it compares favorably with other PSIs. Thus, diclofenac is safer and better tolerated than the two most commonly used PSIs, aspirin and indomethacin. In particular, diclofenac had fewer GI side effects and absent or markedly reduced CNS side effects that are common to aspirin (tinnitus and deafness) and indomethacin (headache and drowsiness). Although not studied as extensively, the renal side effects (papillary necrosis, acute renal failure, and so forth) are reportedly less common with diclofenac. The characteristics of equal or greater efficacy as other PSIs with decreased toxicity have made diclofenac the number one drug of choice for the treatment of inflammatory disease worldwide. Even though its availability in the United States is more recent (1988), it has become the second most utilized PSI in current use for treatment of rheumatoid arthritis and allied conditions.

Availability and Dosage. Diclofenac is available in 25, 50, and 75 mg enteric-coated tablets. In rheumatoid arthritis, the recommended oral dosage is 150 – 200 mg/day in divided doses (50 mg three to four times per day or 75 mg two times per day). In osteoarthritis, the recommended dosage is 100 – 150 mg/day (50 mg two to three times per day or 75 mg two times per day). In ankylosing spondylitis, the recommended dosage is 100–125 mg/day (25 mg four times per day with an additional bedtime 25 mg dose if necessary).

PROPRIONIC ACIDS

The proprionic acid NSAIDs are almost identical in action to other NSAIDs.

The proprionic acid derivatives are a group of NSAIDs that share all the properties of the acetic acid PSIs, including rapid absorption, peak plasma concentrations within 1–2 hours, almost total binding to plasma proteins, and renal elimination as glucuronide or other conjugates of the free acid and its metabolites. In contrast to other acetic acids, naproxen is of singular interest, because its plasma peak concentration occurs at 2–4 hours with a half-life of 13 hours, permitting twice-daily dosage (see Table 28–5). The pharmacological indications, side effects, and drug interactions are identical to the acetic acid derivatives with the notable exceptions described later. For the most part they are equal to aspirin in potency or are intermediate in potency between aspirin and the more potent acetic acids.

Ibuprofen

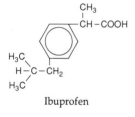

Ibuprofen

Pharmacological Actions and Therapeutic Indications. Ibuprofen was among the first proprionic acid PSIs that were introduced in 1974. Like diclofenac and certain other PSIs, it accumulates in synovial fluid for a prolonged time after plasma levels decrease, which peak in 1–2 hours. Although the side effects on the GI tract are not uncommon (including peptic ulceration), they reportedly occur with a lesser frequency than with aspirin and indomethacin. Ibuprofen is effective for the symptomatic treatment of rheumatoid arthritis, osteoarthritis, and as an analgesic in the relief of musculoskeletal pain; it effectively relieves primary dysmenorrhea, where it reduces PG levels in menstrual fluid and inhibits uterine contractions. Its effectiveness in relieving dysmenorrhea has led to extensive over-the-counter nonprescription use of ibuprofen for self-medication of dysmenorrhea.

Availability and Dosage. Ibuprofen is available in 300, 400, 600, and 800 mg tablets. For rheumatoid and osteoarthritis, the recommended divided daily dose is 1200–3200 mg (300, 400, 600, 800 mg, three to four times per day) tailored to the patient's response and appearance of side effects.

In the treatment of dysmenorrhea, 200–400 mg four to six times per day is recommended (over-the-counter preparations are available in 200 mg tablets) until symptomatic relief occurs. The same dose is recommended for analgesic use in conditions other than dysmenorrhea.

Naproxen

Pharmacological Actions and Therapeutic Indications. Naproxen is one of the more potent PSIs among the proprionic acid derivatives; it is 10–20 times more potent than aspirin. Naproxen also possesses two unique characteristics that have been utilized in more effective anti-inflammatory therapy. In the first place, as previously mentioned the prolonged half-life of naproxen allows for twice-daily dosing. Second, naproxen has potent inhibitory properties on leukocyte migration (as colchicine, see Chapter 59), which may explain its success in the treatment of acute gouty arthritis. Naproxen undergoes 6-demethylation and is excreted as conjugates of this metabolite and the free acid. As with other PSIs, a small percentage (less than 1%) appears in the milk of lactating mothers. Toleration of GI side

Naproxen

effects and CNS side effects is reportedly better than indomethacin, but the whole spectrum of side effects has been observed with naproxen as with other PSIs.

Naproxen is an effective agent for the treatment of rheumatoid arthritis, juvenile arthritis, osteoarthritis, ankylosing spondylitis, acute tendonitis and bursitis, acute gouty arthritis, and as an analgesic, such as in dysmenorrhea.

Availability and Dosage. Naproxen is available as the free acid (NAPROSYN) in 250, 375, and 500 mg tablets as well as an oral suspension (250 mg/10 ml). Naproxen sodium (ANAPROX) is available as 275 or 550 mg tablets (equivalent to 250 or 500 mg naproxen, respectively). For rheumatoid arthritis, osteoarthritis, and ankylosing spondylitis, the recommended daily dosage is 500–1000 mg NAPROSYN (250–500 mg, two times per day) or 550–1100 ANAPROX (275–550 mg two times per day). Dose adjustments are according to symptom relief or side effects at 1–2 week intervals, not to exceed 1500 mg/day for NAPROSYN or 1650 mg/day for ANAPROX. For juvenile arthritis, the recommended daily dosage is 10 mg/kg given in divided doses two times per day.

For acute gouty arthritis, the recommended dose of NAPROSYN is 750 mg followed by 250 mg every 8 hours and that of ANAPROX is 825 mg followed by 275 mg every 8 hours—until the attack subsides. As an analgesic, such as for dysmenorrhea and acute tendinitis and bursitis, the usual dose of NAPROSYN is initially 500 mg followed by 250 mg every 6–8 hours, not to exceed 1250 mg daily.

Fenoprofen

Pharmacological Actions and Therapeutic Indications. Fenoprofen shares the same pharmacological effects and side effects as the other aspirin-like PSIs. It is indicated for acute "flares" and chronic symptomatic pain relief in rheumatoid arthritis and osteoarthritis. Like ibuprofen, fenoprofen is also effective as an analgesic for postpartum and dental pain and in the postoperative management of surgical pain. The incidence of GI and other side effects is also reportedly lower than those of aspirin and indomethacin.

Availability and Dosage. Fenoprofen is available in 200 and 300 mg pulvules and 600 mg tablets. The recommended daily oral dosage for rheumatoid and osteoarthritis is 1200–2400 mg (300–600 mg three to four times per day), not to exceed 3200 mg. Again, adjustments in individual dose depend on symptomatic benefit and the occurrence of side effects.

Ketoprofen

Pharmacological Actions and Therapeutic Indications. Ketoprofen possesses PG synthesis inhibitory properties common to PSIs, but it also inhibits LT production and has antibradykinin activity and lysosomal membrane-stabilizing actions. About 60% of the drug is excreted as glycuronide conjugates of hydroxylated metabolites and the unchanged compound. Ketoprofen can be used for the chronic treatment of rheumatoid arthritis and osteoarthritis.

Availability and Dosage. Ketoprofen is available for oral use in 25, 50, and 75 mg capsules. The recommended daily dosage for rheumatoid arthritis and osteoarthritis is 150–300 mg given in divided doses three to four times per day with milk, food, or antacids (as with other PSIs). The recommended dose for dysmenorrhea is 25–50 mg three to four times per day for optimal clinical response with minimal side effects.

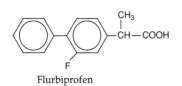

Flurbiprofen

Flurbiprofen

Pharmacological Actions and Therapeutic Indications. Although extensively used for years on a worldwide basis, flurbiprofen is among the more recently introduced (1989) PSIs in the United States. It exhibits all the classic anti-inflammatory and side effects of other PSIs. Ninety percent of flurbiprofen is excreted as conjugates of hydroxylated metabolites and the unchanged compound. Flurbiprofen is effective for the long-term management of rheumatoid arthritis and osteoarthritis.

Availability and Dosage. Flurbiprofen is available for oral use in 50 and 100 mg tablets. The recommended dosage is 200–300 mg daily in divided doses (three to four times per day), adjusted according to clinical response or side effects. The largest recommended single dose is 100 mg in a multidose regimen.

FENAMIC ACIDS

Pharmacological Actions and Therapeutic Indications. The fenamates are derivatives of *N*-phenyl-anthranilic acid and include a group of such compounds of which only *mefenamic acid* and *meclofenamate* are available in the United States. The fenamates have not received wide clinical acceptance for chronic treatment of inflammatory disorders because of their high incidence of GI side effects, particularly diarrhea, which may be protracted and severe.

Mefenamic acid and meclofenamate are potent PSIs. Meclofenamate possesses the property of $PGF_{2\alpha}$ antagonism, in this case of isolated bronchial smooth muscle contraction. The drugs are excreted in the urine (60%) as glucuronide metabolite conjugates and in the feces (40%) as unconjugated metabolites.

Although meclofenamate has an approved use for treatment of rheumatoid arthritis and osteoarthritis (see Table 28–5), the high incidence of diarrhea (10–30%) with bowel inflammation and at times steatorrhea precludes its overall effectiveness in these disorders. Therefore, meclofenamate is not recommended as initial treatment for rheumatoid arthritis and osteoarthritis. It is not indicated for use in children. Fenamic acid has an accepted use as a short-term analgesic (e.g., as treatment for dysmenorrhea), and treatment regimens should not exceed 1 week.

Availability and Dosage. Mefenamic acid is available in 250 mg capsules. For short-term analgesia and relief of dysmenorrhea, the recommended initial dose is 500 mg followed by 250 mg four times per day with antacids, food, or milk, not to exceed 1 week (dysmenorrhea usually 2–3 days).

Sodium meclofenamate is available in 50 and 100 mg mefenamic acid equivalent capsules. For rheumatoid arthritis, the recommended daily dose is 200–400 mg given in divided doses three to four times per day.

OXICAMS

Piroxicam

Pharmacological Actions and Therapeutic Indications. All the previously mentioned PSIs, including the salicylates, are carboxylic acids, whereas the oxicams are benzothiazines possessing an enolic 4-hydroxy substituent. Because of an active enterohepatic circulation, it has a uniquely prolonged half life (30–85 hours) that permits single daily dosing (20 mg) to achieve a plateau of therapeutic blood levels (3–8 μg/ml) after 7–10 days. At this point, daily drug elimination is equal to daily oral intake. Elimination is renal (65%) and fecal (35%) as glucuronide conjugates of the free acid and hydroxylated metabolites.

Piroxicam has potent anti-inflammatory, analgesic, and antipyretic activities derived primarily from its PG synthetase inhibitory properties. It is indicated for the chronic management of rheumatoid arthritis and osteoarthritis. In this regard, it is therapeutically equivalent or superior to aspirin and indomethacin with reportedly greater tolerance. However, once-a-day dosing results in maximal compliance, which is probably a major reason for its therapeutic effectiveness. The most prominent side effects are GI, occurring in about 20% of treated patients.

Piroxicam

Availability and Dosage. Piroxicam is available in 10 and 20 mg capsules. Recommended daily dosage is 20 mg as a single dose or 10 mg two times per day. Maximal effect is not evident for 1–2 weeks, when steady state concentrations are reached. Accordingly, therapeutic assessment of efficacy should be delayed for 10–14 days.

PYRAZOLONES

Phenylbutazone

Phenylbutazone was the first nonsteroid anti-inflammatory agent marketed in the United States (1952) following the introduction of aspirin 40 years earlier. The discovery of this potent agent took place 10 years before the isolation and identification of the PGs and 20 years prior to the observation that aspirin and aspirin-like drugs (including phenylbutazone) exert their effects by PG synthesis inhibition. The clinical experience with phenylbutazone provided the impetus for research leading to the introduction of all subsequent PSIs.

Phenylbutazone

Pharmacological Actions and Therapeutic Indications. Phenylbutazone is an enolic acid related closely to aminopyrine, antipyrene, and oxyphenbutazone. Following rapid absorption, it reaches peak plasma concentrations in 2–3 hours and is eliminated primarily by the kidneys as glucuronide conjugates of the hydroxylated metabolites and free acid. Phenylbutazone shares all the side effects of the PSIs, but in addition, it has its own specific actions (such as its uricosuric action in humans) and at times lethal toxic reactions unique to itself; these include agranulocytosis, leukopenia, thrombocytopenia, thrombotic thrombocytopenic purpura, nephrotic syndrome, and optic neuritis. The incidence and severity of these reactions, coupled with its potent sodium-retaining properties, contraindicate its use in patients with hypertension and cardiac, renal, or hepatic disease. In fact, phenylbutazone should never be used as the initial drug of choice; it is appropriate *only* after other PSIs have been tried, and even then only for short-term management of acute severe inflammatory reactions such as acute gouty arthritis. Even short-term treatment (4–5 days) has been associated with toxicity, and the patient should be warned to immediately report occurrences of sore throat, fever, and rash or mouth lesions, and a complete blood count should be obtained.

Availability and Dosage. Phenylbutazone is available in 100 mg tablets and capsules. For acute gouty arthritis, the recommended dosage is 400 mg initially, followed by 100 mg every 4 hours until the acute episode subsides.

This is usually within 4 days, but the drug should never be given for periods longer than 1 week.

SIDE EFFECTS COMMON TO PROSTAGLANDIN SYNTHETASE INHIBITORS

The burgeoning appearance of PSIs in the past 10–15 years with more similarities than differences (despite promotional claims) has resulted in confusion and uncertainty for the physician weighing options to provide the optimal treatment for a wide spectrum of inflammatory disorders in any individual patient. Generally, it can be safely stated that the risk of *any* and *all* side effects should be considered to be equal among all PSIs in any given patient undergoing PSI therapy. In the individual patient, the therapeutic response and risk of serious side effects are totally unpredictable, and the ultimate selection of the proper agent rests on the experience, knowledge, and judgment of the prescribing physician. Given the potential serious side effects of all PSIs, subsequent medical care and detailed follow-up must be total and complete.

There are a multitude of side effects common to all PSIs. The most potentially lethal are GI, renal, hypersensitivity, and bleeding reactions.

> The major side effects common to all PSIs are GI, renal, hypersensitivity, and bleeding.

Gastrointestinal Side Effects

Among the most commonly encountered side effects during long-term PSI administration are GI symptoms. These include dyspepsia, epigastric pain, nausea, vomiting, flatulence, abdominal cramps, which can be associated with peptic ulceration and massive GI hemorrhage, and ulceration. The true prevalence of these symptoms with any given PSIs is almost impossible to determine, but individual symptoms for all PSIs have been reported to be in the range of 5–10% with a frequency of total GI symptoms of 20–60% for aspirin. A similarly high prevalence exists for indomethacin and phenylbutazone, which has led to discontinuence of medication in about 20% of patients on these PSIs. Although somewhat lower total frequencies have been reported with other PSIs (10–25%), individual patients with GI symptoms to one PSI tend to show similar symptom vulnerability when placed on a different medication. In general, the proprionic acids show a lower incidence of GI side effects. The GI side effects of PSIs have been the subject of several recent reviews (Butt et al, 1988).

> The major GI side effects are epigastric pain, peptic ulceration, and GI hemorrhage.

Although symptomatic peptic ulceration with and without GI hemorrhage and perforation occurs reportedly in about 1% of all patients during PSI treatment, more recent studies indicate that the incidence of bleeding is much higher with asymptomatic GI ulcers, where bleeding with anemia was as high as 40% (Butt et al, 1988). The patients at higher risk include the elderly, those taking high and prolonged doses, and those with a history of previous ulcers. In patients presenting with GI bleeding, a history of occurrence of previous ingestion of PSIs is extremely high, approaching 60%. In fact, many practicing gastroenterologists, when confronted with severe GI bleeding, claim it is almost invariably associated with prior ingestion of PSIs or alcohol, or both; the combination of the two is potentially lethal. Because peptic ulceration with and without bleeding can occur in *any* patient receiving PSI treatment, and not just those with a prior history of ulcer diathesis, the FDA in the United States in 1989 required that package inserts for all PSIs include the following warning, which also serves as an accurate and concise state of the art summary of the status of the GI tract and PSIs:

Serious gastrointestinal toxicity such as bleeding, ulceration, and perforation, can occur at any time, with or without warning symptoms, in patients treated chronically with NSAID (nonsteroidal anti-inflammatory drug) therapy. Although minor upper gastro-intestinal problems, such as dyspepsia, are common, usually developing early in ther-apy, physicians should remain alert for ulceration and bleeding in patients treated chronically with NSAIDs even in the absence of previous GI tract symptoms. In pa-tients observed in clinical trials of several months to two years duration, symptomatic upper GI ulcers, gross bleeding or perforation appear to occur in approximately 1% of patients treated for 3–6 months, and in about 2–4% of patients treated for one year. Physicians should inform patients about the signs and/or symptoms of serious GI toxicity and what steps to take if they occur.

FDA warning

Studies to date have not identified any subset of patients not at risk of developing peptic ulcerations and bleeding. Except for a prior history of serious GI events and other risk factors known to be associated with peptic ulcer disease, such as alcoholism, smoking etc., no risk factors (e.g., age, sex) have been associated with increased risk. Elderly or debilitated patients seem to tolerate ulceration or bleeding less well than other individuals and most spontaneous reports of fatal GI events are in this popula-tion. Studies to date are inconclusive concerning the relative risk of various NSAIDs in causing such reactions. High doses of any NSAID probably carry a greater risk of these reactions, although controlled clinical trials showing this do not exist in most cases. In considering the use of relatively large doses (within the recommended dosage range), sufficient benefit should be anticipated to offset the potential increased risk of GI toxicity.

The mechanism whereby PSIs exert their GI side effects is largely by PG synthesis inhibition. The effects of PGE_2 on the GI tract include (1) increased intestinal motility; (2) inhibition of basal and stimulated (e.g., pentagastrin, food) gastric hydrochloric acid secretion; (3) experimental prevention of peptic ulceration induced by PSIs, steroids, and pyloric liga-tion; and (4) cytoprotection.

The antiacid secretory effects of some naturally occurring PGs, when administered parenterally, have been well established in animals and humans. The importance of endogenous PGs in modulating mucosal de-fense mechanisms is derived from the observation that PSIs damage gastric mucosa, whereas exogenous PGs in nonantisecretory dosages protect the mucosa from damage by NSAIDs and a wide variety of other noxious agents. This phenomenon was termed *cytoprotection*. In fact, some investi-gators reported that in patients with peptic ulcer disease, the gastric, but generally not the duodenal, mucosa synthesizes smaller amounts of arachi-donic metabolites than does the gastric mucosa in controls. It has been suggested that PGs exert their protective effect by preventing the vascular responses to noxious agents. However, $PGF_{2\alpha}$, which is a vasoconstrictor, also demonstrates similar protective effects to vasodilatory PGE_2, indicat-ing changes in blood flow are not the only causes whereby PGs exert their protective effects. Although the precise mechanisms of PGs' cytoprotec-tion remain to be solved, several experimental studies suggest the possible role of an increase in mucosal phospholipid, stimulation of sodium and chloride transport, stabilization of lysozomes, maintenance of mucosal sulfhydryl groups and stimulation of cyclic AMP, which are supposed to maintain initial mucosal resistance or affect mucosal repair.

The mechanism of antiacid effects of PGs include inhibition of gastric HCl secretion and cytoprotection.

Because the anti-inflammatory and toxic effects may be related to cyclooxygenase inhibition, which is shared by all PSIs, it can be concluded that similar toxic effects will be seen with all PSIs when administered in dosages sufficient to result in anti-inflammatory actions. When intolerance to one PSI develops, another PSI may be substituted, but at the risk of losing therapeutic efficacy or continuing toxicity. Alternatively, the side effects may be diminished by the use of antacids or histamine (H_2)-receptor antagonist, such as cimetidine, while continuing PSI therapy. The use of enteric-coated salicylates or nonacetylated salicylates may provide satis-

Misoprostol is an orally active analog of PGE$_1$, used to prevent the GI side effects of PSIs.

A major renal side effect of PGs is elevation of blood pressure.

Under hypovolemic conditions, renal blood flow is supported by PGs.

factory alternatives also. However, in patients who have experienced major GI toxicity, such as massive bleeding or active peptic ulcers, PSI administration is contraindicated, and non-PSI treatment should be instituted.

An orally active analog of PGE$_1$, misoprostol (CYTOTEC), has been introduced for prevention of hyperchlorhydria, gastric bleeding, and ulceration. Because PGs normally exert a cytoprotective effect on the gastric mucosa, and because this effect is reduced or abolished following administration of PSIs, the rationale for gastric PGE replacement during PSI treatment is obvious. Studies to date indicate that during chronic PSI treatment, oral administration of misoprostol (100–200 g four times per day) reduced gastric ulceration from 22% to 1–5%, which was associated with a significant reduction in fecal blood loss. There was no effect on the efficacy of anti-inflammatory effects of the PSIs. However, there was also no effect in prevention of duodenal ulceration or abdominal pain. The main side effect of misoprostol is diarrhea (14–40%). The drug is contraindicated in pregnant women because miscarriage may be induced.

Renal Side Effects

Renal PGs (especially PGE$_2$) have been shown to participate in many important renal physiological processes, such as autoregulation of renal blood flow and glomerular filtration, modulation of renin release, and the renal handling of sodium and water. The renal side effects of PSI administration include hypertension, azotemia with oliguria progressing to acute renal failure, hyponatremia and hyperkalemia, edema, papillary necrosis, interstitial nephritis, and the nephrotic syndrome. To understand and attempt to prevent these serious and at times life-threatening events, it is important to understand the rationale behind the discovery of the renal PGs and the normal role of the renal PGs in renal function.

The renal PGs (PGA$_2$, PGE$_2$, and PGF$_{2\alpha}$) were discovered and identified in the 1960s (Lee et al, 1963, 1967) as the result of a search for renal vasodepressor substances that might underlie the antihypertensive endocrine function of the kidney. According to this hypothesis, hypertension may reflect a deficiency of vasodepressor compounds, allowing pressor axes (e.g., renin-angiotensin, sympathetic nervous system) to act unopposed, leading to the development of hypertension with normal levels of pressor activity. It is not surprising, therefore, that PSI administration may result in blood pressure elevation in susceptible individuals. This can be severe and, if not recognized and PSI treatment decreased or stopped, can lead to cardiovascular complications common to patients with untreated essential hypertension not receiving PSIs. For the most part, the elevation in blood pressure with PSIs is mild, as shown in Figure 28–3, averaging 5–10 mmHg, a rise overlooked often in routine office measurements. The lack of uniformly higher blood pressure elevations may be explained in part by the additional actions of PSIs in concomitantly decreasing prohypertensive renal renin production leading to low plasma renin and urinary aldosterone levels (Fig. 28–3). In fact, PSI administration to normal subjects may lead to clinical and laboratory findings almost identical with low renin hypertension (low plasma renin, hypoaldosteronism, low urinary PGE$_2$ excretion, hyponatremia, and hyperkalemia). It is entirely unpredictable when mild or severe hypertension (or no effect) will develop in any given patient treated with PSIs; thus, all patients need close follow-up with frequent blood pressure determinations.

With the exception of hypertension, most of the detrimental effects of PSIs on renal function occur in a setting of hypovolemia with decreased

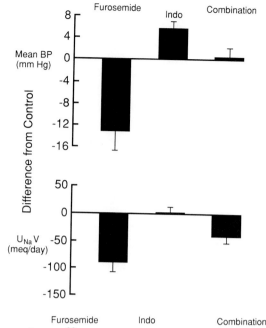

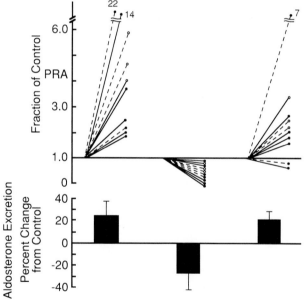

Figure 28-3

Effect of furosemide (80 mg every 8 hours for 4 days), indomethacin (50 mg every 6 hours for 4 days), and combined furosemide and indomethacin in three normal subjects *(open circles)* and seven patients with essential hypertension *(closed circles)* on blood pressure, sodium excretion, plasma renin activity (PRA), and urinary aldosterone. The bar graphs show the mean of cumulative 4-day periods. Results are expressed as mean ± standard error. All results statistically significant except for combined treatment on blood pressure and the effect of indomethacin on daily urinary sodium excretion. (From Patak RV, Mookerjee BK, Bentzel CJ, et al: Antagonism of the effects of furosemide by indomethacin in normal and hypertensive man. Prostaglandins 10:649–659, 1975.)

effective intravascular volume and high renin levels. Although PGE_2 increases renal blood flow, glomerular filtration rate, and sodium excretion, renal function, including renal blood flow, is not normally dependent on PGs; therefore, PG synthesis inhibition in such individuals with normal kidney function is without renal effects. However, any condition leading to decreased plasma and effective intravascular volume results in decreased renal blood flow. This can be illustrated by the hypovolemic state induced by reduced sodium intake when glomerular filtration rate estimated as creatinine clearance or inulin clearance decreases by 12–15%, respectively.

Volume contraction caused by sodium deprivation activates vasopressor mechanism, such as the adrenergic and renal renin-angiotensin system. Angiotensin II, a potent vasoconstrictor, stimulates aldosterone secretion from the adrenal cortex, which in turn appropriately increases renal so-

Under hypovolemic conditions, PSI administration may cause acute renal failure.

Figure 28-4

Hypothetical schema whereby volume depletion may lead to renin-angiotensin release and physiological antagonism of angiotensin II antinatriuretic and hypertensive actions. (From Lee JB: Prostaglandins and the renin-angiotensin axis. Clin Nephrol 14:159–163, 1980.)

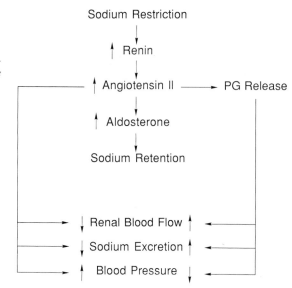

A second renal side effect is edema.

dium reabsorption. Angiotensin II (as well as vasopressin and catecholamines) also stimulates renal PGE_2 synthesis under these conditions, which by its vasodilatory and natriuretic activity counteracts the vasoconstrictor and antinatriuretic influences of angiotensin II (Fig. 28–4). At this point, basal renal blood flow and sodium excretion is supported in large part by continued renal PGE_2 production. Inhibition of PG synthesis by PSIs in this situation can reduce basal renal blood flow below levels critical for maintenance of normal function leading to azotemia, oliguria, and acute tubular necrosis. Clinical hypovolemic conditions in which PSI usage may result in this serious sequence of events include sodium restriction, diuretic therapy, posthemodialysis, existing renal disease, and edematous states where effective intravascular volume and renal blood flow are compromised (e.g., congestive heart failure, cirrhosis, and nephrotic syndrome). Therefore, close monitoring of the cardiovascular states and renal function is imperative in such patients receiving PSIs.

An important renal side effect of PSIs is sodium retention associated with edema in 10–25% of patients. Because PGE_2 has a direct inhibitory effect on renal tubular sodium transport, the effect of PSIs has been attributed to increased sodium chloride reabsorption. This effect may occur independently from the decrease in glomerular filtration rate and renal blood flow known to occur with PSIs. Severe hyperkalemia and hyponatremia may be observed also, which are believed to be secondary to PG synthesis suppression, leading to hyporeninemia and hypoaldosteronism.

An additional renal effect of PSIs is an increase in maximal urinary concentration and a decrease in free water clearance (PGEs inhibit vasopressin-induced water reabsorption), which is the rationale for use of PSIs in nephrogenic diabetes insipidus. Thus, dilutional hyponatremia may be observed in PSI-treated patients.

Other nephrotoxic effects of PSIs that may or may not be related to PG synthesis inhibition are papillary necrosis and interstitial nephritis with and without nephrotic syndrome. Paradoxically, PSI has been employed in the treatment of nephrotic syndrome, which produces a decrease in massive proteinuria, the result of PSI-induced decreases in glomerular filtration rate. However, deterioration of renal function may occur in this instance with production of irreversible azotemia and renal failure. The renal syndromes associated with PSIs (NSAIDs) have been reviewed extensively (Clive and Stoff, 1984).

Hypersensitivity Reactions

These have been discussed in the section on salicylates. Patients who have aspirin-exacerbated rhinosinusitis, nasal polyps, and bronchial asthma show cross-reactivity with other PSIs, which are contraindicated under these conditions. The mechanism is believed to be by PSI increase in slow-reacting substance A (bronchoconstrictor LTs as discussed earlier), following allergen challenge. In addition, PSIs may selectively inhibit bronchodilatory PGs, allowing an enhanced channeling of arachidonic acid into bronchoconstricting LTs. The demonstration of rare but lethal acute anaphylactic reactions with cardiorespiratory collapse to one PSI is an absolute contraindication to the use of any other PSI, because hypersensitivity cross-reactions are common.

Hypersensitivity reactions to PSIs

Other Side Effects

One of the most common effects of PSI administration is CNS symptoms, including headache (10–25%), drowsiness, dizziness, depression, and fatigue. As outlined in the discussion of the side effects of aspirin, prolongation of the bleeding and prothrombin times may be induced by PSIs, leading to serious hemorrhagic diatheses in susceptible patients (e.g., hemophilia, patients undergoing surgery).

Abnormal borderline elevations in hepatic function tests (serum glutamic-pyruvic transaminase, SGPT; serum glutamic-oxaloacetic transaminase, SGOT) may occur in about 15% of patients receiving PSI treatment. In less than 1% of patients, these may progress to frankly elevated levels, and in rare instances fatal hepatic reactions with jaundice and hepatitis have occurred. In instances where hepatic function tests do not stabilize or are associated with systemic hypersensitivity reactions such as rash or eosinophilia, the PSI should be stopped immediately.

Miscellaneous side effects of PSIs

Blurred vision with corneal depositions and macular changes have been reported in some patients on prolonged PSI treatment regimens. Other more rare side effects have been reported but are not discussed further here.

Because the effects of PSIs on the fetus during human pregnancy is unknown, and because PSIs appear in the milk of lactating mothers, its use in pregnancy and during nursing is not recommended. In fact, use of PSIs during the last trimester of pregnancy may be regarded as an absolute contraindication, because premature closure of the ductus arteriosus and delayed parturition (postmaturity) may occur with serious sequelae.

DRUG INTERACTIONS WITH PROSTAGLANDIN SYNTHETASE INHIBITORS

Diuretics and Antihypertensive Drugs

The first observation that PSIs blunt or abolish the diuretic or vasodepressor effects of antihypertensive medications was Patak and associates' (1975) observance that indomethacin inhibits the natriuretic and blood pressure–lowering effects of furosemide in hypertensive humans. It is evident from Figure 28–3 that furosemide administration alone lowered mean blood pressure by 10–20 mmHg, which was associated with enhanced renal sodium elimination and elevation in plasma renin and aldosterone. Indomethacin alone caused a slight rise in blood pressure, no change in sodium excretion, and marked suppression of plasma renin and aldosterone. The blood pressure–lowering effect of furosemide was abolished completely and sodium excretion blunted by 50% with concomitant indomethacin administration, although plasma renin and aldosterone

The natriuretic and hypotensive effects of diuretics are inhibited by PSIs.

were increased to comparable levels as those observed with furosemide alone. In subsequent animal studies, it was demonstrated that the natriuretic effect of furosemide was the result of a direct effect of furosemide in stimulating renal PGE_2 synthesis. This effect was associated with a marked rise in *in vitro* papillary PGE_2 synthesis and urinary PGE_2 excretion. Prior administration of indomethacin markedly reduced furosemide-induced natriuresis, renal PGE_2 synthesis, and urinary PGE_2 excretion.

The observation that PG synthesis inhibition of renal PG synthesis produced a drastic reduction in the antihypertensive and natriuretic effects of the loop diuretic furosemide has been extended to many other antihypertensive drugs and diuretic compounds. These include β-adrenergic blocking agents, thiazide diuretics, prazosin, and captopril. The attenuation of natriuretic and hypotensive effects of diuretic and antihypertensive drugs has been demonstrated with aspirin, indomethacin, flurbiprofen, piroxicam, diclofenac, and naproxen.

Because almost any PSI may interfere with the actions of a wide variety of antihypertensive and diuretic agents, patients should be monitored closely regarding the effectiveness of these drugs when concomitantly receiving PSIs. Generally, this includes patients with hypertension and diseases associated with edema (congestive heart failure, cirrhosis, and nephrosis).

Other Drug Interactions

Because they prolong bleeding time, PSIs must be used with caution in anticoagulated patients.

Although many PSIs do not alter the prothrombin time in patients receiving coumarin anticoagulants, they may prolong bleeding time by virtue of their inhibitory effects on platelet aggregation. This, coupled with the fact that PSIs displace warfarin from plasma protein-binding sites, indicates that caution and close monitoring should be exerted in patients on anticoagulant therapy receiving PSIs.

Aspirin has been shown to displace other PSIs from plasma-binding sites, leading to unpredictable therapeutic results. There is no reason, therefore, for the use of combined PSI administration for treatment of inflammatory disorders. On the other hand, gold and steroids have been shown to have beneficial and additive actions combined with PSIs in certain individual patients with rheumatoid arthritis.

Caution should be exercised in the combined use of PSIs with lithium (potentiation of lithium toxicity), methotrexate (potentiation of effects of methotrexate), probenecid (heightened PSI effects requiring dosage reduction), and potassium-sparing diuretics such as triamterine (sudden hyperkalemia and renal failure). Although PSIs may displace oral hypoglycemic agents from plasma protein-binding sites, there appears to be only minimal clinically relevant drug effects from this interaction.

Non–Prostaglandin Synthetase Inhibitors

The non-PSIs are a heterogeneous group of drugs with either solely analgesic-antipyretic effects (para-aminophenols) or anti-inflammatory actions in rheumatoid arthritis or gout (see Table 28–3). The mechanism of their action is uncertain but does not involve PG synthesis inhibition. The para-aminophenols, gold, and levamisole are discussed in this chapter. The other non-PSIs are discussed more appropriately elsewhere in the text.

PARA-AMINOPHENOLS

Historical Aspects. The para-aminophenols are aminobenzenes derived from acetanilid, which was discovered originally to have antipyretic activity in 1886 by Cahn and Hepp. However, its extreme toxicity stimulated a search for other structurally similar compounds, which led to the formulation of phenacetin and acetaminophen. Phenacetin was utilized extensively in a wide variety of analgesic mixtures, but its causal role in analgesic-abuse nephropathy led to its withdrawal from the market. Subsequent use of nonphenacetin analgesic-antipyretic mixtures resulted in a dramatic decline in analgesic-abuse renal failure, which had reached an alarming incidence (10–15%).

Acetaminophen is the active metabolite of both acetanilid and phenacetin. It was first used by von Mering in 1893 and has been available as a nonprescription drug in the United States since 1955.

Chemistry, Metabolism, and Excretion. Following ingestion, acetaminophen is rapidly and completely absorbed, reaching a peak plasma concentration in 30–60 minutes with a plasma half-life of 2 hours. Acetaminophen, unlike PSIs, is only slightly bound to plasma proteins. It is extensively metabolized by hepatic microsomal enzymes to glucuronide and sulfate conjugates, which are almost entirely excreted by the kidney within 24 hours. An important (albeit quantitatively minor) metabolite of acetaminophen is the hydroxylated metabolite N-acetyl-benzoquinone, which reacts with and depletes renal and hepatic glutathione following acetaminophen ingestion in toxic doses.

Normally, phenacetin is metabolized to acetaminophen, its active metabolite and many other metabolites, some of which are toxic and produce methemoglobin and erythrocyte hemolysis. Because phenacetin is no longer readily available for analgesic-antipyretic use, it is not discussed further.

Pharmacological Actions, Side Effects, and Therapeutic Indications. Acetaminophen is only a weak PSI. It possesses literally no anti-inflammatory reaction but displays analgesic-antipyretic activity roughly equivalent to that of aspirin. Little is known of the mechanism of the analgesic properties of acetaminophen, although its major actions are believed to be on the CNS rather than in the periphery.

There are few side effects of acetaminophen at the usual dosage (325–650 mg three to four times per day) when taken infrequently and for short time durations. However, when taken in massive doses or for prolonged periods (daily or weekly for years), serious hepatic or renal side effects have been reported. With massive overdose (10–15 g), hepatic toxicity may occur, which is potentially lethal in doses of 20–25 g. The onset of acetaminophen hepatitis occurs within 2–3 days and is manifest by nausea, vomiting, fever, and malaise followed by jaundice and the classic signs of liver failure. Liver function tests are typically abnormal (elevated transaminases, hyperbilirubinemia, and prolonged prothrombin time). Pathologically, biopsy specimens show central lobular necrosis. Hepatic failure may be accompanied by acute renal failure. Minimal hepatic damage can be expected with acetaminophen plasma levels in the range of 120 μg/ml 4 hours after ingestion and severe damage with plasma levels in excess of 200 μg/ml 4 hours after ingestion. Treatment should be immediate with supportive measures, gastric lavage, induction of emesis with ipecac, and a full course of sulfhydryl replacement. All these measures are most effective if performed within 4 hours of treatment. Sulfhydryl replacement with replenishment of glutathione stores may be accomplished by oral administration of N-acetylcysteine (MUCOMIST) with an initial loading dose of 140 mg/kg followed by 70 mg/kg every 4 hours for 17 doses (for emergency information the Rocky Mountain Poison Center, Denver, Colorado, may be called at 1–800–525–6115).

Although the use of phenacetin, a major precursor of acetaminophen,

Phenacetin

Acetaminophen

Acetaminophen: Metabolism

Acetaminophen: Major side effects include hepatic toxicity, interstitial nephritis, and papillary necrosis.

has been curtailed because of serious renal side effects, including interstitial nephritis and papillary necrosis, only more recently have the renal side effects of acetaminophen been reported in large-scale epidemiological studies. These studies, which need confirmation, clearly reveal that self-prescribed daily use of acetaminophen in usual therapeutic dosage for 1 or more years for headache, backache, arthritis, or nonspecific indications may be associated with a threefold risk of renal disease when compared to nonusers or matched controls without renal disease (serum creatinine: less than 1.5 mg/dl). Although comparable figures are not available in the United States, the incidence of analgesic-associated nephropathy in Australia is reportedly 13% despite complete withdrawal of phenacetin from the market. Whether this significant and serious side effect of prolonged analgesic use is attributable to acetaminophen, ibuprofen, or other analgesic agents is unknown. *Nevertheless, prolonged, indiscriminate daily use of acetaminophen for trivial somatic complaints should be strongly discouraged until further experience is gained with the potentially serious renal side effects of this commonly used non-PSI.*

Acetaminophen is effective for relief of headache, dysmenorrhea, myalgias, neuralgias, fever, and where aspirin and other PSIs are contraindicated (e.g., GI side effects, renal symptoms, and bleeding disorders).

Availability and Dosage. Acetaminophen is available over-the-counter under a host of trade names (ANACIN-3, DATRIL, TEMPRA, PANADOL, TYLENOL, and so forth) in tablets or capsules of 160, 325, 500, and 650 mg. Preparations also include chewable tablets, elixirs, solutions, wafers, and suppositories. Combinations with other analgesic, antihistaminic, and antisecretory agents (e.g., aspirin, caffeine, phenyltoloxamine) are also available (ANACIN, EXCEDRIN EXTRA-STRENGTH, PERCOGESIC, and so forth). Combinations with codeine (15, 30, 60 mg) have proved useful for the relief of more severe pain (e.g., postdental extraction, postminor surgery, neuralgias), although drug dependence on codeine is a hazard on prolonged usage. The usual adult dose of acetaminophen is similar to aspirin (650 mg three to four times per day), with a total daily dose not to exceed 4000 mg. A physician should be consulted if no relief is obtained after 7–10 days.

ANTIRHEUMATOID ARTHRITIS AGENTS

Gold

Gold: Metabolism

Chemistry, Metabolism, and Excretion. Gold salts have been in use for over 60 years in the treatment of rheumatoid arthritis. Their particular value lies in the fact that, unlike the other NSAIDs, gold has been shown to retard the progression of bone and articular destruction. Chemically, gold linked to sulfur is rendered water-soluble by linkage to hydrophylic compounds (glucose, sodium malate). The three most commonly utilized preparations are gold sodium thiomalate, aurothioglucose, and auranofin.

Following intramuscular (IM) administration of gold (sodium thiomalate and aurothioglucose), peak plasma concentrations occur in 2–6 hours with an initial plasma half-life of about 1 week. However, with extended treatment and prolonged accumulation, the plasma half-life is extended for weeks. Gold is bound to plasma protein (95%) during the first 7 days but may be transported in sizable amounts by erythrocytes after this time period. Gold accumulates in many tissues, including synovial membrane, macrophages, skin, and hepatic and renal tubular cells, where it can persist for years. Gold is eliminated by the kidneys (60%) and in the feces (40%). Following oral administration of auranofin, about 25% of the gold is absorbed. The terminal plasma half-life is about 26 days. The renal and hepatic excretion rates are comparable to the IM preparations. It is obvious that the accumulation of gold and its elimination are slow processes that result in delayed therapeutic responses.

Pharmacological Actions, Side Effects, and Therapeutic Indications. The mechanism whereby gold suppresses the chronic inflammatory response and retards cartilage and bone destruction is unclear. The accumulation of gold in macrophages depresses macrophage activity, migration, and immune responses. Its accumulation in the synovial cells reaches concentrations five to ten times that of other tissues, probably accounting for its preferential anti-inflammatory activity in chronic rheumatoid arthritis.

Gold therapy *(chrysotherapy)* is indicated in the treatment of active rheumatoid arthritis, which remains active after a course of PSI treatment for several months. Side effects of parenteral administration include a host of systemic reactions, the most common of which is dermatitis (15–25%) and skin pigmentation with pruritus, which can lead to exfoliative dermatitis and alopecia. Stomatitis is also a common side effect. Other serious parenteral effects include renal reactions (proteinuria, hematuria, and nephrotic syndrome) and more rarely hematological reactions (anemia, leukopenia, and thrombocytopenia). Hypersensitivity reactions ("nitroid" effects with flushing, dizziness, and sweating) have been reported as well as overt anaphylactic reactions. Encephalitis, enterocolitis, peripheral neuropathy, hepatitis, and pulmonary infiltrates are more uncommon side effects from gold administration. The oral preparation auranofin exhibits all the side effects mentioned earlier but with lesser incidence and severity. However, with auranofin, GI disturbances are common, particularly diarrhea.

> Gold: Major side effects include dermatitis, stomatitis, and renal dysfunction.

Gold treatment is contraindicated in patients with diabetes mellitus, renal disease, enterocolitis, hepatic dysfunction, congestive heart failure, hypertension, blood dyscrasias, recent hepatitis, recent irradiation, a history of prior gold intolerance, and allergic reactions. Gold treatment is not advised in pregnant or lactating women.

Side effects of gold administration are minimized by withholding gold therapy until the side effects disappear. Regular examination of the skin, buccal mucosa, and urine (for red blood cells and albumin) together with blood counts should be performed before each injection or at regular intervals. Treatment of side effects includes gold therapy cessation and the use of glucocorticoids for severe renal, dermatological, and hematological reactions.

Availability and Dosage. Gold sodium thiomalate (MYOCHRYSINE) is available in 25 and 50 mg/ml ampules. Aurothioglucose (SOLGANAL) is available in a 10 ml multiple-dose vial (50 mg/ml). Auranofin (RIDAURA) is available in 3 mg capsules.

The usual parenteral dosage is 10 mg IM the first week, 25 mg the second and third weeks, followed by 50 mg at weekly intervals for a total dose of 1000 mg or until symptoms abate at a lower cumulative dose. If a favorable therapeutic response is evident after 1000 mg, and side effects are absent or minimal, therapy can be extended indefinitely at intervals of 1 month. A beneficial response may not be evident for months. The weekly dose of gold should not exceed 100 mg in resistant cases. The recommended oral dosage with auranofin is 6 mg/day, increasing to a maximal dosage of 9 mg/day if a favorable response is not evident after 6 months.

Levamisole

Levamisole is of interest because it is an antihelminthic drug that has been tried experimentally in rheumatic disorders where it apparently restores the immune response by increasing macrophage chemotaxis and T lymphocyte function. Paradoxically, this immune enhancement appears to be beneficial in rheumatoid arthritis where dermatitis, leukopenia and thrombocytopenia, and nausea and vomiting have been reported as side effects.

Following absorption, levamisole reaches peak plasma levels in 2 hours with a half-life of 4 hours. The drug is metabolized by the liver and is eliminated mainly by the kidney. At present, it is not available in the United States for treatment.

Cost Considerations

There are wide variations in cost for the identical NSAIDs.

Cost considerations for NSAID usage are extremely important and relevant for both nonprescription and prescription preparations. In the calendar year 1988, for example, approximately 6800 tons of aspirin were marketed in the United States, which amounts to over 19 billion tablets having a marketing value of 1.1 billion dollars. Comparable figures for acetaminophen are 5800 tons, amounting to over 16 billion tablets and a market value of 925 million dollars. For ibuprofen, approximately 2200 tons were manufactured, amounting to over 5 billion tablets with a market value of 500 million dollars. These figures exclude the more potent prescription anti-inflammatory agents listed in Table 28–5, but they do serve to indicate that the analgesic–antipyretic–anti-inflammatory market is staggering in its size and can be considered a giant multibillion dollar industry in excess of 2.5 billion dollars per annum. Although the figures are given for 1988 and vary somewhat at the time of publication, the relative values persist in roughly the same absolute range.

The cost to the individual of the *same* preparation and chemical formulation is strikingly variable. For generic aspirin, ST. JOSEPH aspirin, and NORWICH aspirin, the cost varies from $1.05 to $1.25/100 tablets. Most other commercial preparations of the identical aspirin compounds with or without caffeine or acetaminophen cost between $5 and $6/100 tablets (e.g., ANACIN, ASCRIPTIN, BAYER, BUFFERIN, DOAN'S, ECOTRIN, EXCEDRIN, EMPIRIN). It is clear that all medical indications being equal, the purchase of generic aspirin or its brand-name equivalent for between $1 and $2/100 tablets should be encouraged.

Table 28–5 summarizes the cost of common prescription remedies for chronic inflammatory disorders such as rheumatoid arthritis. Again, it is evident that whenever indicated, tolerated, and of benefit, generic aspirin (written by prescription) is the drug of choice for the treatment of rheumatoid arthritis from a purely cost standpoint. The remaining anti-inflammatory compounds are from 6 to 25 times the cost of aspirin. It is obvious that with cost variability so great for a class of PSIs with essentially the same beneficial effects, side effects, and risks, judicious selection of any agent by the physician should include cost factors as well as medical indications and contraindications.

ACKNOWLEDGMENTS

The authors acknowledge the valuable contributions and advice of Bruce Mosher, Peterson Drug Stores, and Joseph W. Stanfield, Westwood Pharmaceuticals Inc.

References

Bergstrom S, Ryhage R, Samuelsson B, Sjovall J: The structure of prostaglandins E, F_1 and F_2. Acta Chem Scand 16:501–502, 1962.

Bergstrom S, Ryhage R, Samuelsson B, Sjovall J: The structures of prostaglandins E_1, F_1 and $F_{1\beta}$. J Biol Chem 238:3555–3564, 1963.

Butt JH, Barthel JS, Moore RA: Clinical spectrum of the gastrointestinal effects of nonsteroidal anti-inflammatory drugs. Am J Med 84 (Suppl 2A):5–14, 1988.

Clive DM, Stoff DM: Renal syndromes associated with nonsteroidal anti-inflammatory drugs. N Engl J Med 310:563–572, 1984.

Ferreira SH, Moncada S, Vane JR: Indomethacin and aspirin abolish prostaglandin release from the spleen. Nature (New Biol) 231:237–239, 1971.

Lee JB, Crawshaw K, Takman BH, et al: The identification of prostaglandins E_2, $F_{2\alpha}$ and A_2 from rabbit kidney medulla. Biochem J 105:1251–1260, 1967.

Lee JB, Hickler RB, Saravis CA, Thorn GW: Sustained depressor effect of renal medullary extract in the normotensive rat. Circulation 26:747, 1962.

Lee JB, Hickler RB, Saravis CA, Thorn GW: Sustained depressor effect of renal medullary extract in the normotensive rat. Circ Res 13:359–366, 1963.

Patak RV, Mookerjee BK, Bentzel CJ, et al: Antagonism of the effects of furosemide by indomethacin in normal and hypertensive man. Prostaglandins 10:649–659, 1975.

Smith JB, Willis AL: Aspirin selectively inhibits prostaglandin production in human platelets. Nature (New Biol) 231:235–236, 1971.

The Steering Committee of the Physicians' Health Study Research Group: Preliminary report: Findings from the aspirin component of the ongoing physicians' health study. N Engl J Med 318:262–264, 1988.

Zurier RB: Prostaglandins and inflammation. *In* Lee JB (ed): Prostaglandins, 91–112. New York: Elsevier, 1982.

29

Treatment of Headache; Ergot Alkaloids

Cedric M. Smith

Most people suffer from headaches.

Therapy to relieve or prevent headaches is usually effective.

Rational and effective therapy is based on (1) accurate diagnosis; (2) identification of trigger or predisposing factors; (3) prevention of occurrence; and (4) aborting the attacks.

Classification of headaches provides an overview of syndromes and mechanisms.

Headache is one of the most common of symptoms and disease syndromes; more than 90% of the adult population have experienced at least a few or many headaches. Although the majority of headaches are infrequent, of minor consequence, time-limited, and discontinue after modest therapy of aspirin or its equivalent, or with no medication at all, some can be incapacitating and recur as often as every day. In a recent large sample of young adults, 57% of the males and 76% of the females had experienced a headache within 4 weeks of being interviewed (Linet et al, 1989). Thus, headaches are not necessarily mild and they are a frequent presenting medical complaint; for example, they were found to be the seventh leading presenting complaint in ambulatory care centers. Usually self-limited, persistent headache is a symptom worthy of attention because it occurs in two thirds of those who are found to have brain tumors; however, a persistent headache is caused by a brain tumor in only approximately one in a thousand patients.

Classification of headaches provides a convenient frame of reference for the consideration of drugs used in treatment of headache, either to prevent them from occurring or to relieve them once they have begun (Table 29–1). Rational therapy of headaches rests on an understanding of the pathophysiology of the syndromes and the factors that aggravate or trigger a headache. Many of the drugs discussed in this chapter have

Table 29–1 OVERVIEW OF CLINICAL CLASSIFICATION OF HEADACHE

I. Migraine
  A. Migraine headache
    Some examples of the various types of migraine headache are
      1. Classic (with aura)
      2. Common (without aura)
      3. Ophthalmoplegic and hemiplegic
      4. Basilar artery migraine
      5. Many other varieties (also included in some classifications are migraine equivalents such as aura without headache or attacks of pain in the abdomen or other sites)
  B. Triggers, predisposing factors for migraine, or similar mechanisms
      1. Familial
      2. Stress—afterward
      3. Change in blood glucose, fasting
      4. Hormonal—premenstrual more frequent than other times in the menstrual cycle
      5. Oversleeping
      6. Dietary factors—high tyramine, chocolate, nuts, citrus juice, aged cheese
      7. Depression
      8. Panic and anxiety disorders
      9. Alcoholic drinks, certain red wines

Table 29–1 *OVERVIEW OF CLINICAL CLASSIFICATION OF HEADACHE Continued*

      10. Bright sunlight
      11. Hypoxia
      12. Carbon monoxide
      13. Drugs—nitroglycerin, marijuana, estrogen, oral contraceptives
      14. Drug withdrawal/rebound—ergotamine, NSAIDs, benzodiazepines, MAOI, caffeine
      15. Collagen disease
      16. Fever
  II. Tension-type (Common, Chronic Recurring Undifferentiated Headache, Muscle Contraction)
    A. Frequently occur in same patients who have migraine
    B. Etiology, predisposing, or confounding factors; see also all the other varied causes of headaches, including:
      1. Depression
      2. Primary sleep disorder—e.g., central or peripheral sleep apnea with periods of hypoxia
      3. Panic and anxiety disorders
      4. Caffeine withdrawal
      5. Benzodiazepine withdrawal
      6. Stress, emotional and psychodynamic factors
      7. Cervical osteoarthritis
      8. Muscle tension
      9. Temporomandibular joint dysfunction
 III. Cluster
    A. Precipitated by alcoholic beverages. Also can be initiated by histamine or nitroglycerin
    B. Occurs almost exclusively (>99.1%) in men
 IV. Miscellaneous Without Structural Lesion
    A. Cold stimulus headache, benign exertional, and headaches associated with sexual activity
  V. Headache Associated with Head Trauma
 VI. Headache Associated with Vascular Disorders
VII. Headache Associated with Nonvascular Intracranial Disorder
VIII. Headache Associated with Substances or Their Withdrawal
    A. Headache induced by acute substance use or exposure
      1. Nitrate/nitrite induced headache
      2. Monosodium glutamate induced
      3. Carbon monoxide induced
      4. Alcohol induced
      5. Other substances
    B. Headache induced by chronic substance use or exposure
      1. Ergotamine induced headache
      2. Analgesic abuse headache
      3. Other substances
    C. Headache from substance withdrawal (acute use)
      1. Alcohol withdrawal headache (hangover)
      2. Other substances
    D. Headache from substance withdrawal (chronic use)
      1. Ergotamine withdrawal headache
      2. Caffeine withdrawal headache
      3. Narcotics abstinence syndrome
      4. Other substances
    E. Headache associated with substances but with uncertain mechanism
      1. Birth control pills or estrogen
      2. Other substances, such as a benzodiazepine
 IX. Headache Associated with Noncephalic Infection
  X. Headache Associated with Metabolic Disorder
    A. Hypoxia
      1. High altitude headache
      2. Hypoxic headache (low pressure environment, pulmonary diseases causing hypoxia)
      3. Sleep apnea headache
    B. Hypercapnia
    C. Mixed hypoxia and hypercapnia
    D. Hypoglycemia
    E. Dialysis
    F. Headache related to other metabolic abnormality
 XI. Headache or Facial Pain Associated with Disorder of Cranium, Neck, Eyes, Ears, Nose, Sinuses, Teeth, Mouth, or Other Facial or Cranial Structures
XII. Cranial Neuralgias, Nerve Trunk Pain, and Deafferentation Pain Including Trigeminal Neuralgia (Tic Douloureux)
XIII. Headache not Classifiable

Adapted and reduced from Olesen J: Classification of headache disorders, cranial neuralgias and facial pain; and a diagnostic criteria for primary headache disorders. Cephalalgia 8 (Suppl 7):35–38, 1988. For many of the classifications only the major heading is reproduced here. Some of the trigger and etiological factors have been added to this classification.

Drugs to be discussed are those used in treatment of migraine, cluster, common (or tension-type) headaches, and in trigeminal and postherpetic neuralgia.

Ergotamine is a standard drug used exclusively in the abortive treatment of migraine headaches.

already been presented in some detail in chapters dealing with nonsteroidal anti-inflammatory agents, adrenergic blocking agents, and calcium channel-blocking agents.

The focus of this chapter is the drug treatments of the two prominent headache syndromes—migraine headaches and tension-type, or common, headaches. Although discussed separately, it should be recognized that most patients seen in office practice and headache clinics have mixed headaches—the common, tension-type headache as well as migraine headaches.

Trigeminal and postherpetic neuralgia can present with facial and head pain; because the therapies of neuralgia contrast with those of other head pain syndromes, these are discussed briefly.

Some ergot alkaloids, such as ergotamine, have essentially unique uses in medicine in the treatment of migraine headaches. Thus, a short section of this chapter is devoted not only to those used for headache, but the ergot alkaloids in general.

Syndromes and Pathophysiology of Common Headaches

Common, tension-type headaches are associated, in only a few patients, with demonstrably increased muscle activity.

The mechanisms underlying tension-type or common headache are currently under some dispute. The names used in the past reflect these differences. Since the 1950s it has been dogma that such headaches were due to sustained contraction of neck muscles, hence the name *muscle contraction headache*. However, sustained muscle contraction cannot be demonstrated in most patients studied, and muscle relaxants are generally ineffective. The other common name has been *tension headache*, referring to fact that headaches appear to accompany psychological tension and stress. Given the absence of compelling data on mechanism, the term *common headache* is used in this chapter to refer to such recurrent nonspecific headaches, the headache suffered occasionally by most people.

Headache is the most frequent symptom of the hangover following consumption of an alcoholic beverage.

Hangover is associated with large ethanol consumption, concurrent consumption of an alcoholic beverage, and the endogenous accumulation of low levels of methanol.

There are, as Table 29–2 indicates, a variety of headache syndromes, many of which have not been studied extensively. Among these syndromes, one of the more prevalent is the *hangovers* that are experienced by most individuals the morning after a night of overindulgence of alcoholic beverages. Headache is perhaps the most common symptom of hangover, but also frequent are nausea, vomiting, tremor, dry mouth, anxiety, depression, guilt, diarrhea, photophobia, sweating, and chills. The headaches are frequently pulsatile and aggravated by movement or bearing down, but they may be simply generalized, steady, and aching in character. The syndrome is complex and is a function of individual differences, amount consumed, and the level of methanol reached consequent to alcohol metabolism (Smith and Barnes, 1983; Jones, 1987).

Drugs Useful in the Treatment of Common Headaches

Primary therapeutic consideration for common and migraine headaches is the determination of the triggers and predisposing factors.

Among the most prevalent predisposing factors is the affective disorder of mood, depression.

The drugs can be divided according to their use into those that are taken to relieve an ongoing headache, *abortive* treatment, and those that are taken chronically to *prevent* the recurrence of the headache. In fact, the primary concern of management of the patient with headache is the determination of the events that can serve to trigger the headaches, the avoidance of such events, and the procedures that can serve to decrease the individual's sensitivity to such triggers. Table 29–1 presents a long list of conditions, situations, or drugs that are rather well-established and predisposing conditions. Prominent among these triggers are specific foods and underlying physiological conditions, including notably the biopsychiatric affective disorder of depression. Depression is present in some 40% of those with migraines, and a prominent symptom of depression is common headache and disordered sleep, but which comes first is difficult to determine. Headache, in a similar fashion, is a common accompaniment of sleep disorders, such as sleep apnea.

Drugs effective for the abortive and prophylactic treatments of the common, so-called undifferentiated headache are considered first, followed by those used in the treatment of common vascular headaches, migraine and cluster headaches.

ABORTIVE TREATMENT OF THE COMMON HEADACHE

The well-known, established drugs that alleviate headache are the nonsteroidal anti-inflammatory drugs (NSAIDs), notably the old agent aspirin (Chapter 28); some of the newer agents, such as ibuprofen, may be found to produce a rapid onset of relief in as little as 15 minutes. In addition to the NSAIDs, acetaminophen has been found to have efficacy essentially equivalent to that of aspirin.

Many of the over-the-counter preparations for headache are combinations of a NSAID or acetaminophen, with caffeine. The caffeine combinations may have somewhat greater effectiveness. The origin of the inclusion of caffeine, along with a wide variety of agents that have fallen out of use, is lost in the history of the varied and complex pharmaceutical preparations, but it is possible that its inclusion may have begun when it was determined that some headaches were caused, at least in part, by the reduction or withdrawal from the usual caffeine consumption, i.e., a caffeine-withdrawal headache. In addition to the side effects of NSAIDs discussed in Chapter 28 is the paradoxical occurrence of headache during the chronic use of NSAIDs. Recurrent headache can be caused by chronic use of either of the two major classes of headache medications—NSAIDs or ergot alkaloids.

Caution should be exercised in the use of combination products, many with highly advertised and promoted names, that contain barbiturates or codeine or so-called muscle relaxants. Such combinations may be truly hazardous. First among the hazards are the lack of awareness of the ingredients, for example, the administration of a combination containing aspirin to patients with aspirin-sensitive asthma, which can result in near fatal consequences. Second, the so-called antianxiety barbiturate or muscle relaxant agents have significant potential for acute or chronic toxicity. In short, headache is one condition that needs to be managed not only for relief of the immediate symptoms; there should be management over time in combination with patient education regarding agents to use and those to avoid.

Severe, acute tension-type or migraine headache can be alleviated by opioids; however, a more appropriate therapy for severe unrelenting headache is the intravenous (IV) administration of chlorpromazine or prochlorperazine; such treatment is warranted only in patients who have severe, incapacitating headaches that do not respond to oral preparations.

PREVENTIVE, PROPHYLACTIC TREATMENTS OF THE COMMON HEADACHE

The primary objective of prophylactic treatment is the identification of the behaviors, situations, and conditions that serve as triggers or predisposing factors for a given individual patient. A partial list of the candidates is presented in Table 29–1. Given that common headache syndromes and migraine syndromes may constitute a continuum, the triggers for migraine listed may well be operative in individuals who fail to exhibit the full migraine syndrome.

Primary therapy to abort an existing headache is aspirin, acetaminophen, or a NSAID such as ibuprofen.

Caffeine may aggravate depression or disturbance of sleep.

Over-the-counter preparations frequently contain caffeine and are on average slightly more effective in relieving headache pain.

Chronic use of most of the agents that are helpful in treating a headache can actually cause headaches—NSAIDs, ergotamine, caffeine.

Avoid trade-named combination medications—most people do not need or benefit from barbiturates; the muscle relaxants sometimes included are not generally effective; codeine or other opioids present added risk to the patient.

Among the most frequently occurring correlates of recurrent headaches is the presence of the affective disorder of depression. Effective alleviation of the depression witnesses the disappearance of the recurrent headaches. In this context, a first-line pharmacotherapy of common headaches is an antidepressant. Of these the most frequently used have been the tricyclic antidepressants such as amitriptyline or imipramine (see Chapter 22).

Thorough work-up and therapy for depression not only potentially prevents subsequent headaches but can also profoundly improve quality of life.

In view of the association with headache of sleep disorders and affective disease, panic disorders, anxiety disorders and substance abuse, including the chronic taking of analgesic drugs, all patients with recurrent headaches deserve not only a thorough diagnostic work-up, but counseling and periodic follow-up that addresses at the least all of the factors and conditions listed in Table 29 – 1. Approximately 90% of patients with headaches can be helped significantly by appropriate therapy; however, at present most patients fail to receive an adequate evaluation and appropriate therapy.

Syndromes and Treatment of Migraine Headaches

Migraine headaches are characterized by the initial vasoconstriction of certain cerebral, retinal, and extracranial blood vessels (associated with an aura), *followed by* vasodilation and the phase of headache.

Migraine headaches involve disturbances of mood and affect, sleep patterns, autonomic blood vessel regulation, and regulation of fluid balance.

Neurotransmitters and mediators known to be intimately involved in migraine headache syndromes are serotonin, norepinephrine, histamine, prostaglandins, substance P, and enkephalins.

Administration of a serotonin agonist has been found to produce a migraine attack.

The same drugs used for common headache may be effective in migraine if given at the outset of an attack.

Migraine headaches are frequently classified among the primary vascular headaches because of (1) the symptoms of throbbing and tenderness along vessels and (2) the sequence of vasoconstriction followed by vasodilation that figures prominently in theories of the migraine pathophysiology. In considering therapy, it needs to be emphasized that migraine disease involves a complex sequence of neurogenic, vascular, neuroendocrine, and fluid balance interactions. Sensory nerves innervating cranial blood vessels are the ultimate source of the pain. These vessels are subject to serotonergic and adrenergic actions, prostaglandin release, alterations in calcium movements involved in the vascular muscle function, alterations in platelet aggregation, and inflammation and edema of vessel walls; in addition, migraine may be associated with systemic retention of water followed by diuresis. Major neural and autonomic nervous systems participate in the pathophysiology of the attack, the response to triggering factors, and the cyclic natural history of the disease. At the least the following endogenous neuroeffective substances are involved intrinsically in the migraine syndrome: serotonin, norepinephrine, histamine, prostaglandins, substance P, and enkephalins.

ABORTIVE TREATMENT OF MIGRAINE HEADACHES

The primary initial therapy for migraine headaches are the same drugs used for common headaches — aspirin, acetaminophen, NSAIDs (such as naproxen or ibuprofen), given alone or perhaps with caffeine. It is the clinical impression that migraine treatment should be started as soon as possible in an attack for the greatest abortive effect.

Ergot Alkaloids

The ergot alkaloid ergotamine is the main standby for the abortive treatment of migraine.

The ergot alkaloids have long-standing credentials as one of the standard types of drug used in the abortive treatment of the migraine attack. The most extensively used of the alkaloids is ergotamine, but dihydroergotamine and ergonovine are probably also effective.

Ergotamine is taken repeatedly every 20 – 30 minutes until relief is obtained or some 6 doses have been taken. Effective doses are associated frequently with side effects of nausea or vomiting, tremor, or cold fingers and toes.

In prescribing ergot preparations it is useful to keep in mind the patient's situation. Most patients will have had prior attacks and are aware of the aura, if any, as well as their characteristic initial symptoms. Frequently occurring with the onset will be visual disturbances and nausea that can progress to brief or protracted vomiting. Under such circumstances, the possible gastrointestinal (GI) side effects of any agent and the route of administration take on important dimensions. Oral administration may not be feasible, or if undertaken might be followed by vomiting, thus confusing the treatment even further. Hence, the agents are available not only for oral administration, but for sublingual, inhalation, intramuscular (IM), and rectal administration.

The *mechanism of action* of the headache-relieving action of the ergot alkaloids is complex and continues to be disputed. For many years it was assumed that their efficacy was due to vasoconstriction, consistent with the knowledge that the headache phase of the migraine attack is accompanied by vasodilation (whereas the aura and initial visual disturbances are associated with vasoconstriction in extracranial and retinal vessels). However, direct vasoconstriction is not a sufficient explanation. The ergot alkaloids have multiple and complex effects on blood vessels and neurons; these actions include direct effects on smooth muscle, as well as agonist and antagonist effects on receptors for serotonin, tryptamine, dopamine, and norepinephrine (illustrated in Table 39–2 in Rall, 1990). At present it is not possible to state which of these actions are most relevant to the alleviation of migraine and other vascular headaches produced by ergotamine; nevertheless, the preponderance of current observations favor an effect on serotonergic systems.

Ergot alkaloids available and useful for abortive treatment of migraine headaches are as follows:

- *ergotamine* — oral, sublingual, inhalation, rectal, or IM preparations (frequently combined with caffeine for increased effects). Prescribed, for example, as ergotamine tartrate, 1 mg tablet orally, repeated every ½ hour if necessary to a maximum of 6 tablets per attack (and a maximum of 10 tablets per week).
- *dihydroergotamine mesylate (DHE 45 Injection)* — used exclusively by the IM or subcutaneous routes. The combined use of IV metoclopramide followed by dihydroergotamine appears to be an effective treatment for the chronic intractable migraine (Raskin, 1986).
- *ergonovine* — orally less effective than ergotamine but less nausea and vomiting.

Ergotamine preparations have unpleasant tastes, and their toxicity includes nausea, vomiting, abdominal cramps, diarrhea, painful uterine contractions, vasoconstriction, coldness, and numbness and tingling in fingers and toes. Large dosages cause thirst, confusion, hallucinations, and unconsciousness; with chronic use, gangrene of the extremities and valvular heart disease have been reported. Ergot alkaloids have an interesting history as agents of mass poisonings and hallucinations (see Chapters 27 and 67).

Another problem associated with the use of ergotamine is the appearance of ergotamine rebound headaches occurring in individuals who use ergotamine on a regular basis. This can be avoided if 2 days are allowed to elapse between repeated uses of ergotamine.

Any of the ergot alkaloids, including ergotamine, are contraindicated in pregnancy and in patients with hypertension, occlusive vascular disease, and liver or kidney disease.

Other drugs that may have utility in aborting the migraine attack include the following:

- *phenothiazines* — chlorpromazine or prochlorperazine given intravenously for severe headache unresponsive to other medications (see Chapter 21).
- *isometheptene mucate* (MIDRIN) — a nonselective α-adrenergic blocking agent given at the onset of an attack. It has not been studied in detail. Its side effects include drowsiness, nausea, and vomiting.

No route of administration of ergotamine is fully satisfactory — oral, sublingual, inhalation, or rectal.

Ergot alkaloids probably act by a combination of direct vasoconstriction, antagonism of specific serotonin receptors, modification of intravascular platelet aggregation. But other neuroeffector systems may contribute — norepinephrine, prostaglandin, or dopamine.

Dihydroergotamine can be given intramuscularly or intravenously if nausea or vomiting precludes oral or other routes of administration.

Ergonovine and dihydroergotamine may be better tolerated than ergotamine, but explicit clinical trials have not been carried out.

Chronic use of ergot alkaloids can be avoided by means of patient education.

Severe, unremitting headaches can respond to chlorpromazine, prochlorperazine, or opioids such as meperidine.

- *propranolol*—has been used at the onset of migraine headaches but is used more frequently as a preventative. Note that propranolol is contraindicated in the presence of ergotamine and *vice versa.*
- *verapamil*—has been reported also to be effective in acute headache; it is given intravenously in dosages of 5–10 mg (see Chapter 31).

For headache-related severe nausea and vomiting, metoclopramide or domperidone are current drugs of choice.

For severe nausea and vomiting, metoclopramide (REGLAN) has been employed with some success; metoclopramide is an antidopaminergic agent with side effects of increased GI absorption of many drugs; it possesses the extrapyramidal and dystonic effects of other dopamine antagonists.

ABORTIVE TREATMENT OF CLUSTER HEADACHES

Cluster headache attacks can be cataclysmic in intensity and the incapacitation they can produce. Treatment is directed generally toward prophylaxis and prevention. Drugs used in migraine are also used in cluster headache, with the emphasis on obtaining the most rapid onset of action possible, such as with dihydroergotamine intramuscularly.

For relief of acute cluster headaches, oxygen inhalation or ergot alkaloids, or both, are given by the most rapidly effective route.

Cluster headaches may be aborted in some 50–70% of cases by inhalation of 100% oxygen administered through a face mask at the rate of 8–10 l/minute for 5–10 minutes.

PROPHYLACTIC TREATMENT OF MIGRAINE SYNDROMES

Chronic administration of propranolol is the therapy of choice for prevention (see Chapter 14).

Prevention of recurrence of headache is *the primary treatment objective for all headaches.*

The chronic administration of NSAIDs has been established recently as effective prophylactic therapy in migraine. Even the physicians taking 1 aspirin tablet (325 mg) every other day in the double-blind Physician's Health Study (Buring et al, 1990) were found to have had 20% fewer recurrences of migraine headaches than those who had received the placebo.

The following have also been found to be effective prophylactic therapies in certain patients:

Drugs from many pharmacological classes have been reported to be effective in at least a portion of individuals with migraine.

- calcium channel blockers (Chapter 32)
- cyproheptadine
- ergotamine
- amitriptyline (Chapter 22)
- clonidine (Chapter 14)
- methysergide (SANSERT; see later)
- other β-adrenergic blockers

An herbal remedy, feverfew, has been found to be effective in migraine prevention, but it is not available commercially in standardized formulations (Murphy et al, 1988).

PREVENTIVE TREATMENT OF CLUSTER HEADACHES

The drug of choice when preventive therapy is indicated is methysergide. Methysergide is a unique agent with established effectiveness. It is thought to act by blocking both the vasoconstriction and inflammatory effects of serotonin. It would be used more extensively except for the fact that it can produce the potentially serious side effect of *retroperitoneal fibrosis,* a potentially irreversible fibrous infiltration around the kidneys and ureters. In severe cases of frequent cluster headaches it is still used, but the chronic

Methysergide is effective prophylactic therapy for migraine and for cluster headaches; however, retroperitoneal fibrosis is a serious life-threatening side effect.

therapy is interrupted every 4 months or more often for a drug holiday of 4–6 weeks. Such intermittent therapy appears to gain appreciable periods of relief without increasing the risk of retroperitoneal fibrosis. This agent represents a good example of the therapeutic dilemma presented by a drug that, although uniquely effective, has the potential of causing an unpredictable, serious side effect.

Drug holidays are one solution to the toxic potential of methysergide.

OTHER USES OF ERGOT ALKALOIDS

Ergonovine and Methyl Ergonovine

Two ergot alkaloids, ergonovine maleate (ERGOTRATE) and methyl ergonovine (METHERGINE), are administered postpartum (IM or sometimes IV) with or immediately after the delivery of the placenta. The drugs cause prompt, sustained contraction of the uterine muscle and thereby reduce the extent of blood loss during the postpartum period. Side effects of such use of ergot alkaloids are infrequent but may include nausea, vomiting, and increased blood pressure.

Ergot alkaloids are obtained from a fungus that infects the grain seed of rye.

Ergot alkaloids are strictly prohibited during pregnancy or labor. For the induction of labor, oxytocin can be used (Chapter 40). (The prostaglandins (PGF_{2a} and PGE_2) produce uterine contractions, but they are not approved for use to induce labor or for therapeutic abortion.)

Unrecognized poisoning by bread made from rye contaminated by ergot has been involved in the mass hysterias of middle and eastern Europe during times of relative famine in the Middle Ages up to the 1800s.

Agents related to ergot alkaloids include bromocriptine, a dopaminergic agonist that has found utility in the treatment of Parkinson's disease (Chapter 24).

Lysergic acid diethylamide (LSD) is a semisynthetic ergot alkaloid with a history of experimental and nonmedical uses (see Chapter 27).

The symptoms of ergot intoxication have been attributed to witchcraft or the intervention of demons or angels. The cause of St. Anthony's fire was ergot poisoning; it has been speculated that the children and witches of Salem, Massachusetts, had consumed ergot-infected rye bread (see Chapter 27).

HEADACHES ASSOCIATED WITH FEVER, HEAD TRAUMA, AND VASCULAR DISORDERS

Many of the headaches associated with these widely varied causes are responsive, at least to some degree, to the nonnarcotic analgesics; if excessively severe, opioids may be required (see Table 29–1, sections V, VI, and VII).

HEADACHES ASSOCIATED WITH SUBSTANCES OR THEIR WITHDRAWAL AND METABOLIC DISORDERS

A variety of drugs can be associated with causing, triggering, or exacerbating headaches. The drug effects range from acute action (such as vasodilators like nitrites or histamine) as well as an acute rebound (hangover due to alcohol), to those associated with chronic use, and with drug withdrawal, such as after cessation of chronic intake of caffeine, benzodiazepines, or ergotamine (see Table 29–1, section VIII).

HEADACHE AND HEAD PAIN OF NEURALGIA

Trigeminal neuralgia is characterized by chronically recurring attacks of severe lancinating pain. Carbamazepine (TEGRETOL) or phenytoin (DILANTIN) has been found to provide moderate relief in some, but not all, patients. For patients who cannot obtain adequate relief, microneurosurgery is sometimes dramatically effective in the relief experienced after the removal of nerve compression by a blood vessel.

Neuralgia is associated with attacks of repetitive discharges along large numbers of sensory nerves. Any drug or procedure that will reduce the occurrence, frequency, or duration of such seizure-like activity can be beneficial.

Neuralgia can be the result also of herpes and herpes zoster. Carbamazepine is employed frequently to relieve such pain. Amitriptyline has

Neuralgia has been relieved by drugs used in treatment of epilepsy—carbamazepine (TEGRETOL) or phenytoin (DILANTIN), by drugs used primarily in depression—amitriptyline and desipramine—and by a drug used primarily as a spice—capsaicin (see Chapter 26).

been reported to be moderately effective in such patients. Studies of desipramine demonstrated its utility and probable preference over amitriptyline, particularly in view of its lesser degree of anticholinergic and sedative effects. Amitriptyline and other tricyclic drugs have analgesic effects that appear to be independent of their antidepressant actions.

Use of Opioids for Severe Common or Vascular Headaches

Opioids may be required to relieve extremely severe, unrelenting headache, but their use sets the stage for repeated doses.

Effective prevention rests on identification of a patient's triggers and predisposing factors.

The principal strategy for the rational use of analgesics to relieve pain is the progression from aspirin or acetaminophen in low dosages and, with inadequate relief, to increase the dosage, add adjuncts, and eventually try preparations that contain low doses of codeine or its equivalent. Codeine-containing preparations are dispensed rather freely by some physicians with the predictable result of the chronic use and escalation of dose by *some* patients. Although some headaches and pains experienced may truly be unrelieved by nonopioid medications, caution is warranted regarding the use of codeine, meperidine (DEMEROL), or other opioids. Once such therapy is initiated, its continuation is likely to be required over months and years because of the recurrent nature of headache syndromes. A better management strategy is the thorough initial diagnostic study, including the detection of triggers and psychiatric conditions, leading to adequate treatment initially. Such an approach would reduce significantly the inappropriate and excessive administration of codeine and meperidine (Chapter 18).

A Look to the Future

Active clinical and basic research and development continues to explore new drugs and therapies for headache, especially recurrent and severe forms. Among the promising leads is sumatriptan, an agent that has been found in controlled trials to be rapidly effective in relieving migraine attacks with far fewer side effects than currently available substances. The manufacturer is reportedly applying for approval to market both an oral and an injectable form of the drug.

References

Blau JN: Migraine: Clinical and Research Aspects. Baltimore: Johns Hopkins University Press, 1987.

Buring JE, Peto R, Hennekens CH: Low-dose aspirin for migraine prophylaxis. JAMA 264:1711–1713, 1990.

Diamond S, Freitag FG: Do non-steroidal anti-inflammatory agents have a role in the treatment of migraine headaches? Drugs 37:755–760, 1989.

Diamond S, Millstein E: Current concepts of migraine therapy. J Clin Pharmacol 28:193–199, 1988.

Diamond S, Solomon GD: Pharmacologic treatment of migraine. Ration Drug Ther 22:1–5, 1988.

Drexler ED: Severe headaches: When to worry, what to do. Postgrad Med 87:164–180, 1990.

Edmeads J: Four steps in managing migraine. Postgrad Med 85:121–134, 1989.

Fozard JR, Gray JA: 5-HT$_{1C}$ receptor activation: A key step in the initiation of migraine? TIPS 10:307–309, 1989.

Glover V, Sandler M: Can the vascular and neurogenic theories of migraine be reconciled. TIPS 10:1–3, 1989.

Jones AW: Elimination half-life of methanol during hangover. Pharmacol Toxicol 60:217–220, 1987.

Jones J, Sklar D, Dougherty J, White W: Randomized double-blind trial of intravenous prochlorperazine for the treatment of acute headache. JAMA 261:1174–1176, 1989.

Kishore-Kumar R, Max MB, Schafer SC, et al: Desipramine relieves postherpetic neuralgia. Clin Pharmacol Ther 47:305–312, 1990.

Kunkel RS: Cluster headache. Pain Management 3:44–51, 1990.

Kunkel RS: Management of migraine. Pain Management 2:156–161, 1989.

Linet MS, Stewart WF, Celentano DD, et al: An epidemiologic study of headache among adolescents and young adults. JAMA 261:2211–2216, 1989.

Murphy JJ, Heptinstall S, Mitchell JRA: Randomized double-blind placebo-controlled trial of feverfew in migraine prevention. Lancet 2:189–192, 1988.

Olesen J: Classification of headache disorders, cranial neuralgias and facial pain; and diagnostic criteria for primary headache disorders. Cephalalgia 8 (Suppl 7):35–38, 1988.

Peatfield R: Drugs and the treatment of migraine. TIPS 9:141–145, 1988.

Peatfield R: Headache. Berlin and Heidelberg: Springer-Verlag, 1986.

Rall TW: Oxytocin, prostaglandins, ergot alkaloids, and other drugs; tocolytic agents. *In* Gilman AG, Rall RW, Nils AS, Taylor P (eds): Goodman and Gilman's The Pharmacological Basis of Therapeutics. New York: Pergamon Press, 1990.

Raskin N: Repetitive intravenous dihydroergotamine as therapy for intractable migraine. Neurology 36:995–997, 1986.

Smith CM, Barnes GM: Signs and symptoms of hangover: Prevalence and relationship to alcohol use. Drug Alcohol Depend 11:249–269, 1983.

Stewart WF, Linet MS, Celentano DD: Migraine headaches and panic attacks. Psychosom Med 41:559–569, 1989.

30

Drugs Used in the Treatment of Gout

Margaret A. Acara

Development of gout in hyperuricemics

Gout is a disease resulting from hyperuricemia. Elevated uric acid levels in the blood result in the deposition of urate crystals leading to acute inflammatory reactions. Tophi, inflamed swellings in subcutaneous tissue, are observed most frequently in the large toe, ankle, or heel but may also be found in other areas such as the wrist, fingers, earlobes, and elbows. Episodes of acute gouty arthritis are excruciatingly painful, requiring prompt treatment. Whereas only a minority of hyperuricemics ever become gouty, all patients with gout have hyperuricemia. When gout does occur it is usually after 20–30 years of hyperuricemia and, if primary in nature, requires a lifetime of commitment to therapy.

Decreased uric acid excretion or increased uric acid synthesis

Primary gout occurs through a direct defect in uric acid production or excretion. Most patients with primary gout exhibit a renal defect, and 10–25% of patients with primary gout have renal stone formation. Secondary gout is associated with hyperuricemia resulting from another disorder. Neoplastic disease, such as leukemia, leads to the breakdown of cellular nucleoproteins and excess formation of uric acid. Lead nephropathy and glycogen storage disease lead to decreased elimination of uric acid. Hyperuricemia may also be induced by drugs that interfere with uric acid excretion.

When blood uric acid reaches the saturation concentration of 7–8 mg/dl, the crystals are phagocytosed by granulocytes, which is accompanied by a release of lysosomal enzymes and acidic substances into synovial fluid. This action leads to a slightly more acidic environment and promotes further crystal precipitation. Because the joints in the extremities have a more acidic environment, they are susceptible areas for deposition.

Deposition of uric acid crystals in joints

Effect of dissociation on crystal form

The pKa of uric acid is 5.75, and at the plasma pH of 7.4 it is 98% dissociated. When the pH of the environment favors dissociation, monosodium urate crystals are formed. At a pH of 4.75, uric acid is 91% undissociated and uric acid crystals form. Thus, in the renal tubule, with its more acidic environment, there is the possibility of the formation of uric acid stones and the development of renal failure.

Approaches for the treatment of gout

There are three pharmacological approaches to the treatment of gout: (1) increase the excretion of uric acid; (2) decrease the synthesis of uric acid; and (3) terminate the inflammatory response. Whether or not and when to treat hyperuricemia itself is controversial, but a blood uric acid level greater than 7 mg/dl may warrant treatment.

Renal Excretion of Uric Acid

The kidney is the major organ for the elimination of uric acid. Two thirds of uric acid cleared from the blood appears in the urine. The remaining third appears in intestinal secretions. The binding of uric acid to plasma proteins is small, less than 10%, and the remainder is filtered freely at the glomerulus. Fractional excretion of uric acid is 0.1, indicating net reabsorption.

Mechanisms for the renal handling of uric acid involve a complex system that includes filtration, reabsorption, and secretion. Bidirectional transport systems are present in the proximal tubule and operate simultaneously. A transporter for uric acid reabsorption is present on the brush border membrane, and one for secretion is situated in the basolateral membrane. Entry of uric acid into the cell is active and saturable and can be competed for by other organic acid molecules. Competition for the secretory transport carrier can result in increased uric acid blood levels, whereas competition for the reabsorptive carrier can result in decreased uric acid blood levels. Because the major direction of uric acid movement is reabsorptive, adequate dosages of drugs that compete for the uric acid transport carriers have the predominant effect of decreasing uric acid reabsorption, increasing its excretion and lowering the blood level.

Uric acid undergoes net reabsorption in the kidney.

Carriers for uric acid transport are present on both basolateral and brush border membranes.

URICOSURIC AGENTS

Uricosuric agents enhance uric acid excretion by inhibiting filtered urate reabsorption in the proximal tubule. Initial treatment with uricosuric agents may be associated with increased amounts of uric acid reaching the kidney and the danger of papillary necrosis. Also, as with all drugs that occupy the organic anion transport system, small doses may raise blood levels. Until drug levels build up to a sufficient concentration to decrease reabsorption, there is a risk of acute gouty attack. Therefore, an agent that prevents the acute attack may be administered before the uricosuric. In addition, a high fluid intake of 3–4 l/day and, in some cases, alkalization of the urine may be useful to prevent uric acid precipitation in the kidney.

Uricosuric agents inhibit uric acid reabsorption.

Requires high fluid intake

Probenecid

The most widely used uricosuric agent is probenecid (BENEMID). It is the prototypical inhibitor of organic anion secretion, but when given in sufficient amounts it interferes with uric acid reabsorption.

Probenecid is bound to plasma proteins, but it is secreted also by the organic acid transport system and thus has a relatively short half-life (6–12 hours). Its occupation of the organic acid transporter may result in interference with the excretion of other drugs that are organic acids and lead to longer half-lives and higher concentrations of these drugs when they are administered simultaneously. In fact, probenecid is used to maintain levels of certain agents whose regular half-lives may be short.

With the exception of patients with renal failure, probenecid is effective in increasing uric acid excretion and lowering hyperuricemia. Some gastrointestinal (GI) irritation and hypersensitivity reactions occur with probenecid, but in general it is well tolerated.

Probenecid is the most widely used uricosuric.

Sulfinpyrazone

Sulfinpyrazone (ANTURAN) is another frequently used uricosuric agent. It is an active metabolite of the anti-inflammatory agent phenylbutazone and, as such, has some anti-inflammatory action. Sulfinpyrazone has the same mechanism of action and characteristics as probenecid, but it is longer acting and more potent. Sulfinpyrazone has become available as an inhibitor of platelet aggregation in the prophylactic treatment of myocardial infarct.

Sulfinpyrazone is longer acting.

Benzbromarone

Benzbromarone has greater potency.

Benzbromarone is a new drug with greater potency than sulfinpyrazone. It is particularly effective in patients with renal dysfunction. Examples of other drugs with uricosuric effects are clofibrate and acetohexamide. Both of these are organic acids, and this effect may be related to inhibition of uric acid reabsorption.

Avoid salicylates in gout.

In general, salicylates antagonize the uricosuric effects of these agents, and they should not be used with uricosuric agents.

Uric Acid Synthesis

Uric acid is the end product of purine metabolism in humans.

Uric acid is the end product of purine metabolism in humans. Humans and great apes do not have the enzyme uricase that converts uric acid to the more water-soluble allantoin. Figure 30–1 shows the final steps in the pathway of purine metabolism. They are the conversion of hypoxanthine and xanthine to uric acid by the enzyme xanthine oxidase.

An average person produces approximately 600–700 mg uric acid/ day. The most common metabolic defect leading to overproduction of uric acid is a deficiency in the enzyme hypoxanthine guanine phosphoribosyl-transferase (HG-PRTase). When this occurs hypoxanthine is not cycled back through inosinic acid and, instead, there is an increased production of xanthine and thereby uric acid.

INHIBITOR OF XANTHINE OXIDASE—ALLOPURINOL

Allopurinol inhibits xanthine oxidase.

There is one major drug used to inhibit the production of uric acid: allopurinol (XYLOPRIM). Allopurinol is a competitive inhibitor of xanthine oxidase. It decreases the level of uric acid and increases the level of its precursors, hypoxanthine and xanthine. Allopurinol is metabolized by xanthine oxidase to oxypurinol, which is an active metabolite that inhibits the same enzyme by forming a reversible complex with it. Chronic administration of allopurinol leads to accumulation of oxypurinol and contributes to its long-term therapeutic use.

Decrease plasma uric acid and increase hypoxanthine and xanthine

Treatment with allopurinol results in a decrease in the plasma level of uric acid and concomitantly its urinary excretion. Because of xanthine oxidase inhibition, there is an increase in plasma levels of the precursors, hypoxanthine and xanthine, and accordingly in their urinary excretion.

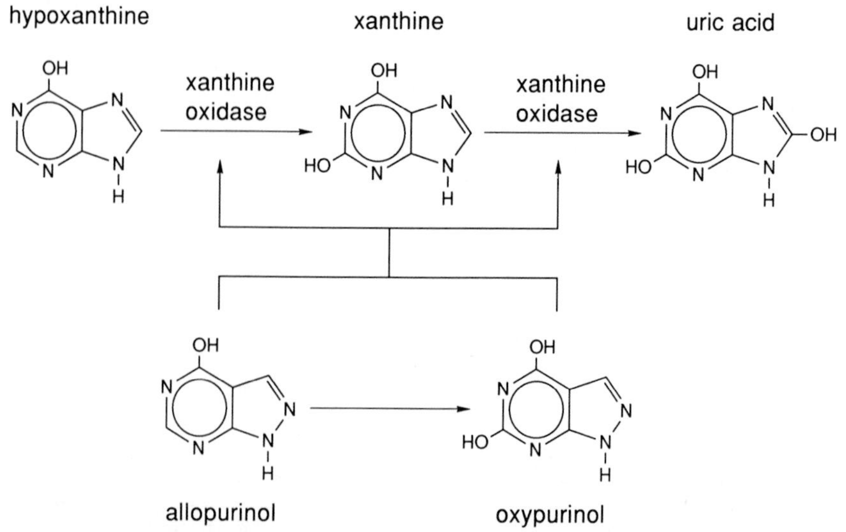

Figure 30–1

Pathway of purine metabolism.

Precipitation of these oxypurines as crystals appears not to be a problem, because they are more soluble than uric acid.

Allopurinol is well absorbed and not well bound to plasma proteins. It is eliminated mainly by metabolism, and its half-life is 2–3 hours. On the other hand, its active metabolite oxypurinol is reabsorbed, and its half-life is much longer, 18–20 hours.

Uricosuric agents are frequently the first approach in the treatment of gout. However, patients who are overproducers of uric acid and those with excessive tophi are candidates for allopurinol therapy. In addition, those who do not respond to uricosuric agents and those with high uric acid levels who have developed renal stones may be treated successfully with allopurinol.

The side effects of allopurinol are somewhat more severe than uricosuric agents (such as probenecid or sulfinpyrazone) and include skin rash, fever, GI upset, and liver toxicity. Therapy with allopurinol, as with the uricosurics, should not be initiated during an acute attack. The initial decrease in plasma uric acid levels causes the mobilization of urate from deposits in the body in sufficient amounts to aggravate the acute attack.

Correction of hyperuricemia is not initiated during acute attack.

The most important drug interaction with allopurinol therapy is that of coadministration of mercaptopurine and azathioprine. The oxidation of these drugs is inhibited by allopurinol, and it is necessary to decrease their dosage by as much as 75% when these agents are administered concomitantly. Allopurinol interferes somewhat with the hepatic microsomal drug-metabolizing enzymes, and caution is required for the administration of drugs metabolized by this system.

Mercaptopurine or azathioprine/allopurinol drug interaction

Because uricosuric agents and allopurinol produce decreased uric acid levels by different mechanisms, their coadministration leads to a more effective therapy to decrease uric acid levels. However, the combined therapy is complicated by the resulting changes in pharmacokinetic profiles. Uricosuric agents increase the urinary clearance of oxypurinol but decrease the excretion of xanthine and hypoxanthine.

Treatment of Gouty Inflammation

Drugs used to treat the inflammation associated with gout are administered not only during the acute attack but also are used prophylactically to prevent the acute attack and in combination with uricosuric agents or allopurinol at the initiation of therapy to decrease the risk of an acute attack of gouty arthritis. Colchicine and indomethacin are the major anti-inflammatory agents used in the treatment of gout, and they differ in their mechanism of action. They are not effective in decreasing uric acid synthesis or reabsorption.

Anti-inflammatory agents treat acute attack.

COLCHICINE

Colchicine is an alkaloid extract of the autumn crocus and has been used for over a century for this purpose. It decreases the release of lactic acid and the movement of granulocytes into the inflamed area, breaking the cycle leading to the inflammatory response. Colchicine is specific for the treatment of gout, and its relief of pain in this disease contributes to the diagnosis. It is not used in other inflammatory disorders.

Colchicine is specific for pain of acute attack.

Therapy with colchicine is begun at the first sign of the acute attack and continued until relief is obtained or until GI reactions appear. A maximum dosage is 6–7 mg. Adverse GI side effects have been observed in 80% of patients treated with colchicine and are the most common cause for changing to another anti-inflammatory agent. Patients learn to titrate the dose of colchicine that they can tolerate based on their GI reactions. Al-

Severe GI side effects

though generally administered by mouth, the drug may be given intravenously and the severe GI reactions avoided.

INDOMETHACIN

Indomethacin inhibits cyclooxygenase and decreases prostaglandin production.

Indomethacin (INDOCIN) is anti-inflammatory, antipyretic, and analgesic. It is useful for the management of the acute attack of gouty arthritis. Indomethacin inhibits the cyclooxygenase enzyme involved in the production of prostaglandins. For this reason it is contraindicated in patients with renal disease in which the prostaglandins are important mediators of renal function. Indomethacin has no effect on uric acid synthesis or excretion. Central nervous system (CNS) effects (headache, vertigo, confusion) and GI effects (nausea, indigestion, vomiting) are included in adverse effects of indomethacin. Ocular effects such as blurred vision and corneal deposits have been reported also.

PHENYLBUTAZONE

Other anti-inflammatory agents

Phenylbutazone (BUTAZOLIDIN) is anti-inflammatory, antipyretic, and analgesic and has some uricosuric effect. However, because of serious side effects its use is reserved for rheumatoid disease that is not controlled by other drugs. The most serious adverse effect is bone marrow depression. Hepatitis, GI disturbances, and sodium and water retention also may occur. Phenylbutazone is highly protein bound and displaces other drugs from plasma protein-binding sites, resulting in potentiation of their effects. Such drugs include oral hypoglycemics, sulfonamides, coumarin-type anticoagulants, and other anti-inflammatory agents. Phenylbutazone also displaces bound thyroid hormone.

Oxyphenbutazone (OXALID) is the principal metabolite of phenylbutazone. It has the same actions, indications, and toxicities as phenylbutazone.

Other nonsteroidal anti-inflammatory drugs, including naproxen, fenoprofen, and ibuprofen, are also effective in the treatment of acute gouty arthritis. Initial administration dosages should be near maximal and gradually tapered as symptoms subside (see Chapter 28).

Occasionally adrenal corticosteroids and corticotropin are used to treat the inflammation associated with acute gouty attacks. However, these drugs are reserved for severe cases and then used only for brief periods of time (up to 3 days).

Diet

A diet low in purines may be of some benefit in decreasing hyperuricemia. However, available drugs are so effective that dietary restrictions may not be necessary. Low purine diets can decrease serum uric acid level by 1 mg/dl.

References

Emerson BT: Urate metabolism and gout—A perspective. Aust NZ J Med 18:319–326, 1988.

Fox IH, Kelley WN: Uric acid and gout. *In* Seldin DW, Giebisch G (eds): The Kidney: Physiology and Pathophysiology. New York: Raven Press, 1985.

German DC, Holmes EW: Hyperuricemia and gout. Adv Rheumatol 70:419–436, 1986.

Van Dyke K: Drugs used in the treatment of gout. *In* Craig CR, Stitzel RE (eds): Modern Pharmacology, 2nd ed. Boston: Little, Brown, 1986.

Cardiovascular System Pharmacology

31

Drugs Affecting Calcium — Regulation and Actions

David J. Triggle

Calcium critical to cellular function

Calcium is a particularly abundant element, making up some 3% of the earth's crust. Calcium is similarly abundant in the human body, being the fifth most common element. The average individual contains approximately 1 kg of calcium, the majority of which is immobilized as the mineral hydroxyapatite in teeth and bones. Only 1–2% of this total amount of calcium is found in the intracellular and extracellular fluids; however, it is upon this small fraction that the critical calcium-mediated processes, including excitation-contraction and stimulus-secretion coupling, underlying cellular excitability depend. In addition to these broad categories of cellular response, calcium plays vital roles in the control of cellular integrity, in the blood coagulation cascade, and in the activation of intracellular and extracellular enzymes controlling protein and phospholipid breakdown.

In 1883 the English physician and physiologist Sidney Ringer (1836–1910) observed the critical role of calcium for the maintenance of cardiac contractility. This finding was rapidly extended by others to show the fundamental roles for calcium in the maintenance of cellular integrity and in the actions of many drugs.

Calcium a key intracellular messenger

Probably several reasons underlie the choice by the cell of calcium as a key cellular messenger. The high extra- to intracellular ratio of calcium concentrations is clearly appropriate for an inwardly directed messenger function, and the coordination chemistry of calcium confers advantages relative to magnesium for the formation of tight complexes of flexible geometry with polyanionic centers. This behavior of calcium is demonstrated in its reaction with the intracellular calcium-binding proteins, including calmodulin, troponin C, and related species that serve as receptors to mediate the functions of messenger calcium. Finally, it has been suggested that this role of calcium was inevitable once cellular energy metabolism was committed to a phosphate currency.

The Regulation of Calcium

Calcium regulated at multiple sites

The multiple roles of calcium in cell and organ function demand that it be a regulated species. In fact, regulation of calcium is achieved at multiple loci by multiple processes (Fig. 31–1). Calcium absorption from food is actively regulated in the gastrointestinal (GI) tract and excretion is actively regulated in the kidney. The major locus of body calcium, that of bone, serves as a bank for deposit or withdrawal of calcium according to supply and demand. These processes are regulated by a triumvirate of hormones, parathyroid hormone (PTH), calcitonin, and vitamin D. In turn the activities of these agents are controlled by the circulating levels of calcium. Thus,

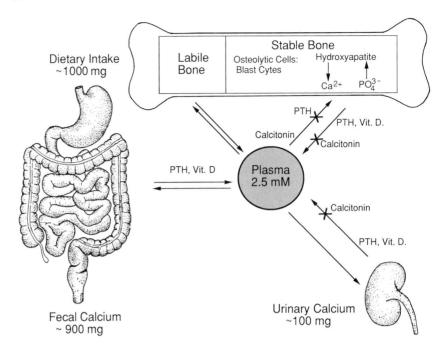

Calcium absorption is regulated by vitamin D, calcitonin, and parathyroid hormone.

a fall in plasma calcium produces a rise in PTH concentration leading to restoration of calcium levels by enhanced mobilization from bone, increased reabsorption in the kidney, and facilitated absorption from the gut. Similar roles are played by vitamin D, particularly in enhanced GI absorption. In contrast, calcitonin secretion is stimulated when the plasma concentration of calcium rises. Calcitonin opposes the actions of PTH and vitamin D and causes deposition of calcium into bone and enhanced urinary excretion. The reciprocal relationships of calcium and PTH, vitamin D, and calcitonin are summarized in Table 31–1. It must be noted that phosphate and calcium metabolism are regulated in coordinate manner. Parathyroid hormone has net opposing actions on serum Ca^{2+} and phosphate levels: it enhances Ca^{2+} and phosphate absorption through the gut, and enhances Ca^{2+} reabsorption but promotes phosphate excretion in the kidney (Table 31–2).

Table 31-1 RELATIONSHIP BETWEEN SERUM CALCIUM AND PARATHYROID HORMONE, CALCITONIN, AND CALCITRIOL

	Hormone Response		
Plasma Signal	*Parathyroid Hormone*	*Calcitonin*	*Calcitriol*
$Ca^{2+} \downarrow$	↑	↓	↑
$Ca^{2+} \uparrow$	↓	↑	

Hormone	**Hormone Change**	**Plasma Ca^{2+} Change**
Parathyroid hormone	↑	↑
	↓	↓
Calcitonin	↑	↓
	↓	↑
Calcitriol	↑	↑
	↓	↓

Table 31-2   THE ACTIONS OF VITAMIN D AND PARATHYROID HORMONE ON PHOSPHATE AND CALCIUM REGULATION IN GUT, KIDNEY, BONE, AND PLASMA

System	Vitamin D	Parathyroid Hormone
Gut	Ca^{2+} absorption ↑ PO_4''' absorption ↑	Ca^{2+} absorption ↑ PO_4''' absorption ↑
Kidney	Ca^{2+} excretion ↓ PO_4''' excretion ↓	Ca^{2+} excretion ↓ PO_4''' excretion ↑
Bone	Ca^{2+} resorption ↑ PO_4''' resorption ↑	Ca^{2+} resorption ↑ PO_4''' resorption ↑
Plasma	$[Ca^{2+}]$ ↑ $[PO_4''']$ ↑	$[Ca^{2+}]$ ↑ $[PO_4''']$ ↓

The concentration of calcium in plasma is maintained at a fairly constant level, approximating 2.5×10^{-3} M (5.0 mEq/l) as a consequence of the balance between intake, storage, and excretion achieved by the cooperative actions of PTH, vitamin D, and calcitonin. Plasma calcium may be considered as three separate fractions: calcium bound to protein (primarily albumin) constitutes approximately 40%; calcium complexed to anions including phosphate and citrate is about 10%; and the remaining fraction represents the free ionized calcium. Distinction between these fractions, particularly the free and protein-bound components, is important to any considerations of the physiological or pathological significance of changes in plasma calcium levels. Both the total calcium level and the ionized fraction of calcium can be altered independently. Increased or decreased serum albumin concentrations result in parallel changes in the total calcium concentrations. An increase in serum pH during, for example, respiratory alkalosis increases the fraction of ionized calcium without affecting total calcium.

Plasma calcium exists at several compartments.

A second set of control processes is exerted at the cell level to ensure that intracellular calcium concentrations and storage are regulated. Although the total concentration of calcium within a cell may be millimolar or higher, most of this is stored within intracellular organelles or tightly bound to intracellular proteins, and the concentration of free calcium in resting nonstimulated cells is low, approximately 10^{-7} to 10^{-8} M. This low concentration of intracellular ionized calcium and the presence of large extracellular and intracellular reservoirs, together with the presence of high affinity calcium-binding proteins (calcium receptors), confers upon calcium the role of an intracellular messenger coupling membrane events to cellular responses.

Control of calcium at the cell membrane

Cellular calcium control is derived from a variety of processes operating at both plasma membrane and intracellular levels (Fig. 31–2). Plasmalemmal calcium channels are controlled by two principal types of signal—chemical and electrical—and are referred to frequently as receptor-operated and potential-dependent channels, respectively. These major categories of plasmalemmal channels are in turn subdivided according to electrophysiologic characteristics and coupling processes between receptor and channel (Fig. 31–3). An electrogenic Na^+:Ca^{2+} exchanger (3 Na^+:1 Ca^{2+}) operates in the plasma membrane and according to membrane potential and relative ionic gradients can move calcium into or out of the cell. During depolarizing conditions the process probably operates primarily as a source of calcium and during polarizing conditions maintains intracellular calcium at a low level. This latter function is shared by the calmodulin-dependent Ca^{2+}-adenosinetriphosphatase (ATPase). At the intracellular level the major storage and mobilization sources of calcium are the endo-

Calcium channels of two major types

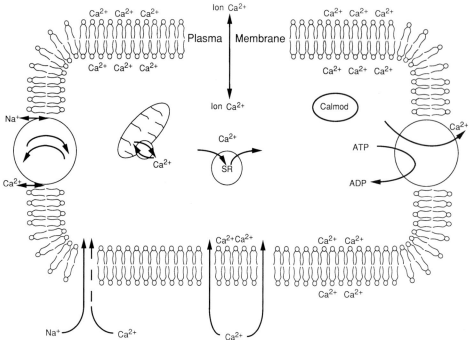

Figure 31–2

The control of calcium regulation at the cellular level. Depicted are the several calcium mobilization and storage processes operating in many cell types. Not all of the processes indicated may operate in any one cell, and the extent to which any process operates is cell-dependent, stimulus-dependent, and time-dependent.

Sarcoplasmic reticulum is a major intracellular store of Ca^{2+}.

plasmic and sarcoplasmic reticulum and the mitochondria. The sarcoplasmic reticulum clearly serves as the dominant source of calcium for excitation-contraction coupling in skeletal muscle, but also contributes in cardiac and smooth muscle despite the importance of extracellular calcium mobilization through plasmalemmal calcium channels in these tissues. The endoplasmic reticulum of nonmotile cells represents the major source of physiologically stored and released calcium and, together with extracellular calcium mobilized through one or more types of plasmalemmal calcium channel, is involved in stimulus-secretion coupling processes of secretory cells.

The mechanisms underlying calcium uptake and release by the endoplasmic and sarcoplasmic reticulum are still being defined, but the Ca^{2+}-ATPase is likely identical or similar in both types of organelle. The release processes probably differ and include direct electrical coupling in skeletal muscle, Ca^{2+}-induced calcium release in heart and inositol-1,4,5-triphosphate (IP3)–induced release in smooth muscle and nonmotile cells.

Figure 31–3

Pathways of cellular calcium mobilization activated by membrane receptor–initiated signals. Depicted are two primary categories of calcium channels, receptor-operated channels (ROC) and potential-dependent channels (PDC), which are associated with specific receptors, A and B. Receptors may be associated with a specific phospholipase C (PLC), itself coupled to a guanine nucleotide (G)–binding protein that generates the intracellular signal inositol-1,4,5-triphosphate ($InsP_3$) from phosphatidylinositol lipids. $InsP_3$, or a derivative, liberates calcium from the endoplasmic/sarcoplasmic reticulum and may serve also to activate calcium entry through the plasmalemmal receptor-operated calcium channels. (See also Chapter 15.)

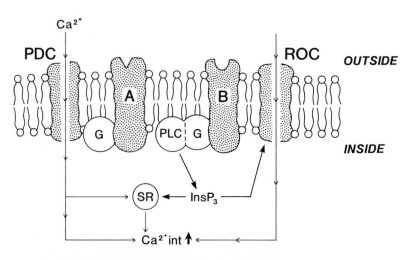

Mitochondria have long been recognized as major sinks for calcium and it has been assumed that they play important roles in the acute regulation of calcium supply and demand. This is no longer thought to be true, and under physiological conditions the role of the mitochondrial transport systems is now believed to be the regulation of matrix calcium concentrations and thus of the matrix-associated calcium-dependent dehydrogenase enzymes. Nonetheless, the low affinity mitochondrial calcium uptake system has an extremely high capacity for calcium that it can precipitate as hydroxyapatite. Thus, the mitochondria function as calcium depots under conditions where the cell is challenged with or overloaded with large amounts of calcium. This is an important safety device, because excessive amounts of calcium are toxic to the cell and, unless sequestered or removed, lead to calcium-induced cell death. With continued cellular calcium loading the mitochondria are eventually damaged irreversibly and cell death occurs.

Ca^{2+} deposition and overloading in mitochondria

The overloading of mitochondria by Ca^{2+} is a major factor in Ca^{2+}-dependent cell death.

Calcium Requirements and Relationship to Other Ions

The recommended daily requirements of calcium range between 360 and 1200 mg/day. The adult requirement is between 800 and 1200 mg/day with supplements of 400 mg/day for pregnant and nursing women. However, calcium intake varies considerably between 200 and 2500 mg/day, and there is concern that dietary calcium deficiencies exist in segments of the population. Until recently this concern was directed largely at aging individuals, particularly postmenopausal females, because of the increased incidence of osteoporosis associated with this population. The loss of both bone mineral and matrix in osteoporosis predisposes to fracture often during minimum trauma. There is little evidence that increased calcium alone past the daily requirements reverses osteoporosis once the process is initiated, but it is suggested that adequate calcium intake and exercise, particularly during the premenopausal phase in females, can substantially ameliorate age-induced osteoporosis. However, other factors are clearly important, including the role of estrogens in preventing bone resorption (see Chapter 42).

The adult daily requirement for Ca^{2+} is approximately 1200 mg/day.

Additional emphasis has been placed on dietary calcium with the reports that calcium-deficient diets are associated with reduced serum concentrations of calcium that are linked to hypertension, and that in some individuals calcium supplementation can serve to reduce elevated blood pressure. There is little doubt, however, that factors other than dietary calcium are involved, including age, parathyroid hormone, calcitonin and renin levels, and the relationship of calcium concentrations to those of other ions.

Calcium deficiency may be associated with hypertension.

Phosphate is an ion of particular importance to calcium metabolism, because hydroxyapatite is a form of calcium phosphate and because calcium and phosphate are coregulated species. Thus, parathyroid hormone actions on the kidney increase tubular reabsorption of calcium and inhibit reabsorption of phosphate, and the active metabolites of vitamin D enhance both calcium and phosphate absorption from the GI tract and enhance renal reabsorption of these ions.

Magnesium, well known for its roles in maintaining the activities of cellular enzymes, notably the ATP-utilizing systems, is being increasingly examined for its direct pharmacological effects, particularly as they relate to calcium. Frequently, the roles of calcium and magnesium are antagonistic, and elevated magnesium can depress calcium-dependent secretory events. A number of dietary and drug procedures, including loop diuretics, aminoglycoside antibiotics and cyclosporine A, can induce renal magnesium loss and hypomagnesemia. In turn, hypomagnesemia may potentiate the effects of calcium-mobilizing or calcium-dependent processes. However, renal magnesium and calcium transport are affected similarly by parathyroid hormone, and dietary magnesium deficiency is associated with a hypocalcemia resistant to calcium supplementation. Dietary studies of magnesium intake in the United States suggest that a significant fraction, perhaps greater than one third, of the population receives inadequate amounts.

A Na⁺: Ca²⁺ exchange process contributes to cellular Ca²⁺ homeostasis.

A relationship between sodium and calcium has long been recognized. The plasmalemmal $Na^+:Ca^{2+}$ exchange is an important contributor to cellular calcium homeostasis, and elevated intracellular sodium increases intracellular calcium concentrations by both depolarizing the cell and activating voltage-dependent calcium channels and by stimulating the $Na^+:Ca^{2+}$ exchange process. These pathways assume particular importance in view of a suspected principal role of dietary sodium in the etiology of essential hypertension.

What is becoming clear is that calcium cannot be treated as an ion in isolation. The requirements for calcium and the regulation of calcium must be viewed in the context of the regulation of the other ions, notably Na^+, K^+, Mg^{2+}, and PO_4^{3-}. These are not independent ions.

Bone Formation and Resorption

The major mineral of bone is hydroxyapatite, $Ca_{10}(PO_4)_6(OH)_2$, which is similar to the mineral fluoroapatite, $Ca_{10}(PO_4)_6F_2$. However, bone material does contain other organic species in addition to the cells whose function is to synthesize and resorb the bone structure in response to physiological and pathological demands. Thus, bone should be regarded as an impure hydroxyapatite.

Osteoblasts, osteoclasts, and osteocytes represent the three major cell types in bone.

The three major cell types in bone are represented by the osteoblasts, osteocytes, and osteoclasts. Osteoblasts are responsible for synthesizing the components of the extracellular bone matrix and for priming this material for mineralization. The osteocytes, which are derived from osteoblasts, are found embedded with the mineralized matrix where they communicate with each other and with the surface osteoblasts through a lattice. This communicating network is important to the processes of mineral exchange between bone and plasma. Osteoclasts, lying at the bone surface, are of a different cell lineage than osteoblasts and the derived osteocytes. Osteoclasts are involved, together with the osteocytes, in the resorption of bone primarily from the labile rather than the mature stable fraction. Collectively, the presence of active bone remodeling and resorption create a dynamic skeleton in which there is considerable and rapid turnover of calcium. The bone mass thus serves as a large and important calcium buffer. Bone remodeling occurs throughout life and serves to minimize the damage caused by routine wear and stress. However, its occurrence past the time of cessation of growth undoubtedly contributes to the progressive loss of skeletal mass with age. Bone is frequently, but incorrectly, viewed as a static entity. In fact, there is a constant metabolic turnover and renewal operating through the activities of the bone cells. Although the principal calcium-mobilizing hormones, parathyroid hormone, calcitonin and vitamin D, are well recognized to have primary effects on these cells, it is increasingly clear that a large number of other agents also exert direct and indirect effects on bone resorption and formation (Table 31–3).

Bone is not a static entity.

Much remains to be learned about the processes of mineralization. The plasma concentrations of calcium and phosphate in the blood exceed the solubility factor of hydroxyapatite, but the factors inducing precipitation remain to be defined fully. It is likely that the organic matrix of bone facilitates precipitation by acting as a nucleating surface; important players

---

Table 31-3 AGENTS THAT REGULATE BONE FORMATION AND RESORPTION

Hormone and Growth Factors	Drugs and Toxic Agents
Activators of bone formation	
Vitamin D metabolites	Phosphate
Insulin	Fluoride
Insulin-like growth factors	
Estrogen	
Anabolic steroids	
Thyroxine	
Inhibitors of bone formation	
Glucocorticoids	Diphosphonates
Activators of bone resorption	
Parathyroid hormone	Endotoxin
Prostaglandins	Retinoids
Transforming growth factor (TGF)	Heparin
Epidermal growth factor (EGF)	Phorbol esters
Inhibitors of bone resorption	
Calcitonin	Mithramycin
Estrogen	Colchicine

---

in this role are collagen and bone-specific proteins including osteocalcin. Matrix vesicles, derived from plasma membranes and found in a variety of mineralizing tissues, are associated with a number of enzymatic activities, including alkaline phosphatase, which have been suggested to be involved in the initial formation of hydroxyapatite.

Additionally, a number of agents affect mineralization. Thus, fluoride enhances bone formation in part by changing the composition of the mineral and in part by changing the activities of osteoblastic processes. The presence of fluoride at a concentration of 1.0 ppm has been established to be of considerable practical significance in the reduction of dental caries with optimum benefits being achieved before and during tooth eruption. However, large doses of fluoride impair mineralization, produce mottling of tooth enamel, and become progressively toxic to the individual. Additional biological actions of fluoride may derive from its ability, as the complex fluoraluminate anion, AlF_4^-, to activate guanine nucleotide (G) proteins that couple many receptors to their effector units. Mineralization is affected also by bisphosphonates including editronate (ethane-1-hydroxy-1, 1-diphosphonic acid, EDHP) that retard bone formation, dissolution, and remodeling by aluminum salts that complex phosphate and by strontium that impairs active vitamin D metabolite formation. Additionally, tetracyclines have a high affinity for calcium and bone mineral deposits in bones and teeth, giving the latter a cosmetically discoloring appearance.

Fluoride ion enhances bone formation.

Defects in Calcium Regulation

Defects in calcium regulation have in principal a variety of origins. Until more recently emphasis has been placed on serum levels of calcium as providing the definition of hypocalcemic and hypercalcemic states. Quite generally calcium is regarded as a controller of cellular excitability, and deficiencies and excesses are associated with increases and decreases, respectively, in cellular excitability. However, the recent ability to measure intracellular levels of ionized calcium has expanded this definition. Decreased levels of serum calcium and increased levels of cystolic calcium have been suggested to accompany the hypertensive state (see Chapter 35).

Hypocalcemia may arise as a consequence of chronic calcium or vitamin D deficiency stemming either from inadequate diet or from inadequate

Hypocalcemia may be associated with Ca^{2+} deficiency, vitamin D deficiency, hypoparathyroidism.

source in the diet. Hypocalcemia may be precipitated by sodium fluoride ingestion or by transfusions with citrated blood. Hypoparathyroidism and pseudohypoparathyroidism and the associated deficiencies of inadequate amounts or inadequate actions of parathyroid hormone result also in hypocalcemic states. Hypocalcemia is associated frequently with advanced renal failure associated with hyperphosphatemia. Acute signs of hypocalcemia include paresthesias, tetany and increased neuromuscular excitability, laryngospasm and enhanced excitability of other smooth muscles, and convulsions.

Hypercalcemia may be associated with vitamin D excess, hyperparathyroidism, immobilization.

Hypercalcemia has as its major causes hyperparathyroidism, cancer, vitamin D excess, and body immobilization. Hyperparathyroidism, in mild or severe forms, is the most common form of hypercalcemia. Milder or less common origins of hypercalcemia include adrenocortical deficiency, hyperthyroidism, and the use of benzothiadiazide diuretics. Hypercalcemia itself may have particularly serious consequences including kidney calcification and loss of function and, in the case of hyperparathyroidism, skeletal loss and fragility. Additionally, there may be general deposition of calcium in other soft tissues including those of the cardiovascular systems. The latter processes of calcification may have serious hemodynamic consequences.

Hypercalcemia may be associated with some forms of cancer.

It has been known for some time that cancer patients, particularly those with solid tumors of the lung and breast, myelomas or head and neck tumors, frequently have significant hypercalcemia. Recent work has suggested that this is attributable to a peptide isolable from the malignant cells with significant homology to parathyroid hormone at the amino terminal region, but of about twice the size. Such homology suggests that this protein may act at parathyroid hormone receptors.

Hormones Regulating Calcium

VITAMIN D

Vitamin D is a steroid hormone.

Vitamin D presents many unusual aspects and more subtle modes of action than have been generally realized. Vitamin D is not actually a vitamin and in normal conditions its inclusion in the diet is probably unnecessary for full health. Rather, vitamin D is a hormone, a steroid derivative, that is synthesized by photochemical reactions in the skin, undergoes a series of activating biochemical reactions, and acts on specific intracellular receptor sites in a wide variety of tissues to provoke as a major response an increased plasma Ca^{2+} concentration. This response is achieved cooperatively with parathyroid hormone and stands in negative feedback relationship to serum calcium concentrations.

7-dehydrocholesterol is the precursor to Vitamin D.

The immediate chemical precursor of vitamin D is 7-dehydrocholesterol, which is present in the skin and undergoes a photochemical transformation in which the bond between C9 and C10 in ring B is broken to yield cholecalciferol or vitamin D_3 (Fig. 31–4). Cholecalciferol is not itself an active Ca^{2+} mobilizing or antirachitic species but requires metabolic activation by two key steps. First, cholecalciferol is hydroxylated at position 25 to yield 25-hydroxy vitamin D_3 or calcifediol. The process of 25-hydroxylation takes place predominantly in the liver by the microsomal hydroxylating system. The second and critical step is conversion to 1,25-dihydroxy vitamin D_3 or calcitriol, the active form of vitamin D. A summary of the several forms of vitamin D is shown in Table 31–4. The 1-hydroxylation step occurs in the kidney, in the distal part of the proximal convoluted tubule, after calcifediol has arrived through the vitamin D-binding globulin. The kidney hydroxylase is a mixed function nicotinamide-adenine dinucleotide (NADPH)-dependent mitochondrial oxidase that represents

Vitamin D_3 is also known as calcitriol.

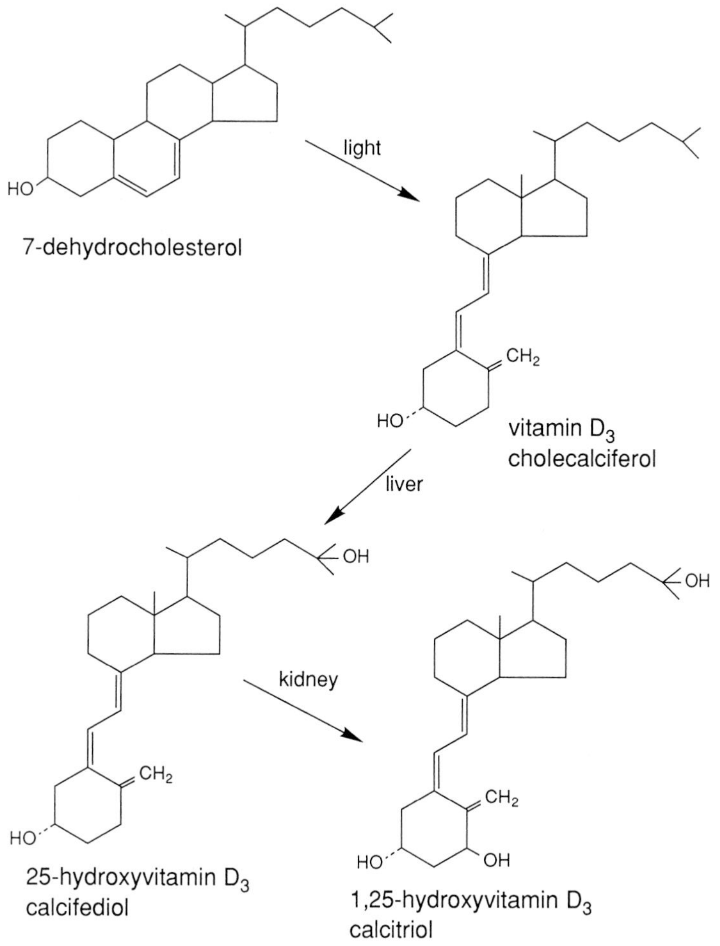

7-dehydrocholesterol

light

vitamin D₃
cholecalciferol

liver

kidney

25-hydroxyvitamin D₃
calcifediol

1,25-hydroxyvitamin D₃
calcitriol

the key regulated stage of the vitamin D biosynthetic system. Activity of the 1-hydroxylase is regulated by several dietary and hormonal factors that are critically linked to the process of Ca^{2+} homeostasis. Dietary or circulating deficiencies of vitamin D, calcium, or phosphate stimulate the activity of the enzyme as do parathyroid hormone, estrogens, growth hormone, and prolactin.

It is likely that growth hormone and prolactin are major physiological regulators of calcitriol production and are particularly important during conditions of growth, pregnancy, and lactation. The role of estrogens likely assumes particular importance in postmenopausal states when their deficiency is important to the development of osteoporosis. High intake of vitamin D or high circulating levels of calcitriol suppresses the activity of the 1-hydroxylase. As noted earlier, calcifediol circulates bound to a specific α-globulin; in this form it is the major circulating form of vitamin D

Growth hormones and prolactin regulate vitamin D_3 production.

Table 31-4 THE SEVERAL FORMS OF VITAMIN D

Chemical Name	Abbreviation	Generic Name
Vitamin D₃	D₃	Cholecalciferol
Vitamin D₂	D₂	Ergocalciferol
25-hydroxyvitamin D	25(HO)D₃	Calcifediol
1,25-hydroxyvitamin D₃	1,25(HO)2D₃	Calcitriol

Vitamin D₃ actions are mediated through a nuclear receptor.

with a half-life of approximately 19 days, considerably longer than the 3- to 5-day half-life of calcitriol.

The actions of calcitriol are mediated analogously to other steroid hormones through interaction with a specific cytosolic receptor. These high-affinity receptors interact subsequently at the calcitriol complex with specific sites in nuclear chromatin where transcription is initiated of genes coding for proteins that regulate calcium and phosphate transport. The receptor protein is found in intestine, kidney, and bone; has a high affinity for calcitriol, K_D 5×10^{-11} M; and has a high specificity. More recently receptor sites for calcitriol have been found in many other tissues, including glandular cells, smooth muscle, neurons, epithelial cells, epidermal cells, secretory cells, and cells of the immune system. It is not clear whether all of the effects of calcitriol in this variety of cell types stem from a primary action on calcium transporting processes. However, this distribution of receptor sites suggests a correspondingly widespread role for vitamin D. Indeed, it may be that calcitriol should be viewed as exerting two primary sets of effects. Actions in the calcium transporting and mobilizing organs, notably the gut, are primarily to increase calcium transport, whereas effects in other organ and cell systems are permissive in nature and may be concerned with a multiplicity of effects.

The physiological role of vitamin D is that of a positive regulator of calcium homeostasis, serving to maintain normal plasma concentrations of calcium and phosphate by promoting their intestinal absorption, increasing their mobilization from bone, and decreasing their excretion by the kidney. The major mechanism of action is enhanced absorption of calcium and phosphate through the gut.

Vitamin D₃ nuclear receptors enjoy widespread distribution.

The actions of vitamin D are mediated through a hormone-receptor complex that regulates gene expression in a manner entirely analogous to that used by the classic steroid hormones. Additionally, the cloning of the vitamin D receptor has revealed its similarity to that of other nuclear receptors, including those for estrogens and thyroid hormone. This receptor enjoys a ubiquitous distribution, suggesting roles of vitamin D additional to mineral mobilization. Indeed, it is now apparent that vitamin D may be considered to regulate the activity of several groups of functions, including classical mineral homeostasis, differentiation events in the immune system and skin, as well as control of DNA replication and cellular proliferation. It has been proposed that vitamin D serves as a master steroid hormone functioning to regulate a genetic differentiation/replication switch.

Vitamin D deficiency leads to nutritional rickets.

Vitamin D is available in a variety of forms, including ergocalciferol (vitamin D₂), calcifediol, and calcitriol, all of which are orally active. Dihydrotachysterol is an analog of vitamin D, which becomes 25-hydroxylated to the active form. The major uses of these agents are in the treatment and cure of nutritional and metabolic rickets, osteomalacia, and in the treatment of hypoparathyroidism. Nutritional rickets, a deficiency of vitamin D, differs from metabolic rickets, which reflects an inability to respond to physiological levels of the vitamin. Metabolic rickets has a variety of origins, including an inborn error of metabolism leading to failure to produce calcitriol from 25-hydroxycholecalciferol, and renal rickets that is associated with renal failure and loss of 1-hydroxylase activity.

PARATHYROID HORMONE

Parathyroid hormone is a polypeptide.

The role of parathyroid hormone and its relationship to serum calcium was first established by MacCallum and Voegtlin in 1909. Parathyroid hormone is a single polypeptide hormone of 84 amino acid residues (Fig.

A

H$_2$N-Ser-Val-Ser-Glu-Ile-Gln-Leu-Met-His-Asn-Leu-Gly-Lys-His-Leu
|
Asn-His-Val-Asp-Gln-Leu-Lys-Arg-Leu-Trp-Glu-Val-Arg-Glu-Met-Ser-Asn
|
Phe-Val-Ala-Leu-Gly-Ala-Pro-Leu-Ala-Pro-Arg-Asp-Ala-Gly-Ser-Gln
|
Lys-Glu-His-Ser-Glu-Val-Leu-Val-Asn-Asp-Glu-Lys-Lys-Arg-Pro-Arg
|
Ser-Leu-Gly-Glu-Ala-Asp-Lys-Ala-Asp-Val-Asp-Val-Leu-Thr-Lys-Ala
|
HO$_2$C-Gln-Ser-Lys
84

B

H$_2$N-Cys-Gly-Asn-Leu-Ser-Thr-Cys-Met-Leu-Gly-Thr-Tyr-Thr
|
Ile-Ala-Thr-Gln-Pro-Phe-Thr-His-Phe-Lys-Asn-Phe-Asp-Gln
|
Gly-Val-Gly-Ala-Pro-CONH$_2$
32

Figure 31–5

Amino acid sequences of (*A*) parathyroid hormone and (*B*) calcitonin.

31–5*A*) that is synthesized as the preprohormone of 115 residues. This peptide is processed by removal of the terminal methionine residues and the 23 amino acid signal sequence that is responsible for translocation through the endoplasmic reticulum. Following further processing the 84 residue hormone is then stored in secretory granules of the parathyroid cells.

The activity of the hormone is associated with the N-terminal sequence of residues 1–34, and the hormone is cleaved between positions 34 and 37 to give the briefly circulating N-terminal and the more persistent, but inactive, C-terminal fragment. Circulating parathyroid hormone is thus a heterogeneous mixture and most assays measure both active and inactive fragments.

Secretion of parathyroid hormone is under the control of plasma calcium that represents the primary control process. A reduction in plasma calcium increases the secretion of the hormone, and if the reduction is persistent there is accompanying hypertrophy of the parathyroid glands. Conversely, hypercalcemia results in a decreased secretion and glandular hypoplasia. It is likely that levels of parathyroid cellular Ca^{2+}, reflecting the plasma levels, regulate growth of the parathyroid cells and their synthesis and secretion of the hormone. This may be achieved through a novel plasmalemmal calcium receptor that mediates calcium permeability to permit cytoplasmic calcium levels to mirror changes in extracellular calcium. Other agents, including catecholamines and vitamin D, also serve to regulate parathyroid hormone release. The inhibitory effects of vitamin D on parathyroid hormone release are likely to be of physiological significance and achieved both indirectly through the effects of calcitriol on plasma calcium and directly through calcitriol interactions with specific receptors on parathyroid cells.

The primary function of parathyroid hormone is to regulate the concentration of plasma calcium; this is achieved by conservation of calcium and elimination of phosphorus. It has been suggested that this reflects a mechanism of adaptation of our basically marine metabolism, where calcium is more abundant than phosphorus, to the opposing mineral distribution found in the terrestrial environment. The primary effects of parathyroid hormone are exerted on the kidney, the bone, and the GI tract (see Table 31–2). In the kidney, parathyroid hormone increases the tubular

Parathyroid hormone release is triggered by a fall in plasma Ca^{2+} levels.

PTH increases kidney tubular reabsorption of Ca^{2+}.

The actions of PTH are mediated through cAMP.

reabsorption of calcium and inhibits the reabsorption of phosphate. Consequently, plasma calcium and phosphate levels rise and fall respectively. Parathyroid hormone affects the secretion of other ions also, notably magnesium, whose excretion rate is reduced with a consequent rise in plasma levels. These effects of parathyroid hormone on ion excretion rates are mediated through a hormone-sensitive adenylate cyclase system. A second effect of parathyroid hormone mediated through the kidney is the enhanced conversion of 25-hydroxycholecalciferol to the active calcitriol. The enhanced production of active vitamin D underlies increased absorption of calcium and phosphate in the GI tract following increases in parathyroid hormone level. The third major locus of activity of parathyroid hormone is at bone where it increases the rate of resorption primarily from the older and more stable fractions. This activity of parathyroid hormone is achieved through stimulation of both osteoclasts and osteoblasts. Thus, the combined effects of this stimulation is the enhancement of both bone turnover and remodeling.

CALCITONIN

Calcitonin is a polypeptide hormone.

The hypocalcemic hormone calcitonin was discovered in 1962 by Copp. Calcitonin is secreted from the parafollicular C cells of the thyroid gland and is a 32-residue peptide with a cysteine disulfide bridge between positions 1 and 7; this bridge is essential for activity (Fig. 31–5B).

Calcitonin secretion is increased by increased plasma Ca^{2+}.

The secretion of calcitonin, like that of parathyroid hormone, is under the control of calcium and is increased or decreased in hypercalcemic or hypocalcemic states, respectively. It is likely that other agents exert physiological control over calcitonin release also. The presence of calcitriol receptors on the C cells suggests that these may represent the direct basis for the enhancing effect of calcitriol on calcitonin release. Additionally, gastrin and cholecystokinin also produce acute increases in calcitonin levels, and this may be related to postfeeding events. The half-life of calcitonin is brief, approximately 10 minutes; the plasma concentration is significantly higher in men than in women and declines further in women following ovarian failure or menopause.

Calcitonin inhibits osteoclast-mediated bone resorption.

The primary hypocalcemic and hypophosphatemic effects of calcitonin are achieved at the level of the bone by a direct inhibitory action on the osteoclast to inhibit the bone resorbing functions of these cells (see also Fig. 31–1 and Table 31–3). These effects oppose those produced by parathyroid hormone but appear to be produced through activation of a hormone-sensitive adenylate cyclase. However, calcitonin should not be regarded in mechanistic terms as an antiparathyroid hormone. An additional action of calcitonin seen on chronic administration is that of a reduction in the number of bone osteoclasts over a period of weeks and months. Calcitonin also acts on the kidney, where it enhances the production of calcitriol. An additional effect of calcitonin, though of unknown significance in terms of calcium homeostasis, is that of central analgesia.

Calcitonin gene-related peptide is located neuronally.

Alternative processing of the calcitonin gene leads to the production of a second mRNA, coding for the 37-residue calcitonin gene-related peptide (CGRP). The calcitonin/CGRP gene complex is composed of at least two genes, referred to as the α and β genes. In humans these genes are located on chromosome 11, between the catalase and the parathyroid hormone genes. CGRP and calcitonin show little homology, are immunologically distinct, and enjoy different distribution; CGRP is distributed primarily in the nervous system. The abundance of CGRP in the central nervous system (CNS) clearly indicates a neurotransmitter or neuromodulator role. The receptors for each peptide are distinct, but there is cross-interaction. There are a number of important differences in the biological activities of the two peptides. Thus, CGRP is a potent vasodilator, but in a number of other respects, including the lowering of serum calcium and the inhibitory effects on feeding and secretion, the effects of both hormones are similar. The factors that regulate the alternative splicing of the calcitonin/CGRP gene are not known, but their elucidation is clearly of considerable importance to an understanding of hormonal regulatory processes.

Defects in Hormonal Calcium Regulation

Abnormalities in hormonal calcium regulation inducing either hypo- or hypercalcemic states, often with accompanying and corresponding changes in phosphate availability, have significant effects on both soft and hard tissue function.

A dramatic and historically well-recognized example of calcium deficiency is that of rickets in children and osteomalacia of adults attributable to vitamin D deficiency. The resultant reduction in intestinal Ca^{2+} and phosphate absorption causes the bone-mobilizing actions of parathyroid hormone to become dominant to maintain plasma levels. This results in a failure in children to mineralize newly formed tissues with consequent bone deformation and in adults a generalized decrease in bone density. The observations in the late nineteenth and early twentieth centuries that a significant fraction of city-dwelling children in the industrialized temperate zones suffered from rickets led, through the work of Mellanby (1919) and Huldschinsky (1919), to the realization that both sunshine and dietary factors were deficient. As a consequence of these early studies, programs of oral supplementation by cod liver oil were initiated followed by the dietary supplementation of foods with added vitamin D. In the United States juvenile rickets is a clinical rarity, but there is evidence for Ca^{2+} deficiencies in some segments of the adult population.

Rickets is a calcium deficiency.

Hypercalcemia may be precipitated by excessive amounts of vitamin D, usually ingested through dietary supplements or through the use of vitamin D in the treatment of hypoparathyroidism. Prolonged hypercalcemia results in initially reversible and subsequently irreversible renal damage, calcification of other soft tissues, including those of the cardiovascular system, and loss of bone mass. In children, hypervitaminosis may be accompanied by complete or significant retardation of growth, and vitamin D toxicity may cause fetal defects, including vitamin hypersensitivity, reduction in parathyroid function, and aortic stenosis.

Vitamin D excess is associated with hypercalcemia.

Deficiencies of parathyroid gland function are associated with increases and decreases in serum calcium levels in hypo- and hyperparathyroidism respectively. Hyperparathyroidism may arise from hypersecretion of the parathyroid glands due to hyperplasia or malignancy and may be secondary to other deficits in calcium homeostasis, including defective intestinal absorption or renal disease. A reduced sensitivity to calcium of parathyroid cells in hyperparathyroidism likely underlies the abnormal parathyroid hormone release in this condition. Hypoparathyroidism arising from surgical procedures or a defect in the parathyroid glands themselves, idiopathic hypoparathyroidism, differs from pseudohypoparathyroidism; in the former the secretion of hormone is absent or reduced, whereas in the latter there is end-organ resistance in the presence of normal or elevated levels of hormone. Accompanying hypoparathyroidism is a reduction in calcitriol levels caused by a reduction in parathyroid hormone–induced calcitriol formation.

Pseudohypoparathyroidism is a receptor-coupling defect.

Pseudohypoparathyroidism reflects a defect in the coupling of para-thyroid hormone receptors to the adenylate cyclase effector systems. Gs-deficient pseudohypoparathyroidism is accompanied by a deficiency in the guanine nucleotide-binding protein Gs. In Type 1a individuals, unusual physical features termed Albright's hereditary osteodystrophy are displayed with a generalized Gs deficiency leading to hyporesponsiveness to many hormones, including thyroid-stimulating hormone (TSH), glucagon, and gonadotropin acting in diverse tissues. This deficiency extends to olfactory dysfunction, because olfaction is also a Gs-dependent process mediated through adenylate cyclase activation. In Type 1b individuals, this deficiency is confined to the kidney, and such individuals are not resistant to the actions of other adenylate cyclase–dependent hormones.

THERAPEUTIC USES OF PARATHYROID HORMONE, VITAMIN D, AND CALCITONIN

Calcitonin reduces hypercalcemia.

Calcitonin is effective in diminishing calcium and phosphate levels in hypercalcemic individuals with hyperparathyroidism, vitamin D excess, excessive Ca^{2+} absorption or ingestion, and malignancies. However, other measures are used also, including prednisone and other glucocorticoids, phosphates including sodium editronate, and mithramycin. Additionally, calcitonin is effective in bone disorders, such as Paget's disease, which are accompanied by extensive skeletal remodeling. Sodium editronate may well be as efficacious in the control of Paget's disease and has the advantage of substantially lower cost. Salmon calcitonin, rather than human or porcine material, is used principally because it has a longer half-life and increased potency. However, resistance following chronic use may develop due to the formation of antibodies.

The major therapeutic uses of vitamin D may be considered in three main areas: nutritional rickets, metabolic rickets, and osteomalacia and hypoparathyroidism. Nutritional rickets is rare in the United States largely because of the general availability of vitamin D-enriched foods. Rickets can be successfully prevented or cured with any of the available vitamin D preparations. Metabolic rickets, including vitamin D-dependent rickets, deficiency of calcitriol formation and chronic renal failure, are treated with calcitriol or dihydrotachysterol or its 25-hydroxy derivative because these agents do not require renal 1-hydroxylation to become activated. Dihydrotachysterol has long been used in the treatment of hypoparathyroidism because it has a more rapid onset of acting than other vitamin D derivatives, but the other agents including calcitriol are effective.

A variety of calcium preparations are also available for the treatment of hypocalcemia, particularly in the control of associated tetany. Calcium chloride, gluconate, and calcium gluceptate can be given intravenously for the most rapid actions, and calcium gluconate, lactate, carbonate, and phosphate are used for oral administration.

Cellular Regulation of Calcium

Various types of Ca^{2+} channels

Calcium entry across the plasma membrane in response to chemical and electrical stimuli represents a major pathway of cellular control of calcium (see Fig. 31–3). The potential-dependent calcium channels, activated and inactivated by depolarizing stimuli generated electrically or chemically, represent the best characterized of the plasmalemmal calcium entry processes, primarily because of the existence of a group of powerfully active therapeutic agents, the calcium channel antagonists effective at this class of ion channel.

CELLULAR CALCIUM ANTAGONISM

Fleckenstein introduced the concept of calcium antagonism based on observations that verapamil mimicked in reversible fashion the effects of calcium withdrawal on cardiac function and that these effects could be overcome by elevation of extracellular calcium. The ability of verapamil, and other agents of the phenylalkylamine class, to produce vasodilatation, coronary and peripheral, and to produce negative inotropic and chronotropic actions could thus be attributed to interference with calcium mobilization for excitation-contraction coupling. Similar properties were observed subsequently for other agents of diverse structural classes, including the 1,4-dihydropyridine nifedipine and the benzothiazepine diltiazem.

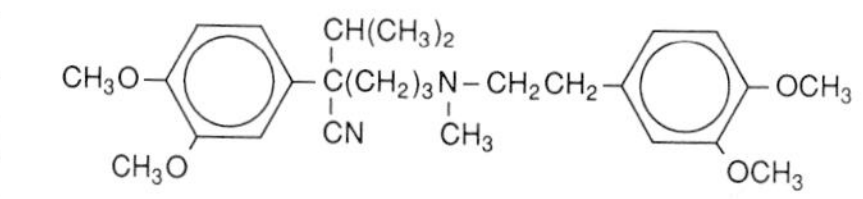

Although many other structures possess to some extent similar properties, major therapeutic attention has focused on the three structural classes referred to variously as calcium antagonists, calcium channel antagonists, calcium entry blockers, or slow channel blockers; they possess the common ability to inhibit calcium current through a major category of voltage-dependent calcium channel. This current underlies the plateau phase of the cardiac action potential in conducting tissue or the slowly rising phase in cardiac pacemaker cells and, although electrophysiologic data is scarce, likely underlies excitation-contraction coupling in much vascular smooth muscle. Therefore, the calcium channel antagonists may be regarded as a subclass of the several groups of agents that should modify calcium metabolism at the sites depicted in Figure 31–1. This consideration is a key component to the determination of the selectivity of action of these agents; they are effective only against those stimuli that provoke calcium mobilization through voltage-dependent calcium channels. Calcium mobilization from intracellular stores or through receptor-operated channels is insensitive or weakly sensitive to these agents.

The major current therapeutic uses of these agents are in the cardiovascular area, in the control of angina in its several forms, the relief of certain arrhythmias (notably supraventricular tachycardia), and in the control of hypertension and some peripheral vascular disorders. Consistent with the chemical heterogeneity of these agents, they are not uniformly effective in the above disorders (Table 31–5). There is currently major

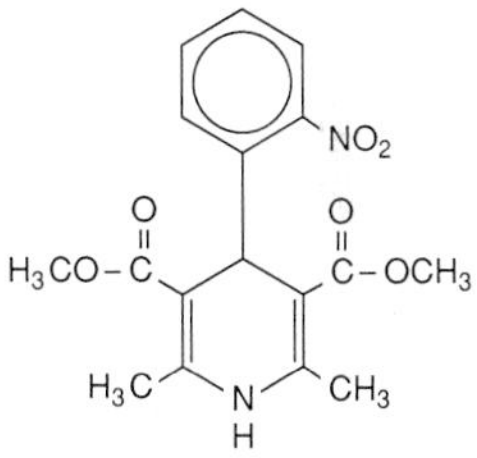

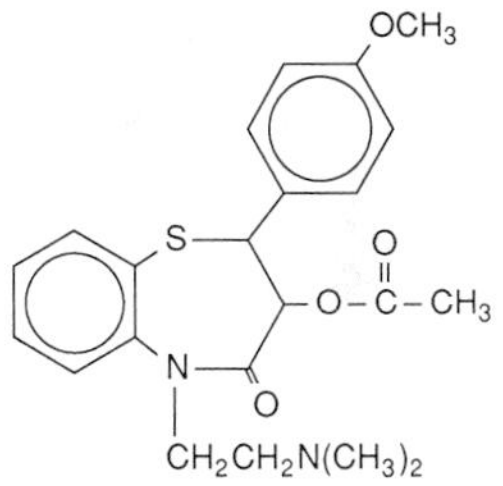

Calcium antagonists

Verapamil

Calcium antagonists block voltage-dependent calcium channels.

Nifedipine

Diltiazem

Table 31–5 CLINICAL USES OF Ca²⁺ CHANNEL ANTAGONISTS

Current Use	Drug*	Potential Use†	Drug*
Myocardial ischemia		Cardiovascular	
Exertional angina	D,N,V	Migraine	V,N
Prinzmetal's angina	D,N,V	Raynaud's disease	N
Unstable angina	D,N,V	Cardioprotection	V,D
Hypertension	D,N,V	Subarachnoid hemorrhage	nimod
Hypertensive emergencies	N	Cerebral insufficiency	nimod
		Pulmonary hypertension	N?
Cardiac arrhythmias		Congestive heart failure	N?
Supraventricular tachycardia	V		
Atrial fibrillation and flutter	V,D	Noncardiovascular	
Hypertropic cardiomyopathy	V	Asthma (exercise-induced)	V,N
		Esophageal motor disorders	N
		Premature labor	N
		Urinary incontinence	N
		Dementia	nimod

* D, diltiazem; N, nifedipine; V, verapamil; nimod, a 1,4-dihydropyridine analog of nifedipine.
† Only a partial listing of potential uses is provided here. The Ca²⁺ channel antagonists have been suggested to be of potential use in virtually all cases in which hyper- or excessive activity of smooth muscle systems is involved.

Table 31–6 ADDITIONAL AND POTENTIAL USES OF CALCIUM CHANNEL ANTAGONISTS

Cardiovascular	Nonvascular Smooth Muscle	Other
Atherosclerosis	Achalasia	Aldosteronism
Congestive heart failure	Asthma	Epilepsy
Erectile impotence	Chronic obstructive lung disease	Motion sickness
Headache	Urinary incontinence	Tinnitus
Headache, cluster, migraine		Vertigo
Intermittent claudication		
Stroke		

Calcium antagonists and cardiovascular disease

$(C_6H_5)_2CH-N$ ... $NCH_2CH=CH-$

Cinnarizine

Calcium antagonists are of different structural types.

$(C_6H_5)_2CHCH_2CH_2NHCHCH_2-$ ... CH_3

Prenylamine

$CH_2CH_2N(C_2H_5)_2$ ... O ... CH_2- ... OCH_3

Caroverine

interest in the potential application of these and future agents to a variety of other disorders of the cardiovascular system, of nonvascular smooth muscle, and of neuronal systems (Table 31–6).

CLASSIFICATION, SITES, AND MECHANISMS OF ACTION OF CALCIUM CHANNEL ANTAGONISTS

Although the calcium channel antagonists share a common mode of action —blockade of voltage-dependent calcium channels—their chemical heterogeneity indicates that they act at different sites to modulate channel function. This is borne out by the existence of specific structure-activity relationships for each category of agents and by the direct demonstration of specific, discrete, but allosterically linked binding site for each category of drug (Fig. 31–6). The recognition that separate sites and mechanisms define calcium channel antagonist properties underlies the relative cardiac:vascular selectivity of these agents, nifedipine and other 1,4-dihydropyridines being dominantly smooth muscle selective, whereas verapamil and diltiazem have both vasodilator and cardiodepressant properties. These distinct selectivities are recognized in the World Health Organization classification where calcium channel selective drugs are categorized as Group I (verapamil-like), Group II (nifedipine-like), and Group III (diltiazem-like). Other agents whose actions are nonselective for calcium channels (see Table 31–6) include the cinnarizine- and flunarizine-like agents

Figure 31–6

Representation of the organization of the specific binding sites for 1,4-dihydropyridines (antagonists and activators), phenylalkylamine, and benzothiazepine categories of calcium channel drugs. The binding sites represent an allosteric association linked one to the other and to the gating and permeation processes of the calcium channel.

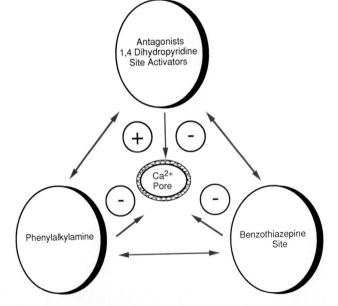

(Group IV), the prenylamine-like (Group V), and the caroverine and perhexiline type (Group VI).

A number of factors probably determine the specific patterns of pharmacologic activity of the calcium channel antagonists. Biochemical evidence indicates that the binding sites for the three major structural classes of agent exist on a single major polypeptide, the sequence of which has now been determined. However, drug interaction with the channel is both frequency- and voltage-dependent whereby drug affinity is determined by selective interactions with the resting, open, or inactivated states of the channel (Fig. 31–7). Additionally, electrophysiologic data indicate that these agents interact at an intracellular locus on the channel. Verapamil and diltiazem, basic molecules significantly charged at physiologic pH, show prominent frequency-dependence, activity increasing with increasing frequency of stimulation, whereas nifedipine and other neutral 1,4-dihydropyridine molecules show increasing activity with decreasing membrane potential. These phenomena likely represent a preferential interaction with the open or inactivated states of the calcium channel whereby charged species access through an open channel state (hydrophilic pathway) and neutral species access through the membrane phase (hydrophobic pathway).

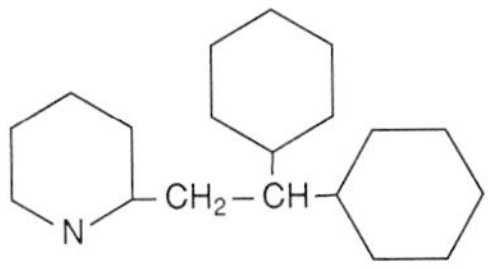

Such considerations of state-dependent interactions (the modulated receptor hypothesis) underlie in large part the relative cardiac:vascular selectivity of these agents and the antiarrhythmic actions of verapamil and diltiazem. It should be noted also that if voltage-dependent channels open briefly, as may be the case for neuronal channels, drugs will appear to be inactive if there is inadequate time to access a state of preferential affinity.

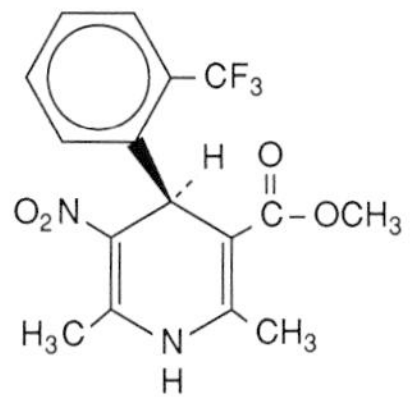

Closely related in structure to nifedipine is a group of 1,4-dihydropyridines, including Bay K 8644, which serve to activate rather than to block the potential-dependent channel. These compounds have properties exactly opposed to those of nifedipine, being vasoconstrictive, hypertensive, and cardiostimulant. The discovery of this group of compounds that maintain the channel in an open state argues against a simple pore-plugging mechanism of action for antagonists. However, such a mechanism may well operate for the inorganic cations including Mn^{2+}, Co^{2+}, Ni^{2+}, Cd^{2+}, and Pb^{2+}, which also serve as channel blockers. The existence of both antagonists and activators of the 1,4-dihydropyridine class that act specifically at calcium channels raises the interesting question of whether, by analogy to the opiate and benzodiazepine receptors, endogenous ligands may exist also for the receptor sites defined by the synthetic drugs.

Calcium antagonists are chemically and pharmacologically heterogeneous.

Perhexiline

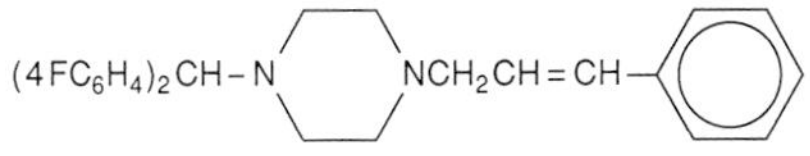

Flunarizine

Calcium antagonists interact with the channel by state-dependent mechanisms.

Bay K 8644

Calcium channel activators of the 1,4-dihydropyridine class

Inorganic cations block Ca^{2+} channels

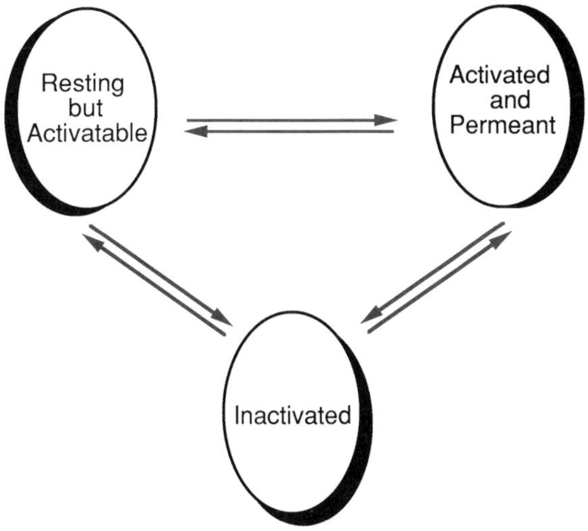

Figure 31–7

The calcium channel, shown schematically, cycling through resting, activated (open), and inactivated states.

Currently, there are no therapeutic indications for calcium channel activators. However, cardioselective agents could prove to be useful positive inotropic agents, and specific secretory cell stimulants could be, for example, insulin-releasing hypoglycemic drugs.

The calcium channel antagonists exert their primary actions at voltage-dependent calcium channels. However, they are not devoid of other pharmacological actions that may contribute to their total pharmacological profile. Both verapamil and diltiazem possess significant local anesthetic properties (approximately equipotent with procaine), and verapamil and D600 are antagonists at several receptors, including α-adrenergic, muscarinic, opiate, and serotonergic. Diltiazem is an inhibitor of $Na^+:Ca^{2+}$ exchange in mitochondria, and 1,4-dihydropyridines have been reported to stimulate the Na^+, K^+-ATPase and Ca^{2+}-ATPase transport systems and to interact with the adenosine transporter. Interactions of phenylalkylamines at other ion channels, including those for sodium and potassium, have been reported also. These actions are all exerted at concentrations higher than those needed to produce calcium channel antagonism, and it is not clear to what extent these properties contribute to the observed therapeutic profile. It is usually assumed that the 1,4-dihydropyridines are the most specific of the agents. However, all compounds are lipophilic and thus may accumulate significantly in the plasma and intracellular membranes where they may modulate excitable systems other than calcium channels.

> Calcium antagonists may work at other pharmacological receptors also.

Pharmacological Properties

The extent to which individual agents of the calcium channel antagonist class affect specific tissues is clearly a major determinant of their selectivity. In the most general terms selectivity depends upon the presence of the appropriately sensitive channel and the extent to which it is activated by the stimulus.

CARDIOVASCULAR EFFECTS

> Calcium antagonists are vasodilators.

All three calcium channel antagonists are vasodilators. Both *in vitro* and *in vivo*, nifedipine is the more potent and verapamil is usually more potent than diltiazem. These properties of coronary and peripheral vascular bed vasodilatation underlie the antianginal and antihypertensive activities of these agents. The vasodilatory properties are most potent in arterial smooth muscle, and there is a reduction in both systolic and diastolic blood pressure. There has been considerable discussion concerning the possible selectivity of these agents for regional vascular beds; it is likely that selectivity occurs primarily as a consequence of the pre-existing degree of tone in different beds or differences in Ca^{2+} channel receptors.

In isolated cardiac muscle these agents inhibit contractility, but the potency sequence is distinct from that observed for vasodilatation with verapamil and diltiazem being more potent or equipotent with nifedipine. *In vivo*, the net effect on cardiac function reflects the balance between direct cardiodepression and cardiostimulation produced by reflex activation (Table 31–7). Thus nifedipine and other 1,4-dihydropyridines produce a net positive chronotropic effect because of their powerful vasodilatory properties. However, this reflex tachycardia usually disappears during chronic treatment, probably because of resetting of the barostats. In contrast, verapamil is a less potent vasodilator than nifedipine and has more prominent cardiodepressant properties. At dosages sufficient to cause vasodilatation any reflex tachycardia is approximately balanced by the negative inotropic, chronotropic, and dromotropic effects of verapamil (see Table 31–7). The cardiodepressant properties of verapamil and diltiazem

> Nifedipine may produce reflex cardiac stimulation.

Table 31-7 ELECTROPHYSIOLOGICAL AND CARDIOVASCULAR PROPERTIES OF Ca²⁺ CHANNEL ANTAGONISTS

Property	Diltiazem	Verapamil	Nifedipine
Heart rate			
Isolated atria	↓	↓	↓
Intact animal	↓	↑↓	↑
Heart contractility	0	↓↑	0,↑
A-V node conduction			
Isolated heart	↓	↓	↓
Intact animal	↓	↓	0
ERP and intervals			
A-V node ERP	↑	↑↑	0
Ventricular ERP	0	0	0
His-Purkinje ERP	0	0	0
P-R interval	↑	↑	0
A-H interval	↑	↑	0
H-V interval	0	0	0
Coronary vessels:			
Tone	↓↓	↓↓	↓↓↓
Flow	↑↑	↑↑	↑↑↑
Peripheral vasodilatation	↑	↑↑	↑↑↑

Code: ↓ decrease; ↑ increase; o, no effect.
ERP, effective refractory period.

are of importance in clinical situations where impaired cardiac function occurs. However, the relatively selective effects of these agents on arterial relative to venous beds and the consequent ventricular unloading likely underlies the increased cardiac output observed following calcium channel antagonist administration.

CARDIOVASCULAR-RELATED EFFECTS

Despite the vasodilatation produced by the calcium channel antagonists they exert comparatively little activation of the renin-angiotensin-aldosterone system, particularly after chronic administration. In this respect they differ significantly from other vasodilators. Their ability to block calcium-dependent processes may prevent the release of aldosterone by angiotensin II. Additionally, these agents also cause diuresis and natriuresis rather than the water and salt retention seen with other classes of vasodilators. The diuretic effects of the calcium channel antagonists can be seen experimentally and clinically and are not simply attributable to changes in renal blood flow. Rather, they may reflect a direct role of calcium and calcium channels in the control of ion and water transport in the kidney.

In vitro these agents are not potent antagonists of platelet aggregation and at therapeutic concentrations exert little effect on release or aggregatory processes. *In vivo* there is some evidence that these agents may impair platelet aggregation and that these effects may arise from drug partitioning into platelet membranes.

Calcium antagonists do not promote water and salt reabsorption.

EFFECTS IN OTHER SYSTEMS

Because voltage-dependent calcium channels are widely distributed it might be anticipated that the actions of the antagonists would be correspondingly broad. Thus, both brain and skeletal muscle possess voltage-dependent calcium channels, but the currently available antagonists are, experimentally or clinically, without the dramatic effects in these systems

Calcium antagonists have little effects on neuronal calcium channels.

that are observed for cardiac and smooth muscle. There are several reasons for these discrepancies. A cell or organ type may not mobilize calcium through the sensitive channels, or the kinetics of channel opening and closing are such as not to permit antagonist equilibration with states of preferential interaction. However, the functional presence of these channels can be detected by the appropriate stimulus such as the 1,4-dihydropyridine activator Bay K 8644. Under such circumstances the effects of calcium channel antagonists can readily be demonstrated.

Calcium channels exist in several different classes.

It is also clear, particularly for neuronal systems, that other categories of calcium channels exist that are distinguishable both electrophysiologically and pharmacologically from the so-called L channels (long lasting and slowly inactivating) that dominate in the cardiovascular system. Other categories of drugs may be found to interact with other channel classes and will likely have a different pharmacological profile from currently available agents. Thus, T channels that open from a negative potential and inactivate rapidly give rise to transient currents and are likely of importance in pacemaking functions. No specific antagonists are yet known. In contrast, N channels appear to be associated specifically with the nervous system, both central and peripheral, and are antagonized potently and specifically by toxins from the *Conus* genus of mollusks.

Therapeutic Applications

ISCHEMIC HEART DISEASE

Ischemic heart disease represents a broad spectrum of disorders from mild manifestations of chronic exercise-induced angina through variant and unstable angina, the latter being frequently prefatory to myocardial infarction. Such ischemic episodes represent the imbalance between oxygen supply and demand brought about by either coronary artery atherosclerosis or by increased coronary artery tone, including arterial spasm. Spasm plays an important contributory role in both variant and unstable angina and may have a number of origins, including local and circulating vasoactive factors superimposed upon enhanced reactivity associated with arterial damage.

Calcium antagonists are used in the several forms of angina.

Diltiazem, verapamil, and nifedipine are all used chronically and acutely in the treatment of the several forms of angina. Nifedipine and diltiazem appear to be approximately equally efficacious in either chronic or acute use, but several reports suggest that verapamil may be somewhat less effective. It is likely that several mechanisms underlie the usefulness of the calcium channel antagonists in angina, including coronary artery dilatation, redistribution of blood flow to ischemic areas, peripheral vasodilatation, reduction of afterload and, with verapamil and diltiazem, lessening of oxygen demand through reduced contractility (see also Chapters 33 and 35).

Use of the calcium channel antagonists during or immediately subsequent to myocardial infarction is potentially beneficial but is still under investigation. Benefits will be expected to arise because of the shifts in oxygen demand:supply balance noted previously and because of the protection of ischemic zones and borders against the detrimental effects of calcium overload. Additionally, verapamil and diltiazem may offer protection also against infarction-induced arrhythmias. Interest is focusing on the use of calcium channel blockers as adjuncts during cardioplegia, the period of ischemia during cardiac surgery.

HYPERTENSION

Calcium antagonists are effective antihypertensive agents.

The use of the calcium channel antagonists for the treatment of hypertension is increasingly clear. Primarily because of their peripheral vasodilatory properties they are being employed more widely in systemic hypertension either alone or in combination with other agents. Combination of nifedipine with β-adrenoceptor antagonists is particularly appropriate because of the initial reflex tachycardia seen frequently with nifedipine alone. Additional indications are for hypertensive crises, for hypertension during pregnancy, and for hypertension during renal disease.

CARDIAC ARRYTHMIAS

Verapamil and diltiazem are experimentally and clinically effective in the treatment of certain categories of cardiac arrythmias, in particular supraventricular tachycardia. However, the clinical experience with verapamil has been significantly more extensive. Although these effects are exerted at the voltage-dependent calcium channel for which nifedipine is also an antagonist, the latter agent is essentially ineffective.

Verapamil is the agent of choice as a class III antiarrythmic agent (see Chapter 33) for terminating episodes of paroxysmal supraventricular tachycardia (PSVT) that involve regions of the heart, principally the atrioventricular (A-V) node, that show calcium channel–dependent slow responses. Approximately 80% of such patients show conversion to sinus rhythm after intravenous (IV) verapamil. Such arrythmias may have a variety of origins, including A-V nodal reentry, accessory pathway reentry (Wolf-Parkinson-White syndrome), and atrial fibrillation and flutter. Verapamil and diltiazem are effective in terminating PSVT; they appear likely to be used prophylactically, but this role is less well investigated. Verapamil may be effective also against digitalis-induced arrythmias and ventricular tachycardia and fibrillation caused by coronary artery spasm, but ventricular arrythmias of other origins are not major therapeutic targets for either verapamil or diltiazem. These agents carry the danger of producing excessive A-V block (see Chapter 33 and Table 33–8).

Verapamil is an effective agent against PSVT.

Nifedipine is not an antiarrhythmic agent.

DOSAGES AND ADMINISTRATION

Nifedipine (PROCARDIA, ADALAT) is available in 10 mg capsules and a delayed release formulation. The usual starting dosage is three capsules daily, once daily for PROCARDIA XL, with subsequent dosage adjustment to achieve the desired level of anginal relief or lowering of blood pressure. Dosages in excess of 180 mg/day are not recommended, and the usual effective dosage range is 30–60 mg/day.

Verapamil (ISOPTIN, CALAN) is available in 5 mg (2 ml) ampules and syringes, 10 mg (4 ml) syringes, and 5 and 10 mg vials for IV administration as well as 80 mg tablets for oral administration. For IV administration the usual starting dosage is 5–10 mg as a bolus repeated after 30 minutes if necessary. For pediatric patients the dosage is reduced to 0.1–0.3 mg/kg body weight. With oral administration the starting dosage is 80 mg three times daily, and the optimal daily dosage for most patients is 320–480 mg daily.

Diltiazem (CARDIZEM) is available for oral administration in 30 mg and 60 mg tablets. The initial dosage is 30 mg four times daily with the usual dosage range being 180–360 mg/day.

PHARMACOKINETICS

There is a broadly similar pattern in the pharmacokinetic behavior of diltiazem, nifedipine, and verapamil. All three agents are well absorbed following oral administration and all are subject to significant first-pass metabolism. Thus, the bioavailability of nifedipine is 50%, diltiazem 40%,

Calcium antagonists are well absorbed.

and verapamil rather lower at 20%. However, with continued administration of verapamil bioavailability increases.

Hepatic metabolism is the dominant inactivation route for all three compounds. The metabolites of nifedipine are pharmacologically inert pyridine carboxylic acids. However, metabolites of both diltiazem (desacetyl- and monomethyldiltiazem) have activity, although substantially less than that of the parent compound. Norverapamil (N-desmethylverapamil), a metabolite of verapamil, is also pharmacologically active.

The agents are all extensively, more than 90%, protein bound in the plasma and all achieve rapid peak plasma concentrations following oral administration. This coincides with the rapid onset of pharmacologic actions; nifedipine and diltiazem achieve peak effects more rapidly than does verapamil. The half-lives of these agents are comparatively short, 3–4 hours, but that for verapamil is significantly increased in patients with liver dysfunction, and this is likely also true for nifedipine and diltiazem. Renal insufficiencies appear to exert little effect on duration or intensity of action of these agents. The relationships between plasma concentrations and hemodynamic effects remain to be established quantitatively.

DRUG COMBINATIONS

The calcium channel antagonists function in angina and hypertension by mechanisms fundamentally different from those employed by the β-adrenoceptor antagonists, the angiotensin-converting enzyme (ACE) inhibitors, and the organic nitrates that are used extensively also in these disorders (see Chapters 35 and 36). Hence, combinations of calcium channel antagonists with these agents may offer certain advantages in providing a second stage of therapy and in reducing the side effects associated with any of the drugs alone.

The combination of nifedipine and β blockers has been studied fairly extensively, because its use will attenuate the initial reflex tachycardia seen with nifedipine alone. Additionally, because nifedipine at vasodilatory dosages does not depress cardiac conduction or contractility, it does not add to the effects of the β blockers. Enhanced hypotension may occur. Combinations of β blockers with verapamil or diltiazem should be employed with caution because of the possibility of A-V block.

Calcium channel antagonists and ACE inhibitors may provide an interesting combination of preload and afterload reduction useful in both hypertension and angina. With nifedipine, the absence of the initial reflex cardiac stimulation and the production of natriuresis and diuresis perhaps adequate to prevent addition of a diuretic to the therapeutic regimen may be a particularly useful combination.

Calcium channel antagonists may be employed with organic nitrates to obtain additional relief in exertional or vasospastic angina. The combination of reductions in both preload and afterload may prove to be particularly advantageous.

Related to the questions of combination therapy is the question of choice of individual agent for anginal therapy. In general, choice is predictable on the basis of the known spectrum of pharmacological and hemodynamic properties of the individual agents. Thus, nitrates and calcium channel antagonists may be used effectively in exertional, variant, and unstable angina and when these states are associated with chronic obstructive pulmonary disease, peripheral vascular disease, or diabetes. Of the calcium channel antagonists nifedipine may be preferable in exertional angina, verapamil or diltiazem may be preferable in unstable angina, and nifedipine is definitely preferable when sinus or A-V node disease is present or

---

Calcium antagonists undergo extensive first-pass metabolism.

Calcium antagonists may be employed in combination with other drugs, including β blockers, nitrates, and ACE inhibitors.

The clinical choice of calcium antagonist in angina depends upon associated symptoms.

where left ventricular dysfunction exists. Among the calcium channel antagonists, nifedipine is the likely agent of choice when angina coexists with hypertension, congestive heart failure, or peripheral vascular disease; verapamil or diltiazem for angina with cardiac arrythmias, save in the presence of nodal disease; and diltiazem may be preferable in angina with cerebral ischemia because of its relatively weak peripheral vasodilatory properties.

CONTRAINDICATIONS AND DRUG INTERACTIONS

The adverse reactions precipitated by the calcium channel antagonists are generally related to their fundamental pharmacological properties, have a generally low incidence, and are usually tolerable or can be accommodated by switching agents. The major side effects of verapamil are, in order of reported frequency of incidence, constipation, dizziness, hypotension, headache, peripheral edema, and bradycardia. For diltiazem, edema, headache, nausea, and dizziness and for nifedipine, dizziness, facial flushing, headache, peripheral edema, hypotension, and nausea are the major side effects reported.

The specific contraindications thus far defined relate generally to the respective cardiac and vascular selectivities of these agents. Verapamil and diltiazem are contraindicated where nodal disease, A-V block, and hypotension exist. Additionally, verapamil is contrainindicated for hypertrophic cardiomyopathy, atrial fibrillation and flutter and a coexisting A-V accessory pathway, and severe left ventricular dysfunction; IV verapamil is contraindicated in patients on β-blocker therapy or with Duchenne's muscular dystrophy. Nifedipine should be used with caution in hypotensive patients.

Verapamil and diltiazem are contraindicated in cardiac disease.

Several known drug interactions exist; many of these are discussed in Chapters 33 and 35. Beta blockers should be used with caution in combination with verapamil and diltiazem because of the possibility of excessive cardiac depression. Inhalational anesthetics depress membrane excitability and may potentiate the actions of the calcium channel antagonists. Verapamil, diltiazem, and nifedipine all increase the serum levels of digoxin; cimetidine increases plasma nifedipine levels; and quinidine may potentiate the hypotensive actions of verapamil. Calcium channel antagonists enhance the activity of neuromuscular blockers of both the competitive and depolarizing classes. Verapamil and diltiazem should be used with caution with such antihypertensive agents as reserpine or α-methyldopa that depress nodal function. Finally, verapamil in an action almost certainly unrelated to its calcium channel–blocking properties can reverse the resistance of tumor cells to such antitumor agents as vincristine or doxorubicin.

Beta blockers should be used cautiously in combination with verapamil or diltiazem.

Calcium antagonists reverse multiple drug resistance in cancer cells.

Calcium Metabolism and Cardiovascular Disease

The control of calcium metabolism is discussed typically in separate fashion at the cellular and organ levels. It is increasingly clear, however, that the regulatory systems are not separate and that alterations in the control of body calcium homeostasis can lead to changes in cellular function and *vice versa*. The communications between the two sets of control processes are clearly critical to physiological function, and alterations likely underlie a number of pathological states. This may be strikingly so for essential hypertension.

Cellular defects in calcium metabolism and consequent increases in intracellular calcium have been presumed by many workers to be associated with the hypertensive state, although it is not clear whether such changes are causal or are secondary to other disturbances of cellular func-

Defects in calcium metabolism are associated with hypertension.

tion. Such a hypothesis accords with the central role of calcium in vascular smooth muscle contraction, accommodates the frequently observed nonspecific hyperreactivity of vascular smooth muscle seen in both experimental and clinical hypertension, is consistent with elevated intracellular calcium levels found in some cell types in hypertension, and is obviously consistent with the effectiveness of calcium channel antagonists as antihypertensive agents (see Chapter 35).

An alternative viewpoint suggests, however, that essential hypertension may be associated with a calcium deficiency rather than with a calcium excess. Consistent with this hypothesis are observations of hypercalciuria, reduced serum calcium levels in hypertension, and several sets of observations that a low dietary calcium uptake is associated with hypertension and that oral calcium loading can reduce blood pressure in both clinical and experimental situations.

These opposing hypotheses suggesting that essential hypertension is associated both with elevated and depressed levels of calcium are not necessarily mutually exclusive nor are they necessarily conflicting. Deficient plasma levels of calcium may be associated with elevated intracellular calcium through the interrelationship of the calcium regulatory systems at both the cellular and body levels and by the association of both sets of control processes with the renin-angiotensin-aldosterone system.

Renin levels in hypertension are known to be an important component of the profile of the hypertensive patient. Renin levels correlate with serum calcium and magnesium, low renin being associated with low calcium and high magnesium. Renin levels appear also to correlate with serum levels of parathyroid hormone, vitamin D, and calcitonin. Parathyroid hormone and vitamin D are highest in the low renin state and calcitonin is highest in the high renin state of hypertension.

Such studies suggest that there is a broad association between the control of calcium metabolism and renin activity in essential hypertension. Furthermore, this interrelationship provides a better understanding of drug therapy according to patient profile. Thus, low renin or low serum calcium predisposes to a hypotensive response following oral calcium loading. Such individuals also show selective benefit with calcium channel blockers, and this beneficial effect in low-renin, volume-dependent hypertensives likely reflects, at least in part, the low serum calcium concentrations. In contrast, high-renin individuals with normal or elevated serum calcium levels respond most beneficially to β blockers or to ACE inhibitors. Because both diuretics and calcium channel blockers can raise serum calcium, as can dietary calcium in low-renin salt-sensitive individuals, a close link may exist between diet and drug therapy in hypertensive individuals.

Both a cellular calcium excess and a serum calcium defect may be associated with hypertension.

Renin levels may correlate directly with serum calcium levels.

PTH and vitamin D levels may be elevated in the low renin state in hypertension.

Summary

In this chapter calcium regulation is examined in a holistic manner. This appears to be particularly appropriate given the considerable biological and therapeutic interests in calcium. Major pharmacological and therapeutic attention is directed currently toward the calcium channel antagonists. The group of compounds, including the clinically available verapamil, nifedipine and diltiazem, represent only the first generation of calcium channel antagonists. Second-generation compounds with improved pharmacokinetic characteristics and enhanced selectivity will be available shortly. These will include the 1,4-dihydropyridines nitrendipine (hypertension), nicardipine and amlodipine (angina and hypertension), nisoldipine (angina), and nimodipine (cerebral vasodilatation). Other, and subsequent, developments will probably include neuron selective agents that act at channel classes distinct from those dominant in the cardiovascular system

Other 1,4-dihydropyridines include nitrendipine, nicardipine, nimodipine, and amlodipine.

and the possible use of calcium channel activators as positive inotropic and secretory agents. Calcium channel antagonism may be also a property of drugs whose therapeutic properties have, in part or in whole, been attributed to other mechanisms of action. Thus, calcium channel antagonism may underlie the neuroleptic properties of the diphenylbutylpiperidines pimozide and fluspirilene and the antidiarrheal effects of loperamide and diphenoxylate. It is likely that disease states will be identified that are associated with specific defects in calcium channel structure and function or that involve immune defects in the channel system.

Calcium antagonism may be associated with the actions of other drug classes.

Important as these potential directions in calcium channel drugs may be, it should not be ignored that the potential dependent calcium channel represents but one of the regulatory pathways of calcium control. Calcium is involved in many fundamentally important events where its movements and mobilization are not controlled by this class of channels. Among such events we may note calcium mobilization through the inositol polyphosphate and excitatory amino acid pathways. Definition of these pathways is likely to be of importance to drug development for the control of, for example, secretory cell function and neuronal ischemia.

Because calcium plays critical roles in cell metabolism from the enthusiasm of fertilization to the finality of cell death from calcium overload, it is to be anticipated that new classes of drugs based on the calcium theme will be an important contributor to human health in the future. These roles of calcium are best appreciated when the ion is viewed as a key regulator of biological function whose properties are expressed in integrated fashion.

Calcium plays multiple roles in cell metabolism.

References

Baker PF (ed): Calcium and Drug Action. New York and Heidelberg: Springer-Verlag, 1987.

Baky S: Verapamil. *In* Scriabine A (ed): New Drugs Annual. Vol 2, 71–101. New York: Raven Press, 1984.

Breimer LH, MacIntyre I, Zaidi M: Peptides from the calcitonin genes: Molecular genetics, structure and function. Biochem J 255:377–390, 1988.

Campbell AK: Intracellular Calcium: Its Universal Role As Regulator. New York: Wiley & Sons, 1983.

Chaffman M, Brogden RN: Diltiazem. Drugs 29:387–454, 1985.

DeLuca HF, Schnoes HK: Vitamin D: Recent advances. Annu Rev Biochem 52:411–439, 1983.

Fleckenstein A: Calcium Antagonism in Heart and Smooth Muscle. Experimental Facts and Therapeutic Prospects. New York: Wiley & Sons, 1983.

Freedman DD, Waters DD: 'Second generation' dihydropyridine calcium antagonists. Greater vascular selectivity and some unique applications. Drugs 34:578–598, 1987.

Inogna KL, Broadus AE: Hypercalcemia of malignancy. Annu Rev Med 38:241–256, 1987.

Janis RA, Silver P, Triggle DJ: Drug action and cellular calcium regulation. Adv Drug Res 16:309–591, 1987.

Klein HO, Kaplinsky E: Digitalis and verapamil in atrial fibrillation and flutter. Is verapamil now the preferred agent? Drugs 31:185–197, 1986.

Laragh JH, Buhler FR (eds): Update on calcium antagonists in hypertension. Parts I and II. J Cardiovasc Pharmacol 9(Suppl 4):S1–S322, 1987.

Laragh JH, Ritz E (eds): Calcium antagonists. J Cardiovasc Pharmacol 10(Suppl 10):S1–S212, 1987.

Levine MM, Kleeman CR: Hypercalcemia: Pathophysiology and treatment. Hosp Pract [Off] 22:93–110, 1987.

Marcus R: Normal and abnormal bone remodeling in man. Annu Rev Med 38:129–141, 1987.

Minghetti PP, Norman AW: 1,25 (OH)2-Vitamin D_3 receptors: Gene regulation and genetic circuitry. FASEB J 2:3043–3053, 1988.

Morad M, Nayler WG (eds): The Calcium Channel: Structure, Function and Implications. Berlin: Springer-Verlag, 1989.

Opie LH: Calcium channel antagonists. Part I: Fundamental properties: Mechanisms of classification, sites of action. Cardiovasc Drugs Ther 1:411–430, 1987.

Opie LH: Calcium channel antagonists. Part II: Use and comparative properties of the three prototypical calcium antagonists in ischemic heart disease, including recommendations based on an analysis of 41 trials. Cardiovasc Drugs Ther 1:461–491, 1988.

Rasmussen H: The calcium messenger system. N Engl J Med 314:1094–1170, 1986.

Resnick LM, Laragh JH, Sealy JE, Alderman MH: Divalent cations in essential hypertension. N Engl J Med 309:888–891, 1983.

Resnick LH, Nicholson JP, Laragh JN: Calcium metabolism in essential hypertension: Relationship to altered renin system activity. Fed Proc 45:2739–2745, 1986.

Scriabine A: Current and potential indications for Ca^{2+} antagonists. Ration Drug Ther 21:1–7, 1987.

Scriabine A, Garthoff B, Kazda S, et al: Nitrendipine. *In* Scriabine A (ed): New Drugs Annual. Vol 2, 37–50. New York: Raven Press, 1984.

Singh BN, Nademanee K, Baky SH: Calcium antagonists. Clinical use in the treatment of arrhythmias. Drugs 25:125–153, 1983.

Snyder SH, Reynolds IJ: Calcium antagonist drug-receptor interactions that clarify therapeutic effects. N Engl J Med 313:995–1002, 1985.

Sorkin EM, Clissold SP, Brogden RN: Nifedipine. Drugs 30:182–274, 1985.

Suva LJ, Winslow SA, Wettenhall REH, et al: A parathyroid hormone-related protein implicated in malignant hypercalcemia: Cloning and expression. Science 237:893–896, 1987.

Tietze KJ, Schwartz ML, Vlasses PH: Calcium anatagonists in cerebral/peripheral vascular disorders. Current status. Drugs 32:531–538, 1987.

Triggle DJ: Calcium channel drugs: Antagonists and activators. ISI Atlas Pharmacol 1:319–324, 1987.

Triggle DJ, Janis RA: Calcium channel ligands. Annu Rev Pharmacol Toxicol 27:347–369, 1987.

Vanhoutte PM: The expert committee of the World Health Organization on classification of calcium antagonists: The viewpoint of the rapporteur. Am J Cardiol 59:3A–8A, 1987.

Young EW, Bukoski RD, McCarron DA: Calcium metabolism in experimental hypertension. Proc Soc Exp Biol Med 187:123–141, 1988.

Treatment of Congestive Heart Failure — Digitalis Glycosides

Claire M. Lathers

Digitalis glycosides are among the most frequently prescribed drugs in the United States. For example, in 1980, digoxin ranked eighth in the number of prescriptions written, digitoxin was sixteenth, and digitalis leaf was twenty third (Doherty, 1985). The recognition of the variability in clinical responses resulting from the pharmacokinetics and drug interaction complexities, in the face of frequent occurrence of digitalis toxicity, makes the therapeutic use challenging indeed. The unusually narrow margin between therapeutic and toxic dosages and serum levels of digitalis mandates that the physician be both knowledgeable about, and attentive to, early symptoms of digitalis toxicity to achieve the best risk : benefit ratio. Recognition of toxicity is imperative because a high mortality ensues when digoxin is continued after the appearance of toxic symptoms.

Digitalis glycosides have served as important research tools in the advancement of knowledge of cardiac muscle contractility, cellular electrophysiology, and membrane ionic fluxes. Animal models of digitalis toxicity have contributed to the understanding of cardiac arrhythmias and the role of the autonomic nervous system in the regulation of cardiac function. The development of antibodies to measure drug levels and to reverse digitalis toxicity has contributed to better patient management. The detection of endogenous digitalis substances has initiated investigations into the neuroendocrine control of blood pressure, cardiac contractility, and electrolyte balance.

This chapter includes the most salient facts about the use of digitalis glycosides, but the reader is referred to recent texts, reviews, and research reports cited in the references.

Early accounts of the use of digitalis derivatives are found in the Ebers Papyrus (1500 BC), in centuries of Chinese writings, in early Roman records (AD 1000), and in the chronicles of the botanist Leonhard Fuchs (1542). In 1785 William Withering published a treatise that introduced digitalis into the clinical practice of medicine by describing the effects of the active ingredient of an "herbal brew" composed of 20 or more herbs contained in Welsh family recipes for the cure of dropsy (edema). Withering's monograph summarized 9 years of systematic observation and contained detailed case presentations of the use of digitalis to treat dropsy and its diuretic actions, with an emphasis on dosage selection, a description of its toxic effects, and a comment on its power over the "motion of the heart." In 1799 John Ferriar concluded that digitalis exerted its primary effect on the heart and a secondary action on the kidney. In 1911 Mackenzie noted its

Digoxin is one of the most frequently prescribed drugs in the United States.

Therapeutic use of glycosides is confounded by

1. variable pharmacokinetics
2. numerous drug interactions
3. narrow therapeutic index

Digoxin toxicity is associated with high mortality.

Glycosides are also used as research tools to study

1. normal cardiac function
2. interaction of autonomic nervous system and arrhythmias
3. antibodies to treat clinical toxicity
4. endogenous digitalis substances

History

History of digitalis glycosides; Withering's contribution

primary beneficial action was in patients with atrial fibrillation; he did not advocate its use for heart patients with congestive heart failure and normal sinus rhythm. In 1938 Cattell and Gold attributed its primary mechanism in relieving congestive heart failure to a direct action to increase the force of contraction. Ongoing research in the twentieth century has established its use for congestive heart failure and supraventricular arrhythmias.

Chemistry

Chemistry of glycosides and semisynthetic derivatives

Digoxin

Structure and activity components of glycosides

Digitoxin

Digitalis and other cardiac glycosides are found in plant extracts and in the venom of some toads. Semisynthetic derivatives, such as acetylstrophanthidin and ASI-222, have also been designed in unsuccessful attempts to improve the therapeutic action while decreasing toxicity. In this chapter, the expressions *digitalis glycosides, digitalis,* or *glycosides* are used to designate the entire group of cardiac glycosides.

The structure of each digitalis glycoside consists of an aglycone or genin conjugated with one to four molecules of sugar. The aglycone or genin moiety contains the pharmacological activity whereas the sugar molecules enhance water solubility and cell penetrability. Thus, the sugar portion of the structure influences glycoside potency and the dose-response relationship. The cyclopentanoperhydrophenanthrene nucleus is attached to an unsaturated lactone ring at C17. Differences among the chemical structures of the various aglycones are due to methyl, hydroxyl, or aldehyde substitutions attached at various positions of the molecule. The combination of the unsaturated lactone ring and the steroid ring imparts cardiotonic activity to the structure. When the lactone ring is saturated, cardiotonic activity is decreased tenfold or more, but the onset of the development of the cardiac action is increased.

Digoxin is the glycoside used mostly; over recent years digitoxin has been less and less prescribed. Both of these have an aglycone with three molecules of digitoxose and 2,6-dideoxyhexose joined in glycoside linkage attached at position 3.

Pharmacokinetics

Pharmacokinetics of glycosides differ with respect to

1. extent of water in solution
2. polarity
3. product formulation
4. half-life
5. protein binding
6. onset of action
7. peak effect
8. therapeutic serum concentration

Differences in the pharmacokinetics and pharmacodynamic properties among the various digitalis glycosides are due to variations in water or lipid solubility and polarity caused by both the diversity in the chemical structure (Table 32–1) and the formulation of the product. Digitoxin is lipid-soluble and thus absorbed completely from the gastrointestinal (GI) tract. It has a half-life of 5–7 days. Digoxin is less lipid-soluble than digitoxin, is not as well absorbed as digitoxin, and possesses a half-life of 1–1½ days. Ouabain lacks lipid solubility and thus is absorbed poorly from the GI tract; it has a rapid onset when given intravenously (IV), and its half-life is 21 hours. The various digitalis preparations exhibit different degrees of binding to plasma proteins: digitoxin 86%; acetyldigitoxin 81–90%; digoxin 10–15%; and ouabain is not bound. Protein binding in blood is not thought to account for the differences in onset or speed of action, but protein

Table 32–1   CARDIAC GLYCOSIDE PREPARATIONS

Agent	GI Absorption	Onset (IV — minutes)	Peak (hours)	Half-Life (days)	Metabolic Path	Digitalizing Dose (IV)	Maintenance Dose (Oral)	Therapeutic Concentration (Serum)
Digoxin	55–75%	15–30	1½–5	1½–2	Renal	0.75–1.0 mg	0.25–0.5 mg	0.2–2.0 ng/ml
Digitoxin	90–100%	25–120	4–12	4–7	Liver	1.0 mg	0.10 mg	10–25 ng/ml
Ouabain	Unreliable	5–10	½–2	<1	Renal, Some GI	0.3–0.5 mg	—	0.4–0.6 ng/ml

Adapted/condensed from Antman EM, Smith TW: Pharmacokinetics of digitalis glycosides. *In* Smith TW (ed): Digitalis Glycosides, Chapter 15, 241–275. Orlando, FL: Grune & Stratton, 1986. Adapted from Smith JW: Drug Therapy: Digitalis glycosides. Reprinted with permission from The New England Journal of Medicine, vol 28, pp 719–722, 1973.

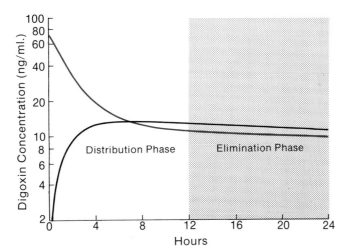

Figure 32-1

Relationship between tissue and plasma digoxin ion concentration after administration of an IV dose of the drug. Concentration in plasma is shown in red; concentration in tissue in black. (Redrawn from Soldin SJ: Digoxin—Issues and controversies. Clin Chem 32:5-12, 1986.)

binding in cardiac tissue may be involved in determining the duration of action of the glycoside. Table 32–1 also summarizes the onset of action, the peak effect, and the therapeutic serum concentration for the clinically important glycosides. Figure 32–1 illustrates the relationship between tissue and plasma digoxin concentration after its IV administration, and Figure 32–2 depicts its distribution in human tissue 5.5 hours after its administration. (Ouabain is mentioned in this chapter not because it is used clinically, which it is not, but because its solubility and pharmacokinetic properties have resulted in its extensive use in research on the mechanisms of action of digitalis.)

Digitoxin is primarily, but not entirely, metabolized in the liver, in contrast to digoxin. Digitoxin also undergoes enterohepatic circulation, is excreted in the bile, and is then reabsorbed. One of the metabolites of digitoxin is digoxin. Although digoxin is more active than digitoxin, it is eliminated more rapidly. Liver disease may increase the half-life of digitoxin. Digoxin, in contrast to digitoxin, is primarily excreted by the kidney; its half-life is increased in patients with renal disease. Because there is, in most patients, a positive correlation between the decrease in creatinine clearance and in the plasma digoxin concentration, pharmacological agents such as vasodilators that change renal perfusion will change the rate of elimination of digoxin. Thus, when using glycoside preparations, patient management requires assessment of renal and liver function.

Distribution of digoxin in human tissue

Rhamnose   Ouabain

Metabolism of glycosides

1. liver disease
2. renal disease
3. drug effects

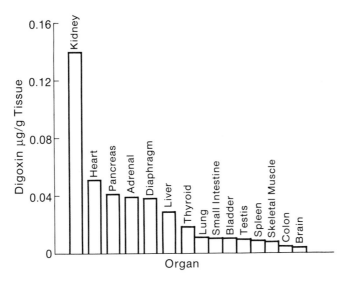

Figure 32-2

Tissue digoxin in a patient who received 1.0 mg of tritium-labeled digoxin 5.5 hours before death. Note concentration in the kidney, the major organ of excretion, and that in heart, diaphragm, and liver. (Redrawn from Doherty JE: Clinical use of digitalis glycosides: An update. Cardiology 72:225-254, 1985. By permission of S. Karger AG, Basel.)

Table 32-2 *CARDIOACTIVITY OF DIGOXIN METABOLITES*

Metabolite	Activity Relative to Digoxin (%)
Dihydrodigoxin	2–6
Dihydrodigoxigenin	2
Digoxigenin	4–21
Digoxigenin mono-digitoxiside	66
Digoxigenin bis-digitoxiside	77

Data from Soldin SJ: Digoxin—Issues and controversies. Clin Chem 32:5–12, 1986.

Digoxin has metabolites with cardioactivity.

Digoxin is metabolized to a number of metabolites that also exhibit cardioactivity (Table 32–2). An additional and important problem associated with the use of digoxin is that different brands of the preparation have significantly different bioavailability characteristics (absorption, metabolism, time course of effects). These differences have caused problems in *digitalizing* (establishing a steady level of digitalis effects or blood level) and maintaining patients properly. These differences in product, in association with the low therapeutic index of this class of agents, necessitates constant patient surveillance.

Mechanism of Action

CONTRACTILE ACTIONS

Pathophysiology of congestive heart failure

The major features of the pathophysiology of congestive heart failure are depicted in Figure 32–3. The failing heart manifests decreased myocardial contractility and catecholamine content; the catecholamine deficit is thought to be due to the inability of synthesis to follow the increased sympathetic activity involved in the compensatory responses to the decreased cardiac output.

Digitalis increases the force of contraction at a given fiber length or tension in papillary preparations.

Digitalis increases the force of contraction at a given fiber length or tension when added to an isolated papillary muscle preparation. When administered *in vivo* it increases ventricular contractility in normal and in failing hearts. This increase in myocardial contractility is called a *positive inotropic effect* (Fig. 32–4).

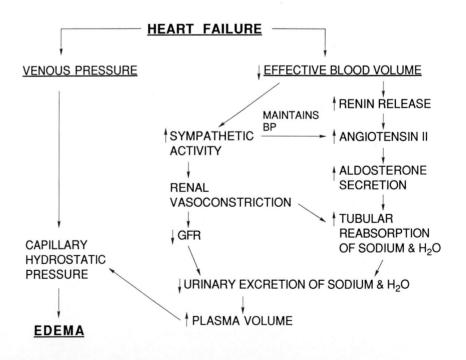

Figure 32-3

Major pathophysiological features of congestive heart failure. (BP = blood pressure; GFR = glomerular filtration rate.)

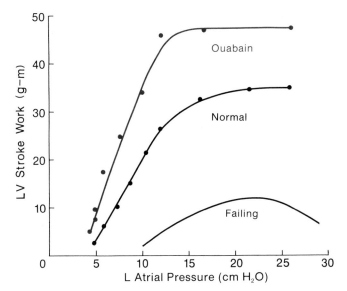

Figure 32–4

The effect of a digitalis glycoside (ouabain) on myocardial function obtained in a normal dog before and after administration of ouabain, 0.05 mg/kg. Left atrial pressure was increased by infusion of blood into the atrium at appropriate rates. The curves labeled *normal* and *ouabain* were obtained experimentally. For comparison, a hypothetical curve for a failing heart has been added. Note that a reduction of atrial pressure from 30 to 10 cmH₂O would increase the work output of the failing heart. The glycoside, by increasing contractility of the heart, shifts the function curve, permitting greater work output at any given atrial pressure. (Redrawn from Cotten MD, Stopp PE: Action of digitalis on the nonfailing heart of the dog. Am J Physiol 192:114, 1958.)

In the normal heart the peak rate of rise of intraventricular pressure and intramyocardial tension during isovolumic contraction is increased by digitalis. The period of isovolumic left ventricular contraction is shortened, whereas the mean systolic ejection rate is increased. In the failing heart, the ability of digitalis to increase myocardial contractility results in an improvement of the impaired circulatory dynamics. Generally, but not always, the stroke volume and cardiac output will be increased and the elevated left ventricular end-diastolic pressure (Fig. 32–5) and volume will be decreased. Contractility of atrial tissue is increased also by the administration of digitalis. The increased atrial contractility increases ventricular filling and thus also contributes to the increased cardiac output.

Digitalis increases peak rate of rise of intraventricular pressure and intramyocardial tension during isovolumic contraction.

In the failing heart, digitalis increases contractility and improves hemodynamics.

Digitalis increases contractility of atrial tissue.

CARDIAC OUTPUT

Digitalis has no effect on or slightly decreases cardiac output in the normal heart. No change results in reflex adjustments in the force of cardiac con-

Digitalis has no effect on or decreases the cardiac output of normal heart.

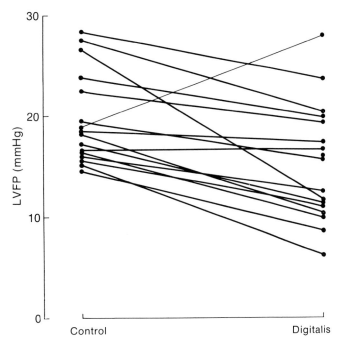

Figure 32–5

Effects of IV digitalis on left ventricular end-diastolic pressure (LVFP) in patients with acute myocardial infarction in whom the preglycoside LVFP was above normal (greater than 12 mmHg). All patients had congestive heart failure without cardiogenic shock. (Redrawn from Mason DT, Amsterdam EA, Lee G: Digitalis glycosides: Clinical pharmacology and therapeutics. *In* Mason DT [ed]: Congestive Heart Failure: Mechanism, Evaluation, and Treatment, 321. New York: Dun-Donnelley, 1976.)

In congestive heart failure, digitalis increases cardiac output.

Digitalis induces a reflex decrease in sympathetic activity.

traction to prevent the decrease in cardiac output that would otherwise occur when digitalis increases afterload by increasing vasoconstriction of the arterial tree. When digitalis is given to an individual in congestive heart failure, the direct myocardial action increases the stroke volume and results in an increase in cardiac output, overcoming the peripheral vasoconstriction action on the arterial vessels. Digitalis induces a reflex decrease in sympathetic activity also, thus reducing afterload, increasing ventricular ejection, and decreasing venoconstriction.

OXYGEN CONSUMPTION

Digitalis enhances contractility and thus myocardial oxygen consumption.

Digitalis actions on the failing heart include decreases in size and wall tension.

Myocardial oxygen consumption is increased after digitalis because of the enhanced contractility. In the normal heart there is no change in the physical size of the heart but wall tension is increased, resulting in increased energy and oxygen requirements. In the failing heart digitalis induces an increase in the stroke volume that results in a decrease in the size and wall tension of the myocardium. The consequence is a decrease in oxygen consumption that compensates for the increase in oxygen consumption associated with the digitalis-induced increase in myocardial contractility.

POSTULATED CELLULAR EXPLANATION OF THE POSITIVE INOTROPIC ACTION

Increased cellular calcium is involved in the role of digitalis-induced inotropic action associated with Na^+/K^+ ATPase inhibition.

The positive inotropic action of digitalis involves calcium; more calcium is available to the myocardial troponin-tropomyosin actomyosin system in the presence of digitalis. Inhibition of cardiac sodium/potassium-activated adenosine triphosphatase (ATPase) enzyme results in an inhibition of the Na^+ pump and results in an increase in the intracellular sodium concentration. This increase in intracellular sodium is thought to displace calcium from the sarcoplasmic reticulum and increase the concentration of intracellular calcium available for excitation-contraction coupling. The resultant increased calcium binding to troponin-tropomyosin activates the actomyosin system and increases myocardial contractility.

The stability of the digitalis sodium/potassium ATPase (Na^+/K^+ ATPase) complex correlates well with the cardiac sensitivity of different species to the inotropic actions of digitalis. It has been suggested that the receptor for digitalis is, in fact, the membrane-bound sodium/potassium ATPase.

Electrophysiological Properties

Digitalis exerts its antiarrhythmic effect by actions primarily exerted on atrial and A-V nodal tissue.

Toxic doses of digitalis may cause A-V block.

SINOATRIAL AND ATRIOVENTRICULAR NODES

Digitalis has little effect on the transmembrane potential at therapeutic concentrations. Nontoxic doses of digitalis exert their antiarrhythmic action primarily on atrial and atrioventricular (A-V) nodal tissue by modifying autonomic neural discharge. Likewise, the indirect action of digitalis on the autonomic nervous system modifies (usually decreases) the rate of impulse formation by the sinoatrial (S-A) node.

Toxic dosages of digitalis may partially depolarize S-A nodal fibers, stopping the generation of action potentials. High concentrations depress conduction of the impulses through the A-V node by first decreasing conduction velocity and increasing the effective refractory period. The conduction changes are associated with decreases in the maximal diastolic potential, the rate of rise of the action potential, and in the amplitude of the action potential at the A-V node.

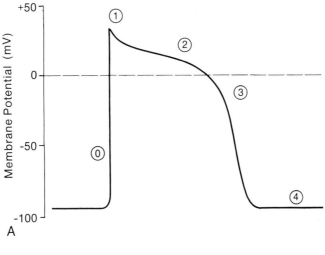

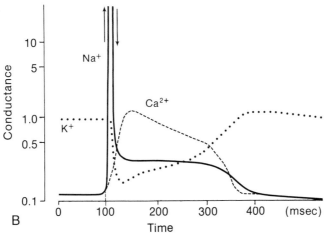

Figure 32–6

A, A schematic diagram of a cardiac transmembrane action potential. Vertical axis is membrane potential in millivolts (mV). Cardiac cells have an electronegative resting membrane potential, which is maintained until a stimulus of sufficient magnitude occurs to lower the resting membrane potential to its threshold potential, which then results in an action potential. Phase 0, or rapid depolarization, results from a rapid influx of sodium into the intracellular space. This is followed by three phases of repolarization. The first (Phase 1) is a short rapid repolarization, followed by a plateau (Phase 2), and finally by a return to its resting membrane potential (Phase 3). *B,* Ionic conductances (mmho/sq cm) for sodium (Na^+), potassium (K^+), and calcium (Ca^{2+}) during these phases.

ATRIAL AND VENTRICULAR MUSCLE FIBERS

The response in the specialized atrial fibers is similar to that observed in Purkinje fibers. After digitalis there is an increase in automaticity due to an enhanced Phase 4 depolarization and the generation of ectopic impulses due to initiation of delayed after-depolarizations.

Digitalis enhances automaticity.

Digitalis-induced changes in the duration of the action potential are similar to those observed in Purkinje fibers. Although the decrease is not marked, it is thought to explain the decrease in the QT interval. Ventricular transmembrane action potentials demonstrate an increase in the slope of the plateau and a decrease in the slope of Phase 3. These changes indicate alterations in the ST segment and in the T wave. Higher dosages of digitalis decrease the resting potential and the amplitude of the action potential in both atrial and ventricular fibers and decrease the maximal role of depolarization during Phase 0. As conduction velocity decreases, inexcitability is produced (Fig. 32–6). Clinically, Phase 4 depolarization in atrial or ventricular muscle fibers does not occur, but delayed after-depolarizations may develop.

Myocardial inexcitability results as digitalis decreases conduction velocity.

Purkinje Fibers

Much of the experimental evidence used to explain the toxic effects of digitalis on the electrical activity of the heart is based on studies of Purkinje fibers. The time of exposure to the glycoside and the concentration used

Figure 32–7

Effects of a digitalis glycoside (ouabain) on the cardiac action potential. The transmembrane potential was determined using conventional 3-M KCl intracellular microelectrodes. Although Phase 3 was accelerated by the glycoside, the maximal diastolic potential after repolarization was less than in the control. (Redrawn from Miura DS, Biedert S: Cellular mechanisms of digitalis action. J Clin Pharmacol 25:490–500, 1985.)

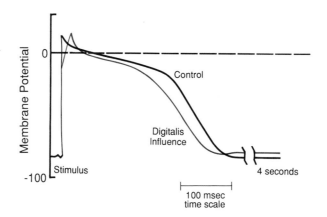

Low dosages of digitalis produce a small increase in the action potential duration of Purkinje fibers.

Digitalis toxicity decreases Vmax and conduction velocity in Purkinje fibers and eventually renders them inexcitable.

The extracellular potassium concentration is a factor involved in determining the action of glycosides on Phase 4 in Purkinje fibers.

Delayed after-depolarization amplitude increases as digitalis toxicity develops.

Digitalis can trigger ectopic beats by two mechanisms

  1. delayed after-depolarizations
  2. enhancement of normal Phase 4 depolarization

determine the effect on the transmembrane action potential and on the resting potential (Fig. 32–7). With low, but not high, rates of stimulation, a small increase in the action potential duration occurs. This is followed by a decrease in the action potential duration due mostly to a shortening of the duration of the Phase 2 plateau. This change is associated generally with an increase in the slope of Phase 4 depolarization and a subsequent decrease in the resting potential or maximal diastolic potential and a further decrease in the action potential duration. Eventually the maximal rate of rise of Phase 0 (Vmax) and the amplitude of the action potential decrease; these changes may be due to the less negative resting potential or because Phase 4 depolarization causes the upstroke of the action potential (Phase 0) to start at a less negative potential. With digitalis toxicity there is a decrease in Vmax and conduction velocity and eventually the Purkinje fibers become inexcitable.

The concentration of extracellular potassium, as well as other factors, determine the action of glycosides on Phase 4 in the Purkinje fibers. Low concentrations of potassium generally cause an increase in the slope of Phase 4, resulting in increased automaticity. At higher levels of potassium, the time course of the change in the membrane potential is different and is associated with the appearance of delayed after-depolarizations (Fig. 32–8). After-depolarizations have also been designated a transient depolarization that appears initially as a subthreshold depolarization early during Phase 4 or as a damped train of after-depolarizations. The amplitude of the after-depolarization increases as digitalis toxicity develops until the threshold for the initiation of an action potential is reached. At this point the delayed after-depolarization initiated by the extra response is also likely to reach the threshold, because the amplitude of the delayed after-depolarization increases as the interval between the action potentials decreases. Thus, digitalis can trigger ectopic beats by two different mechanisms: (1) the development of delayed after-depolarizations, and (2) the enhancement of normal Phase 4 depolarization.

The precise mechanisms by which digitalis glycosides exert their direct effects to alter the transmembrane potential of cardiac fibers is still under study. Low levels of digitalis do not influence the fast inward sodium current. Thus, the increase in the action potential duration observed with low concentrations of digitalis may be due to inhibition of sodium/potassium ATPase. The inhibition of the pump and the resultant decrease in the outward sodium current produces a modest decrease in the resting potential and an increase in the slope of diastolic depolarization. The extracellular potassium concentration in the interfiber spaces transiently increases during each action potential because of the potassium efflux from the cardiac fibers. This increase is magnified when the sodium/potassium pump is inhibited by a glycoside. The increased extracellular potassium

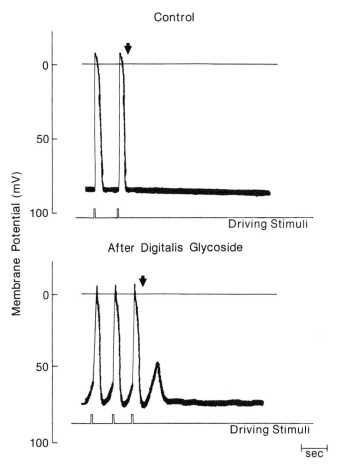

Control

After Digitalis Glycoside

Driving Stimuli

Driving Stimuli

sec

Figure 32–8

Digitalis-induced changes in Phase 4 depolarization. The top panel is the control Purkinje fiber superfused with Tyrode's solution. The drive stimuli are discontinued at the *arrows,* and electrical quiescence follows. The *bottom panel* was recorded after 35 minutes of superfusion with 2×10^{-7} M ouabain. Phase 4 depolarization is occurring, and discontinuation of the driving stimuli *(arrow)* is followed by a delayed after-depolarization and subsequent electrical quiescence. (Adapted from Rosen MR, Wit AL, Hoffman BF: Electrophysiology and pharmacology of cardiac arrhythmias. IV. Cardiac antiarrhythmic and toxic effects of digitalis. Am Heart J 89:391, 1975.)

increases the time to the onset of repolarization by increasing membrane permeability to potassium. Because there is a small decrease in the resting potential, conduction velocity may increase slightly.

As the concentration of digitalis increases, the decrease in pump activity produces an additional lowering of the resting potential, and both the potassium equilibrium potential and the resting potential decline as the extracellular potassium concentration increases. The internal sodium concentration increases the sodium equilibrium potential and prolongs the action potential amplitude decrease. The increase in the slow inward current shifts the action potential plateau to more positive potentials and prolongs the action potential duration. It is assumed that toward the end of the plateau the total outward current is increased enough to offset the change in the slow inward current, because the action potential is actually shortened; three contributory factors are thought to be involved:

1. An elevation of the internal calcium concentration speeds up the inactivation of the slow inward current and increases the outward current carried by potassium.

2. As the pump is further inhibited, the external potassium concentration increases even more during each action potential and thus speeds the onset of repolarization.

3. As toxicity develops, Phase 0 is depressed because of

   a. a greater loss of the resting potential and the voltage-dependent inactivation of the sodium channels;

   b. the greater increase in the internal sodium concentration; and

   c. the direct action of the glycoside to modify the voltage dependence of sodium channel inactivation.

Low levels of digitalis may increase action potential duration by inhibition of Na^+/K^+ ATPase, resulting in

1. a decrease in outward Na^+ current
2. decrease in the resting potential
3. increase in the slope of diastolic depolarization
4. increased extracellular K^+, which increases the time to the onset of repolarization by increasing membrane permeability to K^+
5. slight increase in conduction velocity (due to the small decrease in the resting potential)

Calcium is involved in the cardiac action potential plateau and changes in conduction velocity.

Conduction velocity decreases because of the reduction in the excitatory currents associated with small action potentials and because of the decrease in the extracellular spread of current produced by calcium at the gap junctions between cardiac fibers. The overall result of these changes is a reduction in the amount of cardiac tissue that can be excited by an action potential at any one time.

Multiple factors are thought to be involved in the cellular electrophysiological changes associated with arrhythmias associated with digitalis toxicity. The automaticity in the Purkinje fibers is thought to be associated with an inward current carried mostly by the sodium ion; the action of digitalis on this current is unknown. It is known that digitalis induces the delayed after-depolarizations by causing a calcium overload that is associated with an oscillatory release and reuptake of calcium by intracellular stores such as the sarcoplasmic reticulum. The oscillatory changes in the internal calcium concentration result in "after-contractions" and a simultaneous transient inward current due to alteration in the exchange of sodium for calcium or from a special sarcolemmal conductance, which then initiates the after-depolarizations. Any increase in the internal calcium concentration causes delayed after-depolarizations and after-contractions. Factors such as blockade of the slow inward channels or a decrease in the external calcium concentration reduces the influx of calcium and decreases or abolishes the delayed after-depolarizations and after-contractions.

Purkinje fibers are more sensitive to digitalis toxicity than are ventricular muscle fibers. The left Purkinje fibers have been shown to be more sensitive to ouabain than the right Purkinje fibers, at least in the dog, and it was concluded that the action of this glycoside was nonuniform. In both Purkinje and ventricular fibers the toxicity develops more quickly if the fibers are stimulated at a faster rate. An increase in the extracellular potassium inhibits the development of digitalis toxicity, whereas an increase in the extracellular calcium concentration facilitates the occurrence of toxicity. An increase in the extracellular potassium may reverse the toxicity by stimulating the pump or by decreasing the binding of digitalis to the sodium/potassium ATPase enzyme.

ELECTROCARDIOGRAPHIC

The primary effects on the electrocardiogram (ECG) of therapeutic dosages and levels of digitalis are PR-interval prolongation, QT shortening, ST depression, and T-wave depression. The effect of digitalis on the ST segment has been referred to as the hockey-stick appearance or as an inverted

---

Side notes (left margin):

Digitalis toxicity increases automaticity in Purkinje fibers.

Digitalis induces delayed after-depolarizations.

Purkinje fibers are more sensitive to digitalis toxicity than are ventricular muscle fibers.

Ouabain exerts a nonuniform action in that left Purkinje fibers are more sensitive than right fibers.

Stimulation of ventricular fibers at a faster rate induces digitalis toxicity more rapidly.

Digitalis in therapeutic doses

1. prolongs the P-R interval
2. shortens the QT interval
3. depresses the ST segment
4. depresses the T wave

Figure 32–9

Electrocardiographic effects of digitalis glycoside. *Top tracing* has been copied from an ECG in a patient receiving digitalis, showing the typical "hockey-stick" appearance of the ST segment. *Bottom tracing* shows coupled ventricular extrasystole. (a = normal QRS complex; b = ventricular extrasystole.) (Redrawn from Joubert PH: Digitalis in clinical practice. S Afr Med J 50:146–152, 1976. This figure has been redrawn from the South African Medical Journal vol 50 dated 31 January 1976, with permission.)

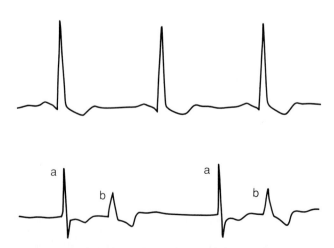

correction mark and may be quite characteristic, especially in the absence of pre-existing T-wave abnormalities (Fig. 32–9).

THE CARDIOVASCULAR SYSTEM

The effects of a digitalis glycoside are the result of multiple actions, including changes in the force of ventricular contraction, heart rate, vascular smooth muscles, reflex hemodynamic status, activity of the autonomic nervous system, and the presence or absence of congestive heart failure. Measurements of the effect of digitalis on arterial blood pressure, cardiac output, heart size, and end-diastolic and venous pressures vary with the presence or absence of anesthesia, exercise, and stress.

BLOOD PRESSURE

The IV injection of cardiac glycosides, especially aglycones, increases arterial pressure due to a direct vasoconstrictive action on peripheral vessels and a central sympathetic or reflex action. Glycosides also alter blood pressure through an action on the autonomic nervous system. The vasoconstriction that occurs through an action on the α-adrenergic receptors occurs in a dose-response fashion. Thus, an IV bolus dose may cause an immediate contraction of the smooth muscle vasculature through the direct action of the glycoside and a slower, prolonged vasoconstriction that can be blocked by α-blocking agents. In a normal individual, mean arterial blood pressure, systemic vascular resistance, and venomotor tone may be moderately increased and forearm blood flow decreased by glycosides. Patients with congestive heart failure respond with reduced peripheral resistance and vasomotor tone. Usually there is no increase in arterial pressure, although it may increase if there is an increased stroke volume.

SMOOTH MUSCLE VEINS

Digitalis acts directly on the smooth muscles of veins to induce constriction. This action is prominent in the hepatic veins and may cause venous pooling in portal vessels.

HEART

Contractility increases due to the direct positive inotropic action of digitalis. Heart rate may decrease moderately, stroke volume increase, and end-systolic ventricular volume decrease slightly. The increase in contractility is countered by the combined effect of increased systemic vascular resistance and decreased heart rate, thus cardiac output generally remains constant or decreases slightly. The decrease in the heart rate is primarily due to a reflex action of arterial baroreceptors to the rate of change and the extent of increase in arterial pressure. Glycosides also exert a direct positive inotropic action with the left ventricle capable of maintaining or increasing stroke volume and maintaining cardiac output without increasing end-diastolic fiber length. The inotropic action persists in spite of increased aortic pressure.

CORONARY CIRCULATION

Therapeutic dosages of digitalis induce little or no direct action on coronary circulation, but after toxic dosages coronary vessels are constricted with a decrease in coronary flow (Fig. 32–10). The autonomically mediated α

Organ/System Pharmacology

Multiple sites are involved in the action of digitalis on the cardiovascular system.

Glycosides modify blood pressure by a direct α-adrenergic vasoconstrictive action on peripheral vessels and by a central sympathetic or reflex action.

Glycosides excite the smooth muscle of veins.

Digitalis inhibits a positive inotropic action on the heart.

Toxic dosages of digitalis constrict coronary vessels.

Figure 32-10

Effects of digitalis glycosides on flow in coronary vessels. Coronary flow (ml/min) was measured in isolated perfused guinea pig Langendorff's heart preparations. Hearts were equilibrated for the first 60 minutes following mounting. At 62 minutes, ouabain (1.37×10^{-6} M) was added to the reservoir bottle containing perfusing media. Untreated controls (n = 14) are shown in black; ouabain-treated hearts are in color. (* — p = 0.02, ** — p = 0.005, *** — p = 0.001.) (Redrawn from Tanz RD, Russell NJ, Banerian SP, Sharp VH: Ouabain-induced tachyarrhythmias and cell damage in isolated perfused guinea pig hearts. I. Protection by propranolol. J Mol Cell Cardiol 14:655, 1982.)

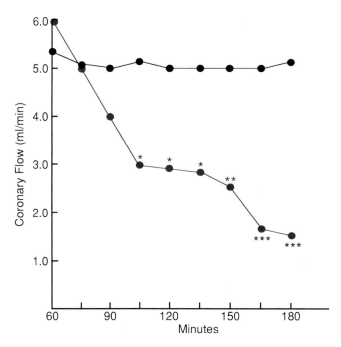

constriction is a dose-related effect that is centrally mediated and that can be blocked by α-blocking agents.

Adverse Effects

Both the ECG and plasma levels must be assessed to determine digitalis toxicity because of the variability among individual plasma levels.

In 1785 Withering estimated the prevalence of digitalis toxicity to be 18–25%. In the 1970s reports suggested that it varied between 20 and 30%; the incidence in the 1980s seemed to be lower, with a prevalence of 6–18%. The detection of digitalis toxicity is confounded by the fact that *digitalis serum levels in patients exhibiting good control of cardiac failure with no toxicity overlap with those obtained in patients manifesting digitalis toxicity (Fig. 32–11). Thus, determining the serum level is important but insufficient; it is also essential to monitor the patient's electrocardiogram and clinical condition.*

Table 32-3 OCCURRENCE OF DIGITALIS-INDUCED ARRHYTHMIAS (n = 926)		
Type of Arrhythmias	**N**	**Percent of all arrhythmias***
Ventricular arrhythmias	567	62
Ventricular premature beats	481	
Ventricular tachycardia	85	
Ventricular fibrillation	1	
A-V block	314	34
Atrial arrhythmias	248	27
Fibrillation, tachycardia, premature beats, flutter		
Junctional rhythms	138	15
S-A arrhythmias	106	12
Tachycardia, bradycardia, arrest, block, wandering pacemaker		
A-V dissociation	92	10

Adapted from Fisch C, Stone JM: *In* Fisch C, Surawicz B (eds): Digitalis, 162–173. Orlando, FL: Grune & Stratton, 1969.
* The percentages add up to more than 100% because a given individual or study may have more than one type of arrhythmia.

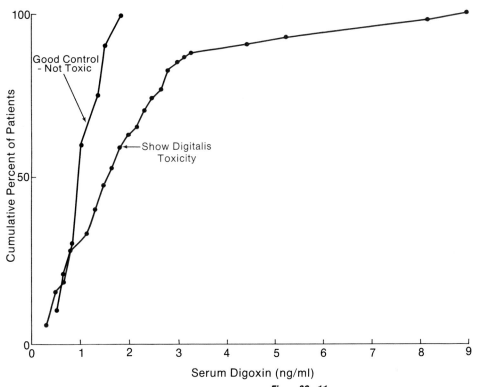

Figure 32 – 11

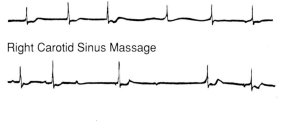

CARDIAC TOXICITY

The more common and most serious forms of digitalis toxicity are those related to alterations in cardiac rate and rhythm. Extrasystoles are the most common cardiac effect and generally originate in the ventricle (Table 32–3; Fig. 32–12; see also Fig. 32–9). Bigeminy and pulsus trigeminus may develop. Younger patients, in particular, may exhibit sinus arrhythmia. Paroxysmal atrial or ventricular tachycardia may be observed. Although the occurrence is unusual, atrial flutter or atrial fibrillation may be associated in individuals with congestive heart failure who previously exhibited a normal sinus rhythm. Other arrhythmias associated with toxicity may include A-V block, A-V junctional tachycardia, pulsus alternans, and atrial standstill (Table 32–3). Death associated with digitalis toxicity is most often due to ventricular fibrillation.

Figure 32 – 11

Relationships between serum digoxin level (abscissa) and digitalis toxicity (ordinate). The "good control—not toxic" curve is a plot of the cumulative percent of patients in good control of their congestive failure and their respective digoxin blood levels. The cumulative frequency plot of the blood levels of those patients who exhibited toxicity is on the right. Note that some patients exhibited toxicity even at very low levels of digoxin, whereas all those in good control without toxicity had levels below 2 ng/ml. (Data from Joubert PH: Digitalis in clinical practice. S Afr Med J 50:146–152, 1976.)

Digitalis toxicity may be associated with atrial or ventricular arrhythmias.

Figure 32 – 12

Electrocardiogram of a 17-year-old woman after she attempted to commit suicide by ingesting 3.0–4.0 mg (30–40 tablets) of digitoxin. The *upper strips,* recorded on the day of ingestion, demonstrate depression of S-A node activity and supraventricular rate after right carotid sinus massage. The *next strip,* recorded on the same day, shows regular sinus rhythm with a rate of 90 beats/minute and a normal PR interval after IV administration of 0.4 mg of atropine sulfate. *Bottom strip,* recorded 4 days after digitoxin ingestion, demonstrates persistent depression of S-A node activity and supraventricular escape complexes. (From Surawicz B, Mortelmans S: Factors affecting individual tolerance to digitalis. *In* Fisch C, Surawicz B [eds]: Digitalis, 127–147. Orlando, FL: Grune & Stratton, 1969.)

Right Carotid Sinus Massage

After 0.4 mg Atropine

4 Days Later

Ventricular arrhythmias induced by digitalis are due to the impairment of cardiac automaticity, leading to parasystole and ventricular tachycardia. The resting membrane potential is lowered at pacemaker sites. Thus, even if an ectopic pacemaker does not drive the heart, electrical conduction through the pacemaker areas is slower than that going through nonpacemaker sites. Thus, re-entrant arrhythmias, including extrasystoles and coupled rhythms, may be initiated. Digitalis also slows conduction within Purkinje fibers. This action may be due to the decrease in the membrane potential associated with inhibition of the sodium/potassium ATPase activity. This may cause slowing of conduction or left and right bundle-branch block simultaneously with the altered cardiac rhythm. The occurrence of both slowed conduction and increased automaticity may initiate potentially lethal ventricular fibrillation.

A faster heart rate in an *in vitro* preparation induces digitalis toxicity more rapidly.

Hearts or *in vitro* preparations driven at faster rates develop digitalis toxicity faster. This may be due to a greater uptake of digitalis into the cardiac tissue, an increased ionic exchange in the presence of inhibition of the sodium/potassium pump, or a postulated increase in calcium ion movement. The last is thought to contribute to the late stage of depolarization of the action potential and to the plateau phase during repolarization. That an alteration in the transmembrane exchange of calcium ions may be involved is suggested by the synergistic actions of calcium and digitalis that produce cardiac arrhythmias. Use of chelating agents or citrate to lower blood calcium levels may abolish digitalis-induced ectopic beats. The calcium ion is thought to be involved in the development of after-depolarizations associated with digitalis-induced toxicity; the greater the concentration of calcium, the more pronounced the oscillatory potentials. Calcium is carried through the membrane slow channels to contribute to a significant inward current during the plateau portion of the cardiac action potential. Agents, such as manganese and verapamil, that block the calcium current through the slow channels decrease or eliminate digitalis-induced arrhythmias. It has been suggested that because the loss of potassium, due to inhibition of sodium/potassium ATPase, may be the basis of digitalis toxicity, potassium may be antagonistic to digitalis intoxication, especially if serum potassium is low. Low levels of potassium enhance oscillating afterpotentials whereas high levels reduce the calcium-induced after-potentials. Thus, the ionic movement of both potassium and calcium are involved in digitalis-induced toxicity.

Calcium ion is involved in after-depolarization associated with digitalis toxicity.

CONTRIBUTION OF THE AUTONOMIC NERVOUS SYSTEM TO THE PRODUCTION OF DIGITALIS TOXICITY

Digitalis induces arrhythmias through a direct action on the heart and by modifying autonomic neural activity.

Digitalis toxicity induces arrhythmias through mechanisms involving both direct actions on the heart and through modifications of the neural activity of both divisions of the autonomic nervous system (Table 32–4). Digitalis

Table 32–4 MECHANISMS OF DIGITALIS TOXICITY

Site of Action of Digoxin	Toxic Electrophysiologic Effect
Sinus node	Antiadrenergic, direct drug effect
Atrium	First-degree direct drug effect, increased automaticity, triggered activity
A-V node	First-degree direct effect, cholinergic
Purkinje fibers and ventricular muscle	Increased automaticity, delayed after-depolarizations, re-entry mechanism

Reprinted by permission of the Western Journal of Medicine. Bhatia SJS: Digitalis toxicity—Turning over a new leaf? 1986, July, 145:74–82.

increases activity of the cardiac vagus nerve resulting in a slowing of the heart rate and the possible initiation of atrial fibrillation or A-V block. Digitalis also alters the activity of the sympathetic nervous system. In the early stages of digitalis toxicity the discharge of the postganglionic cardiac sympathetic branches becomes nonuniform, i.e., activity in some fibers is increased while simultaneously there are decreases or no changes in others. This nonuniform discharge is probably due to glycoside action on multiple sites within the adrenergic nervous system, i.e., pre- and postganglionic fibers, the postganglionic adrenergic nerve terminal, adrenal catecholamines, baroreceptors, and the central nervous system (CNS), including brainstem regions of the area postrema and the nucleus tractus solitarius. The nonuniform neural discharge imposes a nonuniform increase in excitability within the myocardium, predisposing it to the development of arrhythmias. As toxicity progresses, an enhanced sympathetic cardiac discharge contributes to the maintenance of arrhythmias; agents such as reserpine, guanethidine, or bretylium that prevent the actions of the adrenergic neural discharge on the heart can protect against arrhythmias induced by digitalis (see Chapter 33).

> Digitalis increases vagal activity and slows the heart.

> Digitalis exhibits a nonuniform action on the discharge of cardiac sympathetic nerves, resulting in the development of ventricular arrhythmias.

CORONARY CONSTRICTION AND TOXICITY

Figure 32–13 depicts a suggested contribution of digitalis-induced coronary constriction to digitalis toxicity. The resultant ischemia/hypoxia induces a number of changes that ultimately result in arrhythmia.

> Digitalis toxicity includes coronary constriction that results in ischemia and hypoxia.

CENTRAL NERVOUS SYSTEM

Eye

Digitalis toxicity includes a variety of visual disturbances including blurred vision, white borders or a halo around dark objects, transitory amblyopia, and changes in color vision. The latter most often include chromatopsia for yellow and green but occasionally for red, brown, and blue. Data obtained in human subjects indicate that differences in the pharmacokinetic parameters of digitalis preparations may influence the degree to which these

> A frequent manifestation of digitalis toxicity is a change in vision.

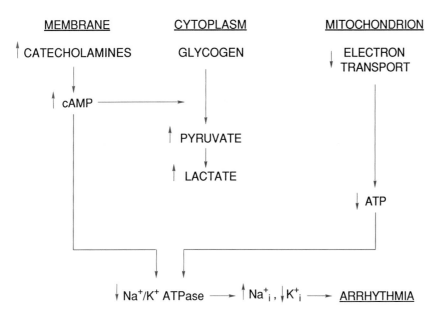

ISCHEMIA/HYPOXIA

Figure 32–13

Proposed mechanism(s) whereby digitalis-induced coronary constriction may contribute to the formation of toxic arrhythmias. (From Tanz RD: Possible contribution of digitalis-induced coronary constriction to toxicity. Am Heart J 111:812–817, 1985.)

Table 32–5   FREQUENCIES OF ERROR SCORES IN COLOR VISION

| Drug | Plasma Digitalis Level | | Volume (L) Distribution | Extent of Plasma Protein Binding (%) |
	Therapeutic	Toxic		
Digoxin	17/28	5/5	840	10–25
Digitoxin	0/13	7/13	38	86
Acetyldigitoxin	0/8	3/8	57.5	81–90

From Haustein KO, Oltmanns G, Rietbrock N, Aiken RG: Differences in color vision impairment caused by digoxin, digitoxin, or pengitoxin. J Cardiovasc Pharmacol 4:536–541, 1982.

Pharmacokinetic properties of different glycosides vary and result in different effects on color vision.

agents produce visual disturbances. The error scores in color vision testing increased as the digitalis glycoside plasma levels increased. Table 32–5 presents the error scores in color vision in patients taking the digitalis preparation indicated. Thus, digoxin altered color discrimination in approximately two thirds (17 of 28) of the patients with therapeutic levels and all of those with toxic levels (5 of 5). Neither digitoxin nor acetyldigitoxin impaired color discrimination in individuals with therapeutic levels. Seven of 13 digitoxin-treated patients and three of eight acetyl-digitoxin-treated patients exhibited disturbances in color vision at toxic levels. It was suggested that these differences may be due to the higher uptake of some glycosides into the retina or to a difference in the concentration of the glycoside within the retina. The latter is determined by the volume of distribution of the glycoside. Thus, digitoxin and acetyldigitoxin have low distribution volumes when compared to digoxin. The differences in the volume of distribution are thought to be related to the variations in the extent of binding to plasma protein found among the glycosides. Of the three glycosides, digoxin would be present in the retina in the highest concentration. Nevertheless, patient complaints of disturbed or yellow vision, or actual tests thereof, provide another warning sign of possible toxicity.

Brain

Central symptoms of digitalis intoxication include headache, fatigue, malaise, and drowsiness.

Patients intoxicated with digitalis may complain of headache, fatigue, malaise, and drowsiness. These complaints are often noted in the early stages of intoxication. Mental confusion and disorientation generally precede the more serious signs of cardiac toxicity and they are a significant hazard, all too frequently unrecognized, in the elderly.

Gastrointestinal

Digitalis may act on the chemoreceptor trigger zone to induce vomiting.

In some, but not all, patients the earliest symptoms of digitalis overdosage include anorexia, nausea, and vomiting due to a central action on the chemoreceptor trigger zone. Anorexia is usually observed first, followed several days later by episodes of nausea and vomiting that may begin and end abruptly and then recur with greater severity. Other reported GI effects include diarrhea and abdominal discomfort or pain that subside several days after the digitalis glycoside is discontinued.

Management of Patients Exhibiting Digitalis Toxicity

As noted earlier, the diagnosis of digitalis intoxication cannot be made from an evaluation of only the glycoside plasma levels, because a great overlap exists among the levels associated with toxic and nontoxic conditions (see Fig. 32–11). The occurrence of arrhythmias in the ECG clearly establishes digitalis-induced toxicity. The plasma potassium level should be ascertained, especially if the patient is taking a diuretic that induces loss of potassium; low potassium levels enhance the likelihood of intoxication (Table 32–6).

Plasma K^+ levels must be monitored when treating digitalis toxicity, especially if a diuretic that induces K^+ loss is also being taken.

Once digitalis intoxication has been established, digitalis and diuretic therapy causing potassium depletion must be discontinued. If the serum potassium levels are low the administration of potassium orally or intravenously may reverse digitalis-induced ectopic rhythms without altering the inotropic actions. The administration of potassium decreases the binding of digitalis to the heart and antagonizes the inhibitory effect of digitalis on the sodium pump. If IV potassium is given, the ECG must be monitored frequently and plasma potassium levels measured before and after the administration of potassium. The use of potassium may be dangerous if the patient has A-V block because potassium depresses A-V conduction, an action synergistic with that of digitalis. Also, if the administration of potassium results in hyperkalemia, this will have a direct depressant action on A-V conduction, contribute to the initiation of arrhythmias, and may produce complete A-V block and cardiac arrest. The administration of potassium may mask warning signals normally detected by the occurrence of less ominous arrhythmias; thus, lethal arrhythmias such as ventricular fibrillation may occur with no initial warning change in the ECG.

If K^+ levels are low in digitalis toxicity, giving K^+ decreases digitalis binding to the heart and antagonizes inhibition of the Na^+/K^+ ATPase pump.

The antiarrhythmic agents that reverse digitalis-induced tachyarrhythmias include phenytoin, lidocaine, β blockers, or procainamide. Low dosages of phenytoin or lidocaine do not exert a depressant action on A-V conduction, and therapeutic dosages do not alter conduction in the His-

Phenytoin, lidocaine, β blockers, or procainamide may be used to treat arrhythmias induced by digitalis.

Table 32–6 FACTORS AFFECTING MYOCARDIAL TOLERANCE TO DIGITALIS

Possible Reasons for Increased Sensitivity	Possible Reasons for Increased Tolerance
Cardiac	
Increased automaticity of ectopic pacemakers	Decreased automaticity of ectopic pacemakers
Heart disease*	High potassium*
Heart surgery*	Antiarrhythmic drugs†
Low potassium*	Vagal stimulation
Chronic lung disease	Decreased vagal or increased sympathetic activity
Catecholamines and sympathetic	Fever, infection, hypoxia
stimulation†	Hyperthyroidism*
Impaired S-A function and A-V conduction	Normal infants and young children
Increased vagal activity	Decreased absorption or unusual losses
Decreased sympathetic activity	Malabsorption
Heart disease*	Dialysis (?)
Heart surgery*	Cardiac bypass (?)
Low potassium*	
High potassium	
Low magnesium	
Impaired degradation or excretion	
Hypothyroidism*	
Renal disease*	
Liver disease	
Premature infants*	
Old age	
Interaction with drugs	
Extracardiac	
Allergy and hypersensitivity	
CNS disorders, such as CVAs	
Low body weight	

Adapted from Surawicz B: Factors affecting tolerance to digitalis. Reprinted with permission from the American College of Cardiology (Journal of the American College of Cardiology, vol. 5, 1985, 69A–81A.).
* Factors that appear to be of greatest practical importance.
† Variable effects.
A-V = atrioventricular; CNS = central nervous system; S-A = sinoatrial node.

Atropine may control digitalis-induced sinus bradycardia.

Monoclonal digoxin-specific antibodies, Fab fragments, bind digoxin and free Na$^+$/K$^+$ ATPase, thus reversing the toxic inotropic actions of digoxin.

Purkinje system slowed by the administration of digitalis. Phenytoin can abolish the ventricular tachycardia associated with toxicity, decreasing the extent of digitalis-induced A-V conduction impairment, yet not interfering with the digitalis' inotropic effect.

Procainamide or propranolol also may be used to treat arrhythmias caused by digitalis, but they may induce complete A-V dissociation, making heart block worse (Table 32–7). Atropine can successfully control digitalis-induced sinus bradycardia, S-A arrest, and second- or third-degree A-V block.

Bretylium should be avoided, because the initial release of catecholamines associated with its administration may aggravate the arrhythmias initiated by digitalis. Likewise, electrical counter-shock releases catecholamines, and fatal ventricular fibrillation may develop in the presence of digitalis-induced arrhythmia. Thus, although cardioversion is used infrequently in digitalis toxicity, when it is employed extreme caution should be used. While reversing the ventricular tachyarrhythmias associated with toxicity, the energy level selected should be minimal at first and increased carefully in an attempt to avoid precipitating ventricular arrhythmia. Lidocaine may also be administered as a pretreatment to prevent the development of ventricular fibrillation. Often the defibrillation is unsuccessful because the myocardium is extremely irritable. In this situation, IV amiodarone may be used (see Chapter 33). If the antiarrhythmic agents discussed earlier fail to reverse life-threatening digitalis toxicity, the monoclonal digoxin-specific antibodies, Fab fragments (Smith, 1985), may be administered. Digoxin has a greater affinity for the antibody and thus binds to the Fab fragment rather than binding to the sodium/potassium ATPase receptor. Thus, digoxin is removed from the receptor site, enters the general circulation, and is readily excreted. Detectable antibodies to the Fab fragments have not been detected in serum and hemodynamic instability does not develop. The use of the digoxin-specific antibodies reverses its positive inotropic action and eliminates its toxic effects on Purkinje fibers and the

Table 32-7 POTENTIAL USES AND TOXICITY OF SECOND-LINE DRUGS FOR DIGOXIN TOXICITY

Drug	May Increase A-V Block	May Increase Ventricular Ectopy	Negative Inotropic Effect	Potential Indications
Procainamide hydrochloride or quinidine	Yes	No	Yes	Ventricular ectopy, ventricular tachycardia, atrial tachycardia with block, AVT
β blockers	Yes	No	Yes	Ventricular ectopy, ventricular tachycardia, atrial tachycardia with block
Verapamil	Yes	No	Yes	Atrial tachycardia with block, AVT, ventricular ectopy, ventricular tachycardia
Amiodarone	Yes	No	Yes	Ventricular tachycardia (refractory dysrhythmia)
Isoproterenol	No	Yes	No	Bradycardia (refractory dysrhythmia)
Bretylium tosylate	No	Yes	No	Ventricular tachycardia, ventricular fibrillation (refractory dysrhythmia)

Reprinted by permission of the Western Journal of Medicine. Bhatia SJS: Digitalis toxicity—Turning over a new leaf? 1986, July, 145:74–82.
A-V = atrioventricular; AVT = nonparoxysmal atrioventricular junctional tachycardia.

A-V node. Once the Fab fragments have been used, it is necessary to re-establish therapeutic effects by retitrating the patient with digitalis.

The digitalis glycosides are employed in the treatment of congestive heart failure and arrhythmias such as atrial fibrillation, atrial flutter, and atrial and A-V nodal paroxysmal tachycardia. In toxic dosages they initiate ventricular arrhythmias. Table 32–6 summarizes the factors that may increase sensitivity and tolerance to digitalis.

Therapeutic Uses

Digitalis is used to treat congestive heart failure, atrial fibrillation and flutter, and atrial and A-V nodal paroxysmal tachycardia.

CONGESTIVE HEART FAILURE

The most common therapeutic use for digitalis glycosides is in the management of heart failure. The management of congestive heart failure is designed to decrease sodium and water intake, reduce the work of the heart, and to employ pharmacologic agents such as digitalis, diuretics, vasodilators, or catecholamines. Some patients, such as those exhibiting advanced ischemic heart disease, may not respond to this regimen or may become refractory to treatment. Patients with heart failure due to valvular, coronary artery, or congenital heart disease should undergo cardiac catheterization to determine whether surgical intervention would lessen or correct the underlying lesion. However, if patients with these lesions have progressed to an advanced state of heart failure, severe disorders of contractility may still be present in spite of surgery.

Congestive heart failure is managed by using various combinations of

1. decreasing Na^+ and water intake
2. digitalis
3. diuretics
4. vasodilators
5. catecholamines

Patients with mild heart failure may be treated acutely with synthetic catecholamines and diuretics. Mild heart failure may respond to digitalis. Moderately severe heart failure may respond to digitalis and a diuretic. A venous vasodilator may be added if continued pulmonary congestion is present. An arterial vasodilator may be used if the patient is weak or if other low-output symptoms are present. Prazosin or an angiotensin-converting enzyme inhibitor may be used if both congestion and weakness are noted. Severe chronic heart failure with a history of nocturnal orthopnea may respond to topical nitroglycerin or intramuscular morphine sulfate. After 2 or 3 days, the latter is discontinued but the topical nitroglycerin may be continued. A loading dose and then a maintenance dose of digitalis may be given; furosemide, ethacrynic acid, or bumetanide may be used also. A potassium-sparing diuretic or a thiazide diuretic may be added. Venous vasodilators may be used if the congestive symptoms are prominent. In the presence of low-output symptoms, arterial vasodilators are employed. The presence of both types of symptoms may respond to a combination of arterial and venous vasodilatory agents such as hydralazine or nitrates, a drug with both actions, or to an angiotensin-converting enzyme inhibitor.

Prazosin or an angiotensin-converting enzyme inhibitor may be used to treat congestive heart failure.

The use of digitalis in patients with myocardial infarction is controversial. Digoxin has been shown to produce a minimal but significant improvement in the ejection fraction without compromising left ventricular perfusion or regional wall motion. However, the benefit of the digitalis-induced increase in contractility may be offset by the resulting bulging of the infarcted and ischemic myocardium. Furthermore, the digoxin-induced increase in peripheral resistance may produce an increase in the afterload, which may counter the inotropic action. Different responses to digitalis may result in different patients with infarctions due to the fact that the overall hemodynamic response is a result of several factors: the direct inotropic action on the myocardium; the consequence of the inotropic action on nonresponsive myocardium; and the variable action on systemic vascular resistance. Pulmonary edema may occur as a result of the increased systemic vascular resistance due to the direct arteriolar vasoconstriction.

Digitalis use in myocardial infarction is controversial.

It is recommended that digitalis should not be used in the patient with infarction if there is no evidence of heart failure. Digitalis and a diuretic may be used in infarction patients if pulmonary congestion is present, although the diuretic can be given alone to ascertain its effects. Digitalis may be used to treat acute pulmonary edema due to infarction, but it is recommended that its use follow the administration of nitroprusside to reduce afterload. Digitalis may be used to control the ventricular rate of patients and its reversion to a normal sinus rhythm in those with infarction or angina with atrial fibrillation or flutter. In general, an increase in arrhythmias will not follow the use of digitalis in those with myocardial infarction.

CARDIOGENIC SHOCK

Digitalis use in the treatment of cardiogenic shock is controversial because digitalis increases the force of contraction in both normal and hypoxic myocardium.

Although digitalis may be used in patients with a normal rhythm and cardiogenic shock due to myocardial infarction, it generally is not. The use of digitalis glycosides in the treatment of cardiogenic shock is controversial because it increases the force of contraction in both normal and hypoxic myocardial tissue. Cardiac oxygen consumption associated with the administration of digitalis is determined by the changes in ventricular volume and contractility. In the failing heart, the decrease in volume and wall tension predominates over the increase in contractility, and cardiac oxygen consumption is usually decreased. (In the normal heart, the increase in contractility is usually greater than the decrease in volume, so oxygen utilization is increased.)

Cardiac O_2 consumption is determined by changes in ventricular volume and contractility.

The use of digitalis in the treatment of chronic heart failure is complicated by the fact that it is not possible to predict which patients may safely have their digoxin discontinued despite continuation of diuretic therapy. It is known that digitalis exhibits a long-term inotropic action in those with a normal sinus rhythm. In clinical studies, the withdrawal of digoxin was associated with clinical deterioration in most patients. Although in some patients with little evidence of failure while taking digoxin, withdrawal was associated with clinical deterioration. However, conflicting studies have concluded that chronic digoxin therapy is of no clinical benefit, because substitution of a placebo for 3 months was not associated with clinical deterioration. Thus, the identification of patients with chronic failure in whom digitalis may safely be discontinued is difficult. If digitalis was initially given to treat acute heart failure associated with myocardial infarctions, pneumonia, or surgery-induced failure and clinical signs of failure have not reappeared, it is generally concluded that the digitalis may be discontinued. Furthermore, some patients may have circulatory failure due to diastolic dysfunction; digitalis is not likely to induce an improvement in patients with failure in the presence of a normal left ventricular ejection fraction.

There is no universal consensus as to whether withdrawal of digoxin in patients with chronic heart failure is associated with clinical deterioration.

ANGIOTENSIN-CONVERTING ENZYME INHIBITION —CAPTOPRIL

The low output and congestion of congestive heart failure are due to changes in the renin-angiotensin-aldosterone system.

ACE inhibitors prevent the formation of active angiotensin from inactive angiotensin.

Alterations of renin-angiotensin-aldosterone regulation explain much of the pathophysiology of congestive heart failure, i.e., symptoms of low output and congestion. Use of an angiotensin-converting enzyme (ACE) inhibitor such as captopril (CAPOTEN) prevents the conversion of inactive angiotensin to active angiotensin (see Chapter 35) and is effective in the treatment of heart failure. The combination of digitalis, captopril, and generally a lower dosage of diuretic may be used to treat moderate severe or severe chronic heart failures in those patients who are not well controlled by digitalis and diuretics. The addition of an ACE inhibitor to the digitalis and diuretic drug regimen has been shown to increase the survival of patients with moderate to severe congestive heart failure. Captopril has been approved for use in the treatment of heart failure in those who have not tolerated digitalis. A recent study established that the use of captopril and diuretics in patients with mild to moderate heart failure improves functional capacity and exercise tolerance better than just diuretics alone and at least as much as the combination of digoxin and a diuretic. Ongoing studies are attempting to assess whether early treatment with an ACE inhibitor can prevent the development of heart failure and decrease mortality in patients recovering from myocardial infarction.

One advantage of the combination of an ACE inhibitor with a diuretic, but no digoxin, is that hypokalemia and ventricular arrhythmias occur less frequently. Unfortunately, one disadvantage of this combination is that hypotension and deterioration of renal function may occur.

ANTIARRHYTHMIC ACTIONS

Digitalis is often used to manage supraventricular arrhythmias including paroxysmal atrial tachycardia, atrial flutter, and shifting the atrial or A-V junctional tachycardia to a normal sinus rhythm, primarily through its effects to increase cholinergic neural activity. Also, sinus node discharges are decreased due to a direct action. Atrial cells are hyperpolarized, and conduction within the atria is increased. Conduction within the A-V node is decreased, and the A-V nodal effective refractory period is increased. The hyperpolarization and decreased slope of Phase 4 in specialized atrial cells explains the slowing or abolition of ectopic activity, as well as slowing of atrial pacemakers competing with the S-A node.

Digitalis also controls ventricular rhythm in patients exhibiting atrial flutter or fibrillation by an indirect autonomic effect that slows conduction and prolongs the effective refractory period in the A-V node; sometimes the atrial flutter or fibrillation is converted to normal sinus rhythm. When this occurs it is most likely that the underlying congestive heart failure with atrial load has initiated the arrhythmias. Premature atrial contractions may be suppressed. In general digitalis does not exhibit an antiarrhythmic action in the ventricles; this is predictable because there is no significant vagal innervation of the conducting system in the ventricles.

Digitalis is used to treat supraventricular arrhythmias, including paroxysmal atrial tachycardia and atrial flutter.

Digitalis does not exert a direct antiarrhythmic action in the ventricles but may indirectly produce an autonomic action on the A-V node and thus control ventricular rhythm.

PEDIATRIC PATIENTS

Therapeutic Aspects

Oral or parenteral digoxin controls congestive heart failure or arrhythmias in children. The feeding schedule does not appear to alter the absorption of digoxin from the GI tract. However, drug administration should be at times other than just before or after feeding because regurgitation or vomiting may cause unpredictable loss of drug. Although digoxin is used to manage infants and children, IV lanatoside C is often used for rapid digitalization, because the onset of action and time to peak effect are similar to those of digoxin. The use of IV digoxin in an emergency situation has an advantage because it allows a smoother transition to parenteral or oral maintenance dosages of digoxin after the emergency situation has been controlled. It is more difficult to make the transition to digoxin maintenance after initial IV lanatoside C because the latter is excreted more rapidly than digoxin and is marketed only in a parenteral dosing form. Suboptimal digoxin serum levels may occur because lanatoside C has a short half-life. It still is not clear whether a loading rather than a maintenance dosage of digoxin should be used when following digitalization with lanatoside C.

Effect of Age on the Action of Digitalis Glycosides

Oral or parenteral digoxin treats congestive heart failure or arrhythmias in children, but oral doses should not be given with feeding so that regurgitation or vomiting is avoided.

Decreased renal function necessitates lower dosages of digoxin in premature and immature infants.

Premature and immature infants require lower dosages of digoxin because of decreased renal function. The dosage regimen must be individualized according to the degree of maturity of the infant. (For a detailed description of dosage regimens for the premature newborn, the full-term neonate, infants, and children, see Wettrell and Andersson, 1986.) As the children get older the digoxin requirements are considerably increased until early teens, although the requirements may vary with different underlying diseases. These differences are thought to be due to altered binding to sodium/potassium ATPase and not to differences in renal function.

Toxic Effects

ECGs obtained in pediatric patients may not exhibit signs of digitalis toxicity even though symptoms of seizures, coma, or respiratory arrest occurred.

At the time that pediatric patients exhibit seizures, coma, and respiratory arrest due to digitalis intoxication, the ECG may reveal only rather innocuous changes. Vagal stimulation leading to sinus arrhythmia is often seen. Visual disturbances similar to those observed in adults have been reported.

Vomiting in an infant taking digitalis requires consideration of whether toxicity is present.

Infants often manifest changes in A-V conduction and atrial ectopic beats and may demonstrate paroxysmal atrial tachycardia with a variable ventricular response. Rarely do ventricular ectopic beats and tachyarrhythmias occur. Sinus slowing, with a rate less than 100 beats/minute due to increased vagal activity, may develop in premature and newborn infants. If a child taking a digitalis preparation begins to vomit, consideration of the possibility of toxicity is warranted. Explanations for the differences between cardiac toxicities observed in the adult and the newborn are unknown.

GERIATRIC PATIENTS

Therapeutic Aspects

Reduced renal function in geriatric patients usually requires a reduction in the digoxin dosage.

Nursing home patients on digitalis, a diuretic, or potassium should be monitored continuously for digitalis toxicity.

The half-life of digoxin may be 50% greater in geriatric patients.

The geriatric population in general has reduced renal function, necessitating a reduction in the dosage of digoxin. Patients on digitalis entering a nursing home may also receive a diuretic or potassium supplement, or both; thus, they must be followed and examined regularly to ensure the maintenance of a therapeutic level and to avoid the occurrence of unrecognized toxicity, *such as gradually increasing dementia.* Blood levels of digoxin and metabolites after a single dose have been reported to be almost twice as high in the geriatric patient as in younger patients; correspondingly, the digoxin half-life can be 50% greater in the elderly than in younger adults.

Toxic Effects

Adverse drug interactions with digitalis and over-the-counter drugs and with prescription medications must be considered when treating geriatric patients.

The elderly patient often takes several other drugs in addition to digitalis, so the possibility of adverse drug interactions with both prescription and over-the-counter preparations must be considered. Digitalis toxicity may develop in the geriatric patient given dosages of digoxin that are well tolerated in younger patients. Suggested explanations for this effect include an age-induced increase in myocardial sensitivity to the normal dosages, higher myocardial levels, hypokalemia due to diuretic or laxative use, a smaller body size, or decreased renal function resulting in an increased half-life for plasma levels of digitalis.

Drug Interactions

The single most frequent cause of digitalis toxicity arises from the concomitant use of digitalis and diuretics that causes the loss of potassium. The latter include thiazide diuretics, ethacrynic acid, furosemide, bumetanide, and acetazolamide. (Diuretics that do not cause the loss of potassium include spironolactone, triamterene, and amiloride.)

The concomitant use of digoxin and quinidine increases serum digoxin levels in more than 90% of the patients. The average serum increase is twofold, with a range from zero to sixfold. The increase in digoxin is due to a decrease in renal and nonrenal clearance and in the volume of distribution. Some digoxin is thought to be displaced from working myocardial-binding sites, but not from Purkinje fibers. The major portion of increased digoxin originates from nonspecific binding sites in skeletal muscle.

Current clinical approaches to the quinidine-digoxin interaction vary, although most physicians lower the amount of digoxin given when quinidine is started and then follow this with a plasma digoxin level within 24–48 hours. The follow-up digoxin dosage is adjusted on the basis of the level. When digoxin is used to control the ventricular response in atrial fibrillation, the reduction of the ventricular rate is used as a clinical guide. In this case the digoxin level does not necessarily have to be reduced when quinidine therapy is instituted.

The simultaneous use of digoxin and the calcium channel blockers is associated with variable effects on the digoxin levels. In more than 90% of the patients, verapamil increases the digoxin levels by decreasing its clearance and, possibly, its volume of distribution. Nifedipine does not appear to alter the digoxin levels, whereas diltiazem induces a small increase. In general, the dosage of digoxin does not need to be adjusted when calcium channel blockers are administered concurrently.

The use of digoxin and amiodarone increases the digoxin level twofold by decreasing clearance; the volume of distribution is not altered. Signs of digoxin toxicity may appear as the plasma digoxin levels increase. In general, the dosage of digoxin is not reduced when amiodarone therapy is started.

Spironolactone inhibits active tubular digoxin secretion, causing an increase in plasma digoxin levels. Likewise, antihypertensive agents may decrease renal blood flow and glomerular flow rate to increase the digoxin serum concentrations.

The absorption of digoxin is decreased by the concurrent administration of antacids, bran, kaolin pectate, cholestyramine resin, cholestipol hydrochloride, activated charcoal, sulfasalazine, neomycin, or para-aminosalicylic acid. If digoxin is given 2 hours prior to these agents, the decreased absorption is minimized. If the interacting agent is withdrawn without decreasing the dosage of digoxin, enhanced absorption and toxicity can occur. Digoxin absorption is decreased by metoclopramide hydrochloride or cathartics, drugs that increase intestinal motility. Cytotoxic drugs that induce malabsorption and mucosal damage decrease the absorption of digoxin. On the other hand, agents such as atropine or propantheline bromide that decrease intestinal motility increase the absorption of digoxin.

> Digitalis toxicity is most frequently caused by the concomitant use with diuretics that cause K^+ loss.

> Increased digoxin levels occur when given with quinidine due to a decrease in renal and nonrenal clearance of digoxin and a decrease in its volume of distribution.

> Verapamil increases plasma digoxin levels; nifedipine does not alter them; and diltiazem induces a small increase.

> Amiodarone increases plasma digoxin levels twofold by decreasing its clearance.

> Spironolactone increases plasma digoxin levels by actively inhibiting tubular digoxin secretion.

> Antihypertensive agents may decrease renal blood flow and glomerular flow rate, resulting in increased digoxin levels.

> Digoxin absorption is decreased by many agents such as antacids, bran, kaolin pectate, and neomycin.

Digitalis Assay and USP Unit

A comparison of the spectrophotometric assay of digoxin and digitoxin with reference standards is required by the United States Pharmacopeia (USP). A bioassay of powdered digitalis to compare the lethal dosage in pigeons with that produced by a reference standard is required. Tablets or capsules of digitalis powder are prescribed by weight or in units. The official USP unit is a potency of 100 mg of the USP digitalis reference standard powder and is approximately equivalent to 0.1 mg digitoxin.

> The USP requires assay of digoxin and digitoxin preparations to prevent unwanted toxicities due to variations in pharmaceutical preparations.

Preparations and Dosages

Digoxin (LANOXIN) is available in a variety of dosage formulations as tablets, capsules, an elixir, and injectable solutions. Digitoxin (CRYSTODIGIN, PURODI-

GIN) and deslanoside (desacetyl-lanatoside C; CEDILANID-D) are also available but have limited use.

Ouabain is not now commercially available in the United States but it is anticipated that the IV product will be reintroduced.

The average digitalizing dosage and usual daily oral maintenance dosage for various glycosides differ.

Table 32–1 summarizes the average digitalizing dosage and the usual daily oral maintenance dosage for various cardiac glycoside preparations. To treat overt heart failure and cardiac enlargement associated with acute myocardial infarction and cardiogenic shock, digoxin is commonly given in an initial loading dose of 0.25 mg or 0.5 mg, followed by daily doses of 0.125–0.25 mg IV or orally.

The renal and electrolyte status and the severity, type, and extent of arrhythmias and underlying disease determines the route and rapidity of administration of a digitalis preparation.

When using digitalis to treat arrhythmias, it is not possible to establish a fixed dosage schedule. The route and rapidity of administration is determined by the renal and electrolyte status of the patient, the severity of the arrhythmia, and the extent of the underlying cardiac disease. Maintenance dosages of digoxin range from 0.25 to 0.5 mg/day, although some patients may require more or less.

New Developments

Since 1785 when William Withering first recognized the benefit of digitalis, it has been the therapeutic basis for the treatment of congestive heart failure. This role has been questioned because its action on left ventricular end-diastolic pressure and cardiac output may be modest or of little value. Studies have yet to demonstrate that overall cardiac performance, i.e., left ventricular filling pressure and cardiac output, is improved even though ventricular contractility is consistently improved. Ongoing research is attempting to develop better inotropic agents.

Researchers are looking for new inotropic drugs, e.g., amrinone, that possess a larger therapeutic index than digitalis.

Much effort has been invested in the development of newer inotropic agents that possess a larger therapeutic index than digitalis. Amrinone (INOCOR) is such a compound. Amrinone is presently available only as an injectable and is used commonly in the critical care setting for the short-term treatment of patients with severe congestive heart failure who are refractory to cardiac glycosides and diuretics. It has been used also as supportive therapy in coronary bypass and surgical transplant patients. Amrinone (0.75 mg/kg, IV) may be injected over 2–3 minutes. An identical second dose may be given again in 30 minutes and followed by a maintenance infusion of 5–10 ug/kg/minute. The daily dosage should not be greater than 10 mg/kg. An oral form has been tested for the treatment of congestive heart failure but has been withdrawn from clinical trials because it induced hypotension, unwanted GI and CNS effects, and thrombocytopenia, arrhythmias, and sudden death and because it did not show long-term efficacy. The impact that amrinone will have on the clinical use of digoxin and other glycosides remains to be seen. It increases the force of atrial and ventricular muscle contraction without increasing the atrial rate *in vitro.*

In normal patients its IV administration produces a positive inotropic effect. The cardiac index is increased and ventricular end-diastolic, pulmonary capillary and right atrial pressures are decreased when given through the same route to digitalized patients with congestive heart failure. Mean heart rate is not altered, and the aortic mean pressure is decreased slightly. In patients with intractable myocardial failure who do not respond to digitalis or diuretics, the cardiac index may be increased and left ventricular ventricular-filling pressure may be decreased. Additional studies will determine ultimately its role in the treatment of congestive heart failure.

In the early 1980s digoxin immunoreactivity was noted in dog and human plasma and urine even though no digoxin had ever been administered. This factor has been termed *endoxin* because it is an endogenous substance that binds to digoxin antibodies. This postulated hormone can cross react in digoxin immunoassays, inhibit Na^+/K^+-ATPase, and cause natriuresis and diuresis. Endoxin should not be confused with atrial natriuretic factors that cause a natriuresis, diuresis, and a fall in blood pressure but do not cross react with digoxin antibodies and do not inhibit Na^+/K^+-ATPase. Correlations between the concentrations of endoxin and the mean arterial blood pressure in normotensive and hypertensive individuals have been found. (Although the etiology of essential hypertension is unknown, the discovery of endoxin and atrial natriuretic factor, substances that alter salt and water content, suggest that future studies may provide a better understanding of the pathogenesis of essential hypertension.)

An endogenous digoxin substance, endoxin, has been detected in human plasma.

References

Antman EM, Smith TW: Digitalis toxicity. Annu Rev Med 36:357–367, 1985.

Bhatia SJS: Digitalis toxicity—Turning over a new leaf. West J Med 145:74–82, 1986.

Bigger JT: Digitalis toxicity. J Clin Pharmacol 25:514–521, 1985.

The Captopril-Digoxin Multicenter Research Group. JAMA 259:539, 1988.

Cattell M, Gold H: Influence of digitalis glycosides on force of contraction of mammalian cardiac muscle. J Pharmacol Exp Ther 62:116–125, 1938.

Cervoni P, Chen PS: The digitalis glycosides. *In* Goldberg PR, Roberts J (eds): Handbook on Pharmacology of Aging, 15–23. Boca Raton, FL: CRC Press, 1983.

The Consensus Trial Study Group. N Engl J Med 316:1429, 1987.

Doherty JE: Clinical use of digitalis glycosides. Cardiology 72:225–254, 1985.

Gillis RA, Quest JA: The role of the nervous system in the cardiovascular effect of digitalis. Pharmacol Rev 31:19–97, 1980.

Graves SW, Brown B, Valdes R: An endogenous digoxin-like substance in patients with renal impairment. Ann Intern Med 99:604–608, 1983.

Han J, Moe GK: Nonuniform recovery of excitability in ventricular muscle. Circ Res 14:44–60, 1964.

Haustein KO, Oltmanns G, Rietbrock N, Aiken RG: Differences in color vision impairment caused by digoxin, digitoxin, or pengitoxin. J Cardiovasc Pharmacol 4:536–541, 1982.

Lathers CM, Kelliher GJ, Roberts J, Beasley AB: Nonuniform cardiac sympathetic nerve discharge: Mechanism for coronary occlusion and digitalis-induced arrhythmia. Circulation 57:1058–1065, 1978.

Lathers CM, Lipka LJ, Klions HA: Controversies in the actions of digitalis substances: Are all digitalis derivatives alike? J Clin Pharmacol 25:501–506, 1985.

Lathers CM, Lipka LJ, Klions HA: Digitalis glycosides: A discussion of the similarities and differences in actions and existing controversies. Rev Clin Basic Pharm 7:1–108, 1988.

Lathers CM, Roberts J: Digitalis toxicity revisited. Life Sci 27:1713–1733, 1980.

Lathers CM, Roberts J, Kelliher GJ: Correlation of ouabain-induced arrhythmia and nonuniformity in the histamine-evoked discharge of cardiac sympathetic nerves. J Pharmacol Exp Ther 203:467–479, 1977.

Mackenzie J: Digitalis. Heart 2:273–386, 1911.

Mancini DM, Keren G, Aogaichi K, et al: Inotropic drugs for the treatment of heart failure. J Clin Pharmacol 25:540–554, 1985.

Mathes S, Gold H, Marsh R, et al: Comparison of the tolerance of adults and children to digitoxin. JAMA 150:191–194, 1952.

Newman TJ, Maskin CS, Dennick LG, et al: Effects of captopril on survival in patients with heart failure. Am J Med 84(Suppl 3A):140–144, 1988.

Okita GT: Dissociation of Na^+, K^+-ATPase inhibition from digitalis inotropy. Fed Proc 36:2225–2230, 1977.

Reiser J, Anderson GJ: Preferential sensitivity of the left canine Purkinje system to cardiac glycosides. Circ Res 49:1043–1054, 1981.

Repke VK, Portius HJ: Uber die identitat der ionenpumpen-ATPase in der zellmembran des herzmuskels mit einem digitalis-rezeptorenzym. Experientia 19:452–458, 1963.

Roberts J, Kelliher GJ, Lathers CM: Minireview. Role of adrenergic influences in digitalis-induced ventricular arrhythmia. Life Sci 18:665–678, 1976.

Runge TM: Clinical implications of differences in pharmacodynamic action of polar and nonpolar cardiac glycosides. Am Heart J 93:248–255, 1977.

Runge TM, Stephens JC, Holden P, et al: Pharmacodynamic distinctions within the cardiac glycoside family. Technical report 73-1-R, Bio-Medical Engineering Research Laboratory, University of Texas at Austin, June, 1973.

Singh S: Clinical pharmacology of digitalis glycosides: A developmental viewpoint. Pediatr Ann 5:578–586, 1976.

Smith TW: New advances in the assessment and treatment of digitalis toxicity. J Clin Pharmacol 25:522–528, 1985.

Smith TW (ed): Digitalis Glycosides, 1–348. Orlando, FL: Grune and Stratton, 1986.

Soldin SJ: Digoxin—Issues and controversies. Clin Chem 32:5–12, 1986.

Steinfeld L, Dimich I: Digitalis: A pediatric viewpoint. *In* Donoso E (ed): Drugs in Cardiology, Vol 1, Part 2, 124. New York: Stratton, Intercontinental, 1975.

Wettrell G, Andersson KE: Cardiovascular drugs II: Digoxin. Ther Drug Monit 8:129–139, 1986.

Withering W: An account of the Foxglove and some of its medicinal uses, Sweeney M (ed). Birmingham, United Kingdom, 1785.

Antiarrhythmic Agents

33

Claire M. Lathers
Daniel K. O'Rourke

The pharmacology and clinical applications of cardiac antiarrhythmic agents have developed at a rapid rate during the 1970s and 1980s, and the rate of development is accelerating. It is expected that many new agents will be introduced for clinical use within the next few years. These advances have been made possible by clinical research techniques such as computer-assisted arrhythmia recognition programs, continuous 24-hour electrocardiographic recordings, and intracardiac electrocardiography. Advances have been attributed also to new basic information about the physiology of arrhythmias, the cellular basis of drug action as well as mechanisms in intact individuals, the physical chemistry of protein binding, and the mode of metabolism of antiarrhythmic agents, plus new techniques to measure the free plasma concentrations of these agents. The combination of all clinical and basic science information has contributed to the conversion of what historically has been an empirically based medication to rational pharmacotherapy. The study of the pharmacology of specific drugs has established the basic mechanisms of action of antiarrhythmic drugs. This chapter provides the foundation for understanding the clinical use of current as well as new drugs when they are introduced.

The normal heart continues beating 60 or more times a minute every minute of every day for a lifetime. Unfortunately, there are diseases in which the fine-tuned sequence of membrane, ionic, electrical, and mechanical events becomes disturbed. A variety of pharmacological agents with differing mechanisms of action have been discovered that can aid in restoring the physiological rhythm of the heart. Nevertheless, the drugs currently available rarely restore the heart to its fully normal condition. None of the agents that are discussed repairs the diseased state; thus, a reasonable hope when these agents are used is a change of the disturbed rhythm to one that has an improved functional capability.

In review, the pumping function of the heart is achieved in the following sequence (Fig. 33–1). Blood enters the right atrium of the heart, returning from the body in its lowered oxygenated state. It passes to the right ventricle through the tricuspid valve. The right ventricle pumps blood to the lungs through the pulmonary arteries; oxygenated blood returns through the pulmonary arteries to the left atrium. The left ventricle pumps blood to the body.

It is helpful to try to understand and to remember the mechanism of action of an antiarrhythmic agent and thus to deduce its indications and

Cardiac Function and Physiology

Knowledge of the physiology of the heart is a prerequisite to understanding the mechanisms of action of antiarrhythmic drugs.

Figure 33–1

Figure 33–1

Schematic of the conduction system of the heart. The sinoatrial (S-A) node serves as the normal pacemaker of the heart. There are four specialized conduction pathways through the atria originating near the S-A node and ending near the A-V node. The atrioventricular (A-V) node is located between the right atrium and the right ventricle just to the right of the interventricular septum. From the node, conduction of excitation proceeds to the ventricles by the His-Purkinje system in the interventricular septum.

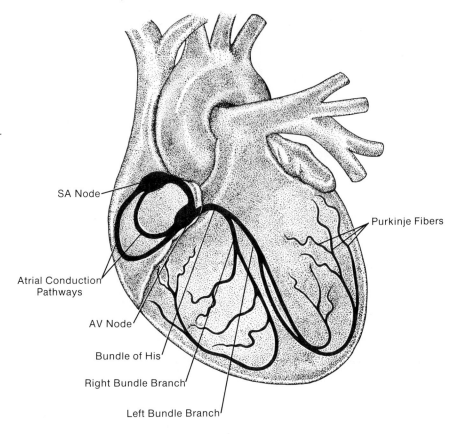

A specialized conduction system links the pacing of the S-A node with ventricles.

side effects, rather than simply memorizing the indications and side effects for each drug—the former fosters greater understanding and usually requires less work.

ELECTROPHYSIOLOGY OF THE HEART AND CLINICAL APPLICATIONS

The normal conduction route of the heart begins with transient depolarization of the tissues of the sinoatrial (S-A) node. This is culminated in an action potential that is conducted through specialized atrial conduction tissue to the atrioventricular (A-V) node. Cells in the A-V node have *slow response action potentials*, a type of action potential characterized by a long duration and conduction time. This long conduction time in the individual A-V node cells is reflected as the A-V node delay. From the A-V node the action potential travels down the bundle of His into the right and left bundle branches splitting into smaller and smaller fibers until it reaches the terminal Purkinje fibers. The latter are in direct contact with the cells of the myocardium, and thus the end response, by means of the propagated transient membrane depolarization, is excitation of the muscle cells of the ventricles.

Cardiac Action Potentials

The cardiac action potential is defined as a change in the transmembrane potential that is conducted and transmitted to immediately adjacent cells. This quality of propagation, also termed *conduction*, is crucial to the description of the function of action potential. With sufficient depolarization, i.e., to above the electrical threshold of the membrane, the characteristic action potential is initiated. Microelectrode recordings from isolated and

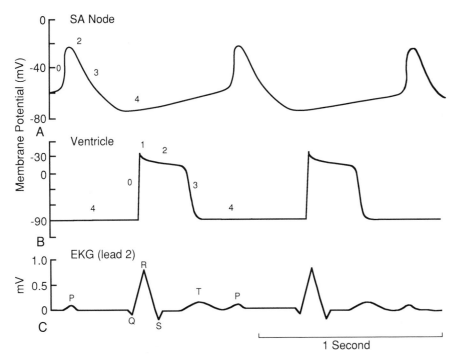

Figure 33-2

The slow and fast action potentials of the heart and the electrocardiogram (EKG, ECG). *A*, The slow action potential that occurs in the S-A node. It is characterized by an unstable, slow depolarization phase 4. Cells with an unstable phase 4 possess automaticity and are potential pacemakers. The cells with the fastest rate of spontaneous depolarization are located in the S-A node and hence are the normal pacers of the heart. Phase 0 is a rapid depolarization that occurs when a membrane voltage equal to the threshold voltage is reached. Phase 1 is the overshoot, and it is usually not seen in slow action potentials. Phase 2 is the plateau period of the action potential; it is very short in this type of action potential. Phase 3 is an increased rate of return to the resting potential—repolarization. Phase 3 merges into phase 4, and the cycle repeats itself.

B, A fast-type action potential as is normally seen in the ventricle. It is characterized by a flat phase 4, an overshoot of phase 1, and a long phase 2 plateau.

C, A schematic ECG. The P wave is

produced by the depolarization of the atria. The inactive period between the P wave and the QRS complex is known as the PR interval and represents the delay at the A-V node. The QRS complex derives from the depolarization of the ventricles. The T wave represents ventricular repolarization.

intact cardiac cells have revealed the presence of two characteristic action potentials. These are illustrated in Figure 33–2. The fast-type action potential is the more ubiquitous of the two and is seen in most atrial and ventricular cells. Its shape is conventionally described as consisting of five phases, 0 through 4, which are defined in terms of ion movement, the membrane potential, the rate and direction in which the membrane potential is changing, and the level of excitability.

The second, slow-type, action potential is seen in pacemaker cells or in those that have the ability to become ectopic pacemakers, i.e., pacemakers located away from the normal pacemaker site. It is characterized by the presence of phase 0, the absence of a phase 1, a short plateau or phase 2, a phase 3 that is more or less continuous with phase 2 and not obviously separate from it, and most prominently an unstable phase 4. This instability of phase 4, i.e., a tendency to undergo gradual and spontaneous depolarization, is the characteristic that causes cells to be pacemaker cells. Antiarrhythmic agents modify these two types of action potentials in predictable ways. Moreover, different cells may be differentially sensitive to the effects of any one drug. Thus, the basis of the pharmacology of antiarrhythmic drugs is the description of the differential effects of the various drugs on these membrane functions.

> Antiarrhythmic agents act to modify cardiac action potentials.

Resting Membrane Potential

The combination of the ubiquitous sodium/potassium pump, i.e., Na^+-K^+ adenosine triphosphatase (ATPase), and the ion permeability characteristic of plasma membranes creates a potassium rich/sodium poor cell interior that results in electochemical gradients. These gradients are made up of two parts. First, there is the tendency for sodium ions to flow into the cell and for the potassium ions to flow out owing to simple diffusion. Second, there is the tendency for the sodium to move into the cell because of an electrical potential that is created. This potential is negative inside of the cell with

> The resting membrane potential is created by ionic pumps and a selectively permeable plasma membrane.

respect to the outside. As a result, there is a constant tendency for positively charged ions to move into the cell. Sodium is the positive ion in highest concentration in the extracellular space. In the steady state situation, the affinity of the interior of the cell for sodium is countered by the impermeability of the plasma membrane to the sodium ion in the resting state plus the action of the sodium pump to regulate internal sodium concentration. With depolarization of the membrane, such as produced by an applied electrical current, an action potential results as the consequence of the transient opening of sodium channels in the plasma membrane.

Gate Theory of Permeability

Figure 33–3 is a schematic representation of the sodium channel, shown in open, phase 0, condition. During phase 0 there is a rapid influx of sodium ions. Functionally, the channel contains two gating systems. The first has been called the *activation* (or M) *gate,* and it opens when the membrane potential of the cell reaches the threshold value. The second, called the *inactivation* (or H) *gate,* closes channels when the potential of the cell starts to become more positive. The protein transmembrane helices labeled "d" in Figure 33–3 are postulated to function as the gating system for sodium channels. These two gates act antagonistically, the first opening channels as the cell begins to depolarize, the second closing as the cell gets more positive.

An analogy with the mousetrap may be useful in explaining the different states of the channel. Fast sodium channels exist in three states just as a mousetrap does. The set stage of the trap is similar to when the activation

> The gate theory describes the transient permeability of the cell for various ions during an action potential.

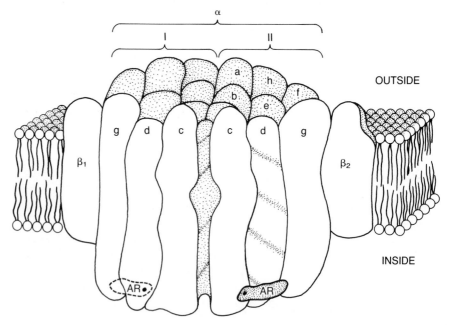

Figure 33–3

Schematic representation of a cross section of a transmembrane sodium channel, shown in the open, sodium conducting condition. The channel is composed of four α proteins (I to IV; I and II are depicted), and associated proteins, β_1 and β_2. Each α unit comprises eight homologous transmembrane polypeptide segments, designated a through h (some authors use Sa through Sh, or segments S1 through S8). The channel lining is thought to be constructed by the association of 4 homologous helical c segments that can form a pore of some 4 Å across. Each segment is presumed to possess a helical arrangement as does each of the closely associated segments. The postulated voltage-sensitive gating system consists of the helical segment d. Membrane depolarization activates the channel by rotation of the charged surface of d, which pulls the g helix in toward the channel, pushing the d segment out, thereby moving the c helices to open, forming the pore.

One of the major sites of the receptors for antiarrhythmic and local anesthetics (in membranes of heart muscle or nerve) lies near or on the gating helices (AR, shown in color), such that binding of a local anesthetic or antiarrhythmic agent reduces or prevents the conformational changes in the transmembrane segments.

The sodium channel is known to exist functionally in the following states: O = open, and conducting sodium ions; C = closed, and not conducting; I = inactivated, and not conducting; and R = resting, and closed, not conducting.

The usual sequence starting from the resting state is (1) resting to activated and opening of channel; (2) opening of channel; followed by (3) inactivation and closing of channel; followed by (4) recovery to resting.

Antiarrhythmic agents (and local anesthetics) have differential affinities to the various states of the sodium channel; and the degrees and the rates of association and dissociation vary among agents. In general, channel activation to the conducting state is associated with accelerated drug binding, and the drugs bind more tightly and with longer duration to activated (and open) and inactivated channels than they do to resting channels. Once bound they preclude the conformational changes of activation. (One explanation for *frequency and use dependence* follows from the selectively greater binding to the activated and inactivated channels than to the resting state.) (Data from Butterworth and Strichartz, 1990; Campbell, 1989; Catterall, 1987; Courtney and Strichartz, 1987; Hogdeghem, 1989; and Montal, 1990.)

gate is closed on the channel — there is no activity, but a little activity on the bait throws the trap. Similarly a minor decrease of potential in the membrane (i.e., toward threshold) opens the channel and initiates the active phase. The active phase of the trap is when the snare wire is swinging to catch the animal. This is a fast phase, and the end condition is different from the position at which the phase began. This is the phase of the channel when both the activation and the inactivation gates are opened and sodium is rushing into the cell. At the end of this phase the intracellular potential of the cell relative to the outside is approximately $+40$ mV, an overshoot beyond the 0 potential difference between inside and outside. The terminal state in the sequence is the inactivated state ("I"). The snare wire on the trap is closed, and no further activity can resume until repolarization and the trap has been reset. Until the channel is reset it is said to be refractory; just as nibbling on the bait of the mousetrap cannot cause the snare wire to release in the inactivated state, a depolarization pulse cannot cause the sodium channel to open.

Depolarization, the *rising phase* of the action potential, has been designated *phase 0*. The potential across the cell begins -80 to -90 mV and changes to a value of $+25$ to $+35$ mV. This phase is associated almost entirely with the rapid increase in the conductance of the membrane to sodium. V_{max} is defined as the maximal rate of phase 0 depolarization; it is the slope of the first upswing of the action potential (see Figs. 32–6 and 33–2). The conduction velocity is directly correlated with V_{max} because the action potential and associated currents are the cause of the progressive depolarization of adjacent membrane areas. Finally, given no other changes in time course of the action potential components, the effective refractory period will be inversely correlated with V_{max}.

Phase 0 is marked by depolarization.

Most investigators conclude that *phase 1, a rapid repolarization,* is the result of an influx of chloride ions and an efflux of potassium ions (see Fig. 32–6); the role and movement of another ion, calcium, has been a matter of some controversy. During phase 1 the potential across the membrane of the cell declines from the peak of approximately $+35$ mV to between 0 and -20 mV.

Phase 1 is an early rapid repolarization.

Phase 2 is called the *plateau phase* because it represents a slowing in the process of repolarization; it appears as a flattening of the action potential tracing. During this plateau there is an influx of calcium and chloride ions. Such movement of oppositely charged ions moving in the same direction would not be expected to result in any appreciable change in the membrane potential and it does not; if anything, there may be a slight repolarization.

Phase 2 is the plateau phase and is maintained by slow channels.

Phase 3 is a continuation of membrane repolarization characterized by a much steeper slope, a *more rapid repolarization.* At this time the fast potassium gates open. There is a slowed calcium ion influx lingering from phase 2. Potassium moves out of the cell in a manner similar to the sodium influx in phase 1.

Phase 3 is a return of rapid repolarization.

The shape and duration of phase 3 dictates the maximal rate that a cell can be activated to produce action potentials; the relative refractory period begins at the termination of phase 3. (In fact, during phase 3 there may be, paradoxically, a brief period of supernormal excitability so that a smaller than normal stimulus results in an action potential.)

Phase 4 has been termed the *resting phase* of the cardiac action potential because there are only small changes in the membrane potential. This is really a misnomer because this time of the cycle is spent re-establishing the ionic disequilibrium of the previous action potential sequence. In the non-automatic cell the membrane potential does not change, whereas automatic cells exhibit a small slow continuous depolarization of the membrane. During this phase the sodium/potassium ATPase pump is exchanging three sodium ions for every two potassium ions. Other ions, including

Phase 4 is the diastolic phase.

calcium and chloride, move across the membrane to establish the resting membrane concentrations. Although only a small percentage of the ions available actually move across the membrane during an action potential depolarization-repolarization sequence, these dramatic changes in the transmembrane potential can be explained by the amount of charge that each ion carries.

Excitability of Myocardial Cells

When the resting membrane potential of a myocardial cell reaches a certain critical voltage, the threshold, the cell responds with both an action potential and eventually contraction. The currents generated by an action potential at one site along the membrane depolarize immediately adjacent areas; thus the depolarization–action potential spreads along the fiber and from cell to adjacent cell. The spread along one cell is *conduction;* the spread from cell to cell is known as *transmission.* The electrophysiological state that the cell is in determines the rate at which the action potential can traverse it; this rate is termed the *conduction velocity.* The excitability of cardiac tissue is defined as the minimal stimulus required to cause excitation, i.e., an action potential. Some authors define it in terms of a single cell, in which case it is proportional to the difference between the resting membrane potential and the threshold potential. Excitability varies greatly among cardiac cells; some respond more slowly and others more rapidly.

Most myocardial cells are excitable and possess the ability to contract.

Threshold Value. Signals from other cells are propagated and transmitted only if the signal is greater than the threshold value. This threshold value can be changed by the activity in the autonomic system and certain antiarrhythmic agents. By making the threshold more positive, it is more difficult for the cell to be stimulated. Inversely, the cell with a depressed threshold is said to be extraexcitable. In pacer cells, lowering the threshold increases the *rate* of discharge.

The action potential is initiated when any process causes the resting membrane potential to reach a critical value known as the threshold.

Partial Depolarization. When the cell is partially refractory and a stimulus reaches it, the membrane potential is raised to the potential of the signal. What qualifies it as an action potential is whether or not it is conducted, that is, whether the signal is conducted along the membrane of a given cell as well as whether it is transmitted to the adjoining cells.

Partial depolarizations result from a stimulus that is refractory or subthreshold.

Conduction Velocity. As the slope of phase 0 decreases (becomes less steep), the conduction velocity of the cell decreases. This means that cells of the A-V node and S-A node with normally slow response action potentials (recall that this type of action potential has a normally low V_{max}) also have slow conduction velocities because conduction time is the inverse of conduction velocity.

Conduction velocity is directly proportional to V_{max}.

Refractoriness. The refractory period is that time in the action potential, from the start of phase 0 to late phase 3, when the cell is less likely to respond with an action potential. Refractoriness exists in different degrees ranging from absolute to relative. During the absolute refractory period, no signal can produce another action potential in the cell. Electrophysiologically, this can be explained by the fact that the electrochemical gradient is insufficient to produce a second phase 0, to open the inactivation gate. (To revive the mousetrap analogy, the trap in this state has been sprung and nothing can cause it to activate again until it has been reset.) During the relative refractory period a larger than normal stimulus is required to initiate a second action potential. In other words, the inactivation gate is at the

Refractoriness describes the altered responses of a cardiac cell to further stimulation.

marginal zone, where the usual stimulus does not result in an action potential; for example, this occurs during the late phase 3 and early phase 4.

There is also a period of the normal cardiac cycle termed the *super normal* period. This phase occurs early in phase 4 and represents a time when the threshold is slightly lower so that a smaller than normal stimulus can initiate an action potential. This is the period of the cell cycle when the cell is most susceptible to low amplitude potentials from sources other than the S-A node and constitutes one of the sources of arrhythmias.

Automaticity. Automaticity, also called *inherent excitability,* is defined as the ability of a cell to self-depolarize. Automatic cells can respond also to adequate stimuli originating outside of the cell. Most cells of the heart have the potential for automaticity, but it is most marked in the S-A node, atrial-specialized conducting fibers, node-His cells (NH cells) at the His/A-V junction, and cells of the His-Purkinje system.

> Automaticity allows the heart to pace itself.

The S-A node contains cells with the greatest automaticity in the normal heart. Rapid conduction along specialized groups of contraction cells spreads the action potential to all parts of the heart. The S-A node acts as the pacemaker because the signal from the S-A node reaches the potential pacers before their own phase 4 depolarizations have reached threshold. Thus, these cells depolarize on the cue from the S-A node and not on their own.

> The S-A node is the natural pacemaker of the heart.

INFLUENCE OF THE AUTONOMIC NERVOUS SYSTEM UPON S-A NODE DEPOLARIZATION

By changing the rate of phase 4 depolarization the rate at which automatic cells depolarize is changed. If these cells are in the S-A node, then the heart rate varies accordingly. The heart rate is under the control of the autonomic nervous system innervating the heart. Norepinephrine is released from the nerve terminals of postganglionic sympathetic nerves, and epinephrine is released from adrenal medullary stores. These catecholamines increase the slope of phase 4 depolarization in the automatic cells, thus increasing the rate at which the heart beats. Catecholamines also increase the automaticity of the other cells of the heart and the contractility of the ventricles, i.e., it has both positive chronotropic and inotropic effects. (*Chronotropic* refers to rate and *inotropic* refers to force of contraction.) Acetylcholine acts by hyperpolarizing the pacemaker cells and by decreasing the slope of the phase 4 depolarization. Both actions slow the rate of the S-A node discharge. The parasympathetic system has only a negative chronotropic effect; it has no inotropic effect on the ventricles. Table 33–1 presents the

> The autonomic system influences the rate of S-A node depolarization.

Table 33–1 RESPONSE OF CARDIAC TISSUE TO ADRENERGIC STIMULATION

| Tissue | Effect* | | Receptor Type |
	Automaticity	Conduction Velocity	
S-A node	+	0	β_1, β_2
Atrial muscle	0	+	β_1, β_2
A-V node	+	+	β_1
His-Purkinje system	+	0	β_1
Ventricular muscle	0	0	β_1

Originally published in Perry RS, Illsley SS: Basic cardiac electrophysiology and mechanisms of antiarrhythmic agents. Am J Hosp Pharm 43:957–974, 1986. © 1986, American Society of Hospital Pharmacists, Inc. All rights reserved. Reprinted with permission.
* + = increase; 0 = no change.

distribution of cardiac β_1 and β_2 receptor types within different areas of the heart and the effect of adrenergic stimulation on automaticity and conduction velocity.

(Studies in experimental animals suggest that the distribution of the β-adrenergic receptors among areas of the heart, i.e., atria, ventricles, septum, and within areas of the left ventricle, is not uniform [Lathers et al, 1986a]. These differences in concentrations in the different areas of the heart may be related to functional differences. The gradation of β adrenoreceptors, increasing in density from the base of the heart to the apex, would allow for a graded increase in contractile force from the base to the apex, thus providing for an efficient emptying of the heart. Thus, drug action or the stimulation of these receptors have variable effects in the case of an arrhythmia, depending on both the type and the site of origin within the heart.)

The ECG and Cardiac Action Potentials

The electrocardiogram (ECG) results from the summation of the cardiac action potentials.

An ECG (or EKG or electrocardiogram) is the recording of potentials from the body surface that is associated with the electrical currents generated by the heart. It reflects only the electrical activity and not necessarily the functionally important pumping. There are times that an almost normal ECG recording can exist with compromised pumping activity of the heart.

The ECG is used primarily for two purposes. The first is to determine the rhythm of the heart. This is useful for detecting arrhythmias, and only one or few standard leads are needed. A second use for the ECG is to locate the source of pathological changes in the heart, and thus multiple lead recording is preferable. A brief review of the electrophysiology behind the ECG is presented. Figure 33–2 correlates the ECG with representative action potentials from different areas of the conduction system.

The first wave seen in the normal ECG is the P wave. This wave represents the action potentials of the S-A node. Following the P wave there is a return to baseline, during which the signal passes from the atria through the A-V node to the ventricles. The vast majority of this PR time is accounted for by the slow processing time of the A-V node. The PR interval is clinically important because it is used for diagnosis and is the assessment of the effects of antiarrhythmic agents; it reflects the spread of the action potentials through the A-V node. The QRS complex corresponds to ventricular depolarization; it is the potential difference between the ECG leads caused by the sum of the electrical current generated by the ventricles. The reason that there are upward and downward deflections noted in the ECG is that the net current detected as a potential difference by the electrodes may be negative or positive. During the QRS complex the atria are normally undergoing repolarization, but the current generated by depolarization of the ventricles is of such greater magnitude that it overwhelms the smaller atrial wave. A return to baseline is followed by the QRS; the ECG cycle ends with the T wave, which signals ventricular repolarization.

Cardiac Arrhythmias

Cardiac arrhythmias normally do not occur because of multiple safeguards against their development.

Three initial conditions oppose the development of irregular or inappropriate heart rate. First, there is one and only one normal pacemaker whose baseline automatic rate exceeds all other potentially automatic cells. This is the S-A node. Wide variations in the rate of discharge of S-A node fibers occur because of the refractory periods and slow rates of depolarization of other automatic cells from discharging even when the sinus rate is slow. Second, action potentials are inhibited from traveling in circles, i.e., exiting the conduction system and then entering again, owing to the refractory periods of the cells in relation to their conduction velocities. Third, because of the delays intrinsic to the action potential sequence in the A-V node, a maximal rate of impulses that can be conducted to the ventricles is established. Therefore, if there is an atrial rhythm that exceeds this maximal rate, the impulses are not conducted in a one-to-one fashion. In spite of these "safety" features, alterations in atrial and S-A automaticity and a phenomenon known as *reentry* can occur, resulting in arrhythmias.

Altered Automaticity of the S-A Node

When the activity of the S-A node is separated from the rest of the heart, the next most rapid pacer takes over pacing of the heart. Pathological conditions such as ischemia, infarction, or an altered chemical milieu caused by certain drugs can cause normally nonautomatic cells to become automatic; that is, they develop an unstable phase 4. For instance, when the potassium concentration is increased in the bathing solution of an isolated Purkinje fiber, the action potential is converted from a fast responder type action potential to a slow responder type action potential. When an area of the heart that contains automatic cells develops a rate of depolarization faster than the S-A node, or when an area becomes isolated from the effects of the S-A node, then this area of cells establishes a pacemaker. Under these conditions the S-A node loses its dominance, and pacing is left to these isolated ectopic pacers. Moreover, if several of these pacers exist simultaneously or if one exists in the ventricles, uncoordinated contractions of the heart may result with the consequence of ineffective pumping action by the heart. The consequences of these arrhythmias could be unstable hemodynamics and a decreased cardiac output.

Altered automaticity explains why the S-A node sometimes loses its dominance, allowing other pacers to take over.

Reentry Arrhythmias

During and immediately following the action potential, the heart is refractory. Refractoriness is referred to generally as the duration of the effective refractory period, which is the minimal interval between two propagating responses. In most cardiac cells the effective refractory period is tied closely to the duration of the action potential, because recovery from inactivation of the sodium channel closely parallels repolarization. The sinus and A-V nodal cells (slow responses) have different characteristics in that refractoriness can outlast full repolarization; this results in the effective refractory period being much longer than the action potential duration. In general, antiarrhythmic drugs prolong the effective refractory period relative to the action potential duration in many types of cardiac cells.

Reentry explains arrhythmias that are not a result of ectopic focal pacemaker.

Reentry refers to the existence of a depolarization that is sustained sufficiently so that it can re-excite a rapidly recovering cell. Such sustained depolarizations occur in cardiac tissue that has been damaged or is ischemic (by storage or slow conduction along at least one pathway). The action potential is conducted so slowly through the damaged areas that by the time it is propagated through a group of cells, the first cell is again prepared to be excited. Electrophysiologically, the cell at the beginning of a reentry loop emerges from its effective refractory period by the time that the last cell is beginning to exhibit an action potential; the result can be viewed as a circle from which the propagated action potential — the *stimulus* — cannot exit. Activity in such a loop can be propagated potentially in all directions (Fig. 33–4), and thus reentry requires multiple pathways.

Figure 33–4

A model for *reentry*. *(A)* A schematic of the normal flow of action potentials through cardiac muscle fibers. *(B)* A *reentry* loop is set up by the presence of unidirectional block resulting from an area that is refractory to transmission in one direction, the antegrade direction, but that conducts a signal in the opposite direction, the retrograde direction, by the time the signal has arrived at the other end of the block. This reentry loop can be maintained for many cycles because, by the time the signal exits one side of the block, the entrance point cells are prepared for another action potential. *(C and D)* Two mechanisms by which pharmacological agents can abolish reentry loops are illustrated. In *C* the block is reduced, so that the signal arriving in the antegrade direction will meet the signal in the retrograde direction, and they extinguish each other. In *D* the block is increased, i.e., the cells remain refractory so long that the retrograde signal arrives when the cells are still refractory.

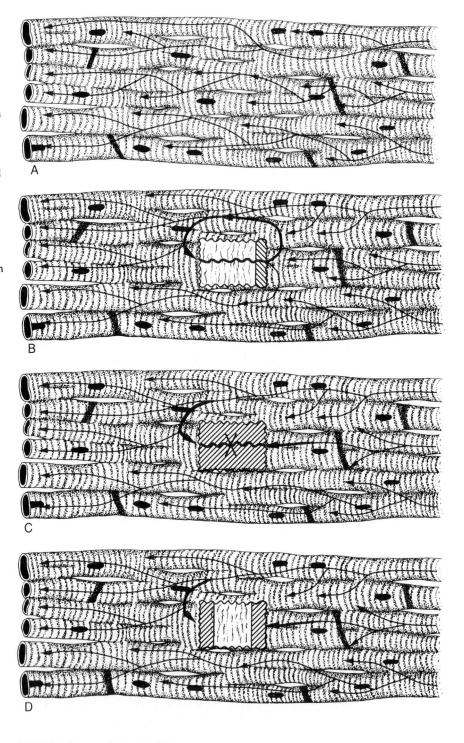

Wolff-Parkinson-White Syndrome

The Wolff-Parkinson-White syndrome explains effects of abnormal electrical connections between the atria and ventricles.

The Wolff-Parkinson-White (WPW) syndrome occurs when there is an accessory electrical connection between the atria and the ventricles. This accessory pathway can be traversed in either direction, resulting in a variety of clinical manifestations, thus the terminology of *syndrome*. If the signal comes from the atria (i.e., an aberrant action potential) then the ventricles begin to contract without the normal A-V node delay. The surface ECG reveals a short PR interval as a result of bypass of the A-V node, whereas insertion of the anomalous pathway into the ventricle causes abnormal ventricular activation with initial slowing of the QRS complex, the so-called delta wave. If the potential arises from within the ventricles, then a

Re-entry Loop

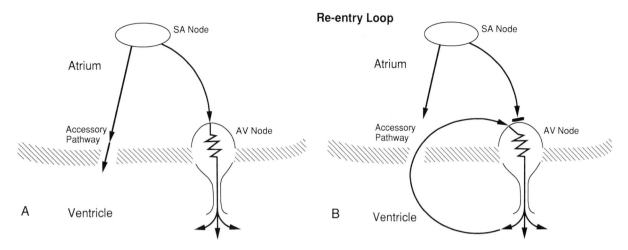

reentry loop may be set up with the A-V node being the unidirectional block (Fig. 33–5). The consequences of this syndrome can be severe: paroxysmal atrial tachycardia (PAT; also called an A-V junctional rhythm); atrial fibrillation; or occasionally, ventricular fibrillation. The WPW syndrome can be treated pharmacologically or by surgical lysis of the pathway.

Torsades de Pointes

Torsades de pointes occurs when a premature ventricular contraction (PVC) falls during the T wave of the preceding beat. It is always associated with a lengthened QT interval that may be congenital or produced by disease or drug. It is a dangerous and unfortunate side effect of several drugs, including phenothiazines, tricyclic antidepressants, procainamide, disopyramide, and quinidine. The rhythm may convert back spontaneously to a sinus rhythm or it may degrade into a ventricular fibrillation (Fig. 33–6).

Figure 33–5

The Wolff-Parkinson-White syndrome. This figure demonstrates how arrhythmias may be set up when there is an accessory pathway present. *(A)* An alternate, accessory, pathway allows the ventricles to be excited without the normal delay time produced by the A-V node. *(B)* A reentry loop is set up; the unidirectional block in this case is the A-V node, and the accessory pathway serves as a conduit for the signal to return to the A-V node, completing the loop.

Torsades de pointes is a ventricular tachycardia/fibrillation associated with an abnormally lengthened QT interval.

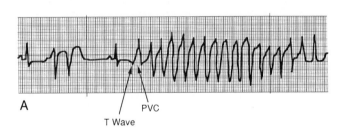

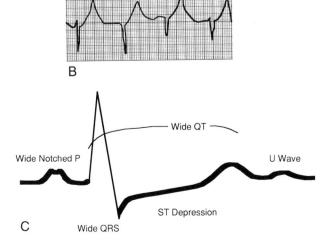

Figure 33–6

Quinidine toxicity and *torsades de pointes*. One of the effects of quinidine toxicity is a lengthening of the QT interval *(A)* and an arrhythmia known as *torsades de pointes* (B). *Torsades de pointes* is characterized by a ventricular tachycardia with an ECG strip that looks as if the QRS peaks were undulating about an axis, a "roller coaster" pattern. This rhythm may terminate itself or it may lead to ventricular fibrillation. *(C)* Schematic summary of the effects of quinidine.

Table 33-2   VAUGHN WILLIAMS CLASSIFICATION OF ANTIARRHYTHMIC DRUGS

Class	Actions	Prototype Agent
I	Inhibits Na^+ transport Reduces dV/dt of phase 0	Quinidine
II	β-adrenergic receptor blockade	Propranolol
III	Prolongs repolarization Alters membrane response	Amiodarone
IV	Calcium channel blockade	Verapamil

From Harrison D: Current classification of antiarrhythmic drugs. Drugs 31:93–95, 1986.

Classification of Antiarrhythmic Agents: A Guide for Their Clinical Use

In view of the different actions on the heart of clinically effective antiarrhythmic agents, attempts have been made to classify them. In 1970 Vaughn Williams published a four-part classification for antiarrhythmic drugs (Table 33–2). (Occasionally a class V category is used; some place digoxin within this category, whereas others insert chloride channel antagonists in this class—see Table 33–2.) Harrison (1986) subdivided class I agents into three subcategories 11 years later (Table 33–3). When referring to these classifications, three points need to be remembered.

1. Drugs are placed in these categories based on their predominant electrophysiological actions, and the classification may not entirely encompass all the mechanisms involved in the antiarrhythmic effects.

2. Drugs within a class do differ, so that one may be effective in a given patient whereas another drug in the same class may not produce a therapeutic action. Furthermore, drugs included within the same class do not necessarily share the same clinical indications nor do they necessarily share common side effects, especially those that have an extracardiac site of origin. Thus, it cannot be categorically stated that because a given patient has "this type of arrhythmia" that a particular drug or class must be used.

3. The presence of heart disease and arrhythmias may, in turn, modify their antiarrhythmic effects because of the changed actions on ischemic myocardium, altered metabolism, hemodynamics, or on the central and autonomic nervous systems.

Class I antiarrhythmic agents act on receptors in the cardiac sodium channels to reduce sodium entry during cardiac membrane depolarization, decrease the rate of rise of phase 0 of the cardiac action potential, necessitate a greater or more negative membrane potential to allow propagation to

Table 33-3   HARRISON MODIFICATION OF CLASS I ANTIARRHYTHMIC AGENTS

Class	Actions	Agents
IA	Slow dV/dt of phase 0; moderate prolongation of repolarization; prolong PR, QRS, and QT intervals	Quinidine, procainamide, disopyramide
IB	Limited effect on dV/dt of phase 0; shorten repolarization; shorten QT in clinical dosages; elevate fibrillation thresholds	Lidocaine, tocainide, mexiletine
IC	Markedly slow dV/dt; little effect on repolarization; markedly prolong PR and QRS on ECG	Encainide, lorcainide, flecainide

From Harrison D: Current classification of antiarrhythmic drugs. Drugs 31:93–95, 1986.

adjacent cells (i.e., increase threshold), and prolong the effective refractory period of fast response fibers. In general, higher plasma concentrations, i.e., higher than those levels usually employed clinically, of class I agents exhibit local anesthetic actions and depress myocardial contractility. Class I drugs suppress normal automaticity in Purkinje fibers and the His bundle and abnormal automaticity in damaged myocardial tissue. Abnormal automaticity is suppressed selectively, allowing the S-A node to become or remain the driving pacemaker.

More specifically, although class IA drugs, with quinidine being the prototype drug, do alter conduction velocities and dV/dt (V_{max}), they exhibit relatively more pronounced effect on the absolute and effective refractory periods of Purkinje and ventricular tissue. Imipramine, a psychoactive agent used in the treatment of depression, also induces electrocardiographic and antiarrhythmic effects similar to those of quinidine and procainamide; thus, it is occasionally classified as a class IA agent.

Quinidine is the prototype class IA drug.

CLASS IA

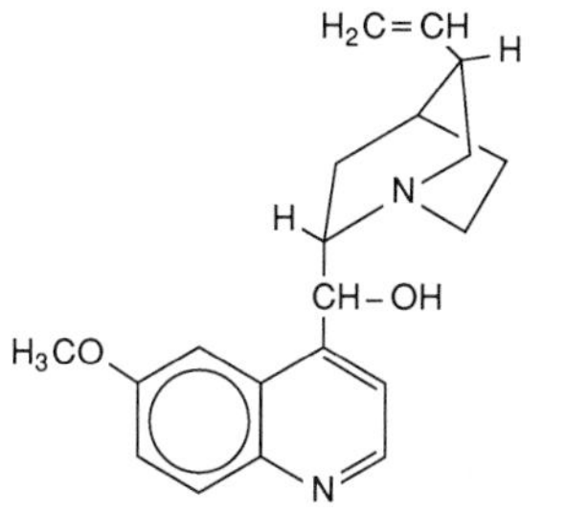

Quinidine 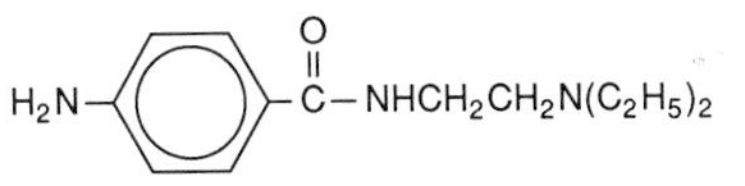   Procainamide 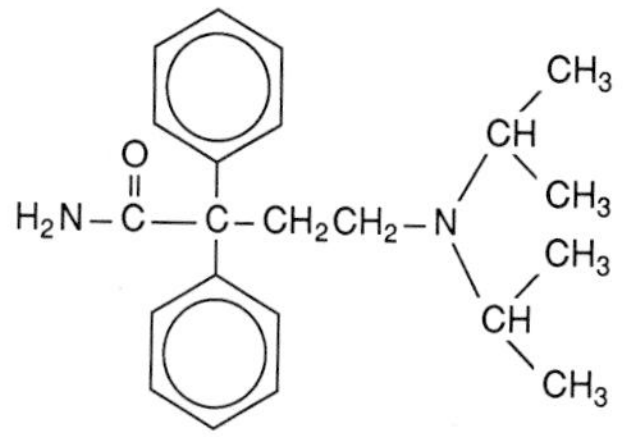   Disopyramide

Drugs included in class IB prototype drugs (lidocaine, phenytoin, tocainide, and mexiletine) exert little effect on conduction velocities and may improve refractoriness, expecially in ischemic areas. They also elevate the threshold for the appearance of fibrillation.

CLASS IB

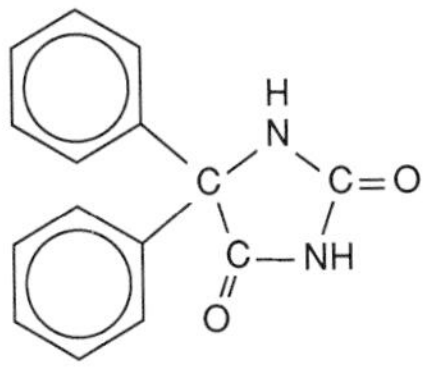

Phenytoin 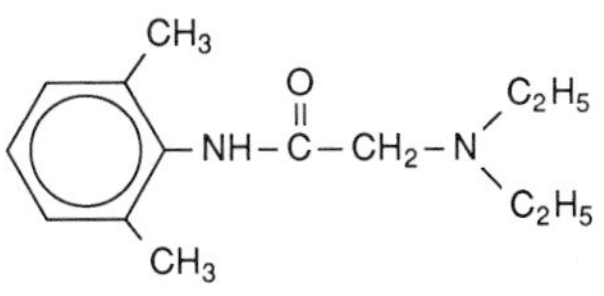   Lidocaine 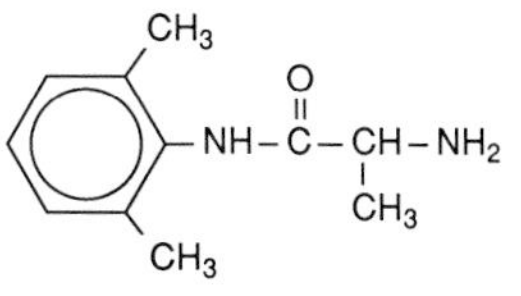   Tocainide 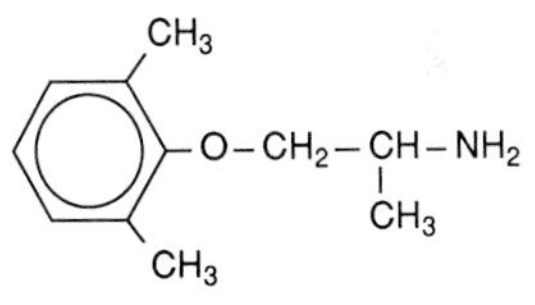   Mexiletine

Agents in the IC class, flecainide and encainide, have a profound effect on His-Purkinje conduction in normal and abnormal myocardium and exhibit a mild to moderate effect on refractoriness.

CLASS IC

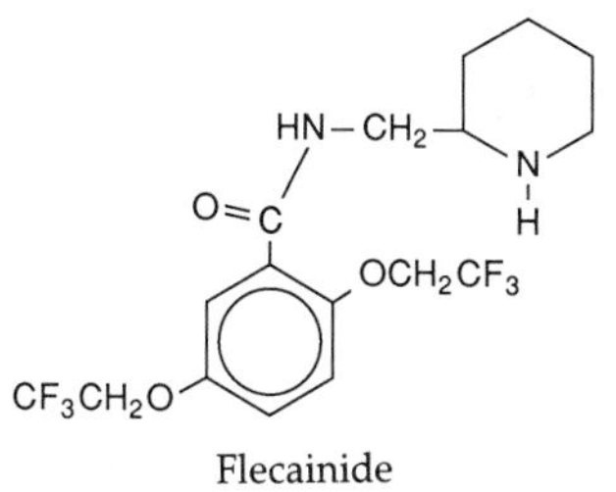

Flecainide 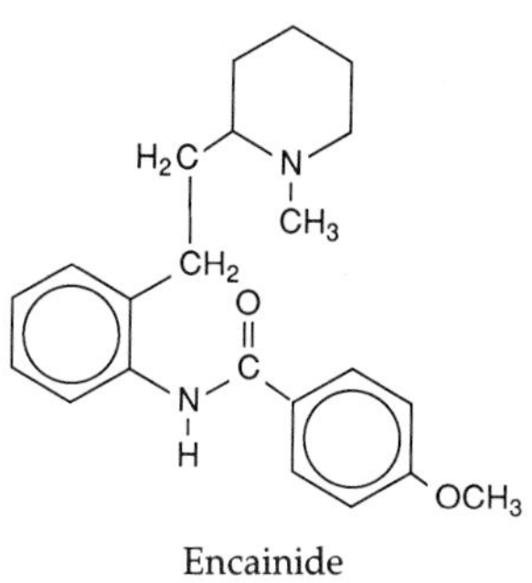   Encainide 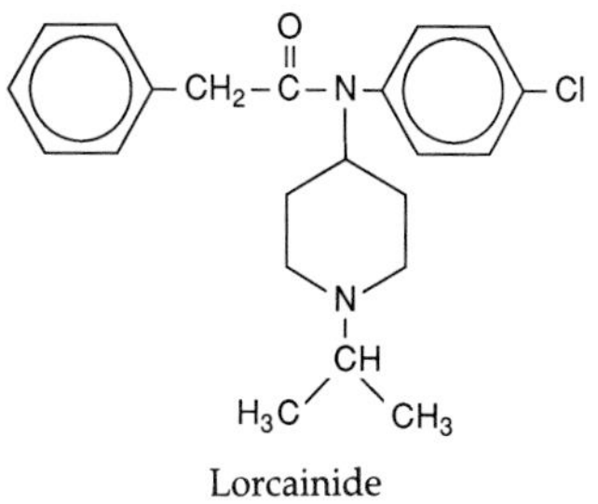   Lorcainide

Electrophysiological observations of the voltage and rate dependency of drug action suggest that classification of class I agents may be based also on the time constants for inactivating Na^+ channels in the cell membrane

Class I agents can be broken into three subgroups based on depolarization speed and action potential duration: fast, intermediate, and slow.

and on the recovery time once the channels are inactivated. The kinetics of the speed of onset of rate-dependent depression of the maximal rate of depolarization (V_{max}) and the action potential duration allow three subgroups to be formed with titles of *fast* (lidocaine, tocainide, and mexiletine), *intermediate* (quinidine, disopyramide, and procainamide), and *slow* (flecainide, encainide, and lorcainide) kinetics. Drugs in the fast category (Harrison IB) share the ability to markedly prolong the effective refractory period relative to the action potential duration, i.e., the action potential duration is shortened. The slow drugs (Harrison IC) exhibit only minor effects on the effective refractory period despite the finding that all three drugs produced a greater depression of the steady state V_{max} than either of the other groups. The drugs classified as intermediate (Harrison IA) induce a small to moderate increase in the effective refractory period relative to the action potential duration, but also significantly prolong the action potential duration. Thus, this classification agrees with the IB, IC, and IA subgroups of Vaughn Williams (1984).

Propranolol is the prototype class II drug.

Class II antiarrhythmic agents are β-blocking agents. Propranolol is a prototype drug in this class. Most competitively block β adrenoceptors and inhibit catecholamine-induced stimulation of cardiac β receptors. Some class II drugs, i.e., propranolol and acebutolol, also produce electrophysiological changes in Purkinje fibers that are similar to those produced by class I agents; this effect has been designated *membrane-stabilizing*. Labetalol blocks both α and β adrenoceptors. Sotalol is a β-blocking agent that possesses electrophysiological actions similar to drugs in class III; thus, it may be categorized as both a class II and a class III agent. The dual action of sotalol supports the concept that the β-blocking property of class II agents may not be the entire explanation of their antiarrhythmic action.

CLASS II

Propranolol

Timolol

Metoprolol

Sotalol

Labetalol

The class III agents sotalol, bretylium, and amiodarone all prolong the duration of the cardiac action potential without changing phase 0 of depolarization or the resting membrane potential and alter the function of sympathetic innervation to the heart. (The antiarrhythmic action of bretylium places it in the class III category rather than with the adrenergic neuronal blocking agents of class II. However, in addition to the evidence suggesting that its antiarrhythmic action is due to a direct action on the heart, other data indicate that its adrenergic neuronal blocking properties also contribute to its antiarrhythmic actions.)

CLASS III

Bretylium

Amiodarone

Drugs included in class IV block the slow inward calcium current (i.e., verapamil, diltiazem, and nifedipine), occurring during phases 0 to 2 of the cardiac action potential. The greatest effect is exerted on slow response cardiac action potentials in the sinus and A-V nodes. The class IV agents, verapamil, diltiazem, and nifedipine, decrease conduction velocity and increase refractoriness in the A-V node; thus, conduction of supraventricular impulses through the A-V node to the ventricle is decreased.

Clinical guidelines have been developed from the Harrison classification allowing prediction of effect of: drugs on specific arrhythmias; appropriate combination of drugs to treat resistant or intractable arrhythmias; side effects; and contraindications of specific syndromes to certain agents (Harrison, 1986). For example, knowing that agents in the IC category profoundly affect conduction, one can predict that these drugs may be used to treat individuals with accessory pathways of conduction, such as those pathways occurring in the Wolff-Parkinson-White syndrome. The clinical effectiveness of these drugs supports this concept, because both antegrade and retrograde conduction velocities in the bypass tracks and in the A-V node are markedly altered. It is possible also to predict that patients with major intraventricular conduction defects would be more likely to have a higher rate of abnormal reactions to drugs that more strongly alter conduction, i.e., class IC. Indeed, high dosages of these agents clinically do induce a marked widening of the QRS duration.

The design of combination antiarrhythmic therapy is possible also using this classification. Patients unable to tolerate high dosages of some antiarrhythmic agents may respond to a combination of lower dosages of drugs from different subgroups to produce additive electrophysiological effects while decreasing unwanted side effects. Thus, a combination of a drug from classes IA and IB may induce a maximal decrease in the likelihood of fibrillation while inducing minimal prolongation of repolarization or alteration in the refractoriness.

The combination of drugs in classes IA and IC is contraindicated because a high incidence of heart block or impaired intraventricular conduction may be produced. Use of the classification suggests also that agents altering repolarization and prolonging the effective and relative refractory periods would be contraindicated in individuals with congenital long QT syndromes. Clinically this prediction has been observed because quinidine increases the likelihood of *torsades de pointes* in such patients (see Fig. 33–6).

GENERAL CONSIDERATIONS OF ANTIARRHYTHMIC AGENTS

In this chapter, as in the book, important details of selection of dosage, formulations, and routes of administration — the recipes of management — are not presented except as they illustrate or emphasize major pharmacological properties or principles. These details are not provided because they lack importance, but because the physician should, before administering any drug, consult the most up-to-date information, such as that provided in current medical literature and in the package insert. This applies in full force to *all* antiarrhythmics, because every one of these agents has serious side effects, including the capability to elicit arrhythmias and the potential to be lethal when used in attempts to ameliorate serious disturbances in cardiac rhythm.

Most of the antiarrhythmic drugs are available in dosage formulations that permit the rapid establishment of effective levels, usually by intravenous (IV) administration. For long-term use oral preparations are preferred

Class IV drugs block calcium current during phases 0 to 2 of the cardiac action potential.

CLASS IV

Verapamil

Class IC agents can be used to treat Wolff-Parkinson-White syndrome.

Antiarrhythmic agents have serious side effects.

and, again, are available in a variety of dosage formulations for most agents. Moreover, in view of usual need to maintain blood levels within a rather narrow range, regular monitoring of levels and cardiac status is the rule. This is especially true whenever drugs other than antiarrhythmic agents are also being used (which is most of the time), when the patient is elderly or quite young, and when the cardiovascular system is not stable. Each of these situations is likely to occur in patients being considered for antiarrhythmic drug therapy.

CRITERIA FOR THE IDEAL ANTIARRHYTHMIC AGENT

Criteria for the ideal antiarrhythmic include (Muhidden and Turner, 1985):

1. effectiveness in the treatment of a well-defined group of arrhythmias;
2. lack of cardiac and extracardiac adverse effects;
3. no clinically significant drug interactions;
4. oral and IV dosing forms, with the oral dose exhibiting minimal first-pass metabolism;
5. no clinically significant genetically determined polymorphic metabolism between subjects;
6. reasonable half-life to allow infrequent dosing with resultant better patient compliance;
7. relatively little "between and within" patient variability in pharmacokinetic properties;
8. a good correlation between its effectiveness and its plasma concentration.

To date no one antiarrhythmic agent meets all these criteria. However, the list may be used to remember advantages and disadvantages of the various drugs.

CLASS IA ANTIARRHYTHMICS

General Characteristics

The class IA drugs contain some of the oldest antiarrhythmics, but their attributes are valuable enough that they are widely used and new class IA agents are being developed. The electrophysiological requirements for an agent in this class are the following: they decrease the slope of phase 0 (the maximum rate of depolarization); increase the repolarization time, thereby producing an increase in the refractory time; increase conduction time by decreasing conduction velocity; and decrease automaticity. They act principally by slowing the fast sodium channels, which decreases the slope of phase 0 of the action potential. Class IA agents are effective in the treatment of atrial and ventricular arrhythmias.

Class IA agents are used to treat atrial and ventricular arrhythmias.

Quinidine

Quinidine is effective for prophylaxis against atrial fibrillation, for the treatment of atrial and ventricular premature contractions, and of ventricular tachycardia.

History. Quinine, the dextrorotatory isomer of quinidine, has been used for hundreds of years to treat moderate pain, fevers, and malaria. It was noticed that patients with malaria who also had atrial fibrillation converted occasionally to normal sinus rhythms when treated with quinine for their malaria. Such an observation led to the investigation for a more potent antiarrhythmic agent from the chinchona plant, the source of quinine. The three principal alkaloids from the plant are quinine, chinchonine, and quinidine. Of the three, quinidine was found to be the most effective in treating atrial fibrillation.

Mechanism of Action. Quinidine works by two separate mechanisms: a direct action of the drug on myocardial cells, and through its indirect anticholinergic actions (atropine-like). This dual mechanism of action is typical of all the antiarrhythmic agents in this class.

The S-A Node and Atrial Myocardium. The effect of normal vagal nerve activity on the S-A node is blocked by quinidine, resulting in an increased rate of depolarization in the cells of the S-A node. In opposition to these effects, quinidine acts directly on atrial myocardium, including the specialized cells of the S-A node, to decrease excitability and membrane responsiveness. These actions result in an increase in the level of threshold of excitation, i.e., a larger stimulus is required to cause excitation; a decrease in V_{max} (recall that this is related directly to conduction velocity); and an increase in the effective refractory period. The direct effects on the atrial tissue result in a decreased S-A node rate, but the net effect on the S-A node is negligible, although there may occasionally be a slight increase in the rate. The atrial tissue has a net decreased conduction velocity and increased refractory period. Automaticity is reduced throughout the atrial tissues, making quinidine effective in relieving atrial tachyarrhythmias.

> Quinidine acts directly on the atrial myocardium to decrease excitability and membrane responsiveness.

A-V Node. The actions of quinidine on the A-V node are due to its anticholinergic actions; because the A-V node is normally under tonic vagal influence, the atropine-like effects of quinidine increase A-V nodal conduction. For this reason quinidine is not used alone in treating atrial arrhythmias with fast rates, because increasing the A-V nodal conduction would increase the ventricular rate to possibly dangerously high levels. This problem is overcome by prior treatment with digitalis (digitalization), which counters the A-V nodal effects of quinidine. (The direct effects of quinidine on the A-V node are just the opposite of its anticholinergic actions. The direct effects include an increase in the effective refractory period and a decrease in the conduction velocity.)

> Digitalis can be used prior to quinidine administration to offset high ventricular rates.

Ventricular Myocardium and Specialized Conduction Tissue. All the effects of quinidine on the ventricles are accounted for by the direct effects of the drug. The direct effects here are the same as those given earlier: decreased automaticity; decreased conduction velocity; and increased effective refractory period. Automaticity is decreased by a decrease in the slope of phase 4 depolarization.

By decreasing conduction velocity and increasing the refractory period, a unidirectional block is converted to a two-way or bidirectional block, thus abolishing the reentry loop (see Fig. 33–3). There is also another action by which quinidine administration operates in both the atria and the ventricle. It has been termed *postrepolarization refractoriness.* The probable mechanism is that the sodium fast gate channel has not reset itself. Although the membrane potential has returned to the resting level, the cell is refractory to further depolarizations, because the sodium fast gates cannot open.

Electrocardiographic Changes. The PR, QRS, and QT intervals are increased. The PR interval, which reflects the speed of the action potentials through the A-V node and represents the sum of three processes, is lengthened with quinidine administration. The second process, the A-V node delay, is decreased. The third process, the His-Purkinje interval, increases after quinidine.

The QRS interval represents the time needed for depolarization of the ventricles. Its increase in duration during quinidine administration is dose-dependent and provides a good measure of therapeutic effects. The QT interval is lengthened more with quinidine administration than with any of the other class IA agents. Lengthening of the QT interval represents a slowing of the repolarization of the ventricles. (An abnormally lengthened QT interval is an ominous sign because it is a sign of quinidine toxicity and is sometimes followed by a rhythm known as *torsades de pointes*. This is a dangerous arrhythmia that can lead to ventricular fibrillation and death.)

Torsades de pointes can lead to ventricular fibrillation and death.

Actions on Other Organ Systems. The antimalarial and antipyretic properties of quinine, although retained in quinidine, are not used clinically. The anticholinergic effects of quinidine on the A-V node are not confined to the heart inasmuch as it blocks the effects of vagal stimulation or acetylcholine. Quinidine also has substantial α-adrenergic blocking activity, which leads to a significant hypotension when administered IV. The combination of the cholinergic blockade and the increased β-adrenergic activity induced by quinidine can increase the sinus rate and enhance A-V nodal conduction in some patients. It is for this reason, and because there is increased risk of toxicity, that quinidine is seldom given IV.

Quinidine is seldom given IV because of its toxicity.

Pharmacokinetics. Quinidine is well absorbed when taken orally (Table 33-4). Approximately 80-90% of the drug is bound by albumin, other plasma proteins, and hemoglobin in erythrocytes principally in the un-

Table 33-4 PHARMACOKINETICS OF ANTIARRHYTHMIC DRUGS

Drug	Inactivation or Route of Elimination (%)	Active Metabolites	Protein Binding (%)	Elimination Half-Life (hour)	Oral Bioavailability (%)
Class IA					
Quinidine	Liver 50-90	Probable	70-95	7-18	70
	Kidney 10-30				
Procainamide	Kidney 30-60	Yes	15	2.5-4.7	75
	Liver 40-70				
Disopyramide	Kidney 36-77	Yes	20-60	7-9	80
	Liver 11-37				
Class IB					
Lidocaine	Liver 90	Yes	40-70	1.5-4	35
Phenytoin	Liver 95	No	85	24	70-100
Mexiletine	Liver 90	No	70	8-24	90
Tocainide	Liver 50-60	No	50	12-15	100
	Kidney 40-50				
Class IC					
Flecainide	Liver 70	No	40	11-30	95
Lorcainide	Liver 98	Yes	85	7.6	80-100
Class II					
Propranolol	90+	No	90+	2-6	~30
Sotalol	Kidney 90	No	0	10-20	100
Class III					
Bretylium	Kidney 70-80	No	?(low)	4-16	20
Amiodarone	Liver 99	Unknown	?(high)	25-55 days	20-50

Adapted from Siddoway LA, Roden DM, Woosley RL: Clinical pharmacology of old and new antiarrhythmic drugs. *In* Josephson ME (ed): Sudden Cardiac Death. Brest AN (editor-in-chief): Cardiovasc Clin 15:199-248, 1985.

charged state. The chief elimination route of quinidine is through metabolism in the liver and elimination through the kidneys, although up to 20% of the parent drug may be eliminated directly through the kidney. Most of the urinary metabolites are hydroxylated at one site only, on the quinoline ring or on the quinuclidine ring. Some metabolite is in the form of the dihydroxy compound. The therapeutic blood level of quinidine is well established (2–4 μg/ml), although slightly higher levels are sometimes necessary; clinical signs of toxicity occur at levels of approximately 8 μg/ml. The pharmacokinetics of the major antiarrhythmics are compared in Table 33–5. Important aspects compared include absorption, protein binding, elimination, and route of excretion.

Therapeutic Uses. Quinidine is used primarily to suppress ventricular ectopic areas and to prevent these areas from causing paroxysmal ventricular tachycardia. It may be used for the maintainence of a regular sinus rhythm after atrial fibrillation has been converted, and although no longer indicated for this purpose, it alone may convert atrial fibrillation. Further, quinidine may be used to prevent the development of paroxysmal supraventricular tachycardia. However, in the A-V nodal form of paroxysmal supraventricular tachycardia, digitalis is tried usually before quinidine because of the significant toxicity of quinidine. (Although the actions of quinidine and procainamide are similar, quinidine is generally preferred for long-term therapy because of a drug-induced lupus syndrome that can develop with procainamide.)

Effect of Age on Pharmacokinetic Parameters. Liver disease significantly increases the half-life of the drug, as would be expected; the effect of renal disease on quinidine levels is less clear. It appears that the normal decrease in renal function that accompanies aging should be accompanied by a decrease in the dosage. However, in states of decreased renal function, including congestive heart failure, there is little change in the quinidine levels. Some of the metabolites of quinidine are thought to be cardioactive.

Adverse Effects, Drug Interactions, Contraindications (Table 33–5). The adverse effects of quinidine therapy involve the gastrointestinal (GI) system, central nervous system (CNS), immune-mediated responses, cardiac toxicity, and interactions with other drugs. The GI side effects of quinidine appear frequently because they can occur after usual therapeutic dosages; these include nausea, vomiting, diarrhea, vague abdominal pain, and loss of appetite.

Nausea and vomiting are GI side effects of quinidine.

A unique complex of side effects associated with toxicity of both quinidine and quinine has received a specific name, *cinchonism*. It is particularly likely to appear after rapid administration or large doses; headaches, tinnitus, visual disturbances, and vertigo characterize cinchonism. The symptoms of cinchonism are so characteristic that every physician should be able to recognize them in a patient being treated with quinidine and should suspect intoxication when they appear. Toxicity may be associated also with headache, diplopia, photophobia, and altered color perception. Immune-mediated responses are less common with quinidine than procainamide, but they do occur and include blood dyscrasias, rashes, fevers, and rarely, anaphylactoid reactions. A hypersensitivity response mounted against quinine is active against quinidine also.

The cardiac toxicity of quinidine has already been mentioned, including the potentially fatal rhythm of *torsades de pointes*. Myasthenia gravis can be aggravated by the action of quinidine at the neuromuscular junction.

Table 33-5 PHARMACOLOGICAL MECHANISMS, EFFECTS, AND TOXICITY OF ANTIARRHYTHMIC AGENTS

Drug	Electrophysiological Effects*				Hemodynamic Properties	Toxicity
	Automaticity	*APD*	*ERP*	*QRS*		
CLASS IA						
Quinidine	−	+	+	+	Negative inotropism Vasodilatation Hypotension	Impaired conduction/asystole Ventricular arrhythmias Gastrointestinal intolerance Cinchonism Thrombocytopenia Drug fever

Procainamide	−	+	0, +	+	Negative inotropism
					Vasodilatation
					Hypotension
						Impaired conduction and
						  ventricular arrhythmias
						Nausea, vomiting
						Agranulocytosis
						Drug-induced systemic lupus
						  erythematosus

Disopyramide	−	+	+	+	Negative inotropism
					Vasodilatation
					Hypotension
					A-V block
						Anticholinergic effects: dry mouth,
						  constipation, urinary retention,
						  blurred vision, psychosis
						Ventricular arrhythmias
						Agranulocytosis

CLASS IB						
Lidocaine	−	−	+	0	No impairment of normal contractility	Drowsiness Respiratory arrest Convulsions Rare — heart block
Phenytoin	−	−	0, −	0	Hypotension and altered heart rate	Nystagmus, ataxia Lethargy Gastrointestinal intolerance Gingival hyperplasia Hirsutism
Mexiletine	−	−	0, +	0	Prolonged conduction Bradycardia Hypotension Cardiac depression	CNS: tremor to convulsions GI: nausea and vomiting Dermatological: photosensitive dermatitis
CLASS IC						

Flecainide	−	−	0	+	Arrhythmias
					Chest pain
						Neurological: dizziness, visual
						  impairment, headache, tremor,
						  paraesthesia
						Gastrointestinal: nausea,
						  constipation, diarrhea, abdomi-
						  nal pain
						Asthenia, fatigue

Encainide	−	−	+	+	Worsening of conduction system
					  disease
					Prolonged H-V interval and QRS
					  complex
					Worsening of ventricular
					  arrhythmias
						Dizziness, ataxia, tremor
						Diplopia
						Nausea
						Metallic taste
						Leg cramps

Lorcainide	−	−	+	+	Prolongation of PR interval and
					  QRS duration
					Worsening conduction disturbances
					Hypotension
						Insomnia with sweating and
						  nightmares
						Dizziness
						Dry mouth
						Flatulence
						Vivid dreams

CLASS II						
Propranolol	0, −	0, −	0, +	0	Negative inotropism Hypotension	Impaired A-V conduction/asystole Bronchospasm Nightmares, insomnia

Table 33-5 PHARMACOLOGICAL MECHANISMS, EFFECTS, AND TOXICITY OF ANTIARRHYTHMIC AGENTS Continued

Drug	Electrophysiological Effects*				Hemodynamic Properties	Toxicity
	Automaticity	APD	ERP	QRS		
CLASS III						
Bretylium	0, +	+	0	0	Hypotension	Gastrointestinal intolerance Parotid swelling
Amiodarone	−	+	+	0	No impairment of normal contractility Hypotension and increased coronary blood flow on IV administration	Photosensitivity Pigmentation Thyroid function abnormalities Corneal microdeposits
CLASS IV						
Verapamil	−		+	0	Negative inotropism Vasodilatation Hypotension	Impaired conduction/asystole Gastrointestinal intolerance Constipation

Adapted from Siddoway LA, Roden DM, Woosley RL: Clinical pharmacology of old and new antiarrhythmic drugs. *In* Josephson ME (ed): Sudden Cardiac Death. Brest AN (editor-in-chief): Cardiovasc Clin 15:199–248, 1985; and Muhiddin KA, Turner P: Is there an ideal antiarrhythmic drug? A review with particular reference to Class I antiarrhythmic agents. Postgrad Med J 61:665–677, 1985.
* Abbreviations: APD = action potential duration; ERP = effective refractory period; − = decreased: + = increased: 0 = no change.

Quinidine interacts with many drugs; only a few are presented here (see also Chapters 64 and 67). Quinidine directly displaces digoxin from its binding sites on the heart and perhaps sites in skeletal muscles; there is also a reduction in the renal clearance of digoxin. Consequently, the dose of digoxin can be reduced by as much as 50% when administered with quinidine. Thus, if a full dose of quinidine is given to a chronically digitalized patient, serious and even life-threatening arrhythmias can occur. Also, if a patient is already toxic to digoxin and thus presents with arrhythmia for which quinidine would otherwise be given, it is dangerous to use quinidine as the antiarrythmic agent. The anticoagulant coumadin is displaced from its plasma protein-binding sites and, therefore, has an increased action to prevent clotting. This may result in excessive bleeding or even hemorrhage. Both quinidine and propranolol exert a negative inotropic action on the heart; because of the possibility of combined cardiac depressant effects, caution is recommended when using both drugs concurrently.

Quinidine displaces digoxin from its binding sites.

Electrolyte and Acid-Base Imbalance Effect on Arrhythmia and Drug Actions. Potassium is the major electrolyte that must be monitored when administering quinidine. Hypokalemic patients taking drugs such as the thiazides are prone to rhythm disorders and are resistant to therapy with quinidine. Hyperkalemia increases the local anesthetic properties of quinidine, so that the decrease in membrane responsiveness is exacerbated.

Potassium levels should be monitored during quinidine administration.

Quinidine is excreted as a weak base, and its excretion is reduced when urinary pH is increased. Thus, the concomitant administration of acetazolamide or sodium bicarbonate may result in increased serum levels of quinidine, which may induce quinidine toxicity. It should be remembered that electrolyte imbalances are common causes or accompaniments of cardiac arrhythmias. Thus, electrolyte imbalances should not only be suspected as causes of arrhythmias but should be corrected before giving most antiarrhythmic drugs, especially in a chronic dose regimen or at unusually high doses.

Contraindications in Heart Block or Congestive Heart Failure. Third-degree heart block (complete) is a contraindication to quinidine therapy because of its intrinsic ability to decrease automaticity; abolishing a ventricular or A-V node pacemaker could cause asystole. Quinidine is also usually not indicated in congestive heart failure because its negative inotropic effect would have disastrous effects on an already depressed heart. In addition, most patients with congestive heart failure are already taking digoxin and thus would be at greater risk for toxicity.

Preparations and Dosages (QUINIDEX, QUINAGLUTE, CARDIOQUIN; QUINI-DINE GLUCONATE). CARDIOQUIN is marketed in 275 mg tablets. Quinidine gluconate sustained-release tablets contain 324 mg. Quinidine can be given orally (PO), IV, or intramuscularly (IM), but the latter two routes are rarely used. The IV route is used infrequently because of the increased chance of toxicity and hypotension. IM injection increases creatinine titers (confusing myocardial infarction dating and therapy), and it causes a great deal of pain at the injection site. Treatment with quinidine should be started at a rather low dosage, for example, 200 mg PO every 6–8 hours, and then tapered upward to achieve effective plasma concentrations. New assays have been developed that are much more sensitive for quinidine and can differentiate the parent drug from its metabolites. These tests may not be available in all centers, and consequently, values vary among laboratories. Quinidine is available in a variety of formulations that vary with respect to absorption rate and GI side effects. The pharmacokinetic differences among the various dosage formulations of quinidine may possibly be detrimental to the patient if the pharmacist or the physician switches quinidine preparations haphazardly.

Procainamide

Procainamide and quinidine have similar uses.

Procainamide is effective generally against the same arrhythmias as quinidine, including singlet PVCs to runs of PVCs; arrhythmias during myocardial infarction; and supraventricular arrhythmias, including supraventricular tachycardias and atrial fibrillation and flutter. In fact, the drugs have indications that overlap so much, one might ask why have two? The answer is that the peculiar human individualities are such that one may respond to one agent and not the other for currently unknown reasons. Further, untoward effects of long-term procainamide administration may make quinidine a better choice in certain patients. But the fact that procainamide can be given IV and then switched to oral medications makes it the drug of choice in some situations.

History. Procaine has been used for many years as a local anesthetic. It was shown that direct application of procaine to the canine heart afforded some protection against induced arrhythmias. The problem with using procaine as an antiarrhythmic is that it is quickly deactivated by plasma cholinesterase, although hepatic metabolism occurs also. Procainamide is the result of a search for an agent that was less susceptible to peripheral breakdown but retained antiarrhythmic actions similar to procaine.

Unlike quinidine, procainamide can be used IV with less risk of hypotension.

Mechanism of Action. The direct effects of procainamide do not differ from quinidine enough to be clinically significant (see Chapter 17). Both agents are local anesthetics; they decrease membrane responsiveness, the slope of phase 0, and automaticity while increasing the effective refractory period. The drugs differ significantly in their indirect effects, pharmacokinetics, and untoward effects. The indirect effects of procainamide are much less significant than are those of quinidine. There is a much weaker anticholinergic effect and there is almost no α-adrenergic blockade; thus it can be given IV with much less risk of hypotension.

Electrocardiographic Changes. The effect of procainamide therapy on the ECG is similar to that of quinidine because of the similarities in their electrophysiological effects. The PR, QRS, and QT intervals are each lengthened. The QRS and QT intervals are increased in a dose-dependent fashion but are somewhat less affected by quinidine. Furthermore, *torsades de pointes* is seen in procainamide therapy, albeit much less commonly than with quinidine therapy. Severe toxicity is manifest usually in the ECG as widening of the QRS, third-degree heart block, and ventricular tachyarrhythmias. Procaine has a more modest effect on the QT and QRS intervals than quinidine, and the sinus rate is unchanged.

Actions on Other Organ Systems. Like quinidine, procainamide causes GI side effects, although they are much less pronounced. These GI effects are nausea and vomiting, anorexia, and diarrhea. The CNS effects are unique for this class and include mental confusion, giddiness, psychosis with hallucinations, depression, and insomnia.

Pharmacokinetics. Procainamide is almost entirely absorbed when taken orally, except when it is administered in a sustained-release formulation. The lower bioavailability of the sustained-release preparations is associated with delayed absorption and a duration of action that exceeds 8 hours. The liver metabolizes procainamide by an acetylation process to *N*-acetyl procainamide (NAPA). The rate at which this process occurs varies markedly, and the population falls into a bimodal distribution of slow and fast acetylators. In fast acetylators the concentrations of NAPA in the plasma may equal or exceed those of the parent compound. It is not known whether slow acetylators have an increased risk of developing the systemic lupus erythematosus–like syndrome; they may be because they are more susceptible to hydralazine-induced lupus. The percentage of liver metabolism to direct excretion of the parent drug by the kidney is approximately 50 : 50.

NAPA—*N*-acetyl procainamide

NAPA is a cardioactive metabolite that is being investigated for its own antiarrhythmic properties. Its characteristic action on the heart puts it in the antiarrhythmic class III. That is, conduction is not affected when NAPA is administered alone, but the refractory periods of both the atria and the ventricles are prolonged, as is the time required for repolarization, represented by the QT interval. NAPA has a longer half-life than does the parent compound and is eliminated primarily by the kidney. It is for these reasons, and the fact that more parent compound is being converted to NAPA, that in states of renal failure the plasma concentration of NAPA may rise to dangerously high levels.

Therapeutic Uses. Procainamide can be used IV, which makes it a more convenient drug to use than quinidine; IV titration can be followed by oral administration for continued use. A major problem with this drug is its potential to produce a syndrome resembling systemic lupus erythematosus with long-term therapy (see Adverse Effects, Contraindications, and Drug Interactions).

Nevertheless, it can be given IV for ventricular tachyarrhythmias resistant to lidocaine therapy. It is an excellent drug for the treatment of tachyarrhythmias in the Wolff-Parkinson-White syndrome.

Effect of Age on Pharmacokinetic Parameters. Because renal function declines with age, the dosage of procainamide may need to be decreased or the dosage interval increased. In class IA procainamide is the drug of choice in the elderly because quinidine has a higher propensity to cause diarrhea in the elderly. Diarrhea can be serious in this age group, especially in view of the effects of hypokalemia on antiarrhythmic drug actions.

Adverse Effects, Contraindications, and Drug Interactions. Procainamide is contraindicated in complete heart block; decreasing the automaticity of a ventricular or A-V nodal pacemaker, when that is the only pacemaker the patient has, only compounds the problems.

Procainamide can exacerbate myasthenia gravis.

Procainamide can cause an exacerbation of myasthenia gravis because of its ability to decrease the release of acetylcholine at skeletal muscle motor nerve endings. Thus, procainamide administration may be hazardous without optimal adjustment of anticholinesterase medications and other precautions.

Known hypersensitivity to the drug or similar compounds, including the local anesthetic procaine, is a contraindication. Because hypersensitivity reactions are the most common side effect noted with the use of procainamide, fever occurring within the first days of therapy may necessitate discontinuance of the drug. Moreover, agranulocytosis may develop within a few weeks.

Procainamide should not be given to patients with supraventricular tachycardias without first pretreating them with digitalis. Just as in the case of quinidine, these drugs can decrease the atrial rates and increase the conduction at the A-V node, thereby causing a paradoxical increase in the ventricular rate. Digitalis-induced block at the A-V node can check this response by the ventricles. Unlike quinidine, procainamide is not associated with cinchonism.

Procainamide can produce a syndrome resembling systemic lupus erythematosus.

A principal adverse effect of procainamide therapy can develop with its long-term use. There is a high percentage of drug-induced lupus, a syndrome similar to authentic lupus erythematosus. Procainamide-induced lupus presents with arthralgias followed by a rash and resolves spontaneously when the drug is withheld. It can be monitored (diagnosed) by performing an assay for antinuclear antibodies (ANA). These can be detected in 80% of patients on long-term procainamide therapy.

More recently, reports have made an association with neutropenia and long-term procainamide administration. The occurrence of neutropenia is rare and is almost always resolved upon discontinuation of the drug, although some fatalities have been reported. For this reason it is recommended that routine complete blood counts (CBCs) with differential white counts be done regularly, as well as close follow-up on any complaints, even if they may seem as insignificant as cold symptoms. Neutropenia is also a rare side effect of quinidine and disopyramide therapy, so other alternatives are not necessarily readily available. Concurrent use of procainamide with quinidine or disopyramide may produce enhanced prolongation of conduction or depression of contractility and hypotension. Anticholinergic agents used concurrently may produce an additive antivagal action on the A-V nodal conduction. Because procainamide reduces acetylcholine release less neuromuscular blocking agents are required for muscle relaxation.

Cardiac and Extracardiac Effects of Toxicity. Kidney, liver, and heart failure can precipitate toxicity if the dosage of the drug is not adjusted. Heart failure decreases perfusion to all organs, including the kidney and the liver. The principal cause for the toxicity is the decreased glomerular filtration rate that accompanies renal failure.

Preparations (PRONESTYL). Procainamide is usually given IV or orally. IM administration is possible, although it rarely offers advantages over the IV route. For therapy a loading dose of 12–17 mg/kg is given over 60 minutes, followed by a maintenance infusion of 2–5 mg/minute. The wide variation in these dosages is needed to accommodate patients in heart failure and renal failure (lower dosages).

Oral therapy is begun with the conventional procainamide hydrochloride preparations every 3–4 hours until the arrhythmia is under control. The patient can be switched then to a sustained-release preparation given every 6 hours.

Disopyramide

Disopyramide was developed in an attempt to find a class IA agent with fewer side effects than quinidine or procainamide. With this drug there is a tradeoff by avoidance of some of the untoward effects of the other class IA agents for some of its own.

Mechanism of Actions. The mechanism of action of disopyramide is the sum of its direct and anticholinergic effects. The direct effects are similar to those of quinidine and procainamide except that it has a large negative inotropic effect that can be quite profound in congestive heart failure. The anticholinergic effects of disopyramide are the most prominent of all the agents in the IA class.

> Disopyramide's anticholinergic effects are the most prominent among all class IA drugs.

Action on Other Organ Systems. The principal actions on other organ systems are secondary to the anticholinergic effects. In addition, disopyramide acts as a vasoconstrictor and therefore significantly increases the afterload on the heart. This effect is much greater than any similar effects noted with quinidine or disopyramide. This effect on the heart, combined with the negative inotropic effect on the drug, can combine to produce frank heart failure in uncompensated or marginally compensated heart failure.

Therapeutic Uses. Disopyramide is effective in suppressing premature ventricular complexes and the potential ventricular tachycardia associated with such ectopic foci. It is not as effective in treating supraventricular tachyarrhythmias as is quinidine or procainamide. The anticholinergic side effects and significant negative inotropic effect make it a poor choice in the elderly.

Pharmacokinetics. Disopyramide is well absorbed when taken orally; however, malabsorptive disorders, diarrhea, and myocardial infarction may significantly decrease the absorption of the drug. About 25% of the drug is removed by a first-pass effect. The binding of the drug to plasma proteins is variable, but averages around 15%. However, the great variability in levels may be managed in the future by assay of free disopyramide plasma levels. Elimination of the drug is achieved partly by metabolism in the liver, producing a number of metabolites, at least one of which is cardioactive but somewhat less active than the parent drug; about half of the parent drug is excreted directly by the kidney.

Effect of Age on Pharmacokinetic Parameters. Disopyramide is eliminated at a decreased rate in the elderly as a result of the decreased renal function in this population. Also, disopyramide has a relative contraindication in the elderly because of its more prominent negative inotropic effect and because it may cause urinary retention by its anticholinergic effects in the face of benign prostatic hypertrophy in elderly men.

> Disopyramide is eliminated at a decreased rate in the elderly.

Adverse Effects and Contraindications. The major adverse reactions to disopyramide come from its anticholinergic side effects; these may be severe enough to mandate discontinuation of the drug. Among the more prominent of these adverse effects are dry mouth, blurred vision, mydriasis, and possible exacerbation of glaucoma, constipation, and urinary retention. Urinary retention is an especially troublesome complication of disopyramide therapy in the elderly male, given the high occurrence of benign prostatic hypertrophy in this population. The CNS effects and the occurrence of drug-induced lupus observed with quinidine and procainamide therapy do not occur or are found rarely with disopyramide therapy. Upon initiation of therapy, ventricular extrasystoles and arrhythmias may be produced. Close observation for these effects in the early stages of therapy are appropriate. The untoward effects of long-term therapy may actually be less than those with quinidine and procainamide.

Cardiac and Extracardiac Effects of Toxicity. Congestive heart failure in uncompensated and marginally compensated cases is produced by the vasoconstrictive and negative inotropic effects of the drug. Its adverse effects on ventricular function can be great in those with pre-existing ventricular failure.

Conduction disturbances may be produced as with the other class IA antiarrhythmics as a result of their local anesthetic effects. If first-degree heart block develops while on disopyramide therapy, the dosage should be reduced; if a block of higher degree develops the drug must be discontinued.

Beneficial and Adverse Effects with Other Drugs. Disopyramide does not increase the blood levels of digoxin as observed with quinidine therapy. It interacts with negative inotropic agents such as β blockers to compound their cardiac depressant effects. Moreover, anticholinergic agents should be used with great caution with disopyramide, because it possesses a cholinergic blocking activity of some 10% as atropine.

Other drugs that have a negative inotropic effect like calcium channel blockers and β blockers should be given with great caution and with consideration of the combined negative inotropic effects of disease and drug.

Contraindications include congestive heart failure and complete heart block.

Contraindications in Heart Block or Congestive Heart Failure. Congestive heart failure and complete heart block (without an artificial pacemaker) are contraindications to the use of disopyramide because of an exacerbation of the syndrome in the former, and in the latter because of the ability of the drug to decrease ventricular pacemakers to produce asystole.

Preparations. Disopyramide is available for oral use as disopyramide phosphate and in controlled-release capsules.

Pirmenol

Pirmenol, another experimental class IA agent, shows promise in suppressing PVCs with few observed side effects.

Pirmenol is an experimental agent that shows promise in its ability to suppress PVCs and may be of use in ventricular tachycardia. It has a long half-life, and there appear to be few side effects at this time.

Electrophysiology. Pirmenol is a class IA agent with an electrophysiological action similar to quinidine. It acts to block the fast sodium channels, thus decreasing the slope of phase 0 and decreasing the conduction velocity.

Pharmacokinetics. When taken orally pirmenol is approximately 87% bioavailable and has not been shown to have a significant first-pass effect.

It is extensively bound to plasma proteins (80–90%), but the drug is removed from the body equally by renal excretion and metabolism. There does not appear to be an active metabolite.

Adverse Effects and Drug Interactions. A decrease in ejection fraction with an increase in the end-diastolic pressure occurs during pirmenol therapy. This may predispose a patient with poorly compensated congestive heart failure to exacerbations with pirmenol therapy. There is a significant increase in the QT interval as seen with the other agents in this class and especially with quinidine. The antiarrhythmic action of pirmenol seems to be independent of the potassium concentration.

Contraindications. Pirmenol will probably be contraindicated in congestive heart failure because of the depressant activity it has on the compromised heart and potential for exacerbation. In complete heart block, as with all class IA agents, there is an absolute contraindication to pirmenol.

CLASS IB ANTIARRHYTHMIC AGENTS

Type IB agents exert little or no effect on V_{max} of phase 0 of normal fibers but depress conduction in fibers with a depressed fast response, decrease the action potential duration, and to a lesser degree, decrease the effective refractory period.

Phenytoin

History. Phenytoin was introduced as an anticonvulsant agent in the 1930s (Chapter 23) and was first used as an antiarrhythmic agent in the 1950s. It is a structural analog of the barbiturates.

> Phenytoin is a class IB agent first used as an antiarrhythmic agent in the 1950s.

Pharmacokinetics. Phenytoin is absorbed completely from the GI tract. It may take up to 12 hours to reach peak plasma levels after the initial oral dose; thus a loading dose is usually given. The relationship between dose and steady state plasma concentrations is not linear, and thus, it is difficult to maintain a consistent plasma concentration (see also Chapter 23).

Mechanisms of Action (see Table 33–5)

Sinoatrial Node. Phenytoin produces little direct change in S-A nodal function. The hypotension associated with its IV administration can reflexly increase sympathetic tone and thus increase the sinus heart rate.

Atria. The action potential duration and effective refractory period are not altered until high concentrations are used. The frequency of stimulation and the extracellular K^+ concentration determine the action of phenytoin on membrane responsiveness. At a normal extracellular K^+ concentration (3–5 nm) phenytoin depresses the rate of phase 0 depolarization. Conduction velocity is unaltered or slightly depressed.

Atrioventricular Node. In isolated preparations, phenytoin has been shown to act directly on the A-V node to facilitate transmission but lacks the anticholinergic actions exhibited by quinidine, procainamide, and disopyramide. Phenytoin decreases the effective refractory period of the node and increases the conduction velocity. Conduction does not seem to be depressed. In a patient intoxicated with digitalis, phenytoin can normalize transmission and decrease the ventricular automaticity associated with intoxication.

Phenytoin decreases the action potential duration.

His-Purkinje System. Phenytoin shortens the action potential duration and the effective refractory period. When membrane responsiveness has been decreased by digitalis toxicity or by hypoxia, phenytoin increases the maximal rate of phase 0 depolarization. At normal extracellular K^+ concentrations, phenytoin does not alter or produce a slight decrease in V_{max} of phase 0 depolarization. The rate of phase 4 depolarization in Purkinje tissue is decreased, as is the rate of discharge of ventricular pacemakers.

Electrocardiographic. Phenytoin may decrease the PR and QT intervals as a result of improved A-V conduction and a shortened action potential duration in ventricular muscle.

Organ/System Pharmacology. Rapid IV administration may induce a transient hypotension, the result of a direct action on the vascular bed and heart to produce peripheral vasodilatation and depression of cardiac contractility. The slow administration of larger dosages produces a dose-related decrease in the left ventricular force, the rate of force development, and cardiac output. Left ventricular end-diastolic pressure increases.

Adverse Effects. Nystagmus appears at phenytoin blood levels greater than 20 μg/ml, ataxia when levels are between 30 and 40 μg/ml, and coma and seizures at concentrations greater than 40 μg/ml (see Table 33–5). Rapid IV administration may produce arrhythmias and asystole, although cardiac toxicity is rarely observed following an oral overdose. Other adverse effects include nausea, vomiting, hyperglycemia, fever, skin rashes, dermatitis, hepatitis, gingival hyperplasia, lymphoid hyperplasia, and hematological abnormalities. Some individuals have a hereditary difference in the enzymes involved in parahydroxylation; they become saturated by concentrations of phenytoin in the therapeutic range and, consequently, may exhibit toxic signs with therapeutic dosages.

Reports indicate a correlation between phenytoin and higher incidences of birth defects.

Reports suggest an association between the use of phenytoin and a higher incidence of birth defects, cleft lip/palate, and heart malformations in children born to these women, although a definite cause and effect relationship has not been established. A *fetal hydantoin embryopathy syndrome* consisting of prenatal growth deficiency, microcephaly, mental deficiency, and coagulopathies have been also reported from observations in neonates. Nevertheless, the great majority of females on an antiepileptic drug deliver normal offspring. Only in those females in whom the severity and frequency of the seizure disorder is not a serious threat should the drug be discontinued prior to and during pregnancy. Even so, minor seizures may constitute a hazard to the fetus. (This is also discussed in Chapter 23.)

In spite of being widely prescribed, few deaths have been reported from an overdose of phenytoin. The deaths that have occurred have been due to idiosyncratic reactions or have occurred during a rapid IV injection. Overdose with phenytoin is treated by focusing on symptomatic and supportive care. Charcoal hemoperfusion, diuresis, and hemodialysis are generally of no benefit. The utility of exchange transfusion is unclear (Mofenson et al, 1986).

Phenytoin is effective in treating atrial and ventricular arrhythmias induced by digitalis toxicity.

Therapeutic Uses. The primary clinical application of phenytoin for arrhythmias is in the treatment of atrial and ventricular arrhythmias induced by digitalis toxicity. Phenytoin is used also as a prophylactic agent to prevent position version arrhythmias, especially in a digitalized patient. It is also effective in the treatment of ventricular arrhythmias occurring in acute myocardial infarction, open-heart surgery, anesthesia, cardiac catheterization, cardioversion, and angiographic studies.

Phenytoin, like lidocaine (discussed later), is much more effective in the treatment of ventricular than supraventricular arrhythmias. Phenytoin is *ineffective* in converting atrial flutter or atrial fibrillation; treating supraventricular arrhythmias not associated with intoxication by digitalis; or preventing sudden coronary death owing to ventricular fibrillation post-myocardial infarction. Phenytoin may increase ventricular rate in patients with atrial flutter or atrial fibrillation. The combination of phenytoin with a β antagonist or with other class I drugs seems to increase its efficacy in the treatment of ventricular arrhythmias (Anderson, 1985).

Drug Interactions (see Chapters 6, 23, and 64). Because 80–90% of plasma phenytoin is bound to protein, a small decrease in binding may increase its therapeutic or toxic actions. Agents such as salicylates, sulfonamides, phenylbutazone, and bilirubin all displace phenytoin from its binding site on plasma protein and thus increase the free plasma level. Free phenytoin levels increase two to three times in uremic patients in spite of the total phenytoin plasma concentrations remaining within the therapeutic range. The metabolism of phenytoin is inhibited by decreased liver function and by drugs such as cimetidine and isoniazid. These drugs induce a marked increase in the half-life and plasma levels of phenytoin. Metabolism of phenytoin is accelerated by microsomal enzyme induction induced by phenobarbital. In addition, phenytoin itself induces the liver enzymes and thus may enhance the metabolism of drugs such as corticosteroids, digitoxin, and methadone.

Preparation and Dosage (DILANTIN). Phenytoin sodium is marketed as capsules and tablets. Because there are significant differences in the bioavailability among the various phenytoin preparations available, it is recommended that patients be treated with the product of a single manufacturer. Phenytoin is also marketed as a sterile solution for parenteral use. The vehicle has a pH of approximately 12 and may cause severe phlebitis unless infused slowly with dilution. The IM route is not used to treat serious arrhythmias because absorption is too unreliable.

The various formulations of phenytoin differ in their bioavailability.

Lidocaine

Lidocaine, a local anesthetic discussed in Chapter 17, was first used as an antiarrhythmic agent in the 1950s and today is the mainstay in the treatment of ventricular arrhythmias in intensive care units. One of its limiting features is its low bioavailability after oral dosing, with one third reaching the circulation because of extensive first-pass hepatic metabolism; consequently, it is always given parenterally (and almost always IV). This limitation has led to the development of newer lidocaine congeners, such as tocainide, that possess oral effectiveness.

Lidocaine is limited by its inability to be administered orally.

Pharmacokinetics. Exponential plasma concentration time curves occur after the IV administration of lidocaine. The initial rapid decline represents the distribution phase and has a half-life of 20 minutes; this initial phase is followed by a slow decline associated with elimination and has a half-life of 2 hours. Five to 7 hours are required to achieve steady state plasma concentrations with a constant infusion of lidocaine. Table 33–4 includes the volume of distribution, the extent of protein binding, oral bioavailability, and other pharmacokinetic properties of lidocaine.

Mechanism of Action—Electrophysiological

S-A Node. Therapeutic concentrations of lidocaine have no effect on sinus rate, unlike procainamide, quinidine, or disopyramide.

Atria. Actions on atria are similar to those of quinidine. Membrane responsiveness, the amplitude of the action potential, and excitability of atrial muscle are decreased by lidocaine, producing a decrease in the conduction velocity. The effective refractory period is slightly increased or unaltered.

A-V Node. Conduction velocity and the effective refractory period are altered to a minimal extent by the usual therapeutic dosages of lidocaine.

His-Purkinje System. The amplitude of the action potential and membrane responsiveness are both decreased. If myocardial ischemia has reduced the resting membrane potential to -70 to -60 mV, blood levels on the high side of the therapeutic range of lidocaine may depress phase 0 depolarization in the Purkinje fibers, which can result in complete blockade of conduction. The action potential duration and effective refractory period are shortened at lower levels of lidocaine than required to alter the same parameters in ventricular muscle. Phase 4 depolarization and the spontaneous discharge rate are decreased by lidocaine; high levels suppress automaticity and eliminate phase 4 depolarization.

Ventricular Muscle. Action potential duration and the effective refractory period are decreased.

Electrocardiographic. Lidocaine may shorten the QT interval but usually does not alter the PR, QRS, and QT intervals.

Organ/System Pharmacology. When lidocaine is used in therapeutic dosages, it rarely induces hemodynamic changes.

Side effects such as drowsiness, muscle twitching, and vertigo may be observed as plasma levels of lidocaine are increased.

Adverse Effects. Therapeutic plasma concentrations range from 1 to 5 μg/ml. As plasma levels of lidocaine increase above a level of 5 μg/ml, drowsiness, muscle twitching, paresthesias, speech disturbances, vertigo, tinnitus, and disorientation may be observed (see Table 33–5). Levels twice that, of 9 μg/ml or more, may be associated with psychosis, respiratory depression, or seizures. Patients receiving lidocaine should be monitored closely because potentially fatal status epilepticus may develop quickly. Such convulsions are dose-related and can be prevented by using a rate of infusion to keep plasma concentrations below 5 μg/ml. Toxic levels may also cause severe bradycardia, sinus arrest, and A-V block.

Treatment of overdosage should focus on the management of the serious cardiovascular effects, the seizures, and the possibility of methemoglobinemia. Seizures may be relatively refractory to therapy, but phenytoin can be employed. There is a likelihood that seizures may still be present after the lidocaine serum levels have fallen below 5 μg/ml, because the metabolite monoethylglylcine xylidide is also a convulsant. If the methemoglobin level is greater than or equal to 30% and is associated with dyspnea, metabolic acidosis, or altered mental status, methylene blue (for treatment of drug-induced methemoglobinemia) and oxygen should be administered. Oxygen transport depends on the maintenance of intracellular hemoglobin in the reduced (Fe^{2+}) state. As the oxidation of hemoglobin to methemoglobin occurs, the heme iron becomes Fe^{3+} and is incapable of binding oxygen. Normal red cells contain less than 1% methemoglobin. If methemoglobin exceeds 1.5 g/dl (10% of the total hemoglobin), individuals will exhibit signs of clinically obvious cyanosis. At levels of approximately 35% the affected person will experience headache, weakness, and breathlessness. Severe toxic methemoglobinemia is treated with methylene blue (2 mg/kg, repeat if needed). Within an hour the methemoglobin level is usually reduced by at least 50%. Hemodialysis is not effective.

Therapeutic Uses. Lidocaine is used almost exclusively to treat ventricular arrhythmias; it is ineffective in the treatment of most supraventricular arrhythmias. In the acute myocardial infarction patient, lidocaine will control ventricular arrhythmias and prevent ventricular fibrillation with little risk, because it lacks significant depressant effects on the cardiovascular system and because the toxic side effects are of short duration. Either lidocaine or phenytoin may be used to treat ventricular arrhythmias associated with digitalis intoxication.

Precautions and Contraindications. The elimination of lidocaine in individuals with congestive heart failure will be delayed. Renal failure does not alter its clearance. Contraindications to the use of lidocaine include severe hepatic dysfunction, a previous history of grand mal seizures following lidocaine, hypersensitivity to amide local anesthetics, or the presence of second- or third-degree heart block. Lidocaine may increase the degree of pre-existing heart block and can depress an idioventricular pacemaker that may be maintaining cardiac rhythm.

> Lidocaine can depress an idioventricular pacemaker.

Lidocaine plasma concentrations may be increased in the elderly because of increased binding to acid-α-1-glycoprotein. These concentrations may not produce toxic effects because unbound drug produces the effect. Nevertheless, the use of lidocaine in patients 70 years of age or older is contraindicated. Table 33–6 summarizes the cardiovascular drugs, including lidocaine, that have been identified as producing an increased risk of adverse effects in the elderly.

Drug Interactions. Lidocaine is metabolized by hepatic microsomes, so any drug increasing or decreasing liver microsomal enzyme activity alters its metabolism. Thus, cimetidine increases lidocaine plasma levels and increases its half-life because of the ability of cimetidine to reduce hepatic

> Drugs affecting liver microsomal enzyme activity alter the metabolism of lidocaine.

Table 33–6 REPRESENTATIVE CARDIOVASCULAR DRUGS EXHIBITING AGE-RELATED ALTERATIONS IN DISPOSITION OR RESPONSE

Drug	Principal Age-Related Factor	Pharmacokinetic Changes*			Comments
		V_d	$t_{1/2}$	Cl	
Digoxin	Renal clearance	↓	↑	↓	Reduce dosage
Lidocaine	Liver clearance	↑	↑	0	Reduce dosage
Procainamide	Renal clearance	--	--	↓	Reduce dosage with compromised renal function and congestive heart failure
Quinidine	Liver and renal clearance	0	↑	↓	Individualize dosage
Disopyramide	Renal clearance: anticholinergic side effects	--	↑	↓	Reduce dosage with compromised renal function; check bowel and bladder function
Tocainide	Renal clearance	--	↑	↓	Reduce dosage with compromised renal function
β blockers, lipid-soluble	Liver clearance	0	↑	↓	Decreased response; individualize dosage
β blockers, water-soluble	Renal clearance	--	↑	↓	Decreased response; individualize dosage

Adapted from Rocci ML, Vlasses PH, Abrams WB: Geriatric clinical pharmacology. Cardiol Clin 4:213, 1986.
* 0 = no significant change; -- = no information or not relevant; ↑ = increased; ↓ = decreased.

blood flow. Pharmacological agents that induce or inhibit the liver P-450 system will also alter lidocaine metabolism. Cimetidine also binds to cytochrome P-450 and thus decreases the activity of the hepatic microsomal mixed-function oxidases. Barbiturates appear to enhance the disposition of lidocaine. Although this has been assumed to be due to induction of hepatic microsomal enzymes, hepatic blood flow is probably the primary determinant of lidocaine disposition. (However, because lidocaine is usually titrated to achieve the desired response, patients are infrequently adversely affected in the event that they are more or less sensitive to the effects of lidocaine.)

Preparations and Dosages (XYLOCAINE). Lidocaine for systemic antiarrhythmic purposes is only administered IV or IM. This injection solution does not contain a preservative, a sympathomimetic, or other vasoconstrictor agent; thus, it is only this preparation that should be used for the IV administration of lidocaine for treating arrhythmias.

When controlling ventricular arrhythmias, an initial IV loading dose no greater than 1.4 mg/kg may be given over 1–3 minutes and may be supplemented over 3–5 minutes with a sustained slower infusion. Care must be exercised to ensure that the rate and total dosages do not exceed recommended amounts, e.g., 200–300 mg in 1 hour. As much as 50% reduction in dosage may be necessary in patients in shock or in those with hepatic disease or heart failure.

An IM administration can provide therapeutic plasma levels within 15 minutes. Every 90 minutes thereafter one half of the initial dose must be given to sustain the therapeutic plasma level. However, administration of lidocaine by this route is painful and results in erratic absorption. Thus, the IM route should be used only when IV access cannot be established.

Future Agents. Newer class IB antiarrhythmic agents have been designed in the hope of finding a lidocaine analog that possesses an antiarrhythmic action when given orally, a long duration of action, and a large therapeutic index. Tocainide and mexiletine are two antiarrhythmic agents that meet some of these criteria.

> Tocainide and mexiletine were developed as an oral alternative to lidocaine.

Tocainide

Chemistry. Tocainide hydrochloride (2-amino-*N*-2, 6-dimethylphenylalaninamide hydrochloride) is a primary amine analog of lidocaine. This alteration of the side chain of lidocaine results in tocainide, which does not undergo appreciable first-pass metabolic degradation in the liver, in contrast to lidocaine. Approximately 10–50% of the tocainide administered is bound to protein. Overall, 50% of tocainide is metabolized in the liver and 40% is excreted in urine.

Pharmacokinetics. Tocainide is well absorbed after oral administration with bioavailability approaching 100% (see Table 33–4). Peak plasma levels occur between 30 minutes and 4 hours after oral dosing. The half-life is approximately 14 hours in normal individuals. The plasma concentration is related directly to the dosage unless administered with food; food decreases the peak plasma concentration but does not decrease the overall bioavailability. To prevent initial high levels, it is recommended that tocainide be taken with meals. The therapeutic plasma concentration ranges between 3 and 7 μg/ml for the base and from 4 to 10 μg/ml of tocainide hydrochloride. No known active metabolites of tocainide have been found. Tocainide is approximately half as potent as lidocaine.

> Tocainide's absorption is excellent; bioavailability is close to 100%.

Mechanism of Action. Tocainide exhibits most of the electrophysiological effects of lidocaine (see Table 33–5). It reduces phase 0 and shortens the effective refractory period of the cardiac action potential.

A-V Node and Atrial and Ventricular Muscle. The effective refractory period is shortened; the predominant effect is observed in the A-V node.

S-A Node. Tocainide exerts little effect on S-A nodal automaticity or intra-cardiac conduction.

Purkinje Fibers. The slope of phase 4 depolarization is reduced. The rate of rise of phase 0 is decreased, and a depression of the amplitude of the action potential occurs.

Electrocardiographic. Tocainide has minimal effects, although the QT interval is shortened.

Organ/System Pharmacology. Tocainide exhibits only a minor effect on cardiac hemodynamics even in patients with cardiac dysfunction.

Adverse Effects. Tocainide has a wider margin of safety than lidocaine, particularly when actions on the CNS are compared. The most common side effects associated with the use of tocainide are GI symptoms and include nausea, vomiting, abdominal pain, anorexia, and constipation. The administration of smaller dosages or concomitant intake with food may minimize these actions. The occurrence of headache, dizziness, paresthesias, and tremor are thought to be more closely correlated with the doses than are the GI side effects. Hypersensitivity reactions, including rash, induction of arrhythmias (Table 33–7) and fatal agranulocytosis, are uncommon. Because agranulocytosis, bone marrow depression, leukopenia, hypoplastic anemia, neutropenia, and thrombocytopenia have also been reported and sequelae such as septicemia and septic shock have been reported with doses in the recommended range, periodic CBCs, especially

Table 33–7 GUIDELINES FOR THE MANAGEMENT OF ARRHYTHMIAS

| Arrhythmia | Acute | | Chronic | |
	First Line	*Alternatives*	*First Line*	*Alternatives*
Atrial premature beats	Usually no treatment		Quinidine	Disopyramide Procainamide
Atrial flutter/fibrillation	Cardioversion Digitalis	Verapamil Propranolol Type IA	Digitalis ± Quinidine	Verapamil Amiodarone
Paroxysmal atrial tachycardia	Verapamil	Digitalis Propranolol	Digitalis Verapamil	Quinidine Amiodarone
A-V nodal tachycardias	Verapamil	Digitalis Propranolol Procainamide	Digitalis Propranolol	Verapamil Type IA Amiodarone
Ventricular premature beats	Lidocaine	Procainamide Quinidine Disopyramide	Quinidine	Procainamide Disopyramide Amiodarone
Ventricular tachycardia	Cardioversion Lidocaine	Procainamide Disopyramide Quinidine Bretylium	Procainamide Disopyramide Quinidine	Amiodarone

during the first 6 months of use, are recommended. Patients with atrial flutter or atrial fibrillation may exhibit an increase in the ventricular rate after the administration of tocainide. In some patients, tocainide has exacerbated congestive heart failure and worsened pre-existent conduction disturbances. IV administration has been reported to induce bradycardia.

Therapeutic Uses. Tocainide suppresses the presence of premature ventricular contractions in 50% of patients exhibiting them chronically and is of benefit in the treatment of ventricular ectopy associated with the early stages of acute myocardial infarction and those associated with postmyocardial infarction. Tocainide is effective for the short-term suppression of ventricular arrhythmias; it appears to be the logical agent to use for chronic oral dosing of patients in whom IV lidocaine resulted in suppression of ventricular tachycardia and ventricular ectopic activity. The majority of patients exhibiting drug-resistant ventricular arrhythmias, including recurrent sustained ventricular tachycardia or fibrillation, respond positively to the administration of tocainide.

In summary, to date tocainide appears to be an orally active antiarrhythmic agent with actions similar to lidocaine; the predictability of its efficacy in patients responsive to lidocaine aids in its clinical use. Patients responsive to lidocaine also respond to tocainide in a majority of cases, whereas failure to respond to lidocaine usually predicts failure to respond to tocainide, although there are exceptions to this. It is effective in the prophylaxis and treatment of patients with refractory or chronic ventricular arrhythmias.

The efficacy of tocainide is approximately that of other drugs in class I, such as quinidine, procainamide, and disopyramide. Although the side effects associated with the use of tocainide are similar in frequency to those reported for quinidine, the unwanted actions of tocainide are often milder and better tolerated, and patients respond well to a change in the dose.

Cautions. The plasma half-life is 12–15 hours and may be increased twofold in patients with renal failure or hepatic disease.

Drug Interactions. To date, drugs that decrease hepatic blood flow and alter hepatic degradative enzymes have not been reported to produce an increase in plasma tocainide, unlike the situation with lidocaine. Interactions of cimetidine, propranolol, and verapamil with tocainide have been looked for but have not been reported. The concomitant administration of metoprolol and tocainide does not alter the time to reach the maximal plasma concentrations, plasma half-lives, and myocardial function. The frequency of adverse reactions in individuals receiving tocainide alone or with digoxin did not vary nor did the plasma digoxin levels increase. No interaction involving the coadministration of warfarin sodium and tocainide has been found.

Preparations and Dosages (TONOCARD). Tocainide is available in 400 or 600 mg tablets. The initial dosage is 400 mg every 8 hours, with the total dose ranging between 1200 and 1800 mg/day given in three doses. A dose of 400–600 mg given every 8–12 hours will usually suppress ventricular arrhythmias.

Mexiletine

Mexiletine was approved as a treatment for ventricular arrhythmia in the United States in 1986.

History. Mexiletine was approved in the United States for the treatment of ventricular arrhythmias in 1986, although it had been commercially avail-

Chapter 33 / Antiarrhythmic Agents **539**

able since 1976 in England. Nevertheless, additional efficacy, toxicity, and pharmacokinetic studies are required to establish its clinical status.

Chemistry, Pharmacokinetics (see Table 33–4), **and Mechanism of Action.** Mexiletine shares many of its electrophysiological effects with lidocaine and tocainide (see Table 33–5). Thus, mexiletine decreases V_{max} and the depolarization threshold of both atrial and ventricular myocardium. Studies in humans indicate that A-V nodal conduction time and refractoriness and His-Purkinje conduction time (HV interval) are increased or unchanged. The ventricular effective refractory period is increased. Mexiletine differs from lidocaine in that it has a relatively greater effect at slower pacing rates.

Adverse Effects. Like other antiarrhythmic drugs, mexiletine has a narrow therapeutic margin, yet a direct correlation with the concentration of mexiletine and observed toxic effects does not seem to exist. Neurological side effects are generally observed at plasma levels greater than 2.0 μg/ml but occasionally develop at levels less than 1.0 μg/ml. Side effects have been reported for a mean of 30% of the patients taking it (range 10–60%), and the drug may have to be discontinued in from 5 to 30% of the patients. The most common side effects are related to the CNS, are dose-related, and occur with both IV and oral dosages. The initial symptom is a fine hand tremor. Ataxia, dizziness, lightheadedness, nystagmus, paresthesias, blurred vision, diplopia, dysarthria, confusion, drowsiness, psychosis, and seizures have been reported.

Sinus bradycardia or conduction abnormalities have been noted in patients with pre-existent conduction disease such as sick sinus syndrome. The rapid IV bolus administration of mexiletine may produce hypotension, QRS widening, and bradycardia. Aggravation of underlying ventricular arrhythmia and mexiletine-induced *torsades de pointes* have been observed.

Therapeutic Uses. Mexiletine is effective in the treatment of premature ventricular contractions not associated with acute myocardial infarction as well as in the prevention of ventricular ectopy in the acute infarction patient or postinfarction. Clinical studies suggest that mexiletine is not effective in the management of drug-refractory inducible ventricular tachycardia. Studies combining quinidine and mexiletine demonstrated a better response in treating ventricular tachycardia, whereas the combination of amiodarone and mexiletine controlled drug-refractory ventricular tachycardia. Used alone, mexiletine is effective in a small number of patients with recurrent ventricular tachycardia; in combination with other antiarrhythmic agents it is more effective in drug-refractory patients.

Precautions and Contraindications. Because mexiletine is primarily (90%) eliminated hepatically, with only 10% of a dose excreted unchanged in the urine, its dose requires adjustment only in patients with severe renal dysfunction, i.e., those with a creatinine clearance less than or equal to 10 ml/minute. Peritoneal dialysis, with or without peritoneal inflammation, does not alter the systemic clearance of mexiletine. In contrast, patients undergoing hemodialysis may require a supplemental dose on the day of dialysis. Conflicting data exist about the use of mexiletine in the patient with congestive heart failure. Preliminary studies indicate that in patients with liver disease the plasma clearance of mexiletine is increased (see Table

Ninety percent of mexiletine is eliminated hepatically.

33–4). Studies of plasma levels after single doses of mexiletine given to acute myocardial infarction patients, many exhibiting signs of left ventricular dysfunction, suggest that the elimination half-life and volume of distribution are increased by approximately 40%.

Preparations and Dosages (MERITIL). Mexiletine hydrochloride is available in the United States in oral capsule dosage form in various strengths.

CLASS IC AGENTS

Class IC agents depress V_{max}, but unlike class IA drugs, they do not cause a significant change in refractoriness or the action potential duration. Unlike class IB drugs, they do not depress V_{max} in a potassium-dependent manner.

Flecainide and encainide are class IC agents.

History. Flecainide and encainide are relatively new antiarrhythmic drugs. Although they are effective for ventricular arrhythmias and are usually well tolerated, some cases have been reported in which worsening of arrhythmias has occurred. Although all antiarrhythmic drugs may cause arrhythmias, flecainide and encainide have been shown to increase the sudden-death rate and total mortality when used to treat asymptomatic or minimally symptomatic ventricular arrhythmias in patients after myocardial infarction. The risk appeared to be similar across all patient subgroups entered in the Cardiac Arrhythmia Suppression Trial and seemed to exist despite the effective suppression of spontaneous ventricular premature beats by these agents. The mechanism of these sudden deaths are unclear, but they have been attributed to the induction of lethal ventricular arrhythmias. In patients with a history of myocardial infarction, it has been recommended that class IC agents be reserved for use in those patients in whom other antiarrhythmic agents are poorly tolerated or not effective (Ruskin, 1989).

Flecainide

Chemistry and Pharmacokinetics. Flecainide was developed through a systematic alteration of procainamide and lidocaine molecules.
Pharmacokinetic parameters are presented in Table 33–4.

Flecainide was derived from an alteration of procainamide and lidocaine molecules.

Mechanism of Action (Table 33–5)

S-A Node. The mean sinus cycle length is usually decreased only slightly; however, it can have unpredictable actions on sinus node automaticity and conduction.

Atria. The maximal rate of depolarization is decreased. The membrane responsiveness curve is shifted to the right. Conduction velocity is decreased.

A-V Node and His-Purkinje Conduction. A-V (AH interval) and His-Purkinje (HV interval) conduction is prolonged by flecainide.

Electrocardiographic. The PR and QRS intervals are prolonged.

Organ/System Pharmacology. Myocardial contractility is decreased slightly after the administration of flecainide. Ejection fraction and the velocity of circumferential fiber shortening decrease after IV dosing, although not all echocardiography studies confirm this slight negative inotropic action (Mueller and Baur, 1986). Blood pressure is not altered. The working capacity of healthy individuals and patients with heart failure is not modified. Thus, to date the data indicate that flecainide has minimal hemodynamic actions.

Adverse Effects. It has been suggested that the main consideration when using flecainide is its potential arrhythmogenic actions (see Table 33–5). Patients treated for sustained ventricular tachycardia, who frequently have heart failure, a history of myocardial infarction, or an episode of cardiac arrest, have been reported to be more prone to a proarrhythmic action. Too rapid administration of an IV loading dose can also induce arrhythmias. Thus, for patients with sustained ventricular tachycardia, flecainide treatment should be initiated in the hospital with rhythm monitoring. For treatment of those with symptomatic congestive heart failure or sinus node dysfunction, even if no history of sustained ventricular tachycardia exists, hospitalization is also recommended. Hospitalization should also be considered for those with significant myocardial dysfunction, i.e., a low ejection fraction.

Arrhythmias can be induced by a rapid administration of an IV loading dose of flecainide.

Other adverse reactions associated with the use of flecainide include visual disturbances, abdominal cramps and distention, flatulence, headache, drowsiness, dry mouth, nausea, and vomiting. Tremors, hot and cold sensations, shortness of breath, and constipation occur less frequently. With continued use of flecainide, most of these side effects disappear.

Experimental and clinical studies confirm that flecainide is beneficial in the treatment of ventricular arrhythmias, including repetitive episodes of ventricular tachycardia and those occurring after acute myocardial infarction. Its beneficial use has been shown in patients with supraventricular re-entry tachycardia and supraventricular extrasystoles. Atrial flutter and atrial fibrillation in patients with Wolff-Parkinson-White syndrome have responded to treatment with flecainide.

Precautions and Contraindications. As discussed earlier, patients with low ejection fraction and sustained ventricular tachycardia are especially prone to flecainide's arrhythmogenic action. Flecainide should be used with caution in individuals with sinus node abnormalities because it exhibits an unpredictable action on sinus node automaticity and conduction. It depresses A-V nodal function, and in patients with pre-existing conduction defects blocks involving the His-Purkinje system may develop. There have been reports of sinus bradycardia, sinus pause, or sinus arrest. Therefore, flecainide should not be used in the setting of pre-existing second- or third-degree A-V heart block, or with bifascicular block unless a pacemaker is present. Flecainide should be used with caution and in reduced dosages in the presence of congestive heart failure.

Drug Interactions. When flecainide and amiodarone are used together, the dosage of flecainide should be decreased by 50% and the patient should be monitored for adverse effects. The concurrent administration of flecainide and digoxin in healthy volunteers induced a transient elevation of the steady state digoxin plasma levels. Six hours later the digoxin levels returned toward baseline. Concurrent dosing with flecainide and propranolol appears to induce less of a decrease in the heart rate than when only propranolol is given; this effect is thought to be due to an anticholinergic action of flecainide. A greater prolongation of the PR interval and a slightly increased reduction in the systolic and diastolic blood pressure occur when propranolol and flecainide are used together.

CLASS II AGENTS: β-ADRENOCEPTOR BLOCKING AGENTS

Class II drugs inhibit the effect of sympathetic stimulation on the heart.

Propranolol

Mechanism of Action and Pharmacokinetics. The antiarrhythmic action of propranolol (see Table 33–5) is generally attributed to a combination of β-adrenergic blockade (thus removing the adrenergic modulation of the heart), an increase in the outward potassium current, and in higher dosages, a depression of sodium current.

Pharmacokinetics of propranolol is discussed in Chapter 14.

> Propranolol blocks the β receptors in the S-A node.

Sinoatrial Node. Propranolol blocks the β receptors in the S-A node and thus prevents adrenergic stimulation from increasing the slope of phase 4 depolarization and increasing the spontaneous firing rate in the sinus node. It is this action that is thought to explain how propranolol decreases the heart rate. In general, the resting heart rate is only slightly decreased, but increases in heart rate induced by exercise or emotion are decreased. If the patient has pre-existing sinus node disease, the heart rate may be greatly decreased by propranolol.

Atria. Propranolol exhibits a local anesthetic action and exerts a quinidine-like action on the atrial membrane action potential. Membrane responsiveness, action potential amplitude, excitability, and conduction velocity are all decreased.

A-V Node. The conduction velocity through the A-V node is decreased, and the A-V nodal refractory period is increased by the propranolol-induced β blockade. This increase in the effective refractory period is thought to explain the antiarrhythmic actions of propranolol.

His-Purkinje System. Therapeutic concentrations of propranolol depress catecholamine-induced automaticity. Membrane responsiveness, the action potential amplitude, and tissue excitability are decreased by propranolol. Conduction velocity is subsequently decreased. All these actions occur at dosages higher than therapeutic concentrations and higher than the dosage required to establish β-adrenoceptor blockade.

Ventricular Muscle. Membrane responsiveness and myocardial excitability is decreased by propranolol. The duration of the action potential is increased only at high plasma concentrations.

Electrocardiographic Action. The PR interval may be increased, the QT interval is shortened, and the QRS complex duration prolonged only after large doses of propranolol have been administered.

Autonomic Nervous System. The establishment of β-adrenoceptor blockade with propranolol does not affect the α-adrenergic receptor or the parasympathetic division of the autonomic nervous system. Experimental data show that some β blockers, such as practolol and metoprolol, depress spontaneous discharge in the cardiac sympathetic nerves whereas others, i.e., timolol or sotalol, do not (Lathers et al, 1986b).

Organ/System Pharmacology. When propranolol blocks the cardiac β-adrenergic receptor it prevents or decreases the effect of stimulating the cardiac sympathetic nerves and catecholamine-induced inotropic and chronotropic actions. Systolic ejection periods at rest and during exercise are increased; this has a tendency to increase myocardial oxygen consumption. The decrease in heart rate and decrease in force of contraction cause a decrease in myocardial oxygen consumption; this effect is the dominant action.

Adverse Effects and Drug Interactions. The unwanted effects associated with the use of any β-blocking agents are the consequence of their ability to block β receptors. The use of a β-blocking agent to control an arrhythmia in the presence of enhanced sympathetic activity may result in hypotension or left ventricular failure. The concomitant use of diuretics, vasodilators, or digitalis may allow the use of chronic oral propranolol in patients with ventricular failure. Interestingly, propranolol-induced heart failure can be reversed immediately by the administration of glucagon.

Hypotension and left ventricular failure are possible adverse effects from propranolol's β-blocking action.

Amrinone, an inotropic agent, will also increase cardiac contractility in the presence of β blockade established by propranolol. It has been noted that propranolol can precipitate left ventricular failure in individuals previously free of heart failure.

The ability of propranolol to decrease A-V conduction may result in bradycardia, A-V block, or asystole. Atropine, IV, may reverse propranolol-induced bradycardia. Ventricular asystole associated with the use of propranolol will respond to mechanical or electrical stimulation but does not respond to the administration of exogenous catecholamines.

The rapid IV infusion of propranolol produces vasodilatation and results in hypotension. Cardiac β-adrenergic receptor blockade and the direct myocardial depression also contribute to the precipitation of hypotension.

Both normal and asthmatic patients may experience bronchospasm and increased airway resistance associated with $β_2$-adrenergic receptor blockade induced by propranolol. Aminophylline, but not isoproterenol, can reverse such propranolol-induced bronchospasm.

Diabetic patients, patients with partial gastrectomy, and children recovering from anesthesia may exhibit hypoglycemia in response to the blockade of the β-receptor–mediated glycogenolysis in skeletal muscle. Finally, fetal cardiac responses to the stress associated with labor and delivery are blocked by the administration of propranolol because it crosses the placental membrane and enters the fetal circulation.

If propranolol is discontinued abruptly in individuals with angina pectoris, cardiac arrhythmias, a worsening of the angina symptoms, or acute myocardial infarction may appear. These effects of discontinuation may be related to the increased cardiac β receptor density associated with chronic dosing with β-blocking agents (Lathers et al, 1986b).

Therapeutic Uses

Supraventricular Arrhythmias. The supraventricular tachyarrhythmias of atrial fibrillation, atrial flutter, and paroxysmal supraventricular tachycardia are the chief indications for the use of propranolol as an antiarrhythmic agent. Propranolol decreases the ventricular rate by eliminating β-adrenergic stimulation of receptors in the A-V node and thus increasing refractoriness of the A-V node. Thus, the therapeutic goal is to decrease the ventricular rate rather than to abolish the arrhythmia; it is unusual if propranolol achieves the latter. Propranolol is often prescribed, in addition to digitalis, for patients who manifest atrial fibrillation or flutter not controlled by digitalis alone. A combination of the mechanisms of action

Propranolol is used primarily to decrease supraventricular tachyarrhythmias.

of the two drugs, i.e., the increased vagal activity induced by digitalis and the establishment of β blockade at the A-V node by propranolol, is thought to explain the beneficial effect of the additive therapy (see Table 33–9).

The combination of propranolol and quinidine is thought to increase the probability of converting atrial fibrillation to a normal sinus rhythm. In the treatment of paroxysmal supraventricular tachycardia of the Wolff-Parkinson-White syndrome, when propranolol alone has failed to control the arrhythmia, the combination relies on the ability of quinidine to increase the refractoriness in A-V tissue and propranolol to increase A-V nodal refractoriness. Propranolol alone is not effective in preventing atrial fibrillation after cardioversion, but a combination with quinidine is more effective than quinidine alone.

Ventricular Arrhythmias. Propranolol is usually not effective in the treatment of ventricular arrhythmias. Propranolol is effective in the treatment of ventricular premature depolarizations in patients with no structural heart disease. Propranolol will also suppress the ventricular arrhythmias associated with exercise, anxiety, pheochromocytoma, or thyrotoxicosis. In the presence of ischemic heart disease, propranolol has been shown to prevent ventricular arrhythmias by decreasing or preventing ischemia. Numerous clinical trials have shown that chronic treatment with β blockers, including propranolol, timolol, metoprolol, or atenolol, reduces the incidence of reinfarction and the mortality in individuals who have survived a myocardial infarction (Fig. 33–7). The precise mechanism of the protection afforded by dosing with chronic β-blocking agents has yet to be determined. The possibility of the occurrence of tachyarrhythmias, angina

Chronic treatment with propranolol has been shown to reduce frequency of reinfarction and mortality.

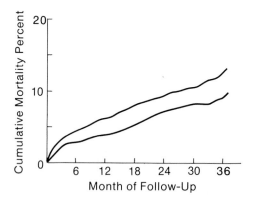

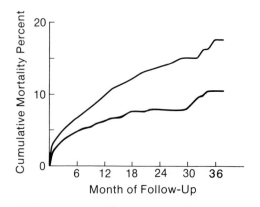

Figure 33–7

Survival rates with treatment with β-blocking agents. *Top:* Results from two different studies, redrawn to be on the same scale. Survival results of β Blocker Heart Attack Trial. A total of 3837 patients were randomized to treatment with propranolol *(color)* or a placebo. After a 3-year follow-up, there was a significant reduction in mortality in those treated with propranolol. (From National Institutes of Health, β Blocker Heart Attack Study Group: A randomized trial of propranolol in patients with acute myocardial infarction. JAMA 247:1707–1714, 1982.) *Bottom:* Multicenter trial with timolol. A total of 1884 patients with myocardial infarctions were randomized to placebo or timolol *(color)* therapy. After an average follow-up of 33 months, there was a significant reduction in mortality in the timolol group. (From Timolol-induced reduction in mortality and reinfarction in patients surviving acute myocardial infarction. Reprinted with permission from The New England Journal of Medicine, 304:801–807, 1981.)

pectoris, or hypertension in the postinfarction period would also justify the use of chronic β-blocking agents.

Digitalis-Induced Arrhythmias. Propranolol can abolish digitalis-induced ventricular arhythmias. This action is attributed to its direct action on the heart and to suppression of central and peripheral sympathetic neural activity. Nevertheless, phenytoin or lidocaine is the drug of choice for treatment of digitalis-induced arrhythmias because the occurrence of adverse effects, including bradycardia, is greater when propranolol is used.

Anesthetic-Induced Arrhythmias. The inhalational anesthetic halothane sensitizes the heart to the arrhythmic effects of exogenous catecholamines and the catecholamines released during surgery in response to stress, increased pCO_2, or hypotension. The cardiac arrhythmias associated with the use of halothane can be effectively suppressed by propranolol.

> Propranolol can suppress cardiac arrhythmias brought about by halothane use.

Preparations and Dosages. Propranolol hydrochloride (INDERAL) is given as 10–40 mg three or four times a day to treat supraventricular arrhythmias. Larger doses (320 mg/day or more) may be necessary to treat ventricular arrhythmias. Propranolol, 1–3 mg IV over several minutes, is used to treat life-threatening arrhythmias or those associated with the administration of anesthesia. Constant hemodynamic and electrocardiographic monitoring is essential during the IV administration of propranolol.

Future Directions

IV administration of a β-blocking agent during the acute phase of myocardial infarction achieves plasma concentrations within the therapeutic range almost immediately, circumventing the lower and less predictable levels associated with oral dosing. However, the beneficial action of a β-blocking agent in the emergency treatment of myocardial infarction may be compromised if the patient exhibits hypotension, congestive heart failure, bradyarrhythmias, or ventricular arrhythmias related to the bradyarrhythmias. Newer ultrashort-acting β-blocking agents (such as esmolol or flestolol) are being tested currently in critically ill patients to determine whether their use eliminates the problems associated with β-blocking agents possessing longer durations of action. The short duration of action offers increased safety when the importance of sympathetic stimulation in maintaining cardiac output may be uncertain (Kirschenbaum et al, 1985).

Compounds such as labetalol, possessing β- and α-adrenergic receptor blocking properties, decrease blood pressure in hypertensive patients by the establishment of β blockade and the induction of vasodilatation. Experimental studies are at present evaluating the possibility that experimental agents such as dilevalol, an isomer of labetalol that possesses more β- than α-blocking properties, may be effective in treating ventricular arrhythmias observed in the postinfarction patient. It has been suggested that the value of this combination is that in the presence of selective β blockade of cardiac receptors, given the high level of sympathetic input associated with infarction, the α receptors may take on a proportionally greater role in the development of infarction.

Animal and human studies are also currently investigating the therapeutic role for pharmacological agents exhibiting α, β, and calcium channel blocking properties. CGS 10078B has been shown to protect against digitalis-induced arrhythmias (Lathers et al, 1987) and to lower blood pressure in normal and hypertensive animals. The therapeutic usefulness of an agent with this combination of mechanisms of action has yet to be clearly established in that the potential for action at multiple sites in the body may also increase unwanted side effects.

Bretylium is a class III agent that prolongs the action potential and increases the effective refractory period.

CLASS III AGENTS

Class III antiarrhythmic agents prolong the action potential duration and increase the effective refractory period.

Bretylium

History. Bretylium, a benzylammonium compound, was marketed initially as an adrenergic neuronal blocking agent to be used in the treatment of hypertension, but the development of tolerance to its antihypertensive effects and its unpredictable oral absorption ultimately precluded its use for hypertension. It is used currently to suppress ventricular fibrillation occurring during clinical emergencies, such as a myocardial infarction, or when the use of other antiarrhythmic agents has failed.

Pharmacokinetics. Bretylium exhibits poor and unpredictable absorption after oral administration.

Mechanism of Action. Bretylium has two actions. It directly modifies the electrical properties of the myocardium, and it depresses adrenergic neuronal transmission following a brief initial period of increased adrenergic amine release.

Autonomic Nervous System Actions. Bretylium is taken up by the adrenergic nerve terminals and stored there. Norepinephrine is released initially from the nerve terminals as the bretylium is taken up. This is manifest often as a proarrhythmic effect on administration. Subsequently, the release of norepinephrine is prevented; this action, in addition to its direct action on the myocardium, has been suggested to contribute to its antiarrhythmic action. Actions on heart rate and blood pressure have not been associated with its antiarrhythmic effect.

Sinoatrial Node (Table 33–5). Only a brief increase in sinus automaticity occurs with the initial release of catecholamines induced by bretylium. As noted earlier, this brief effect can transiently worsen arrhythmias. This increase in automaticity is followed by no change or a decrease.

Atria. The atrial action potential is prolonged, causing a prolongation of the effective refractory period in the atrial muscle.

Atrioventricular Node. Conduction velocity may be increased and the A-V nodal refractory period may be decreased. The initial catecholamine release improves A-V transmission to the extent that acceleration of the ventricular rate may develop. The consequence is that bretylium cannot be used to treat atrial flutter or fibrillation.

His-Purkinje System. Bretylium increases the firing rate of Purkinje fibers *in vitro* and may induce firing in quiescent fibers. The conduction rate in Purkinje fibers is not altered. The duration of the Purkinje action potential is prolonged.

Ventricular Muscle. The diastolic electrical current threshold is not altered noticeably by bretylium. However, the ventricular fibrillation threshold is increased significantly in both normal and ischemic hearts; this action is greater than that induced by other antiarrhythmic agents. The electrical threshold for successful defibrillation is lowered by bretylium, whereas the success rate for defibrillation is increased. The conduction rate in ventricular muscle is not altered by bretylium. The duration of ventricular muscle fiber action potential is prolonged.

In normal and ischemic hearts, bretylium increases the ventricular fibrillation threshold.

Membrane responsiveness of Purkinje fibers or ventricular muscle is unaltered.

Organ/System Pharmacology. An increase in catecholamine activity, manifested by phase 4 depolarization, an increase in automaticity, and a transient increase in arterial pressure, occurs immediately following its administration. This is followed by a decrease in arterial blood pressure consistent with adrenergic neuronal blockade. The hypotensive effect develops between 1 and 2 hours after the administration of bretylium. Standing upright increases the magnitude of the hypotension, and it is maximal during exercise in an upright position.

Heart Rate and Rhythm. In normal humans bretylium affects the ECG only by increasing the normal sinus rate. The initial increase in heart rate induced by bretylium generally returns to normal or is decreased. The PR and QT intervals are increased, but the duration of the QRS complex is not altered. If there is an initial increase in the force of myocardial contractility initiated by the catecholamine release, it is followed usually by a decrease in the force of contraction as adrenergic neuronal blockade is established. The initiation of ventricular arrhythmias caused by the release of catecholamines have been reported in animals anesthetized with halothane.

Adverse Effects. The major adverse effects associated with the use of bretylium relate to its modification of adrenergic function. The initial catecholamine release may increase blood pressure and heart rate transiently; 10–15% of patients exhibit a transient increase in ventricular ectopy. Only a few patients develop sustained ventricular tachycardia or fibrillation. The catecholamines released also may cause anxiety, excitement, flushing, substernal pressure sensation, headache, or angina pectoris. Nasal congestion and conjunctival suffusion may be observed 1–2 hours after its acute administration.

Modification of adrenergic function is bretylium's primary adverse effect.

The IV use of bretylium to treat acute arrhythmias is associated with profound, long-lasting hypotension resulting from the peripheral vasodilatation. About 10% of patients will require discontinuation of bretylium because of hypotension. Parotid pain has also been reported following chronic oral dosing. Rapid IV administration may initiate nausea and vomiting. Irritation at the injection site has followed its IM administration. The safety of bretylium in pregnant females or in children has not been determined.

Therapeutic Uses. The only clinical use for bretylium is within the intensive care unit to treat life-threatening ventricular fibrillation or other ventricular arrhythmias (especially ventricular tachycardia) that have not responded favorably to lidocaine or procainamide, or to repeated direct current (DC) countershock. Bretylium appears to be effective in up to 70% of patients exhibiting ventricular fibrillation refractory to all other drugs. Ventricular tachycardia or ventricular premature depolarizations do not

Clinical use of bretylium is limited to treating life-threatening ventricular arrhythmias in the intensive care unit.

respond generally until 6 or more hours after the administration of the bretylium. Patients with recurrent ventricular fibrillation have responded to IV bretylium for 24–48 hours followed by oral bretylium. Its administration is limited at present to no longer than 5 days.

Precautions. If the patient has a disease associated with a fixed cardiac output, e.g., severe aortic stenosis or pulmonary hypertension, the expected increase in cardiac output from compensating for the peripheral vasodilatation may not occur. It is recommended that bretylium be used only if necessary in these decreased states and that vasoconstrictor amines be given to support blood pressure if this is necessary. However, because ventricular fibrillation is lethal, bretylium may be required in spite of the presence of other clinical problems.

Future Directions. The clinical use of bretylium has prompted examination of other pharmacological agents possessing similar electrophysiological actions. Bethandine is one example that possesses better absorption following oral administration. Clofilium, meobentine, and UM 360 are quaternary ammonium compounds that possess less ganglionic action than bretylium. Amiodarone is a long-acting class III agent. Beta-blocking agents such as sotalol also exhibit similar antifibrillatory actions. It is anticipated that the clinical use of bretylium and similar agents will increase as clinical experience with these agents more clearly defines their potential advantages and disadvantages.

Preparations and Dosages. Bretylium (BRETYLOL) is approved only for short-term IV or IM administration. For example, during cardiac resuscitation a dose of 5 mg/kg of the undiluted solution may be infused IV over 10–30 minutes. This dose may be given again at intervals of 15–30 minutes with the total dose not to exceed 30 mg/kg over a 6- to 8-hour period.

Amiodarone

Amiodarone (see Tables 33–4 and 33–5) is an antiarrhythmic that possesses some of the pharmacological properties of bretylium, e.g., it slows repolarization in myocardial fibers and increases the ventricular fibrillation threshold. It is unique with a half-life of 25 to 55 days. IV administration suppresses supraventricular and ventricular tachyarrhythmias.

Amiodarone has a half-life of 25–55 days.

Pharmacokinetics. Amiodarone exhibits a slow onset of action. This makes it difficult to evaluate its efficacy, or lack thereof, as well as the efficacy of other drugs that may be used adjunctively. Amiodarone exhibits an oral bioavailability between 20 and 50%, is thought to be highly bound to plasma proteins, possesses an elimination half-life of 25–55 days, and is inactivated primarily by the liver (see Table 33–4). The long half-life means that some of the manifestations of its toxicity or adverse effects may be long-lasting, even if its administration is stopped.

Mechanism of Action

Cardiac Electrophysiological Action. S-A conduction may be slowed and the sinus rate decreased. Ventricular, atrial, and A-V nodal effective refractory periods are lengthened. The ventricular action potential is prolonged, and the ventricular fibrillation threshold is increased. AH and HV intervals are increased (see Table 33–5).

Organ/System Pharmacology. Acute administration induces a mild, transient depression in systemic vascular resistance and left ventricular function.

Adverse Effects. Asymptomatic corneal microdeposits have been reported in almost all patients administered amiodarone; peripheral neuropathy or hypothyroidism (Chapter 39) have been reported. Other reported side effects include pulmonary fibrosis, slowing of His bundle conduction, lightheadedness, and bluish-gray tint in the skin. As amiodarone has been used more widely and in more diverse patient populations, serious thyroid, pulmonary, and cardiovascular reactions have been reported. Amiodarone therapy is associated with a variable incidence of hypo- and hyperthyroidism; the mechanism of these effects is unknown. Amiodarone blocks the peripheral conversion of T_4 to T_3, resulting in elevated serum levels of total T_4, free T_4, and inactive reverse T_3. Serum levels of T_3 decline.

Interstitial pneumonitis, pulmonary fibrosis, and associated changes in pulmonary function have been associated with the use of amiodarone. It is desirable to carry out pulmonary function tests and chest x-rays prior to initiation of therapy with amiodarone and during follow-up examinations. (The pulmonary function test may be viewed as a defensive practice to reduce the risk of questions of malpractice, in the unfortunate event that a patient develops potentially fatal pulmonary fibrosis during therapy with amiodarone.) Amiodarone may impair myocardial contractility; cause symptomatic sinus bradycardia, S-A block, or sinus arrest requiring cardiac pacing; or induce ventricular tachycardia or fibrillation. The frequency of these reactions varies considerably in different studies, and the differences among studies cannot be explained on the basis of different dosages or modes of administration. A consensus on the status of amiodarone awaits thorough evaluation of its long-term toxicity.

Therapeutic Uses

Indications
Amiodarone appears to be an agent effective in the prevention of sudden death. It may be used in the long-term management of individuals with recurrent ventricular tachycardia or ventricular fibrillation and in those patients with atrial fibrillation associated with the Wolff-Parkinson-White syndrome.

Precautions and Contraindications. Amiodarone is only used to treat life-threatening arrhythmias because of its substantial toxicity. It produces several potentially fatal toxicities, including pulmonary toxicity, liver injury, and exacerbation of the arrhythmia by making it less well tolerated or more difficult to reverse. Even in patients at high risk of arrhythmic death in whom the toxicity of amiodarone is an acceptable risk, its use may be associated with major management problems. IV amiodarone may cause significant drops in blood pressure and urinary flow in patients with impaired left ventricular function. In addition, infusions into peripheral veins have resulted in venous thrombosis.

The therapeutic and toxic actions may be present for weeks after the amiodarone has been discontinued. This may be due to its long half-life or to active metabolites. Metabolism occurs in the liver, and the desethyl derivative accumulates with chronic administration; the biological activity of this metabolite is not known.

Preparation and Dosages (CORDARONE). Amiodarone comes as 200 mg tablets; loading dosages are required, and individual titration is essential

Amiodarone appears to effectively prevent sudden death, but its substantial toxicity limits its use.

because a uniform, optional dosage schedule has not been determined. To treat ventricular fibrillation or unstable ventricular tachycardia in a hospital setting, loading doses of 800–1600 mg/day are required, continued for 1–3 weeks until a desirable response is obtained. When the arrhythmias are controlled, or if side effects supervene, the dose is decreased to 600–800 mg/day for 1 month and eventually reduced to the maintenance dose of 400 mg/day.

CLASS IV AGENTS

Verapamil

Although calcium exerts a role in the genesis of arrhythmias, the calcium channel blockers exhibit disparate actions, and no uniform antiarrhythmic effect can be attributed to them (see Chapter 31).

Mechanism of Action

Verapamil is a calcium channel blocker (class IV agent).

Sinoatrial Node. In normal S-A nodal cells, spontaneous phase 4 depolarization depends on deactivation of an outward K^+ and a slow inward current carried by Na^+ and Ca^{2+} ions. The rate of rise and slope of the slow diastolic depolarization, the maximal diastolic potential, and the membrane potential at the peak of depolarization are reduced by verapamil. The result is a decrease in the heart rate.

Atria. Verapamil has no effect on normal atria. Spontaneous diastolic activity in diseased atrial tissue, tested after obtaining it in surgery, was inhibited by verapamil. This action could explain how verapamil suppresses supraventricular arrhythmias.

A-V Node. Verapamil decreases conduction through the A-V node and increases the A-V nodal refractory period consistent with the fact that depolarization in the A-V node is dependent on an inward slow Ca^{2+} current (see Table 31–7).

His-Purkinje System. Verapamil decreases the rate of phase 4 spontaneous depolarization in cardiac Purkinje fibers. It will block the delayed after-depolarizations and triggered activity associated with intoxication by digitalis.

Electrocardiographic Actions. The PR interval is increased and heart rate is decreased by verapamil.

Organ/System Pharmacology. Changes in blood pressure, heart rate, peripheral vascular resistance, left ventricular end-diastolic pressure, or contractility generally do not occur with antiarrhythmic dosages of verapamil; if they do occur after IV dosing, they do not last long.

Verapamil appears to be well tolerated by the body.

Adverse Effects. In general, verapamil is well tolerated, with only 1% of the patients requiring discontinuation because of unwanted side effects. Bradycardia, transient asystole, constipation, hypotension, initiation of or worsening of heart failure, and the induction of arrhythmia have been noted. Some patients complain also of headache, dizziness, nausea, skin reactions, and dyspnea. Although less than 1% of patients may have life-threatening adverse responses to verapamil, these reactions do occur and include rapid ventricular rate in atrial flutter/fibrillation; marked hypotension; or extreme bradycardia/asystole. Therefore, it is necessary to monitor the initial IV use of verapamil and to have resuscitation facilities immediately available.

Therapeutic Uses. Verapamil is the drug of first choice to treat paroxysmal supraventricular tachycardia due to A-V nodal reentry or to abnormal A-V conduction (Wolff-Parkinson-White syndrome or concealed bypass tracts). Verapamil also decreases the ventricular response to atrial flutter or fibrillation. Table 33 – 8 summarizes the efficacy of verapamil, nifedipine, and diltiazem in the treatment of arrhythmias and other disorders.

Precautions and Contraindications. Verapamil should be used with caution or should not be used in patients exhibiting sick sinus syndrome without an artificial pacemaker or in patients with A-V conduction abnormalities. The same is true for patients with severe congestive heart failure or those requiring β-blocking agents or disopyramide. The use of verapamil to treat digitalis-induced delayed after-depolarizations and triggered activity is risky, because additional A-V block may be induced and automaticity in the His-Purkinje fibers may be suppressed.

Drug Interactions. Disopyramide should not be given 48 hours or less before, or 24 hours after, verapamil. Flecainide and verapamil may have additive effects on myocardial contractility, A-V conduction, and repolarization. Hypotension has occurred when quinidine and verapamil were given to those with hypertrophic cardiomyopathy. Verapamil may lower lithium levels, yet it may increase carbamazine levels resulting in diplopia, headache, ataxia, or dizziness. The oral bioavailability of verapamil is reduced by rifampin, whereas phenobarbital increases the clearance of verapamil. Verapamil may increase the effects of inhalation anesthetics as well as depolarizing neuromuscular blocking agents (discussed further in Chapter 31).

Preparations and Dosages. Verapamil hydrochloride (CALAN, ISOPTIN) is given orally to treat angina and to prevent supraventricular tachycardia. IV

Table 33 – 8 EFFICACY OF THE CALCIUM ANTAGONISTS IN VARIOUS CARDIOVASCULAR DISORDERS

Drug	Very Effective	Somewhat Effective	Possibly Effective	Ineffective or Deleterious*
Verapamil	Paroxysmal supraventricular tachycardia, atrial fibrillation and flutter. Hypertrophic cardiomyopathy Variant angina, angina of effort, unstable angina	Mild-moderate systemic hypertension	Ventricular tachyarrhythmias	Pulmonary hypertension Unloading agent in CHF Raynaud's phenomenon or disease
Nifedipine	Mild-moderate systemic hypertension Pulmonary hypertension Variant angina, angina of effort (especially combined with a β blocker), unstable angina	Unloading agent in CHF Raynaud's phenomenon or disease	Selected patients with hypertrophic cardiomyopathy Migraine headache	Supraventricular or ventricular tachyarrhythmias
Diltiazem	Variant angina, angina of effort		Supraventricular tachyarrhythmias Pulmonary hypertension	Untested in systemic hypertension, Raynaud's disease, or hypertrophic cardiomyopathy

From Winniford MD, Hillis LD: Calcium antagonists in patients with cardiovascular disease. Medicine 64(1):61 – 73, © by Williams & Wilkins, 1985.
* Abbreviation: CHF = congestive heart failure.

Table 33-9 REPRESENTATIVE ANTIARRHYTHMIC COMBINATIONS WITH PROBABLE CLINICAL UTILITY

Combination	Uses	Comments
Digitalis and β blocker or verapamil	Resistant supraventricular tachyarrhythmias with rapid A-V conduction	Potentiation of A-V nodal effects of each drug alone
Digitalis and class I antiarrhythmic	Supraventricular tachycardias; for conversion/ maintenance ?Selected efficacy in ventricular arrhythmia	Digitalis antagonizes vagolytic effects of class I drugs on A-V node
Mexiletine and quinidine (classes IB and IA)	Refractory ventricular arrhythmias (monitor assessment)	Decreased dosage, toxicity of each drug, increased efficacy Other combinations of class IB (lidocaine, tocainide, or phenytoin) with quinidine or other class IA may be tried
β blocker and class I drug	Post-MI ventricular arrhythmia (despite β blocker) Other resistant ventricular arrhythmias Conversion of atrial fibrillation and maintenance therapy Other supraventricular arrhythmias Acute MI, IV with lidocaine	Under study for post-MI arrhythmias β blocker may decrease toxicity of class I drug
Amiodarone and class I drug	Initial management of resistant ventricular arrhythmias during amiodarone loading	Caution with quinidine (QT prolongation, torsades) May discontinue concomitant therapy after 1–2 months
Amiodarone and digitalis, propranolol or verapamil	Initial management of resistant supraventricular arrhythmias during amiodarone loading	Caution must be used (additive effects) May discontinue concomitant therapy after 1–2 months

From Anderson JL: Rationale of combination antiarrhythmic drug therapy. *In* Dreifus LS (ed): Cardiac Arrhythmias: Electrophysiologic Techniques and Management. Brest AN (editor-in-chief): Cardiovasc Clin 16:307–327, 1985.

dosing may decrease the required time of onset. IV infusions can be employed effectively for supraventricular tachyarrhythmias.

CLASS V AGENTS

Digitalis Glycosides

Digitalis glycosides are used to treat congestive heart failure and atrial tachyarrhythmias.

The digitalis glycosides are used commonly in the management of congestive heart failure and atrial tachyarrhythmias. The antiarrhythmic effect results from an action on the atria and A-V node and a complex interaction of glycosides on the autonomic nervous system and cardiac cells. Table 33–9 summarizes the combination of antiarrhythmic agents such as quinidine, propranolol, or verapamil with digitalis to treat atrial fibrillation/flutter, paroxysmal supraventricular tachycardias, and the sick sinus syndrome.

General References

Anderson JL: Rationale of combination antiarrhythmic drug therapy. Cardiovasc Clin 16:307–327, 1985.

Butterworth JF, Strichartz GR: Molecular mechanism of local anesthesia: A review. Anesthesiology 72:711–734, 1990.

Campbell TJ: Subclassification of class I antiarrhythmic drugs. *In* Vaughan Williams EM (ed): Antiarrhythmic Drugs, 135–156. New York: Springer-Verlag, 1989.

Catterall WA: Structure and function of voltage-sensitive ion channels. Science 242:50–61, 1987.

Chiale PA, Przybylski J, Halpern MS, et al: Comparative effects of ajmaline on intermittent bundle branch block and Wolff-Parkinson-White syndrome. Am J Cardiol 39:651–657, 1977.

Courtney KR, Strichartz GR: Structural elements which determine local anesthetic activity. *In* Strichartz GR (ed): Local Anesthetics, 47–94. New York: Springer-Verlag, 1987.

Drugs for cardiac arrhythmias. Med Lett Drugs Ther 33:55–60, 1991.

Dunn M: Clinical use of amiodarone. Heart Lung 14:407–411, 1985.

Garfein OB (ed): Annals of the New York Academy of Sciences, Clinical Pharmacology of Cardiac Antiarrhythmic Agents: Classical and Current Concepts Reevaluated, Vol 432, 1–321. New York: The New York Academy of Sciences, 1984.

Harrison DC: Current classification of antiarrhythmic drugs as a guide to their rational clinical use. Drugs 31:93–95, 1986.

Hogdeghem LM: Interaction of class I drugs with the cardiac sodium channel. *In* Vaughan Williams EM (ed): Antiarrhythmic Drugs, 157–174. New York: Springer-Verlag, 1989.

Kirshenbaum JM, Kloner RA, Antman EA, Braunwald E: Use of an ultrashort-acting beta blocker in patients with acute myocardial ischemia. Circulation 72:873–880, 1985.

Lathers CM, Gerard-Ciminera JL, Baskin SI, et al: Role of the adrenergic nerve terminal in digitalis-induced cardiac toxicity: A study of the effects of pharmacological and surgical denervation. J Cardiovas Pharmacol 4:91–98, 1982.

Lathers CM, Levin RM, Spivey WH: Regional distribution of myocardial beta-adrenoceptors in the cat. Eur J Pharmacol 130:111–117, 1986a.

Lathers CM, Spivey WH, Suter LE, et al: The effect of acute and chronic administration of timolol on cardiac sympathetic neural discharge, arrhythmia, and beta adrenergic receptor density associated with coronary occlusion in the cat. Life Sci 39:2121–2141, 1986b.

Lathers CM, Tumer N, Frame VB, Roberts J: Protection of CGS 10078B against ouabain-induced arrhythmia in the cat. Pharmacology 35:35–46, 1987.

Mofenson H, Caraccio TR, Schauben J: Poisoning by antidysrhythmic drugs. Pediatr Toxicol 33:723–738, 1986.

Montal M: Molecular anatomy and molecular design of channel proteins. FASEB J 4:2623–2635, 1990.

Morganroth J: Encainide for ventricular arrhythmias: Placebo-controlled and standard comparison trials. Am J Cardiol 58:74C–82C, 1986.

Morganroth J, Nestico PF, Horowitz LN: A review of the uses and limitations of tocainide—A class IB antiarrhythmic agent. Am Heart J 110:856–863, 1985.

Mueller RA, Baur HR: Flecainide: A new antiarrhythmic drug. Clin Cardiol 9:1–5, 1986.

Muhiddin KA, Turner P: Is there an ideal antiarrhythmic drug? A review—with particular reference to class I antiarrhythmic agents. Postgrad Med J 61:665–678, 1985.

National Institutes of Health, β Blocker Heart Attack Study Group: A randomized trial of propranolol in patients with acute myocardial infarction. JAMA 247:1704–1714, 1982.

Nestico PF, Morganroth J: Cardiac arrhythmias in the elderly: Antiarrhythmic drug treatment. Geriatric Cardiol 4:285–303, 1986.

Perry RS, Illsley SS: Basic cardiac electrophysiology and mechanisms of antiarrhythmic agents. Am J Hosp Pharm 43:957–974, 1986.

Phillips HR: Hemodynamic effects of the antiarrhythmic drug pirmenol. Clin Pharmacol Ther 32:235–239, 1982.

Podrid PJ: The role of antiarrhythmic drugs in prevention of sudden cardiac death. Cardiovasc Clin 15:265–286, 1985.

Pool PE: Treatment of supraventricular arrhythmias with encainide. Am J Cardiol 58:55C–57C, 1986.

Ruskin JN: The cardiac arrhythmia suppression trial (CAST). N Engl J Med 321:386–389, 1989.

Schraeder BJ, Bauman JL: Mexiletine: A new type I antiarrhythmic agent. Drug Intell Clin Pharm 20:255–260, 1986.

Vaughn Williams EM: Classification of antiarrhythmic drugs. *In* Sandoe E, Flensted-Jansen E, Olesen KH (eds): Symposium on Cardiac Arrhythmias, 449–472. Sweden: Ab Astra Sodertalje, 1970.

Vaughn Williams EM: A classification of antiarrhythmic actions reassessed after a decade of new drugs. J Clin Pharmacol 24:129–147, 1984.

Winniford MD, Hillis LD: Calcium antagonists in patients with cardiovascular disease. Medicine 64:61–73, 1985.

Woosley RL: Antiarrhythmic drugs. Annu Rev Pharmacol Toxicol 31:427–455, 1991.

34

Renal Pharmacology — Diuretics

Margaret A. Acara

The kidney regulates urinary electrolyte and fluid excretion.

The kidney maintains the volume and composition of body fluids within narrow limits. This organ has been programmed to fine-tune the concentrations of electrolytes and other substances present in extra- and intracellular fluid compartments, so that they are appropriate to support normal body function. The kidney performs its regulatory functions through the processes of filtration, reabsorption, secretion, and metabolism. These functions also govern drug excretion, and this aspect of renal pharmacology is addressed.

Diuretics change electrolyte and fluid excretion so that a more normal composition of body fluids is achieved.

Pharmacological agents that alter renal function are useful in disease states in which composition and volume of body fluids are abnormal; the major category of these agents is diuretics. The goal of diuretic therapy is to achieve a more normal composition of body fluids and thereby maintain normal physiological/cellular function. An understanding of renal function and fluid balance is required for the understanding of the mechanism of action of agents that alter the excretion of water and electrolytes.

Correction of fluid and electrolyte imbalances occurs at the level of the kidney, which responds to the composition of the plasma.

The three major fluid compartments of the body — plasma, interstitial fluid, and intracellular fluid — are in continual turnover. Whereas circulating plasma is most immediately subject to influxes and effluxes of water and electrolytes, intracellular and interstitial spaces also respond quickly to changes in volume and composition of plasma. Imbalances are reflected generally in the plasma or extracellular fluid compartment, which is monitored and adjusted continually by the kidney. Disturbances or changes in volume, composition, distribution, or a combination of these may result in alteration of the relative sizes of the fluid compartments along with changes in their respective electrolyte concentrations. The cause of fluid and electrolyte disorders varies, but the therapeutic approach must involve the kidney because it controls electrolyte and water excretion.

Figure 34–1 illustrates the overall function of the nephron and the mechanisms associated with sodium reabsorption. These are described in the following paragraphs.

Salt and Water Balance

In 1 day the two kidneys of a normal adult receive over 1700 l of blood (about 1200 ml/minute or 660 ml/minute plasma flow). It filters through the glomeruli 180 l/day or 125 ml/min (20% of the entering plasma volume) containing 25,200 mEq sodium/day. An ultrafiltrate containing electrolytes and other low-molecular-weight solutes is formed through this process. The essentially protein-free filtrate contains all the filterable solutes in concentrations equal to their nonprotein-bound fractions in the aqueous phase of the plasma. As fluid is forced through the glomerular

A protein-free filtrate is formed at the glomerulus, and the unfiltered protein in the plasma maintains oncotic pressure.

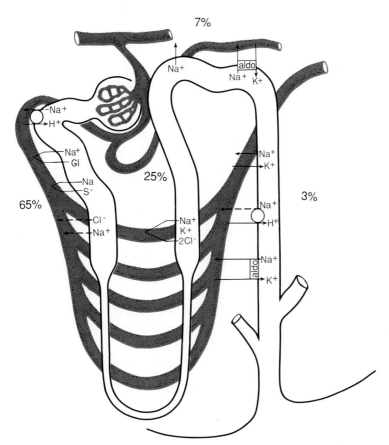

7%

25%

65%

3%

Na+

aldo
Na+   K+

-Na+
H+

Na+
Gl

Na
S-

Cl-
Na+

Na+
K+

Na+
K+
2Cl-

Na+
H+

aldo Na+
K+

Figure 34–1

Diagram of a nephron indicating tubular sites for sodium reabsorption, the capacity of the different segments, and the mechanisms for sodium entry into the cell at each site. Sodium is actively transported out of the cell across the basolateral membrane into the blood by the sodium/potassium pump. In the proximal tubule, approximately 65% of filtered sodium is reabsorbed through (1) countertransport with hydrogen, (2) cotransport with glucose (G1) or neutral organic solutes, (3) cotransport with nonchloride anions, (4) diffusion following a chloride gradient. In the thick ascending limb, approximately 25% of filtered sodium is reabsorbed through the electroneutral cotransport of one K^+, one Na^+, and two Cl^-. In the distal convoluted tubule, approximately 7% of filtered sodium is reabsorbed against an electrochemical gradient, through a sodium chloride cotransport. In the late distal tubule, approximately 3% of filtered sodium is reabsorbed mainly through sodium/potassium exchange, some of which is under aldosterone control. The sodium/hydrogen exchange in the distal tubule is associated primarily with urine acidification.

endothelium, the plasma proteins remain in the vasculature, maintaining oncotic pressure (the sum of the protein osmotic pressure and the osmotic pressure of obligate cations). The hydrostatic pressure from the heart is the major force for the filtration, and the differences in pressure between the afferent and efferent arterioles along with the permeability of the filtering membranes regulate the filtered load. The glomerular filtration rate (GFR) is expressed as the unit volume of fluid passing through the glomerulus per unit time (generally in milliliters per minute).

After the fluid is filtered at the glomerulus, it is processed by the tubules, which normally reabsorb greater than 99% of the filtrate; the composition of the reabsorbed filtrate approximates the composition of the extracellular fluid. Sodium is the major electrolyte of the extracellular compartment, and the mechanisms for its reabsorption are associated with the recapturing of filtrate.

Glomerular tubular balance describes the concept that changes in GFR are compensated for by parallel changes in tubular reabsorption of sodium (an increase in GFR is accompanied by an increase in the absolute amount of sodium reabsorbed, whereas the fraction of sodium reabsorbed by the tubule remains the same). This is true for excretion also; when GFR increases, the amount of sodium excreted increases also but fractional excretion remains the same. Water and electrolyte excretion can be regulated by changing either tubular reabsorption or glomerular filtration rate. In general, clinically useful diuretic agents have tubular actions that inhibit reabsorption, although secondary effects may alter GFR.

As the filtrate proceeds along the tubule, tubular reabsorption takes place because tubular cells move certain solutes and water back into the postglomerular peritubular capillaries. Cells, in particular segments of the

Less than 1% of filtered sodium is excreted, or greater than 99% of filtered sodium is reabsorbed.

Glomerular-tubular balance: An increase in GFR is accompanied by an increase in the amount of sodium excreted or reabsorbed and *vice versa*, but the percent excreted or reabsorbed remains the same.

Particular nephron segments are associated with particular electrolyte transport mechanisms.

Sodium enters the cell passively across the brush border membrane and is moved actively into the blood across the basolateral membrane by the sodium/potassium exchange pump.

nephron, are associated with mechanisms for the movement of particular ions. These mechanisms differ according to which other electrolytes are involved in the reabsorptive process for sodium and in which segment they are located.

In the reabsorptive process, sodium passively enters the tubule cell across the brush border or luminal membrane, down an electrochemical gradient. There are five mechanisms established for sodium entry into the cell from tubule fluid: (1) *per se* entry of sodium; (2) carrier-mediated cotransport with organic solutes such as sugars and amino acids; (3) carrier-mediated cotransport (one sodium, one potassium, and two chloride ions); (4) carrier-mediated cotransport of one sodium and one chloride ion; and (5) carrier-mediated countertransport with hydrogen. Sodium also may diffuse back into peritubular capillaries by paracellular pathways. Sodium moves against a concentration gradient from the cell into the blood through an active transport mechanism at the basolateral membrane. This transport system is the sodium/potassium exchange pump fueled by adenosine triphosphate (ATP), which moves sodium out of the cell and potassium into it.

Most diuretics act primarily on sodium movement in a single segment of a nephron. However, the urinary electrolyte excretion profile reflects the combined action on all nephron segments.

Reabsorptive Processes in Particular Nephron Segments

Sixty to 70% of filtrate is reabsorbed in the proximal tubule.

The early proximal tubule has sodium cotransport with organic solutes or nonchloride anions as well as sodium/hydrogen exchange mechanisms.

Carbonic anhydrase in the proximal tubule facilitates sodium/hydrogen exchange.

The proximal tubule reabsorbs 60–70% of the filtered load, and this reabsorption involves mechanisms 2, 3, and 5 above, which link sodium reabsorption to the reabsorption of other substances. In the early part of the proximal tubule, sodium is reabsorbed preferentially without chloride. The three identified pathways for this reabsorption are (1) cotransport with neutral organic solutes such as glucose and amino acids; (2) cotransport with nonchloride anions—acetate, phosphate, citrate, and lactate; and (3) sodium and bicarbonate transport linked to hydrogen ion secretion.

The reabsorption of sodium bicarbonate occurs primarily in the early proximal tubule (Fig. 34–2). In this process a hydrogen ion combines with bicarbonate in the filtrate and forms carbonic acid. Carbonic anhydrase is abundant in the brush border of the proximal tubular cell, and in its presence luminal carbonic acid is dehydrated to CO_2 and water. The uncharged CO_2 diffuses freely across the luminal membrane into the tubular cell, where it is hydrated to carbonic acid. This acid dissociates to yield a hydrogen ion that may be secreted back into the lumen in exchange for a sodium, which may exit across the peritubular membrane of the cell with a bicarbonate anion. The net effect of this process is the reabsorption of filtered sodium bicarbonate and the secretion of a hydrogen ion. Both the hydration and the dehydration reactions are under the control of carbonic anhydrase, whereas the ionic dissociation of H_2CO_3 occurs spontaneously. There are several different forms of the carbonic anhydrase enzyme, which exist in great excess in tissues. It is necessary to inhibit more than 99% before a physiological effect is observed. Most forms of carbonic anhydrase are subject to inhibition by sulfonamides, which comprise a number of diuretic compounds.

Blood to tubule fluid gradient in the late proximal tubule favors chloride reabsorption, and sodium follows chloride.

The reabsorption of sodium bicarbonate and water early in the proximal tubule results in an increase in the concentration of chloride in the later proximal tubule fluid. Thus, there is a chloride gradient favoring its movement into the peritubular capillary. This segment is highly permeable to chloride, and reabsorption of chloride occurs. Sodium follows chloride to maintain electrical neutrality, and water accompanies the solutes by osmotic obligation.

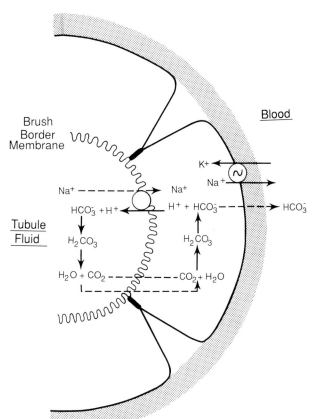

Figure 34–2

Sodium/hydrogen exchange and carbonic anhydrase. Sodium enters the tubule cell in exchange for a hydrogen, which has been generated by dissociation of carbonic acid produced from CO_2 and H_2O by the hydration action of carbonic anhydrase inside the cell. Carbonic anhydrase, associated with the brush border, also catalyzes the dehydration reaction of carbonic acid to CO_2 and H_2O.

The largest amount of total filtrate is reabsorbed in the proximal tubule, and the anionic components reabsorbed include 80–90% of the filtered bicarbonate and phosphate, and most of the filtered chloride. The proximal tubule is freely permeable to water, and reabsorption at this site is isotonic. Fluid leaving the proximal tubule has the same osmolality as that of plasma.

> Proximal tubule reabsorption of filtrate is isotonic.

Although some diuretics directly inhibit sodium reabsorption in the proximal tubule, the most useful diuretics have their major site of action distal to this. Because the loop of Henle has a high capacity for sodium reabsorption, the sodium that is inhibited from being reabsorbed in the proximal tubule can be reabsorbed almost completely at more distal sites. This process negates the effect of proximally active diuretics. Carbonic anhydrase inhibitors, which act by decreasing the generation of a hydrogen ion for sodium/hydrogen exchange, have their major site of action in the proximal tubule because that is where the enzyme is mainly localized. The pars recta leads to the descending limb of the loop of Henle and active transport processes have not been demonstrated in this limb segment.

In the thick ascending limb of the loop of Henle, sodium reabsorption occurs through the electroneutral cotransport of a potassium ion, a sodium ion, and two chloride ions from the lumen of the tubule into the tubule cell (Fig. 34–3). The Na^+-K^+-$2Cl^-$ cotransporter in the apical membrane facilitates the entry of these ions from the lumen. Thus, transepithelial NaCl movement is secondary active transport, driven by the inward gradient for sodium across the apical cell membrane. The driving force for this transport is again the action of sodium/potassium ATPase, which serves to maintain high intracellular potassium. The existence of potassium conductance in the apical membrane allows potassium to recycle to the Na^+-K^+-$2Cl^-$ cotransporter, whereas the existence of chloride conductance in the basolateral membrane allows chloride to exit from the cell. This allows net

> Electroneutral cotransport of 1 Na^+, 1 K^+, and 2 Cl^- from tubule fluid to cell

Figure 34–3

Mechanism for sodium reabsorption in the thick ascending limb: cotransport of one K⁺, one Na⁺, and two Cl⁻. Sodium and potassium enter the cell along with two chloride ions. Potassium recycles through conductance across the apical membrane to the cotransporter, and chloride conductance occurs across the basolateral membrane.

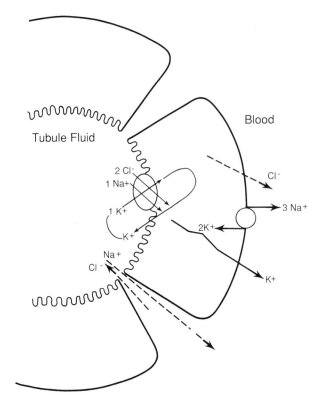

K⁺ is recycled across the brush border luminal membrane.

The thick ascending limb is impermeable to water.

reabsorption of Na^+ and Cl^- ions against their concentration gradients, and the potassium ion is thought to be quickly recycled to maintain this activity. One Na^+, 2 Cl^-, and 1 K^+ cotransported across the luminal membrane and K^+ being recycled across the luminal membrane generate a lumen-positive transepithelial potential difference. An important aspect of reabsorption of filtrate in the ascending limb is that this segment is impermeable to water. The unreabsorbed water remains in the tubule, and fluid leaving the thick ascending limb, the principal diluting site, is hypotonic compared with plasma. The movement of solute into the interstitium contributes to the interstitial osmolality and acts as an osmotic force for water reabsorption in the presence of antidiuretic hormone in the concentration of urine through the counter-current multiplier action of the kidney. Diuretics that act at this site interfere with the development of a concentrated interstitium and may lead to an isotonic urine.

PROSTAGLANDINS AND MEDULLARY WASHOUT

Vasodilation by prostaglandins leads to medullary washout.

The concept of medullary washout is related to the contribution of the vasa recta in establishing a concentration gradient from cortex to medulla to permit formation of a concentrated urine. Because vasa recta act as passive conduits for the equilibration of osmolar solutes in the interstitium, the rate of flow through these vessels plays an important role. The greater the flow rate through the medullary region, the less time there is for the blood to equilibrate with the more concentrated interstitium. Osmolar solutes are picked up and carried away, effectively diluting the medullary interstitium.

The dynamics of blood flow through the medullary region is in part under the control of prostaglandins, particularly prostaglandin E_2. PGE_2 acts as a medullary vasodilator to promote blood flow to this region. Although the mechanisms are not worked out clearly, the interactions between the prostaglandin-induced medullary vasodilation and the ability of loop diuretics to increase prostaglandin concentrations in the medulla provide at least circumstantial evidence for a contribution of this system to a diuretic effect. That is, the inability to establish as concentrated an interstitium in the presence of PGE_2 interferes with the formation of negative and positive free water and contributes to the diuresis.

The thick ascending limb ends and the early distal tubule begins at the macula densa. This is that portion of the nephron where the tubule returns to touch upon the glomerulus from which it originates. It is referred to as the juxtaglomerular apparatus and is involved in the release of renin. The distal tubule extends from the macula densa to a site where other distal tubules come together to form cortical collecting tubules. Sodium is actively reabsorbed against an electrochemical gradient in the distal convoluted tubule (early distal tubule), and provides the driving force for passive potassium entry into the lumen. Calcium is reabsorbed here also by an active sodium-independent mechanism. In the absence of antidiuretic hormone (ADH), late distal tubular sites are also water-impermeable, and sodium reabsorption is largely independent of water reabsorption, leading to further dilution of the tubular fluid. Carbonic anhydrase activity is present in this nephron segment, but its inhibition here does not appear to produce a significant diuresis. The function of this enzyme in the distal tubule is related primarily to the sodium/hydrogen exchange that participates in urine acidification. The flow rate of tubule fluid through this segment and the production of hydrogen ion are major factors for regulating potassium excretion in the urine.

Active reabsorption of sodium and chloride occurs in the cortical collecting tubule. This segment is also impermeable to water so that some urinary dilution takes place. Potassium secretion under the control of mineralocorticoids occurs here. Aldosterone stimulates distal tubular sodium reabsorption and potassium secretion. The collecting tubule becomes more permeable to water in response to ADH, and in the medullary collecting tubule solute-free water is reabsorbed toward a hypertonic interstitium.

Exchange sites for sodium reabsorption and potassium secretion in the distal and collecting tubules regulate the amount of potassium excreted in the urine. Almost all of the filtered potassium is reabsorbed in the proximal tubule, and variations in urinary potassium reflect the activities of these distal segments. Potassium excretion will increase in response to (1) increased amounts of sodium reaching these sodium/potassium exchange sites and (2) increased levels of circulating aldosterone. There are two major ways for increased amounts of sodium to reach the distal tubule. One is inhibition of sodium reabsorption at a more proximal site and the other is an increased flow rate through the distal tubule.

RENIN-ANGIOTENSIN-ALDOSTERONE

The fact that potassium is reabsorbed in the distal tubule with and without aldosterone stimulation is the reason for the use of two types of potassium-sparing diuretics, one of which is dependent on the presence of aldosterone. The other acts on a sodium/potassium exchange mechanism that is not related to aldosterone. Aldosterone stimulates both potassium and hydrogen ion excretion in exchange for sodium. This steroidal hormone enters the distal tubule cell and binds to cytoplasmic receptors. This complex interacts eventually with the nucleus to cause the encoding of new mRNA, which directs the synthesis of new aldosterone-induced proteins

---

Side notes:

The juxtaglomerular apparatus occurs where the tubule touches back upon the glomerulus from which it originates.

Carbonic anhydrase in distal tubule important in urine acidification

Aldosterone stimulates distal tubule sodium reabsorption and potassium secretion in distal tubule.

Exchange sites

Potassium excretion increases in response to increased amounts of sodium reaching distal tubule and increased levels of aldosterone.

Potassium is reabsorbed in distal tubule using aldosterone-dependent or aldosterone-independent mechanisms.

Renin release increases angiotensin II levels.

Major stimulus for renin release is a falling perfusion pressure.

(AIPs). These increase sodium reabsorption in an as-yet unclearly defined manner. Aldosterone itself is released from the zona glomerulosa in response to stimulation by angiotensin II or III. The concentration of angiotensin is in turn regulated by plasma renin levels. The major stimulus for renin release from the juxtamedullary apparatus (that portion of the nephron in which the distal tubule touches back upon the glomerulus from which it originates) is a falling renal perfusion pressure. This stimulus is eventually overcome by aldosterone-increased sodium reabsorption and subsequent volume expansion. Other stimuli for renin release include increased sympathetic innervation and increased amounts of chloride reaching the macula densa.

Another major action of angiotensin II is renal and systemic vasoconstriction. Inhibition of the enzyme that produces angiotensin II (known as angiotensin-converting enzyme, ACE, and also as peptidyldipeptidase or kininase II) is an important therapeutic approach in the treatment of hypertension, particularly renovascular hypertension.

VASOPRESSIN (ANTIDIURETIC HORMONE)

The ability to form a concentrated urine is dependent upon circulating levels of ADH and the development of an osmotic gradient of increasing concentration from cortex to medulla. This gradient results in part from the cotransport of $1Na^+$, $2Cl^-$, and $1K^+$ in the thick ascending limb. Figure 34–4 describes the relative osmolarities attained in the tubule lumen and in the vasa recta of the various zones of the kidney. The arrows depict the direction of movement of sodium and water in different nephron segments and in the descending and ascending vasa recta, which tend to equilibrate passively with the tubule fluid and interstitium. It is likely our future understanding will include additional participation of the thin limb of the loop of Henle as well as biological signals resulting in increases or decreases in intracellular organic osmolar solutes. This discussion includes only the participation of sodium chloride and water.

Vasopressin acts on the distal tubule and collecting duct to increase the water permeability of the cell membranes in these segments. Under the

Figure 34–4

Concentrating mechanism in the kidney. As tubule fluid flows through the nephron (left side of figure) and blood through the vasa recta (right side of figure), the osmolality increases as the inner medulla is reached and then decreases as fluid moves back toward the cortex. Sodium and chloride are moved into the interstitium without water in the thick ascending limb, creating a slightly higher interstitial osmolality. Water from the descending limb moves toward this osmotic force, and sodium chloride moves into the descending limb. Reabsorbed fluid is carried off in the vasa recta, where alteration of flow rate affects the amount reabsorbed. (Modified from Koushanpour E, Kriz W: Renal Physiology— Principles, Structure, and Function. 2nd ed. New York: Springer-Verlag, 1986.)

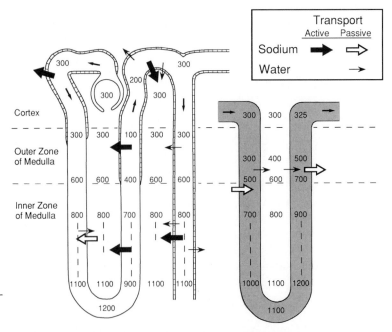

condition of a concentrated interstitium, water is reabsorbed toward an osmotic driving force. This force was set up by the reabsorption of sodium and chloride without water in the thick ascending limb of the loop of Henle. In conjunction with vasopressin, the osmotic gradient (increasing from cortex to papilla) permits the formation of a concentrated urine. The reabsorption of sodium and chloride without water in the thick ascending limb contributes a part of the driving force that results in the production of both positive and negative free water. Diuretics that interfere with reabsorption of sodium and chloride in the thick ascending limb produce the largest diuretic effect and interfere with the production of both positive and negative free water.

Free water is an operational concept that describes the ability of the diluting segment to dilute and of the concentrating segment to concentrate. Both concentration and dilution result from the cotransport of sodium, potassium, and chloride in the ascending limb. Arithmetically, it is equal to urine flow rate minus osmolar clearance and is expressed in units of milliliter per minute. *Positive free water* is formed by the removal of sodium and chloride from the tubular fluid without the removal of water, and this results in a hypotonic fluid reaching the early distal tubule. This part of the nephron where salt is reabsorbed without water is designated the diluting segment. *Negative free water* is water that is reabsorbed primarily in the medullary collecting tubules in the presence of vasopressin and toward an osmotically concentrated interstitium. This portion of the nephron is called the concentrating segment.

If the reabsorption of sodium chloride in the cortical diluting segment is inhibited, there is a decrease in the production of positive free water. If sodium chloride reabsorption in the medullary diluting segment is inhibited, there is not only a decrease in positive free water but also a decrease in the osmotic driving force. Thus, the force drawing water into the interstitium in the presence of vasopressin is decreased and so is negative free water production.

The major stimulus for vasopressin release is an increasing plasma osmolarity, and the response of increased water reabsorption decreases plasma osmolarity back toward normal. The increasing plasma osmolarity is sensed by the supraoptic nuclei of the hypothalamus, and the message is transmitted through a neurophysin to the posterior pituitary, from which vasopressin is released. The cellular action of vasopressin includes binding of the hormone to an adenyl cyclase–activated membrane receptor on the basolateral membrane. These tubule receptors have been designated V_2 receptors (as opposed to the vascular or V_1 receptors for vasopressin). Cyclic adenosine monophosphate (AMP) activates a protein kinase that phosphorylates membrane proteins, resulting in a more water-permeable state on the brush border membrane. Development of V_2 antagonists may provide another approach to diuretic therapy.

As with most hormones, the endocrine disorders associated with abnormal levels of ADH relate to the activity of the gland or the response of the target organ. Diabetes insipidus is the disease related to hyposecretion of vasopressin or hyporesponsivity of the target sites, the distal tubules, and collecting ducts. An insufficient amount of water is reabsorbed and hypovolemia ensues. SIADH, syndrome of inappropriate antidiuretic hormone secretion, is related to hypersecretion of vasopressin or hyperresponsivity of the receptors and is characterized by hypervolemia (see Chapter 40). A paradoxical use of diuretics occurs in the treatment of hypovolemic, nephrogenic diabetes insipidus (negative water balance). The rationale for this is based on a decreased delivery of filtrate to the diluting segment and is discussed under Thiazides.

Vasopressin permits water to be reabsorbed toward a concentrated interstitium.

Positive free water is formed by the removal of salt without water in diluting segment.

Negative free water is reabsorbed from the medullary collecting tubules (concentrating segment).

ATRIAL NATRIURETIC FACTOR

ANF has hypotensive and natriuretic effects.

This hormone is secreted by specific granules in the atria of the heart, particularly the right atrium, in response to an increasing vascular volume. Atrial natriuretic factor (ANF; atrial natriuretic peptide; atriopeptin) has been isolated and characterized to contain between 21 and 33 amino acids; the most potent human natriuretic peptide has 28. In general, its effects are hypotensive and natriuretic. There are numerous reports on the differential selectivity of the hypotensive effects in various vascular beds; the mechanisms of natriuresis include both an inhibition of sodium reabsorption and an increase in GFR. ANF increases vascular permeability, decreases cardiac output and blood volume, increases hematocrit, and circulates in abnormally high levels in congestive heart failure. It is fairly conclusive that ANF produces responses opposite to those that occur within the renin-angiotensin-aldosterone system. Manipulations of the release, activation, and deactivation of this hormone and the development of therapeutic analogs may hold the key to future approaches for the treatment of cardiovascular disease.

VOLUME HOMEOSTASIS AND BLOOD PRESSURE

Hydrostatic and oncotic pressure changes across proximal tubule affect fluid balance.

Hemodynamic mechanisms themselves may contribute to salt and water loss or retention. Changes in hydrostatic or oncotic pressures, particularly at the level of the proximal tubule, can act to readjust volume and pressure to normal by either retention or loss of fluid. In the volume-loaded state, hydrostatic pressure has a positive force and oncotic pressure a negative force for elimination of fluid. The outward pressure in the peritubular capillary acts to retard reabsorption from the tubule fluid. In addition, a relatively low oncotic pressure does not favor fluid reabsorption. Thus, increases in arterial pressure cause natriuresis and diuresis, which in turn tend to reduce extracellular fluid volume and help to counteract the increases in pressure. When volume and blood pressure are decreasing, the kidneys decrease sodium and water excretion, thereby increasing extracellular fluid volume; this helps to restore volume and pressure to normal. It is thought that inasmuch as arterial pressure is determined by the blood volume and the vascular compliance, the kidney, by regulating fluid and electrolyte loss, is involved in determining the level of arterial pressure.

Edema

In edema, fluid accumulates in interstitial spaces.

Edema is an excessive accumulation of fluid in the interstitial space. Alteration of cardiac, renal, hepatic, or endocrine function may be of primary importance in the etiology of the edema state. In these pathological states, widespread swelling of most interstitial tissues occurs. The distribution of edematous fluid can be explained by simple physical forces, that is, an imbalance in hydrostatic and oncotic pressures across the capillary wall. Changes in Starling forces across the capillary in the direction of increased systemic venous hydrostatic pressure and decreased plasma oncotic pressure promote loss of fluid from the vascular system. Under the condition of increased hydrostatic pressure, there is increased outward movement of water and diffusive solutes from the capillary, and the decreased oncotic pressure does not draw a balanced volume of fluid back. Thus, the loss of fluid to the interstitium exceeds the rate of absorption from it. This accumulation represents retention of both water and sodium chloride as an isotonic solution. The distention of capillaries that occurs in positive volume states is also contributory to the distribution of edematous fluid through leaky capillaries. Proteins may be lost from the vasculature and accumulate in the interstitium, further contributing to the decreased oncotic pressure and edema formation.

Increased hydrostatic pressure or decreased oncotic pressure contributes to edema.

The decreased excretion (or increased retention) of sodium is the renal defect that is focused upon in the treatment of these disease states. When accumulation of edematous fluid compromises the vascular system through an inadequate circulating volume, the normal renal responses continue to contribute to sodium retention. A decrease in the effective circulating volume is sensed by the juxtaglomerular apparatus as a decrease in perfusion pressure, and renin is released. This leads to the formation of angiotensin II and an increase in aldosterone release that increases sodium reabsorption in the distal tubule. The retention of sodium is associated with the retention of fluid that is redistributed subsequently as additional edematous fluid in a vicious-circle fashion. Decreases in GFR, occurring because of a compromised circulatory system not accompanied by a decrease in sodium reabsorption, result in glomerular tubular imbalance and contribute to sodium retention. The following are disease states in which a vicious circle needs to be interrupted to resolve the problem.

Therapy focused on correcting sodium retention

Decreased renal perfusion activates renin-angiotensin-aldosterone cycle.

Edematous disease states

Congestive Heart Failure. Eventually in the development of congestive heart failure a point is reached at which the myocardium no longer responds to an increased end-diastolic volume with an increased force of contraction. This leads to the pooling of blood proximal to the heart, distention of peripheral blood vessels and loss of protein through leaky capillaries, accumulation of edematous fluid, and a decrease in the effective circulating blood volume. The progression is toward decreased renal perfusion pressure, increased release of renin, and eventually increased aldosterone levels with consequent sodium retention.

Backward heart failure occurs when one or the other ventricle fails to discharge its contents normally, the end-diastolic volume of the ventricle rises, the pressures and volumes in the atrium and venous system behind the failing ventricle become elevated, and retention of sodium and water occurs as a consequence of the elevation of systemic venous and capillary pressures and the resultant transudation of fluid into the interstitium. In constrast, in forward heart failure the clinical manifestations result directly from an inadequate discharge of blood into the arterial system. Salt and water retention, then, is a consequence of diminished renal perfusion and excessive proximal tubular sodium reabsorption and of excessive distal tubular reabsorption, through activation of the renin-angiotensin-aldosterone system.

Liver Disease. The inability of the liver to function normally leads to a damming of blood proximal to the liver, distention of splanchnic vessels, and the formation of ascites in the peritoneum. Secondary aldosteronism may occur because of the inability of the liver to metabolize this hormone. A decrease in the synthesis of plasma proteins by the liver will decrease albumin and, subsequently, oncotic pressure. These effects further compromise the circulatory system.

Nephrotic Syndrome. Glomerular nephritis exists in this syndrome, and glomerular membranes permit the loss of proteins into the tubule, which are excreted subsequently into the urine. The loss of plasma proteins decreases the oncotic pressure, and the circulatory system is again compromised with the resulting activation of the renin-angiotensin-aldosterone system.

Pulmonary Edema. Acute left ventricular failure leads to increased end-systolic and end-diastolic volume, resulting in increases in pressure in pulmonary veins and capillaries. Fluid accumulates in the pulmonary interstitium and causes resistance in the airways. This may be a severe, acute situation and require immediate treatment.

Diuretics increase loss of salt and water and thus decrease plasma volume.

None of the disease states mentioned earlier is cured by the use of diuretics but, in each case, diuretics can alleviate the symptoms by increasing sodium and water excretion by the kidney. They do not act on the edema fluid directly. As salt and water are lost from the vascular compartment through the action of these drugs on the kidney, additional fluid is drawn out of the edematous interstitium and into the vascular system for subsequent elimination. The diuretic-induced loss of salt and water lowers intravascular hydrostatic pressure and increases plasma oncotic pressure enough so that Starling forces favor absorption of edematous fluid back into the intravascular space. The edema is alleviated, and a new steady state for sodium and water balance is achieved. Volume contraction and weight loss accompany the increased salt and water excretion. A major goal of diuretic therapy is to produce a degree of negative sodium chloride balance that results in a decrease of excess extracellular fluid volume without compromising the circulating blood volume.

Diuretics decrease hydrostatic pressure and increase oncotic pressure.

Nonedematous disease states

Nonedematous States. The reabsorption of substances like potassium, calcium, magnesium, phosphate, bicarbonate, and glucose may be linked to that of sodium during conditions of increased or decreased reabsorption. The manipulation of certain diuretics to alter in one way or another the excretion of these substances has become useful in certain nonedematous states.

Diuretics are frequently drugs of choice in the treatment of mild to moderate hypertension. The precise mechanism by which diuretics lower blood pressure remains uncertain. During the initial days or weeks of therapy, diuretics cause natriuresis and reduction in the plasma and extracellular fluid volume and cardiac output. This leads to a modest weight loss and reduction in blood pressure. Eventually blood volume expands, but not to the pretreatment level. However, with little change in cardiac output, there is a decrease in total peripheral resistance. High salt intake reverses the decrease in blood pressure produced by the diuretics, indicating that sodium may be associated with the hypertension (see Chapter 35).

Thiazide diuretics are of benefit in the treatment of nephrogenic diabetes insipidus and SIADH and sometimes in acute renal failure.

Abnormalities in plasma calcium levels in either direction may be corrected with appropriate diuretic therapy. Hypercalcemia is corrected by loop diuretics, which increase calcium excretion by preventing its reabsorption. On the other hand, thiazide diuretics increase calcium reabsorption and are helpful in preventing hypercalciuric stone formation.

Renal Excretion of Drugs

CLEARANCE MEASUREMENTS OF RENAL FUNCTION AND DRUG EXCRETION

Clearance techniques are useful in the measurement of kidney function and drug excretion.

Clearance is the measurement of the effectiveness of the removal of a substance from the blood. It is expressed as rate of removal in volume per unit time (usually milliliters per minute). When applied to the kidney, as in renal clearance, it expresses the contribution of this organ to plasma clearance. Clearance techniques are useful in the measurement of whole kidney function and the effects of systemic factors or substances on this function. Clearance techniques permit the measurements of glomerular filtration rate, renal plasma flow, and the net rates of excretion and reabsorption of drugs.

Renal function and drug excretion

In the conventional measurement of renal clearance, timed urine samples are obtained and the excretion rate of the compound under study in amount per minute is divided by its plasma concentration to determine the volume of plasma from which it was derived. The traditional formula for clearance is UV/P, where U is the concentration of compound in urine, V is urine flow rate, and P is the concentration of compound in plasma.

It is necessary at the outset to define clearance in relation to the compartments observed in the method of calculation. Clearance by the whole kidney includes the amount of substance that was lost from the blood to the organ, as well as to the urine, and is appropriately designated renal clearance. Clearance that describes loss to urine only may be appropriately designated urinary clearance. However, there is a lack of consensus in nomenclature, and agreed-upon designations need to be reached. The distinction between renal clearance and urinary clearance is frequently overlooked.

Renal clearance is calculated as the product of the extraction ratio and renal plasma flow (RPF) and is expressed as milliliters per minute. It represents the total volume of blood from which a substance, S, has been removed by the kidney in 1 minute. Renal clearance, or $R\,Cl_s = E \times RPF$, where the extraction ratio $E = (A - V)/A$, and A and V represent the concentrations of S in arterial and venous plasma, respectively. Information from renal clearance studies describes the integrated functions of the whole kidney. Renal clearance is the net contribution of the kidney to removal of a substance from the plasma and accounts for all pathways of disposition of S in the kidney: what appears in the urine; what is metabolized by the kidney; and what is stored in the kidney.

Urinary clearance, on the other hand, describes the clearance of the substance attributable to the urine only and does not account for the disposition of the substance in other renal compartments. Urinary clearance uses the traditional clearance calculation to express the volume of plasma that contained the amount of S that was excreted in the urine in 1 minute: $U\,Cl_s = UV/P$, where U and P represent the concentrations of S in urine and plasma respectively and V is the urine flow rate. It is only when a substance is neither metabolized nor stored in the kidney that its renal clearance is equal to its urinary clearance. This is true for those substances used to measure renal plasma flow, e.g., *p*-aminohippuric acid (PAH), and those used to measure glomerular filtration rate, e.g., inulin. It also follows that the difference between renal clearance and urinary clearance represents storage and metabolism by the kidney.

Total action of kidney on compounds is not reflected in urinary clearance.

Values for either renal or urinary clearance may range from zero for a substance that does not undergo metabolism, storage, or excretion by the kidney to a value equal to the RPF for a substance that is completely transferred into the urine from the blood in a single pass through the kidney.

Kidney metabolizes many organic compounds.

The fractional excretion (FE) of a substance (S) is the ratio of the urinary clearance of S, calculated as $U\,Cl_s$, to the GFR. A *ratio greater than 1.0* indicates that there has been tubular addition of S from blood to tubule fluid, and a secretory component resulting in net excretion. A *ratio less than 1.0* is generally interpreted to indicate movement of S from tubule fluid back into blood, and a reabsorptive component resulting in net reabsorption. The qualification occurs because the procedure does not account for a metabolic component, and a ratio less than 1.0 simply indicates disappearance from tubule fluid.

Fractional excretion of a compound indicates addition to or removal from tubule fluid.

Because the majority of drugs are eliminated at least in part by the kidney, there are important renal mechanisms that play a role in determining the concentration of drug in the plasma. The actions of the kidney that

Renal mechanisms regulating drug levels in plasma

affect the amount of drug in the plasma are hemodynamic, metabolic, and transport related. These are the same mechanisms that regulate the plasma concentrations of endogenous substances. When kidney function is abnormal, these mechanisms are altered and the plasma concentrations of drugs (particularly those whose main route of elimination is by the kidney) become abnormal. Situations in which the monitoring of plasma drug concentrations is important are when the drug administered has a narrow margin of safety, renal failure, and polypharmacy.

The kidney normally has an unusual susceptibility to undesirable chemical insults. It receives a large amount of cardiac output, and through filtration and transport processes renal tubular cells can be exposed to large amounts of drugs and chemical substances. Both peritubular membranes (exposed to the blood) and brush border membranes (exposed to tubular fluid) are vulnerable. In addition, because of concentrating mechanisms, drugs and chemicals can become 100–1000 times more concentrated in tubule fluid.

Amount of filtered drug is dependent upon GFR and plasma protein binding.

The amount of drug reaching the kidney is determined by renal plasma flow. This is calculated as plasma flow in milliliters per minute times the concentration of drug in plasma in milligrams per milliliter and is expressed as milligrams per minute. Renal plasma flow is also a major determinant of the GFR. Approximately 20% of the blood that reaches the kidney is filtered by it. The amount of drug filtered is determined by the GFR and the degree of plasma protein binding of the drug. The protein-bound portion of the drug is not filtered, and only the free drug is present in the ultrafiltrate. The portion of drug that is filtered may remain in the tubule to be excreted in the urine, or the drug may be reabsorbed through either passive or active processes.

Nonionic back-diffusion in distal tubule; pH and pK_a

Many drugs undergo nonionic passive back-diffusion in the distal tubule. As filtrate moves along the tubule, water is reabsorbed. This results in the drug's becoming more concentrated in the tubule fluid, and a gradient is created that favors back-diffusion. This process occurs for most part in the distal tubule, because water reabsorption prior to this site has resulted in a large concentration gradient from tubule fluid to blood.

Because it is in their nonionized form that drugs cross cell membranes, the pK_a of the drug and the pH of the tubule fluid govern the movement of drug back into peritubular capillaries. Numerous drugs are either weak acids or weak bases and exist in a mixture of ionic and nonionic forms depending upon their dissociation constant and the pH of their environment. Weak acids are relatively nonionized in acid urine, and reabsorption is favored. Weak bases are nonionized in alkaline urine, and reabsorption is favored. This same principle is taken advantage of when toxic levels of weak acids are reached and rapid elimination is important, such as in salicylate poisoning. In this case the urine is made alkaline (e.g., by sodium bicarbonate or acetazolamide) and the salicylate becomes ionized and not reabsorbable. Therefore, its excretion is increased. The opposite of these events occurs for weak bases. Reabsorption of the nonionized form of weak bases is favored in an alkaline tubule fluid, and their excretion as charged molecules is favored in an acid urine. These physicochemical features of nonionic passive back-diffusion have significant effects on the half-life of a drug.

Back-diffusion affects half-life of drug.

Alter half-life of drug by altering pH of tubule fluid.

Increased renal excretion of drugs by interference with nonionic back-diffusion is reasonably achievable when the pK_a of the drug falls within an attainable urine pH range. Urine pH may be decreased to 5.0 using acidifying salts and increased to 8.0. Forced alkaline diuresis can result in an enhancement of phenobarbitol excretion by as much as 50%. Forced acid diuresis can increase excretion of weak bases such as amphetamine. The

GFR governs the amount of drug within the tubule that is capable of being excreted by this maneuver. However, if decreased renal function is present, there is little to be gained by these procedures.

The blood that is not filtered enters the postglomerular peritubular capillary system carrying both free and bound drug. An equilibrium exists between the protein-bound and free portions of the drug, and free drug is able to bind to receptors or carriers located on the tubule cell. Substances bind to these carriers and are moved by active transport systems from the postglomerular peritubular capillary system across the tubule cell into the lumen of the tubule. Separate excretory transport systems exist for organic acids and organic bases. These systems are saturable and are identified by their ability to be inhibited by prototypical competitors; probenecid inhibits the organic anion transport system and quinine or mepiperphenidol inhibits the organic cation system. PAH, an organic acid, is used frequently to measure renal plasma flow, because at concentrations less than its transport maximum, all of the compound that reaches the transport system in the proximal tubule is secreted by it. TEA (tetraethylammonium) is the organic cation that is comparable to PAH in this regard. The use of a specific inhibitor to prolong the half-life of a drug that is excreted rapidly is an accepted strategy. The most frequently cited version of this procedure is the use of probenecid to maintain plasma levels of penicillin.

Pathways also exist for the active reabsorption of organic compounds in the proximal tubule, and two of these systems have been well studied: glucose reabsorption and amino acid reabsorption. It seems probable that any drugs analogous in structure to these will be handled in a similar manner. Frequently, these mechanisms for reabsorption are linked to a biotransformation of the substrate being reabsorbed. For example, glucose is metabolized to glucose-6-phosphate as it moves across the luminal membrane into the cell. Another endogenous compound, choline, is transformed to its oxidized metabolite, betaine, during its transit from lumen to blood. Elucidation of the mechanisms of reabsorption of organic compounds awaits future investigation.

It needs to be pointed out that substances may be actively transported in both directions by carrier-mediated mechanisms in the proximal tubule. The best example of this is the handling of uric acid. In humans, uric acid has a fractional excretion of 0.1 and so undergoes net reabsorption. However, the direction of its movement depends on the species that is being studied. Any drug that occupies the organic acid transport system has the potential of affecting the plasma concentration of uric acid. For example, the thiazide diuretics ethacrynic acid and furosemide can inhibit the excretion of uric acid and contribute to the production of hyperuricemia. On the other hand, probenecid is used as a uricosuric agent to inhibit the reabsorption of uric acid and decrease hyperuricemia. Other drugs also occupy the systems that handle uric acid.

As noted for the reabsorptive process for glucose and choline, a metabolic step is necessary for returning the molecule to the blood. In the secretory process for certain organic ions, biotransformation is also important. In fact, the kidney plays a major role in the metabolism of many drugs. With regard to the secretory process, the action of certain enzymes can transform a molecule to a more polar and water-soluble metabolite. Glucuronidation is a good example of this. Synthesis of glucuronide conjugates by the enzyme uridine diphosphate glucuronyl transferase acts to enhance drug excretion. Sulfate conjugation also increases the excretion of a substance, although on a quantitatively smaller scale than glucuronidation. *N*-oxidation of meperidine by the kidney contributes to its excretion.

Binding of drug to plasma proteins and transport carriers

Active reabsorption of organic compounds occurs in proximal tubule.

Reabsorption is linked frequently to biotransformation.

Bidirectional transport of uric acid

Drug biotransformations in the kidney

DRUG EXCRETION IN RENAL FAILURE

A patient with renal failure may be undergoing treatment for more than one medical problem and therefore may be receiving a number of medications. The kidney is the major organ for drug excretion, and renal dysfunction leads to abnormal excretion and metabolism of drugs. Many separate functions may go wrong. There is little or no urine along with reduced RPF and GFR. Acute renal failure may be caused by many things: hypotension in response to trauma, blood loss, myocardial infarction, septicemia, or nephrotoxins. Patients with poor renal function have inappropriate responses to ordinary doses of many drugs. The reason for the inappropriate responses may be an abnormality in absorption, distribution, metabolism, or excretion of the prescribed medication that has resulted in an inappropriate plasma concentration, or it could be a change in the sensitivity of the target tissue to the drug. The effect of uremia itself to induce alterations in receptor environment may result in untoward effects of drugs. Drug prescribing in renal failure is difficult and potentially dangerous. Studious drug selection and careful dose modification are essential for successful drug therapy.

> Drug prescribing in renal failure is complicated.

Hemodynamic factors that affect drug elimination by the kidney are renal blood flow and GFR. When these are decreased, as in renal failure, the amount of drug reaching the kidney, the amount of drug filtered, and thus the amount of drug excreted are all decreased. This situation leads to plasma drug concentrations that are higher than desired.

> Plasma drug concentrations are higher than desired.

A complicating feature of drug excretion in renal failure is the changes that occur, sometimes in unpredictable fashion, in protein binding. There is generally a decreased binding of drugs, especially highly bound acidic drugs such as furosemide. An additional factor to be considered is that in certain conditions, such as the nephrotic syndrome, hypoalbuminemia may be present or the ratio of different globulin fractions changes and a new binding picture emerges. In uremia there may be an alteration of the binding sites themselves, or certain compounds present in uremia may compete with drugs for binding. The usual outcome is that more free drug is present in plasma than would normally have been predicted. For those drugs that are excreted by carrier transport systems in the proximal tubule, an alteration in the binding to carrier may occur, most likely contributing to a decreased excretion of the agent.

> Protein-binding profiles are unpredictable.

Alterations in drug metabolism are still more complicated. The uremic state has differential effects on enzyme systems and may lead to increased or decreased formation of drug metabolites. Some oxidations that occur in the endoplasmic reticulum of the liver are accelerated in uremia (e.g., oxidation of phenytoin). If the metabolic step leads to an active metabolite, the result is a more intense effect of the drug. The CNS depressant meperidine is metabolized to normeperidine by the liver and to meperidine N-oxide by the kidney. In renal failure more normeperidine than normal is formed because the renal metabolic route is not functioning. The outcome is more severe CNS toxicity from higher levels of normeperidine.

> Routes of drug metabolisms may change.

Certain guidelines should be used in an effort to avoid adverse drug reactions in patients with renal failure. The obvious one is not to prescribe drugs unless they are clearly indicated. When a drug dosage needs to be modified, the GFR, determined by endogenous creatinine clearance, may be used as an indicator. The half-life of a drug increases as the GFR decreases. In general the loading or initial dose should be the usual dose because the immediate therapeutic effect may be important. However, if volume depletion exists, it may be necessary to decrease the initial dose of certain drugs that have a narrow therapeutic index (e.g., digoxin).

> Modification of drug dosage

DRUGS CONTRAINDICATED IN RENAL FAILURE

Two classes of drugs in particular are associated with significant adverse effects when administered to patients in renal failure. These are NSAIDs (nonsteroidal anti-inflammatory drugs) and ACE inhibitors. Both of these types of drugs act to further compromise the already existing renal failure and for this reason are clearly contraindicated in this setting.

NSAIDs are cyclooxygenase inhibitors and decrease the production of prostaglandins. Prostaglandin-associated renal vasodilation is particularly important in maintaining renal blood flow during renal failure. The system does not appear to be as important when kidney function is normal. The administration of NSAIDs prevents the prostaglandin-induced maintenance of blood flow in renal failure.

NSAIDs are contraindicated in renal failure.

Glomerular filtration is maintained in part by the pressure difference across the glomerulus, and this is controlled in part by the degree of vasoconstriction in the afferent and efferent arterioles. Angiotensin II apparently has a greater effect to constrict the efferent arteriole than the afferent arteriole and in doing so enhances the GFR. The administration of ACE inhibitors prevents the efferent vasoconstriction and decreases GFR and tubule flow rate.

ACE inhibitors in renal failure

Diuretics

A diuretic is any substance that produces an increase in urine volume. Ingestion of large volumes of fluid increases urine output, and this generally occurs through an increase in volume in the vascular compartment, which causes an increase in renal plasma flow and an increase in glomerular filtration rate. As noted earlier, glomerular tubular balance demands that increases in GFR result in increases in urine volume and sodium excretion. However, pharmacological agents currently useful as diuretics do not produce their effect by increasing GFR. Our present armamentarium of diuretic drugs consists of compounds that act on certain sites along the nephron to interfere with the particular sodium reabsorptive pathways located there. The resulting natriuresis and diuresis are therefore tubular effects, and in general, a decrease in the amount of sodium reabsorbed obligates a decrease in the amount of tubule fluid reabsorbed.

The effect produced by diuretics, increased loss of salt and water, is a useful therapy for diseases associated with positive sodium balance. In general, these are disease states associated with edema. Diuretics act by stimulating renal sodium excretion to the point that excretion exceeds intake and edema fluid is mobilized. With the exception of a new class of diuretics, the vasopressin (V_2) antagonists, or *aquaretics*, modern diuretic drugs act by inhibiting renal tubular solute reabsorption at distinct nephron sites. Fluid follows solute and diuresis ensues.

In general, currently useful diuretics act directly on the tubule.

In addition to changes in electrolyte excretion, there are hemodynamic effects that may contribute also to the characteristic effects of a particular diuretic. The initial mobilization of edema fluid can be associated with increases in RPF and GFR but, as therapy continues, the decreasing circulating volume may be associated with a decrease in renal hemodynamics.

Secondary hemodynamic effects occur.

Certain pharmacological agents are capable of increasing renal plasma flow and glomerular filtration rate, thereby increasing the filtered load of sodium leading to increased sodium excretion. Xanthine derivatives increase renal blood flow through afferent arteriolar vasodilation. Dopamine decreases renal vascular resistance and thereby increases renal blood flow. Dobutamine increases cardiac contractility and cardiac output, and digitalis glycosides act similarly, increasing cardiac output with the resulting increased renal perfusion. However, these agents are not generally used as diuretics not only because they tend to be inconsistent in their natriuretic/ diuretic effects but also because the disorder that is being treated is associated with increased reabsorption at the level of the tubule. Thus, drugs that counteract sodium retention by acting at the reabsorptive event are the major ones to be considered.

Most effective diuretics now in use are organic anions. This structural feature confers particular pharmacokinetic characteristics. Such agents are tightly bound to plasma proteins and filtered at the glomerulus in only negligible amounts. They are moved across the tubule cell from the post-glomerular peritubular capillary blood into the lumen by the active organic acid transport system in the straight segment of the proximal tubule. They travel in the lumen to their tubular site of action, and their concentration in the lumen determines the diuretic response. Therefore, in order for the diuretic to reach its site of action adequate renal function must exist.

Although attempts have been made to classify diuretic agents according to their chemical structure, this is of limited value in understanding their renal action. Compounds with similar structures may result in diureses with different profiles of electrolyte excretion. On the other hand, structurally dissimilar diuretics may result in similar electrolyte excretion. A more useful classification is achieved according to the major site of action of a particular diuretic, and this is the traditional procedure for placing a diuretic into a particular class. Because inhibition of sodium reabsorption in a particular nephron segment affects electrolyte excretion in a particular manner, this classification is based upon the tubule segment at which a diuretic exerts its major effect. The nephron site at which a particular class of diuretic acts confers the relative potency to other classes of diuretics. It may be the determining factor also for some side effects and other thera-

Most diuretics are secreted by proximal tubule and travel in lumen to site of action.

Classification is according to tubule segment upon which they act.

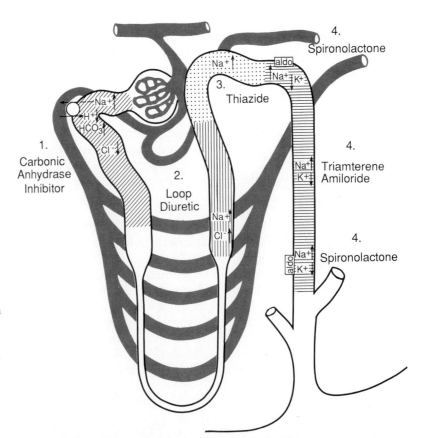

Figure 34–5

Sites at which different classes of diuretics act and the effect on particular electrolytes at that site. (1) Carbonic anhydrase inhibition results in a decrease in hydrogen and chloride ions and an increase in sodium and bicarbonate ions in the proximal tubule. (2) Loop diuretics result in an increase in sodium and chloride ions in the thick ascending limb. (3) Thiazides interfere with the reabsorption of sodium in the early (convoluted) distal tubule. (4) Spironolactone, triamterene, and amiloride result in increased sodium and decreased potassium concentrations in the late distal tubule.

peutic features. The following is the classification arising from the action of diuretics on particular sites in the tubule: Site 1 is the proximal tubule, Site 2 is the thick ascending limb of Henle's loop, Site 3 is the early distal tubule or cortical portion of the diluting segment, and Site 4 is the late distal and early collecting tubule. This is the order for discussion because it continues to provide the basis of our understanding of the mechanism of action of the different classes of diuretics (Fig. 34–5).

Diuretics That Act on the Proximal Tubule (Carbonic Anhydrase Inhibitors)

History and Chemistry. Carbonic anhydrase was first identified in red blood cells. Subsequently, it was found to exist in great excess in tissue, and it is known now to exist in several different forms in kidney, stomach, pancreas, eye, and central nervous system (CNS). The carbonic anhydrase inhibitors were developed to inhibit the enzyme associated with hydrogen transport in various tissues, and this effect on the kidney was observed to be associated with the production of a diuresis.

Carbonic anhydrases are inhibited by sulfonamides, and when sulfanilamide was introduced into therapy, its diuretic potential was observed. Subsequently, a number of sulfonamides were tested for their ability to inhibit this enzyme, and acetazolamide was the most successful clinically. Its usefulness as a diuretic was limited because inhibition of the renal enzyme results in refractoriness to the drug and only a modest diuretic effect.

Mechanism of Action. The only diuretics with their *major* site of action on the proximal tubule segment of the nephron are those that inhibit carbonic anhydrase. Whereas other classes of diuretics may have some proximal tubule action, their major activity lies in other nephron segments. Carbonic anhydrase is present both in the tubule lumen and in the cytoplasm of the tubule cell. It is not clear which of these sites are inhibited in producing the associated diuresis.

Site 1—proximal tubule

ACETAZOLAMIDE

Acetazolamide (DIAMOX) is the prototypical carbonic anhydrase inhibitor. Its mechanism of action as a diuretic can be completely accounted for by noncompetitive inhibition of renal carbonic anhydrase. When this enzyme is inhibited, there is a decreased generation of hydrogen ion to exchange for sodium and less sodium enters the tubule cell. A decrease in the hydrogen ion concentration in the lumen results in a decrease in the hydration of bicarbonate to carbonic acid and in its subsequent dissociation to carbon dioxide and water. It is as carbon dioxide and water that diffusion back into the cell occurs. The bicarbonate ion itself does not readily diffuse back across the cell. It remains in the lumen and is excreted along with sodium.

The sodium and water that were not reabsorbed in the early proximal tubule reach the late proximal tubule and prevent the normal differential increase in late proximal tubule chloride. This decreases the diffusion gradient that is normally present for the passive reabsorption of sodium chloride and water. Most of the sodium and chloride escaping from the proximal tubule are reabsorbed subsequently in the ascending limb. However, there is an increase in the delivery of sodium bicarbonate to the distal tubule. Here bicarbonate acts as a nonreabsorbable anion and increases sodium and potassium excretion. Fractional excretion of sodium reaches 3–5% of the filtered load. Bicarbonate, which is only minimally reabsorbed in the more distal nephron, is increased in excretion by as much as 30% of

CH_3CONH — S — SO_2NH_2
N —— N
Acetazolamide

Inhibition of carbonic anhydrase and sodium/hydrogen exchange

Increased urinary bicarbonate and
production of alkaline urine

the filtered load. The fractional excretion of potassium may increase up to 70%, and this is related to the delivery of increased sodium and large amounts of nonreabsorbable bicarbonate to the distal sodium/potassium exchange area. Urine volume increases, and the normally acid urine becomes alkaline as a result of the presence of large amounts of bicarbonate. Sodium and potassium excretion parallels the loss of bicarbonate, whereas the urinary concentration of chloride decreases.

Hyperchloremic metabolic acidosis

The excretion of bicarbonate instead of chloride leads to the development of hyperchloremic metabolic acidosis. This is analogous to the proximal bicarbonate wasting that occurs in proximal renal tubular acidosis. In an acid environment the effect of carbonic anhydrase inhibitors is decreased or absent so that refractoriness to the diuretic develops within a few days.

Thiazides have minor carbonic anhydrase
inhibitory effect.

Although thiazide diuretics also inhibit carbonic anhydrase, this is not considered the principal mechanism of their diuretic activity, and their carbonic anhydrase inhibitory potencies differ from their diuretic potencies. Also, the electrolyte excretory profile observed after administration of the thiazide diuretics differs greatly from electrolyte excretion observed after the administration of carbonic anhydrase inhibitors. The loop diuretics furosemide, bumetanide, and piretanide (but not ethacrynic acid) also have some inhibitory effect on carbonic anhydrase, but this is a minor factor in the production of diuresis.

Acetazolamide is a weak diuretic.

Therapeutic Uses. Acetazolamide is never a first-choice diuretic. It is chosen as a diuretic when the addition of a proximally acting agent to the therapeutic regimen is warranted. It is used primarily in patients with pre-existing metabolic alkalosis, such as those with congestive heart failure who have been treated previously with more distally acting diuretics. Its proximal action is taken advantage of when it is given along with a distally acting diuretic to produce a sequential blockade.

Carbonic anhydrase inhibitors have found a place in the therapy of some disorders that are unrelated to renal function. They have been used effectively in the treatment of grand and petit mal epilepsy. Movement of sodium into cerebral spinal fluid (CSF) is associated with carbonic anhydrase activity of glial and choroid plexus cells. Inhibition of this enzyme decreases sodium entry into the CSF and the rate of CSF formation.

Nondiuretic uses

In the eye, inhibition of carbonic anhydrase lowers the rate of formation of aqueous humor by 45–60%. The decreased fluid formation translates to a reduction in intraocular pressure. Acetazolamide, methazolamide, dichlorphenamide, and ethoxzolamide have been used for the treatment of wide angle and chronic glaucoma and to reduce intraocular pressure following cataract surgery. When used for these conditions the agents are given systemically because their limited lipid solubility restricts their transcorneal permeability. In addition, acetazolamide has been found to be effective in preventing or reducing the severity of acute mountain sickness, although its side effects may limit its usefulness.

The alkaline diuresis that occurs with the use of carbonic anhydrase inhibitors is taken advantage of in the treatment of overdose and poisoning with agents that are organic acids such as salicylates or phenobarbital. When given for this purpose, acetazolamide may be given intravenously to more quickly counteract the toxicity. The production of an increased volume of alkaline urine facilitates the renal elimination of uric acid also, and for this reason it is useful sometimes to treat the hyperuricemia associated with gout.

Adverse Effects. Only a few toxic effects have been observed with carbonic anhydrase inhibitors, and the most notable of these is the loss of potassium leading to hypokalemia. This occurs through the delivery of increased amounts of sodium to the distal tubule along with the nonreabsorbable anion bicarbonate. More potassium exchanges for the increased sodium and stays with the bicarbonate anion. Acetazolamide and other carbonic anhydrase inhibitors apparently have the curious ability to alter taste sensitivity and to eliminate the tingle of carbonated drinks.

In large doses acetazolamide may produce drowsiness and paresthesias. Hypersensitivity reactions are rare and when they do occur they consist of fever, skin reactions, bone-marrow depression, and sulfonamide-like renal lesions. Decreases in urinary citrate may lead to calculus formation and ureteral colic. Because teratogenic effects have been demonstrated in animals, these drugs should not be used in pregnant women.

Drug Interactions. Thyroidal iodine uptake may be depressed by acetazolamide, and this should be taken into consideration when a patient on acetazolamide is undergoing treatment for thyroid disorders. The alkalization of the urine that is associated with the use of these diuretics may interfere with the action of the urinary tract antiseptic methenamine. Coadministration of phenytoin has been reported to result in drug-induced osteomalacia.

Preparations and Pharmacokinetics. Other carbonic anhydrase inhibitors are benzolamide, methazolamide (NEPTAZANE), and dichlorphenamide (DARANIDE). Methazolamide, a derivative of acetazolamide, is used only for glaucoma.

Acetazolamide has excellent bioavailability and reaches its peak plasma concentration within 2 hours following oral administration. It has a half-life of 13 hours and is eliminated unchanged in the urine. Because it is an organic acid diuretic, it is tightly bound to plasma proteins, undergoes negligible filtration, and is secreted by the proximal tubule organic acid transport system.

Acetazolamide, at 20 mg/kg, has been observed to completely inhibit carbonic anhydrase activity. The oral dose effective in humans is 250–500 mg/day. When used as a diuretic, it is given once a day or every other day. When prescribed for its metabolic acidosis effects, it is given every 8 hours. For chronic simple glaucoma, 250–1000 mg is given in divided doses.

History and Chemistry. The first loop diuretics were the organic mercurials. Their usefulness was noted in the sixteenth century when Paracelsus observed that calomel (mercurous chloride) increased urine output and alleviated the symptoms of congestive heart failure. Merbaphen, another organic mercurial, was used originally in the treatment of syphilis when its diuretic properties were observed. Subsequently, a less toxic mercurial, mersalyl, was introduced. Its success as a diuretic led to the development of a number of other organic mercurial agents for this purpose.

Loop or High-Ceiling Diuretics

The general formula for organic mercurial diuretics is RCH (OY) CH_2Hg^+ in which the Y is an alkyl group and the R a bulkier organic moiety. Although there is some dispute, the most generally accepted theory of mercurial action is that a dissociation of the carbon-mercury bond occurs, and the mercury ion combines with a sulfhydryl group associated with a receptor on the thick ascending limb of Henle's loop—the mercury ion theory. The combined disadvantages of (1) the need to administer mercurials by intramuscular injection and (2) the development of refractoriness to the drug due to the development of hypochloremic alkalosis led

Furosemide

Ethacrynic acid

Bumetanide

Actions at Site 2—thick ascending limb of Henle's loop—produce greatest diuretic effect

Inhibit 1 Na$^+$, 1 K$^+$, 2 Cl$^-$ cotransport

Decrease positive and negative free water formation

to their abandonment when orally effective loop diuretics became available.

The loop diuretics furosemide and ethacrynic acid emerged on the therapeutic scene about the same time in the early 1960s. Ethacrynic acid was developed in the United States and furosemide in Germany. Ethacrynic acid contains an activated double bond attached to a moiety containing a carboxylic acid group. Furosemide resulted from investigations of a series of 5-sulfamoylanthranilic acid derivatives substituted on the aromatic amino group. Furosemide is 4-chloro-*N*-furfuryl-5-sulfamoyl-anthranilic acid. Bumetanide, 3-(butylamino)-4-phenoxy-5-sulfamoyl-benzoic acid, was introduced more recently; it is structurally related to furosemide.

Mechanism of Action. These agents act on the thick ascending limb of Henle's loop (Site 2) and, for that reason, they are the most effective diuretics. The most commonly used loop diuretic is furosemide. All the loop diuretics are capable of producing a diuresis that is 25% of the filtered load. They are called *loop* diuretics because they act at a site immediately distal to the loop of Henle, and they are called *high-ceiling* because they produce the greatest diuretic effect. In this chapter they are referred to with the more commonly used term *loop*.

Loop diuretics consist of a group of compounds dissimilar in chemical structure but similar in mechanism and site of action. They inhibit sodium chloride reabsorption at the high-capacity site in the ascending limb of the loop of Henle (Site 2). Solute and water, which are prevented from being reabsorbed there, are passed on to the distal tubule. In the distal tubule, there is a limited capacity for sodium reabsorption, which cannot compensate for the inhibitory effect on sodium chloride reabsorption in the ascending limb.

There has been some controversy in the past as to whether sodium or chloride is the actively transported ion in this segment. Recent studies show that active sodium transport provides the driving force for reabsorption. The sodium/potassium pump in the peritubular membrane moves sodium out of the cell and maintains a large electrochemical sodium gradient across the luminal membrane. This gradient provides the driving force for the coupled entry of chloride and potassium. This cotransport system moves one sodium cation, one potassium cation, and two chloride anions in an electroneutral process into the cell from the tubule fluid. A cotransport system implies that the individual flows of the cotransported ions are tightly coupled with each other at a fixed stoichiometry. The system has been shown to be inhibited by furosemide, bumetanide, and the cysteine adduct of ethacrynic acid, and this inhibition is strongly correlated to the diuretic effect.

Loop diuretics decrease both positive and negative free water production by inhibiting removal of sodium chloride from the lumen, which leaves the lumen less dilute; and by the same step (inhibition of the co-transport of one sodium, two chloride, one potassium) preventing addition of sodium chloride to the interstitium, which decreases the osmotic force of the interstitium. The inhibition of sodium chloride reabsorption in the ascending limb delivers more salt to the early distal tubule and decreases the dilution of the urine and thereby positive free water formation. The same action decreases the osmotic gradient in the medullary portion of the kidney, which is the force for water reabsorption under the influence of ADH, so that less water is capable of being reabsorbed (negative free water formation). Thus, positive free water (urine dilution) and negative free water (urine concentration) are affected.

Loop diuretics produce a dose-dependent diuresis that is characterized by increases in the excretion of water, sodium, chloride, potassium, calcium, and magnesium. There is washout of the renal medulla with decreased hypertonicity of the inner zones of the kidney. The increased potassium excretion, which can lead to hypokalemia, is mostly due to the increase in volume flow rate through the distal tubule and the increased delivery of sodium to the sodium/potassium exchange site in the distal tubule.

Certain hemodynamic effects are characteristic of loop diuretics. One of these is an increase in venous capacitance. The increased renal vasodilation produced by a decrease in renal vascular resistance permits an increase in renal blood flow. The increase in renal blood flow is primarily in the inner cortical and medullary blood flows, and this is important for the diuresis induced by these agents. Increased medullary flow leads to washout and medullary hypertonicity and decreases water reabsorption in the collecting duct, leading to the excretion of a more dilute urine. Much evidence indicates that this is a prostaglandin-associated process. Both furosemide and ethacrynic acid can lead to increased amounts of the vasodilator PGE_2 by inhibiting the enzyme prostaglandin dehydrogenase. PGE_2 acts directly also on the medullary thick ascending limb to inhibit chloride transport.

Furosemide and ethacrynic acid appear to interfere with tubuloglomerular feedback so that the decrease in GFR associated with increased distal delivery of fluid does not occur generally. They inhibit chloride flux into the macula densa cells, thereby abolishing tubuloglomerular feedback and preventing the expected decrease in GFR secondary to enhanced tubular flow rate.

Biochemical effects of furosemide and ethacrynic acid include inhibition of membrane transport ATPase, inhibition of glycolysis and mitochondrial respiration, and inhibition of the microsomal calcium pump. Furosemide, unlike ethacrynic acid, has some carbonic anhydrase inhibitory activity. Both furosemide and ethacrynic acid inhibit adenylate cyclase and prostaglandin dehydrogenase. The effects of bumetanide are similar to those of furosemide.

Therapeutic Uses. Loop diuretics are commonly used in the treatment of edema of cardiac, hepatic, or renal origin. Because of the potency of these drugs, initial dosages are recommended to be relatively low. Also because of their potency, they are sometimes useful in the early stages of renal failure. This action has been suggested to be related to their ability to increase renal prostaglandin levels. Although these drugs are effective in renal impairment, when GFRs are as low as 2 ml/minute, higher than normal dosages may be needed to achieve diuresis. In order to be effective, loop diuretics must be secreted by the proximal tubule and travel to their luminal site of action. This means that some degree of renal function must exist.

Their rapid action and high potency have made them the drugs of choice also in left heart failure leading to pulmonary edema. Even before the onset of diuretic action, furosemide decreases left ventricular filling pressure and increases venous capacitance. Hemodynamics seem to improve before significant diuresis has occurred. Diuresis then contributes to a further reduction in filling pressure. Because pulmonary edema is an acute situation requiring immediate treatment, furosemide is administered intravenously and is effective within 10 minutes. When furosemide is used to treat pulmonary edema, frequent intravenous doses should be administered so that the urine flow rate can be titrated to the desired level and rapid volume depletion avoided.

Another acute situation that is efficiently counteracted by furosemide

---

Marginal notes:

Renal medullary washout

Increased venous capacitance and decreased renal vascular resistance

Interference with tubuloglomerular feedback

Used in treatment of edema of cardiac, renal, hepatic, or pulmonary origin and also bumetanide is hypercalcemic crisis. The ability of these drugs to inhibit calcium reabsorption by the thick ascending limb of Henle makes them useful in this condition. Because the transport of calcium is an active process, apparently independent of the activity of sodium/potassium ATPase, the calciuria is not a result of inhibition of this enzyme. When furosemide is used for hypercalcemic crisis, it is necessary to replace the large urinary losses of other electrolytes, particularly sodium and chloride.

Adverse Effects. The major toxic effect of the loop diuretics is fluid and electrolyte imbalance due to overdiuresis. The loss of electrolytes and volume contraction can lead secondarily to problems such as hypovolemia, hyponatremia, hypokalemia, hyperuricemia, and hyperglycemia.

Ototoxicity

Diuretic-induced ototoxicity is associated with this class of diuretic and may be due to the alteration of electrolyte composition in the inner ear. The potential for ototoxicity for the three major loop diuretics is in the order of ethacrynic acid > furosemide > bumetanide. In general, this is a reversible adverse effect that disappears upon withdrawal of the drug. However, permanent hearing loss has been reported with ethacrynic acid.

Hyperuricemia

Hyperuricemia may be associated with contraction of plasma volume but is attributed also to the ability of most loop diuretics to interfere with the excretion of uric acid by the organic acid excretory transport system in the proximal tubule. This may be a problem in patients who have a predisposition to gout, in whom loop diuretics should be used cautiously.

Glucose intolerance

A decrease in glucose tolerance has been reported but occurs to a lesser extent than it does with the thiazides. The rationale for its occurrence is unclear, but it may be associated with diuretic-induced hypokalemia or insulin activity.

Drug Interactions. Because of the potential for ototoxicity, drugs with similar potential, such as aminoglycoside antibiotics, should not be coadministered with loop diuretics. These organic acid drugs are significantly bound to plasma albumin and may compete for protein binding with similarly bound drugs such as warfarin and clofibrate. Increased cephaloridine nephrotoxicity has been noted with furosemide, and careful use of cephalosporin is recommended.

Pharmacokinetics

Preparations and Pharmacokinetics. In general loop diuretics have a wide dosage range and maintain their potency in impaired renal function. They have a steep dose-response curve and a rapid onset of action. All loop diuretics are absorbed quickly, with peak concentrations attained within 0.5–2 hours. Their half-lives are approximately 1–2 hours and their onset of action is 30–90 minutes. Although they are extensively bound to plasma proteins, they have strong affinity for the organic acid excretory transporter, and this accounts for their relatively short half-lives.

Furosemide is excreted unchanged in the urine by secretion in the proximal tubule, mostly within 4 hours of an oral dose. One third of ethacrynic acid is excreted in the bile and the remainder by the kidney. The urinary products of ethacrynic acid are divided equally into three fractions: unchanged drug, a cysteine conjugate, and an undetermined metabolite. It appears that the major diuretic action of ethacrynic acid is through its cysteine conjugate.

Clinically, furosemide has two advantages over ethacrynic acid. It has a broader dose-response curve, which allows greater accuracy in titrating a dose to a particular patient, and there are fewer gastrointestinal (GI) side effects. Bumetanide is structurally related to furosemide. It is comparable to furosemide in its activity and maximal effect but is considerably more potent on a weight basis.

Other loop diuretics that have reached the market more recently and have a more prolonged action than those previously mentioned are piretanide, muzolimine, and xipamide. They differ from each other mainly in their pharmacokinetics. The potency of piretanide is intermediate to furosemide and bumetanide. Muzolimine and xipamide also have longer durations of action. Muzolimine has a half-life of approximately 13 hours and only negligible amounts are excreted in the urine.

Furosemide (LASIX), ethacrynic acid (EDECRIN), and bumetanide (BUMEX) are available for oral and parenteral administration. Because these are potent diuretics it is advisable to initiate therapy with small dosages and build up to the desired effect. It has been proposed that the safest and most effective administration for chronic treatment with loop diuretics is alternate-day therapy or intermittent dosing for 3–4 days followed by 1- to 2-day rest periods.

History and Chemistry. The diuretic effects of acetazolamide, a sulfonamide, led to the search for other sulfonamides with this property but without a carbonic anhydrase inhibitory component in order to avoid adverse effects on acid-base balance. The first orally active and clinically useful thiazide diuretic was chlorothiazide (6-chloro-2H-1,2,4-benzothiadiazine-7-sulfonamide 1,1-dioxide). An alkyl group in position 3 results in decreased activity as does methyl substitution on the ring nitrogen at position 2 or 4. One of the most widely used thiazide diuretics, hydrochlorothiazide (6-chloro-3,4-dihydro-2H-1,2,4-benzothiadiazine-7-sulfonamide 1,1-dioxide) was synthesized in 1958 and found to have 10–20 times the potency of chlorothiazide. Alkyl substitution at position 3 confers additional lipid solubility and may be directly related to thiazide effectiveness.

Mechanism of Action. How thiazide diuretics act is understood incompletely. They inhibit sodium chloride reabsorption in the distal convoluted tubule, which they reach after secretion by the organic acid transport system in the proximal tubule. Their chloruretic potency suggests specific interference with chloride reabsorption in the early distal convoluted tubule, where urine is hypotonic. Because thiazides inhibit sodium and chloride reabsorption at this cortical diluting segment (Site 3), they have a relatively moderate potency and lead to excretion of 5–8% of the filtered load.

Action at the cortical diluting site decreases the production of positive free water, because sodium is prevented from being reabsorbed and remains in the tubule fluid. Thiazide diuretics do not interfere with negative free water production because they have no effect on medullary sodium reabsorption that contributes to the osmolar gradient for water reabsorption.

Although they were synthesized as an outgrowth of the carbonic anhydrase inhibitors, they increase the excretion of sodium and chloride in similar quantities unrelated to carbonic anhydrase inhibition. In fact, their potency as diuretics is related inversely to their potency as carbonic anhydrase inhibitors, and there is no thiazide that is equal to acetazolamide in its ability to inhibit the enzyme. The diuresis occurring with thiazide diuretics is associated with increased water, sodium, potassium, chloride, bicarbonate, and phosphate excretion.

Resistance to thiazides may develop with their chronic use. This decreased effectiveness is associated with compensatory sodium reabsorption at a site either more distal or more proximal to that inhibited by the thiazides. Delivery of more sodium to the sodium/potassium exchange site more distal in the tubule stimulates sodium reabsorption there. Contraction of plasma volume as a result of continued diuresis may decrease the filtered

Thiazides

Hydrochlorothiazide

Site 3—cortical diluting segment

Inhibit Na^+, Cl^- cotransport

Decrease positive free water production

Resistance to thiazides through compensatory reabsorption of Na^+

load, and a larger proportion of the filtrate is reabsorbed in the proximal tubule and thick ascending limb. The disadvantages of thiazide therapy include a relatively low potency, and resistance to their effects occurs with renal impairment. Thiazides are of no value in patients with glomerular filtration rates less than 25–30 ml/minute.

In general, the hemodynamic effects of the thiazides include an increase in renal vascular resistance, a decrease in renal blood flow, and a decrease in GFR. It is thought that the decrease in GFR is associated with an increase in intratubular pressure and that tubuloglomerular feedback may play an important role in their hemodynamic effects.

Therapeutic Uses. Thiazide diuretics are used in the management of chronic cardiac decompensation in mild to moderate congestive heart failure (in general, right heart failure). They are effective also in the treatment of edema caused by chronic hepatic or renal disease. Their effects are more gradual than those of the more potent loop diuretics, and they do not have the great propensity to cause electrolyte imbalance.

Used in moderate congestive heart failure, chronic hepatic or renal disease

In the treatment of hypertension, thiazide diuretics have long been the mainstay of initial therapy. Their beneficial hypotensive effects are present even after the edema fluid has been removed. Administration of thiazides results in increased excretion of salt and water accompanied by weight loss and a slightly negative state of sodium balance. As treatment continues the antihypertensive effect persists even though a return toward sodium balance occurs. With little decrease in cardiac output, there is a decrease in total peripheral resistance, and it is not yet clear how this relates to sodium balance. Along with salt restriction, administration of these drugs is frequently a sufficient measure to control mild to moderate hypertension. Because this is usually long-term therapy, periodic assessment of the patient by means of laboratory measurements, particularly serum potassium levels, is required.

Useful in hypertension

Diazoxide (HYPERSTAT) is related chemically to the thiazides and is employed in hypertensive emergencies. It is administered intravenously and rapidly lowers blood pressure. It has no carbonic anhydrase inhibitory or diuretic effects. On the contrary, its use frequently leads to fluid retention as well as hyperglycemia.

The use of the thiazide diuretics in the treatment of diabetes insipidus appears paradoxical, and the explanation of the mechanism is less than satisfactory. In this condition, chronic treatment with thiazides results in a fall in urine volume and a rise in urine osmolarity. The diuretic-induced contraction of blood volume is associated with a decrease in filtration rate and increased proximal reabsorption of filtered load. This results in a decrease in the delivery of fluid to the distal nephron. More of the filtrate is reabsorbed than would occur without the thiazide. The patient is not cured, but a better water balance is achieved.

Used in nephrogenic diabetes insipidus

Thiazide diuretics are the only diuretics that increase the reabsorption of calcium. Because of this, their chronic administration has been found effective in the treatment of hypercalciuric renal stones. Thiazides increase calcium reabsorption from the lumen and prevent the build-up of calcium deposits in the tubule. The action of thiazides at the luminal side of the early distal tubule dissociates the reabsorption of sodium and calcium, decreasing sodium and increasing calcium reabsorption by a mechanism that remains unclear.

Increase in calcium reabsorption

Adverse Effects. As with all diuretics that act proximal to the distal tubule site for sodium/potassium exchange, the development of hypokalemia is a major risk. An increase in sodium reaching this segment is the main cause

Hypokalemia

of potassium loss in the urine.

There is carbonic anhydrase activity associated with the thiazides, and this contributes to the kaliuresis through the presence of increased bicarbonate in the distal tubule acting as a nonreabsorbable anion. However, inhibition of carbonic anhydrase is variable and not the main mechanism for potassium loss. The clearly dangerous situation occurs when therapy includes cardiac glycosides. The diuretic-induced hypokalemia can sensitize the heart to digitalis-induced arrhythmias. It should also be kept in mind that kaliuresis may result in metabolic alkalosis.

Chronic administration of thiazide diuretics can result in hyperuricemia. Two mechanisms for this side effect have been proposed and are the same as with furosemide. The organic acid structure of the thiazides places them in the group of compounds that are secreted from blood to lumen by the transport system for organic acids in the proximal tubule. There is a secretory component involved in the renal handling of uric acid that uses this system also, and inhibition of uric acid secretion by the thiazides may result in hyperuricemia. In addition, the contraction of plasma volume that accompanies diuresis may serve also to increase uric acid reabsorption in the proximal tubule.

Hyperuricemia

Hyperglycemia has been noted during thiazide therapy, and this diabetogenic effect is reversible. The mechanism for this effect is not established. It has been suggested that the diuretic-induced volume contraction contributes to the hyperglycemia, and that the hypokalemia resulting from the use of thiazides alters the effect of insulin. It has been proposed also that the thiazide compound may interfere with the release of insulin.

Glucose intolerance

The decrease in calcium excretion, while beneficial in one respect, requires guarding against the development of hypercalcemia and its attendant serious side effects. During long-term treatment, serum calcium should be monitored.

Hypercalcemia

Preparations and Pharmacokinetics. There are many structural variations of the thiazide diuretics. However, they are all capable of producing the same maximal effect and thus have the same intrinsic activity. There is therapeutic cross resistance among them, in that if one thiazide is not effective, it is unlikely another one will be.

Hydrochlorothiazide (ESIDRIX, HYDRODIURIL, ORETIC) is the prototypical short-acting thiazide, and chlorthalidone (HYGROTON) is the prototypical long-acting agent. Thiazides begin to act in 1–2 hours. They vary widely in their duration of action and in their plasma half-lives. Differences appear to be proportional to plasma protein binding and the degree of reabsorption in the renal tubule. The half-lives of *bendrofluazide, hydrochlorothiazide, hydroflumethiazide,* and *polythiazide* are 3, 10, 17, and 26 hours, respectively. Being organic acids the thiazides undergo active secretion by the proximal tubule. Most compounds are excreted rapidly by the kidneys within 3–6 hours after oral administration. The various thiazides differ in their degree of metabolism. Hydrochlorothiazide is excreted unchanged, whereas polythiazide is metabolized extensively. Lipid solubility is a major determinant of their potency.

Chlorthalidone

THIAZIDE-LIKE AGENTS

Quinazolinones (quinethazone, metolazone, chlorthalidone) have a carbonyl group instead of the ring sulfone in their structure. They act in the same segment of the nephron as the thiazides, although they are structurally different. Their activity as diuretics and their electrolyte excretion profile are similar to the thiazides. Quinethazone is orally active within 2 hours with an 18–24 hour duration of action.

Thiazide-like diuretics

Chlorthalidone is similar to thiazide diuretics except for its prolonged half-life. Peak plasma concentrations occur in 2–4 hours. Its prolonged half-life of several days has been attributed to its strong binding to red blood cells. It is about 70 times more potent than hydrochlorothiazide in inhibiting carbonic anhydrase, and in higher dosages it increases renal excretion of bicarbonate. It is excreted mainly unchanged by the kidney.

The nonthiazide agent *metolazone* (DIULO, ZAROXOLYN) acts at the same site as the thiazides in the distal nephron. Metolazone is long acting and retains its effect in the presence of renal impairment, which thiazides do not generally do. Also, it has a minor proximal tubule effect on phosphate-linked sodium reabsorption that may be useful in sequential blockage. Metolazone has an onset of action of 1 hour and a duration of action similar to quinethazone. It has been designated as both a loop diuretic and a thiazide diuretic.

Indapamide (LOZOL) belongs to a class of diuretics that are indoline derivatives. It is similar in structure to furosemide and bumetanide but different in that it has a prolonged diuretic action. It has the ability to provoke natriuresis despite renal impairment. In addition, indapamide has a vasodilator antihypertensive effect that is independent of any induced natriuresis. It is metabolized extensively and only 5% of the unchanged drug is excreted in the urine. Indapamide is 80% bound to plasma proteins and is concentrated in red blood cells.

There is a considerable variation in the cost of the different thiazide preparations and this should be considered when choosing one of them. These agents are taken for a prolonged duration of time. If cost is not a problem, then a thiazide with a long half-life would improve patient compliance.

Potassium-Sparing Diuretics/Agents Acting on Distal and Collecting Tubules

Spironolactone

Triamterene

Amiloride

History and Chemistry. There are three major drugs that act on the distal tubule and collecting duct, and they are all distinctly different in structure: spironolactone (a steroid), triamterene (an organic acid), and amiloride (an organic base).

Spironolactone is a steroidal analog of the natural hormone aldosterone. It was synthesized in the 1950s in the search for compounds that were aldosterone antagonists. A number of 17-spirolactone analogs were synthesized, and spironolactone (7α-acetylthio-3-oxo-17α-pregn-4-ene-$21,17\beta$-carbolactone acid-γ-lactone) was found orally active and useful.

Triamterene (2,4,7-triamino-6-phenylpteridine) is a pteridine that was originally synthesized as a folic acid antagonist. It was discovered to have diuretic activity in 1961, and this initiated further studies to examine the potential for this type of agent as a diuretic. It was found to be active in both normal and adrenalectomized rats, indicating that aldosterone antagonism was not its major mechanism of action. Diuretic activity is limited to analogs with only small changes in the phenyl ring.

Amiloride (*N*-amidino-3,5-diamino-6-chloropyrazinecarboxamide) has the same pharmacological action as that of triamterene. However, it is a pyrazinoylguanidine, and although there is some chemical resemblance to triamterene, the specific similarities are not related to diuretic activity. It also emerged from screening procedures for folic acid analogs. The introduction of the amino group in position 5 of compounds related to *N*-amidino-3-amino-6-bromopyrazinecarboxamide increased the excretion of sodium and chloride and not of potassium.

Mechanism of Action. The mechanism of action of this class of diuretics is to inhibit the distal sodium/potassium exchange (Site 4). These agents have relatively minor diuretic effects and lead to an excretion of only 2–3%

of filtered sodium and chloride owing to the small delivery of water and solutes to this area.

Site 4—distal and collecting tubules, mild diuresis

This class of potassium-sparing diuretics is divided into two types, and this division is based upon their effectiveness in the presence of aldosterone. Some, but not all, of the sodium/potassium exchange in the distal tubule is aldosterone-controlled, and this is interfered with by competitive inhibitors of this hormone, of which spironolactone is the major drug. The aldosterone-independent sodium/potassium exchange is interfered with by agents that directly block uptake of sodium into the tubule cell. The two major drugs in this category are triamterene and amiloride.

Spironolactone is a competitive antagonist for the aldosterone receptor in the cortical collecting tubules. The aldosterone receptor is a soluble, cytoplasmic protein that appears to exist in two allosteric forms. Spironolactone binds to the receptor and prevents it from assuming the active conformation. The subsequent biochemical chain of events leading to the synthesis of physiologically active transport proteins is stopped. The metabolite canrenone is also an active antagonist of aldosterone. Antagonism of aldosterone causes sodium excretion and potassium conservation. Spironolactone is effective when mineralocorticoid activity is high but has little activity in the absence of aldosterone. Because it is a competitive inhibitor, its action is overcome by higher concentrations of aldosterone. It is not effective in adrenalectomized patients or in individuals on a high sodium diet. It also increases calcium excretion through a direct effect on tubular transport.

Aldosterone-dependent: spironolactone

Binds to aldosterone receptor

Both amiloride and triamterene act on the distal tubule at an aldosterone-independent site to inhibit sodium/potassium exchange that occurs in response to a voltage-dependent process. Triamterene is effective from the peritubular side and irreversibly inhibits the transbasolateral potential difference in the collecting duct. Amiloride acts at the luminal surface of the tubule cell and reversibly inhibits transluminal potential difference in the distal tubule and collecting duct, resulting in a decrease in sodium permeability and a natriuresis without potassium loss. Diuresis includes an increased excretion of sodium accompanied by chloride and a moderate loss of fluid. There is little if any loss of potassium.

Aldosterone-independent: triamterene and amiloride

Decrease potassium excretion

Because potassium loss by distal tubule secretion is associated with the use of more proximally acting diuretics, drugs that interfere with the distal action prevent this loss, and potassium is retained. A slight alkalization of the urine occurs with the use of these diuretics, and this is caused by the inhibition of hydrogen ion secretion in the distal tubule. The mechanism for this inhibition is unknown, although it is known that these compounds do not inhibit carbonic anhydrase.

Therapeutic Uses. Although potassium-sparing diuretics may be used alone, their ability to protect against potassium loss has made them beneficial as adjunct therapy with other, more effective diuretics. They are used primarily in combination with the more proximally acting diuretics to block the kaliuresis that such agents routinely cause. These agents conserve both hydrogen and potassium and so tend to counteract the metabolic alkalosis obtained when sodium and potassium are excreted with chloride (as with the loop diuretics).

Adjunct to other diuretics

Spironolactone has been found to be effective in the treatment of primary aldosteronism. It may be useful in the treatment of heart failure, because hyperaldosteronism is commonly seen in this condition. Hypokalemia and alkalosis are counteracted also by this drug.

Spironolactone in hyperaldosteronism

Adverse Effects. Chronic use of this class of diuretic has the potential to produce hyperkalemia, and this is clearly associated with their mechanism of action. However, diuretic-induced hyperkalemia is not a common occurrence.

Although spironolactone was widely used once for the treatment of hypertension, it has lost popularity because of its side effects, which include hyperkalemia and gynecomastia. Spironolactone, as well as triamterene and amiloride, has the potential to induce hyperchloremic acidosis.

Preparations and Pharmacokinetics. Spironolactone, which begins to act in 8 hours, is almost wholly metabolized to canrenone and canrenoate, which are active, and its overall effect extends over several days. The metabolites have a plasma half-life of 17–22 hours, and the effect of any change in dosage will not peak for 3–4 days. Both triamterene (DYRENIUM) and amiloride (MIDAMOR) have considerably shorter half-lives than spironolactone.

Triamterene has an onset of action within 2 hours and a half-life of 2–4 hours. Thus, there is a need for multiple daily doses. Whereas the *p*-hydroxy metabolite of triamterene is pharmacologically active, the sulfate ester of the metabolite accounts for most of the diuretic activity. Most of the dose is excreted as the active metabolite.

Triamterene excreted mostly metabolized

Amiloride is pharmacologically similar to triamterene but is a stronger base and more water-soluble than triamterene. It is secreted into the proximal tubule fluid by the organic base pathway, and drugs that are organic bases may interfere with its excretion. After oral administration, only 20% of amiloride is absorbed and ultimately excreted unchanged by the kidney. Its half-life is approximately 6 hours, and that is when diuretic activity reaches a peak; its effects are over within 24 hours. Its use is associated with a moderate increase in urinary pH.

Amiloride excreted mostly unchanged

Azolimine, an investigational drug, was discovered in a search for a nonsteroidal antagonist of the renal effects of aldosterone. Its potassium-sparing natriuretic activity has both an aldosterone-antagonist component and an aldosterone-independent component.

Drug Interactions. None of these agents (amiloride, triamterene, and spironolactone) should be prescribed together, because this combination therapy has been observed to produce an unexpectedly high degree of hyperkalemia.

Osmotic Diuretics

Mechanism of Action. Substances that act as diuretics by contributing to the osmotic force of the tubule fluid have no cellular receptor and are not clearly identified as acting in a particular segment of the nephron. Their mechanism of action as diuretics is to contribute nonabsorbable osmolar particles to the tubule fluid and obligate water to remain with the extra solute. The presence of additional solute and the resulting increase in tubule fluid flow rate interfere with reabsorption of filtrate and with normal urinary concentration and can result in the excretion of large amounts of solute and water. Effective osmotic diuretics are given intravenously and contribute to the osmolarity of the plasma. Because they are freely filterable at the glomerulus and undergo limited reabsorption, they also contribute to the osmolality of the tubular fluid and interfere with reabsorption throughout the nephron. Whereas sodium and water are inhibited in the proximal tubule, there is also a major effect to reduce water and sodium reabsorption in the loop of Henle. In part, this may be attributed to a decrease in the osmolar solute concentration of the medulla with a concomitant decrease in water reabsorption from the thin ascending limb of Henle's loop.

Increased osmotic force in tubule fluid retains water.

Mannitol is the most commonly used osmotic diuretic. It is a metabolically inert hexose sugar that is poorly permeant into cells. Administration of isotonic or hypertonic solutions of mannitol results in increased total renal plasma flow as well as medullary and papillary plasma flow. Urine flow increases as does excretion of sodium, potassium, chloride, bicarbonate, calcium, and magnesium.

$$CH_2OH$$
$$|$$
$$HOCH$$
$$|$$
$$HOCH$$
$$|$$
$$HCOH$$
$$|$$
$$HCOH$$
$$|$$
$$CH_2OH$$

Mannitol

Therapeutic Uses. The main use of osmotic diuretics is related to increased urine flow and not mobilization of generalized edema fluid. Osmotic agents are not used therapeutically for the mobilization of edema fluid associated with congestive heart failure, hepatic failure, or the nephrotic syndrome. In these conditions addition of osmolar particles to the plasma may contribute to the edema rather than alleviate it, and expansion of the extracellular fluid is an undesirable hazard. In congestive heart failure, the heart is already faced with more work than it can perform, and additional volume load would compromise its efforts further.

Major use related to increasing urine flow rate

Osmotic diuretics are used to prevent acute renal failure, and this is a clear and important indication. When the GFR falls, there is a more complete reabsorption of tubular fluid, and this may lead to anuria. During surgical procedures when a large loss of blood is anticipated, patients may be primed with intravenous fluids and mannitol to maintain a diuresis throughout the surgery and during the immediate postoperative period.

Acute renal failure

Maintenance of tubule flow also prevents precipitation of toxins in the kidney. In certain situations, toxins can reach high concentrations in the tubules. A decreased tubular fluid volume favors the precipitation of compounds with low solubility, and this may cause physical damage. In cases of drug overdosage in which the kidney is the major route of elimination for the substance, increasing urine flow rate will increase the excretion of the drug.

Toxin precipitation in kidney—drug overdosage

The contribution of mannitol to the extracellular fluid compartment makes it useful in conditions that require dehydration of cells. Increases in intraocular and intracranial pressure can be alleviated by the use of mannitol. Water is drawn toward the osmotically active solute in the plasma.

Expansion of extracellular fluid volume

Adverse Effects. Administration of osmolar solutes may contribute to extracellular osmolarity and is accompanied by expansion of the extracellular fluid volume. In a patient with congestive heart failure, this is hazardous and contraindicated. Mannitol infusion should be terminated if a patient develops signs of progressive renal failure, heart failure, or pulmonary congestion. Otherwise, headache, nausea, and vomiting are relatively common complaints.

Preparations and Pharmacokinetics. Mannitol (OSMITROL) is available for intravenous administration in concentrations of 5–25%. The adult dose for diuresis ranges from 50 to 200 g over a 24-hour infusion period. When used for the prevention of acute renal failure during surgery or for the treatment of oliguria, the total adult dose is 50–100 g.

Other osmotic diuretics are urea (UREAPHIL), glycerin (GLYROL, OSMO-GLYN), and isosorbide (ISMOTIC). The latter two are used primarily in ophthalmological procedures, and there is little diuretic effect.

XANTHINES

Other Diuretics

Although it has been known for some time that ingestion of xanthine compounds (e.g., caffeine, theobromine) results in a diuresis, they are generally not prescribed for this purpose. However, they are the most common over-the-counter diuretics. They are weak diuretics compared with the thiazides, and their primary mechanism of action is not established. It has been demonstrated that they have both hemodynamic and tubular effects. Xanthines have a cardiac stimulatory effect and produce renal arteriolar vasodilation leading to increases in RBF and GFR. They also decrease sodium and chloride reabsorption at the level of the tubule, although the exact site is not known. Theophylline is commonly used as a bronchodilator, and its concomitant diuretic action should be kept in mind.

URICOSURIC DIURETICS

Hyperuricemia is not an uncommon occurrence with diuretic therapy, and many patients who require diuretic therapy are also candidates for antihyperuricemic agents. A pharmacological agent that would increase uric excretion along with electrolytes and water would have clear therapeutic value.

Ticrynafen (tienilic acid) is a substituted derivative of ethacrynic acid and is similar in action to the thiazides with the exception that it decreases plasma uric acid. Popular for a short time, it was withdrawn from most world markets because of an idiosyncratic reaction that results in liver damage.

Indacrinone is an analog of ethacrynic acid; it does not react with sulfhydryl groups but is still natriuretic. Both optical isomers are active as diuretics but the (+) enantiomer has the major uricosuric activity. It is secreted by the proximal tubule in a probenecid-sensitive manner, and its diuretic action is more prolonged than that of furosemide or ethacrynic acid. It inhibits proximal tubule reabsorption of uric acid and the reabsorption of sodium and chloride in the ascending limb. Sodium excretion reaches its peak in 2–4 hours with a duration of 8 hours, and proportionally more sodium is lost than potassium.

AQUARETICS

This is a class of diuretics that is infrequently referred to but that may have use in diseases associated with abnormal vasopressin activity. These agents are unlike the traditional diuretics in that they increase the excretion of water only and not of electrolytes. They are antagonists of the vasopressin (V_2) receptor and interfere with the action of this hormone. Decinine, an alkaloid extracted from the Lythraceae plant family, and the antibiotic demeclocycline are examples. Other vasopressin receptor antagonists are being developed and may find future use in disorders such as SIADH.

V_2 receptor antagonists

Combination Therapy

Sequential blockade

The ability of different classes of diuretics to produce a diuresis through action at different nephron segments provides the rationale for effective and appropriate combination therapy. Therapy based on the principle of sequential blockade is frequently useful when a patient develops resistance to one diuretic or when it is desirable to counteract potassium loss by adding a Site 4–acting drug.

Perhaps the most common combination of diuretic agents is that of Site 2– or 3–acting agents with a Site 4–acting agent. In this way the common side effect of loop and thiazide diuretics, potassium loss, may be avoided. The combination of diuretics that act at Sites 2 and 3 produces an additive effect also. A thiazide plus a loop diuretic can produce a diuresis greater than that attainable with either agent alone.

The Site 1 – acting diuretic acetazolamide is given in combination with loop diuretics in patients refractory to the latter. It is thought that refractoriness to loop diuretics is due to avid proximal tubule reabsorption of solute. This compensatory reabsorption of filtered solute results in the delivery of only small amounts of sodium chloride to the more distal segments and little diuresis. The addition of acetazolamide to inhibit proximal reabsorption "flushes" the solute load to the loop of Henle, where its reabsorption can now be blocked by the loop diuretic, with a resulting significant natriuresis.

Interference with compensatory reabsorption

SODIUM

Particular Ions Affected by Diuretic Therapy

Diuretic-induced hyponatremia is usually mild and clinically innocuous, but occasionally it is severe. Impaired renal conservation of sodium can be associated with chronic administration of diuretics. There is a reduced delivery of filtrate to the diluting sites caused by volume depletion – induced reductions in GFR and stimulation of isotonic proximal tubule reabsorption. The following drugs have the potential to induce hyponatremia, and therefore their coadministration with diuretics should be cautious:

Drug-induced hyponatremia

- drugs that stimulate thirst, such as antihistamines, anticholinergics, phenothiazines, butyrophenones, thioxanthene derivatives, and tricyclic antidepressants;
- drugs that stimulate ADH release, such as acetylcholine, barbiturates, carbamazepine, clofibrate, isoprenaline, morphine, nicotine, and vincristine;
- drugs that enhance ADH-like actions, such as chlorpropamide, tolbutamide, phenformin, oxytocin, nonsteroidal anti-inflammatory drugs, and paracetamol;
- drugs impairing renal dilution acting by unknown mechanisms, such as cyclophosphamide, amitriptyline, thiothixene, fluphenazine, monoamine oxidase inhibitors, and adrenocorticotropic hormone.

POTASSIUM

Potassium loss in the urine is an inevitable consequence of effective action by loop and thiazide diuretics that increase flow rate and deliver more sodium to the distal nephron. In addition, contraction of extracellular fluid volume may cause secondary hyperaldosteronism. Potassium depletion can interfere with renal tubular function, impair glucose tolerance and, in severe cases, impede contraction of skeletal muscle. Considerable controversy exists as to whether treatment is indicated for the typically mild hypokalemia (serum K = 3.0 – 3.5 mEq/l) that occurs with diuretic therapy. Extracellular hypokalemia can exist with little change in intracellular potassium concentrations. When hypokalemia requires treatment, either a potassium supplement or a potassium-sparing agent is added. It should be noted that most table salt substitutes contain potassium.

Treatment of hypokalemia

Prevention of hypokalemia by dietary means is difficult. The use of oral potassium supplements has problems of tolerance and compliance and is less effective than the use of potassium-sparing diuretics. Amiloride seems to have more predictable effects than the other potassium-sparing agents and, when combined with hydrochlorothiazide, it provides a more balanced diuretic therapy.

Certain patients are at particular risk if not treated for hypokalemia. Patients in whom diuretic-induced potassium loss may be harmful include those who have high circulating aldosterone levels (they already are excreting too much potassium); those on digoxin (low potassium enhances

At-risk patients in hypokalemia

excitability of myocardium and potentiates the arrhythmogenic action of the cardiac glycosides); those on high doses of long-acting diuretics (they may already be potassium-depleted); those receiving coincidental therapy with corticosteroids, carbenoxolone, or potent purgatives (these agents may further contribute to the hypokalemia); those who are diabetic (hypokalemia impairs glucose tolerance); and those who are elderly or chronically sick (they are particularly susceptible to the effects of low potassium).

Hyperkalemia in elderly

The elderly are especially vulnerable to potassium depletion. Their diets may be lower in potassium content, and their body potassium stores are decreased (*pari passu* with decreased lean body mass). Renal conservation of potassium during diuretic therapy may be less effective than in younger individuals, and polymedicine is more likely in the elderly so that more than one potassium-losing drug may be included in their medications. Increased risk of digoxin intoxication or likelihood of cardiac arrhythmias is always of concern.

The risk of hyperkalemia is also high in diabetic patients, who often have primary potassium-excreting defects due to coexistent aldosterone deficiencies. Hyperkalemia is difficult to produce by the administration of oral potassium supplements when renal function is normal, and it is also uncommon with the use of potassium-sparing agents, alone or with a thiazide, provided that renal function is normal. However, use of potassium-sparing agents in patients with renal impairment is likely to produce hyperkalemia.

MAGNESIUM

Thiazides increase and K-sparing diuretics decrease magnesium excretion.

The thiazides and loop diuretics also enhance the excretion of magnesium, whereas the potassium-sparing agents conserve this ion. Magnesium depletion is common during long-term diuretic therapy, especially when loop diuretics are used. Potassium-sparing agents have been shown to conserve magnesium, and this makes them a preferred diuretic in elderly individuals.

CALCIUM

Loop diuretics increase and thiazides decrease calcium excretion.

Diuretics have important effects on renal calcium handling. Significant amounts of calcium are reabsorbed ordinarily in the ascending limb of the loop of Henle. Because furosemide inhibits calcium transport at this site it is used in combination with rapid saline administration for the acute therapy of hypercalcemia. Thiazides retain calcium and have been used to prevent the formation of recurrent renal calculi and to prevent osteoporosis. Hypercalcemia is a rare complication of thiazide use, and it has been proposed that the mild volume depletion induced by the thiazides stimulates calcium reabsorption in the proximal tubule and loop of Henle in parallel with sodium reabsorption. Spironolactone and amiloride have also been shown to increase urinary calcium. This has led to the use of these agents in the treatment of calcium nephrolithiasis.

URIC ACID

Hyperuricemia occurs because of contraction of plasma volume and inhibition of uric acid excretion.

Up to 65–70% of patients treated with diuretics develop hyperuricemia. Although this may be associated with contraction of extracellular fluid volume, inhibition of uric acid excretion may be responsible also. Clinical gout rarely occurs and then only in susceptible individuals.

Adverse effects of diuretics may be mechanical, metabolic, or toxic and can usually be avoided by judicious management. Toxic effects are relatively rare. Metabolic effects include electrolyte changes, impairment of glucose tolerance, and increased serum uric acid and lipids. These are not of sufficient clinical significance to outweigh the long record of efficacy and safety of diuretic therapy.

Excretion of chloride with sodium and potassium results in increased serum bicarbonate concentrations. Thiazide and loop diuretics also increase renal hydrogen-ion excretion. These factors may all lead to the development of metabolic alkalosis. Amiloride conserves potassium and hydrogen ions and tends to counteract metabolic alkalosis when administered with a thiazide or loop diuretic.

In elderly patients it is best to avoid a loop diuretic when a thiazide would be adequate because of the possibility of urinary incontinence. Loop diuretics should be avoided in the treatment of elderly hypertensive patients except in those with renal failure. These agents may also be unnecessary, especially as maintenance therapy, in the management of certain elderly patients with congestive heart failure.

Diuretics may alter the serum levels of various lipid fractions. Chlorthalidone and thiazides appear to produce an increase in total serum cholesterol levels of 5–10% and in triglyceride levels of 10–28%. Furosemide and piretanide have similar effects, but indapamide and spironolactone do not. The mechanisms of these changes in lipid metabolism are not clear, although they seem to be potentiated by the development of glucose intolerance.

Resistance to a particular diuretic may develop because of an impaired delivery of the drug to its site of action or because of a decreased delivery of sodium to the site of action of the diuretic. Decreased sodium delivery may be associated with a decreased GFR or increased proximal sodium reabsorption. There may be increased reabsorption of solute at sites distal to the site of action of the diuretic. Impaired secretion of diuretics into the renal tubular lumen from blood may also result in reduced diuretic effect.

SALT RESTRICTION

An apparent resistance to therapy may occur because of salt ingestion. During diuretic therapy it is not unusual for the patient to develop salt hunger and to increase salt intake. The consequence of this is the blunting of the diuretic or antihypertensive effect of the drug. If sodium intake is too high, diuretics may achieve their pharmacological effect, increased excretion of salt and water, without effecting a weight loss. Thus, it is necessary to control salt intake. A salt-restricted diet should be prescribed for patients on diuretics. A recommended dietary intake is 100 mEq/day, which amounts to about 6 g/day. A normal salt intake is about 9 g/day. The low-salt diet contributes to establishing a negative sodium balance in order to mobilize edema fluid.

General Adverse Effects of Diuretics

Careful management of diuretic therapy may avoid many adverse effects.

Development of metabolic alkalosis

Loop diuretics in elderly

Resistance to Diuretic Therapy

Impaired delivery of diuretic to site of action

Salt ingestion blunts diuretic effect.

General References

Acara M, Carr EA Jr, Terry EN: Probenecid inhibition of renal excretion of dyphylline in chicken, rat and man. J Pharm Pharmacol 39:527–530, 1988.

Braunwald E: Disorders of myocardial function. In Peterdorf RG, Adams RD, Braunwald E, et al (eds): Harrison's Principles of Internal Medicine, 1343–1353. New York: McGraw-Hill Book Co, 1983.

Eknoyan G, Martinez-Maldonado M (eds): The Physiological Basis of Diuretic Therapy in Clinical Medicine. Orlando, FL: Grune & Stratton, 1986.

Graber M, Kelleher S: Side effects of acetazolamide: The champagne blues. Am J Med 84:979–980, 1988.

High altitude sickness. Med Lett Drugs Ther 30:89–91, 1988.

Koushanpour E, Kriz W: Renal Physiology—Principles, Structure, and Function. 2nd ed. New York: Springer-Verlag, 1986.

Lohr JW, McReynolds J, Grimaldi T, Acara M: Effect of acute and chronic hypernatremia on myoinositol and sorbitol in rat brain and kidney. Life Sci 43:271–276, 1988.

Puschett JB: Edema formation and diuretic usage. *In* Puschett JB, Greenberg A (eds): The Diuretic Manual. New York: Elsevier Science, 1985.

Springate JE, Van Liew JB, Feld L, et al: Diuretic and natriuretic effects of sorbinil, an aldose reductase inhibitor. Pharmacol Res 23:279–283, 1991.

Weiner IW: Diuretics and other agents employed in the mobilization of edema fluid. *In* Gilman AG, Rall TW, Nies AS, Taylor P (eds): Goodman and Gilman's The Pharmacological Basis of Therapeutics, 8th ed, 713–731. New York: Macmillan Publishing Co, 1990.

Weiner IW: Inhibitors of tubular transport of organic compounds. *In* Gilman AG, Rall TW, Nies AS, Taylor P (eds): Goodman and Gilman's the Pharmacological Basis of Therapeutics, 8th ed, 743–748. New York: Macmillan Publishing Co, 1990.

Drugs Used in the Treatment of Hypertension

35

David B. Case

Elevated arterial pressure, or hypertension, is now recognized as one of the most significant risk factors in the development and progression of cardiovascular disease. Numerous studies have demonstrated the close association between untreated hypertension and the occurrence of cardiac hypertrophy and congestive failure, stroke, retinopathy, dissecting aneurysm, progressive renal failure, coronary artery disease, peripheral vascular disease, and their related complications. Until the period beginning around 1970, however, only severe hypertension was treated systematically, usually in the clinical setting of some hemodynamic emergency such as encephalopathy or congestive heart failure. In 1967, the Veterans Administration (VA) Cooperative Study Group on Antihypertensive Agents reported for the first time controlled study data demonstrating that reduction of diastolic pressures from the range of 105 mmHg or more significantly diminished the prevalence of stroke, congestive heart failure, renal failure, and dissecting aneurysm. Subsequently, the Hypertension Detection and Follow-up Program (1979, 1982, 1984), the Australian Medical Research Council, and the Multiple Risk Factor Intervention Trial have indicated similar benefits in subgroups of different levels of severity and other characteristics (summarized in the 1988 report of the Joint National Committee).

Although the data regarding the cardiovascular benefit of treating hypertension are established for most of the complications of the condition (e.g., stroke, renal failure, congestive cardiac failure), there is a paucity of evidence from the large-scale clinical trials for the benefit in coronary artery disease, specifically reduction of myocardial infarction. That the antihypertensive treatment of these trials did not directly reduce coronary thrombotic events yet did reduce thrombotic stroke remains enigmatic.

Clinical importance of hypertension

Definition of Hypertension

Hypertension refers only to elevated arterial pressure. There is a common popular, yet false, notion that it is associated with a stressed state of mind. The mechanisms by which blood pressure becomes elevated are multiple and often interacting. Therefore, it should not be assumed that any two hypertensive people share common mechanisms for their elevated pressure. For that reason, neither should it be expected that they will respond similarly to a given drug treatment. In clinical practice, terms that define the predominant physiological mechanisms are used informally to characterize the nature of the treatment. For example, the terms *salt-sensitive, renin-dependent,* and *hyperadrenergic* are used commonly but have not worked their way into recommended treatment strategies.

The risk of hypertension is determined by the severity.

589

Hypertension is defined in terms of its severity, its association with underlying causes or related conditions, its association with age and racial groups, and in terms of possible mechanisms responsible for maintaining the elevated arterial pressure. The most common form of hypertension is termed *essential hypertension* and is diagnosed usually on the basis of the presence of a family member with hypertension and a history of gradual onset, beginning with a *labile phase*. This labile phase, often characterized by increased sympathetic activity and periodic elevations of diastolic pressures, occurs during the third and fourth decades before becoming established as a fixed elevation of diastolic and systolic pressures. There is little evidence to justify drug treatment of labile hypertension at the present time.

SEVERITY

Mild Hypertension

Mild hypertension

An average pressure of 140–159/90–104 mmHg is the most common level and is found in 80% or more of all hypertensive patients. Although the World Health Organization (WHO) defines this as *borderline*, it has become common practice to refer to this level as *mild*, particularly in people below the age of 50 years. The value of treatment in this group is usually judged in the light of overall cardiovascular risk and coexisting disease. For example, mild hypertension is usually treated when it occurs with congestive heart failure.

The prognosis for this group is the best and may not be substantially higher than in nonhypertensive people unless coupled with other risk factors. The focus for treatment in this group is to use nonpharmacological treatments initially (weight reduction, reduced salt diet, reduced alcohol intake, stress reduction, and others). If these measures are not adequate or applicable, drug therapy is used based on the best clinical information available for that patient.

Moderate Hypertension

Moderate and severe forms of hypertension

Moderate hypertension embraces average levels of 161–179/105–119 mmHg. In addition to the considerations given to mild hypertension, search for secondary forms of hypertension such as renal artery stenosis may be more justifiably undertaken. Therapy in the clinically stable patient should be delayed until diagnostic testing is complete, because drug treatment may significantly hinder testing.

Severe Hypertension

Severe hypertension corresponds to blood pressure levels above 180/120 mmHg, is associated with the greatest degree of risk, and deserves immediate diagnostic efforts and prompt treatment. If the patient is stable, the condition is termed an *urgency*; if there is an immediate risk of cardiovascular complications or death, then the term *emergency* is used. Urgent conditions should be treated within 24 hours, usually with potent orally active drugs.

Malignant Phase

This is the most serious hypertensive condition, characterized by severe levels of blood pressure (usually greater than 180/120 mmHg) in association with advanced retinopathy, specifically hemorrhages, exudates, and papilledema. There may be associated encephalopathy, congestive heart failure, or stroke. Treatment is begun as soon as possible, often with intravenous (IV) drugs.

SECONDARY FORMS OF HYPERTENSION

These are a group of medical conditions in which there is a specific, often correctable or curable cause for the hypertension. The common forms of secondary hypertension are shown in Table 35–1 along with the commonly used drug treatments used to stabilize the condition in preparation for surgery or a procedure or even for long-term treatment. It should be kept in mind that with newer and better drugs for hypertension, the urgency or even need to treat with risky procedures must be balanced against the clinical stability of the patient on the best pharmacotherapy.

ISOLATED SYSTOLIC HYPERTENSION

In a number of individuals, systolic pressure may exceed 160 mmHg, whereas diastolic pressure is less than 95 mmHg. This so-called isolated systolic hypertension occurs in more than 20% of people over the age of 70 and has been commonly associated with decreased compliance of the arterial tree. In addition, associations of isolated systolic hypertension in this age group have been made with baroreceptor dysfunction and increased stroke and heart attack. The clinical significance in younger people without arteriosclerosis remains relatively obscure. At the present time, several major studies are underway to determine the rationale to treat this entity. The first SHEPS (systolic hypertension in the elderly) has yielded results suggesting the value of treatment.

ASSOCIATED CONDITIONS WITH HYPERTENSION

A number of diseases are associated with a rise in blood pressure, although the interlinking pathophysiology is not always understood. These include vasculitic diseases such as systemic lupus erythematosis, scleroderma, and polyarteritis; endocrinopathies such as hyperthyroidism, hypothyroidism, and acromegaly; and chronic and acute renal glomerular and tubular diseases. Aside from treatment of the underlying condition, antihypertensive drug therapy is often required.

Underlying Causes and Related Conditions

Secondary forms of hypertension

Isolated systolic hypertension

Table 35–1 SECONDARY FORMS OF HYPERTENSION

Condition	Specific Drug Therapy	Definitive Therapy
Renal artery stenosis	Converting-enzyme inhibitor Angiotensin analog	Angioplasty Surgery
Pheochromocytoma	Phenoxybenzamine Labetalol Prazosin, terazosin Metyrosine β blocker	Surgery
Aldosterone-producing adenoma	Spironolactone Amiloride Triamterene α blocker	Surgery
Hyperplastic adrenal	Same as for aldosterone-producing adenoma	No surgery
Coarctation of aorta	β blocker	Surgery

In addition to these medical conditions, a patient's age, sex, race, and coexisting but unrelated medical conditions are particularly relevant in the individualized selection of his or her initial and subsequent therapy.

General Strategy for Drug Treatment of Hypertension

Stepped care: an early approach to treatment

Individualization of therapeutic choices

Tailoring and timing of dosage

Relationship of diuretics, low sodium diets, and drug responses

Substitution for ineffective therapy, not addition

Nonresponders to drug therapy may have a secondary form

Based on the success of the large-scale clinical trials that established the basis for treatment of mild and moderate hypertension, a scheme for treatment based on the initial use of diuretics was devised and referred to as *stepped care.* This scheme involved the sequential addition of antiadrenergic agents to a thiazide diuretic, and later of vasodilators and other drugs if pressure failed to respond. Although revised afterward, the methods of stepped care do not take into account all of the personal and clinical variables needed to select initial therapy. The general guidelines are listed:

1. One agent known to be effective as a monotherapy and compatible with the general and medical condition of the patient should be selected. In addition, considerations such as once-daily dosing, low rate of possible side effects, and cost enhance the opportunities for compliance.

2. The starting dose should be low, allowing for the possibility of an exaggerated response. Several weeks or even longer should be allowed for equilibration and homeostatic adjustments. The goal of therapy is to reduce resting diastolic pressure below 90 mmHg, or as low as can be tolerated without side effects. In most established hypertension, however, weeks to months are required to establish and maintain a lower baseline pressure. For that reason, advances in dosage should be gradual and monitored carefully.

3. Low sodium intake potentiates the effectiveness of most antihypertensive drugs, particularly converting enzyme inhibitors and adrenergic blockers. The first orally active diuretics such as chlorothiazide and hydrochlorothiazide were developed at a time when few people were able to reduce dietary sodium chloride intake. Addition of diuretic to the regimen of patients unable to maintain a low sodium intake enhanced efficacy. A number of antiadrenergics and converting enzyme inhibitors have been marketed as fixed combinations with standard thiazide diuretics for convenience. Although potent and long-acting diuretics such as chlorthalidone have been developed, the American diet has been steadily declining in sodium intake over the past decade, leading to a new concern about diuretic therapy. The combination of potent diuretics with a low sodium diet entails the risk of excessive extracellular fluid volume depletion, thereby leading to hemoconcentration, azotemia, hyperuricemia, hyperreninemia, hyperaldosteronemia, and eventually hypokalemia.

4. Multidrug therapy may result from the stepped care approach in those patients failing to respond to a diuretic and step-two or step-three drugs. Drugs are added on despite their relative ineffectiveness. An alternative approach is to substitute another drug for an ineffective one, instead of adding to it. This latter approach eventually leads to the use of fewer and only effective antihypertensive drugs.

5. Patients not responding to usual doses of standard antihypertensive drugs may need to be investigated for secondary forms of hypertension.

Specific Strategies for the Treatment of Hypertension

Many of the drugs available today are sufficiently potent to be used as initial monotherapy for mild and moderate hypertension. The list of choice monotherapies includes diuretics, β-adrenergic blockers, converting enzyme inhibitors, calcium entry blockers, and some α-adrenergic blockers.

Drugs that are seldomly used first or alone include direct vasodilators, hydralazine, and minoxidil as well as some of the older sympathetic blockers. It has become customary to base the initial selection of drug on the clinical characteristics of each patient.

A summary of drugs used to treat hypertension is shown in Table 35–2, which categorizes groups of drugs according to what is believed to be their predominant antihypertensive mechanism. Further analysis reveals that all of the antihypertensive drugs produce a number of pharmacological actions to which there are both acute and chronic adjustments by the individual being treated. It is indeed the net effect of these opposing homeostatic reflexes that prevents antihypertensive agents from lowering pressure to a greater extent.

    A number of the drugs discussed in this chapter are included in other chapters, for example, diuretics (Chapter 34) and calcium antagonists (Chapter 31).

Drugs Used to Treat Hypertension

DIURETICS

Thiazides and Related Compounds

Although thiazides (benzothiadiazines) and related compounds have become the most widely used drugs to treat hypertension, recent attention has been paid to their metabolic side effects (increases in blood sugar and

---

Table 35–2   ORAL DRUGS USED TO TREAT HYPERTENSION

Diuretics (see Table 35–3)

Sympathetic Nervous System Inhibitors
Drugs acting principally on the central nervous system
  Methyldopa (Aldomet)
  Clonidine (Catapres)
  Guanabenz (Wytensin)
  Guanfacine (Tenex)
Drugs that inhibit catecholamine synthesis
  Metyrosine (Demser)
Drugs depleting norepinephrine stores
  Reserpine and rauwolfia alkaloids
Peripheral α-adrenergic blockers
  Phenoxybenzamine (Dibenzylene)
  Prazosin (Minipress)
  Terazosin (Hytrin)
  Doxazosin (Cardura)
Adrenergic neuron blockers
  Guanethidine (Ismelin) (Esimil)
  Guanadrel (Hylorel)
Combined alpha-beta adrenergic blockers
  Labetalol (Normodyne, Trandate)

Beta-adrenergic Blockers (see Table 35–4)

Vasodilators
Direct vasodilators
  Hydralazine (Apresoline)
  Minoxidil (Loniten)
Angiotensin converting enzyme inhibitors
  Captopril (Capoten)
  Enalapril (Vasotec)
  Lisinopril (Prinivil, Zestril)
Calcium entry blockers
  Verapamil (Calan, Isopton, Verelan)
  Diltiazem (Cardiazem)
  Nifedipine (Procardia)
  Nicardipine (Cardene)

Thiazides are commonly combined with other drugs.

cholesterol, reductions in serum potassium) to bring their common or first-line use into question. Thiazide diuretics have a long record of use and have proved to be generally safe, well tolerated, and relatively inexpensive. Thiazides may be combined with almost all antihypertensive drugs to potentiate the antihypertensive effect by reversing secondary sodium chloride and water retention. Thiazides are commonly combined with potassium-sparing diuretics so that the dosages and side effects of each drug can be reduced. Most thiazides and related compounds are believed to be equally effective in comparable doses. For their history, chemistry, and mechanisms of action see Chapter 34.

Mechanism of Action

Acute effects of diuretics

Acute Actions of Diuretics. Diuretics block sodium, chloride, and water reabsorption in the thick ascending limb of Henle, the cortical diluting segment, or further in the distal tubule. The net acute effect is sustained salt and water loss, contraction of extracellular fluid volume (ECFV), decreased cardiac output, and reduced glomerular filtration rate (GFR) and renal blood flow. Initially, systolic pressure declines somewhat more than diastolic. These acute changes lead to increased renin release and aldosterone secretion that work to limit the antihypertensive effects of ECFV depletion and to potentiate the urinary loss of potassium.

Chronic effects of diuretics

Chronic Action of Diuretics. Over the course of continued treatment, however, cardiac index usually returns back toward pretreatment levels as may the GFR. Studies of blood and plasma volume in patients on long-term diuretics show an average of 5% or less reduction in ECFV. This observation has led to the hypothesis that the mechanism of action in hypertension initially involves reduction in plasma volume, followed by hemodynamic adjustments to the consequent reduction in preload or right ventricular filling pressures. These adjustments may take the form of reduced adrenergic tone. In addition, some diuretics may have direct vasodilatory effects (such as indapamide) or produce vasodilation by alteration of intracellular cation content of vascular smooth muscle. That ECFV depletion is a significant factor in the chronic antihypertensive response is supported by the facts that sodium chloride repletion reverses the antihypertensive effects and that plasma renin activity and aldosterone excretion, sensitive indicators of arterial blood volume, remain elevated during diuretic therapy.

Role of dietary salt in response to diuretic

Relationship of Sodium Chloride Intake to Diuretic Therapy. In more recent years, there have been major public health measures to reduce the salt intake in the American diet, particularly in those people with conditions such as hypertension. Thus, the dosages of a diuretic used must be selected carefully in light of the reported or measured salt intake. The combination of a low-salt diet and a diuretic creates the potential hazard of excessive volume depletion, hypokalemia, azotemia, and hemoconcentration. This may be particularly relevant in the elderly, whose total food and therefore salt intake is relatively low. In general, long-acting diuretics can be administered in the usual daily doses with the expectation that the normal sodium intake can be followed. Salt restriction sufficient to reduce blood pressure requires a constant vigilance and dogged consistency difficult for all but a few individuals who can adhere to a daily diet of only natural and fresh foods and who choose not to dine in restaurants nor eat ethnic or regional foods, most of which contain large amounts of salt.

Differences Among the Antihypertensive Diuretics (Table 35–3; see also Table 35–2).

Table 35-3 ORAL ANTIHYPERTENSIVE DIURETICS

Group	Dosage	Trade Name
Thiazides		
Bendroflumethiazide	2.5–5 mg/day	Naturetin
Benzthiazide	25–50 mg/day	Aquatag, Exna, Proaqua*
Chlorothiazide	250–500 mg/day	Diuril*
Cyclothiazide	1–2 mg/day	Anhydron
Hydrochlorothiazide	25–50 mg/day	Hydrodiuril, Esidrix, Oretic*
Hydroflumethiazide	25–50 mg/day	Diucardin, Saluron*
Methyclothiazide	2.5–5 mg/day	Aquatensen, Enduron*
Polythiazide	2–4 mg/day	Renese
Trichlormethiazide	2–4 mg/day	Metahydrin, Naqua*
Thiazide-like Diuretics		
Chlorthalidone	25–50 mg/day	Hygroton, Thalitone*
Indapamide	2.5–5 mg/day	Lozol
Metolazone	2.5–5 mg/day	Diulo, Zaroxolyn
Quinethazone	50–100 mg/day	Hydromox
Potassium-sparing Diuretics		
Amiloride	5–10 mg/day	Midamor
Spironolactone	25–200 mg/day	Aldactone*
Triamterene	50–100 mg/day	Dyrenium
Loop Diuretics		
Bumetanide	0.5–10 mg/day	Bumex
Ethacrynic acid	25–200 mg/day	Edecrin
Furosemide	20–400 mg/day	Lasix*

* Available in generic form.

THIAZIDES AND THE THIAZIDE-LIKE DIURETICS. The most commonly used diuretics in nonazotemic, nonedematous patients are the thiazides and their related compounds. For practical purposes, most of these compounds produce the same antihypertensive effects and have approximately the same profile of adverse effects. The thiazides are given once or twice daily, whereas the thiazide-like compounds such as chlorthalidone, indapamide, and metolozone are long-acting and therefore given only once daily. More recently, studies have indicated that indapamide and metolozone may be more effective in patients with mild azotemia. Indapamide may have fewer adverse metabolic effects such as raising blood sugar or serum cholesterol. Potassium supplements are commonly given with thiazides. A dose of thiazide reaches a plateau effect after 6–12 weeks. Relatively few patients require more than 50 mg of hydrochlorothiazide or 25 mg of chlorthalidone; raising the dose further increases the occurrence of drug-induced hyperglycemia, hypercholesterolemia, hyperuricemia, and hypokalemia.

Thiazide diuretics

LOOP DIURETICS. Loop diuretics are relatively ineffective as antihypertensive drugs except in patients with renal insufficiency. When given to nonazotemic patients, multiple daily doses are required to sustain a volume-depleting action. In some patients with advanced renal disease, a dose of 160–300 mg/day is needed to promote adequate diuresis. However, these large doses may lead to damage to the eighth cranial nerve or produce significant metabolic abnormalities. Unlike thiazides that may raise serum and ionized calcium, loop diuretics promote calcium excretion and have been used to treat hypercalcemic states.

Loop diuretics

POTASSIUM-SPARING DIURETICS. These agents are relatively weak as diuretics and are most often used in combinations with hydrochlorothiazide to antagonize the potassium wasting of the thiazide and to add to the antihypertensive effect. Mild hypertension in the nonazotemic diabetic or predia-

Potassium-sparing diuretics

betic may be more successful with potassium-sparing diuretics because, unlike thiazides, they do not raise blood glucose nor elevate low-density lipoproteins.

For organ system pharmacology and adverse effects of thiazides, please refer to Chapter 34.

Sympathetic Nervous System Inhibitors

Drugs or surgical procedures that block postganglionic adrenergic transmission reduce blood pressure by vasodilation from the reduction of tonic neural vasoconstriction. Adrenergic blockers of either the central or the peripheral nervous system produce similar hemodynamic responses; that is, greater reduction of seated and standing blood pressure than supine resulting from a greater contribution of sympathetic tone to upright posture. Even though these drugs are effective for most forms of hypertension, there is little evidence to support the concept that chronic essential hypertension is principally maintained by increased adrenergic tone. However, increased sympathetic tone may be generated by direct vasodilators' effect on baroreceptors, ECFV depletion by diuretics, or physiological or exaggerated responses to exercise or emotion. In this way, sympatholytic drugs may be complementary therapy to other drugs or recurrent physiological states.

Hemodynamic Effects

Hemodynamic effects of adrenergic blockage

Interruption of neurogenic arterial vasoconstriction reduces total peripheral vascular resistance. In addition, the baroreceptor-mediated compensatory increase in heart rate in response to vasodilation is blunted. Adrenergic blockers also reduce venous tone and, therefore, lower right heart or preload pressures by venous pooling. In turn, this reduces cardiac output and may lead to postural hypotension. The reduction in cardiac output, along with diminished contractility and heart rate, if not accompanied by a significant arterial vasodilation, could theoretically lead to impaired cardiac performance. In reality, the reduction in afterload or arterial pressure usually more than adequately offsets these effects. However, renal blood flow and GFR may decline, and some degree of sodium chloride retention commonly occurs. Both salt retention and the direct effect of the adrenergic blockers generally reduce normal or elevated plasma renin activity, an indicator of the activity of the renin system in blood pressure maintenance.

Pharmacological Action of Adrenergic Inhibitors

Effects of adrenergic inhibitors

Ultimately, the principal action of adrenergic inhibitors is to reduce activity at the site of the postganglionic nerve terminals that locally synthesize and store the major neurotransmitter norepinephrine (NE) (see Chapter 14). In the presynaptic nerve terminal, tyrosine is transported actively into the axoplasm, converted to dopa and then to dopamine. Dopamine is taken up into storage vesicles, where it is converted to NE by the enzyme dopamine β-hydroxylase (DBH). Any free NE outside of the storage granule is destroyed quickly by the enzyme monoamine oxidase (MAO). Upon nerve stimulation, calcium influx into the nerve terminal triggers degranulation of NE vesicles into the synaptic cleft, where it is free to engage postsynaptic α and β receptors and lead to arteriolar vasoconstriction. NE also can engage α receptors on the presynaptic nerve ending to inhibit further NE release. Most of the released NE is rapidly taken back into the presynaptic nerve terminal for recycling. The remainder is destroyed by the enzyme catechol O-methyl transferase (COMT). Inhibition of steps of the sympathetic nerve function to reduce blood pressure may occur by several different mechanisms:

1. reduction of sympathetic nerve traffic from the central nervous system (CNS)—centrally acting α-2 agonists (methyldopa, clonidine, guanabenz, guanadrel, guanfacine).

2. blockade of NE synthesis (α-methyl paratyrosine).

3. depletion of NE in granules (reserpine and rauwolfia alkaloids).

4. prevention of NE release (bethanidine, debrisoquin, and guanethidine).

5. blockade of presynaptic receptors regulating NE release (methyldopa).

6. blockade of postsynaptic receptors (phenoxybenzamine, prazosin, terazosin, doxazosin).

DRUGS ACTING PRINCIPALLY IN THE CENTRAL NERVOUS SYSTEM

Alpha Methyldopa

History and Chemistry. Methyldopa was first shown to have antihypertensive properties in 1960 when given to treat malignant carcinoid. It is a synthetic phenylalanine derivative related to dopa developed as an inhibitor of L-aromatic amino acid decarboxylase to decrease serotonin production.

Mechanism of Action. Initially, it was thought that methyldopa led to a depletion of NE from peripheral nerve terminals by its action to block decarboxylation of dopa *in vitro*. Later theories held that methyldopa was converted to α-methyl NE in peripheral nerve endings and was released as a false neurotransmitter instead of NE. Currently, most evidence supports the idea that α-methyl NE formed in the brain is a potent α_2 adrenergic agonist that reduces central vasoconstrictor outflow.

Organ System Pharmacology. Absorption of oral methyldopa is variable, with bioavailability ranging between 25 and 50%. After an oral dose, peak plasma levels occur in 2–3 hours, with a half-life of 3–4 hours ($t_{\frac{1}{2}}$ after IV administration is 1.4–1.8 hours). There is no correlation between plasma levels and antihypertensive effect. Methyldopa is eliminated as active drug (63%) or its conjugates by excretion in urine. Some of the active metabolites are excreted slowly in patients with renal failure. Therefore, the dose is reduced in conditions of hepatic and renal dysfunction. Excretion of urinary metanephrine, a screening test for pheochromocytoma, is interfered with by methyldopa. Urinary vanillylmandelic acid (VMA) is not affected, however.

Dose is reduced in renal and hepatic failure.

Physiological Actions. Methyldopa reduces total peripheral resistance but produces minimal changes in cardiac output and heart rate. Both supine and orthostatic pressures are reduced, and despite significant lowering of pressure, renal, cerebral, and coronary blood flow are well maintained. Plasma renin activity usually declines, if elevated initially.

Adverse Effects. The most frequent side effects reported are sedation, postural hypotension, dizziness, nasal congestion, sexual impotence, dry mouth, depression, and headache. Although these may abate somewhat over time, the availability of newer agents with fewer unpleasant side effects has led to a trend away from initiating therapy with this agent. A

Side effects are common.

series of other less common side effects may also occur: sodium chloride and water retention, a reversible malabsorption syndrome (with abnormal biopsy) of the small bowel, positive Coombs' test with and without hemolytic anemia, increases in liver enzymes (chemical hepatitis), and a severe febrile reaction with fevers up to 104 degrees. In addition, methyldopa may decrease the levels of high-density lipoproteins (HDL) and be associated with gynecomastia, leukopenia, thrombocytopenia, hypersensitivity myocarditis, colitis, pancreatitis, lichenoid reactions, and to an extrapyramidal syndrome resembling Parkinson's disease. Finally, as is found with other central α_2 agonists such as clonidine, there is a syndrome of blood pressure rebound after withdrawal of drug beginning 48–96 hours after the last dose, lasting 1–2 days. For that reason, the dose of methyldopa should be tapered upon discontinuation or a peripheral α blocker introduced temporarily in patients with a history of severe hypertension or coexisting cardiovascular disease.

Therapeutic Uses. Although methyldopa is an effective antihypertensive drug, its usefulness is limited by its relatively unfavorable side-effect profile, as compared with more recently developed agents of comparable or greater efficacy. Methyldopa has been used to treat mild, moderate, and severe *essential hypertension.* Because the drug commonly produces salt and water retention, pseudotolerance may develop as a result of expansion of ECFV. Thus, diuretics are often needed to maintain reduction of blood pressure and to prevent edema formation. Methyldopa has been used extensively in hypertension associated with *renal disease* or *renal failure* in reduced doses, because a desirable hypotensive effect can be achieved without further compromise of renal function and without significant orthostatic fall in pressure. In the past, IV methyldopa was used to treat *hypertensive crises,* including malignant hypertension. The use of methyldopa in severe hypertension is limited by the marked sedation and other CNS effects induced by the IV agent, thereby obscuring critical neurological signs and symptoms.

Methyldopa is used in renal failure.

Drug Interactions. The following drug interactions have been described with methyldopa: *tricyclic antidepressants* and *MAO inhibitors* may blunt or prevent the antihypertensive effects of methyldopa; *sympathomimetic amines* such as found in cold remedies, asthma preparations, and amphetamine-like drugs may reverse the antihypertensive effects; methyldopa may undermine the effectiveness of levodopa used to treat Parkinson's disease; a paradoxical rise in blood pressure has been observed when *phenothiazines* and methyldopa were used together; the toxicities of *lithium* and *haloperidol* are increased when used with methyldopa; *barbiturates* increase the metabolic clearance of methyldopa and shorten its half-life; finally, the combination of methyldopa with *other antihypertensive drugs and diuretics* may produce excessive hypotension.

Multiple drug interactions

Preparation and Dosages. Methyldopa is available in tablets of 125, 250, and 500 mg, in an oral suspension of 250 mg/5 ml, and in injectable solution of methyldopate HCl of 50 mg/ml. The initial dose in adults is 250 mg two or three times daily; dose may be increased at weekly intervals, although a diuretic is usually added after the initial dose if not already present. The usual daily dose ranges between 500 and 1500 mg/day. More recent studies have suggested that the drug be given as a single daily dose at bedtime to obviate the problems with sedation and orthostasis seen with morning administration. Little additional effects are noted with doses greater than 2000 mg/day. The pediatric or small person dose is 10 mg/kg daily with a maximum of 65 mg/kg. The IV preparation is given in boluses of 100–500 mg or 10–40 mg/kg every 6–8 hours; this preparation requires de-esterification, a process of some variation among patients leading to nonuniform antihypertensive effects. Methyldopa is available as a brand name product and as a generic product, both of which may contain bisulfites. Methyldopa is also marketed in fixed combinations with thiazides.

Summary. Methyldopa was one of the first widely used antiadrenergic antihypertensive drugs, reducing blood pressure by inhibition of the outflow of CNS vasoconstrictor tone. The use of methyldopa has declined recently because of its side-effect profile in comparison with recently developed drugs of the same and other categories.

Clonidine

History and Chemistry. Clonidine was developed as a nasal decongestant and was discovered to be an antihypertensive drug by accident when it both reduced blood pressure and cleared the nasal passages of an employee of Boehringer Ingelheim. Subsequently, the drug was developed and introduced in Germany in 1966 and in the United States in 1974.

Mechanism of Action. Clonidine acts as a central α_2 partial agonist in the hypothalamus and the medulla oblongata, thereby reducing central sympathetic outflow. In addition, and unlike methyldopa, clonidine as a partial α agonist acts peripherally on presynaptic nerve endings to reduce NE release. The partial agonism is also expressed when clonidine is given IV; initially, there is a rise in pressure before a more gradual decline occurs.

Physiological Actions. Following oral administration, blood pressure falls along with decreases in total peripheral resistance, cardiac output, and heart rate. Normal or elevated levels of plasma renin activity also fall. Cardiac output may return to pretreatment levels over time, but heart rate and peripheral resistance remain decreased. Clonidine lowers both supine and upright blood pressure with little orthostatic hypotension. Renal and coronary vascular resistances are reduced, but renal plasma flow and GFR remain unchanged even with substantial reductions in pressure. By enhancing vagal tone, clonidine may aggravate bradycardia in patients with sinus node dysfunction and may prolong atrioventricular (A-V) conduction when given with digitalis preparations.

Renal blood flow is conserved by clonidine.

Organ System Pharmacology. Clonidine is rapidly and nearly completely absorbed after oral administration and is more than 75% bioavailable. Peak plasma concentrations occur in 1–3 hours, although the antihypertensive effects may be noticed within 30 minutes. There is a correlation between blood pressure reduction and plasma drug levels under 2.0 ng/ml. Maximal effects occur at dose levels under 0.6 mg/day; doses greater than 1.2 mg/day may have a paradoxical effect and raise pressure. The volume of distribution is 1.2 l/kg, and the plasma half-life is about 9 hours. Clonidine is lipid-soluble and achieves good levels in the CNS. Approximately one half of an oral dose of clonidine is metabolized in the liver to inactive metabolites; the remainder is excreted unchanged by the kidneys. Thus, the dual route of excretion permits use in lower dose in patients with renal failure. Clearance of the drug is about 3 ml/minute/kg.

Maximal dose of 1.2 mg/day

Adverse Effects. Dry mouth (xerostomia) and drowsiness occur in half of all patients treated with clonidine but diminish somewhat over time. Nonetheless, 7–10% of patients discontinue treatment because of adverse effects. A variety of other side effects have been reported to occur relatively infrequently: constipation (4%), dizziness (15%), nausea or gastric upset (5%), fatigue, weight gain, gynecomastia, pruritis, pruritic or allergic rash, thinning of hair, sexual impotence, urinary retention, sleep disturbances (insomnia, nightmares), anxiety, depression, congestive heart failure, ventricular arrhythmias, parotid pain, chemical hepatitis, edema and fluid retention, and others.

Clonidine-Withdrawal Syndrome. Abrupt withdrawal of clonidine has produced in patients with moderate or severe hypertension a rebound hypertensive crisis similar in clinical characteristics to the picture seen with pheochromocytoma. Approximately 12–24 hours after the last dose, blood pressure rises, often to levels much higher than pretreatment and into the range of moderate to severe hypertension in association with tachycardia, headache, abdominal pain, sweating, anxiety, and occasionally angina or palpitations. The most severe symptoms usually subside in 24 hours, but the syndrome may persist for a week. A similar syndrome of withdrawal has been described for each of the other central α agonists, with time constants proportional to the half-lives of the drugs. Although the syndrome is uncommon, it can appear to be life-threatening. The manifestations are more pronounced in individuals with underlying moderate or severe hypertension on larger doses of clonidine. However, severe cases have been reported with doses as low as 0.6 mg/day. Concurrent treatment with a β blocker markedly potentiates the withdrawal syndrome because of the α-stimulating action of β blockade. Both plasma and urinary catecholamine levels increase during withdrawal.

> **Clonidine withdrawal**

Clonidine withdrawal can be prevented by gradually tapering the dose down over several weeks to doses as low as 0.05 mg/day. β blockers should be tapered to discontinuance before withdrawing clonidine. Selection for clonidine therapy should be based on potential excellent compliance. Peripheral α blockers such as prazosin, terazosin, or doxazosin or the α-β blocker labetalol may also be given as clonidine is withdrawn or they may be given in the event that withdrawal has begun.

Therapeutic Uses. Clonidine is used to treat mild, moderate, or severe hypertension, usually in combination with a diuretic. Because of the withdrawal syndrome, poorly compliant patients should be treated with other agents. Clonidine may be used to reduce pressure promptly in hypertensive urgencies. A clonidine suppression test has been used to pretreat patients undergoing screening for pheochromocytoma to reduce background nonadrenal NE release. Clonidine has also been used to treat other withdrawal syndromes such as that from opiates or nicotine.

> **Clonidine used in hypertensive emergencies and diagnosis of pheochromocytoma**

Drug Interactions. Clonidine combines favorably with diuretics and direct vasodilators to reduce severe refractory hypertension, particularly when β-adrenergic blockers cannot be used. Tricyclic antidepressants, naloxone, tolazoline, and MAO inhibitors may reverse the antihypertensive effects of clonidine. Additive depressant effects have been reported when clonidine was combined with barbiturates, ethanol, and various tranquilizers.

Preparations and Dosage. Clonidine is supplied in tablets of 0.1, 0.2, and 0.3 mg alone or in combination with chlorthalidone. It is also available in a transdermal patch that delivers 0.1–0.3 mg/day for 7 days. The usual initial dosage is 0.1 mg given once daily at bedtime in patients with mild hypertension, with dose increments of 0.1 mg/day at weekly intervals. For patients requiring higher doses, two or three times daily dose can be given, with the majority at bedtime. Doses greater than 1.2 mg/day are seldom needed and may, in fact, produce paradoxical rises in pressure.

> **Clonidine transdermal patch**

Summary. Clonidine is a potent antihypertensive agent limited, as is methyldopa, by significant adverse effects — principally those in the CNS. Because of its potency, it can be administered once weekly through an efficient transdermal system in patients found to tolerate the drug well orally.

Guanabenz

History, Chemistry, and Mechanism of Action. Guanabenz acetate is a guanadine derivative whose principal mechanism of action is similar to clonidine as a central α_2 agonist inhibiting sympathetic outflow from the brain. In addition, it has a slight peripheral ganglioplegic action similar to guanethidine.

Pharmacology. Guanabenz is about 75% bioavailable and about 90% protein-bound. Nearly all of the drug is metabolized; less than 1% unchanged drug is found in the urine. Peak action of the drug occurs 2–4 hours after oral ingestion. The plasma half-life varies from about 6–12 hours; the antihypertensive effect usually wanes gradually over 10 hours.

Plasma half-life is long — 16–20 hours.

Preparations. Guanabenz acetate is available in 4 and 8 mg tablets, usually administered twice daily. The maximal recommended dose is 32 mg/day.

Guanfacine

History, Chemistry, Mechanism of Action. Guanfacine is a guanadine derivative that lowers blood pressure by a mechanism similar to clonidine and guanabenz, that is, by inhibiting central sympathetic outflow through the activation of central α_2 adrenergic receptors. Its therapeutic uses and effectiveness, adverse effects, and drug interactions are, for practical purposes, the same as clonidine and guanabenz.

Pharmacology. Guanfacine is more than 90% absorbed and has a plasma half-life of 16–20 hours, thereby allowing once-daily dosing. Guanfacine is eliminated both as unmetabolized drug and partially after hydroxylation by renal excretion. However, plasma concentrations and antihypertensive actions are not potentiated in patients with renal insufficiency. Because part of guanfacine is metabolized by the hepatic microsomal system, chronic phenobarbital use results in a shortened plasma half-life.

Adverse Effects. Like other central α agonists, guanfacine has been associated with a rebound or withdrawal phenomenon. However, because of the long duration of action of the drug, the onset of withdrawal develops 2–7 days after cessation of therapy.

Preparations and Dosages. Guanfacine is available in 1 mg tablets that are usually administered once daily at bedtime. Most of the studies done with this drug were carried out in patients already or subsequently treated with diuretics as well. Most patients respond to a dose of 3 mg/day or less.

DRUGS THAT INHIBIT CATECHOLAMINE SYNTHESIS

Metyrosine

Introduction, Mechanism of Action. Metyrosine (α-methyl tyrosine) inhibits tyrosine hydroxylase, the principal rate-limiting step in catecholamine biosynthesis, thereby blocking the conversion of tyrosine to dopa. Its

Metyrosine is used in malignant pheochromocytosis.

use has been restricted to patients with pheochromocytoma because of its demonstrated potency and effectiveness in suppressing urinary catecholamine and catecholamine-metabolite excretion while controlling the clinical expression of the underlying condition. Metyrosine has been used alone or with other antiadrenergic drugs to prepare patients for surgery and, in some cases where surgery was not elected, as long-term therapy. In the absence of data comparing the effectiveness and safety of metyrosine with conventional α and β blockade, metyrosine has been used generally as an adjunct to conventional therapy, particularly in large or malignant tumors or those refractory to drug control.

Adverse Effects. Metyrosine usually produces significant side effects and, therefore, is not chosen for treatment of essential hypertension. CNS side effects predominate: sedation, anxiety, depression, confusion, hallucinations, disorientation, and others. Agitation, insomnia, and hypomania may occur after the drug has been withdrawn following removal of the pheochromocytoma. In about 10% of patients, extrapyramidal movements may occur.

Gastrointestinal (GI) side effects may also occur: diarrhea (10%), which may necessitate cessation of therapy; nausea, vomiting, anorexia, and abdominal pain.

Increased renal stone formation has been reported to occur in association with increased urinary sediment and cells. This complication is less likely to occur when patients are prepared for operation with salt and water loading to prevent postoperative hypotension.

Other side effects include gynecomastia, galactorrhea, sexual impotence, increased prolactin levels, eosinophilia, liver enzyme elevations, hypersensitivity reactions, dry mouth, and nasal stuffiness.

Pharmacokinetics. Metyrosine is well absorbed from the GI tract and excreted unchanged in the urine. Maximal effect from a given dose of drug occurs after 1–3 days. Conversely, 3–5 days are needed to wash out drug effects as estimated by urinary catecholamine and metanephrine excretion.

Phenoxybenzamine is used concurrently.

Preparations and Dosage. The drug is manufactured in 250 mg capsules. The initial dosage is 250 mg four times daily, which is increased to a maximum of 4000 mg/day according to blood pressure and heart rate control and stability. At least 5–7 days of therapy are required before adequate blockade can be established. Generally, phenoxybenzamine is used concurrently. At the time of surgery, phentolamine, or preferably sodium nitroprusside, is used to modulate swings in blood pressure when the tumor is manipulated. If the tumor produces arrhythmias, β-blockers or other specific antiarrythmic drugs are given.

DRUGS DEPLETING NOREPINEPHRINE STORES

Reserpine and Rauwolfia Alkaloids

The medicinal use of plants similar to rauwolfia dates back to ancient Hindu culture. It was not until the 1950s that the potential use for the root of the plant was explored, despite reports of 20 years earlier detailing the previous application in psychoses and hypertension. At this time, reserpine became widely used as one of the few available antiadrenergic drugs, despite its well-recognized adverse effect profile. In fact, reserpine was used in combination with other drugs in the landmark antihypertensive trials of the VA (1967), which established the value of lowering blood pressure on cardiovascular health. However successful in lowering blood pressure in these trials and in practice, the use of reserpine produced such prominent side effects that drugs now used to lower blood pressure must be defended in terms of how they affect the quality of life.

Mechanism of Action. Reserpine produces a prompt, slowly reversible depletion of catecholamine and 5-hydroxytryptamine stores in postganglionic nerves, the brain, and to a lesser extent in the adrenal medulla. Reserpine prevents the uptake of NE into storage granules in neurons by inhibiting an adenosine/triphosphate (ATP)-Mg–dependent uptake mechanism in most likely an irreversible manner (Chapter 14). Impairment of adrenergic neuronal function becomes significant after a 30% depletion of normal stores. Because tissue catecholamines are restored slowly, only small daily doses are required to produce long-term deletion. Although reserpine has prominent CNS side effects, the antihypertensive action is attributed principally to depletion of catecholamines from peripheral sympathetic nerve terminals.

> Reserpine depletes catecholamines from nerve terminals.

Reserpine produces a characteristic hemodynamic profile: slowed heart rate, reduced cardiac output, and mild orthostatic hypotension. Total peripheral resistance is reduced in the supine position. In addition to these effects, reserpine leads to sedation and an attitude of indifference, much like that described for phenothiazines. Extrapyramidal effects may be observed as the dosage is increased.

Pharmacology. Reserpine is well absorbed from the GI tract and is often given with food to lessen gastric upset. The drug binds to biogenic amine storage sites and is taken up readily in fat tissue and brain. There is no correlation between blood levels and effects. Peak antihypertensive response may take up to 3 or 4 weeks. The drug is metabolized but is excreted largely in the urine.

Adverse Effects. The most serious side effect is *mental depression.* Initially, when doses as low as 0.25 mg daily were used, suicidal depression was observed, more so when doses of 0.5 mg or more were given. As a consequence, the bulk of experience with reserpine in clinical trials has been in combination with diuretics and other drugs so that doses as low as 0.125 mg/day were used. Besides depression, reserpine may produce a variety of other CNS side effects: nightmares, vivid dreams, drowsiness, sedation, dizziness, vertigo, headache, extrapyramidal movements, and reduced threshold for seizures.

> CNS and other side effects limit current use of reserpine.

Some of the side effects of rauwolfia alkaloids are related to a marked increase in vagal tone. GI reactions are common and include anorexia, nausea, vomiting, *activation of peptic ulcer (increased gastric acid production and motility),* increased salivation, and abdominal cramps related to increased GI tone.

Prominent among cardiovascular effects are *slowing of the sinus node action potentials* and, therefore, heart rate, ventricular arrhythmias, *salt and water retention,* congestive heart failure, hypotension, and syncope.

Additional side effects include weight gain, fever, arthralgias, myalgias, muscular dyskinesias, bronchospasm, respiratory depression, rash, purpura, lupus-like syndrome, increased prolactin secretion with associated *sexual impotence* and gynecomastia.

Drug Interactions. When combined with diuretics, adrenergic blockers, and other vasodilators, reserpine may induce an *additive antihypertensive effect.* Reserpine may induce a *severe hypertensive response* when given to a

> Drug interactions are limiting factor in reserpine use.

patient *on an MAO inhibitor. Arrhythmias* have been described when reserpine was added to digitalis or Class I antiarrhythmics. *Hypotensive reactions* have been observed when patients on reserpine received inhalant anesthetic agents. Concurrent use of reserpine and tricyclic antidepressants nullifies the antihypertensive effects and leads to CNS excitement. Reserpine in levodopa-treated patients may worsen the *extrapyramidal movement disorder* and lead to *orthostatic hypotension.* Reserpine may lead to *excessive sedation* if combined with CNS depressants such as barbiturates or minor tranquilizers.

Preparations and Dosages. The usual dose of reserpine is 0.1 mg given once daily, in combination with a thiazide diuretic or a direct vasodilator such as hydralazine. Doses higher than 0.25 mg/day are likely to produce significant side effects. Other rauwolfia preparations include rauwolfia serpentina, alseroxylon, deserpidine, and rescinnamine.

Summary. Before modern drugs, reserpine and rauwolfia alkaloid were important antihypertensive drugs, particularly in patients with moderate and severe hypertension. At the present time, except in unusual circumstances, drugs with better side-effect profiles are preferred. Patients established on reserpine and rauwolfia preparations may need to be cycled off the drug periodically to ensure that subtle depression is not being induced.

PERIPHERAL BETA-ADRENERGIC BLOCKERS

Alpha receptors are found in most blood vessels and are in highest concentration in the arterioles of skin, kidney, and mucosal surfaces. Alpha blockers antagonize the vasoconstrictor effects of neurogenic α stimulation and also circulating catecholamines and, therefore, reduce blood pressure by decreasing total peripheral resistance (Chapter 14).

Alpha receptors are classified as α_1 and α_2. Alpha$_1$ are found only on the postsynaptic membranes, whereas α_2 are on both the post- and the presynaptic areas. Alpha stimulation of the presynaptic receptors activates a negative feedback loop for NE release. Of the peripheral α blockers, phentolamine blocks both α_1 and α_2 receptors, whereas prazosin, terazosin, doxazosin, and phenoxybenzamine are more selective blockers of the postsynaptic α_1 receptors.

Phentolamine

Action and Uses. Phentolamine is a short-acting, rapid onset of action, competitive α blocker that is given IV in selected clinical emergencies in which α-induced vasoconstriction is likely to be dominant. These situations include pheochromocytoma (including preparation for surgery), withdrawal of clonidine or other potent central α-agonists, or institution of a MAO inhibitor along with tyramine or some sympathomimetic amine. In the past, phentolamine was used in the diagnosis of pheochromocytoma. However, chemical methods for urinary and blood catecholamines and imaging methods have improved sufficiently to make phentolamine tests relatively nonspecific and obsolete.

The action of phentolamine in lowering blood pressure is due both to its α-blocking properties and to a direct vasodilatory action that raises heart rate by baroreflex stimulation. Phentolamine increases cardiac output and renal blood flow acutely but may also provoke a supraventricular tachyarrhythmia or angina.

Dosage and Preparations. Phentolamine is available in ampules containing 5 mg powder to which sterile diluent is added. Doses of 5–20 mg are given as IV boluses. Alternatively, an infusion may be given starting at the rate of 1 mg/minute.

Phenoxybenzamine

Action and Uses. Phenoxybenzamine is an irreversible blocker of α receptors whose use has been largely limited to preparing patients with pheochromocytomas for surgery. It has also been used to treat inoperable patients with pheochromocytoma and men with chronic prostatism. Phenoxybenzamine may produce reflex tachycardia, orthostatic hypotension, and some salt and water retention. Other side effects such as nasal congestion, nausea, vomiting, diarrhea, impaired ejaculation, and stress incontinence limit the drug's acceptability in the treatment of essential hypertension.

Phenoxybenzamine is used principally for treatment of pheochromocytoma.

Dosage and Preparations. Phenoxybenzamine is available in 10 mg capsules. The dose must be individualized but is usually in the range of 30–60 mg/day in pheochromocytoma.

Prazosin

Introduction and Mechanism of Action. Prazosin is a quinazoline derivative that acts through blockade of postsynaptic α_1 receptors. Because it has little effect on α_2 receptors, prazosin does not produce augmented presynaptic release of NE and, therefore, produces little or no change in heart rate. The drug lowers arterial pressure and acts as a venodilator so that cardiac output is not increased; in congestive heart failure associated with hypertension, cardiac output is improved. Upright blood pressure is lowered somewhat more than supine pressure. Renal blood flow is increased or unchanged by prazosin even in renal failure. Prazosin may reduce plasma renin activity.

Pharmacology. Prazosin is absorbed readily but variably (45–70%) after an oral dose, reaching peak blood levels in 1–3 hours. The absorption is not retarded or enhanced by the food. Plasma half-life is 3–4 hours but may be prolonged in liver disease, congestive heart failure, and in the elderly. The drug is more than 95% bound to albumin, and the volume of distribution is 0.5 l/kg in hypertensive subjects. Prazosin undergoes first-pass metabolism in the liver, where about 90% of it is later conjugated and demethylated and excreted into bile.

Adverse Effects. The most common side effect is first-dose postural hypotension that has led to syncope and loss of consciousness. This appears to occur more frequently in patients who have been salt-depleted on diuretics, who are on other antihypertensive agents, or those given doses larger than 1 mg. The first-dose phenomenon may be preceded or accompanied by rapid supraventricular tachycardia. In most patients, the orthostatic hypotension and dizziness abates over several weeks but may be persistent in some for long periods of time. In order to prevent this, it is recommended that the first dose be limited to 1 mg, which is administered at bedtime so that the patient is recumbent when the drug reaches peak action.

The first dose of prazosin may cause hypotension.

Other side effects include dry mouth, salt and water retention, nasal congestion, headache, palpitations, nightmares, sexual dysfunction, lethargy, drowsiness, nervousness, and constipation. Less common adverse effects include urinary frequency and incontinence, priapism, allergic skin reactions, and polyarthritis. Prazosin lowers total cholesterol and low-density lipoproteins, raises high-density lipoproteins, and does not affect carbohydrate metabolism.

Preparation and Dosage. Prazosin is available in 1, 2, and 5 mg capsules. The first 1 mg dose is given at bedtime with instructions about getting up at night carefully. Additional precautions may need to be taken for elderly patients or those with angina or cerebrovascular disease. The dose may be increased to 20 mg daily or more in two or three divided doses. The action may be potentiated by addition of diuretic.

Terazosin

Action and Uses. Terazosin is a postsynaptic α_1 blocker similar chemically to prazosin. Terazosin differs from prazosin by having a longer half-life and a slower onset of action. These features allow for once-daily dosing and, presumably, a lesser incidence of first-dose hypotension.

Dosage and Preparations. Terazosin is available in 1, 2, and 5 mg tablets taken once or twice daily.

Doxazosin

Action and Uses. Doxazosin, like prazosin and terazosin, is a quinazoline acting as a postsynaptic α_1 competitive antagonist. The adverse effect profile is similar to that of terazosin and includes "first-dose" orthostatic hypotension and syncope.

Pharmacokinetics. Peak plasma levels of doxazosin occur 2–3 hours after the first dose, with extensive first-pass hepatic metabolism. The elimination of doxazosin is slow, with a terminal half-life of about 22 hours. The maximal antihypertensive effects are observed 2–6 hours after an oral dose.

Dosage and Preparations. Starting doxazosin is best reserved until after several days off diuretic or off a low sodium diet. The usual initial dose is 1 mg, given once daily at bedtime. Doses larger than 4 mg have a greater association with postural hypotension.

GANGLION BLOCKERS

Trimethaphan

Although oral ganglion-blocking agents, such as the veratrum aklyoids, are no longer used as antihypertensive drugs, there is occasional use of the IV ganglion blocker trimethaphan camsylate. Like nitroprusside, trimethaphan always lowers blood pressure, but unlike nitroprusside, some degree of head-up position is needed to achieve maximal orthostatic effect. Trimethaphan is given by continuous IV infusion for dissecting aortic aneurysm, acute hypertensive pulmonary edema, subarachnoid hemorrhage, and other critical hypertensive conditions (see also Chapter 12).

ADRENERGIC NEURON BLOCKERS

Guanethidine

Mechanism of Action. Guanethidine reduces blood pressure by inhibiting postganglionic nerve release of NE to sympathetic stimulation and also indirectly by leading to the depletion of neuronal sympathetic amines. Guanethidine is taken up and stored in adrenergic nerves, leading to their depletion of NE (see Chapter 14 and Fig. 14–13). Guanethidine reduces cardiac output by a direct effect on the heart (negative chronotropic and inotropic effects) and by reducing venous tone and, therefore, venous return. The action on arterioles to vasodilate and lead to reduced total peripheral resistance comes about principally in the upright position. Regional blood flow in the hepatic and renal beds is not reduced unless significant postural hypotension occurs. Retention of salt and water is common with guanethidine, however, and may necessitate diuretic treatment to maintain effectiveness (so-called pseudotolerance).

Pharmacology. Less than 30% of an oral dose of guanethidine reaches the circulation. The drug, partially metabolized by the liver, and its metabolites are eliminated rapidly by renal excretion. Guanethidine has a long half-life in the body because it is stored in nerves and may take 2 weeks or more to be cleared.

Adverse Effects. The principal side effect of guanethidine is really its effect, postural hypotension. In fact, levels of hypertension may be relatively unchanged in the supine position. Severe and symptomatic orthostatic hypotension may occur with the drug used alone, particularly when there are other stimuli for vasodilation such as alcohol, exercise, warm environment, dehydration, or other vasodilator drugs. Serious orthostatic hypotension can occur in patients with autonomic neuropathy as found in diabetes mellitus. Because of its negative effects on cardiac output and its action to promote salt and water retention, guanethidine may worsen congestive heart failure, particularly in supine patients whose blood pressures are not being lowered. Weakness, diarrhea, retrograde ejaculation, impotence, fatigue, tremors, and parotid tenderness have been reported to occur also. Guanethidine may trigger a hypertensive crisis in a patient with pheochromocytoma by producing increased sensitivity to circulating catecholamines (like a type of denervation hypersensitivity).

Guanethidine produces postural hypotension.

Therapeutic Uses. Guanethidine is rarely prescribed. Even when there were few choices of antihypertensive drugs, guanethidine was often considered a last-choice drug in view of its limited antihypertensive effect (upright) and because of the frequency and severity of side effects. The drug is included because there are still a few patients being treated with the drug whose therapy has not been updated.

Drug Interactions. All of the tricyclic antidepressants block the effect of guanethidine by inhibiting the nerve uptake of drug. Phenothiazines also antagonize the action of guanethidine. Sympathomimetic amines, such as those found in typical cold remedies, may produce a significant pressor effect in the supine position and should be avoided.

Tricyclic antidepressants and phenothiazines block the hypertensive effect of guanethidine.

Preparations and Dosages. Guanethidine is available in 10 mg and 25 mg tablets. The usual starting dose is 10 mg given once daily, which may be increased in increments of 10 mg at weekly intervals for increased effect. Addition of a diuretic potentiates the effects. The maximal dose used is 100 mg/day.

Guanadrel

Mechanism of Action. Guanadrel sulfate reduces blood pressure by the same mechanism as guanethidine. Like guanethidine, it does not enter or act through the CNS.

Pharmacology. Guanadrel is rapidly absorbed with peak plasma levels attained in about 2 hours and the maximal hypotensive effect in 4–6 hours after oral ingestion. The total half-life of the drug is 10 hours; as a two-compartment system, however, there are 1–4 hours for the α phase and 5–45 hours for the β phase. About half of an oral dose is excreted unchanged in the urine.

Adverse Effects, Therapeutic Uses, Drug Interactions. For practical purposes, these are the same as guanethidine.

Preparations and Dosages. Guanadrel is available in 10 mg and 25 mg doses. The drug may be given in one or two daily doses in increments of 10 mg. The dose is advanced at weekly intervals.

COMBINED ALPHA- AND BETA-ADRENERGIC BLOCKERS

Labetalol

Labetalol reduces heart rate only modestly.

Mechanism of Action. Labetalol is principally a competitive antagonist of α_1 receptors but also blocks with lesser potency β_1 and β_2 receptors. The β-blocking action is characterized by intrinsic sympathomimetic activity on β_2 receptors. Labetalol also inhibits the reuptake of NE into adrenergic nerve terminals. Because of its α- and β-blocking activity, the net effects represent a combination of both features. When given IV, labetalol, in contrast to pure β-blockers, reduces blood pressure immediately with only a modest reduction in heart rate. Over time, however, labetalol may reduce heart rate further, decreasing contractility and A-V conduction. Even though a partial β_2 agonist, labetalol may still lead to bronchospasm in sensitive asthmatic patients. Labetalol is effective in renin-dependent and nonrenin-dependent forms of hypertension and does not adversely affect the lipid profile. The antihypertensive effect might be attenuated by sodium and water retention, which can be relieved by diuretic treatment.

Pharmacology. Labetalol is only about 25% bioavailable due to extensive first-pass hepatic glucuronidation. The bioavailability is enhanced in patients with liver disease and those taking cimetidine. The plasma half-life is about 6 hours. Because only 5% of the drug is excreted unchanged in the urine, labetalol is given in the same dosages in renal insufficiency. Because labetalol treatment markedly increases excretion of what are measured as catecholamines in the urine, the drug should be withheld until testing for pheochromocytoma is completed.

Adverse Effects. In general, labetalol is well tolerated provided that dosing is carried out gradually and carefully. Dry mouth and orthostatic hypotension are relatively common but usually mild if the drug is taken with food to delay absorption. Other side effects, similar to those of β blockers but somewhat less severe, include nausea, diarrhea, abdominal pain, nervousness, fatigue, nasal congestion, erectile impotence, muscle cramps, paresthesias of the hands or scalp, alopecia, depression, vivid dreams, nightmares, bronchospasm, disturbed A-V conduction, bradycardia, palpitations, and facial flushing. Patients on labetalol have developed antinuclear and antimitochondrial antibodies. Although there have been a number of associated skin reactions, a well-defined lupus syndrome is rare. Hepatic dysfunction, also noted rarely, is characterized by cholestatic jaundice and elevated liver enzymes.

Therapeutic Uses. IV labetalol is a versatile antihypertensive agent useful in treating hypertensive crises and also in patients who cannot take medication orally. The drug has been popular in controlling hypertension pre-, intra-, and postoperatively, particularly in patients after myocardial infarction, coronary bypass or angioplasty, withdrawal from clonidine, or in pheochromocytoma. Oral labetalol, also effective in a wide variety of different forms of hypertension, has been useful in situations where α blockade was sought with the orthostatic hypotension attenuated by the β_1 blocking effect. The drug has been tested successfully in subgroups of hypertensives with chronic lung disease, renal insufficiency, diabetes, and congestive heart failure.

> Labetalol can be used in place of an α blocker.

Preparations and Dosages. Labetalol is available in 100, 200, and 300 mg tablets that are usually taken two or three times daily with meals. Doses as low as 50 mg may be suitable in older patients who are more sensitive. Doses as large as 3000–4000 mg/day have been used in refractory hypertension. IV labetalol is given in 5–20 mg increments slowly over 5 minutes in emergencies. An IV infusion may be used to follow bolus injections in solutions of 200 mg/250 ml to achieve a delivery of about 2 mg/minute.

> Labetalol is available in IV form.

β-ADRENERGIC BLOCKERS

Introduction and History. Although originally intended for treatment of cardiac arrhythmias and angina pectoris, β-adrenergic blockers have become most widely used in practice as antihypertensive mediction. Beta receptors are located throughout the vascular tree, in the heart, in the bronchi, in most parenchymal organs, in the brain, in adipose tissue, and other locations. Because β-receptor agonists produce peripheral vasodilation, it was envisioned that pronethalol, an early β-receptor blocker, would not lower blood pressure and might actually raise it. Nonetheless, the drug actually lowered pressure in some hypertensive subjects. Because pronethalol had some unusual toxicity, the principal early studies of the effects of β blockade in hypertension were done using propranalol. Propranalol was first approved for the treatment of angina and in 1979 for hypertension.

Mechanism of Action. The exact mechanisms by which β blockers reduce blood pressure in hypertension remain complex and incompletely understood; there is general agreement that several interacting mechanisms are involved in the net effect on pressure. Several theories have been advanced attributing the blood pressure–lowering action to the effects of the drug to one of three major mechanisms. A summary of these theories follows.

Cardiac Theory. Beta blockers antagonize both the cardiac (β_1) and the noncardiac (β_2) receptors. Blockade of β_1 receptors leads to negative chronotropic (decreased heart rate) and negative inotropic (contractility) effects, producing a maximal reduction of cardiac output of about 15%. A reduction in cardiac output would theoretically lower pressure provided that there were no corresponding change in peripheral vascular resistance. IV propranalol, however, produces an immediate and uniform reduction in cardiac output but does not immediately reduce blood pressure; in fact, arterial pressure may actually rise acutely. This initial lack of change or rise in blood pressure has been attributed to an abrupt *rise* in peripheral vascular resistance induced by the β-blocker by reflex neurogenic tone (unopposed α_1 tone) or tissue vascular autoregulation in opposition to the reduction in cardiac output. Over time, even as long as 6 months, peripheral

> Beta blockers initially raise peripheral resistance.

vascular resistance declines parallel to the reduction in blood pressure, returning toward initial baseline levels. This abatement in resistance is not well understood by mechanism but does occur in patients responding to therapy. The changes in the actions of angiotensin II do not appear to be the exclusive factor responsible for the long-term change in blood pressure, as described by the next theory.

Renin Theory. Release of renin, the enzyme-initiating the generation of angiotensin II, is under direct β-adrenergic control. Thus, β blockers predictably suppress plasma renin activity and have been shown to be preferentially effective in reducing pressure in hypertensive subjects with elevated or even normal renin levels in contrast to those with low levels. However, blockade of angiotensin II cannot be the only mechanism, because IV β blockers immediately suppress renin but do not lower pressure. Moreover, β blockers do not suppress aldosterone excretion, principally under angiotensin II control, except in accelerated or malignant-phase hypertension. However, reduction of angiotensin II levels may be related to the slow attenuation of vascular resistance through mechanisms involving the CNS and the baroreflexes. High doses of β blockers, in addition, may lower blood pressure by these latter mechanisms in patients with low renin levels.

CNS Theory. Beta blockers may produce specific changes in the CNS that may contribute to their antihypertensive actions. The antihypertensive action observed at higher drug doses appears to be hemodynamically different from that at lower doses because upright pressures fall with high doses and rise wth lower doses. It is of interest that β-blocker–induced side effects on the CNS appear to be more prominent with increasing lipid solubility of the agent, corresponding to greater brain penetration. However, the relevance of a CNS effect in lower doses has been questioned because β blockers of widely different lipid solubility lower blood pressure in responsive subjects equally well.

Thus, the antihypertensive effects of β blockers appear to represent the net physiological effects of reduction in cardiac output, compensatory or reflex peripheral vascular resistance to the change in cardiac output that attenuates over time in responders, suppression of the renin-angiotensin system, and to a modest extent the suppression of the CNS preganglionic nerve traffic.

Pharmacology. Although all of the available β blockers have affinity for β-adrenergic receptors, their pharmacological actions differ by having additional properties: membrane-stabilizing activity, partial agonism (also called intrinsic sympathomimetic activity, ISA), selectivity for β_1 receptors (also called cardioselectivity), α-blocking properties, and lipid solubilities.

The pharmacological properties of the individual agents are shown in Table 35–4.

Adverse Effects. The most common side effects are caused by β-adrenergic blockade and therefore are dose-related. Bradycardia and congestive heart failure are the most common cardiac side effects; A-V dissociation and aggravation of A-V block may also occur but rarely.

Peripheral vascular disease may worsen with β blockade, particularly Raynaud's phenomenon and claudication. This is believed to be related to the reduction in cardiac output along with the reflex increase in peripheral vasomotor tone. Cold hands are a common side effect; actual gangrene is

Beta blockers suppress baroreceptor-mediated renin release.

Lipid-soluble β blockers have an effect on the CNS.

Table 35-4 PHARMACOLOGICAL PROPERTIES OF β-ADRENERGIC BLOCKING DRUGS

Beta Blocker	Beta Blocking Potency Compared with Propranolol = 1	Local Anesthetic Properties	Membrane-Stabilizing Properties	Lipid Solubility*	Absorption; % Bioavailable	Metabolism; First-pass Hepatic	Active Metabolites	Plasma Half-life (hour)	Elimination	Usual Daily Dosage
Beta₁ and beta₂ (nonselective) blockers										
Propranolol (Inderal)	1	Yes	Yes	Yes 3.65	Good; 30+	Extensive; yes	Yes	1-5	Urine	40-160 mg two to three times/day; reduce in liver failure
Nadolol (Corgard)	0.5	No	No	No 0.71	Incomplete; 30	Little; no	No	16-20	Unchanged in urine	20-80 mg once; decrease in renal failure
Timolol (Blocadren)	10	Yes	No	Yes 2.10	Good; 50	Extensive; yes	No	4	Urine	5-10 mg once or twice
Penbutalol (Levatol)			No		Complete	Yes	No	5	Urine	20 mg once
Beta₂ (cardioselective)										
Metoprolol (Lopressor)	0.5	Weak	No	Yes 2.15	Good, rapid; 50	Up to 90% (hydroxylated); yes	No	3-4	Urine	50-100 mg once or twice
Atenolol (Tenormin)	1	No	Weak	No 0.23	Incomplete; 40	Little; no	No	6-8	Unchanged in urine	50-100 mg once or twice; decrease in renal failure
Betaxolol (Kerlone)	4	Weak	Weak	No	Good; 89%	Yes; small	No	14-22	Urine	10-20 mg once
Partial agonist (with ISA)										
Pindolol (Visken)	5	Weak	Weak	Some 1.75	Good; 75	50%; little	No	3-4	Urine	5-10 mg two to three times/day
Acebutolol (Sectral)	0.3	Yes	Yes	Some 1.87	Good; 40		Yes	3-4		400-800 mg once or twice
Carteolol (Cartrol)	10	No	No	Low	Good; 85%	<30%	Yes	6	Urine	2.5-10 mg once

* Log partition coefficient octanol/water.

rare. There is only modest evidence to suggest that cardioselective β blockers reduce the occurrence of these side effects.

Although symptoms of angina pectoris are likely to improve on β blockade, withdrawal of β blockers may precipitate anginal attacks, ventricular arrhythmias, or even sudden death if the withdrawal is abrupt. Large dosages of β blockers may raise blood pressure, particularly in the presence of α agonists. For example, blood pressure overshoots have been described in patients on β blockers during clonidine or methyldopa withdrawal and with underlying pheochromocytoma.

All β blockers, even combined α-β blockers, increase airway resistance and can aggravate asthma or bronchospasm. However, there is some evidence to support the safe use of low-dose cardioselective β blockers in patients with chronic obstructive pulmonary disease.

All β blockers can worsen asthma.

Beta blockers exert prominent metabolic effects that are relevant in hypertensive patients. Increases in the range of 20-30% of triglycerides or low-density lipoproteins and decreases of approximately 5% in high-density lipoproteins have been described for most β blockers. Beta blockers with degrees of intrinsic sympathomimetic activity or partial agonism may exhibit lesser or no effects on lipoproteins. Pindolol, for example, may actually raise high-density lipoproteins. Beta blockers block the adrenergic

Beta blockers reduce high-density lipoproteins.

response (tachycardia, nervousness) to hypoglycemia, leaving diabetics without the usual warning signal of a dropping blood sugar. In addition, studies with β blockers indicate a general rise in blood sugar on long-term therapy, perhaps due to blockade of β_2 stimulated insulin release.

A number of other side effects have been described, including nausea, vomiting, and diarrhea, as a vagomimetic effect. Lipid-soluble β blockers (see Table 35–4) in particular may produce CNS side effects such as depression, nervousness, lassitude, nightmares, insomnia, and hallucinations. Sexual impotence has also been a reported side effect.

Therapeutic Uses. Beta blockers may be used in mild hypertension as well as in severe or even malignant-phase hypertension. Currently, β blockers are often a preferred choice in patients having another indication for the use of a β blocker: supraventricular or ventricular arrhythmias, angina pectoris, postmyocardial infarction, migraine, hypertropic obstructive cardiomyopathies, hyperthyroidism, panic attacks, benign essential tremor, or others. Beta blockers are commonly combined with vasodilators that may induce tachycardia and increase renin release, which attenuate the antihypertensive effect. Even though β blockers do not produce sodium and water retention, they are often combined with diuretics with or without vasodilators for added effectiveness.

> Beta blockers do not produce sodium and water retention.

Beta blockers are used in pheochromocytoma after α blockade has been established to control excess β adrenergic catecholamine activity. In selected populations such as those characterized by low plasma renin levels (black race, elderly diabetics), β blockers are generally less effective than α blockers or diuretics. In fact, β blockers may produce rises in blood pressure in some of these groups. This has been attributed to the increased peripheral vascular resistance due to unopposed α tone that is elicited during acute β blockade.

For preparation and dosages see Table 35–4.

Vasodilators

DIRECT VASODILATORS

Hydralazine

Mechanism of Action. Hydralazine acts directly on arteriolar smooth muscle to induce relaxation with little or no effect on veins. The intracellular mechanism involves the activation of guanylate cyclase and the accumulation of intracellular cyclic guanosine monophosphate (GMP). Regional vascular beds appear to react to hydralazine with differing sensitivity, the renal, splanchnic, and coronary arteries dilate more than those in the muscles or skin. Heart rate and contractility increase due to baroreflex stimulation and to direct effects on the myocardium and CNS. These cardiac reactions, however, along with stimulation of plasma renin activity and sodium and water retention, tend to reverse the antihypertensive action of the drug. As a consequence, hydralazine is used usually in combination with an adrenergic blocker (usually a β blocker) and a diuretic.

> Hydralazine relaxes arterial smooth muscle only.

> Hydralazine increases heart rate and produces sodium and water retention.

Pharmacology. Although hydralazine is rapidly and almost completely absorbed from the GI system, it is highly metabolized by N-acetylation but also glucuronidation and hydroxylation. Genetically slow acetylators develop higher serum levels than fast acetylators and, therefore, are more prone to having dose-related side effects. Hydralazine has a relatively short half-life of about 2.2–2.6 hours. Peak concentrations in plasma are found 30–120 minutes after dosing, with a total duration of effect of 6–8 hours.

Hydralazine is also available in parenteral form. When given intramuscularly (IM) or IV, blood pressure begins to fall in about 10–20 minutes, which lasts for 2–5 hours. The drug is nearly 90% protein-bound.

Adverse Effects. If hydralazine were given alone, it would produce unacceptable headache, tachycardia, and other manifestations of baroreflex stimulation and marked sodium and water retention. These features would aggravate angina pectoris, congestive heart failure, and other conditions. Other side effects include diarrhea, constipation, nasal congestion, flushing, and rashes. A lupus-like syndrome has been described with doses of hydralazine greater than 200 mg/day consisting of fever, myalgias, arthalgias, splenomegaly, and edema in association with a positive antinuclear antibody test. Although this rheumatoid-like picture subsides when the drug is withdrawn within 6 months in the majority, a few patients experience persistence of symptoms for more than 8 years.

> Large doses of hydralazine may produce a lupus-like syndrome.

Therapeutic Uses. The use of hydralazine has decreased in recent years because of the availability of newer agents of greater potency and safety that can be used as once-daily administered monotherapies. The potential potency of hydralazine is also restricted by the limitation of the dose to 200 mg/day in order to prevent toxicity. Nonetheless, so-called triple therapy using hydralazine, β blocker, and diuretic is still employed as a reference standard in the treatment of severe forms of hypertension. Although usually requiring a diuretic, hydralazine may be used occasionally without an adrenergic blocker in patients with bradycardia or baroreflex insensitivity. Hydralazine is still used parenterally in pre-eclampsia and eclampsia and hypertensive crises not complicated by ischemic heart disease.

> Hydralazine is used for pre-eclampsia and eclampsia.

Preparations and Dosage. The usual oral dosage is 75–200 mg daily in two to four divided doses, depending on the severity. The parenteral preparation contains 20 mg/ml and is given in 5–10 mg doses at intervals of 20 minutes. Hydralazine is also available in combination products containing thiazide diuretic or reserpine compound, or both.

Minoxidil

Mechanism of Action. Minoxidil is a potent direct vasodilator whose mechanism of action is believed to be the same as hydralazine. However, minoxidil is a significantly more potent antihypertensive agent and has a longer duration of action than hydralazine. As a result, the direct arteriolar vasodilation in the absence of venodilation leads to a marked increase in reflex sympathetic activity and in sodium and water retention. Because of its potency, minoxidil has been used in severe and malignant forms of hypertension as well as treatment-resistant hypertension, usually in combination with a β blocker and a loop diuretic. More recently, because minoxidil (and the diuretic used with it) stimulates plasma renin levels, a rationale has been developed to combine minoxidil with a converting enzyme inhibitor to permit lower dosages of minoxidil to be used and to blunt the hypokalemia resulting from angiotensin-mediated aldosterone release.

> Minoxidil is used for severe or refractory hypertension.

Pharmacology. Minoxidil is promptly and nearly completely absorbed by the GI system, being about 90% bioavailable. Maximal arteriolar dilation occurs within 2–3 hours, with peak plasma levels in about 1 hour after an oral dose. Although the plasma half-life is estimated to be 4.2 hours, the vasodilation effects of minoxidil may last for up to 1–3 days. Minoxidil is metabolized extensively by the liver (glucuronidation). The inactive metabolites of minoxidil and the free drug itself (12%) are excreted in the urine.

Minoxidil produces significant sodium and water retention.

Adverse Effects. Marked sodium and water retention leading to weight gain and edema occurs commonly, especially in patients with azotemia. This usually requires a potent diuretic such as furosemide, ethacrynic acid, or bumetanide to control. If not balanced adequately with a diuretic, the antinatriuresis so produced may precipitate congestive heart failure. With the use of these diuretics, hypokalemia, hyperuricemia, hyperglycemia, and other complications of loop diuretics may occur. In addition, a small fraction of patients on chronic hemodialysis develop pericardial effusions related to the uremic state and fluid retention, requiring special clinical and echocardiographic surveillance.

Reflex sympathetic cardiac stimulation is common and, if not countered by an adrenergic blocker, may precipitate tachyarrhythmias and angina pectoris. Flattening or inversion of T waves with increased QRS voltage are often observed on the electrocardiogram. These reversible changes may revert to normal with continued therapy. There are few reports of myocardial fibrosis and necrosis in papillary muscles in patients on long-term minoxidil treatment. Marked orthostatic hypotension may occur if minoxidil is used in combination with α blockers or ganglionic blockers, but not commonly with β blockers. There have been questions raised about whether minoxidil may lead to or aggravate pulmonary hypertension.

Minoxidil produces increased hair growth.

Hypertrichosis occurs in most patients after 1 month's treatment, presumably because of the regional increase in cutaneous blood flow. A topical form of minoxidil is currently available as a treatment for androgenic alopecia and other forms of baldness. Hair growth related to oral minoxidil is most conspicuous on the face, although it occurs over the entire body. The skin may darken and wrinkle as well. These features are not well tolerated in women and children, even with attentive use of depilatories. These changes are not related to any endocrine disorder and are partially reversible over time even when the drug is continued.

Other rare or unusual side effects include nausea, headache, fatigue, skin rashes, Stevens-Johnson syndrome, breast tenderness, antinuclear antibody formation, and thrombocytopenia.

Therapeutic Uses. The current use of minoxidil is reserved for treatment of severe, drug-resistant forms of hypertension. In light of the availability of newer potent hypertensive agents with significantly better adverse effect profiles, minoxidil is rarely used.

Preparation and Dosages. Minoxidil is available in 2.5 and 10 mg tablets. The usual starting dose is 2.5–5.0 mg, advancing to a maximum of 100 mg daily. The dose may be reduced by the balanced addition of a diuretic, β blocker, and converting enzyme inhibitor.

Diazoxide

Diazoxide is used for hypertensive emergencies.

Mechanism of Action. Used only for hypertensive emergencies, diazoxide is an IV nondiuretic thiazide that, like minoxidil, acts directly on arterioles and, as a result, has a marked antinatriuretic effect.

Pharmacology. Diazoxide is highly bound to plasma proteins and has a half-life of about 30 hours with an indefinite duration of action. The drug is about two thirds metabolized by the liver to inactive metabolites; the remainder is excreted in the urine. Peak plasma levels occur 3–5 minutes after injection, which decline over 4–12 hours.

Adverse Effects. The hemodynamic side-effect profile of diazoxide is similar to that of hydralazine and minoxidil. In addition, diazoxide may produce marked hyperglycemia and hyperosmolarity. Loop diuretics, given concomitantly, may aggravate this. Headache, nausea, vomiting, flushing, hypersensitive reactions, altered smell and taste, salivation, local pain and irritation at the site of injection, and hemolytic episodes have been described.

Diazoxide may produce hyperglycemia.

Therapeutic Uses. Diazoxide is used only for hypertensive emergencies such as malignant hypertension, encephalopathy, and severe hypertension associated with renal parenchymal disease. Because the drug increases ejection fraction and velocity, it is unsuitable in patients with dissecting aneurysms and ischemic coronary artery disease. In addition, because the drug may produce precipitous declines in pressure, it is also unsuitable for those patients with cerebrovascular disease with the risk of stroke or blindness. The drug should not be used in patients with pheochromocytoma or arteriovenous malformations. Currently, preference has been given to IV sodium nitroprusside, labetalol, converting enzyme inhibitors, and calcium channel blockers for treatment of hypertensive emergencies. Because diazoxide stops uterine contractions, it is not a good choice in eclampsia.

Diazoxide may produce precipitous drops in blood pressure.

Preparations and Dosages. Diazoxide is available for IV use in 20 ml ampules containing 300 mg. The drug may be given in small successive IV boluses of 0.5–1.0 mg/kg at intervals of 15–20 seconds or by slow IV infusion. Diuretic and adrenergic blockers are usually also needed.

Sodium Nitroprusside

Mechanism of Action. Sodium nitroprusside is used in IV solutions for the treatment of hypertensive emergencies. Unlike hydralazine, minoxidil, and diazoxide, nitroprusside produces both arteriolar and venous dilatation. The mechanism appears to be the same as for organic nitrates, that is, interfering with the intracellular flux of calcium. Because nitroprusside dilates both resistance and capacitance vessels, the net cardiac effects are modest or no increase in heart rate, decreased myocardial workload, and maintained coronary blood flow. Nitroprusside maintains renal blood flow and glomerular filtration, yet markedly increases plasma renin activity.

IV nitroprusside treats severe hypertension.

Pharmacology. Nitroprusside has almost an immediate onset of action that becomes maximal in 1–2 minutes. The half-life is short; turning down the rate of infusion leads to a rise in pressure within 30 seconds. The ferrous ion in the nitroprusside binds to sulfhydryl groups in red cells (hemoglobin) and other tissues, producing cyanide ions that are promptly reduced to thiocyanate by the liver enzyme rhodanese. Thiocyanate is excreted in the urine with a half-life of 4–7 days in patients with normal renal function.

Adverse Effects. The most frequent adverse effect is hypotension, which usually is a result of inexperience. Thus, nausea, vomiting, headache, sweating, restlessness, chest pain, confusion, and palpitations are not uncommon when initial levels of hypertension are lowered rapidly. These may be avoided by slow and careful titration of the IV infusion.

If nitroprusside is used for days, thiocyanate toxicity may develop, particularly when renal function is impaired or large doses are used. Signs of toxicity include confusion, disorientation, muscle twitching, delirium, or

Thiocyanate toxicity may result from nitroprusside.

overtly psychotic behavior. Serum levels of thiocyanate are generally monitored regularly and maintained below 10 mg/dl. Thiocyanate levels can be reduced by infusing sodium thiosulfate or hydroxycobalamin.

Other, less common adverse effects include hypothyroidism, reduced platelet count, and increase in intracranial pressure in patients with mass lesions or metabolic encephalopathy.

Rebound hypertension is commonly described with the use of nitroprusside and is believed to be related to the high levels of plasma renin activity and, therefore, angiotensin II. When removing patients from nitroprusside, it has become customary to dovetail a β blocker, which suppresses renin release, or an angiotensin-converting enzyme inhibitor, which blocks angiotensin II synthesis.

Therapeutic Uses. Nitroprusside has become the first choice in the treatment of most life-threatening hypertensive emergencies. The features that are most useful are (1) rapid onset of action, (2) consistently effective, (3) acceptable toxicity that can be monitored, (4) easy and precise titration, and (5) favorable hemodynamic response. If a dissecting aneurysm is present, β blockade should be added to reduce heart rate and ejection velocity. The drug is commonly used in the operative management of pheochromocytoma in the presence of adrenergic blockade because of its rapid titratability.

Preparations and Dosages. Nitroprusside is usually made in a 50 mg/5 ml solution. A final solution of 50 mg in 500 ml of 5% dextrose in water yields a solution of 100 μg/ml. The usual rates of infusion are between *0.5 and 10 μg/kg body weight/minute.* After the solution is prepared, it should be covered with aluminum foil to prevent light from inactivating the solution and changed daily. It has become the standard of practice in most intensive care units to infuse nitroprusside with a special infusion pump and to monitor arterial pressure directly.

ANGIOTENSIN-CONVERTING ENZYME INHIBITORS

Angiotensin-converting-enzyme inhibitors act principally by blocking the renin-angiotensin-aldosterone system.

Introduction, History, and Mechanism of Action. Angiotensin-converting enzyme (ACE) inhibitors were developed to produce a specific blockade of the renin-angiotensin-aldosterone system.

Renin is a protease secreted by granular juxtaglomerular cells within the wall of the afferent arterioles of the renal glomeruli. This glycoprotein, with a half-life of about 30–60 minutes, catalyzes the generation of the decapeptide angiotensin I from a hepatic-synthesized substrate angiotensinogen. Angiotensin I, which is largely vasoinactive, is converted to an octapeptide angiotensin II in the presence of pulmonary and nonpulmonary tissue-bound ACE. Angiotensin II raises arterial pressure principally by arteriolar vasoconstriction, by a direct action to decrease renal sodium and water excretion, by stimulating the CNS, and by stimulation of the secretion of aldosterone by the adrenal cortex.

The renin-angiotensin-aldosterone system plays a significant role in the maintenance of normal hemodynamics and in electrolyte and water balance. Physiological changes such as upright posture, stress, and low sodium diet increase renin release to restore pressure-volume relationships. Conversely, high sodium diet, decreased β-sympathetic activity, and supine posture suppress renin release in normal healthy people. Pathological conditions such as hemorrhage, renal ischemia, and injury to the kidney also lead to increased renin release and to hypertension.

In people with essential hypertension, approximately 15% have increased plasma renin activity when referenced with normal or increased sodium balance. Of these, a fraction have increased heart rate or other evidence for increased sympathetic nervous system activity as a likely stimulus for increased renin release. Similar high renin values are also seen in most patients with renovascular hypertension, about one third of those with renal parenchymal disease or obstructive nephropathy, and in nearly all with accelerated or malignant-phase hypertension.

About one half of all patients with essential hypertension have normal plasma renin activity. It has been argued that having normal levels of this pressor hormone in the presence of elevated blood pressure is evidence for a disregulated negative feedback system.

The remaining one third of patients with essential hypertension have low plasma renin activity even when sodium-depleted. However, diuretics can usually stimulate volume depletion and increase renin release so that the blood pressure becomes renin-dependent.

Although converting enzyme inhibitors reduce blood pressure by several mechanisms, the principal effects are believed to be due to the reduction of angiotensin II. This results in arteriolar dilation with reduction of total peripheral resistance, increased urinary sodium and water excretion through both a direct action on the efferent glomeruli and reduction of aldosterone secretion, and reduced central sympathetic outflow. The converting enzyme is also involved in the degradation of the potent local tissue vasodilator hormone bradykinin. However, there is no evidence to suggest that accumulation of bradykinin is related to the long-term antihypertensive effect. Heart rate, stroke volume, and cardiac output in hypertensive subjects without heart failure remain unchanged or slightly increased. Systolic pressure may decline as a result of increased compliance of large arteries.

In patients with congestive heart failure, converting enzyme inhibitors reduce pulmonary vascular resistance, pulmonary capillary wedge pressure, and mean arterial and right atrial pressures. In addition, left ventricular volume and filling pressures are reduced with increased cardiac output, cardiac index, stroke work, and stroke volume. Heart rate is unchanged or reduced. There may be an increase in renal blood flow due to reduced vascular resistance across the renal bed. The resulting decrease in body fluid volume along with decreased venous tone/increased venous capacitance (probably resulting from decreased adrenergic drive related to the congestive heart failure) reduces the preload stress on the heart. Despite relatively low resultant levels of arterial pressure, cerebral and coronary blood flow is well maintained.

Captopril

Pharmacology. Oral captopril is absorbed rapidly and 60–75% bioavailable. There have been some data to indicate that absorption may be either decreased or delayed by food in the upper intestine. Although this seldom has been shown to reduce effectiveness, the drug is usually given before meals. The onset of action occurs within 15 minutes in the postabsorptive state and reaches a peak action after 60–90 minutes. The duration of effect is dose-related but is usually between 2 and 8 hours. After the drug is withdrawn, blood pressure may remain reduced for days to weeks afterward, even though there is no evidence for residual drug stored.

Captopril is distributed rapidly in most body tissues except for the CNS. Approximately 25–30% of captopril is bound to albumin, and the

Captopril dose is reduced in renal insufficiency.

The triphasic response to captopril

volume of distribution is about 0.7 l/kg. About one half of the absorbed dose of captopril is metabolized to either a disulfide dimer or a cysteine disulfide, which with the parent drug is excreted principally in the urine. Excretion is prolonged in patients with renal disease. Therefore, the elimination half-life is less than 2 hours in patients with normal renal function, 20–40 hours in patients with decreased renal function, and up to 6.5 days in anuric subjects.

In patients with severe hypertension, a triphasic response curve has been described in the first few weeks of treatment. Blood pressure may fall significantly after the first dose yet, despite continuation of an adequate dosage, rises back toward pretreatment levels after 6–16 hours. Blood pressure then gradually decreases again over the succeeding 1–2 weeks. The mechanism for this period of resistance during initial therapy is unknown but does imply the need to use temporarily an additional drug in severe or crisis-level hypertension. In addition, it implies the need to wait at least 2 weeks after starting captopril before changing the dosage or adding another drug in more stable patients.

Adverse Effects. Although captopril is now recognized to be well tolerated and safe, the drug's safety was impugned during development as a result of the use of excessive dosages in the earliest clinical trials. A rash, occasionally with pruritis, may occur during the first few days or after an increase in dosage. It may be accompanied by fever, arthralgia, and eosinophilia and be urticarial in presentation. Also described are taste disturbances, persistent cough, and, rarely, neutropenia. The leukopenia develops gradually over the first few months of therapy and may cause agranulocytosis rarely if the decline in neutrophils is not detected. In addition, captopril may cause lymphadenopathy, anemia in children, a positive antinuclear antibody test, and a false-positive test for urine acetone. Proteinuria has been observed in low frequency (less than 2% on high dosages) in patients with and without underlying renovascular disease. Risk factors for neutropenia and proteinuria are the presence of a collagen vascular disease, dosages of captopril more than 150 mg/day, and decreased renal function. The proteinuria may begin after months of therapy and may have an associated nephrotic syndrome. The proteinuria usually reverses with withdrawal or continuation of the drug.

Hypotension following the first dose has been described as a consequence of prior sodium depletion. Thus, the drug is usually used first and the antihypertensive effect amplified by the addition of a diuretic. Alternatively, patients may take a diuretic "holiday."

Increases in blood urea nitrogen and serum creatinine occur, particularly in patients with renal parenchymal or vascular disease. These changes are attributable to the induced reduction in efferent glomerular arteriolar tone that reduces filtration and intraglomerular pressure. This latter effect has been found to be potentially valuable in conserving glomeruli from obsolescence in chronic renal disease. Therefore, the apparent reduction in renal function with captopril is tolerated in order to achieve long-term conservation of renal function. In patients with bilateral renovascular hypertension or solitary kidney renovascular disease, captopril may induce renal failure, particularly if there has been antecedent diuretic-induced sodium depletion.

Captopril conserves potassium.

Captopril usually raises serum potassium due to its blockade of angiotensin-stimulated aldosterone. Clinically important hyperkalemia with captopril has been described when the drug was used with a potassium-conserving diuretic or potassium chloride supplementation, particularly in patients with renal disease.

Cholestatic jaundice, headache, and insomnia have been reported but are rare. Captopril should not be given during pregnancy because there have been instances of fetal resorption, growth retardation, and hypotension at birth.

Therapeutic Uses. Orally administered captopril is effective in both mild and severe forms of renin-dependent hypertension. Because of the absence of side effects in the majority of patients, it is often used as a first agent. The antihypertensive effect is amplified by the use of a diuretic. Captopril may be combined with other forms of antihypertensive additively. The drug is particularly effective in renovascular and malignant hypertension and relatively ineffective when used alone in low renin forms of hypertension.

Drug Interactions. Neurological disturbances have occurred in patients taking captopril and cimetidine together. Indomethacin and aspirin antagonize the antihypertensive effect of captopril.

Dosage and Preparations. Captopril is available in 12.5, 25, 50, and 100 mg tablets. The usual starting dosage in hypertension is 25 mg twice daily. The drug may be increased to 50 mg three times daily before addition of a diuretic. Captopril is also available in combination with hydrochlorothiazide.

Enalapril

Mechanism of Action. The mechanism of action of enalapril as an antihypertensive agent is the same as that of captopril.

Pharmacology. Enalapril is a phosphinic acid ester that is absorbed rapidly even in the presence of food and is metabolized extensively by the liver. The drug is about 40% bioavailable. Enalapril is hydrolyzed to the active dicarboxylic acid enalaprilat. Enalapril reaches peak plasma concentrations and action 3–6 hours after oral ingestion. Because of its long duration of action, enalapril is used either once or twice daily. The accumulation half-life following multiple dosages is 11 hours and is increased with decreased renal function.

Adverse Effects. The side effects of enalapril are similar to those of captopril except that rash and taste disturbances are less common with enalapril. Enalapril may cause headache, nausea, dizziness, diarrhea, or angioedema. A dry persistent cough may occur and necessitate termination of therapy.

Dry cough may occur with converting-enzyme inhibitors.

Therapeutic Uses. Enalapril has the same spectrum of uses as captopril. Because enalapril is available in IV solution, it may be used for hypertensive emergencies or when oral administration is not feasible.

Preparations and Dosages. Enalapril is available in 5, 10, and 20 mg tablets. The usual starting dosage is 5 mg once daily, and doses of up to 40 mg have been used with safety.

Lisinopril

Pharmacology. Lisinopril is the lysine analog of enalapril and, therefore, similar in characteristics. In contrast to enalapril, lisinopril does not require conversion by the liver to the active form. Approximately 25% of lisinopril is absorbed after an oral dose, with maximal serum concentrations being achieved after 7 hours. Lisinopril is not bound to plasma proteins and is excreted unchanged in the urine; its serum half-life is approximately 12 hours. Bioavailability is not affected by food or other drugs and is decreased in congestive heart failure. Because of its long half-life, lisinopril is usually given just once daily.

Adverse effects and therapeutic uses are the same as those of enalapril.

Dosage and Administration. Lisinopril is available in 5, 10, and 20 mg tablets. The usual starting dosage is 5–10 mg once daily.

CALCIUM CHANNEL ANTAGONISTS

Calcium antagonists or channel blockers block the intracellular movement of calcium into arteriolar smooth muscle and cardiac cells and may inhibit the mobilization of calcium from within these cells. The pharmacology, adverse effects, general therapeutic uses, and drug interactions of these agents are discussed in detail in Chapter 31. This section reviews the information related to the treatment of hypertension.

Verapamil

Pharmacological Actions. Verapamil produces both smooth muscle relaxation and nonspecific sympatheetic antagonism. In humans, verapamil slows A-V and S-A nodal conduction, thereby reducing heart rate as well as lowering blood pressure. Verapamil is significantly less potent as a vasodilator than diltiazem or the dihydropyridines. Thus, dosages large enough to reduce moderate or severe hypertension are likely to produce some degree of cardiac depression. Verapamil has a negative inotropic effect on cardiac output and blunts reflex sympathetic compensation. This cardiac effect may become relevant clinically in those with borderline or poorly compensated cardiac failure and in those taking other cardiac depressant drugs such as β-adrenergic blockers or certain antiarrhythmics.

> Verapamil reduces blood pressure and heart rate.

Therapeutic Uses. Verapamil is useful in mild hypertension, particularly when there is coexisting angina pectoris or another indication for the drug. There is conflicting data as to whether diuretics are additive with verapamil.

Diltiazem

Pharmacological Actions. Diltiazem is similar to verapamil in its pharmacological properties but differs slightly in that it is somewhat more potent as an arteriolar vasodilator. There appears to be somewhat less action on enteric smooth muscle.

Therapeutic Uses and Drug Interactions. Diltiazem is used in mild and moderate hypertension, often as a first-line agent when angina pectoris is also present. There is evidence to suggest that diuretics are additive with diltiazem, but the drug is not suitable for combination with a β blocker.

Nifedipine

Pharmacological Action. Nifedipine differs from verapamil and diltiazem by being a more potent arteriolar vasodilator and by having less cardiac actions. This combination leads usually to a slight increase in heart rate that offsets the slight negative inotropic effect on the heart. The myocardial depressant effect may become evident, however, when cardiac function is severely compromised or when other cardiac depresssant drugs are given concurrently.

Therapeutic Uses. Nifedipine can be used to treat all degrees of hypertension but is particularly useful for moderate-to-severe forms, including patients with angina pectoris. It may be combined successfully with a β blocker to reduce side effects as well as to amplify the antihypertensive and antianginal effects. Nifedipine may be given sublingually (by breaking the capsule) for rapid onset of action. This is particularly useful in hypertensive urgencies and emergencies.

Nifedipine may be used to treat all forms of hypertension.

Nicardipine

Pharmacology. Nicardipine is similar to nifedipine but does not, in the reported clinical trials, prolong A-V conduction. The drug is rapidly and completely absorbed and begins to act within 20 minutes, reaching a peak action between 30 and 120 minutes. Nicardipine undergoes first-pass hepatic metabolism and is about 35% bioavailable. Food may diminish the absorption of the drug. Terminal plasma half-life is about 9 hours. About 65% of the drug or metabolites is recovered in the urine and 35% in the feces.

References

General: On Treatment of Hypertension

Case DB: Patient population as consideration for antihypertensive therapy. *In* Hollenberg NK (ed.): Management of Hypertension: A Multifactorial Approach, 101–120. London: Butterworths, 1987.

Croog SH, Levine S, Testa MA, et al: The effects of antihypertensive therapy on the quality of life. N Engl J Med 314:1657–1664, 1986.

Frohlich ED: Newer concepts in antihypertensive drugs. Prog Cardiovasc Dis 20:385–402, 1978.

Gifford RW Jr: Drug combinations as rational antihypertensive therapy. Arch Intern Med 133:1053–1057, 1974.

Hypertension Detection and Follow-Up Program Cooperative Research Group: Effect of antihypertensive drug treatment on mortality in presence of resting electrocardiographic abnormalities on baseline: HDFP experience. Circulation 70:996–1003, 1984.

Hypertension Detection and Follow-Up Program Cooperative Research Group: Five-year findings of hypertension detection and follow-up program: I. Reduction in mortality of persons with high blood pressure, including mild hypertension. JAMA 242:2562–2571, 1979.

Hypertension Detection and Follow-Up Program Cooperative Research Group: Five-year findings of hypertension detection and follow-up program: II. Mortality by race, sex and age. JAMA 242:2572–2577, 1979.

Hypertension Detection and Follow-Up Program Cooperative Research Group: Five-year findings of hypertension detection and follow-up program: III. Reduction in stroke incidence among persons with high blood pressure. JAMA 247:633–638, 1982.

Messerli FH (ed): Cardiovascular Drug Therapy. Philadelphia: WB Saunders Co, 1990.

The 1988 report of the Joint National Committee on Detection, Evaluation, and Treatment of High Blood Pressure. US Department of Health and Human Services. NIH Publication No. 88–1088. Also published in Arch Intern Med 148:1023–1038, 1988.

Diuretic Treatment of Hypertension

Fries ED: How diuretics lower blood pressure. Am Heart J 106:185–187, 1983.

Tweeddale MG, Ogilvie RI, Ruedy J: Antihypertensive and biochemical effects of chlorthalidone. Clin Pharmacol Ther 22:519–527, 1977.

Sympatholytic Drugs

Buhler FR, Laragh JH, Baer L, et al: Propranolol inhibition of renin secretion. N Engl J Med 287:1209–1214, 1972.

Das PK, Parratt Jr: Myocardial and hemodynamic effects of phentolamine. Br J Pharmacol 41:437–444, 1971.

Frishman WH: Drug therapy: Atenolol and timolol, two new systemic beta-adrenoceptor antagonists. N Engl J Med 306:1456–1462, 1982.

Frishman WH: Nadolol: A new beta-adrenoreceptor antagonist. N Engl J Med 305:678–682, 1981.

Frishman WH: Pindolol: A new beta-adrenoceptor antagonist with partial agonist activity. N Engl J Med 308:940–944, 1983.

Furst CI: The biochemistry of guanethidine. Adv Drug Res 4:133–161, 1967.

Graham RM, Pettinger WA: Drug therapy: Prazosin. N Engl J Med 300:232–236, 1979.

Khatri IM, Levinson P, Notargiacoma A, Friess ED: Initial and long-term effects of prazosin on sympathetic vasopressor responses in essential hypertension. Am J Cardiol 55:1015–1018, 1985.

Koch-Weser J: Metoprolol. N Engl J Med 301:698–703, 1979.

McMartin C, Simpson P: The absorption and metabolism of guanethidine in hypertensive patients requiring different doses of the drug. Clin Pharmacol Ther 12:73–77, 1971.

Rosei EA, Brown JJ, Lever AI, et al: Treatment of phaeochromocytoma and of clonidine withdrawal hypertension with labetalol. Br J Clin Pharmacol 3:809–815, 1976.

Sen G, Bose KC: *Rauwolfia serpentina*, a new Indian drug for insanity and high blood pressure. Indian Med World 2:194–201, 1931.

van Zwieten PA: Basic pharmacology of alpha-adrenoceptor antagonists and hybrid drugs. J Hyperten 6 (Suppl 2):S3–S11, 1988.

Wallen JD, et al: Labetalol: Current research and therapeutic status. Arch Intern Med 143:485–490, 1983.

Wilson DJ, Wallin JD, Vlachakis ND, et al: Intravenous labetalol in treatment of severe hypertension and hypertensive emergencies. Am J Med 75 (Suppl 4A): 95–102, 1983.

Converting Enzyme Inhibitors

Kostis JB: Angiotensin-converting enzyme inhibitors: emerging differences and new compounds. Am J Hypertens 2:57–64, 1989.

Kubo SH, Cody RJ: Clinical pharmacokinetics of the angiotensin converting enzyme inhibitors. Clin Pharmacokinet 10:377–391, 1985.

Vidt D, Bravo EL, Fouad FM: Captopril. N Engl J Med 306:214–219, 1982.

Calcium Channel Antagonists

Frishman WH, Weinberg P, Peled H, et al: Calcium entry blockers for treatment of severe hypertension and hypertensive crisis. Am J Med 77 (Suppl 2B):35–45, 1984.

Vasodilators

Klotman PE, Grim CE, Weinberger MH, Judson WE: Effects of minoxidil on pulmonary and systemic hemodynamics in hypertensive man. Circulation 55:394–400, 1977.

Tarazi RC, Dustan HP, Bravo EL, et al: Vasodilating drugs: Contrasting hemodynamic effects. Clin Sci Mol Med 51 (Suppl 3):575–578, 1976.

Other Drugs

Burns JJ, Salvador RA, Lemberger L: Metabolic blockade by methoxamine and its analogs. Ann NY Acad Sci 139:833–840, 1967.

Crout JR, Brown B Jr: Anesthetic management of phaeochromocytoma: The value of phenoxybenzamine and methoxyflurane. Anesthesiology 30:29–36, 1969.

36

Drugs Used in the Treatment of Angina Pectoris

Dennis M. Higgins
Cedric M. Smith

Angina pectoris—paroxysmal pain in the chest

Angina is not a disease; rather, as the word indicates, it is one of the most prominent and well-known symptoms of myocardial ischemia. Attacks of angina can be brought on by a variety of conditions that perturb the relationship between myocardial oxygen supply and demand. For example, angina may occur with aortic stenosis or hypertrophic cardiomyopathy. However, the most common cause of angina is coronary artery disease. Angina is manifested usually as severe, transient, retrosternal pain that sometimes radiates to the left arm, back, or jaw. It is frequently accompanied by fear, anxiety, feelings of suffocation, and a sensation of tightening of the chest. However, as with many symptoms, there is a great deal of individual variation in the intensity and quality of pain, and some ischemic episodes may occur without prominent symptoms. The exact mechanisms that cause the discharge of sensory nerves and that translate ischemia into pain are unknown.

Myocardial Oxygen Supply and Demand in Angina

Angina occurs when the heart muscle demand for oxygen exceeds supply.

Drug therapy of coronary heart disease aims to (1) decrease consumption of oxygen by the heart or (2) alter oxygen delivery to heart muscle tissues.

Myocardial contractility, rate of contraction, wall tension

The heart extracts most of the oxygen carried by its blood supply.

Angina occurs when the myocardial demand for oxygen exceeds the supply provided by the coronary arteries. The goal of antianginal therapy is to re-establish an appropriate balance by reducing myocardial oxygen consumption or increasing oxygen supply. There are three determinants of myocardial oxygen demand. The first is the contractile state of the heart. The more forcefully the heart contracts, the more energy it uses and the more adenosine triphosphate (ATP) it requires. In particular, when the heart is under the influence of catecholamines, its inotropic state and oxygen demand are increased. The second determinant is cardiac rate; generally the faster the heart beats, the more oxygen it consumes. The third determinant of myocardial oxygen demand is wall tension. For a given rate and inotropic state, increased wall tension causes the myocardium to use more oxygen in order to generate a particular pressure. Wall tension is the product of the intraventricular pressure and radius, and the latter is related directly to the volume of blood in the ventricle. Thus, a heart enlarged by high ventricular-filling pressures requires more oxygen. Two types of wall tension are recognized: preload is the tension during ventricular filling, and afterload is the tension during systole. Both types of tension can be altered by antianginal drugs.

The myocardial oxygen supply is determined by both the arteriovenous difference in oxygen tension and the coronary blood flow. Typically, the heart extracts a large fraction (~70%) of the oxygen presented to it, and this high efficiency is changed little by exertion or drugs. Therefore, it is not a major site of therapeutic intervention. Most of the changes in myocardial oxygen supply reflect changes in coronary blood flow. Coronary blood flow is determined by both the perfusion pressure and the resistance within the coronary artery bed. The latter is subject to metabolic autoregulation; increases in myocardial oxygen demand, such as those brought on by exertion, lead to the release of endogenous vasodilators, such as adenosine. These metabolically released vasodilators, in turn, cause decreases in the tone of arteriolar resistance vessels, thereby allowing increased coronary blood flow.

Coronary blood flow—roles of pressure, resistance, and arterial vasodilatation or constriction

Another important determinant of myocardial oxygen supply that is subject to regulation by antianginal drugs is the distribution of coronary blood flow. Because the large coronary arteries are located on the epicardial surface, subendocardial tissue is near the end of the supply line. In addition, the decrease in coronary blood flow that occurs during the generation of systolic tension is not uniform across the ventricular wall; rather, it is greatest in subendocardial tissue and least in the epicardium. Thus, subendocardial tissue is especially vulnerable to ischemic insult.

Angina caused by diseases of coronary arteries may be subdivided into two types: *typical* and *variant*. Typical (classic, exertional) angina is brought on by conditions that increase myocardial oxygen consumption, such as physical exertion, emotional stress, exposure to cold, or eating large meals. It is associated with a depressed ST segment on the electrocardiogram (ECG), indicating subendocardial ischemia. Typical angina occurs in patients with significant atherosclerotic lesions of epicardial coronary arteries. The relationship of such lesions to stress-induced angina is illustrated in Figure 36–1. In normal individuals, increased myocardial activity leads to metabolic dilation of the most significant resistance vessels, the arterioles. Thus, with increased exertion myocardial blood flow may increase severalfold. With atherosclerosis there is a narrowing of the lumen of large epicardial arteries. This imposes another source of resistance into the coronary circulation; therefore, it limits the extent to which blood flow can be augmented to meet increased metabolic demands and leads to exertional ischemia.

Pathophysiology and Treatment of Typical Angina

Typical and *variant* angina

Atherosclerosis limits the ability of coronary flow to increase to meet metabolic demand.

Pharmacological treatment of typical angina is directed first to the relief of acute pain and then to the prevention of its recurrence. Nitroglyc-

Treatment of the acute pain, and treatment directed to prevention of its recurrence

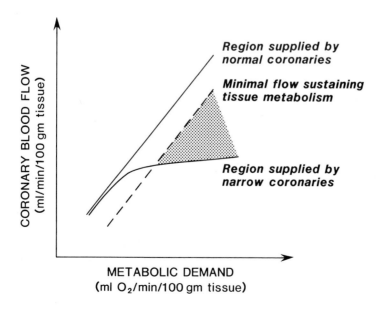

CORONARY BLOOD FLOW (ml/min/100 gm tissue)

METABOLIC DEMAND (ml O_2/min/100 gm tissue)

Region supplied by normal coronaries

Minimal flow sustaining tissue metabolism

Region supplied by narrow coronaries

Figure 36–1

Relationship between coronary blood flow (Y axis) and the myocardial metabolic activity (X axis). In the absence of occlusive coronary disease *(color solid line)*, metabolically induced arteriolar dilation augments coronary flow above the minimal levels necessary to sustain tissue metabolism *(dashed line)*. Where coronary vessels are narrowed *(black solid line)*, increasing metabolic demands evoke progressively smaller increases in coronary flow as the coronary flow rate approaches the limiting values imposed by large, fixed proximal resistances; eventually the flow rate falls below that necessary to support the augmented metabolic activity and ischemia *(shaded region)* ensues. (Redrawn from Goldstein RE, Epstein SE: Medical management of patients with angina pectoris. Prog Cardiovasc 14:360–398, 1972.)

Nitroglycerin—the *prototype* nitrate drug

erin administered sublingually is used for the treatment of acute anginal attacks; patients typically experience relief within 2–5 minutes. The antianginal effects of nitroglycerin involve both decreases in myocardial oxygen consumption and changes in coronary oxygen supply, as discussed later. The prophylactic treatment of angina can be accomplished with long-acting organic nitrate preparations, β-adrenergic blocking drugs, or calcium antagonists; all three classes of drugs can reduce the frequency and severity of anginal attacks. The mechanisms of action of the first two classes of drugs are discussed in this chapter, whereas the antianginal effects of calcium channel blockers are discussed in Chapter 31. The pharmacological treatment of exertional angina should be part of a comprehensive plan designed to reduce factors (such as smoking, obesity, hypertension) and conditions (large meals, exposure to cold, excessive exertion) that may aggravate angina.

Prophylaxis of angina: nitrates, β-adrenergic antagonists, or calcium channel antagonists

Conditions aggravating typical angina.

Variant Angina

Variant angina is *not* related to exertion.

Variation angina is caused by a coronary artery spasm.

Variant angina treated with nitroglycerin or calcium channel–blocking agents

Variant (spastic, Prinzmetal's) angina differs from classic angina in both its etiology and its treatment. Variant angina develops typically at rest rather than during physical exertion; it frequently follows a diurnal rhythm, often occurring in the early morning. Thus, variant angina is not associated with an increased cardiac demand for oxygen; rather, the cause of Prinzmetal's angina appears to be a spasm of one or more coronary arteries. This spasm is often, but not always, associated with atheromatous coronary artery disease. Coronary spasm reduces the myocardial oxygen supply leading to a transmural myocardial ischemia and an elevation of the electrocardiographic ST segment. A variety of mediators, including norepinephrine, serotonin, and thromboxanes are suspected of playing a role in variant angina, but there is still uncertainty regarding the exact cause of the arterial spasms. It is known, however, that the vasoconstrictor ergonovine maleate (Chapter 29) can often precipitate spasms in patients with Prinzmetal's angina; this drug is sometimes used as a provocative test.

The therapeutic goal in the treatment of acute variant angina is to relax the coronary artery spasm; this is most readily accomplished with sublingual nitroglycerin. Long-term prophylactic therapy usually employs either organic nitrates or calcium channel antagonists. In contrast to the treatment of typical angina, β-adrenergic blocking agents are not useful for variant angina. Stimulation of coronary β receptors can lead to vasodilation, and removal of such an influence has the potential to make vasospasms worse.

Organic Nitrates

All nitrates have the same mechanism of action.

O-NO$_2$ is the critical moiety.

Active substances are the metabolites—nitric oxide (NO) or nitrosothiols

STRUCTURES AND MECHANISM OF ACTION

Four organic nitrates are used in the treatment of angina: nitroglycerin (glyceryl trinitrate), pentaerythritol tetranitrate, erythrityl tetranitrate, and isosorbide dinitrate (Table 36–1). The structures of these compounds are shown in Table 36–1. All of these compounds are polyol esters of nitric acid, and all are highly lipid-soluble. The O-NO$_2$ moieties are critical for drug efficacy, and their removal results in inactive compounds. The prototype and most thoroughly investigated member of this group of drugs is nitroglycerin; the other three agents are thought to act by an identical mechanism, differing only in their pharmacokinetic properties (as shown later, and in Table 36–1).

The organic nitrates undergo metabolic activation to yield a short-lived, reactive intermediate(s) that is responsible for their biological activity. Endothelial cells secrete the mediator EDRF (endothelium-derived relaxing factor), which is either NO (nitric oxide) or a closely related

Table 36–1 NITRATES

Drug	Structure	Route of Administration	Dosage (and Regimen)
Nitroglycerin (Nitro-bid, Nitrostat, others)	$H_2C-O-NO_2$ $HC-O-NO_2$ $H_2C-O-NO_2$	Sublingual Buccal Oral	0.3–0.6 mg (prn) 1–2 mg tid 2.5–6.5 mg tid

		Transdermal (some available products)
		  Ointment (2%)
		  Nitrodisc
		  Nitro-Dur
		  Transderm-Nitro
		  Deponit
			
			1.5–5 sq cm q 4–6 hours
			8–16 sq cm/day
			5–30 sq cm/day
			2.5–15 mg/day
			16–32 sq cm/day

		Nasal spray	0.4 mg/dose
Isosorbide dinitrate (Isordil, Sorbitrate, others)		Sublingual Oral (sustained release)	2.5–10 mg q 3 hours 20–80 mg bid/tid
Pentaerythritol tetranitrate (Peritrate, others)	O_2N-O-H_2C CH_2-O-NO_2 C O_2N-O-H_2C CH_2-O-NO_2	Oral	10–60 mg q 6 hours
Erythrityl tetranitrate (Cardilate)	$H_2C-O-NO_2$ $HC-O-NO_2$ $HC-O-NO_2$ $H_2C-O-NO_2$	Sublingual	5–15 mg q 6 hours

metabolite, a nitrosothiol. EDRF diffuses from endothelial cells to vascular smooth muscle cells and therein activates the enzyme guanylate cyclase. Activation of this enzyme and the generation of cyclic guanosine monophosphate (cGMP) leads subsequently to the relaxation of the vascular smooth muscle. Nitroglycerin is taken up by smooth muscle and reacts with intracellular sulfhydryl groups to liberate nitrosothiols; thereby, it mimics the effects of the naturally occurring vasodilator EDRF. This mechanism of action is the cause of the marked tissue specificity of nitroglycerin; it relaxes smooth muscle (both vascular and nonvascular) but is essentially devoid of activity in other structures, including cardiac and skeletal muscle.

Nitrate actions mimic those of EDRF.

ANTIANGINAL EFFECTS

The administration of nitroglycerin alters both myocardial oxygen consumption and supply. Although there is some controversy, the former is probably more important than the latter in treatment of typical angina. The ability of nitroglycerin to relax vascular smooth muscle is the basis of its use in the treatment of variant angina.

Table 36–2 presents the effects of nitroglycerin on patients with coronary artery disease. The most prominent effect of nitroglycerin is to cause a large (in the case of these patients ~30%) decrease in cardiac work. This decrease in cardiac work reduces myocardial oxygen demand, bringing it more in line with supply and thereby alleviating ischemia. Nitroglycerin has no direct effect on cardiac muscle and does not directly elicit changes in either rate or the inotropic state. Rather, the drug-induced change in car-

Nitroglycerin decreases cardiac oxygen consumption.

No direct effects on cardiac muscle

Table 36–2 EFFECT OF NITROGLYCERIN ON THE PULMONARY AND SYSTEMIC CIRCULATION IN PATIENTS WITH CORONARY ARTERY DISEASE

| Patient | Age | Body surface area (sq m) | Heart rate per minute | Cardiac output (l/minute/sq m) | Pressures (mmHg) Brachial artery | | | Pulmonary artery mean | Right atrial mean | Pulmonary capillary mean | Ventricular Work (kg/minute /sq m) | | Coronary Flow (ml/minute) | | |
					Systolic mean	Mean	Diastolic mean				Left	Right	Per 100 g	Per left ventricle	Per 100 g/minute
1	68	1.5	63*	2.5	130	105	90	—	—	—	4.1	—	74	88	8.2
			79†	1.7	105	90	85	—	—	—	2.3	—	76	90	7.8
2	37	1.8	77	3.5	100	87	80	—	—	—	4.6	—	94	118	10.4
			66	2.5	52	48	44	—	—	—	1.6	—	48	61	5.3
3	42	1.7	75	2.9	102	85	82	—	—	—	3.8	—	90	129	7.7
			75	2.7	90	83	81	—	—	—	3.1	—	88	126	7.2
4	54	1.8	90	3.5	108	102	90	21	5	12	4.8	0.76	85	133	10.5
			97	3.4	100	95	88	16	—	8	4.3	0.70	78	122	9.3
5	52	1.5	81	2.7	122	107	98	—	—	—	4.4	—	93	100	10.8
			115	3.3	92	87	79	—	—	—	4.1	—	85	92	11.1
6	51	1.6	75	2.9	106	85	81	16	4	10	4.2	0.88	55	69	5.1
			56	2.8	92	75	71	14	2	8	3.5	0.60	40	50	3.5
7	44	1.7	88	3.5	134	95	90	23	3	15	6.1	0.94	81	119	10.3
			85	2.0	100	82	75	19	—	—	2.6	0.49	69	101	8.1
Average	50	1.6	78	3.1	115	95	87	20	4	12	4.6	0.86	82	108	9.0
			82	2.6	90	80	75	18	2	8	3.1	0.60	69	92	7.5
Change (%)			+5	−16	−22	−16	−14	−10	−50	−33	−33	−31	−16	−15	−17

Adapted from Gorlin R, Brachfield N, MacLeod C, Bopp P: Effect of nitroglycerin on the coronary circulation in patients with coronary artery disease or increased left ventricular work. Circulation 19:705–718, 1959, by permission of the American Heart Association, Inc.
* Before nitroglycerin.
† After nitroglycerin.

diac work reflects a decrease in wall tension caused by the relaxation of vascular smooth muscle. Nitroglycerin can decrease tone in both capacitance and resistance vessels; however, at low dosages, the former is more prominent. Relaxation of venous capacitance vessels leads to pooling of blood and decreased venous return. This, in turn, leads to decreased diastolic-filling pressures and volumes, reducing preload. This effect is complemented frequently by a modest decrease in systemic arterial pressure, reducing afterload.

Potential for hypotension, reflex tachycardia, increased pulse pressure

High dosages of nitroglycerin, which cause a prominent reduction in blood pressure, may elicit reflex tachycardia (see, for example, Patient 5 in Table 36–2). This undesirable side effect may outweigh the beneficial effects of reductions in wall tension on myocardial oxygen consumption; it may aggravate ischemia.

As a vasodilator, nitroglycerin is capable of causing the relaxation of both the large epicardial conductance vessels and the smaller arteriolar resistance vessels. By themselves, such actions would tend to increase coronary blood flow. However, they are counteracted by two other effects of nitroglycerin. First, the decrease in blood pressure caused by nitroglycerin reduces the driving force for blood flow through the coronary arterial bed. Second, because nitroglycerin reduces myocardial oxygen consumption, its administration can cause a decrease in metabolically driven arteriolar vasodilation. Thus, as a consequence of autoregulatory phenomena, there is usually little or no decrease in the tone of resistance vessels during sustained exposure to nitroglycerin. The net result of these interactions is that, although administration of high dosages of nitroglycerin may cause increases initially in coronary blood flow, sustained exposure is usually associated with a decrease in this parameter (see Table 36–2).

Although the actions of nitroglycerin on arteriolar resistance vessels are transient, this drug causes a sustained relaxation of smooth muscle in the large epicardial coronary arteries. This action is critical in relieving the spasms of variant angina; it is probably also significant in exertional angina. In normal individuals, the large coronary arteries are conductance vessels that usually do not offer significant resistance to flow. Thus, their dilatation has little hemodynamic effect. However, in patients with atherosclerosis, the narrowing of the lumen of some of the epicardial arteries represents a significant resistance to myocardial blood flow, particularly in times of stress when there is maximal dilatation of arterioles. Under these conditions, even modest changes in the lumen of the diseased vessels can lead to improved local perfusion of distal ischemic subendocardial areas. Because not all vessels need to be involved, this regional improvement of perfusion can occur in the absence of an increase in total coronary blood flow. The improved regional perfusion of subendocardial tissue is probably complemented by two other actions of nitroglycerin: its ability to dilate collateral vessels and to decrease left ventricular diastolic-filling pressure. The latter action enhances the diastolic perfusion upon which subendocardial tissue is critically dependent.

Sustained relaxation of epicardial coronary arteries

TOXICITY AND UNTOWARD RESPONSES

The most important side effects of the organic nitrates are cardiovascular. Because they cause venodilatation, these agents may cause orthostatic hypotension; this symptom is usually alleviated by repositioning to facilitate venous return. High doses may also cause hypotension leading to reflex increases in sympathetic tone to pacemaker tissue (with tachycardia) and ventricular muscle (with increased force of contraction and arrhythmic actions); each of such actions may aggravate ischemia. Organic nitrates may cause headaches during the first few days of administration; these headaches usually subside within a few days, especially if the dose is decreased. Organic nitrates can affect nonvascular, as well as vascular, smooth muscle, thereby producing bronchodilatation or relaxation of the muscles of the biliary tract.

Risk of orthostatic hypotension; reflex consequences of hypotension; reflex tachycardia; headaches

Nitrates relax many smooth muscles such as veins, bronchi, biliary tract, and ureters.

TOLERANCE TO ORGANIC NITRATES

Chronic administration of long-acting nitrates can lead to tolerance and an attenuation of their beneficial effects. The mechanism of the tolerance may involve depletion of the sulfhydryl groups necessary for the generation of nitrosothiols. Currently, the best procedures for avoiding tolerance development include using the lowest effective doses and interrupting otherwise continuous administration with a daily nitrate-free interval.

This attenuation or tolerance to the hemodynamic and antianginal effects can appear within 12 hours with high, sustained administration and is thus primarily a concern with the long-acting oral preparations; it usually does not occur with intermittent administration of the short-acting substances such as nitroglycerin. Although the use of intermittent therapy avoids the development of tolerance, it may expose the patient to "silent"

Another drug that exhibits tolerance

Avoid tolerance by a nitrate-free interval.

Tolerance may appear within 12 hours!

or symptomatic episodes of angina during the nitrate-free interval. The overall benefit/risk relationships of the long-acting agents has yet to be defined specifically; it may be that the clinical efficacy of the long-acting nitrates is greatest in those patients with large numbers of spontaneously occurring angina episodes.

Because of these problems, long-acting nitrates are not frequently used as the primary prophylactic therapy of patients with angina. Nevertheless, the nitrates can be effectively combined with β-blocking agents such as propranolol. In contrast, their combination with calcium channel blocking agents should be done very cautiously, because hypotension may become a problem.

Nitrates can be combined with propranolol, but usually not with calcium channel blockers.

PHARMACOKINETICS AND PREPARATIONS

The clinically used agents are listed in Table 36–1. All active compounds have the sequence of $C-O-NO_2$ or $C-O-NO$, and most active compounds have several of these functional groups. Thus, the family known as organic nitrates are polyolesters of either nitric acid ($C-O-NO_2$, organic nitrates), or nitrous acid ($C-O-NO$, organic nitrites).

A useful characteristic of these drugs is their rapid absorption through mucosal surfaces. Hence, they are compounded as tablets, creams, and ointments to be administered through the skin, sublingually, or orally.

Rapid absorption through mucosa

Nitroglycerin is the prototype agent and its actions and uses have been described in detail. Others include *isosorbide dinitrate, pentaerythritol tetranitrate*, and *erythrityl tetranitrate*, which are somewhat more effective given orally than nitroglycerin. All have the same basic mechanism of action, and they all have roughly the same pharmacokinetics after absorption, as well as the same mechanisms of inactivation.

As discussed earlier, the organic nitrates undergo metabolic activation to yield short-lived, reactive intermediates that are responsible for their biological activity: NO or closely related metabolites (nitrosothiols), that mimic the effects of the naturally occurring vasodilator EDRF. This mechanism of action is the cause of the marked tissue specificity of nitrates' actions on smooth muscle (both vascular and nonvascular).

Inactive denitrated metabolites

The metabolic inactivation of the nitrates initially involves their biotransformation by reductive hydrolysis by hepatic glutathione organic nitrate reductase to form more water-soluble denitrated compounds and inorganic nitrite. The denitrated metabolites are relatively inactive. This hepatic metabolism is rapid and efficient; thus, these compounds are subject to a marked first-pass effect of metabolism by the liver.

Large first-pass effect

The sublingual route is employed with nitroglycerin, isosorbide dinitrate, and erythrityl tetranitrate (see Table 36–1); this route has the advantage in that most of the drug bypasses the liver initially, and the half-life is a function of the rate of drug delivery to the liver. The intensity of the drug's actions parallels the plasma concentrations. For example, after sublingual administration of nitroglycerin, the maximal effect is obtained in approximately 5 minutes, and the duration of action is a short 20–30 minutes.

Sublingual nitroglycerin acts within minutes and lasts 20–30 minutes.

Sublingual administration is used to alleviate acute angina attacks of both typical and variant types. It is also used for "immediate prophylaxis," that is, given at the onset of a stressful situation that could be expected to give rise to angina.

A number of sustained-release preparations are available; some of these are listed in Table 36–1. Topical nitroglycerin ointment provides for the gradual absorption of the drug over several hours, which permits a more prolonged prophylactic action.

Orally administered organic nitrate regimens have been designed with the purpose of providing prolonged prophylaxis against attacks of angina. However, the effectiveness of many of these regimens has been questioned. The lack of consistent efficacy of oral preparations may be the consequence of the fact that upon absorption, these drugs pass through the liver and thus high doses are needed. Such high doses are more likely to cause side effects and the development of tolerance.

Oral absorption is more variable and less predictable.

(Inhalation has been used with amyl nitrite; however, because the dose and levels are hard to control, it is rarely used clinically. It and some related compounds have been drugs of abuse that have been claimed by some to produce a brief augmentation of sexual excitement—possibly as a subjective interpretation of the faintness and confusion consequent to hypotension and cerebral hypoxia).

OTHER THERAPEUTIC USES

Nitrates are used in congestive heart failure to reduce preload and afterload. They are also being investigated under a similar rationale in the treatment of myocardial infarcts.

Beta-adrenergic blocking agents, such as propranolol, are used in the prophylactic treatment of typical angina. Chronic administration of these agents reduces the severity and frequency of attacks of angina. They also increase exercise tolerance.

Beta-Adrenergic Blocking Agents in the Treatment of Typical Angina

One of propranolol's uses is for typical angina.

Typical angina occurs during times of stress. Stress leads also to the activation of the sympathetic nervous system with the concomitant release of catecholamines. Catecholamines activate cardiac β receptors, increasing rate and contractility; the administration of β-adrenergic blocking drugs attenuates such stress- and exercise-induced changes in two of the primary determinants of myocardial oxygen consumption. Propranolol also decreases systemic arterial pressure (see Chapter 14), which would tend to favorably influence wall tension. The beneficial effects of propranolol are partially offset by two other of its actions: it prolongs the duration of the systolic ejection period and can increase preload. However, the net effect of these interactions is usually a substantial decrease in myocardial oxygen consumption. Although propranolol does not increase coronary blood flow, there is some evidence that it may allow a favorable redistribution of blood flow during exercise, allowing better perfusion of subendocardial tissue.

Propranolol decreases the cardiac response to exercise.

Propranolol does *not* increase coronary blood flow.

The untoward effects and pharmacokinetics of β-adrenergic blocking drugs are described in Chapter 14.

CALCIUM CHANNEL ANTAGONISTS AND COMBINATIONS

Calcium channel antagonists, especially verapamil and diltiazem, are used frequently as monotherapy of angina, as discussed in Chapter 31, or they may be combined with a β-blocking agent such as propranolol. In contrast, although nitrates are not frequently used as the primary prophylactic therapy of patients with angina, they are sometimes combined with β-blocking agents such as propranolol, but usually not with calcium channel antagonists, because the combination may produce hypotension.

References

Abrams J: Nitroglycerin and long-acting nitrates. N Engl J Med 302:1234–1237, 1980.

Coronary heart disease. *In* Andreoli TE, Carpenter CCJ, Plum F, Smith LH Jr (eds): Cecil Essentials of Medicine. 2nd ed. Philadelphia: WB Saunders Co, 1990.

Flaherty JT: Nitrate tolerance. A review of the evidence. Drugs 37:523–550, 1989.

Goldstein RE, Epstein SE: Medical management of patients with angina pectoris. Prog Cardiovasc Dis 14:360–398, 1972.

Gorlin R, Brachfield N, MacLeod C, Bopp P: Effect of nitroglycerin on the coronary circulation in patients with coronary artery disease or increased left ventricular work. Circulation 19:705–718, 1959.

Murad F: Drugs used for the treatment of angina: Organic nitrates, calcium-channel blockers, and β-adrenergic antagonists. In Gilman AG, Rall TW, Nies AS, Taylor P (eds): Goodman and Gilman's The Pharmacologic Basis of Therapeutics. 8th ed. New York: Pergamon Press, 1990.

Antihyperlipidemic Agents

37

Robert Scheig

Hyperlipidemia and atherosclerosis continue to be important medical concerns, especially with respect to their relevance as risk factors for coronary artery disease. This chapter reviews lipoprotein metabolism to establish the basis for the rational approach to the utilization of different drugs in the therapy of hyperlipidemias.

Nicotinic acid and gemfibrozil are the current drugs of choice for the treatment of hypertriglyceridemia. Nicotinic acid or resin therapy reduce serum cholesterol and low-density lipoprotein–cholesterol (LDL-C) levels and have been shown to reduce the incidence of coronary events. Probucol and lovastatin are effective in reducing serum cholesterol and LDL-C levels, but they have not been shown to decrease atherosclerotic events. In one large study, gemfibrozil reduced the incidence of coronary heart disease in patients with hypercholesterolemia, presumably by increasing high-density lipoprotein–cholesterol (HDL-C) levels, whereas there was little change in the levels of LDL-C.

The Consensus Development Conference on Lowering Blood Cholesterol to Prevent Heart Disease sponsored by the National Institutes of Health in 1984 (Consensus Development Conference, 1985) and updated in 1987 (National Cholesterol Education Program, 1988) focused attention on the risk of hypercholesterolemia, specifically high levels of LDL-C in the development of atherosclerosis, and the need to develop screening programs for its detection and on the indications for therapy. Low levels of HDL-C are an additional and independent risk factor for the development of atherosclerosis (Miller, 1980). Among the complications of atherosclerosis, coronary artery disease itself causes some 500,000 deaths each year in the United States; over 5 million patients are symptomatic at any one time; and the disease costs over $60 billion annually in direct and indirect costs. Thus, therapy that improves serum lipoprotein levels and that reduces the risk of coronary artery disease has become an important medical concern.

Hypertriglyceridemia, although not a risk factor in the development of atherosclerosis, is a risk factor in the development of pancreatitis when serum levels rise above 1000 mg/dl (Cameron et al, 1974).

In this chapter, lipoprotein metabolism is reviewed so that a rational approach to drug therapy can be developed. Each drug currently in common use is then discussed.

CHYLOMICRONS

Chylomicrons are formed in the small intestinal mucosa from dietary triglycerides, cholesterol, and fat-soluble vitamins (Fig. 37–1). The triglycer-

Lipoprotein Function and Metabolism

633

Figure 37–1

Dietary triglycerides and cholesterol are absorbed from the gut into lymphatics as chylomicrons. Most of the triglycerides are hydrolyzed by lipoprotein lipase, and the fatty acids released are taken up by striated muscle and adipose tissue. The chylomicron remnant is recognized in receptors present only in the liver. Thus dietary cholesterol goes directly to the liver, as does the remaining dietary triglycerides.

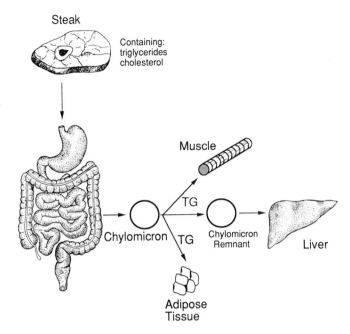

Chylomicrons as carriers

ides are hydrolyzed by an enzyme, lipoprotein lipase, principally found in capillaries supplying striated muscle and adipose tissue. The chylomicron remnant particle is recognized by specific receptors located in hepatocytes. This receptor is different from the low-density lipoprotein (LDL) receptor and is not regulated by cellular cholesterol concentrations. The triglycerides in the remnant particle are either oxidized or used for very low density lipoprotein (VLDL) formation. The absorbed dietary cholesterol is either used by the cell for membrane formation, incorporated into VLDL, or excreted in the bile. In summary, chylomicrons are carriers of energy from dietary triglycerides to striated muscle and adipose tissue and deliver dietary cholesterol and fat-soluble vitamins directly to the liver.

VERY LOW DENSITY LIPOPROTEINS

VLDL are manufactured in the liver, and triglycerides are their major constituent (Fig. 37–2). The fatty acids in the triglycerides are derived from chylomicron remnants, from circulating free fatty acids released from triglycerides contained in adipose tissue stores, or from fatty acids synthesized by the liver. The liver synthesizes fatty acids from acetyl CoA derived from the metabolism of carbohydrates, fats, ethanol, and most amino acids. Thus, excess calories can be converted to triglycerides, which are secreted by the liver as VLDL and utilized, after hydrolysis by lipoprotein lipase, by striated muscle and adipose tissue. As triglycerides are lost from VLDL, considerable remodeling occurs, including the addition of cholesterol from the high-density lipoproteins (HDL), and LDL are formed as a consequence. Thus, the two major functions of VLDL are to deliver energy derived from any calorie-containing source to striated muscle and adipose tissue and to serve as the precursor of LDL.

LOW-DENSITY LIPOPROTEINS

Cholesterol used in the synthesis of cell membranes derives from acetyl CoA and low-density lipoproteins.

LDL are the carriers of cholesterol, which is required by all animal cells for membrane formation. Each cell contains receptors that recognize and bind apoprotein B found in LDL. After binding, parts of the cell membrane pinch off, and the vesicles thus formed deliver cholesterol to the interior. When

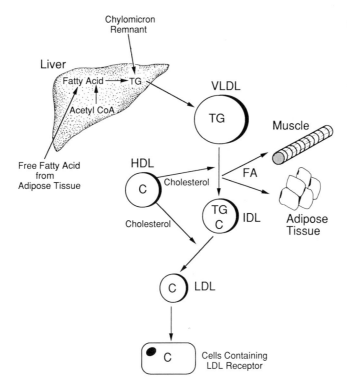

Figure 37–2

VLDL, made in the liver, consists primarily of triglycerides made from fatty acids synthesized *de novo* or from adipose tissue or from triglycerides in the chylomicron remnant. Most of the triglycerides are hydrolyzed by lipoprotein lipase, and the fatty acids released are taken up by striated muscle and adipose tissue. In the remodeling, cholesterol is gained from HDL with the formation of IDL and LDL. These lipoproteins can then be taken up by any cell containing the LDL receptor.

there is an excess of cholesterol in the cell compared with need, LDL receptor synthesis decreases; and when the intracellular levels of cholesterol fall, more receptors are synthesized. Each cell also manufactures its own cholesterol from acetyl CoA. This synthesis is regulated at the rate-limiting step that is the conversion of hydroxymethylglutaryl CoA to mevalonate catalyzed by hydroxymethyl glutaryl CoA reductase (HMG-CoA reductase). The activity of this enzyme is suppressed when cholesterol accumulates in the cell and increases when there is a paucity of cholesterol.

HIGH-DENSITY LIPOPROTEINS

HDL, in addition to being the source of cholesterol for LDL formation, appear to be responsible for reverse cholesterol transport. HDL are often called the scavenger lipoproteins, because they bring cholesterol through peripheral circulation to the liver where it is either excreted in the bile or converted to bile salts, which are excreted subsequently in the bile.

The source of LDL cholesterol is HDL.

Individuals with total serum cholesterol levels between 200–239 mg/dl are considered to have a borderline high risk and those over 240 mg/dl a high risk for the development of atherosclerosis (National Cholesterol Education Program, 1988). If LDL-C measurements are used, levels between 130–159 mg/dl are considered borderline and those over 160 mg/dl considered to place the patient at high risk. Diet is considered a critical aspect of therapy in all cases, because the major cause of hypercholesterolemia is thought to be the excess calories in the usual American diet that results in an overproduction of VLDL and LDL. A major additional factor is the excess cholesterol in chylomicron remnants coming to the liver that results in a decrease in receptor synthesis. Therefore, dietary alterations primarily consist of reducing the total number of calories if the patient is overweight and decreasing fat intake to 30% of total calories with about one third derived from polyunsaturated, one third from monounsaturated,

Diet Therapy

Diet is a critical concern whenever there is excessive level of cholesterol.

This diet is now recommended for everyone.

and one third from saturated fatty acids. Daily cholesterol intake should be less than 300 mg. When there is failure of diet to at least lower cholesterol to the borderline risk level or when additional risk factors are present even though the cholesterol level is only borderline, drug therapy is clearly indicated. It has been shown that for each 1% fall in serum cholesterol there is a 2% decrease in the incidence of coronary artery disease (Lipid Research Clinics Program, 1984). Hypertriglyceridemia should be treated if hypercholesterolemia is also present, because by lowering VLDL, LDL may frequently be lowered also. Finally, patients with fasting serum triglycerides above 500 mg/dl in the absence of hypercholesterolemia should be treated in order to prevent pancreatitis.

Hypertriglyceridemia or hypercholesterolemia are indications for therapy.

Drug Therapy

Nicotinic acid (niacin) is not only a vitamin but a therapeutic drug for hyperlipidemias.

Nicotinic acid

NICOTINIC ACID

Nicotinic acid (niacin), the vitamin known to prevent pellagra, has been used in large doses to decrease cholesterol for over 30 years. The mechanism of action is in part due to inhibition of cyclic adenosine monophosphate (AMP) accumulation in adipose tissue, which decreases the activity of triglyceride lipase. This causes a decreased release of free fatty acids by adipose tissue and thereby a decreased formation of VLDL and LDL. Nicotinic acid is useful, therefore, in the therapy of both hypercholesterolemia and hypertriglyceridemia. The drug is readily absorbed and distributed to all tissues. Its major symptomatic side effects are intense flushing, pruritus, and headache. These usually disappear after a few weeks of therapy and can be alleviated by 160–325 mg aspirin/day because these side effects are prostaglandin-mediated. Nausea, vomiting, diarrhea, and rarely, peptic ulceration are less common side effects.

Because abnormalities of liver function, hyperglycemia, and hyperuricemia occur not infrequently with nicotinic acid treatment, these must be evaluated at the start of therapy and monitored periodically thereafter. Nicotinic acid is especially useful in patients with hypertriglyceridemia or in those with hypercholesterolemia and concomitant hypertriglyceridemia. It is one of the two drugs that has been shown to reduce recurrent myocardial infarction, decrease the progression of atheroma formation, and increase long-term survival (Canner et al, 1986; Blankenhorn et al, 1987). Supplied in tablets of 50–500 mg, the starting dosage is 50–100 mg three times daily taken with meals to prevent gastritis. The dosage should be increased each week by 100 mg three times daily until a final dosage of 500–1000 mg three times daily is reached. With this regimen a 15% lowering of serum cholesterol can be anticipated.

The two drugs reducing myocardial infarctions are nicotinic acid and cholestyramine.

RESINS

Resins are unique agents that act as adsorbents inside the GI lumen.

Cholestyramine (QUESTRAN) and colestipol (COLESTID) are chloride salts of basic anion exchange resins. These resins are not absorbed from the gastrointestinal (GI) tract. They avidly bind anions, including bile acids. By interrupting the enterohepatic circulation of bile acids, the liver increases its catabolism of cholesterol to bile acids, and the cholesterol level in the hepatocyte falls. As a consequence there is both an increase in LDL receptor synthesis and an increase in cholesterol synthesis by the HMG-CoA reductase pathway. Fortunately the effect on LDL receptor synthesis is the greater of the two. Because of this and because the liver contains about 70% of the body's LDL receptors, serum LDL levels fall. The major disadvantages of these agents are the difficulty in swallowing the granules and the development of a variety of GI complaints, especially bloating and constipation. Thus, compliance is a problem. Palatability is improved by making a slurry with fruit juice or mixing with applesauce. Rarely, hypoprothrombinemia due to vitamin K deficiency, reduced serum folate levels, and hyperchloremic acidosis have been reported. Because the resins can bind many anions, anionic medications such as digitalis, thyroxine or warfarin, patients should take other drugs at least 1 hour before, or 4 hours after, the resin. The resins commonly cause an increase in serum triglyceride levels and, obviously, are ineffective in patients with biliary obstruction.

Cholestyramine is supplied in bulk with a scoop or, for twice the price, premeasured in a packet. Each packet contains 4 g of anhydrous cholestyramine resin. The most common dosage is 8–16 g for breakfast, after which the largest concentration of bile salts is discharged into the gut because they have accumulated overnight in the gallbladder, and another 4–8 g at lunch. Colestipol is supplied in bulk with a scoop or in packets, each packet or scoop containing 5 g of the resin. The dosage is 10–20 g for breakfast and 5–10 g for lunch. On the average, a 15–20% reduction of serum cholesterol can be obtained with resin therapy. When resin plus nicotinic acid is combined, a 26% reduction has been obtained associated with a decreased progression of coronary atherosclerosis (Blankenhorn et al, 1987). Resin alone also decreases the incidence of coronary artery disease (Lipid Research Clinics Program, 1984).

LOVASTATIN

Lovastatin (MEVACOR), isolated from a strain of *Aspergillus terreus,* is hydrolyzed after oral ingestion from an inactive lactone to an active hydroxy acid that is a potent inhibitor of HMG-CoA reductase. Lovastatin decreases LDL-C by decreasing the hepatic contribution of cholesterol for VLDL and therefore LDL formation; it also increases LDL-receptor synthesis by lowering intracellular cholesterol levels. Interestingly, lovastatin has no effect on steroidogenesis. About 30% of the oral dosage of lovastatin is absorbed and 10% is excreted in urine and the remainder in feces. The latter represents both unabsorbed drug and that excreted in bile. Because of extensive first-pass extraction by the liver, less than 5% of the oral dose reaches the general circulation. Single daily dosages are more effective when taken at night rather than morning, perhaps because cholesterol is synthesized mainly at night. Plasma concentrations of total inhibitors are higher when administration is with a meal rather than when fasting.

Food and Drug Administration (FDA) approval of lovastatin occurred in 1987; there is still limited experience with the drug and studies are not yet available about its effect on atherosclerosis. Because it crosses the placenta, the drug is currently contraindicated during pregnancy and lactation. Liver function should be monitored every 4–6 weeks because about 2% of patients develop threefold or more elevations in serum transaminases that, fortunately, return to normal on discontinuation of the drug. Myalgia with transient elevations in creatinine phosphokinase has been seen in about 0.5% of the patient population, often in patients concomitantly receiving immunosuppressive therapy or gemfibrozil. Severe rhabdomyolysis precipitating acute renal failure has been reported in cardiac transplant patients receiving immunosuppressive medication including cyclosporine. Currently it is uncertain whether lovastatin causes lens opacities, but baseline and yearly slit lamp examinations are recommended.

Lovastatin is supplied in 20 mg tablets, and the daily dosage is 20–80 mg given with the evening meal. A 15–40% reduction in serum cholesterol can be expected. If combined with a resin, even greater reductions have been noted (Illingworth, 1984; Thompson et al, 1986).

The major problem with resins is poor compliance.

Lovastatin

Lovastatin is a good example of a drug that undergoes a large first-pass extraction by the liver.

A central clinical and personal question is does the risk of serious side effects with lovastatin balance the potential benefits?

PROBUCOL

Probucol is also a potent antioxidant.

Lipoproteins containing oxidized lipids are more avidly taken up by atheromas than those not oxidized.

Probucol

Probucol (LORELCO) is a lipophilic substituted di-t-butylphenol with a chemical structure unlike other cholesterol-lowering agents. It appears to increase the fractional catabolic rate of LDL by enhancing nonreceptor-mediated pathways. It prevents oxidation of fatty acids in lipoproteins, which decreases the ability of endothelial cells to take up LDL. Although it decreases HDL-C, it apparently does so by reducing the size of HDL particles. Small HDL particles are capable of enhanced removal of cholesterol from peripheral depots. Supporting evidence for this enhanced reverse transport is the observation that probucol therapy successfully causes the disappearance of tendinous and tuberous xanthomas.

Absorption of probucol is variable and is better when administered with food. With continuous administration blood levels increase gradually until reaching a rather constant level after 3–4 months. Because of its lipophilic nature it takes 6 months after cessation of therapy for blood levels to fall 80% from the peak.

Adverse reactions are rare. Diarrhea and flatulence are the most common side effects. In animal studies prolongation of the Q-T interval on electrocardiogram (ECG) has been seen but does not appear to be a major problem in humans. Drug interactions have not been reported.

Probucol is supplied as a 250 mg tablet, and the dosage is 500 mg twice daily taken with the morning and evening meal. A 12–18% reduction in serum cholesterol can be anticipated, and the effects of long-term administration or combination therapy with a resin may be even better (McCaughan, 1981). The effectiveness of probucol in altering the incidence of coronary events is not yet known.

FIBRIC ACID DERIVATIVES

Gemfibrozil is a current drug of choice and eventual place in therapy awaits the results of more studies.

New agents for the treatment of hyperlipidemias can be anticipated in view of the importance of coronary artery disease and active research.

Gemfibrozil (LOPID) and clofibrate (ATROMID-S) are fibric acid derivatives useful in reducing serum triglyceride levels in patients with high levels of VLDL. Gemfibrozil has been shown also to reduce the mortality from coronary artery disease, presumably by raising the level of HDL-C, because its effect on LDL-C is small and variable (Frick et al, 1987). Gemfibrozil inhibits hydrolysis of triglycerides in adipose tissue and reduces hepatic extraction of free fatty acids. It also lowers VLDL by inhibiting synthesis and increasing clearance of apoB.

Gemfibrozil is well absorbed from the GI tract, has a plasma half-life of about 1.5 hours, and does not accumulate with continued use. It is excreted mainly in urine as a glucuronide conjugate. Severe hepatic or renal disease are contraindications, and the drug paradoxically causes a pronounced rise in serum lipid levels in primary biliary cirrhosis. Because of structural similarities to clofibrate, which is known to increase gallstone formation, gemfibrozil should be used with caution in patients with biliary tract disease. Occasional liver function abnormalities have been reported and anticoagulant dosage may have to be reduced. GI side effects are the most frequent symptomatic complications.

Gemfibrozil is supplied as 300-mg and 600-mg capsules, and the usual dosage is 600 mg 30 minutes before the morning and evening meal. A 40–45% fall in serum triglyceride level can be anticipated as well as a 20–25% rise in HDL-C. Clofibrate is used little because it has not been shown to reduce cardiovascular events, and in long-term studies, it increases mortality because of noncardiovascular causes, especially malignancy, postcholecystectomy complications, and pancreatitis.

References

Blankenhorn DH, Nessim SA, Johnson RL, et al: Beneficial effects of combined colestipol-niacin therapy on coronary atherosclerosis and coronary venous bypass grafts. JAMA 257:3233–3240, 1987.

Cameron JL, Capuzzi DM, Zuidema GD, Margolis S: Acute pancreatitis with hyperlipemia. Am J Med 56:482–487, 1974.

Canner PL, Berge KG, Wenger NK, et al: Fifteen-year mortality in coronary drug project patients: Long-term benefit with niacin. J Am Coll Cardiol 8:1245–1255, 1986.

Consensus Development Conference: Lowering blood cholesterol to prevent heart disease. JAMA 253:2080–2086, 1985.

Frick MH, Elo O, Haapa K, et al: Helsinki heart study: Primary-prevention trial with gemfibrozil in middle-aged men with dyslipidemia. N Engl J Med 317:1237–1245, 1987.

Illingworth DR: Mevinolin plus colestipol in therapy for severe heterozygous familial hypercholesterolemia. Ann Intern Med 101:598–604, 1984.

Lipid Research Clinics Program: The lipid research clinics coronary primary prevention trial results. JAMA 251:351–373, 1984.

McCaughan D: The long-term effects of probucol on serum lipid levels. Arch Intern Med 141:1428–1432, 1981.

Miller GJ: High-density lipoproteins and atherosclerosis. Annu Rev Med 31:97–108, 1980.

National Cholesterol Education Program (Goodman DS, chairman): Report of the Expert Panel on Detection, Evaluation, and Treatment of High Blood Cholesterol in Adults. Arch Intern Med 148:36–69, 1988.

Thompson GR, Ford J, Jenkinson M, Trayner I: Efficacy of mevinolin as adjuvant therapy for refractory familial hypercholesterolemia. Q J Med New Series 60 232:803–811, 1986.

Endocrine System Pharmacology

Introduction to Endocrine System Pharmacology

38

Paul J. Davis

Endocrine pharmacology has consisted traditionally of replacement hormonal therapy for patients with specific endocrine gland failure, such as insulin administration to diabetic patients or thyroid hormone in hypothyroid states. However, the 1980s enlightened the theory and practice of endocrine pharmacology in several important areas. These areas include the mechanisms of hormone action at the molecular level, increasingly sophisticated structure-activity analysis of hormone molecules, the description of previously unrecognized biological factors that may be classified as hormones, expanded therapeutic roles for hormones, and innovative methods of hormone synthesis or hormone formulation that facilitate the practice of medicine.

Hormone Action at the Molecular Level

Polypeptide hormones such as corticotropin (ACTH) and parathyroid hormone (PTH) act at specific receptor sites on the surface (plasma membrane) of target organ cells to regulate the synthesis of one or more specific products by these cells. The event of binding of ligand (hormone) to cell surface receptor is transduced to an intracellular signal such as cyclic adenosine monophosphate (AMP) or calcium or both, which results ultimately in target cell activation, e.g., cortisol secretion by the adrenal cortex (ACTH action) or osteoclast activity (PTH action). Signal transduction by polypeptide hormones at the plasma membrane may involve the phosphatidylinositol pathway or hormone receptor phosphorylation. The insulin receptor is an enzyme (kinase) that undergoes phosphorylation to initiate hormone action in insulin-sensitive cells.

Kinase initiates hormone action in insulin-sensitive cells.

Steroid hormones—corticosteroids and gonadal hormones—are usually viewed as having little activity at the cell surface and ultimately express their actions through specific binding proteins (receptors) that interact with hormone response elements of genes of target cells. Thyroid hormone also acts largely by this nuclear mechanism. The response elements for various hormones may be structurally similar, e.g., the corticosteroid and thyroid hormone nuclear receptors have structural homologies and are part of a superfamily of nuclear proteins now recognized as oncogene products (c-*erb*-A family). Vitamin A analogs (retinoids) interact with similar nuclear proteins. These hormone response elements bind to DNA to cause changes in the rates of transcription of specific genes. The amino acid sequence of these receptors is important to understand since such understanding may permit the manipulation of the action of hormones.

Steroid hormones express their actions through receptors that interact with the hormone response elements of target cells.

643

Structure-Activity Relationships of Hormones

Intact animal or *in vitro* models of hormone action and sophisticated analyses of hormone structure, such as by x-ray diffraction analysis (crystallography), have permitted the development of synthetic molecules with pharmacological actions that mimic those of endogenous hormones but that may have more desirable pharmacokinetic profiles. The realization, for example, that the amino terminal 24 amino acids of ACTH conferred biological activity on the molecule, whereas the carboxy terminal 15 amino acid peptide was immunoreactive, encouraged the development of a commercial product that consisted of the α 1–24 amino acids (cosyntropin). This molecule is a diagnostic agent of low immunogenic potential compared to the intact, 39 amino acid moiety. 1-deamino-8-D-arginine vasopressin (DDAVP) is a synthetic vasopressin (antidiuretic hormone, ADH) analog that has a longer half-life than vasopressin and that can be administered intranasally rather than by injection. Octreotide is a synthetic octapeptide analog of somatostatin that has a more favorable pharmacokinetic profile than its parent compound, can be administered orally, and is effective in the treatment of acromegaly, malignant carcinoid, and other hormone-secreting tumors.

Newly Recognized Cellular Factors With Hormonal Functions

Hormones are secreted into the circulation as highly specialized products of specific tissues. A number of peptides and lipids have been described that are important to cell-to-cell or tissue-to-tissue communication. Cytokines, such as the interleukins, are important to the activation of defensive cells or to cell growth (growth factors). Prostaglandins are lipids that were recognized decades ago to be produced by a variety of tissues and to have multiple roles. Erythropoietin is a hematopoietic hormone that originates in the kidney; the human gene for this polypeptide hormone has been cloned, facilitating the large-scale synthesis of this hormone for clinical use. Other biological substances observed more recently to have clinically important hormonal functions are the family of atrial natriuretic peptides and certain vitamin A analogs (retinoids).

Expanded Clinical Roles for Hormones

For decades, glucocorticoids have been used as anti-inflammatory agents.

Glucocorticoids administered in larger than replacement dosages have been recognized for decades as effective anti-inflammatory agents. More recent examples of new clinical applications for well-characterized hormones are the use of androgens to modify the course of hereditary angioneurotic edema and the use of prostaglandins (misoprostol) to reduce the risk of peptic ulcer disease in specific clinical settings.

New Means of Production, New Formulations, and Varied Routes of Administration of Hormones

Recombinant DNA technology has expedited the production of polypeptide hormones.

Recombinant DNA technology has expedited the production of human insulin, human growth hormone, and erythropoietin for clinical use. This means of production leads to primary structures of polypeptide hormones that are identical to those of the authentic biological product. However, because posttranslational processing of these substances in humans prior to hormonal secretion is not identical to that in the coliform bacteria transfected with the genes for the hormones, the recombinant product may not be identical to the native hormone in terms of secondary or tertiary structure.

DDAVP is an example of a new (and desirable) formulation of a hormone, and a variety of steroid hormone analogs have been synthesized to take advantage of the anti-inflammatory qualities of the steroid structure. Transdermal administration of estrogen and intranasal application of hormones (such as DDAVP) are alternative routes of administration that have attractive pharmacokinetic advantages or facilitate patient compliance.

Thyroid Hormones and Drugs That Affect the Thyroid

39

Edward A. Carr, Jr.
Stephen W. Spaulding

The thyroid gland, like other endocrine organs, may secrete too little or too much hormone. Effective pharmacological therapies for both hypo- and hyperfunction were achieved for the thyroid before any other endocrine gland.

HISTORY

Noting that Betancourt and Serrano of Lisbon had reported improvement in a myxedematous patient after transplantation of a sheep thyroid gland under her breast, Murray (1891) found it "reasonable to suppose that the same amount of improvement might be obtained by simply injecting an extract of the thyroid gland," a procedure that Vassale (1890) had already reported effective in thyroidectomized dogs. Murray soaked chopped sheep thyroid in phenolized glycerine for 24 hours, filtered it through a sterilized handkerchief, and injected it into a myxedematous woman. Repeated injections, using a fresh gland extract each week, brought about convincing clinical improvement. It was found subsequently that preparations from thyroid tissue could also be successfully administered to hypothyroid patients by mouth. The use of such galenical preparations for the treatment of hypothyroidism is no longer recommended, although various preparations containing thyroglobulin are still on the market. They have been replaced by the pure hormones L-thyroxine (T_4) and triiodothyronine (T_3).

GENESIS AND FATE OF THYROID HORMONES

The thyroid gland normally concentrates the iodide ion about 30-fold relative to the iodide concentration in the plasma. Under stimulation by thyrotropin (thyroid-stimulating hormone, TSH) the gland may achieve iodide concentrations as high as 200 times the concentration in plasma. After this first trapping step, the iodide is oxidized by a peroxidase, permitting iodination of tyrosyl moieties in thyroglobulin (organification), producing mono- and diiodotyrosyl residues. Following this second step, certain of the iodotyrosyl residues transfer their phenolic ring, coupling it to other iodotyrosine residues in the thyroglobulin, to form di-, tri-, or tetraiodothyronine (Fig. 39–1). Whereas diiodothyronine (T_2) is inactive as a hormone, both triiodothyronine (T_3) and tetraiodothyronine (T_4) (thyroxine) are active once they are released from the thyroglobulin molecule. The

Thyroid Hormones

The thyroid traps, organifies, and couples iodide to thyroglobulin. T_3 and T_4 are released into the circulation after proteolysis of the thyroglobulin.

645

Figure 39–1

Tyrosine, thyronine, and their iodinated derivatives.

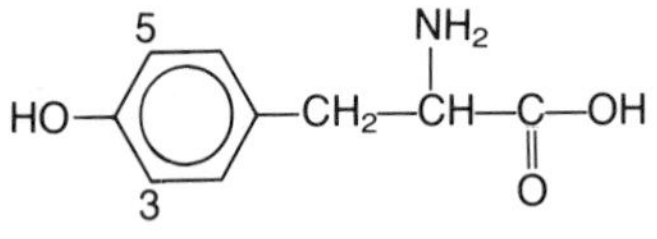

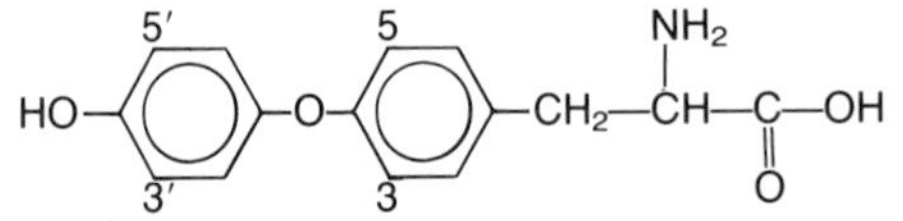

	3	5	3'	5'
Tyrosine	H	H		
Monoiodotyrosine	I	H		
Diiodotyrosine	I	I		
Thyronine	H	H	H	H
3,3'-diiodothyronine (T$_2$)	I	H	I	H
3',3,5-triiodothyronine (T$_3$)	I	I	I	H
3',5',3-triiodothyronine ("reverse T$_3$")	I	H	I	I
Thyroxine (T$_4$)	I	I	I	I

iodinated thyroglobulin is stored in the follicular colloid awaiting the fourth step, in which lysosomal enzymes hydrolyze thyroglobulin and release the T$_4$ and T$_3$ into the blood. This proteolysis also liberates mono- and diiodotyrosine residues that escaped the third, coupling step. These unused iodine-containing building blocks do not go to waste completely, however, for a dehalogenase in the gland removes their iodine atoms, thus providing an efficient scavenging mechanism to retain iodine in the thyroid for reuse. The normal thyroid produces 80–90 μg of T$_4$ and about 30 μg of T$_3$ (Refetoff and Larson, 1989), or about 70 μg of hormonal iodine daily (Riggs, 1952). In the course of secreting thyroid hormones, the gland also releases a small amount of thyroglobulin itself into the plasma. The normally low circulating concentration of thyroglobulin is increased in some pathological conditions.

The control of thyroid function by TSH is discussed in detail in Chapter 40. Serum thyroxine levels are principally responsible for the negative feedback control of TSH secretion by the pituitary. TSH stimulates each of the steps in the formation and secretion of thyroid hormones, many of its actions being mediated by cyclic adenosine monophosphate. Prolonged TSH stimulation of the thyroid leads to goiter formation, a generalized hypertrophy and hyperplasia of both thyroidal follicular cells and stroma. In the common form of clinical hyperthyroidism (Graves' disease), the hyperactivity of the gland is not due to TSH excess, however, but reflects the presence of antibodies to the TSH receptor. These thyroid-stimulating immunoglobulins act as agonists at the TSH receptor and are not subject to feedback control by thyroid hormone.

Only 1/3000 of the circulating thyroxine is unbound.

The majority of the T$_4$ and T$_3$ in the plasma is tightly bound to a specific globulin, thyroxine-binding globulin (TBG). The normal total T$_4$ (bound plus free) concentration in plasma is 4–11 μg/dl (50–140 nmol/l) and the ratio, bound T$_4$/free T$_4$, is about 3000:1, giving a normal mean free T$_4$ concentration of approximately 2 ng/dl (25 pmol/l). The normal total T$_3$ concentration in the plasma is 100–150 ng/dl (1.5–2.3 nmol/l) and the ratio, bound T$_3$/free T$_3$, is approximately 300:1, giving a normal mean free T$_3$ concentration of approximately 0.4 ng/dl (6 pmol/l) (The Committee on Nomenclature of the American Thyroid Association, 1987). Thyroid hormones in serum also bind in lesser amounts to albumin and to transthyretin (thyroxine-binding prealbumin or TBPA), a protein migrating as prealbumin on electrophoresis.

Estrogens increase and androgens decrease the amount of TBG produced by the liver. Thus, estrogens increase total serum levels of T_3 and T_4 above normal, whereas androgens have the opposite effect. For example, a woman receiving oral contraceptives transiently increases the fraction of T_4 bound in her plasma, but her hypothalamic-pituitary-thyroid axis then responds to the fall in free hormone concentration by increasing thyroid hormone secretion, restoring free T_4 to normal levels and resulting in an increased *total* plasma T_4 concentration. Therefore, the serum T_4 value would erroneously suggest hyperthyroidism, but this can be excluded either by measuring the free T_4 concentration directly or, more commonly, by obtaining a test that estimates the degree of saturation of TBG. Drugs such as salicylates can compete with thyroid hormone for binding sites on serum-binding proteins, thus also affecting the bound-to-free ratio of hormones.

> Administration of estrogens or androgens can affect total thyroxine concentration in the plasma.

Thyroid hormones undergo extensive biotransformation in the body. Deiodination of the thyronine rings as well as deamination and decarboxylation of the side chain occur, and conjugation of the phenolic hydroxyl with sulfate and glucuronide further expand the known metabolites. Deiodination is an especially important pathway physiologically, because the deiodination of T_4 can either produce the more active substance, T_3 (by 5'-deiodination of the outer ring), or produce the inactive substance, reverse T_3 (by 5-deiodination of the inner ring). Deiodination of the inner ring of T_3 also inactivates it, forming T_2 (see Fig. 39–1). Decreased caloric intake and a variety of drugs can inhibit these deiodinating pathways. Clinically important effects on deiodination have been observed with propylthiouracil, glucocorticoids, and certain iodinated roentgenographic contrast media, such as iopanoate.

> Deiodination can either activate T_4 (by forming T_3) or inactivate it (by forming reverse T_3). Deiodination of T_3 inactivates it (by forming T_2).

The principal source of T_3 in the plasma is not the hormone released from the thyroid, but is T_3 arising from the deiodination of T_4 in the peripheral tissues. Therefore, administration of adequate amounts of exogenous T_4 to a hypothyroid individual can restore not only the plasma T_4 but also the plasma T_3 concentrations to normal levels.

> Normally most of the circulating T_3 is produced by peripheral deiodination of T_4.

The iodide released during deiodination of the hormones in the peripheral tissues returns for the most part to the plasma, where the thyroid gland must compete again for the iodide with its formidable antagonist, the kidney. The thyroid has a normal plasma iodide clearance of about 15 ml/minute, but this value is subject to wide variations and may increase 15-fold in chronic iodine deficiency. This ability to adapt to iodine deficiency gives the thyroid an advantage over the kidney, despite the latter's greater clearance, which does not change from a fairly constant 35 ml/minute.

Although deiodinated metabolites represent the major pathway for eliminating thyroid hormones, some conjugated hormone is excreted in the bile and urine. Inhibitors of deiodination increase the amount of metabolism through this route. Transplacental transfer of thyroid hormones is another, albeit limited, route of elimination in a pregnant woman.

MECHANISMS OF ACTION OF THYROID HORMONE

Thyroid hormone affects most of the tissues in the body and is particularly critical for normal growth and development of the brain. The actions of thyroid hormone are complex, because most of the processes affected are influenced also by energetic substrates, drugs and other hormones, particularly adrenergic agents. (For example, thyroid hormone is required for expression of the uncoupling protein in brown fat that is regulated by norepinephrine in adaptation to cold.) Thyroid hormone also affects several other pathways involving thermogenesis; it increases both lipogenesis and lipolysis, as well as influencing adenosine triphosphatase (ATPase) activities in a variety of tissues.

ACTIONS OF THYROID HORMONES AT THE MOLECULAR LEVEL

There are several different nuclear receptors for thyroid hormone.

Proteins that bind thyroid hormone have been found in the cell nucleus, the cytoplasm, and various cell membranes. Some of this binding probably reflects sites of hormone metabolism, whereas other binding represents specific sites of action. Nuclear thyroid hormone receptors are part of the superfamily of genes that also include receptors for the glucocorticoids, mineralocorticoids, vitamin D, and retinoic acid. These receptor proteins are all characterized by a DNA-binding region that is closely conserved phylogenically, plus a variable amino terminal region that is responsible for the binding of specific hormones. There are several forms of nuclear thyroid hormone receptor, some resulting from alternative mRNA splicing of a gene, whereas others are the products of additional receptor genes. The receptors' affinities for DNA appear to be similar, but their affinities for thyroid hormone are different. Their relative expression appears to vary according to the tissue and the stage of development being studied. The level of thyroid hormone itself can modulate the receptor transcript formed, because the high-affinity form of thyroid hormone receptor found in the rat pituitary displays down-regulation in response to thyroid hormone (Hodin et al, 1989).

Thyroid hormone affects gene transcription, mRNA processing, and stabilization.

Thyroid hormone plays a leading role in regulating the expression of a few tissue-specific genes, such as the TSH gene in the pituitary. Thyroid hormone also plays a supporting role in regulating the expression of numerous housekeeping genes that are required on a day-to-day basis. Thyroid hormone affects at least three different gene-regulatory mechanisms: (1) it interacts with protein receptors that bind to 5′ upstream sequences (so-called thyroid response elements, or TREs), affecting gene expression of tissue-specific genes; (2) it regulates the stability of specific messenger RNAs; and (3) it can affect mRNA transcript-processing of some genes.

Clinical Manifestations of Hyperthyroidism (Thyrotoxicosis)

The typical thyrotoxic patient appears hot, thin, nervous, and short of breath. These symptoms reflect the direct effects of thyroid hormone excess on many organs, plus responses of organs compensating for increased metabolic activity elsewhere in the body. The basal metabolism of many energetic substrates is increased, reflecting increased tissue functions in some instances, and decreased efficiency in others. The flushed skin reflects in part the need to dissipate the increased production of heat. Despite increased appetite (and more frequent defecation), most hyperthyroid patients lose weight. Bone and muscle turnover is increased. Muscle weakness is a common complaint; increased mitochondrial enzyme activity, particularly in the slow muscle fibers, may play a role. The muscle tremor that is also observed frequently can be ameliorated with β-adrenergic blocking drugs. The bounding pulse reflects an increase in cardiac output, in part due to the increased demand for oxygen in peripheral tissues, and possibly to an increased responsiveness to catecholamines (circulating catecholamine levels actually tend to be low). Thyroid hormone levels alter the proportion of β myosin ATPase in ventricular cells, and the basal contractility of cardiac muscles is increased in hyperthyroidism.

Clinical Manifestations of Hypothyroidism (Myxedema)

Hypothyroid patients are generally sluggish, reflecting the hypometabolic state of many organs. They often complain of feeling cold. It should be noted that not all the signs of hypothyroidism are simply the opposite of those observed in hyperthyroidism. For example, hypothyroid patients commonly have a puffy face and doughy skin. This myxedema reflects the mucinous infiltration of connective tissue in many organs and is caused by overproduction of glycosaminoglycans that would be suppressed by normal levels of thyroid hormone. The important effects of thyroid hormone on fetal and neonatal development are discussed later.

Many but not all of the clinical manifestations of hypothyroidism are the opposite of those found in hyperthyroidism.

Levothyroxine Sodium Tablets

Levothyroxine sodium tablets (e.g., SYNTHROID) are the preferred drug and dosage form for the treatment of most patients with hypothyroidism. Levothyroxine sodium is also available in a lyophilized preparation that may be reconstituted for intravenous (IV) or intramuscular (IM) injection when oral therapy is impossible.

Liothyronine Sodium Tablets

Liothyronine sodium tablets (e.g., CYTOMEL) represent the oral dosage form of triiodothyronine. T_3 has approximately three times the potency of T_4. Because of its shorter half-life and higher peak serum levels, T_3 is not used generally for long-term therapy.

Liotrix Tablets

Liotrix tablets contain a mixture of L-thyroxine sodium and liothyronine sodium in a 4:1 ratio. Although this combination has a theoretical advantage because it more closely simulates endogenous thyroidal production of thyroid hormones, liotrix has not been shown to have a significant clinical advantage over levothyroxine sodium alone. Preparations containing thyroglobulin, e.g., thyroid tablets (also termed *desiccated thyroid*) or pure thyroglobulin tablets, contain a variable amount of thyroid hormones requiring chemical and biological standardization; they are no longer recommended.

ABSORPTION AND ELIMINATION

When thyroid hormones are given by mouth for replacement therapy, bioavailability can vary somewhat among preparations, but a reasonable approximation is 70%. Absorption is reduced if resins like cholestyramine are also being administered. After absorption from the gut, the fate of exogenous thyroid hormones is similar to that of endogenous hormones. After administration of a single dose of thyroxine to a severely hypothyroid patient, the onset of such clinically observable metabolic effects as increased body temperature, heart rate, and warmth of the skin is slow and does not reach maximum for 7–10 days after administration. Even IV administration does not substantially reduce the lag in these effects. If

Preparations for the Treatment of Hypothyroidism

maintenance thyroxine therapy is discontinued abruptly in a hypothyroid patient the former hypometabolic state reappears gradually, a situation that can mislead the patient into thinking the disease is cured. Thyroxine disappears from the blood with a half-life of about 1 week, but the half-life of clinical effects, reflecting what is happening in the tissues, is closer to 2 weeks. Because T_4 is converted in the peripheral tissues to T_3, it is not surprising that administration of the latter hormone has a more rapid onset of effect. The peak effect of a single dose of T_3 occurs about 2 days after administration, and the disappearance of effect has a half-life of about a week.

Clinical Use. Thyroid hormones have therapeutic, prophylactic, and diagnostic uses. The therapeutic uses include replacement and suppressive therapy.

Replacement Therapy. Treatment of severe long-standing hypothyroidism should be initiated usually with small dosages, e.g., 25 μg of levothyroxine by mouth daily, with increments of 25 μg every 2–3 weeks until the proper maintenance dosage is reached (usually in the range of 100–250 μg daily; there is wide individual variability). The metabolic status of a patient receiving exogenous thyroid hormone greatly influences the response; a severely hypothyroid patient, abruptly given a full replacement dose of hormone, may suffer the onset or worsening of heart failure or even acute myocardial infarction. Even if severe consequences do not ensue, the patient may feel worse initially rather than better after such abrupt therapy. Elderly patients may require very cautious initiation of therapy, e.g., 12.5 μg/day, although, as in other patients, consideration must be given also to the dangers of undertreated hypothyroidism.

> Abrupt administration of a full replacement dose of thyroid hormone may precipitate cardiac complications in hypothyroid patients.

Some patients, once euthyroid, can tolerate a much larger dosage of hormone than they could when hypothyroidism was present. This tolerance could occur because any drug eliminated by first-order kinetics has, by definition, an increased rate of elimination when there is increased concentration in the compartment from which elimination takes place. However, an additional factor for thyroid hormone is its ability to increase many metabolic processes, including those controlling its own absorption and biotransformation. Certain disorders, e.g., angina and adrenal cortical insufficiency, may be partially alleviated by hypothyroidism and thus be exacerbated by thyroid hormone replacement therapy unless the other disorders are recognized and treated. Cautious administration of thyroid hormone to a hypothyroid patient with angina may improve his or her well-being without increasing the angina if cardiac function improves, but careful adjustment of the antianginal medications is usually necessary (see Chapter 36). Giving thyroid hormone therapy *before* initiating adrenal cortical hormone replacement in a patient suffering from a combined deficiency of the adrenal and thyroid can precipitate a life-threatening crisis of adrenal insufficiency. In such patients it is essential to treat the adrenal insufficiency first, before initiating thyroid hormone replacement.

> If adrenal insufficiency exists, it should be treated before giving thyroid replacement.

Replacement therapy generally needs to be lifelong except for treatment of the transient hypothyroidism that can occur with subacute thyroiditis. Every patient receiving replacement therapy should be checked periodically to make sure that the serum TSH level (by an ultrasensitive assay) is in the normal range, because requirements for hormone can change without obvious changes in clinical symptomatology.

There are two special situations in which replacement therapy should be vigorous from the onset. In congenital hypothyroidism (cretinism) the child is born already suffering from the effects of intrauterine deprivation of thyroid hormone. The normal fetus depends on his or her own thyroid

> Aggressive treatment of neonatal hypothyroidism is important.

function during the latter part of gestation to maintain euthyroidism. If this function is absent, transplacental passage of thyroid hormone from a euthyroid mother only partly compensates for this deficit (Vulma et al, 1989). Thus, a hypothyroid fetus suffers significant retardation of brain and bone development during gestation and is, of course, totally deprived of the maternal supply of hormone after birth. Therefore, it is essential to diagnose hypothyroidism immediately after birth. Although neonatal hypothyroidism is fairly uncommon (1 : 4000), it represents a situation in which prompt neonatal therapy may prevent a lifelong disaster. Screening of all newborns by measuring T_4 concentration in an eluate of blood spots on filter paper is emphatically recommended. If the T_4 concentration is below normal, further studies, including TSH determinations, should be performed. Therapy of neonatal hypothyroidism should be initiated at once, with frequent readjustment of the dosage on the basis of careful clinical monitoring. Generally a child receives approximately one half the adult dosage by the age of 1 year. Immediate postnatal therapy greatly increases the likelihood of satisfactory mental development. If treatment is delayed, normal physical development may still occur but complete mental development may not be achieved and full replacement therapy can precipitate behavioral problems.

A second indication for rapid initial treatment is the rare condition of myxedema coma. Here, despite the attendant risk, initial IV therapy with a high dosage of L-thyroxine or triiodothyronine is indicated (e.g., 150–500 μg of sodium levothyroxine), together with therapy for accompanying problems such as infection and electrolyte disturbances. Because of its faster onset of effect, triiodothyronine might be theoretically preferable to thyroxine in the treatment of myxedema coma, but clear clinical evidence of such an advantage is lacking.

> In myxedema coma the risk of giving abrupt replacement therapy must be accepted.

The use of thyroid hormone to treat obesity, sluggishness, and other ill-defined complaints in patients who are *not* hypothyroid is neither safe nor effective and should not be condoned.

Suppressive Therapy. Even with an adequate intake of iodine, some individuals, especially women during late adolescence or pregnancy, develop goiters, possibly as the combined result of an increased demand for thyroid hormone and a mild intrathyroidal metabolic defect or subclinical thyroiditis. If goiter has only been present for a short time, the gland usually returns to normal size when the patient is given exogenous thyroid hormone in dosages adequate to suppress TSH secretion. Long-standing goiters and those with an element of non–TSH-dependent enlargement are not likely to return to normal size with suppressive therapy, particularly if they have developed fibrosis and calcification.

> Suppression of TSH by thyroid hormone can be clinically useful.

Suppressive therapy for euthyroid patients who have a thyroid nodule is controversial. Administration of thyroid hormone for 3–6 months may cause a benign nodule to regress, whereas a malignant nodule is not likely to do so. However, such a clinical test does not distinguish unequivocally between the two, and a trial of suppressive therapy should not be allowed to delay other tests for possible malignancy, e.g., fine needle aspiration biopsy.

Prophylactic Use. If a benign goiter in a euthyroid patient has become so large that it requires subtotal thyroidectomy, the postoperative thyroid tissue still may be subject to the same factors that initially caused the goiter to grow. To decrease the chance of recurrence due to TSH stimulation, some physicians believe lifelong thyroid replacement therapy is advisable.

Diagnostic Use. Occasionally it is difficult to distinguish between the nervous individual whose thyroid function test results are at the upper limit of normal and the moderately hyperthyroid individual with Graves' disease. One diagnostic approach that is still used occasionally is the administration of large doses of exogenous liothyronine for several days. This does not decrease thyroid function in Graves' disease, because TSH secretion has already been suppressed by the excessive thyroid hormone secreted by the now autonomous gland. Therefore, thyroid function tests such as radioiodine uptake are not depressed. In contrast, a euthyroid individual with a relatively high radioiodine uptake shows a significant decrease in uptake after several days' administration of exogenous hormone. The need to give large doses of thyroid hormone makes this test risky in patients with poor cardiac status.

Adverse Effects. Because most of the abnormalities observed in the neuromuscular, cardiovascular, and gastrointestinal (GI) systems of a hyperthyroid patient are the result of an endogenous overdose of thyroid hormone, the administration of excessive doses of exogenous thyroid hormone produces similar effects. The danger of too rapid conversion of a severely hypothyroid patient to euthyroidism and the need for special caution when hypothyroidism is accompanied by certain other conditions, e.g., angina, are discussed earlier. Chronic overreplacement, even with a dose that causes no obvious thyrotoxic symptoms, can still be hazardous, because its long-term effects may include early epiphyseal closure in children and osteoporosis in adults.

Drugs Used in the Treatment of Hyperthyroidism (Antithyroid Drugs)

HISTORY

Although the administration of iodine to patients who are already hyperthyroid would appear to be irrational, Plummer (1923) reported good results with iodine used as an adjunct to surgical treatment of their thyrotoxicosis. Preoperative iodine therapy became standard practice and undoubtedly increased the safety of thyroid surgery. A major advance in medical therapy occurred in 1943 after animal studies had shown that certain thioureylenes interfere with the synthesis of thyroid hormone, when Astwood introduced thioureylene drugs for the treatment of hyperthyroidism.

INHIBITORY EFFECTS OF VARIOUS COMPOUNDS ON THE THYROID GLAND

Various drugs interfere with one or more steps in the formation and secretion of thyroid hormones by the gland. Thiocyanate and perchlorate ions interfere with the first, iodide-trapping step of hormonogenesis. Their toxicity makes them unsuitable for chronic administration, although perchlorate is useful occasionally in determining that a diseased thyroid is capable of concentrating iodide but cannot organify it (the perchlorate flush test). Thioureylenes, which inhibit the organification step, are the major antithyroid drugs. Several other drugs, e.g., aminoglutethimide, phenylbutazone and some sulfonamides, have a weak effect on this step, but their effects are neither strong nor reliable enough to make them clinically useful in hyperthyroidism. Although some iodine intake is critical for the formation of thyroid hormones, large doses of iodine inhibit formation of iodotyrosines temporarily (the Wolff-Chaikoff effect). This response provides an intrinsic homeostatic mechanism that avoids overproduction of hormone. Both iodide and lithium ions also inhibit the secretion of the hormones from the gland (Wartofsky et al, 1970; Spaulding et al, 1972). The way in which either ion exerts this effect is unknown, but apparently the hyperthyroid gland is more sensitive to the inhibiting effect of these ions than the normal gland. Lithium is not recommended for routine therapy, because of both its narrow therapeutic/toxic ratio and its lesser efficacy. The therapeutic use of iodine is discussed later.

THIOUREYLENE DRUGS

The thioureylene (thionamide) drugs (Fig. 39–2) are the antithyroid drugs of choice. Their most important mechanism of action is interference with the second stage of thyroid hormone formation, i.e., the mono- and diiodination of tyrosyl residues (so-called organification of iodine). Iodine in its reduced form, i.e., the iodide ion, does not react with tyrosine to form iodotyrosines. It is generally believed that the peroxidase that catalyses the iodination of tyrosines in the thyroid gland does so by oxidizing the iodide ion to some more reactive form, which then can form iodotyrosines. The thioureylene drugs interfere with this process in some still uncertain way. Thioureylenes also interfere with the third, coupling step in thyroid hormone synthesis. In the peripheral tissues, propylthiouracil has an additional antithyroid effect: it inhibits the conversion of thyroxine to triiodothyronine by inhibiting certain deiodinases. Methimazole does not have this effect. Thioureylenes also may affect thyroid immunoregulatory mechanisms.

> The most important effect of thioureylene drugs is to block the organification of iodide in the thyroid gland.

Preparations

Propylthiouracil Tablets. Propylthiouracil (PTU) is well absorbed after oral administration and is widely distributed in body tissues. Of special interest is its accumulation in the thyroid gland. Although the drug's half-life in the plasma is only about 1.5 hours, the effect on the thyroid gland lasts longer. The usual schedule of administration is three to four times per day. Propylthiouracil is metabolized extensively; its metabolites (of which the glucuronide is the most important) together with a small amount of the parent drug are excreted in the urine. Transplacental transfer of propylthiouracil and its excretion in breast milk are discussed later.

Methimazole Tablets (TAPAZOLE). This drug is also well absorbed, is widely distributed in body tissues, and accumulates in the thyroid gland. Its plasma half-life is 4–9 hours but its effect on the thyroid gland lasts longer. Nevertheless, methimazole is commonly administered on a schedule of three times per day. Metabolites of methimazole plus a small amount of parent drug appear in the urine. Transplacental transfer of methimazole and its excretion in breast milk is discussed later.

Carbimazole, which is commonly used abroad for the treatment of hyperthyroidism, is rapidly and almost completely converted to methimazole in humans; its subsequent fate in the body is the same as that of methimazole.

Clinical Use of Thioureylene Drugs. The sole established clinical indication for these drugs is the treatment of hyperthyroidism. There are three

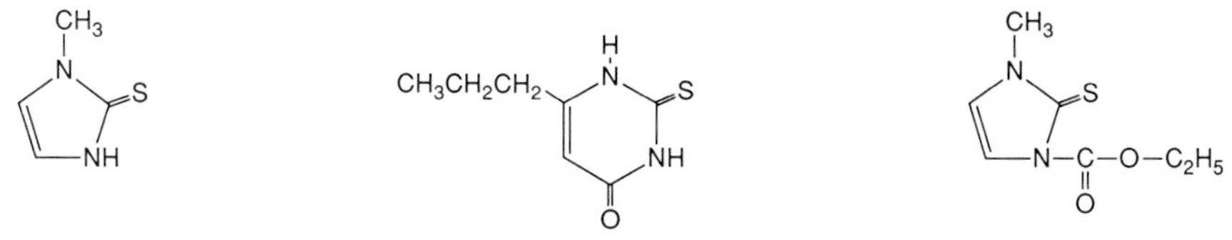

Methimazole   Propylthiouracil   Carbimazole

Figure 39–2
Thioureylene drugs in clinical use.

possible therapeutic strategies for treating hyperthyroidism, and the role of the thioureylene drug depends upon the strategy chosen.

In the Most Common Approach, the Drug Plays the Central Role. It is given in full dosages (e.g., 200 mg propylthiouracil three times daily) until euthyroidism is established. The intrathyroidal block of hormone synthesis produced by the drugs does not prevent any hormone already present in the gland from being secreted and does not cancel the effect of hormone already in the blood and peripheral tissues at the time treatment began. Therefore, the patient becomes euthyroid only gradually, usually over a 1–2-month period. Although the previously noted inhibitory effect of propylthiouracil, but not methimazole, on the conversion of T_4 to T_3 in the periphery gives the former drug a theoretical advantage of faster effect, there is no good evidence for a clinically significant difference between the two drugs in this respect. After euthyroidism is induced, the dosage of the drug needs to be adjusted (e.g., 50–100 mg propylthiouracil two to four times daily) to maintain the euthyroid state. The maintenance dose is usually lower than the initial dose, once the patient is euthyroid; if the initial dose were continued, the patient would gradually become hypothyroid.

At the conclusion of treatment (generally 1–2 years), the drug is discontinued and the patient observed at regular intervals. Such therapy avoids surgery and does not entail exposure to radiation, but a significant number of patients relapse after drug therapy is discontinued. The reported percentage of patients achieving a permanent remission with such therapy varies widely in different published series, ranging from 14% (Wartofsky, 1973) to 76% (Slingerland and Burrows, 1979). If this type of therapy is elected, both patient and physician must be prepared to commit a considerable length of time to it, because most thyroidologists believe that shortening the course of therapy to a period of only a few months increases the likelihood of relapse. Patients who relapse require retreatment, either with the drug or, more commonly, by one of the other modalities.

Because the thioureylene drugs simply interfere with the formation and utilization of thyroid hormone, the intriguing question is not why some patients relapse after treatment stops, but rather why any patients remain in permanent remission. The answer seems to lie in the autoimmune nature of Graves' disease. One suggestion is that an organ-specific defect in suppressor T cells occurs in Graves' disease and that hyperthyroidism itself has an adverse affect on suppressor T-cell function, thus creating a vicious circle that is broken by restoring euthyroidism. Another possible explanation is that gradual development of chronic thyroiditis may be a common spontaneous event in longstanding Graves' disease, leading not only to euthyroidism but often to eventual hypothyroidism. Some believe that partial ablative treatment by surgery or radioactive iodine may unmask and accelerate this process (Wood and Ingbar, 1979).

If Surgical Removal of Most of the Hyperfunctioning Thyroid Is the Treatment Strategy Chosen, the Patient Should Still Be Rendered Euthyroid Before the Operation Takes Place. Any stress, especially the stress of surgery, in a hyperthyroid patient may precipitate an alarming and potentially fatal exacerbation of the hyperthyroid state, the so-called thyroid crisis or thyroid storm. Therefore a hyperthyroid patient for whom surgical treatment is planned should still be treated with a thioureylene drug until euthyroidism is achieved and surgery can be performed safely. However, if a hyperthyroid patient develops a pressing indication for emergency surgery (e.g., acute appendicitis), and it is impossible to wait until euthyroid-

The dose of the thioureylene must be adjusted periodically as hyperthyroidism comes under control.

Many patients treated solely by a thioureylene drug relapse after treatment stops.

Uncontrolled hyperthyroidism increases the risk of surgery.

ism is achieved, use of a β-adrenergic blocking drug and of iodide are rational measures to decrease the risk of thyroid crisis. Corticosteroid drugs may be also useful in preparing a hyperthyroid patient for surgery. The availability of these drugs for the occasional emergency situation should not, however, lure physicians away from the prudent course of delaying elective surgery until a hyperthyroid patient becomes euthyroid.

If the Primary Treatment Strategy Is Radioactive Iodine (RAI), Thioureylenes Are Less Routinely Administered Before Treatment. Some physicians do control hyperthyroid patients with a thioureylene drug initially, even if RAI is planned as the definitive treatment. This approach has special merit if a patient is severely thyrotoxic or if there is significant cardiovascular disease, to avoid the temporary exacerbation of thyrotoxicosis that sometimes follows administration of radioiodine.

If a thioureylene has been used prior to administration of radioiodine, the thioureylene drug must be discontinued several days before administration of the radioiodine, in order to permit incorporation of the latter into hormones in the gland. If incorporation were blocked by the presence of the thioureylene, the radioiodine would leave the thyroid quickly, and the usual dose would be insufficient. The radioisotope of iodine used in treatment is iodine-131 (^{131}I). In contrast to surgical treatment of thyrotoxicosis, the antithyroid effect of the radiation on the thyroid gland is not immediate, and several months may elapse before a euthyroid state is reached. Because of this additional delay, some physicians administer radioactive iodine to mildly or moderately thyrotoxic patients without spending time on prior administration of a thioureylene drug. If this plan is used, some physicians subsequently institute therapy with a thioureylene drug, beginning 1 or 2 weeks *after* administration of the radioiodine in order to make the patient euthyroid somewhat more quickly. Once the radiation has had time to exert its effect, the thioureylene drug is discontinued. However, even though the drug effect is more rapid than the radiation effect, the former takes a number of weeks before euthyroidism is achieved in most patients, so the use of a thioureylene drug as a temporary measure after radioiodine has not been adopted routinely.

Successful treatment of Graves' disease by any modality relieves those clinical features, e.g., nervousness, tachycardia, heart intolerance, that result from excessive secretion of thyroid hormone. However, certain manifestations of Graves' disease, particularly some eye signs, are not the result of high tissue hormone levels but are independent immunological manifestations of the disease. Therefore treatment of the hyperthyroidism does not have predictable effects on these other manifestations of Graves' disease, and exophthalmos, for example, may diminish, remain stationary, or grow worse when the patient is made euthyroid.

Adverse Effects of Thioureylene Drugs and Contraindications

Allergic reactions, most commonly skin rash and pruritus, may occur. Less commonly one or more components of the serum sickness syndrome, i.e., fever, arthritis, lymphadenopathy or peripheral neuropathy, may occur. Other serious disorders occasionally attributable to these drugs include thrombocytopenia, jaundice, polyarteritis nodosa, and systemic lupus erythematosus. A rare effect is hypoprothrombinemia severe enough to cause dangerous bleeding.

The effect of these drugs on the white blood cells deserves special mention. A modest leukopenia, e.g., to about 4000 white cells/cu mm in

Rarely, agranulocytosis may occur during thioureylene therapy.

the peripheral blood, is common. However, occasional patients suffer the life-threatening complication of agranulocytosis, with a precipitous drop in the white blood count and virtual disappearance of all granulocytes. As this reaction may occur without warning, routine serial white blood counts offer little protection. Patients receiving thioureylene drugs should be instructed to report immediately to their physician the onset of severe pharyngitis or any other infection that suggests sudden loss of white cell defenses. The incidence of minor toxic effects, chiefly skin rashes, is about 3% with propylthiouracil and about 5% with methimazole. Major adverse effects (chiefly but not exclusively agranulocytosis) have an incidence of approximately 0.3% with either drug.

Prolonged use of these drugs without periodic monitoring of serum T_4 or TSH levels, or both, may result in hypothyroidism, which is reversible on discontinuation of the drug.

A thioureylene drug should not be given to a patient known to be allergic to that drug. A patient allergic to one thioureylene compound does not inevitably suffer a cross-reaction to another such compound, but the risk of a cross-reaction is high enough to make it undesirable to prescribe, for example, methimazole in a patient who has already suffered a significant allergic reaction to propylthiouracil, unless there is a pressing indication for continuing antithyroid drug treatment. In particular, it is dangerous to reinstitute any thioureylene therapy in a patient who has suffered an episode of agranulocytosis caused by a thioureylene drug.

Propylthiouracil is not contraindicated in pregnancy but special precautions must be taken in treating a pregnant hyperthyroid woman.

These drugs are not contraindicated in a hyperthyroid pregnant woman, but care must be taken to use the lowest dose that will maintain euthyroidism. Note that pregnancy itself alters certain indicators of thyroid function and often provides a temporary amelioration of the hyperthyroid state. Propylthiouracil crosses the placenta less than methimazole and is generally preferred in the treatment of hyperthyroidism in pregnancy. To lessen the risk of hypothyroidism and goiter in the newborn infant still further, the thioureylene drug should be discontinued shortly before the expected delivery date. With this regimen, the risks of neonatal hypothyroidism or obstruction of the newborn's trachea by a goiter are low, but prompt clinical and biochemical examination of the thyroid status of a newborn is still indicated whenever the mother has received any treatment for hyperthyroidism during pregnancy. Neonatal hyperthyroidism, although rare, must always be kept in mind as a possibility in an infant born of a mother who has ever had Graves' disease, whether she is thyrotoxic at the time of delivery or not. Although elevated thyroxine levels in the blood of thyrotoxic mothers increase transplacental thyroxine transfer (Carr et al, 1959), it is probably the transplacental passage of thyroid-stimulating immunoglobulins that determines whether the infant of a mother with Graves' disease will be thyrotoxic or not, rather than the transfer of thyroxine. If the mother has been receiving thioureylene treatment during pregnancy, neonatal thyrotoxicosis may not become clinically evident for several days, when the antithyroid medication but *not* the maternal thyroid-stimulating antibodies have disappeared from the infant's circulation. The treatment of neonatal thyrotoxicosis is discussed later. Nursing mothers should probably not receive thioureylene drugs. If it is essential to administer a thioureylene drug to a nursing mother, propylthiouracil may be preferable to methimazole because of lesser excretion in the milk.

IODIDE

Iodine is readily absorbed from the gut. If ingested as the iodide ion, it is absorbed as such, whereas ingested iodate or elemental iodine is reduced in the gut and enters the blood as iodide. The administration of iodine can produce several markedly different effects on the thyroid gland. Depending on the circumstances, iodine may (1) *prevent goiter and hypothyroidism* in areas of dietary iodine deficiency, (2) *precipitate hyperthyroidism* in occasional euthyroid individuals, (3) *cause goiter and even hypothyroidism* in occasional euthyroid individuals, or (4) *restore euthyroidism* in hyperthyroid patients.

Stable iodine (^{127}I) has divergent effects on the thyroid gland.

Prevention of Goiter and Hypothyroidism

Iodine is in low abundance on the surface of the earth when compared with many other biologically essential elements. Thus, the thyroid gland's ability to take up iodide and store thyroid hormone is critical for its ability to maintain euthyroidism. Chronic deficiency in dietary iodine intake can lead to hypothyroidism, expressed in its most severe form as endemic cretinism. Supplementing the dietary supply of iodine, e.g., by providing iodized salt, is important prophylaxis in areas of the world where the iodine content of food and water is low; otherwise the overworked thyroid gland enlarges and some individuals develop goitrous hypothyroidism. In other individuals compensatory enlargement of the thyroid gland may maintain the euthyroid state if the iodine deficiency is not too severe, because the thyroid becomes substantially more efficient in uptake of iodide ion from the blood.

A chronic dietary deficit in iodine can cause hypothyroidism, including cretinism.

Precipitation of Hyperthyroidism

Occasionally hyperthyroidism occurs following administration of iodine to a previously euthyroid but iodine-deficient patient (Iod Basedow). Replenishment of dietary iodine normally reverses the compensatory increase in the avidity of the gland for iodine, but an occasional patient's thyroid may fail to decrease the activity of the iodide pump after the iodine supply becomes plentiful. This phenomenon was noted almost immediately after Coindet used iodide for goiter in Geneva in 1820, and administration of iodine to goitrous individuals remained controversial thereafter owing to the occasional development of hyperthyroidism. Marine and Kimball's (1921) population studies in Akron, where they gave a small dose of iodine to goiter-prone school children, demonstrated its clear efficacy against endemic goiter. Nonetheless, introduction of iodine for prophylaxis of endemic goiter in various countries has been followed consistently by an increase in the incidence of hyperthyroidism for a few years subsequently.

Administration of iodine to iodine-deficient patients can sometimes induce hyperthyroidism.

In the Western world, chronic exposure to excessive amounts of iodine may become a more significant problem than sporadic iodine deficiency. The ability of the normal thyroid to defend itself against excessive concentrations of iodine by inhibiting formation and release of thyroid hormones enables most individuals to remain euthyroid even after receiving large amounts of inorganic iodine (e.g., in cough mixtures) or of organic iodine (e.g., in x-ray contrast media or in drugs such as amiodarone, which contains 49% iodine). However, a small but significant number of individuals may respond to iodine excess by developing hyperthyroidism. Thus, the control mechanisms for thyroid hormone synthesis, although adequate for most situations, may be overcome occasionally by oversupply of iodine to some patients with no previously known thyroid abnormality.

Occurrence of Goiter and Hypothyroidism

The most surprising of iodine's effects, however, is the occurrence of *hypothyroidism* in some patients receiving excessive amounts of iodine, an effect particularly common in patients with thyroiditis. Here, in contrast to the

Iodine can cause hypothyroidism, particularly in patients with thyroiditis.

euthyroid individual who responds to iodine with hyperthyroidism, an occasional euthyroid individual is *too* sensitive to the inhibitory effects of iodine and cannot escape from the Wolff-Chaikoff effect. In such individuals, the interference with thyroid hormone formation and secretion first causes compensatory enlargement of the thyroid gland (iodide goiter) and may eventually lead to hypothyroidism. The treatment is simple once the cause is recognized: discontinue the offending source of iodide.

Large amounts of iodide, if given to a pregnant woman, create a risk of neonatal goiter.

Restoration of Euthyroidism

The inhibitory effect of iodine on thyroid hormone secretion is much more reliable and dramatic in hyperthyroid than in euthyroid individuals, and occurs with much lower dosages of iodine in the former. Therefore, iodine may be used as adjunctive short-term therapy of hyperthyroidism in selected circumstances.

Preparations

Potassium Iodide Solution (Saturated Solution of KI, or SSKI) contains 1 g of potassium iodide/ml.

Sodium Iodide is available in bulk. In the treatment of a thyroid crisis, sodium iodide may be dissolved, sterilized, and administered IV starting 1 hour after thioureylene therapy has begun. However, the effect of iodine in thyrotoxicosis is still not rapid enough to give the IV route any striking advantage if the oral route is available in this situation.

Strong Iodine Solution (LUGOL'S SOLUTION) contains elemental iodine (5%) and potassium iodide (10%).

Clinical Use of Stable (Nonradioactive) Iodine (Iodine-127) in Treatment of Hyperthyroidism

Iodine is not recommended as a sole treatment of thyrotoxicosis. Whereas thioureylenes eventually convert the hypermetabolic state of most thyrotoxic patients to a completely euthyroid state, the effect of iodine on thyrotoxic patients is usually transient and incomplete. Even if rendered fully euthyroid by iodine, a thyrotoxic patient may "escape" from its inhibitory effect if long-term iodine therapy is attempted. In certain pressing circumstances, however, it is important to take advantage of the effect of iodine in thyrotoxicosis, which usually begins within 24 hours and reaches its maximum in about 10–14 days. Even though not immediate, this is a more rapid effect than the thioureylene drugs produce and therefore is useful in emergencies. One such emergency is the aforementioned thyroid crisis, in which a hyperthyroid patient develops hyperthermia and sometimes cardiovascular collapse. This poorly understood phenomenon may result from stress, such as an intercurrent illness, and is not simply due to high levels of thyroid hormone *per se*. Even in this situation, thioureylene therapy should be instituted about 1 hour before the first dose of iodine is administered. (If iodine were to be given before the first dose of thioureylene drug, the thyroid gland would avidly incorporate the iodine into thyroid hormones, because it is usually iodine-depleted. Once present in thyroglobulin, the iodine is beyond the reach of the thioureylene's blocking effect on hormone synthesis.)

Even the effect of iodine is not rapid enough to be completely satisfactory in the management of thyroid crisis. Patients whose symptoms of

In treatment of a thyroid crisis, iodide should be administered shortly *after* giving a thioureylene. A glucocorticoid and a β-adrenergic blocking drug should be administered also.

thyrotoxicosis are so severe that the combined thioureylene/iodine regimen described here is necessary must be treated also with other adjunctive measures, including a β-adrenergic blocking drug such as propranolol to control the tachycardia and a glucocorticoid drug. Both the glucocorticoid and propylthiouracil (but not methimazole) have the additional effect of inhibiting, at least partially, the conversion of T_4 to T_3.

Neonatal thyrotoxicosis represents another emergency situation in which administration of propylthiouracil, followed by iodine, may be indicated. Adjunctive measures include propranolol and careful attention to nutrition and fluid balance, which are important in all thyrotoxic patients but are critical issues in these severely ill infants. Neonatal thyrotoxicosis is fortunately self-limited and, if death is prevented, the infant usually becomes euthyroid and requires no further treatment after several weeks, when the maternal thyroid-stimulating immunoglobulins have disappeared.

Iodine has still another effect on the thyroid gland that can be put to beneficial use. Iodine administration causes the hyperplastic, highly vascular, colloid-depleted thyroid gland of Graves' disease to undergo involution, i.e., to become somewhat less hyperplastic and vascular, and to accumulate more colloid. The thioureylene drugs, on the other hand, apparently do not have such a direct effect on vascularity. If surgery is elected as the treatment for a case of thyrotoxicosis, the marked vascularity of the Graves' disease gland can increase the difficulty and danger of the operation. Therefore, administration of iodine for 7–10 days before subtotal thyroidectomy is an important adjunct to thioureylene therapy; although the latter drug prevents iodine incorporation into hormone, it does not appear to prevent the iodine from decreasing the vascularity of the gland.

Iodine is often used as a preoperative adjuvant in Graves' disease.

Individuals who have been exposed to massive amounts of radionuclides after nuclear reactor accidents such as that occurring at Chernobyl, U.S.S.R., in 1986 are exposed, *inter alia*, to variable amounts of radioactive iodine. If stable iodine is administered soon after such exposure, the stable iodine lowers the specific activity of the iodide pool in the patient's body and decreases the net thyroidal uptake of radioactive iodine. Thus, both the absorbed radiation dose to the thyroid gland and the duration of stay of radioactive iodine in the body are decreased. The American Thyroid Association has recommended that sodium iodide be given to individuals exposed to radioactive iodine in the event of a reactor accident if the individual's thyroid exposure is expected to be 100 rads (1 Gy) or more; for children and pregnant women the recommended action level is 50 rads (0.5 Gy). It is now known that thyroid exposure in countries other than the western Soviet Union was generally below 0.01 Gy as a result of the Chernobyl accident, but this was unclear at the time. Uncertainty forced health authorities in nearby countries to decide on a course of action before the magnitude of exposure was known. In Poland the decision was made to administer a single dose of Strong Iodine Solution to all individuals up to the age of 17.

Administration of stable iodide reduces the thyroidal uptake of radioiodine.

Adverse Effects

Adverse effects of iodine are not uncommon. In the past, when iodide preparations were used much more commonly (and less rationally) for a variety of diseases, a number of patients developed skin reactions (iododerma) and, rarely, even exfoliative dermatitis. Other reactions, including angioedema, vasculitis and drug fever, have been reported. The iodide ion is secreted into tears, saliva, gastric juice, and bronchial secretions and it is sometimes employed as an expectorant. In some individuals, iodine provokes the syndrome termed *iodism* with irritation of the eyes, nose, and throat and symptoms resembling a bad cold, as well as an unpleasant taste in the mouth; GI and respiratory symptoms are also possible.

Adverse effects of organic iodine-containing compounds used as roentgenographic contrast media are discussed in Chapter 6.

RADIOACTIVE ISOTOPES OF IODINE (RADIOIODINE)

Iodine-131 has a physical half-life of 8 days. It is accumulated by the thyroid gland in the same manner as stable iodine. Iodine-131 emits both β particles and γ rays; the β particles provide about 90% of the absorbed radiation dose to the thyroid gland from this isotope, whereas the more penetrating γ radiation of ^{131}I is useful in permitting external detection, i.e., for diagnostic uptake studies and thyroid scans. However, a different isotope, ^{123}I, which has a half-life of 13 hours and which subjects the thyroid (and total body) to less radiation, is the isotope of choice for clinical *diagnostic* tests of thyroidal iodine metabolism. The therapeutic indications for ^{131}I are carcinoma of the thyroid gland and hyperthyroidism.

If a thyroid carcinoma retains the ability to concentrate iodide, ^{131}I therapy is useful.

In the treatment of thyroid carcinoma it is generally advisable to begin surgically with as complete a thyroidectomy as possible (including removal of the largest possible amount of the neoplasm itself), creating a temporary hypothyroid state. The consequent increase in TSH secretion then stimulates iodine uptake by the remaining tissue, both normal and neoplastic, provided the latter is differentiated sufficiently to concentrate iodine. If a subsequent thyroid scintigram shows evidence of persisting thyroid malignancy or residual uptake in the normal thyroid bed, a large therapeutic dose, up to 200 mCi (7.4 GBq), is then given. After an appropriate interval, e.g., several days to a week, the patient's hypothyroid state is relieved by administration of replacement doses of thyroid hormone. For a detailed discussion of such management, including the times when additional treatment with ^{131}I is indicated, specialized texts should be consulted. Immediate adverse effects may include manifestations of acute radiation sickness, including nausea, salivary and nonsalivary gland neck pain, and transient marrow suppression. As the iodide ion is excreted in the urine, pooling of urine in a cystocele or delayed emptying of the bladder because of outlet obstruction must be prevented to avoid radiation cystitis. Care must be taken in disposing of any vomitus, because I$^-$ is also secreted by the salivary glands and the gastric mucosa. Long-term adverse effects are related to the amount of whole body irradiation received, but in those patients whose thyroid carcinoma takes up significant amounts of radioiodine, the benefit of treating the thyroid cancer outweighs the risks of leukemia, because even distant metastases may be ablated in such patients. When extensive pulmonary metastases are treated repeatedly with large dosages of ^{131}I, pulmonary fibrosis results occasionally.

Administration of radioactive iodine (^{131}I) is an effective treatment of hyperthyroidism.

The doses of radioiodine used for the treatment of hyperthyroidism are much smaller, generally in the range of 10–20 mCi (370–740 MBq) depending upon the percent of administered dose taken up by the individual patient's thyroid gland and the size of the gland. The patient should understand that radioiodine therapy is likely to render her or him hypothyroid sometime in the future. If the first dosage proves insufficient and retreatment is necessary, the subsequent dosage must be readjusted, because both the uptake of iodine and the gland's sensitivity to the radiation are likely to be lower than at the time of the first dosage.

Adverse effects can include radiation thyroiditis, which is seldom severe, and a temporary exacerbation of hyperthyroidism after administration of the ^{131}I, which is caused by increased efflux of thyroid hormones from the radiation-damaged gland. In patients with concomitant coronary artery disease, cardiac complications may be lessened by concurrent administration of a β-adrenergic blocking drug.

The possible risk of developing leukemia or thyroid cancer as late effects of radioiodine treatment of thyrotoxicosis has been reviewed extensively. A follow-up study in which 22,000 patients who had received ^{131}I treatment for hyperthyroidism were compared with 14,000 whose hyperthyroidism had been treated surgically or with antithyroid drugs showed that the ^{131}I-treated patients had no significant increase in the incidence of leukemia above that occurring in Graves' disease given other forms of therapy (Saenger et al, 1968). Similarly, there is no good evidence that the treatment of hyperthyroidism with ^{131}I significantly increases the risk of subsequent development of thyroid cancer. ^{131}I therapy is less commonly administered to children or to women planning to become pregnant soon, in view of the small amount of data thus far available concerning possible genetic risks in these groups.

> The incidence of thyroid cancer and leukemia in Graves' disease has not been increased by ^{131}I therapy.

Hypothyroidism develops at about an equal rate during the first post-treatment year in patients treated surgically and those treated with ^{131}I, but in subsequent years the incidence of hypothyroidism in patients who were treated with ^{131}I steadily increases when compared with the incidence in those who received surgical treatment (Sridama et al, 1984) (Fig. 39–3). A suggested explanation for the steady increase in hypothyroidism years after ^{131}I therapy is that subtle radiation effects on thyroid cells, resulting in eventual cell death, may not become important until many cell divisions have occurred. In contrast, surgical damage to thyroid tissue is more likely to lead to prompt death of the damaged cells.

> Most hyperthyroid patients treated with ^{131}I eventually become hypothyroid.

Radioiodine therapy is usually the preferred treatment for adult hyperthyroid patients and for those who are poor surgical risks or who have recurrent hyperthyroidism after previous surgical treatment. Radioiodine therapy is indicated also for hyperthyroid patients who have relapsed after antithyroid drug therapy or (rarely) who have failed to achieve euthyroidism after an adequate trial of such drugs, as well as for those who suffer a significant adverse effect of a thioureylene drug that forces discontinuation

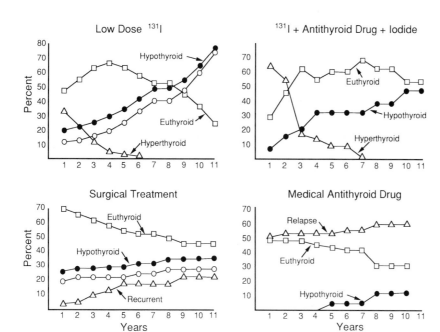

Figure 39–3

Cumulative incidence of permanent hypothyroidism *(open circles)*, permanent plus probable hypothyroidism *(solid circles)*, relapse or continued hyperthyroidism *(triangles)*, and euthyroidism *(squares)*, after various treatments. (From Sridama V, McCormick M, Kaplan EL, et al: Long-term follow-up study of compensated low-dose ^{131}I therapy for Graves' disease. N Engl J Med 311:426–432, 1984.)

of the drug. Except for the obvious contraindication of pregnancy, some thyroidologists consider radioiodine the initial therapy of choice for most adult hyperthyroid patients.

OTHER AGENTS

Beta-adrenergic blocking drugs, which can suppress some of the signs and symptoms of hyperthyroidism, are not used as definitive therapy of this disorder. However, if no contraindications such as asthma or heart failure exist, these drugs are used by some physicians as adjunctive treatment during early therapy or in preparing hyperthyroid patients for surgery. The use of these drugs in certain emergency situations has been discussed earlier.

DRUG INTERACTIONS

Drugs commonly affecting thyroid hormone synthesis or metabolism are listed in Table 39–1. The use of thioureylenes in combination with stable or radioactive iodine and the need for the proper sequence of administration have been discussed earlier. Unwanted interactions occasionally occur. For example, when a euthyroid individual who is receiving lithium for a psychiatric disorder is also given iodine-containing medication, the additive effect may lead to goiter or even hypothyroidism.

The effects of several drugs can be modified by the thyroid status of the patient. For example, hypothyroid patients are sensitive to central nervous system depressants, e.g., narcotics. The responsiveness to digoxin can be increased in hypothyroidism and decreased in hyperthyroidism. Thus, heart failure in hyperthyroid patients responds poorly to digoxin, but a cardiac glycoside may become more effective after restoration of euthyroidism. In contrast, oral anticoagulants are less effective in hypothyroid patients, whereas hyperthyroid patients are more responsive than normal individuals. If a hypothyroid patient is well controlled by a given dosage of oral anticoagulant, restoration of euthyroidism makes the patient more sensitive to the anticoagulant, probably by increasing metabolism of some clotting factors, so a reduction in the dosage of anticoagulant may be necessary to avoid hemorrhage.

The clearance of theophylline and certain β-adrenergic blocking drugs such as propranolol and metoprolol is decreased in hypothyroidism. Requirements for insulin and oral hypoglycemic agents may be increased in hyperthyroid diabetic patients and decreased in hypothyroid diabetics. Hyperthyroid patients may be more sensitive to the effects of tricyclic antidepressant drugs than are euthyroid individuals.

Table 39–1   DRUGS INTERFERING WITH THYROID HORMONE SYNTHESIS OR AFFECTING ITS ABSORPTION OR METABOLISM

Intrathyroidal	
Iodide transport	ClO_4^-, TcO_4^-, SCN^-, high iodide intake
Organification of iodide	Propylthiouracil, methimazole, some sulfonamides, SCN^-, phenylbutazone
Coupling of iodotyrosyls	Propylthiouracil, methimazole, some sulfonamides
Thyronine release	I^-, Li^+
Dehalogenase	Nitrotyrosines
Absorption and Peripheral Metabolism	
Inhibition of intestinal absorption	Cholestyramine, other resins, soy flour
Inhibition of peripheral deiodination	Propylthiouracil, glucocorticoids, iopanoate and other iodine-containing x-ray contrast agents
Induction of catabolic microsomal enzymes	Phenobarbital

References

Astwood EB: Treatment of hyperthyroidism with thiourea and thiouracil. JAMA 122:78–80, 1943.

Carr EA Jr, Beierwaltes WH, Raman G, et al: The effect of maternal thyroid function on fetal thyroid function and development. J Clin Endocrinol 19:1–18, 1959.

Committee on Nomenclature of the American Thyroid Association: Revised nomenclature for tests of thyroid hormones and thyroid related proteins in serum. J Clin Endocrinol Metab 64:1089–1094, 1987.

Hodin RA, Lazar MA, Wintman BI et al: Identification of a thyroid hormone receptor that is pituitary-specific. Science 244:76–79, 1989.

Marine D, Kimball OP: The prevention of simple goiter in man. JAMA 77:1068–1070, 1921.

Murray GB: Note on the treatment of myxoedema by hypodermic injections of an extract of the thyroid gland of a sheep. Br Med J 2:796–797, 1891.

Plummer HS: Results of administering iodine to patients having exophthalmic goiter. JAMA 80:1955, 1923.

Refetoff S, Larson PR: Transport, cellular uptake, and metabolism of thyroid hormone. *In* deGroot LJ, Besser GM, Cahill GF Jr et al (eds): Endocrinology, 2nd ed, 541–561. Philadelphia: WB Saunders, 1989.

Riggs DS: Quantitative aspects of iodine metabolism in man. Pharmacol Rev 4:284–370, 1952.

Saenger EI, Thoma GE, Tompkins EA: Incidence of leukemia following treatment of hyperthyroidism. JAMA 205:855–862, 1968.

Slingerland DW, Burrows BA: Long-term antithyroid treatment in hyperthyroidism. JAMA 242:2408–2410, 1979.

Spaulding SW, Burrow GN, Bermudez F, Himmelhoch JM: The inhibitory effect of lithium on thyroid hormone release in both euthyroid and hyperthyroid subjects. J Clin Endocrinol Metab 35:905–911, 1972.

Sridama V, McCormick M, Kaplan EL, et al: Long-term follow-up study of compensated low-dose ^{131}I therapy for Graves' disease. N Engl J Med 311:426–432, 1984.

Vassale G: Intorno agli effetti dell'iniezione intravenosa di succo di tiroide nei cani operati di estirpazione della tiroide. Rivista Sperimentale di Freniatria Reggio-Emilia 16:439–455, 1890.

Vulma T, Gons MH, de Vijlder JJM: Maternal fetal transfer of thyroxine in congenital hypothyroidism due to a total organification defect or thyroid agenesis. N Engl J Med 321:13–16, 1989.

Wartofsky L: Low remission rate after therapy for Graves' disease. JAMA 226:1083–1088, 1973.

Wartofsky L, Ransil BJ, Ingbar SM: Inhibition by iodine of the release of thyroxine from the thyroid gland of patients with thyrotoxicosis. J Clin Invest 49:78–86, 1970.

Wolff J, Chaikoff IL: Plasma inorganic iodine as a homeostatic regulation of thyroid function. J Biol Chem 174:555–564, 1948.

Wood LC, Ingbar SM: Hypothyroidism as a late sequela in patients with Graves' disease treated with antithyroid drugs. J Clin Invest 64:1429–1436, 1979.

40

Pituitary Hormones

Steven M. Simasko

The pituitary gland resides in the sella turcica and is attached to an area of the hypothalamus known as the *median eminence* by the infundibular stalk. It plays a key role in integrating outputs from the central nervous system to peripheral endocrine organs and target tissues. The gland can be divided into two parts, the anterior pituitary (or adenohypophysis), which makes up 75% of the mass of the pituitary, and the posterior pituitary (or neurohypophysis), which makes up 25% of the mass of the pituitary. These two regions of the gland have different embryological origins and function in slightly different manners.

Anterior Pituitary

The secretory behavior of pituitary cells is profoundly influenced by hormones that are released by the hypothalamus.

The anterior pituitary is formed from ectodermal cells that pinch off from the oral cavity to form Rathke's pouch. This mass of cells migrates cranially until it comes into contact with the infundibulum upon which it begins to proliferate into the cells of the anterior pituitary. These cells do not receive direct innervation from the central nervous system. However, their secretory behavior is profoundly influenced by hormones that are released in the median eminence. Blood from the superior hypophyseal artery enters a portal system in the median eminence that then drains into the hypophyseal vein. The blood in the hypophyseal vein, rich in hypothalamic-releasing and -inhibiting hormones, then bathes the cells of the anterior pituitary through a secondary portal system. The cells of the human anterior pituitary are known to secrete at least ten active hormones. In this chapter the therapeutic manipulations of the six most important of these hormones are considered. These are growth hormone (GH), prolactin (PRL), thyrotropin (or thyroid-stimulating hormone, TSH), follicle-stimulating hormone (FSH), luteinizing hormone (LH), and adrenocorticotropin (ACTH). Table 40–1 presents a summary of the anterior pituitary hormones.

Hormones of the anterior pituitary can be divided into three major groups based on structural similarities: those related to GH (GH and PRL), those related to TSH (TSH, FSH, and LH), and those of the pro-opiomelanocortin family (ACTH, melanocyte-stimulating hormones, and lipotropins). GH and PRL are both large single-chain proteins that have about 20% amino acid sequence homology. Because the exact amino acid sequences of these hormones are species-specific, they are more properly abbreviated as hGH and hPRL; the lowercase letter standing for *hormone of human origin*. In addition, a hormone of placental origin, placental lactogen (or chorionic somatotropin), has a very high sequence homology to GH. GH and PRL are secreted from somatotrophs and lactotrophs, respectively. Evidence has suggested that a subtype of cell exists that secretes both GH

Table 40–1   HORMONES OF THE ANTERIOR PITUITARY

Hormone	Structure	Pituitary Cell Type (% of Pituitary)	Hypothalamic-Releasing Hormone*	Hypothalamic-Inhibiting Hormone	Target Tissue	Target Tissue Hormone
Growth hormone	Single chain, 191 amino acids	Somatotrophs (40–50)	GHRH	Somatostatin	Liver, muscle, fat	IGF-I‡
Prolactin	Single chain, 198 amino acids	Lactotrophs (10–25)	?PRF ?TRH	Dopamine ?PRIF†	Mammary gland	
Thyrotropin	Two chains, glycoprotein	Thyrotrophs (3–5)	TRH		Thyroid	Thyroxine
Follicle-stimulating hormone	Two chains, glycoprotein	Gonadotrophs (10–15)	GnRH		Gonads (female—granulosa cells) (male—Sertoli cells)	Estradiol Inhibin
Luteinizing hormone	Two chains, glycoprotein	Gonadotrophs (10–15)	GnRH		Gonads (female–theca cells) (male—Leydig cells)	Androgens Testosterone
Adrenocorticotropin	Single chain, 39 amino acids	Corticotrophs (15–20)	CRH		Adrenal cortex	Cortisol

* GHRH = growth hormone–releasing hormone; PRF = prolactin-releasing factor; TRH = thyrotropin-releasing hormone; GnRH = gonadotropin-releasing hormone; CRH = corticotro-pin-releasing hormone.
† PRIF = prolactin release–inhibiting factor.
‡ IGF-I = insulin-like growth factor I.

and PRL (somatolactotrophs). The hypothalamus stimulates the release of GH by secretion of growth hormone–releasing hormone (GHRH) and inhibits the release of GH by secretion of somatostatin (SS; somatotropin-release–inhibiting hormone, SRIH). Prolactin is unique among the pituitary hormones in that in the absence of hypothalamic input (e.g., pituitary stalk transection), PRL levels increase. This suggests that there is a spontaneous release of PRL that is suppressed by hypothalamic input. The main inhibitor of PRL release is thought to be dopamine released in the median eminence by tuberoinfundibular dopaminergic neurons. In addition, an inhibitory protein factor has been suggested, although the physiological significance of such a factor remains controversial. A PRL-releasing factor has also been hypothesized to exist. Several candidate hormones have been shown to increase PRL release (thyrotropin-releasing hormone, OXY, vasoactive intestinal peptide, neurotensin, and angiotensin-II), but whether any of these hormones are physiologically relevant PRL-releasing factors has not been firmly established.

The second family of pituitary hormones are TSH, FSH, and LH. These hormones consist of two polypeptide chains, an α chain of 89 amino acids that are nearly identical among these hormones (and are functionally interchangeable), and homologous but nonidentical β chains. In addition, these proteins have extensive carbohydrate moieties that are essential for biological activity. A hormone of placental origin, chorionic gonadotropin (CG), is also related to this family of hormones. All these hormones are important regulators of peripheral endocrine tissues. Thyrotropin stimulates the thyroid gland to produce thyroid hormone, whereas FSH, LH, and CG regulate the activity of the gonads. Because of the gonadal actions of FSH, LH, and CG, these hormones are also referred to as *gonadotropins.* Thyrotropin is produced in thyrotrophs. Thyrotrophs release TSH in response to thyrotropin-releasing hormone (TRH). SS has been shown to inhibit TSH release, but this is thought to be more of pharmacological interest than of physiological significance. FSH and LH are produced in gonadotrophs. It has been shown by immunohistochemical techniques that some gonadotrophs produce only FSH, others produce only LH, and yet another type produces both FSH and LH. How LH and FSH are independently regulated is unknown; however, in many cases the release of these hormones is parallel. Gonadotrophs are stimulated by the hypothalamic release of luteinizing hormone–releasing hormone (LHRH). After many years of unsuccessful efforts to isolate a separate FSH-releasing hormone, it has become generally accepted that LHRH releases both gonadotropins and thus has been renamed *gonadotropin-releasing hormone* (GnRH). There are no known inhibitory hormones released by the hypothalamus that influence gonadotroph function.

The third group of hormones are those of the pro-opiomelanocortin family. This family includes ACTH, α and β melanocyte-stimulating hormone (MSH), and β and γ lipotropin. Within the amino acid sequence of β lipotropin is the sequence of β endorphin, an endogenous opiate-like compound. These hormones are related to each other through a pentapeptide sequence that is common to all and because they are synthesized on a common precursor molecule pro-opiomelanocortin. Although actions can be attributed to MSHs and lipotropins, the physiological importance of these actions in humans would appear to be slight. These peptides are produced by corticotrophs. Corticotrophs are stimulated to release ACTH by corticotropin-releasing hormone (CRH). No hypothalamic inhibitory hormone is known to act on corticotrophs.

With one exception (dopamine), all the hypothalamic and pituitary hormones are proteins. These range in length from a three–amino acid peptide (TRH) to proteins that contain almost 200 amino acids (GH and PRL). Because of this similarity, certain generalizations can be made about the biosynthesis, release, pharmacokinetics, and actions of these hormones. All are coded by particular genes, and their biosynthesis occurs through standard protein synthetic mechanisms. However, there are particular posttranslational processing events unique to each hormone. All are stored in secretory granules, and their release is mediated by vesicle fusion events. All are thought to be unbound in the plasma, and they are relatively rapidly inactivated (half-lives of a few minutes except for glycosylated hormones, which have slightly longer half-lives). The receptors for these hormones are on the plasma membranes of target cells, and in many cases, the initial intracellular events that occur after receptor activation are known to be mediated by either cyclic adenosine monophosphate (cAMP) or activation of phosphatidylinositide (PIP_2) turnover. Finally, hormonal products from peripheral target tissues act on the hypophyseal system to decrease release of these pituitary trophic factors. In some instances this negative feedback regulation is straightforward and can be used as the basis for diagnostic testing (TSH and ACTH), whereas in others it is complex and still not fully understood (gonadotropins).

Therapeutic interventions that utilize hypothalamic and pituitary hormones can be categorized into three general areas: (1) diagnostic; (2) replacement; and (3) control of excess secretion. Because of the proteinaceous nature of these hormones, in many cases it has been difficult to obtain amounts large enough to use therapeutically. In some cases, replacement with peripheral target organ hormone is more economical (glucocorticoids and thyroid hormone). In other cases, hormones from biological sources are used (gonadotropins). Until 1985, hGH for therapeutic application was isolated from the pituitaries of deceased humans; however, recombinant DNA techniques have now progressed to the point at which this hormone is made by biosynthetic methods. Another difficulty with these hormones has been their short half-lives in plasma. Several analogs of these hormones resistant to degradation have been synthesized and are now beginning to be explored for their therapeutic potential.

With one exception (dopamine), all hypothalamic and pituitary hormones are proteins.

Therapeutic interventions that utilize hypothalamic and pituitary hormones can be categorized into three general areas:

1. diagnostic;
2. replacement; and
3. control of excess secretion.

GROWTH HORMONE

Chemistry. Human GH is a single 191–amino acid peptide chain that contains two internal disulfide bonds. The molecular weight of GH is about 22,000 daltons; however, a hormone twice the predicted size of GH has been found in the plasma and pituitary by radioimmunoassays. The "big" form of GH is less biologically active than "small" GH. About 70% of the GH detected in plasma is the small variety. In addition, a 20,000-dalton fragment of GH has been shown to be biologically active. Initially this fragment was thought to be devoid of the metabolic effects of GH, but more recent investigations, using a biosynthetically produced 20,000-dalton fragment, show this fragment to possess some of the metabolic actions of GH. Only GHs from primate species have been found to be active in humans. As a result, GH isolated from human cadavers has been used therapeutically. This practice has been stopped because of several reports of Creutzfeldt-Jakob disease that have appeared in GH-treated patients years after the treatment was terminated. Two biosynthetic GHs are now marketed: somatotropin (HUMATROPE), which has the identical amino acid sequence as endogenous human GH, and somatrem (PROTROPIN), which has an extra methionine on the amino terminal end of human GH.

Physiology. GH has two major actions: increased growth and metabolic alterations. The increased growth is a generalized event that affects almost all tissues of the body. Of particular importance is the effect on long bone growth because this will determine final adult height. If the epiphyses of the bone have closed, GH does not produce any increase in bone length but causes bones to thicken. The growth-promoting actions of GH are indirectly mediated through the generation of somatomedins produced by nearly all tissues, although the liver is the largest source (>90%). It has been shown that several somatomedins are identical to growth factors isolated through different lines of research. In particular, somatomedin C, the most important somatomedin, is identical to insulin-like growth factor I (IGF-I).

The metabolic actions of GH are mediated by a direct action of GH on the liver, muscle, and adipocytes. The initial actions of GH have been described as insulin-like (i.e., there is an increase in glucose utilization and antilypolysis). These effects are only seen in tissues that have not been recently exposed to GH (e.g., hypophysectomized animals), and thus their physiological significance is questionable. Several hours after exposure to GH anti-insulin–like effects are observed. These include impaired glucose utilization and increased lypolysis. GH also produces a decreased sensitivity to the actions of insulin. This latter action can eventually lead to a diabetic state in individuals exposed to excessive GH. These late effects of GH require the presence of glucocorticoids and are blocked by protein synthesis inhibitors. The net result of the metabolic actions of GH is to shift the body to the utilization of fats as a fuel. The growth-promoting effects of GH also lead to a positive nitrogen balance (decreased urinary urea) owing to the increased protein synthesis required in growth.

Several factors regulate the secretion of GH both by direct actions on somatotrophs and by influences at the hypothalamic level. Sleep, exercise, and stress stimulate GH secretion, presumably through higher brain centers impinging on hypothalamic neurons containing GHRH and SS. IGF-I acts to decrease GH release at the level of both the pituitary and the hypothalamus. Androgens act synergistically with GH to promote growth. Excessive glucocorticoids inhibit the actions of GH. Protein stimulates GH

Growth hormone has two major actions: increased growth and metabolic alterations.

release, whereas carbohydrates inhibit GH release. Finally, GH cannot produce its growth-promoting activity without the presence of thyroid hormone.

The most prominent use of GH is replacement therapy in children who lack GH.

Therapeutic Use. The most prominent use of GH is replacement therapy in children who lack GH. Individuals who only lack GH do not suffer from a life-threatening condition. If GH is not replaced, these individuals grow into properly proportioned adults of short stature (dwarfs). An important aspect to the therapeutic use of GH is the determination of appropriate therapeutic situations. GH therapy intended to increase height is only useful in individuals who do not have closed epiphyses. The proper diagnosis of GH deficiency usually requires both low basal levels of circulating GH and negative response to a provocative challenge (GHRH, arginine infusion, or onset of sleep). Care must be taken in the interpretation of basal levels of GH because the hormone is released in a pulsatile manner and plasma levels can fluctuate significantly. Previously, when GH for therapeutic use was isolated from human sources, the scarcity of the hormone forced careful selection of patients and only those with extreme deficiencies of GH gained access to GH therapy. With the advent of biosynthetically produced GH, supplies are virtually limitless, although therapy is still extremely expensive. Because GH deficiency occurs on a continuum rather than absolutely, the selection of patients for GH therapy has become an important ethical issue. Although serious side effects from treatment are rare, the expense and potential unknown effects that may appear years later argue for a conservative selection of patients.

GH therapy has also been used in adults who have a GH deficiency. In these individuals significant increases in lean body mass have been achieved as a result of the metabolic actions of GH.

GH is given by intramuscular or subcutaneous injection three times weekly. The half-life of intravenously injected GH is 20–25 minutes; however, the actions of GH last much longer. Part of this is due to the long half-life of IGF-I (4–5 hours), which circulates bound to carrier proteins. In some individuals antibodies against GH form after treatment has begun. This is more significant with somatrem (hGH with an extra amino acid, 30% of cases) than with somatotropin (2% of cases). The immunoneutralization of GH can usually be overcome by increasing the dosage. In many cases the lack of GH is associated with a generalized hypopituitarism. Because of the importance of thyroid hormone and glucocorticoids in the actions of GH, it is important to stabilize these endocrine functions before GH therapy is started. Patients on GH therapy should be routinely monitored for diabetes (owing to the anti-insulin actions of GH) and hypothyroidism (owing to suppression of TSH release by elevated hypothalamic release of SS).

A subset of dwarfs (Laron-type dwarfs) have been identified who have normal or elevated levels of immunoreactive GH yet exhibit symptoms of GH deficiency. GH in these individuals is biologically active. The defect in these individuals has been shown to be an inactive GH receptor. These individuals have no circulating IGF-I and are resistant to the actions of exogenously given GH.

Growth Hormone–Releasing Hormone

Chemistry. GHRH is the most recently isolated hypothalamic-releasing hormone. The isolation was achieved by the use of GHRH-releasing tumors of pancreatic origin. This work resulted in the isolation of two different factors, a 44–amino acid peptide and a 40–amino acid peptide, both of which are active. It has been shown that the 44–amino acid factor is endogenous to human hypothalamic tissue. Truncated GHRH (amino acids 1–29) has been found to be biologically active.

Physiology. GHRH acts on the somatotrophs of the anterior pituitary to release GH.

Therapeutic Use. Synthetic GHRH is available. The only current use of GHRH is for diagnostic tests of the pituitary to determine the functional capacity of somatotrophs. A potential therapeutic use of GHRH is in treatment of GH-deficient patients in whom the deficiency is produced by hypothalamic inadequacy.

Somatostatin

Chemistry. GH-release inhibitory activity was first found during attempts to isolate a GH-releasing factor. This hormone, called *somatotropin-release–inhibiting hormone* (SRIH) or *somatostatin* (SS), is a 14–amino acid peptide with one internal disulfide bond. Since the discovery of SS in the hypothalamus, several other tissues have been shown to contain this hormone, most notably the gastrointestinal tract and pancreas. Somatostatin has been found to have an inhibitory effect on hormone secretion in both these tissues. A 28–amino acid peptide that contains the sequence for SS within its structure (prosomatostatin or SS-28) has also been isolated from intestine and brain. Prosomatostatin has been shown to be more potent than SS in several bioassays. Structure-activity studies of SS analogs have shown that amino acids 7–10 in native SS (PHE-TRP-LYS-THR) are the essential portion of the peptide for retention of SS-like activity. An 8–amino acid analog of SS that contains this core, octreotide (SANDOSTATIN), has been approved for therapeutic use (Fig. 40–1).

Physiology. The action of SS can be summarized as inhibition of hormone secretion. In the pituitary, SS is an important physiological regulator of GH secretion. At higher concentrations, SS can also inhibit the release of other anterior pituitary hormones (TSH, ACTH, and PRL), but this is not thought to be important physiologically. In the pancreas, SS inhibits the release of both glucagon and insulin, although it is about 50 times more potent on glucagon secretion. In other parts of the gastrointestinal tract SS has been shown to inhibit the release of secretin, renin, vasoactive intestinal peptide

The action of SS can be summarized as inhibition of hormone secretion.

Somatostatin

```
ALA — GLY — CYS — LYS — ASN — PHE — PHE
              |                           \
              S                           TRP
              |                           |
              S                           LYS
              |                          /
            CYS — SER — THR — PHE — THR
```

Octreotide

```
          D — PHE — CYS — PHE
                    |        \
                    S      D —TRP
                    |        |
                    S       LYS
                    |      /
         THR — ol — CYS — THR
```

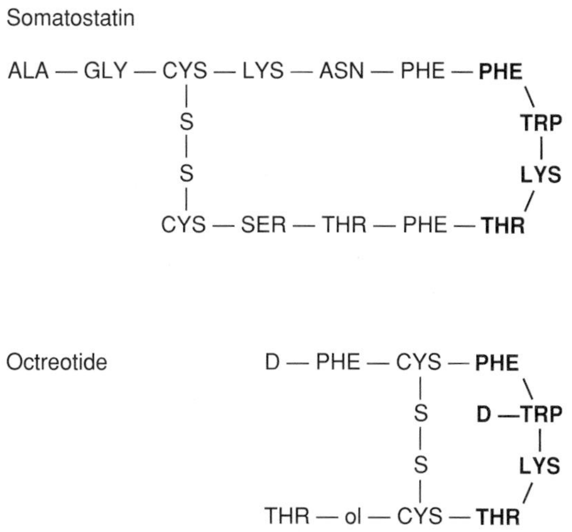

Figure 40–1

Comparison of the amino acid sequence of somatostatin and the long-acting somatostatin agonist octreotide. The essential core of the peptides is indicated in color.

(VIP), and motilin. In addition, SS is a potent inhibitor of gastric acid secretion and gastric mucosal blood flow.

Therapeutic Use. The therapeutic usefulness of SS is limited by its short half-life (3 minutes), its need to be administered intravenously, its broad range of actions on hormone secretion, and a rebound hypersecretion that occurs on cessation of SS infusion. On the other hand, octreotide has a relatively long half-life (50 minutes), is active subcutaneously, preferentially inhibits GH secretion over insulin secretion, and does not cause a rebound hypersecretion on cessation of treatment. This latter effect is thought to be due to the long half-life of octreotide that results in a slow decrease in plasma levels.

Octreotide has been approved for use in the treatment of metastatic carcinoid, in which it is effective in inhibiting the diarrhea and flushing associated with this disease, and in VIP-secreting tumors, in which it is effective in inhibiting the diarrhea associated with this disease and restoring plasma electrolyte balance. Octreotide has also been shown to be effective in the treatment of acromegaly. Almost all acromegalic patients respond to octreotide with a decrease in circulating GH, and tumor shrinkage occurs in about 50% of those treated. Some success has also been reported in reducing discharge from TSH-secreting tumors, ectopic ACTH secretion, and ACTH secretion in Nelson's syndrome. Adverse reactions to prolonged octreotide therapy are similar to effects produced by SS-secreting tumors. These include steatorrhea, diabetes mellitus, and cholelithiasis. These effects are a result of the well-characterized actions of SS to decrease exocrine pancreas secretion, inhibit insulin secretion, and prevent gallbladder contractions.

PROLACTIN

Chemistry. PRL is a 198–amino acid peptide with two internal disulfide bonds, related to GH. As with GH, "big" and "small" forms of PRL have been shown to exist.

Physiology. PRL plays an essential role in stimulating milk production in the mammary gland. The plasma level of PRL becomes progressively elevated during pregnancy (as does the level of placental lactogen). The actions of PRL and placental lactogen are important for adequate development of the mammary glands during pregnancy. During pregnancy, lactation is suppressed by the high levels of estrogen and progesterone. With the delivery of the placenta, sex steroid levels rapidly decline and the lactogenic effects of PRL become expressed. Stimulation of the nipple during breast-feeding activates a neuronal reflex arc that results in the release of PRL from the pituitary. Thus each feeding session provides continued hormonal support for the production of milk.

PRL also has effects on the gonads. In some species PRL is luteotropic and in some it is luteolytic. In humans PRL suppresses gonadal function. The degree to which this is due to suppression of gonadotropin release from the pituitary or to an action directly on the gonads remains controversial. Elevated PRL in women who are breast-feeding usually results in suppression of menses.

The primary control of PRL release is a continuous inhibitory tone produced by the release of dopamine from the hypothalamus. A common side effect in the therapeutic use of dopamine blockers is elevated PRL levels. Other potential hypothalamic influences on PRL release are discussed in the introductory section of this chapter. It has also been shown that estrogens increase PRL release. In rodents the PRL surge on the evening of proestrus in an important component to the overall estrus cycle. However, in humans PRL levels do not change during the normal menstrual cycle.

PRL is not available for clinical use. However, PRL-secreting adenomas are a common pituitary dysfunction. Symptoms in females include amenorrhea, galactorrhea, infertility, and hypogonadism. Symptoms in males include infertility, impotence, and galactorrhea. The effect of dopaminergic agonists to suppress PRL release is exploited in the therapy of PRL-secreting adenomas.

The effect of dopaminergic agonists to suppress PRL release is exploited in the therapy of PRL-secreting adenomas.

Therapeutic Use of Bromocriptine. Bromocriptine (PARLODEL) is an ergot derivative that has agonist effects on dopamine receptors. Activation of dopamine receptors on lactotrophs leads to an inhibition of PRL secretion. Bromocriptine also stimulates GH release in normal subjects. For reasons that are not yet apparent, bromocriptine has also been shown to decrease GH release in acromegalics.

Bromocriptine has gained wide usage in the treatment of hyperprolactinemia due to PRL-secreting adenomas. Bromocriptine is successful in restoring menses and preventing galactorrhea in about 75% of patients. Relief of symptoms may be rapid (days) or may require many months. Reduction in tumor size has also been noted. Tumor growth, galactorrhea, and amenorrhea usually return on cessation of treatment. Definitive relief of symptoms usually requires surgical removal of the tumor.

Bromocriptine is also of use in preventing breast engorgement after parturition in women who elect not to breast-feed. It is recommended that such use be restricted to cases of significant engorgement. A rebound effect occurs in about 30% of women once therapy is stopped.

Bromocriptine has also been used alone or in combination with pituitary irradiation or surgery in cases of acromegaly. Bromocriptine may be of use in reducing tumor size and controlling symptoms before and after surgical intervention.

Bromocriptine may also be effective in the treatment of Parkinson's disease. This use of bromocriptine is recommended as an adjuvant in those patients who are beginning to deteriorate on levodopa therapy.

For treatment of hyperprolactinemia PARLODEL (bromocriptine) is given orally once a day. Additional tablets are added to the regimen every 3–7 days until therapeutic benefit is achieved. Adverse reactions with bromocriptine are relatively common. These include nausea, headache, dizziness, fatigue, lightheadedness, vomiting, and diarrhea. Care should be given to those patients receiving antihypertensive medications because bromocriptine also lowers blood pressure. Incidence of spontaneous abortions or birth defects in mothers who have taken bromocriptine for a portion of their pregnancy is no greater than that expected in the general population.

THYROTROPIN

Chemistry. Thyrotropin or TSH consists of two amino acid chains (α has 89 amino acids and β has 115 amino acids) that are glycosylated. The α chain is nearly identical to the α chain in FSH and LH. Specificity of thyroid stimulatory activity resides in the β chain.

Physiology. Thyrotropin stimulates the thyroid gland by increasing cAMP levels. The thyroid gland responds to TSH both by increasing thyroid hormone production and by proliferating. Thyrotropin secretion is increased by TRH and is suppressed by thyroid hormone.

Therapeutic Use. Thyrotropin from bovine sources has been used to test thyroid function; however, this test has been largely supplanted by use of a sensitive radioimmunoassay for TSH levels in conjunction with the TRH stimulation test.

Thyrotropin-Releasing Hormone

Chemistry. TRH was the first hypothalamic-releasing factor isolated and structurally resolved. This is due in part to the simple structure of TRH, a tripeptide with a carboxy terminal pyroglutamyl and an amino terminal prolinamide.

Physiology. TRH is released by the hypothalamus and causes thyrotrophs of the pituitary to increase TSH release. In addition, TRH has been found to increase PRL and GH release, but the physiological significance of these actions is questionable. TRH has been shown to exert its actions in the pituitary through receptor-mediated increases in phosphoinositide turnover. TRH has also been found to exist in a variety of brain areas outside the hypothalamus and in several peripheral organs including the pancreas, gastrointestinal tract, and prostate. TRH has been found to exert a variety of effects that do not require an intact pituitary-thyroid axis and are not mimicked by TSH or thyroid hormone. These include general arousal effects, increases in blood pressure and heart rate, increased respiration, gastrointestinal effects (increased motility and acid secretion), and a hyperthermic effect.

The primary clinical use of TRH is as a diagnostic tool to assess thyroid function.

Therapeutic Use. The primary clinical use of TRH (protirelin, RELEFACT TRH) is as a diagnostic tool to assess thyroid function. The TRH stimulation test can provide useful information in the assessment of secondary versus tertiary hypothyroidism and in the evaluation of the effectiveness of thyroid therapy in patients with nodular or diffuse goiter and patients on thyroid replacement therapy.

Interpretation of the TRH stimulation test requires an understanding of the negative feedback control of TSH release by thyroid hormone. Patients with primary (thyroid) hypothyroidism have elevated basal TSH levels due to lack of thyroid hormone action on the pituitary. Patients with secondary (pituitary) hypothyroidism have normal to low basal TSH levels and a blunted increase in TSH in response to a TRH challenge. Patients with tertiary (hypothalamic) hypothyroidism have normal to low basal TSH levels and a potentiated increase in TSH in response to a TRH challenge.

The adequacy of thyroid hormone therapy for the suppression of TSH release in patients with nodular or diffuse goiter can be evaluated with a TRH stimulation test. If thyroid hormone therapy is adequate, TSH levels should be low and a TRH challenge should result in a blunted TSH release. The adequacy of thyroid hormone replacement therapy in hypothyroid patients can also be evaluated with a TRH stimulation test. If thyroid hormone replacement is adequate, a TRH challenge will produce a normal or slightly blunted TSH release.

Adverse reactions occur in about 50% of tested patients. These reactions are usually minor and persist for only a few minutes. Most important are changes in blood pressure (hypertension and hypotension), which can be significant. In addition, headache, lightheadedness, nausea, abdominal discomfort, and urge to urinate occur. Leakage may also occur in lactating women.

The extraendocrine effects of TRH have prompted investigations into the application of TRH or TRH analogs in several therapeutic situations such as motor neuron diseases, spinal cord injury, circulatory shock, and Alzheimer's disease. However, no clear therapeutic interventions have yet been identified.

GONADOTROPINS

Chemistry. FSH and LH consist of two glycosylated peptide chains. The α subunits contain 89 amino acids and are virtually identical to each other and to the α subunit of TSH. The biological specificity of these hormones is contained in the β subunit. In both FSH and LH the β subunits are 115 amino acids in length. In addition to the pituitary gonadotropins, a gonadotropin of similar structure is released by the placenta. Human chorionic gonadotropin (hCG) consists of an α subunit of 92 amino acids and a β subunit of 145 amino acids. The β subunit of hCG is virtually identical to the β subunit of LH except for a 30–amino acid addition to the carboxy terminal end. The predominant effects of hCG are similar to LH, although weak FSH-like activity is present. These hormones are heavily glycosylated, and the carbohydrate moieties are essential for biological activity but not for receptor binding. The high degree of glycosylation also increases the plasma half-life. Owing to the high degree of glycosylation, the biosynthesis of these hormones by recombinant DNA in bacterial expression systems is not possible; however, success has been achieved with mammalian cell cultures, and biosynthetic gonadotropins should soon become available. Currently, gonadotropins isolated from human urine are used for therapeutic purposes. These include menotropins (PERGONAL), a mixture of FSH and LH isolated from the urine of postmenopausal women; urofollitrophin (METRODIN), a preparation from the urine of postmenopausal women in which the FSH activity has been purified; and hCG (PREGNYL, PROFASI), a preparation of hCG from the urine of pregnant women.

> The gonadotropins are heavily glycosylated, and the carbohydrate moieties are essential for biological activity.

Physiology. The targets of the gonadotropins are the gonads, and because of the sex-based differences in gonadal function, the actions of the gonadotropins in males and females must be considered separately. However, in both males and females the molecular mechanisms of FSH and LH action, as well as hCG, are thought to be mediated by increases in cAMP.

The only cells within the male gonad that express LH receptors are the interstitial cells of Leydig. In the presence of LH, these cells increase production of androgenic steroids, of which testosterone is the most important. FSH increases the potency of LH on Leydig cells, although this must be an indirect action because Leydig cells do not express FSH receptors. Through mechanisms that are not completely understood, stimulation of the Sertoli cells of the seminiferous tubules by FSH, in the presence of testosterone, promotes spermatogenesis. FSH stimulates Sertoli cells to produce several protein products including androgen-binding protein, which is necessary for maintaining high concentrations of testosterone in the gonads, and various growth factors, including IGF-I. Spermatogenesis can be maintained in the testes without FSH if high local concentrations of testosterone are maintained. However, previous maturation of the seminiferous tubules with FSH is required.

In the female, the effects of gonadotropins are dependent on the phase of the menstrual cycle. In the early follicular phase, LH stimulates the theca cells to increase steroidogenesis, which results in production of progesterone and testosterone. Androgenic steroids produced by the theca cell diffuse into the adjacent granulosa cells where they are converted to estradiol by aromatase activity. Under stimulation of FSH and estradiol, immature follicles begin to develop. By mechanisms not understood, one follicle becomes dominant and suppresses the development of neighboring follicles. As the follicle matures, the granulosa cells become more responsive to FSH and continue to increase the production of estradiol even though plasma FSH levels decline slightly. Near the time of ovulation, the granulosa cells of the dominant follicle begin to lose FSH receptors and develop LH receptors. The midcycle surge of LH from the pituitary (see later) induces the rupture of the mature follicle and release of the ovum. The remnants of the follicle then develop into the corpus luteum, which, under stimulation of LH, produces elevated progesterone levels. The elevation of progesterone levels relative to estradiol levels in the luteal phase of the cycle is due to a decrease in the relative amounts of aromatase activity present in the luteinized granulosa and theca cells. If implantation occurs, the primitive trophoblasts begin to secrete hCG. CG rescues the corpus luteum, so that plasma progesterone levels are maintained until the placenta begins adequate production of this hormone.

In the male, LH is negatively regulated by testosterone. This action of testosterone would appear to be predominantly mediated by a decrease in the frequency of GnRH pulses from the hypothalamus without changes in pulse amplitude. A direct action of testosterone to decrease gonadotroph responsiveness to GnRH has also been observed. In contrast, testosterone has only minor effects on FSH secretion. Inhibin, a protein hormone released by Sertoli cells, is thought to be the primary regulator of FSH secretion. Inhibin has been shown to act directly on gonadotrophs to decrease FSH secretion.

The regulation of gonadotropin release in the female is complex owing to both negative and positive feedback of estradiol.

In contrast to the relatively simple negative feedback control of gonadotropin release in the male, the regulation of gonadotropin release in the female is complex and not easily comprehended. The complexity is due to both negative and positive feedback effects of estradiol. In the follicular phase, estradiol is thought to decrease the amplitude of GnRH pulses from the hypothalamus without changing frequency. In addition, estradiol acts directly on the gonadotrophs to decrease the amount of gonadotropins released to a given challenge of GnRH. This is thought to occur by a shift in the packaging of gonadotropins from a readily releasable pool to a storage pool. These actions lead to a suppression of LH and FSH release but an increase in the stores of these hormones in the gonadotrophs. A second event that occurs is continued pulsatile release of GnRH from the hypothalamus, leading to an increase in GnRH receptors on gonadotrophs (i.e., a "self-priming" event). At a point in the late follicular phase when the plasma estradiol level exceeds a particular threshold, there is a recruitment of gonadotropins from the storage pool into the releasable pool. This, in combination with an increased sensitivity to GnRH due to the increase in GnRH receptors, results in a surge of LH and, to a lesser extent, FSH release. The surge of LH induces ovulation. During the luteal phase the presence of progesterone is thought to decrease pulse frequency, which results in the loss of GnRH receptors on gonadotrophs (i.e., the "self-priming" event requires a particular frequency of GnRH stimulation). Decreases in GnRH receptors lead to a decrease in the responsiveness of gonadotrophs to GnRH and a fall in plasma FSH and LH levels. As discussed later, the pulsatile nature of GnRH release is an important physiological concept in the therapeutic use of GnRH analogs.

Therapeutic Use. Therapeutic use of gonadotropins should only be attempted by those physicians familiar with infertility problems and the criteria for selection of patients. The primary therapeutic application of gonadotropins (menotropins and hCG) is the treatment of infertility in females due to hypogonadotropic anovulation and in males due to hypogonadotropic hypogonadism. In both cases it is important to determine that gonadal failure is secondary to pituitary or hypothalamic failure. This can be ascertained by low to nonexistent plasma sex steroid levels concomitant with low to nonexistent plasma gonadotropin levels. Urofollitrophin (FSH) has been found useful in induction of follicle maturation in women with polycystic ovarian disease who have an elevated plasma LH/FSH ratio. Urofollitrophin has also been used for induction of multiple oocytes in patients participating in *in vitro* fertilization programs. Preparations of hCG may be helpful in cryptorchidism that is not due to anatomical blockage.

In anovulatory hypogonadic women, the therapeutic regimen is designed to mimic the natural menstrual cycle. Menotropins are given for 7–12 days to stimulate follicle development, followed by a single large dose of hCG to initiate ovulation. Major adverse reactions include ovarian enlargement, which may lead to ovarian hyperstimulation syndrome; pulmonary complications (atelectasis and acute respiratory distress syndrome); and cardiovascular complications (thrombosis and embolism).

In hypogonadotropic hypogonadic males, treatment for 4–6 months with a preparation of hCG to elevate serum testosterone levels is recommended prior to combined menotropin/hCG therapy. Combined menotropin/hCG therapy should proceed for at least 3–4 months before examination of the ejaculate for spermatozoa, as it takes approximately 74 days for the human male germ cell to develop into spermatozoa. Potential adverse reactions include fluid retention as a result of increased androgen production.

Treatment with hCG for cryptorchidism not due to anatomical blockage is usually performed between the ages of 4 and 9. Although descent produced with hCG treatment is frequently temporary, a positive response is usually a good predictor of eventual permanent descent during puberty. Use of hCG in prepubertal boys may result in the induction of precocious puberty. Therapy should be halted if any pubertal signs are observed.

The therapeutic regimen with gonadotropins is designed to mimic the natural menstrual cycle.

Gonadotropin-Releasing Hormone

Chemistry. GnRH is a 10–amino acid peptide, and synthetically produced GnRH is available (gonadorelin hydrochloride, FACTREL). An analog of GnRH (leuprolide acetate, LUPRON), in which glycyl at position 6 has been replaced with D-leucyl and the carboxy terminal glycinamide has been removed, is also available (Fig. 40–2). The major advantage of leuprolide is an increased potency due in part to an increased plasma half-life.

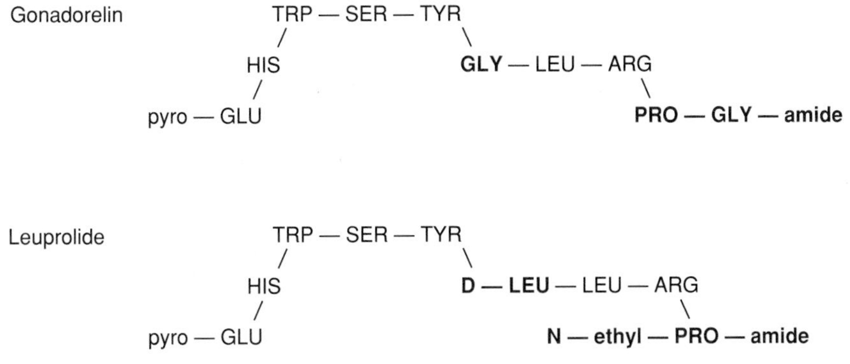

Figure 40–2

Comparison of the amino acid sequence of GnRH and the long-acting GnRH agonist leuprolide. Differences are indicated in color.

Physiology. The only confirmed action of GnRH is the release of gonadotropins from the pituitary. As with all hypothalamic-releasing hormones, GnRH is found in many areas of the brain outside the hypothalamus and has been shown to exert effects on neuronal behavior. A possible role for GnRH in control of reproductive behaviors has been suggested.

GnRH is released from the hypothalamus in pulses that occur approximately once an hour. Pulse frequency is important in the actions of GnRH. If the frequency is too slow or too fast, the actions of GnRH are diminished. Estradiol has been shown to decrease pulse amplitude without altering pulse frequency, whereas testosterone and progesterone decrease pulse frequency without changing pulse amplitude. Opiates also produce an inhibitory effect on GnRH release.

The importance of the pulsatile nature of GnRH release to its action permits use of GnRH both as a stimulator and as an inhibitor of gonadotroph function.

Therapeutic Use. Both GnRH agonists and GnRH antagonists have been synthesized. However, therapeutic application of antagonists has been disappointing because they rapidly lose their effectiveness. This is most likely due to compensatory increases in GnRH release that eventually overcomes the block produced by the antagonists. On the other hand, the pulsatile nature of GnRH release in maintenance of GnRH action permits the use of GnRH agonists both as stimulators of gonadotroph function and as inhibitors of gonadotroph function, depending on the regimen of therapy. For example, nighttime hourly injections of GnRH were shown to be capable of inducing puberty, whereas constant infusions of GnRH were ineffective. On the other hand, constant infusion of GnRH agonists suppresses gonadal function in several circumstances.

Synthetic GnRH is approved for diagnostic use in the assessment of gonadotroph function. Leuprolide is approved for use in prostate cancer for which orchiectomy or estrogen therapy is either not tolerated or unacceptable to the patient. During the first week of leuprolide therapy testosterone levels rise, which may exacerbate symptoms. This is followed by a decrease below pretreatment levels that is maintained as long as treatment is maintained. Upon termination of treatment, pituitary function recovers and testosterone levels return to pretreatment values. Leuprolide is not orally active and has a half-life of 3 hours. A depot preparation has been developed (LUPRON DEPOT) that is administered intramuscularly once a month.

Other applications of GnRH agonists have been in the treatment of precocious puberty, infertility, as a contraceptive, and in other sex hormone–dependent conditions (for example, breast cancer and endometriosis). Many of these uses have only recently begun, and clinical trials are still necessary to evaluate whether GnRH agonist treatment produces significant improvements over existing therapies. The use of GnRH agonists to suppress pituitary function in precocious puberty appears to be a significant medical advancement. Promising results have also been obtained in the use of GnRH agonists to suppress pituitary function during procedures designed to induce multiple oocyte release for *in vitro* fertilization.

ADRENOCORTICOTROPIN

Chemistry. ACTH is a 39–amino acid peptide that is produced by the proteolytic cleavage of a larger precursor molecule known as *pro-opio-melanocortin* (POMC). The amino end of POMC gives rise to ACTH, which can be further cleaved to release α-MSH. The carboxy terminal of POMC gives rise to β lipotropin. β lipotropin can be further cleaved to produce γ lipotropin and β endorphin. Within γ lipotropin is the sequence of β-MSH, and within β endorphin is the sequence of several additional opiate-like peptides (γ and α endorphin and met-enkephalin). It is thought that the final proteolytic processing of POMC occurs within the secretory granule, thus β lipotropin and β endorphin are secreted along with ACTH. The physiological significance of circulating β lipotropin and β endorphin in humans is unknown. Amino terminal fragments of ACTH retain biological activity. ACTH for therapeutic use is available from purified sources (corticotropin, ACTHAR) or produced synthetically (ACTH$_{1-24}$, cosyntropin, CORTROSYN).

Physiology. ACTH stimulates the adrenal cortex to release cortisol, corticosterone, aldosterone, and weak androgenic steroids. In addition, adrenal hypertrophy and hyperplasia occur. These actions are mediated by increases in cAMP. The steroidogenic effects are produced by an increase in the conversion of cholesterol to pregnenolone, the rate-limiting step in steroid biosynthesis.

Plasma levels of ACTH vary on a 24-hour cycle, with the highest level occurring in the early morning. In addition, multiple forms of stress immediately stimulate release of ACTH. ACTH release is mediated primarily by an increase in CRH release from the hypothalamus and, to a lesser extent, by β adrenergic receptor activation on corticotrophs by epinephrine released from the adrenals. In addition, vasopressin has been shown to increase ACTH release. Glucocorticoids feed back to decrease ACTH release. Somatostatin has been shown to decrease ACTH release; however, this is not thought to be physiologically relevant.

> Multiple forms of stress immediately stimulate release of ACTH.

Therapeutic Use. Preparations of ACTH are used for the diagnosis of adrenocorticoid function and therapeutically for conditions responsive to glucocorticoid therapy. Adrenal insufficiency can be determined by a failure of an intravenous challenge of ACTH to produce an increase in plasma glucocorticoids. Separation of primary (adrenal) from secondary (pituitary) insufficiency can be made by determination of plasma levels of ACTH (elevated in primary but suppressed in secondary). In secondary adrenal insufficiency, prolonged stimulation of the adrenal cortex with ACTH may be required before significant increases in plasma cortisol levels are achieved.

Therapeutic use of ACTH is based on its ability to release glucocorticoids. It is only helpful in those patients with adequate adrenal function. Its effects tend to be less predictable than exogenous glucocorticoids; however, some clinicians report superior results with ACTH over glucocorticoids, particularly concerning acute exacerbations of multiple sclerosis. The short duration of action (plasma half-life less than 20 minutes) and route of administration (subcutaneous or intramuscular) make therapeutic use inconvenient. Excessive use may result in significant elevations of mineralocorticoids, with resultant increases in sodium and water retention. Other side effects of prolonged use are a result of excess glucocorticoids. Use of ACTH is contraindicated in those situations for which glucocorticoids are contraindicated.

Corticotropin-Releasing Hormone

Chemistry. CRH is a 41–amino acid peptide that is expressed in many parts of the nervous system as well as peripheral organs such as the pituitary, adrenal, and testis. The highest concentrations of CRH are found in the hypothalamus, where it has been localized to neurons that reside in the paraventricular nucleus and project to the median eminence.

Physiology. The best-understood action of CRH is its ability to regulate ACTH release from the pituitary. CRH is thought to cause secretion of

ACTH from corticotrophs through the production of cAMP. It has also been suggested that CRH in the pituitary may function in a paracrine manner to regulate ACTH release. In addition, intraventricularly injected CRH induces a general behavioral activation while inhibiting specific behaviors such as feeding and sexual activity.

Therapeutic Use. Synthetic CRH is available and is only used for diagnostic testing of pituitary function. Cushing's disease of pituitary origin can be distinguished from that due to ectopic ACTH production by a CRH stimulation test. In Cushing's disease of pituitary origin, CRH usually produces an elevation of plasma ACTH, whereas ectopic ACTH production does not respond to CRH.

Posterior Pituitary

The posterior pituitary is formed by a downpouching of the floor of the third ventricle. The cell bodies of the neurons that make up the neurohypophysis reside in the supraoptic and paraventricular nuclei of the hypothalamus. These neurons send axons through the infundibulum that terminate in the lobe of the posterior pituitary. The hormones of the posterior pituitary, antidiuretic hormone (ADH; arginine vasopressin, AVP) and oxytocin (OXY), are released directly from these nerve terminals into the blood supplied by the inferior hypophyseal artery. The hormones of the posterior pituitary are summarized in Table 40–2.

VASOPRESSIN (ANTIDIURETIC HORMONE)

Chemistry. Vasopressin (AVP; antidiuretic hormone, ADH) is a 9–amino acid peptide with an internal disulfide bond between cysteines at position 1 and position 6 and a carboxy terminal glycinamide (Fig. 40–3). The integrity of the ring structure and the carboxy terminal amide are important for the potency of AVP. Vasopressin is synthesized in the cell bodies of magnocellular neurons of the paraventricular and supraoptic nuclei and transported in neurosecretory vesicles to the posterior lobe of the pituitary, from which it is released into the circulation. During transit to the posterior pituitary the prohormone is processed into three moieties: AVP, a 39–amino acid glycoprotein, and a 10,000-dalton protein called *neurophysin.* Both the glycoprotein and neurophysin are released into the circulation; however, their function is not known. The half-life of AVP in the circulation is 10–20 minutes. Synthetic AVP is available in an injectable preparation (PITRESSIN) and as a long-acting suspension for intramuscular administration (vasopressin tannate, PITRESSIN TANNATE IN OIL). In addition, an analog of AVP (desmopressin, DDAVP) that has a circulating half-life about five times longer than native AVP is available as an injectable preparation and for intranasal application.

Table 40–2 HORMONES OF THE POSTERIOR PITUITARY

Hormone	Structure	Location of Cell Body	Stimulus for Release	Target Tissue
Vasopressin or antidiuretic hormone	Single chain, 9 amino acids	Paraventricular nucleus, supraoptic nucleus	High plasma osmolarity, low plasma volume	Collecting ducts of kidney, small arterioles and venules
Oxytocin	Single chain, 9 amino acids	Paraventricular nucleus, supraoptic nucleus	Stimulation of nipple, parturition	Myoepithelial cells of breast, myometrium

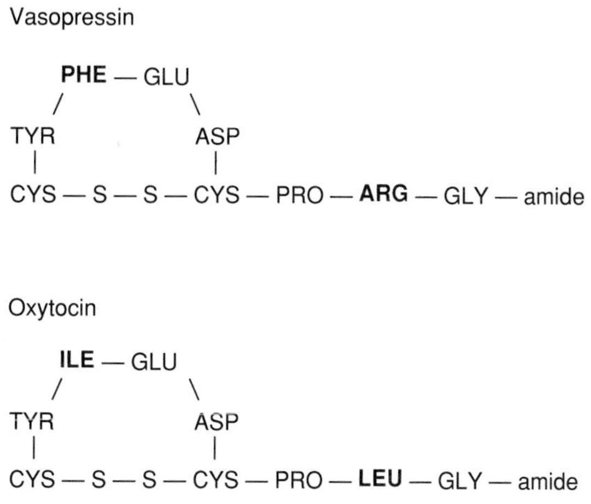

Vasopressin

```
        PHE — GLU
       /          \
    TYR            ASP
     |              |
    CYS — S — S — CYS — PRO — ARG — GLY — amide
```

Figure 40–3

Amino acid sequence of vasopressin and oxytocin. Differences in amino acid sequence are indicated in color.

Oxytocin

```
        ILE — GLU
       /          \
    TYR            ASP
     |              |
    CYS — S — S — CYS — PRO — LEU — GLY — amide
```

Physiology. AVP has two major peripheral actions. In the kidneys AVP reduces urine formation. This is accomplished primarily by increasing water reuptake in the late distal tubules and collecting ducts. Because of this action AVP is also known as *antidiuretic hormone* (ADH). This action is mediated by activation of V_2 receptors that result in elevated intracellular cAMP.

The second action of AVP is on the vasculature, where it is the most potent circulating vasoconstrictor known. Small venules and arterioles are more sensitive than large veins and arteries. This vasoconstriction leads to an increase in total vascular resistance, which in turn leads to a decrease in cardiac output mediated through the baroreceptor reflex. Because of the compensatory decrease in cardiac output, overall blood pressure tends to show little change. Not all vascular beds are equally sensitive to AVP. Although blood flow to the skin and skeletal muscles is very much reduced, blood flow to the kidney and liver is not changed. Blood flow to other tissues decreases in proportion to the decrease in cardiac output. In addition to shifting regional blood flow, the increase in small arteriole resistance produced by AVP leads to a decrease in capillary and venule pressure. This decrease in pressure produces a net absorption of fluids from the interstitial space, resulting in an increase in blood volume. The vascular effects of AVP are mediated by the V_1 receptor, which is thought to work through increases in PIP_2 turnover. The vasoconstrictor actions of AVP require higher concentrations of AVP than that required for actions in the kidneys.

The primary stimuli for AVP release are plasma osmolarity and plasma volume, with osmolarity more sensitive than volume. An increase of plasma osmolarity as small as 1–2%, sensed by brain osmoreceptors thought to reside in the organum vasculosum, elicits a prompt release of AVP. Plasma volume is sensed by stretch receptors on the arterial side in the carotid sinus and aortic arch and on the venous side in the atria and the thoracic veins.

AVP has also been localized to many brain structures outside of the hypothalamic-pituitary axis. The precise function of AVP in these extrahypothalamic areas remains controversial. Control of cardiovascular function through modulation of the autonomic nervous system has been suggested, as well as a possible role in memory consolidation.

Therapeutic Use. The primary therapeutic use of AVP (PITRESSIN and DDAVP) is hormone replacement therapy in central diabetes insipidus and the control of polyuria caused by head trauma. PITRESSIN may be given subcutaneously or intramuscularly at 3- to 4-hour intervals or intranasally

AVP is the most potent circulating vasoconstrictor known.

on cotton pledgets, by nasal spray, or by dropper. Overdosage results in water intoxication, of which the symptoms are drowsiness, listlessness, and headaches that eventually develop into coma and convulsions. Other adverse reactions include abdominal cramps, nausea, vomiting, tremor, vertigo, headaches, and sweating. AVP must be used with caution in the presence of epilepsy, migraine, asthma, heart failure, or other conditions in which rapid increases in plasma volume may precipitate an adverse reaction.

Other approved uses of PITRESSIN include prevention and treatment of postoperative abdominal distention and in abdominal roentgenography to dispel interfering gas shadows. Desmopressin is approved for the treatment of hemophilia A and type I von Willebrand's disease in which it has been shown to be effective in raising plasma levels of Factor VIII activity. AVP has also been tested in the treatment of variceal hemorrhage for which it is thought that an AVP-mediated reduction in portal pressure results in a decrease in variceal pressure, leading to termination of bleeding. Although AVP has been shown to be effective in reducing variceal bleeding, the long-term outlook for AVP-treated patients is no better than for those not given AVP.

OXYTOCIN

Chemistry. OXY is a 9–amino acid peptide related to AVP in that the amino acid sequence is identical except that phenylalanine at position 3 and arginine at position 8 in AVP are replaced with isoleucine and leucine, respectively (see Fig. 40–3). Like AVP, OXY is also synthesized in cell bodies of neurons in the paraventricular and supraoptic nuclei and transported in neurosecretory vesicles to the posterior pituitary from which it is released into the circulation. There does not appear to be any overlap in AVP-containing neurons and OXY-containing neurons. An OXY-specific neurophysin is also released with OXY; however, a moiety analogous to the 39–amino acid glycoprotein in the AVP-containing neurons is not present. OXY has a half-life in plasma of 1–6 minutes. A synthetically produced OXY is available (PITOCIN) in an injectable form. Although OXY is synthetically produced and free of AVP contamination, due to the similar sequence homology between OXY and AVP, OXY does have AVP-like actions at high concentrations.

Physiology. OXY plays an integral role in lactation. Stimulation of the nipple results in the activation of a neural reflex arc that ultimately produces the release of OXY from the posterior pituitary and PRL from the anterior pituitary. Whereas PRL acts on the epithelial cells of the alveoli to increase milk production, OXY causes the myoepithelial cells to contract, thus expelling the contents from the lumen of the alveoli into the lobuloalveolar ducts. Many lobuloalveolar ducts converge to form a single lactiferous duct, which carries the milk to the surface of the nipple.

OXY causes contraction of uterine myometrium during parturition.

A second action of OXY is to cause contraction of the uterine myometrium during parturition. During pregnancy the myometrium and decidua increase their sensitivity to OXY by increases in OXY receptor numbers. Although OXY release is an essential component in human parturition, it is not thought to be involved in the initiation of labor.

As with AVP, OXY is also found in areas of the central nervous system outside the hypothalamus. Whereas AVP is thought to play a role in memory consolidation, OXY has been shown to have an opposite effect.

Therapeutic Use. PITOCIN is used prepartum for the induction of labor, in ongoing labor to augment uterine contractions, and in the management of abortion to aid in the expulsion of uterine contents. PITOCIN may also be used postpartum to control uterine bleeding. During parturition PITOCIN is given intravenously, starting at 1 mU/minute. The dose is increased in steps of 1 mU/minute every 15 minutes until the desired response is achieved. At term, rates exceeding 9–10 mU/minute are rarely required; however, in preterm labor higher concentrations may be required owing to lower uterine sensitivity. Continuous monitoring of uterine responses and for potential fetal distress is essential during PITOCIN administration. Adverse reactions of the mother include severe hypertensive episodes, subarachnoid hemorrhage, and rupture of the uterus. Prolonged administration at high concentrations may lead to significant water retention owing to AVP-like effects.

General References

Growth Hormone

Amselem S, Duquesnoy P, Attree OP, et al: Laron dwarfism and mutations of the growth hormone-receptor gene. N Engl J Med 321:989–995, 1989.

Brown P: Human growth hormone therapy and Creutzfeldt-Jakob disease: A drama in three acts. Pediatrics 81:85–92, 1988.

Davidson MB: Effects of growth hormone on carbohydrate and lipid metabolism. Endocrine Rev 8:115–131, 1987.

Froesch ER, Schmid C, Schwander J, Zapf J: Actions of insulin-like growth factors. Annu Rev Physiol 47:443–467, 1985.

Lamberts SWJ: The role of somatostatin in the regulation of anterior pituitary hormone secretion and the use of its analogs in the treatment of human pituitary tumors. Endocrine Rev 9:417–436, 1988.

Lantos J, Siegler M, Cuttler L: Ethical issues in growth hormone therapy. JAMA 261:1020–1024, 1989.

Salomon F, Cuneo RC, Hesp R, Sonksen PH: The effects of treatment with recombinant human growth hormone on body composition and metabolism in adults with growth hormone deficiency. N Engl J Med 321:1797–1803, 1989.

Prolactin

Jaffe RB: Pathological alterations in prolactin production. *In* Yen SSC, Jaffe RB (eds): Reproductive Endocrinology, 2nd ed, 546–570. Philadelphia: WB Saunders Co, 1986.

Molitch ME: Management of prolactinomas. Annu Rev Med 40:225–232, 1989.

Yen SSC: Prolactin in human reproduction. *In* Yen SSC, Jaffe RB (eds): Reproductive Endocrinology, 2nd ed, 237–263. Philadelphia: WB Saunders Co, 1986.

Thyrotropin

Carr D, McLeod DT, Parry G, Thornes HM: Fine adjustment of thyroxine replacement dosage: Comparison of the thyrotrophin releasing hormone test using a sensitive thyrotrophin assay with measurement of free thyroid hormones and clinical assessment. Clin Endocrinol 28:325–333, 1988.

Griffiths EC: Clinical applications of thyrotrophin-releasing hormone. Clin Sci 73:449–457, 1987.

Gonadotropins

Bardin CW: Pituitary-testicular axis. *In* Yen SSC, Jaffe RB (eds): Reproductive Endocrinology, 2nd ed, 177–199. Philadelphia: WB Saunders Co, 1986.

Boepple PA, Mansfield MJ, Wierman ME, et al: Use of a potent, long-acting agonist of gonadotropin-releasing hormone in the treatment of precocious puberty. Endocrine Rev 7:24–33, 1986.

Burger HG, Baker HWG: The treatment of infertility. Annu Rev Med 38:29–40, 1987.

Catt KJ, Pierce JG: Gonadotropic hormones of the adenohypophysis. *In* Yen SSC, Jaffe RB (eds): Reproductive Endocrinology, 2nd ed, 75–114. Philadelphia: WB Saunders Co, 1986.

Liu L, Banks SM, Barnes KM, Sherins RJ: Two-year comparison of testicular responses to pulsatile gonadotropin-releasing hormone and exogenous gonadotropins from the inception of therapy in men with isolated hypogonadotropic hypogonadism. J Clin Endocrinol Metab 67:1140–1145, 1988.

Macnamee MC, Taylor PJ, Howles CM, et al: Short-term luteinizing hormone–releasing hormone agonist treatment: Prospective trial of a novel ovarian stimulation regimen for in vitro fertilization. Fertil Steril 52:264–269, 1989.

Yen SSC: The human menstrual cycle. *In* Yen SSC, Jaffe RB (eds): Reproductive Endocrinology, 2nd ed, 200–236. Philadelphia: WB Saunders Co, 1986.

Adrenocorticotropin

Axelrod J, Reisine TD: Stress hormones: Their interaction and regulation. Science 224:452–459, 1984.

Carter JL, Rodriguez M: Immunosuppressive treatment of multiple sclerosis. Mayo Clin Proc 64:664–669, 1989.

Krieger DT, Liotta AS, Brownstein MJ, Zimmerman EA: ACTH, β-lipotropin, and related peptides in brain, pituitary, and blood. Recent Prog Horm Res 36:277–336, 1980.

Posterior Pituitary

Cardozo L, Pearce JM: Oxytocin in active-phase abnormalities of labor: A randomized study. Obstet Gynecol 75:152–157, 1990.

Cowley AW, Liard JF: Cardiovascular actions of vasopressin. *In* Gash DM, Boer GJ (eds): Vasopressin, 389–434. New York: Plenum Press, 1987.

North WG: Biosynthesis of vasopressin and neurophysins. *In* Gash DM, Boer GJ (eds): Vasopressin, 176–210. New York: Plenum Press, 1987.

Stump DL, Hardin TC: The use of vasopressin in the treatment of upper gastrointestinal haemorrhage. Drugs 39:38–53, 1990.

Valtin H: Physiological effects of vasopressin on the kidney. *In* Gash DM, Boer GJ (eds): Vasopressin, 369–388. New York: Plenum Press, 1987.

Androgens

41

Christina Wang
Ronald S. Swerdloff

Testosterone is the most important sex steroid in men. Over 95% of testosterone is secreted by the Leydig cells of the testes under the stimulation of luteinizing hormone (LH) from the pituitary gland. Approximately 7 mg/day of testosterone is produced by the testes in a young male. In addition, small amounts of the potent androgen 5-α-dihydrotestosterone and the androgen precursor androstenedione are also secreted by the testes. Androgens circulate in women in much lower concentrations than those seen in men. The production rate of testosterone in women is 0.3 mg/day and that of androstenedione is 3.5 mg/day. Approximately 60% of androgen action in the female is the result of production of androgen or androgen precursors from the adrenal, and the remainder of the action comes from the ovary. Although the ovary in premenopausal women is not a major source of testosterone secretion, it does secrete large amounts of androstenedione, which is converted in the periphery to testosterone. The ovarian secretion of androgens comes from the theca and stromal cells of the ovary and is under the regulation of LH. The adrenal is the source of large amounts of androgen precursors, such as dehydroepiandrosterone, dehydroepiandrosterone sulfate, and androstenedione. The adrenal secretion of androgens and androgen precursors is under the regulation of pituitary adrenocorticotropic hormone (ACTH) and possibly other putative pituitary hormones (corticoadrenal-stimulating hormone, CASH).

Testosterone is transported in blood bound to plasma proteins. It circulates tightly bound to a β globulin, sex hormone–binding globulin (SHBG); loosely bound to albumin; or as a free (unbound) form. The free and albumin-bound forms of testosterone are available in target tissues for full biological activity. Adult women have about twice the plasma concentration of SHBG as adult men. This is because the liver production of SHBG is stimulated by estrogens and inhibited by androgens. In men about 3% of testosterone is free, 67% bound to albumin, and 30% bound to SHBG. In contrast, in women about 2% of testosterone is free, 40% bound to albumin, and 58% bound to SHBG. Thus the proportion of testosterone available for biological action at the target tissue is much higher in males than in females.

Testosterone exerts its androgenic effects directly on the target tissues or through the conversion to 5α-dihydrotestosterone by the enzyme 5α-reductase. In the skin, 5α-dihydrotestosterone is further metabolized to 3α-androstanediol and its glucuronide, which is a sensitive marker of peripheral androgen action. The actions of testosterone and 5α-dihydrotestosterone are mediated by specific androgen receptors present in the

Androgen Physiology

Testosterone is the most important sex steroid in men; the average male produces 7 mg/day.

Adrenocorticotropic hormone (ACTH)

Sex hormone–binding globulin (SHBG)

The male has a higher proportion of testosterone available for biological activity than the female has.

683

androgen target tissues. Androgen receptor contents vary in some tissues during different stages of development. For example, the androgen receptor is present in the penis during childhood but disappears in adulthood. Testosterone is also converted to estradiol by the aromatase enzyme, and some of the androgen effects (mammary gland, adipose tissue) are mediated by estradiol binding to the estrogen receptors.

The biological actions of androgens on target tissues are listed in Table 41–1. The action of testosterone on target tissues depends on the age and stage of development of the male. Testosterone is required during early fetal life for the differentiation of the wolffian ducts, the external genitalia, and the brain. As indicated in the table, masculinization of the external genitalia and stimulation of the accessory sex glands (e.g., prostate) require the conversion of testosterone to dihydrotestosterone at the tissue site of action. During puberty and adolescence, testosterone together with growth hormone is responsible for the pubertal growth spurt. At puberty testosterone stimulates epiphyseal closure, laryngeal enlargement, enlargement of the penis, rugation of the scrotum, and the appearance of sexual hair. During adulthood, androgens are required for maintenance of normal libido and potency, secondary sex characteristics, muscle mass, and prevention of loss of bone mass. One of the most important functions of testosterone is to initiate and maintain spermatogenesis. It is important to note that very high levels of testosterone within the testis are required for its action. The administration of exogenous androgen will not have stimulatory effects on the germ cells and will inhibit spermatogenesis and sperm production by the negative feedback action on LH secretion and intratesticular testosterone production.

> Testosterone and growth hormone are responsible for the pubertal growth spurt.

> Testosterone initiates and maintains spermatogenesis.

Table 41–1 ANDROGEN TARGET TISSUES AND BIOLOGICAL ACTIONS

Target Tissues	Biological Actions
Hypothalamus	Negative feedback on gonadotropin-releasing hormone secretion
Pituitary	Negative feedback on LH and follicle-stimulating hormone secretion
Reproductive tissues	
Seminiferous tubules, Seminal vesicles, Epididymis, Vas deferens (Testosterone-dependent)	Initiation and maintenance of spermatogenesis
Prostate, Penis, Scrotum (Dihydrotestosterone-dependent)	Differentiation and development of the male accessory ducts and external genitalia
Nonreproductive tissues	
Liver (enzymes/lipoprotein)	Stimulation or suppression of protein synthesis
Kidney	Stimulation of erythropoietin, which indirectly increases hematopoiesis
Hematopoietic system	Direct stimulation of growth of stem cells; indirect stimulation by erythropoietin
Central nervous system	Facilitation of libido and sexual function; male aggressive behavior
Muscle	Development of muscle mass and strength
Skin, sebaceous gland, and hair (dihydrotestosterone-dependent)	Stimulation of growth of beard, axillary, and pubic hair, increase in temporal hair recession and balding; increase in sebum secretion
Bone/cartilage	Promotion of epiphyseal fusion; Maintenance of bone mass
Larynx and vocal cords	Enlargement of larynx and thickening of vocal cords; deepening of voice
Mammary glands (estrogen-dependent)	Development of gynecomastia affected by ratio of androgen to estrogen

The actions of androgens have traditionally been classified as *androgenic* or *anabolic*. All effects that cause growth of the male reproductive tract or development of secondary sex characteristics are termed *androgenic*, whereas the effects on nonreproductive tissue — e.g., muscle, liver, bone, bone marrow — are termed *anabolic*. Although early studies suggested that there might be two independent actions of the same class of androgens, subsequent experiments showed that these are organ-specific responses and that all androgens act through the same molecular mechanisms. All androgens have both androgenic and anabolic actions. Most of the pharmacological anabolic androgens can be used for replacement therapy in hypogonadal men. The one exception may be danazol. This 17α-alkylated testosterone is particularly effective in suppressing gonadotropin secretion but relatively ineffective in other anabolic or androgenic actions. However, if female infants are exposed to danazol *in utero*, masculinization can occur.

> Androgenic effects involve the growth of the male reproductive tract and the development of secondary sex characteristics. Anabolic effects refer to the nonreproductive tissue.

> Exposing female infants to danazol *in utero* can cause masculinization.

Impaired testicular secretion of androgen leads to hypogonadism and infertility. Clinical features of androgen deficiency depend on the degree of deficiency, the age of onset of the dysfunction, and the relative sensitivity of the androgen-sensitive tissues (see Table 41–1). Deficiency of androgens occurring in early fetal life leads to pseudohermaphroditism. The clinical spectrum ranges from mild hypospadias to female external genitalia. Androgen deficiency during late fetal development is associated with unambiguous male genitalia but small phallus (micropenis). The development of hypogonadism during childhood results in failure of pubertal development and eunuchoidal proportions. Lack of androgens (and estrogens) causes delayed fusion of the epiphysis and continued long bone growth. This results in arm span being greater than height and the lower segment of the body being longer than the upper segment. Androgen deficiencies occurring after puberty result in decrease in facial, axillary, and pubic hair, decrease in libido and potency, loss of muscle bulk, and decrease in testis size. Gynecomastia occurs in some patients with androgen deficiency and reflects a decreased testosterone-to-estradiol ratio. In the assessment of body hair, the physician must take into account the patient's ethnic background. Orientals, Native Americans, and blacks frequently do not shave everyday. Caucasian men usually have pectoral, back, and flank hair in addition to axillary and pubic hair.

Androgen excess occurs in boys with precocious puberty due to central (hypothalamic-pituitary) causes, testicular and adrenal tumors, and non-gonadotropin-mediated Leydig's cell hyperstimulation (familial testotoxicosis). The use of antiandrogens and androgen synthesis blockers in these conditions are discussed later in this chapter.

Androgen excess in females leading to hirsutism or virilism may be due to ovarian or adrenal causes. As in the male, the ethnic background and the family history must be taken into consideration in a female patient with hirsutism. Most patients with hirsutism have an unexplained idiopathic increased androgen secretion or increased peripheral conversion of androstenedione and testosterone to dihydrotestosterone. The second most common cause of increased hair growth in the female is the polycystic ovary syndrome. Other less common causes include Cushing's syndrome, adult-onset nonclassical congenital adrenal hyperplasia, androgen-producing tumors of the ovary or the adrenal, and ovarian hyperthecosis.

Disorders of Androgen Secretion

> Fetal androgen deficiency leads to pseudohermaphroditism.

Androgen Preparations and Their Pharmacology

When unmodified testosterone is administered orally, it is rapidly absorbed into the portal blood, and after the first-pass degradation by the liver, very small amounts of testosterone reach the systemic circulation. Similarly,

Chemical modifications of testosterone retard the rate of absorption.

Testosterone enanthate, methyltestosterone, and nandrolone are three common modifications of testosterone's chemical structure.

when testosterone is administered parenterally, it is absorbed from the injection site and rapidly degraded, so that the effective androgen levels are not sustained in the plasma. To circumvent this problem, chemical modifications of testosterone are required to retard the rate of absorption and catabolism. The common modifications of the chemical structure of testosterone are (1) esterification of the 17-β-hydroxyl group (e.g., testosterone enanthate); (2) alkylation at the 17-α-position (e.g., methyltestosterone); and (3) changes in the ring structure of testosterone (e.g., 19-norandrogen; nandrolone) (Fig. 41–1). Specific examples of available agents within these classes are shown in Table 41–2. More recent developments include the preparation of orally active micronized testosterone and testosterone cyclodextrins, the incorporation of testosterone into skin patches, and testosterone linked to polylactide-co-glycolide microcapsules for intramuscular injections.

ORAL

Alkylated derivatives of testosterone are metabolized slowly by the liver.

The alkylated derivatives of testosterone are effective when administered orally or buccally because they are slowly metabolized by the liver. They pass through the liver to reach the systemic circulation and produce effective plasma concentrations. Usually these drugs are administered on a daily basis. The alkyl groups are not removed, and most likely these 17α-alkylated steroids act unmodified in the target tissue. These alkylated compounds are potentially hepatotoxic and cause more metabolic side effects than do testosterone esters, and they should not be prescribed except for special indications such as hereditary angioneurotic edema.

Mesterolone is a weak androgen that does not suppress gonadotropin secretion.

Other alterations in the ring structure include alkylation at the 1 position. The resultant steroid mesterolone is a weak androgen that does not

Table 41–2 SOME PREPARATIONS OF ANDROGENS

Generic Name	Trade Name	Route of Administration	Dose	Supplier
Alpha-Alkylated Androgens				
Methyltestosterone	Android	Buccal or oral	5, 10, 25 mg/tablet	ICN
	Metandren			CIBA
	Testred	Oral	10 mg/capsule	ICN
Fluoxymesterone	Android F	Oral	10 mg/tablet	ICN
	Halotestin		2, 5, 10 mg/tablet	Upjohn
	Oreton		10 mg/tablet	Schering
Oxymetholone	Anadrol	Oral	50 mg/tablet	Syntex
Oxandrolone	Anavar	Oral	2.5 mg/tablet	Searle
Stanozolol	Winstrol	Oral	2 mg/tablet	Winthrop
Danazol	Danocrine	Oral	50, 100, 200 mg/tablet	Winthrop
Testosterone Esters				
Testosterone undecanoate*	Andriol	Oral	40 mg/tablet	Organon
Testosterone enanthate	Delatestryl	Intramuscular injection	200 mg/ml	Squibb
Testosterone cypionate	DEPO-Testosterone	Intramuscular injection	100, 200 mg/ml	Upjohn
	Testred		200 mg/ml	ICN
Modified Ring Structure				
Mesterolone*	Androviron	Oral	25 mg/day	Schering
	Proviron			AG
Nandrolone phenpropionate	Durabalin	Intramuscular injection	25–50 mg/ml	Organon
Nandrolone decanoate	Deca-Durabolin	Injection	50–200 mg/ml	Organon

* Not available in the United States.

suppress gonadotropin secretion. Testosterone undecanoate ester is so nonpolar that it is absorbed into the lymphatics. As a result, it can maintain normal androgen levels after oral administration. The drug must be taken three times per day because of its short duration of action. The testosterone levels achieved tend to be variable within the same subject and between subjects. Although widely used in Europe and Asia, testosterone undecanoate is not available in the United States.

Orally active testosterone preparations under development include micronized testosterone and testosterone cyclodextrin preparation. When micronized testosterone is administered in large amounts, a small proportion of the steroid escapes the first pass, and adequate blood levels can be obtained. Similarly, testosterone cyclodextrin preparations are rapidly absorbed orally and cleared quickly. Both preparations must be administered several times a day, and testosterone pulses occur after each dose.

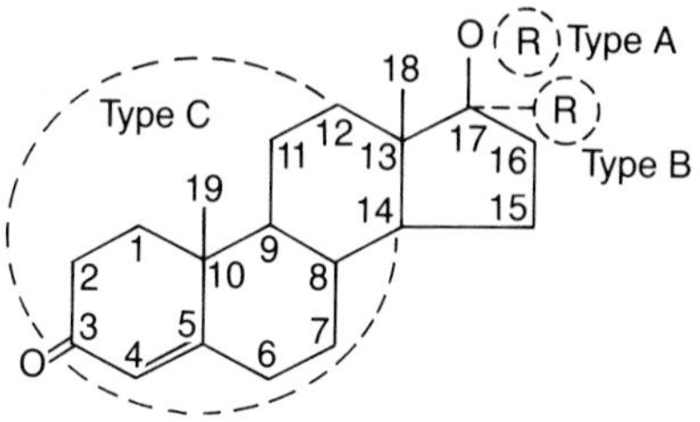

PARENTERAL

The parenteral route of administration of testosterone is the one most commonly used for androgen replacement. Testosterone esters are lipophilic and are absorbed slowly when injected as an oil depot. These agents are of sufficient potency to achieve therapeutic effect without other significant side effects. The most commonly used testosterone ester is testosterone enanthate. After an intramuscular injection of 200 mg of testosterone enanthate in oil, peak supraphysiological levels of testosterone are reached rapidly within 1–3 days. The testosterone levels gradually decrease and reach baseline levels over the next 10–14 days (Fig. 41–2). Most hypogonadal men respond well to self-administration of intramuscular injections of testosterone enanthate 150–200 mg every 2 or 3 weeks. Occasionally, emotional lability and mood swings occur a few days prior to each injection. For these patients, 100 mg of testosterone enanthate can be administered every week. Testosterone cypionate has essentially the same pharmacokinetics and bioavailability as those of testosterone enanthate and can be used effectively as androgen replacement therapy.

Because of the occurrence of the initial peak of testosterone after each

Figure 41–1

Categories of androgens commonly used pharmacologically. Type A, esterified androgens; type B, 17α-alkylated androgens; type C, androgens with alterations of the steroid nucleus. (Redrawn from Wilson JD: Androgen abuse by athletes. Endocr Rev 9[2]:181–199, 1988, © by The Endocrine Society.)

Injections of testosterone are used to treat hypogonadal men.

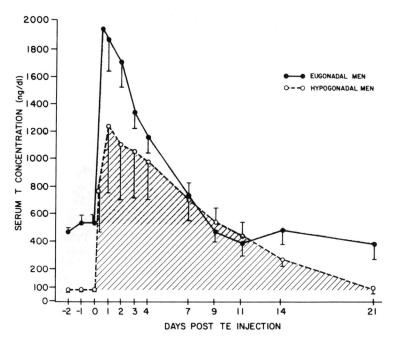

Figure 41–2

Mean and standard error of testosterone (T) levels in eugonadal and hypogonadal men before and at various time intervals after an intramuscular injection of 200 mg of testosterone enanthate (TE). (From Sokol RZ, Palacios A, Campfield LA, et al: Comparison of the kinetics of injectable testosterone in eugonadal and hypogonadal men. Fertil Steril 37:425, 1982. Reproduced with permission of the publisher, The American Fertility Society.)

Testosterone-trans-4-n-butylcyclohexyl-carboxylate has a half-life of 63 days (in nonhuman primates).

injection, long-acting esters of testosterone are currently under development for use in clinical medicine. One of these is testosterone-trans-4-n-butylcyclohexyl-carboxylate, which has a half-life of 63 days as opposed to 6 days for testosterone enanthate (in primates). Testosterone in polylactide-co-glycolide microspheres can be given by intramuscular route and can sustain testosterone levels for over 70 days. These longer-acting testosterone preparations, capable of maintaining androgen levels within the physiological range without the initial burst, will probably be the agents of choice for androgen replacement in the near future.

TRANSDERMAL

Transdermal patches help hypogonadal men maintain normal testosterone levels.

Testosterone incorporated into transdermal delivery systems (40 or 60 sq cm) are worn as patches on the scrotum. These patches are changed daily. They can maintain normal testosterone levels when applied to hypogonadal men. Dihydrotestosterone levels are above the normal range, but the significance of a high dihydrotestosterone-to-testosterone ratio is unknown. These patches will be available in the United States in the near future.

IMPLANTS

Subcutaneous implants of testosterone pellets require a minor surgical procedure.

Testosterone can be administered as subcutaneous implants. The pellets (400–600 mg of testosterone in four to six pellets) maintain testosterone levels within the physiological range for about 4–6 months. A minor surgical procedure involving a local anesthesia is required to insert the pellets by a trained physician. Sometimes extrusion of the pellets can occur from the injection site, and fibroses around the pellets make removal difficult.

Androgen Replacement Therapy

Androgens are used primarily to treat hypogonadism.

Androgens do not reverse infertility.

The indications for androgen treatment are shown in Table 41–3. The primary use of androgens is for the treatment of hypogonadism. Patients with primary testicular failure must be treated with androgens to relieve their clinical symptoms and signs. Response to androgen replacement therapy is monitored by improvement in the clinical features of hypogonadism. Improvements in sexual function, frequency of shaving, secondary sexual characteristics and general well-being occur rapidly after the initiation of treatment. It is often useful to monitor nadir and peak testosterone levels during the start of therapy and in patients who do not show adequate clinical response. Androgen treatment will not reverse their infertility.

Table 41-3 INDICATIONS FOR ANDROGEN THERAPY	
Definite	Male hypogonadism
Probable or possible	Micropenis in children
	Constitutional delayed puberty
	Aging men (with evidence of androgen deficiency)
	Male contraception
	Hereditary angioneurotic edema
Dubious or controversial	Hematological disorders such as aplastic anemia, myelofibrosis with myeloid metaplasia, hemolytic anemia, autoimmune thrombocytopenia, and leukopenia
	Improvement of nitrogen balance in non–androgen-deficient catabolic state
	Improvement of libido in hypogonadal women
Not indicated	Anemia associated with renal failure
	Improvement of muscle strength and endurance in athletes and body builders

Patients with hypogonadotropic hypogonadism are also treated with androgens because of the ease of administration and low cost. If patients with hypogonadotropic hypogonadism desire fertility, human chorionic gonadotropin with human menopausal gonadotropin or pulsatile gonadotropin-releasing hormone (GnRH) injections or infusions may be given to induce spermatogenesis and fertility. Prior treatment with testosterone does not jeopardize the chances of fertility in these patients with hypogonadotropic hypogonadism.

In children with micropenis, a short course of low-dose androgen therapy is often tried. In adolescent boys with constitutional delay of puberty in whom the psychological effects of delayed puberty are significant, short-term treatment with testosterone enanthate for 3–4 months may be indicated.

For children with micropenis and adolescent boys with delayed puberty, low-dose androgen therapy is tried.

Total and free testosterone levels decrease with age. A decrease in sexual function is often observed in older men. It has not been proved that androgen therapy in older men will improve sexual function or prevent bone and muscle loss. At present, it is not known whether androgen replacement therapy will improve the quality of life of aging men. The possible beneficial effect of androgens must be balanced against the possible adverse effects on lipids, prostate, and sleep-related breathing disorders.

In endocrine approaches to male contraception, when spermatogenesis is inhibited by suppression of hypothalamus and pituitary resulting in suppression of both LH and follicle-stimulating hormone (FSH), androgen supplementation is always required. Examples of experimental male contraceptives include androgens given alone or combined with progestagens or GnRH analogs. In these regimes, androgens function both to suppress sperm production by inhibiting gonadotropins and to provide physiological androgen replacement.

In hereditary angioneurotic edema, anabolic steroids such as stanozolol and danazol have been used to prevent attacks. These anabolic steroids increase the synthesis of complement 1 inhibitor, which is deficient in these patients. Because of the known side effects of these agents, they are not recommended for use in pregnant women and children with this hereditary disorder.

Anabolic steroids have been used to treat hereditary angioneurotic edema.

The role of androgens in the treatment of hematological disorders remains controversial. Treatment of hypoplastic anemia with androgens may be tried for 3–6 months, but in responders treatment has to be continued for a much longer period. The reader should refer to other sections for the use of androgens in myelofibrosis, autoimmune thrombocytopenia, and hemolytic anemia (see Chapters 46 and 59). Because of the availability of recombinant human erythropoietin with its more specific action and its lack of side effects, androgens should not be used for patients with anemia associated with chronic renal failure.

Androgens have been used in clinical situations, such as trauma or chronic illness, in which the patient is in a negative nitrogen balance. The long-term results are generally disappointing.

In postmenopausal women, small doses of androgens have been used together with estrogen-progestagen supplementation for improvement of libido. However, controlled trials showing a definite improvement in sexual drive after androgen therapy are lacking. Higher doses of androgens are associated with hirsutism and virilization in women.

There is an increasing trend toward the use of androgenic steroids by athletes and body builders. The pattern of androgen use by athletes involves the intermittent and cyclical administration of pharmacological doses of a combination of oral and parenteral agents. These unprescribed

Body builders and athletes have been using androgenic steroids increasingly.

It is not clear whether the administration of androgens enhances athletic performance in eugonadol men.

The toxic side effects of supraphysiological doses of androgens include gynecomastia, hepatic toxicity, polycythemia, HDL lowering, and suppression of spermatogenesis.

androgens may include huge doses of drugs, including veterinary agents that either are potentially toxic or have not been tested in humans. Androgens increase muscle mass and strength in women and prepubertal children. In normal adult men, it is not clear whether the administration of additional androgens enhances athletic performances. Most information is anecdotal; however, a number of studies have been performed. Double-blind studies either are in conflict or have not shown beneficial effects on athletic performance in postpubertal males. Even in those studies in which increased strength and performance were seen, the changes induced by these agents were small; thus documentation of clinically significant improvements in muscle strength and endurance may be difficult. Despite the controversy, some physicians have argued that changes in performance justify use of these agents by some high-performance, competitive athletes. Most physicians, however, believe that the unsupervised use of androgens and high-dose androgen treatment impose some risk of undesired toxic effects. The toxic side effects of virilization in the female and premature bone closure in prepubertal children should preclude androgen use in athletes in these groups. In addition, the long-term abuse of supraphysiological doses of a combination of androgens in men may lead to gynecomastia, hepatic toxicity, polycythemia, lipid changes (lowering of high-density lipoprotein, HDL), and suppression of spermatogenesis. These toxic side effects are sufficient to discourage use of androgens for nonmedical reasons in people of all ages, even adult men.

Adverse Effects

Acne and oily skin are frequently experienced by patients undergoing androgen supplementation.

Other adverse effects include weight gain, suppression of spermatogenesis, decrease in testicular size, and virilization in women and prepubertal children.

In general, testosterone and its esters have fewer side effects than the 17α-alkylated androgens. Acne and increased oiliness of skin are frequently experienced by patients at the initiation of androgen supplementation. Because testosterone is metabolized to estradiol, gynecomastia may develop. The gynecomastia is often mild, and treatment is unnecessary. Most patients will gain weight when administered androgens. The weight gain is related to water retention, increased blood volume, and increased lean body mass. All patients given exogenous androgen therapy will have suppression of spermatogenesis. Some patients will notice a decrease in testicular size. The decrease in sperm production and seminiferous tubule volume is a consequence of the suppression of LH and FSH. Androgens will cause virilization in women and prepubertal children. In addition, androgens promote premature epiphyseal closure in children. For these reasons, androgens should not be used in women and in children of both sexes except for specific indications as discussed previously.

HEPATIC DYSFUNCTION

Hepatic disorders are not observed with testosterone but are observed with the 17α-alkylated androgens.

Changes in liver function and hepatic disorders are not observed with testosterone or its esters. The 17α-alkylated androgens can produce liver dysfunction including cholestasis and elevation of plasma alkaline phosphatase and conjugated bilirubin. Methyltestosterone causes cholestatic jaundice with little parenchymal liver damage. Recovery is usually rapid after drug discontinuation. Peliosis hepatis or hepatic tumors rarely occur and only when high pharmacologic doses of androgens are used to treat conditions such as refractory aplastic anemia. Since most of these reports involve conditions that are associated with increased incidence of neoplasms, the implications of such reports for the treatment of hypogonadal men remains controversial.

LIPID CHANGES

When a 17α-alkylated androgen, stanozolol, is administered to normal men, HDL cholesterol, apolipoprotein A-I and A-II levels are decreased, and low-density lipoprotein (LDL) cholesterol and apolipoprotein B levels are increased. These changes in lipid profiles have been identified as risk factors for coronary atherosclerosis. Such changes in lipid profile may not be associated with testosterone esters such as testosterone enanthate perhaps because some of the testosterone is converted to estrogens that have the opposite effects on lipid profile than do androgens. Another explanation for the difference on lipid profiles may be that the orally active anabolic steroids have a first-pass effect on the liver, leading to effects on lipids not apparent with the parenterally administered testosterone esters. More data are needed in larger groups of men to determine whether the testosterone esters are truly free of adverse effects on lipid profiles.

Administration of stanozolol, a 17α-alkylated androgen, decreases HDL cholesterol levels and increases LDL levels in normal men.

HEMATOPOIESIS AND FIBRINOLYSIS

Androgens cause small increases in hemoglobin, hematocrit, and total red cell count when administered to normal or hypogonadal men. Androgens stimulate erythropoietin production by the kidneys. Androgens may also have a direct effect on the bone marrow stem cells. Clinically significant polycythemia is uncommon in hypogonadal men given androgen replacement except in patients prone to develop polycythemia, e.g., those with chronic obstructive pulmonary disease or sleep apnea.

Androgens cause small increases in hemoglobin, hematocrit, and total red cell count.

The 17α-alkylated androgens, stanozolol and danazol, have been given to men with coagulation disorders. Although small increases of clotting factors are recorded, these anabolic steroids increase fibrinolysis and antithrombin III levels (a natural anticoagulant). The net effect was that increased bleeding episodes were observed. The increase in fibrinolysis may counterbalance the negative effects of lipid profiles on the risk of coronary heart disease.

Administration of stanozolol and danazol may increase fibrinolysis and antithrombin III levels.

RESPIRATORY PROBLEMS

In hypogonadal men treated with androgen replacement, sleep-related breathing disorders have been reported. In patients with obesity and chronic obstructive airway disease, the physician should question the patient about sleep-related breathing disorders before the commencement of androgen replacement.

Sleep-related breathing disorders have been reported in hypogonadal men treated with androgens.

CARBOHYDRATE METABOLISM

Although there are reports of androgen-induced mild resistance to insulin action, the usual doses of testosterone esters, when given to normal men, are not associated with changes in glucose or insulin levels. There have been reports of adverse effects on glucose control in diabetic patients given androgen replacement.

PROSTATE PROBLEMS

Benign prostatic hypertrophy (BPH) and prostate cancer rarely occur in men who developed androgen deficiency prior to puberty. Despite this fact, there is no clear evidence to indicate that androgen replacement given to men who become hypogonadal after puberty will increase the risk of prostatic disease. For all adult men, especially older men, on long-term androgen therapy, regular rectal examinations must be performed. If there is a suspicion of prostatic enlargement, a transrectal prostatic ultrasound should be performed, and prostate-specific antigen levels should be monitored.

PSYCHOSEXUAL PROBLEMS

Changes in psychosexual behavior can occur in prepubertal boys given testosterone replacement.

In prepubertal boys given testosterone replacement, changes in psychosexual behavior may occur. To avoid these problems, small dosages of testosterone enanthate (25–50 mg) every 3–4 weeks are administered at the initiation of androgen therapy. After 6 months or a year, the testosterone dosage can be increased to 50–100 mg every 3–4 weeks for the next 2 years and further increased to the adult replacement dosage as necessary. Frequent erections can occur at the start of androgen therapy. Priapism is uncommon. Psychosexual problems usually decrease with time.

Antiandrogens

Antiandrogens interfere with the action of androgens at target tissues.

Spironolactone, a weak antiandrogen, has been used to treat women with hirsutism.

The antiandrogens exert their effect by interfering with the action of androgens at the target tissues. These include the mineralocorticoid antagonist spironolactone and the pure antiandrogens cyproterone and flutamide. The other groups of drugs are inhibitors of androgen biosynthesis including ketoconazole and the newly developed finasteride. The indications for antiandrogen therapy are listed in Table 41–4. The weak antiandrogen spironolactone has been used for the treatment of hirsutism (women). Originally developed for male hypersexuality, cyproterone acetate, the antiandrogen with progestational activity, has been used extensively for the treatment of women with hirsutism and boys with precocious puberty. Flutamide has been tested in clinical studies alone or in combination with a potent GnRH agonist as hormonal therapy for metastatic advanced prostatic cancer. Finasteride has been shown to decrease prostate size in animals and humans and is potentially useful in the treatment of hirsutism, BPH, and carcinoma of the prostate.

SPIRONOLACTONE

Spironolactone, an aldosterone antagonist, blocks androgen action by occupying specific androgen receptors in the target tissues and by inhibiting androgen synthesis.

The aldosterone antagonist spironolactone has been found to have weak antiandrogen properties. It inhibits the cytochrome P-450 enzyme system, which is required for the synthesis of androgens. It also interferes with the action of androgens by occupying the specific androgen receptors in the target tissues. Clinical studies have shown that spironolactone reduced the hair density and diameter in patients with hirsutism. The dose of spironolactone used is 100 mg/day orally. Although spironolactone is associated with menstrual disturbances when given to normal females, it can induce normal menstrual periods in patients with anovulatory hyperandrogenism.

Table 41–4 INDICATIONS FOR ANTIANDROGEN THERAPY
Hirsutism/virilism in females
Benign prostatic hypertrophy
Advanced prostatic cancer
Hypersexuality
Gonadotropin-independent precocious puberty in boys (familial testotoxicosis)
(Not recommended for control of precocious puberty in both girls and boys because of the availability of gonadotropin-releasing hormone analogs.)

CYPROTERONE AND CYPROTERONE ACETATE

The pure antiandrogen cyproterone interferes with androgen binding to the nuclei receptor at the target tissue. Peripheral testosterone and gonadotropin levels are not suppressed but often elevated in patients given the drug. Its acetate derivative has both antiandrogen and strong progestational effects; the latter activity suppresses the secretion of gonadotropins, which secondarily decrease testosterone biosynthesis. Cyproterone acetate is widely used in Europe for the treatment of hirsutism. It is administered at an oral dose of 50 mg in combination with estrogens on days 5–25 of the menstrual cycle for the treatment of hirsutism. A much reduced dose of 2 mg of cyproterone acetate in combination with estrogens is available for the treatment of mild hirsutism and acne. Because of its suppressive effects on gonadotropins, cyproterone acetate has been used for the arrest of puberty in gonadotropin-dependent (central) precocious puberty. Although pubertal development is arrested, bone maturation usually continues, leading to reduction in final height. GnRH agonist is more effective in the treatment of central precocious puberty because its greater effectiveness in suppressing gonadotropin secretion results in arrest of secondary sexual development and skeletal maturation. The estimated final height of the children is, therefore, not compromised. Cyproterone acetate has also been used in Europe to treat advanced prostate cancer, although use of GnRH analogs with or without antiandrogens appears to be the preferred medical therapy. Cyproterone acetate sometimes causes hepatic dysfunction; despite its widespread use in other countries, the drug is not approved for use by the Food and Drug Administration (FDA) in the United States.

> Cyproterone acetate is used widely in Europe to treat hirsutism.

> Cyproterone acetate can cause hepatic dysfunction and has not been approved for use in the United States.

FLUTAMIDE

Flutamide is a nonsteroidal antiandrogen that blocks androgen action at the target tissue. In humans, flutamide, like pure cyproterone, leads to elevated serum levels of testosterone and LH. It has been used as an investigational drug alone or in combination with GnRH agonists for the treatment of advanced prostatic cancer to achieve complete androgen blockade. The common side effect is gynecomastia. Very occasionally, flutamide may cause hematological disorders such as methemoglobinemia.

> Flutamide can be used for the treatment of prostatic cancer.

KETOCONAZOLE

Ketoconazole, an orally administered imidazole used for treatment of fungal infections, blocks adrenal and testicular androgen biosynthesis. Ketoconazole directly inhibits the cytochrome system of steroidogenic enzyme primarily on the enzyme C17–20 lyase and cholesterol side-chain cleavage enzymes. Ketoconazole has been shown to be effective in the treatment of gonadotropin-independent precocious puberty (familial testotoxicosis). The initial dose used for the suppression of precocious puberty is 3 mg/kg body weight/day. Ketoconazole has also been used for advanced prostatic cancer. The drug may cause some significant side effects when used in dosages in excess of 600 mg/day. These include transient adrenal suppression, nausea, vomiting, anemia, and elevated liver enzymes.

> Ketoconazole, an antifungal agent, decreases androgen biosynthesis.

> Adverse side effects of ketoconazole include transient adrenal suppression, nausea, vomiting, anemia, and elevated liver enzymes.

FINASTERIDE

Finasteride is a specific inhibitor of 5α-reductase that converts testosterone to 5α-dihydrotestosterone. It has been shown to be effective in reducing

Pilot studies of finasteride administration to patients with BPH showed reductions in prostatic volume and increased urinary flow.

prostate size in dogs and rats. In human, finasteride causes dose-dependent decreases in serum 5α-dihydrotestosterone as well as its metabolites, 3α-androstanediol glucuronide and androsterone glucuronide. Preliminary studies demonstrated no decrease in serum levels of testosterone and little change in serum FSH and LH levels. Pilot studies of finasteride in patients with BPH demonstrated reductions in prostatic volume and increases in urinary flow. This experimental drug is potentially useful in dihydrotestosterone-dependent disease conditions such as BPH, prostatic cancer, hirsutism, and virilism.

References

Androgens

Amuss SS: The role of androgens in the treatment of hematologic disorders. Adv Intern Med 34:191, 1989.

Cantrill JA, Dewis P, Large DM, et al: Which testosterone replacement therapy? Clin Endocrinol (Oxf) 21:97, 1984.

Mooradian AD, Morley JE, Korenman SG: Biological actions of androgens. Endocr Rev 9:181, 1984.

Snyder PJ, Lawrence DA: Treatment of male hypogonadism with testosterone enanthate. J Clin Endocrinol Metab 51:1335, 1980.

Sokol RZ, Palacios A, Campfield LA, et al: Comparison of the kinetics of injectable testosterone in eugonadal and hypogonadal men. Fertil Steril 37:425, 1982.

Swerdloff RS, Sokol RZ: Manifestations of androgen deficiency and effects of androgen therapy. *In* Steinberger E, Frajese G, Steinberger A (eds): Reproductive Medicine, 39–53. New York: Raven Press, 1986.

Wilson JD: Androgen abuse by athletes. Endocr Rev 9:181, 1988.

Antiandrogens

Ghormley GJ, Stoner C, Rittmester RS, et al: Effects of finasteride, a 5 alpha-reductase inhibitor on circulating androgens in male volunteers. J Clin Endocrinol Metab 70:1136, 1990.

Holland FG, Fishman L, Bailey JD, Frazekers ATA: Ketoconazole in the management of precocious puberty not responsive to LHRH-analogue therapy. N Engl J Med 312:1023, 1985.

Neuman F: Pharmacology and potential use of cyproterone acetate. Horm Metab Res 9:1, 1977.

Shapiro G, Evron S: A novel use of spironolactone: Treatment of hirsutism. J Clin Endocrinol Metab 51:429, 1980.

Sogani P, Fair WR: Treatment of advanced prostatic cancer. Urol Clin North Am 14:2, 1987.

Estrogens and Progestins

42

Lynnette K. Nieman
D. Lynn Loriaux

The cyclical secretion of hormones by the ovary is responsible for the development and maintenance of female sexual characteristics and function. The importance of the ovary to these processes has been recognized since antiquity, as shown by the use of ovariotomy for contraception by the ancient Egyptians. The hormonal control of reproductive function was not understood, however, until the early twentieth century, and the isolation of the ovarian hormones was not accomplished until the 1930s (Fieser and Fieser, 1959).

The existence of ovarian hormones was demonstrated independently in 1900 by Knauer and Halban, who showed that transplantation of ovarian tissue prevented uterine atrophy in sexually mature castrated animals and allowed normal sexual development in immature castrated animals. Frankel demonstrated the importance of the corpus luteum in 1903 by showing that its removal caused abortion. In 1906 Marshall and Jolly showed that injections of ovarian extracts induced estrus in castrated animals. The publication of the vaginal smear test for estrus by Papanicolaou and Stockard in 1917 suggested a bioassay method that could be used to evaluate putative estrogenic substances.

In 1923 Allen and Doisy showed that a cell-free extract of graafian follicles (but not the corpus luteum) stimulated the growth of vaginal epithelium in the castrated rat, establishing that the active principle is a chemical substance. The urine of menstruating and pregnant women was shown subsequently to contain estrogenic substances as well. This was a boon to the investigators attempting to isolate the active principle(s), and they turned to urine as a source of large quantities of raw material. Estrone was crystallized from the urine of pregnant women by Doisy in 1929. Butenandt published its chemical structure in the same year. Estriol was characterized by Marseian in 1930, and 17β estradiol was isolated from 4 tons of sow ovaries by MacCorquodale in 1935.

The contemporaneous effort to characterize the hormone(s) regulating gestation was advanced in 1928 when Corner and Allen established that the corpus luteum was the source of a hormone that prepares the uterus for implantation. This hormone, progesterone, like estradiol, was not abundant in urine. It was isolated from sow ovaries nearly simultaneously by four laboratories in 1934. The difficulty of the isolation is illustrated by Butenandt's report that the ovaries of 50,000 sows were required for the purification of 20 mg of progestin. Shortly thereafter, Slotta proposed the correct chemical structure of progesterone and Butenandt reported its complete synthesis.

> Hormonal control of reproductive function was not understood until the early twentieth century.

695

DES was the first estrogen that could be readily synthesized.

By 1935 estradiol and progesterone could be synthesized (at high cost) from natural intermediates. Unfortunately these hormones lost biological activity when given by mouth. The first orally active estrogen was discovered in 1938, when Dodds found that a nonsteroidal compound, diethylstilbestrol (DES), had potent estrogenic activity when given by mouth. This was the first estrogen that could be readily synthesized.

The understanding of two important structure-function relationships contributed to the subsequent synthesis of a variety of clinically useful substituted steroids. First, the Schering Corporation discovered in 1938 that substitution of an ethinyl group at the C17 position of testosterone yielded an orally active compound. Second, Ehrenstein showed in 1944 that the inactive compound isoprogesterone could be made into an active progestin by removing the C19 methyl group. This led to the synthesis of a number of C19-norsteroids. The practical application of these principles resulted in the synthesis of an orally active estrogen, ethinyl estradiol, and an orally active progestin, norethindrone (17α-ethinyl, 19-nortestosterone).

The understanding of the physiology of these hormones progressed also. The ability of progesterone to inhibit ovulation was noted by Makpeace in 1940. One year later Sturgis and Albright reported the successful use of estradiol to inhibit ovulation in patients with dysmenorrhea. These studies foreshadowed the contraceptive trials of Pincus in the early 1950s.

The synthesis of steroids was facilitated by the discovery by Marker that the roots of the Mexican yam, cabeza de negra, contained diosgenin. This naturally occurring steroid has a structure that is a suitable starting point for the large-scale synthesis of a variety of steroidal compounds at a lower cost. Meanwhile, efforts to produce steroids by total synthesis continued and culminated in 1963 with the first total synthesis of 19-nor-steroids.

Total steroid synthesis was achieved in 1963.

Estrogens

CHEMISTRY

Structure

The basic steroidal structure is shown in Figure 42–1. By convention the carbon atoms are numbered and the rings are alphabetized as shown. The removal of successive carbons leads to the prototypic skeleton for the major classes of steroid hormones: C21, pregnane, the progestins; C19, androstane, the androgens; and C18, estrane, the estrogens. A saturated ring structure is indicated by the suffix -ane and an unsaturated one by the

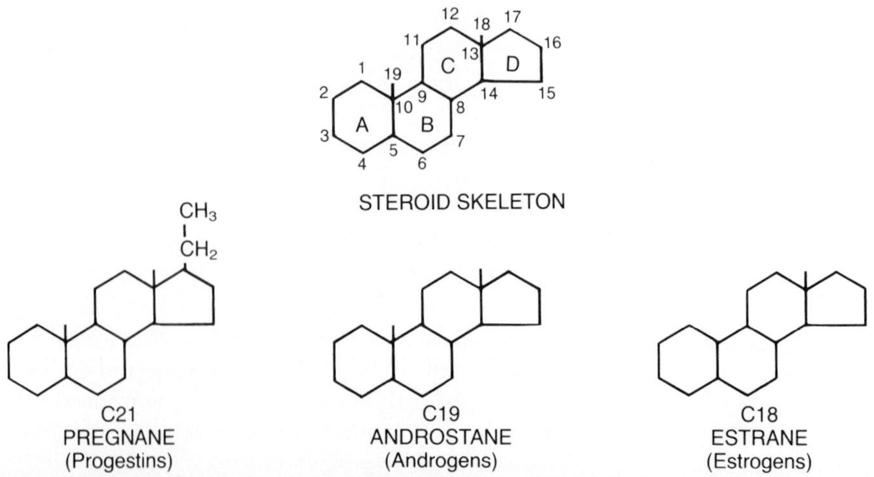

STEROID SKELETON

C21
PREGNANE
(Progestins)

C19
ANDROSTANE
(Androgens)

C18
ESTRANE
(Estrogens)

Figure 42–1

Structure of the steroid hormones.

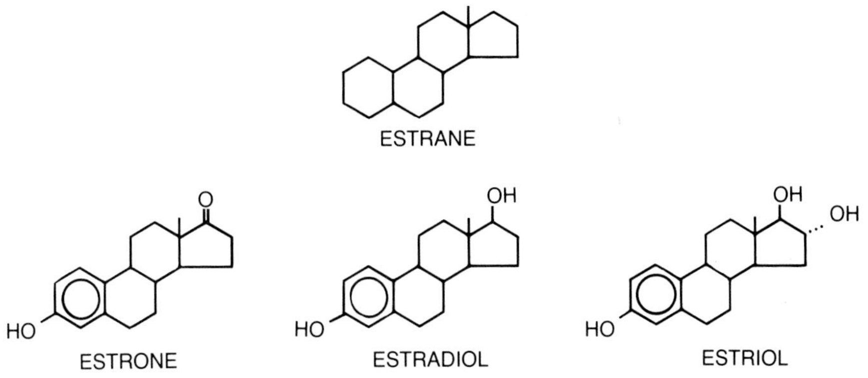

Figure 42-2

Structure of estrane, the prototypic estrogen, and the three major estrogens in women: estrone, estradiol, and estriol.

suffix -ene. The position of a single double bond is indicated by the numbers of the two carbons. Side chains or substitutions at a variety of sites may occur naturally or can be synthesized. Those side chains that project below the plane of the molecule are said to be in the α position and are indicated with a dotted line. Those projecting above the molecule are said to be in the β position and are drawn graphically by a heavy line. Ring keto groups are indicated by the suffixes -one, -dione, and so forth, and ring hydroxyl groups by the suffixes -ol, -diol, and so forth. Thus, this chemical nomenclature can be used to name and identify all steroids by their basic carbon skeleton and by the site and position of substitutions. Many steroids also have a shorter or trivial name that is used more commonly because the chemical nomenclature is cumbersome.

Estrogens can be naturally occurring or synthetic steroids or nonsteroidal compounds having estrogenic activity. All natural estrogens are steroids, including estrone, estradiol, and estriol (Fig. 42-2), as well as preparations of conjugated estrogens derived from the urine of pregnant mares. Synthetic estrogens may be steroidal or nonsteroidal. All steroidal estrogens are derived from an 18 carbon estrane skeleton, with an unsaturated A ring and a phenolic hydroxyl group at C3, a methyl group at C13, and an oxygen (ketone or hydroxyl) at C17 of the estrane skeleton. Structural changes at these positions can affect biological properties. Examples include the shift of the C17 hydroxyl group from β to α position, which eliminates nearly all biological activity, and the substitution of an ethinyl group at C17, which allows the compounds to be orally active.

Production

The ovary is the primary source of estrogens in normally cycling women. Estradiol, the most potent of the naturally occurring estrogens in women, is the major secretory product of the ovary. During the early follicular phase, estradiol secretion is similar from both ovaries. Later, estradiol derives largely from the ovary containing the dominant follicle. Similarly, in the luteal phase, the predominant estradiol secretion is from the ovary containing the corpus luteum.

Estrone is synthesized by the ovaries and can be derived also from estradiol by oxidation in the liver. Androstenedione is aromatized to estrone in peripheral tissues such as fat, liver, the skeletal muscles, hypothalamus, and hair follicles. The conversion of androstenedione to estrone is dependent on the availability of the substrate and increases with age and body mass. Thus, in the menstruating woman, the ovary is the primary source of both estradiol and estrone, whereas peripheral production contributes a small amount (approximately 25%) of circulating estrone. In men and postmenopausal women, peripheral aromatization of adrenal andro-

Estradiol is the most potent naturally occurring estrogen in women.

stenedione to estrone is the major source of estrogen. The testis is an additional source of estrogen in men. Estriol is produced in the liver and conjugated there. Little free estriol exists in the plasma (less than 10 pg/ml in nonpregnant women).

Estrogen production increases dramatically during pregnancy. The synthesis of estrogens in pregnancy is unique in that nearly all the androgenic precursors of estriol and about 50% of those for estradiol are derived from fetal adrenal precursors, DHA, and 16α-hydroxy-DHA. These compounds are aromatized in the placenta, and the estrogens are secreted preferentially into the maternal blood stream.

Sex hormone–binding globulin (SHBG)

Estrogens are weakly bound in plasma to albumin and more tightly to sex hormone–binding globulin (SHBG). Estriol is less well bound than estradiol or estrone. Approximately one half of the estrogens in blood are conjugated.

MECHANISM OF ACTION

Hormones bind to receptors — low-capacity binding proteins probably located in the nucleus.

Estrogens, like other steroids, diffuse freely and rapidly into cells. Estrogen-sensitive organs, or target tissues, contain specific high-affinity, low-capacity binding proteins called *receptors.* Although early work suggested that these receptors were located in the cytosol, more recent reports suggest that they reside primarily in the nucleus. The hormone binds to the receptor, and the hormone-receptor complex binds to acceptor sites at or near DNA sites that initiate mRNA synthesis. Protein formation is one of the earliest measurable effects of estrogen on its target cell and occurs within the first 6 hours of exposure. DNA replication and cell division are promoted within 24 hours. Long-term exposure to estrogens results, therefore, in tissue growth.

The potency of various estrogenic compounds is proportional to the length of time that the hormone-receptor complex is in the cell nucleus. Estriol has the shortest (1 – 4 hours) transit time after a single injection and a short-lived biological effect, leading to its classification as a weak estrogen. However, chronic exposure to estriol leads to a biological effect between that of estradiol and that of estrone. Estrone, estradiol, and DES have intermediate length nuclear retention (6 – 24 hours). The triphenylethylene derivatives (nafoxidine, tamoxifen) have the longest nuclear retention (24 – 48 hours). These compounds act as agonists when given as a single dose in the absence of estradiol, and as antagonists when administered on a chronic basis in the presence of estradiol, presumably because of a decrease in receptor number and a subsequent reduction in mRNA transcription.

Estradiol receptors characterize hormonally dependent tumors. This has led to the use of hormones or hormone antagonists as chemotherapeutic agents. When compared with autonomous tumors, hormone-dependent breast carcinomas take up more estrogen, have more receptors, and respond better to hormonal chemotherapy. The receptor content of the excised tumor has been used, therefore, to predict the subsequent response to hormonal ablation therapy.

ORGAN AND SYSTEMIC PHARMACOLOGY

Absorption, Distribution, Elimination

Estrogens are absorbed readily through the gastrointestinal (GI) tract and are delivered as a bolus to the portal system. The natural unconjugated estrogens are converted primarily to estrone in this process. They subsequently undergo hepatic conjugation and enterohepatic circulation. Therefore, the oral administration of estrone, estradiol, or estriol results in increased serum estrone levels. The conjugated estrogens, some synthetic derivatives of the natural estrogens, and the nonsteroidal estrogens are degraded more slowly and retain biological activity when given orally.

Estrogens are absorbed efficiently through the skin and mucous membranes. The rate of absorption is affected, however, by the vehicle by which the estrogen is delivered. Vaginal administration of estradiol as a saline suspension or micronized tablet results in prompt absorption, whereas absorption is decreased after administration of estradiol as a cream. Local and topical administration of estrogens results generally in absorption and systemic effects. The enterohepatic circulation does not affect estrogens given by a nonoral route, and their subsequent biological action is related to their metabolism and intrinsic potency.

Because estrogens are poorly soluble in water, they are injected as a crystalline aqueous suspension or as a solution in oil. Both are rapidly absorbed, leading to high peak plasma concentrations, a potential disadvantage. The rate of absorption can be decreased by esterification or polymerization of the estrogen.

The metabolism of exogenously administered estrogens is similar to that of the endogenous hormones. Estradiol and estrone are metabolized in the liver to more water-soluble, less protein-bound substances by hydroxylation (at the 16α and C2 positions) and conjugation with sulfuric or glucuronic acid. These compounds are excreted by the kidney. Hepatic hydroxylation is catalyzed by microsomal enzymes and is affected by drugs that induce these enzymes. Estriol has little biliary excretion or metabolic transformation and is excreted more rapidly and quantitatively in the urine. Estrone sulfate, a major metabolite of estradiol, is cleared slowly because it is tightly bound to albumin.

BIOLOGICAL EFFECTS

The primary function of estrogen is to develop and support the reproductive processes in women. Estrogen is necessary to the development and maintenance of normal secondary sexual characteristics, including the growth and maintenance of the uterus, vagina, and fallopian tubes; enlargement of the breasts; maturation of the skeleton; and maintenance of the tone and elasticity of the skin.

Estrogen develops and supports the female reproductive process.

The size and number of cells in the endometrium and myometrium increase under the influence of estrogens, leading to proliferation and regeneration of the endometrial layer. The number and length of the straight tubular endometrial glands increase also. Estrogens stimulate mitosis in the endometrial glands and stroma and promote growth of the spiral arterioles.

Estrogens affect the uterine cervix by increasing the cell height of the cervical mucosa and promoting the formation, amount, and elasticity of cervical mucus. The labia minora become thicker and larger. The vagina elongates and increases in elasticity, rugation, and distensibility. Estrogens induce fluid transudation across the vaginal mucosa and formation of the superficial layer of cornified cells. Estrogens also maintain the elasticity and tone of the urogenital structures and support the growth of axillary and pubic hair.

Extragenital effects of estrogen include the promotion of a female distribution of fat and body hair. Estrogens stimulate growth of the mammary ducts, resulting in breast enlargement.

Estrogens affect bone maturation in a biphasic dose-dependent manner. At low dosages there is an initial stimulation of bone growth, but with

Estrogens affect the body configuration of women.

chronic high dosages there is an acceleration of epiphyseal fusion. This influences the body configuration of women, resulting in narrower shoulders, wider hips, and shorter height compared with men.

Estrogens promote minor salt and fluid retention, which may result in edema.

Estrogens suppress follicle-stimulating hormone (FSH) secretion by the pituitary gland as a result of feedback inhibition. The effect on luteinizing hormone (LH) is more complex and may result in an increase or decrease in LH concentration, depending on the amount and pattern of estrogen levels.

Hepatic lipid metabolism is affected by estrogens. Total cholesterol and low-density lipoprotein (LDL) cholesterol decrease, whereas total triglycerides and high-density lipoprotein (HDL) cholesterol increase, especially HDL2 and its apolipoproteins A1 and A2. These effects depend on the dose, type of estrogen, and route of administration. The greatest effect appears after the oral administration of synthetic estrogens such as ethinyl estradiol, and little effect has been noted with transdermal administration of estradiol. The changes in hepatic lipid metabolism may not be explained entirely by the first-pass effect because vaginal and oral administration of equivalent dosages of conjugated estrogens had similar effects on blood lipid levels. It is important to note that progestins may antagonize this estrogenic effect.

Estrogens have androgenic properties. They decrease the rate of prostatic growth, decrease libido, and decrease sebaceous gland activity. When estrogens are present in sufficient quantity, they cause gynecomastia.

ADVERSE EFFECTS

Nausea is the most common side effect of estrogen administration. At conventional replacement dosages this complaint seldom interferes with eating, and no weight loss is seen. It may be worse in the morning and usually decreases with continued administration of the drug. With increasing dosage, however, this may progress to anorexia and vomiting.

Breast engorgement, endometrial hyperplasia, and bleeding are also common side effects of estrogen administration.

The side effects of estrogens differ according to the type and dosage of estrogen that is given and whether or not progestins are given concomitantly. The following sections report the effects seen with estrogen replacement therapy. Most studies of the effects of estrogen replacement therapy reflect the use of conjugated estrogens at a daily dosage of 0.625 or 1.25 mg. The side effects of contraceptive agents may differ because other estrogens and higher dosages are commonly used in combination with a progestin. These are discussed in a later section.

Nausea, breast engorgement, endometrial hyperplasia, and bleeding are common adverse effects of estrogen administration.

Breast Neoplasia

The breast is an estrogen-sensitive organ. The risk of developing breast cancer is increased by early menarche and late menopause and decreased by early oophorectomy. Several animal models suggest that estrogen may induce breast cancer in the presence of other cocarcinogens of a viral, chemical, or radiation nature. Taken together, these data suggest that endogenous estrogen may play a role in the etiology of breast cancer and have raised concern about the use of estrogen in menopausal women. Many of the studies that have examined this issue are methodologically flawed, and unfortunately, no clear-cut answer has been obtained. Most well-designed studies, however, either fail to show a relationship between estrogen replacement therapy and breast cancer or suggest a small increased relative risk that may not be significant (Wingo et al, 1987). This issue has not been resolved, and certain aspects deserve further study. These include questions of the effects of the dose and duration of estrogen replacement therapy, history of oophorectomy, and the risk for older women with a family history of breast cancer. The potentially beneficial addition of progesterone has been advocated by some investigators and deserves further consideration.

Genital Malignancy and Abnormalities

Endometrial Cancer. The relationship between estrogen and the development of endometrial carcinoma has been suggested by several different lines of investigation (Gambrell, 1986). The likelihood of endometrial cancer is increased by exposure to excess unopposed endogenous estrogen, either from estrogen-producing tumors or from increased peripheral conversion of androstenedione to estrone in obese, postmenopausal women.

Exogenous estrogen administration has been associated also with endometrial cancer. The use of DES for estrogen replacement has been implicated in the development of endometrial cancer in some patients with Turner's syndrome. Epidemiological studies in women receiving estrogen replacement therapy have supported this hypothesis. One study reported that the incidence of endometrial cancer in eight areas of the United States was stable from 1930 to 1970 (Weiss et al, 1976). At that time it increased, coincident with increased United States sales of estrogens. Another study showed a parallel increase in endometrial cancer and estrogen sales in the San Francisco Bay area between 1969 to 1975, followed by a decline in estrogen treatment and endometrial cancer cases between 1975 and 1979. Numerous retrospective case-control studies published since 1975 have indicated that postmenopausal exposure to estrogens for more than 1 year results in a 2–12-fold increased relative risk for endometrial cancer (reviewed by Peterson et al, 1987). A relation between the dose and the duration of estrogen use has been shown, the risk being increased after 1–4 years of estrogen use and rising with the duration of use.

The addition of progesterone to estrogen replacement therapy appears to decrease the risk of endometrial hyperplasia and endometrial cancer to equal to or below that in women receiving no hormonal treatment. Studies suggest that the optimal regimen to prevent hyperplasia consists of 12–13 days of progestogen treatment each month when estrogens are administered (Sturdee et al, 1978; Whitehead et al, 1982).

> Studies indicate that the addition of progesterone to estrogen replacement therapy decreases the risk of endometrial hyperplasia.

Genital Abnormalities. Exposure to DES *in utero* has caused urogenital tract abnormalities and reproductive problems in both male and female offspring. Two thirds of women exposed to DES *in utero* have epithelial changes in the vagina and cervix. Many DES-exposed women have structural abnormalities of the uterine cavity as demonstrated by hysterosalpingography. Clear cell carcinoma of the vagina occurs in less than 0.1% of exposed female offspring, peaking at age 19 and decreasing to low levels by age 30 (Food and Drug Administration [FDA] Drug Bulletin, 1978). Functional abnormalities include an increased incidence of first and second trimester miscarriages, ectopic pregnancy, and premature delivery. Data are not available for other estrogens given in pregnancy, but the presumption is that they would have similar effects. If a patient becomes pregnant while using estrogens or if estrogens are inadvertently prescribed to a pregnant patient, they should be discontinued and the woman should be informed of the potential hazards to the fetus.

Cardiovascular

The effects of estrogen on the cardiovascular system are complex.

The effects of estrogens on the cardiovascular system are complex and contradictory. For example, the risk of death from cardiovascular disease is much higher in men than in premenopausal women, suggesting a protective effect of endogenous estrogen. In contrast, pharmacological dosages of estrogen (conjugated estrogen or DES, 5 mg/day) given to men for cancer treatment appear to increase the risk of cardiovascular events and thromboembolism. Lower dosages of estrogens given to women for contraception also appear to increase the cardiovascular mortality rate.

The results of studies of cardiovascular disease risk in postmenopausal women receiving estrogen replacement therapy are conflicting (Henderson et al, 1985). More recent case-control studies have suggested a decreased risk of fatal and nonfatal myocardial infarction in women receiving estrogen replacement therapy, with a relative risk ranging from 0.33 to 0.90 (reviewed by Bush and Barrett-Connor, 1985). Another study demonstrated a similar protective effect of estrogen replacement on coronary artery stenosis as diagnosed by catheterization, with estrogen users having a relative risk of 0.44 (Sullivan et al, 1988). However, two studies have suggested an increased risk of coronary artery disease (Gordon et al, 1978) or cerebrovascular accident (The Boston Collaborative Drug Surveillance Program, 1974) in postmenopausal women taking estrogens.

The beneficial effect of estrogens is assumed to be related to a decrease in total and LDL cholesterol and to an increase in HDL cholesterol. Most of the patients in these series were taking conjugated estrogens and no progestin. The addition of progestins, especially of the 19-nor series, may reverse the beneficial effects on lipids seen with estrogen replacement. Few data are available to judge whether progestins counteract the beneficial effects of estrogens on cardiovascular events.

Blood pressure does not appear to be affected by estrogen therapy.

There is no apparent increase in thromboembolism in women receiving estrogen replacement therapy (conjugated estrogens in dosages up to 1.25 mg/day), and most series do not report an increase in stroke. Blood pressure, on average, appears to be unaffected by estrogen therapy, although both increases and decreases have been reported.

Liver and Gallbladder

High dosages of oral estrogens have been reported to elevate hepatocellular enzyme levels and, less commonly, cause cholestatic jaundice. The risk of gallstones is increased with oral contraceptive use; as yet this remains a theoretical risk for women taking replacement dosages of estrogens. Oral contraceptive use is associated with the development of hepatocellular adenomas, a benign liver tumor that is highly vascular and may hemorrhage with serious consequences. This complication has not been reported with the use of replacement dosages of estrogen.

Oral contraceptive use increases gallstone risk.

Estrogens enhance hepatic protein production.

Estrogens enhance the hepatic production of a variety of proteins. These include the carrier proteins corticosteroid-binding globulin (CBG), SHBG, thyroid-binding globulin (TBG), transferrin, and ceruloplasmin. Although this is not hazardous, it does influence the results of laboratory tests used to determine the levels of substances bound to these proteins. Estrogens also increase the hepatic synthesis of other proteins that may contribute to disease processes. These include clotting factors, angiotensinogen, and lipids.

Central Nervous System

Estrogens may precipitate headaches and should be stopped if migraine headaches begin or increase or if a new headache pattern emerges. Depression may occur also with the use of conjugated estrogens.

Effects on Laboratory Tests

Estrogens stimulate the hepatic synthesis and secretion of a variety of proteins, including SHBG, CBG, and TBG, as well as clotting factors (especially VII and X). As a result, the quantity of the bound hormone increases and the total amount of hormone as measured by radioimmunoassay increases, whereas the unbound or free fraction of the hormone is unchanged. A radioimmunoassay method that measures the total circulating hormone gives a result that may be increased above the normal range, perhaps giving the false impression that the free concentration of hormone is elevated as well. This effect is not counteracted by the addition of progestin to the treatment regimen.

THERAPEUTIC USES

Hormonal Replacement Therapy

In a young woman with a failure to pubesce, estrogen alone may be used to produce the changes of early puberty. Patients benefiting from such a strategy include those with primary ovarian failure and those with hypogonadotropic hypogonadism due to hypopituitarism or luteinizing hormone–releasing hormone (LH-RH) deficiency. If the epiphyses have not fused, ethinyl estradiol therapy should be initiated at low dosages (100 ng/kg/day) to promote the growth of the long bones. The breasts and endometrium do not respond to this dose of estrogen (Ross et al, 1983). If the bones have fused, therapy can be initiated at a higher dosage (200–800 ng/kg/day) to promote breast development and feminization. Progestins should be added at the time of the first breakthrough bleeding episode to induce cyclical withdrawal bleeding.

> Estrogen can produce the changes of early puberty.

Estrogen therapy is useful also for treating symptoms of estrogen deficiency, especialy vasomotor instability, in the castrated or climacteric woman. Vasomotor symptoms occur in as many as 85% of climacteric women. These include hot flushes (a subjective sense of heat with a red facial flush), dizziness, nausea, headaches, palpitations, diaphoresis, and night sweats. These symptoms commonly occur at night, resulting in sleep disturbance.

The vagina, urethra, and bladder trigone undergo atrophy as a result of estrogen deficiency, resulting in dyspareunia, vaginitis, and abacterial urethritis (dysuria, frequency, urgency, and nocturia). These symptoms improve with estrogen replacement therapy, and some investigators advocate that estrogens be given before atrophy occurs.

Estrogens have not been shown to be useful in the treatment of menopausal depression and should not be used for that indication alone.

> Estrogen has not been shown effective in treating menopausal depression.

The usefulness of estrogens in the prevention of postmenopausal osteoporosis is controversial. It appears that initiation of estrogen replacement therapy close in time to the onset of amenorrhea may retard further bone loss and development or progression of osteopenia (Hunt, 1987). Case-control and other retrospective studies suggest that the long-term use of estrogen in postmenopausal women may decrease the risk of fracture by up to 50%, especially if therapy is started within 5 years of the last menses (Hutchinson et al, 1979; Weiss et al, 1980; Ettinger et al, 1985). Prospective studies are necessary, however, to show that the eventual fracture rate is decreased by this approach. When considering the use of estrogen replacement therapy, other risk factors for osteoporosis such as dietary intake of calcium, exercise, and weight should be modified. Further studies are needed to determine the optimal dosage and timing of estrogen treatment in the prevention of osteopenia.

Taken together, these data suggest that long-term use of estrogen in climacteric women ameliorates vasomotor and urogenital climacteric complaints and may yield a decreased risk of fracture and cardiovascular disease. The major long-term risk of postmenopausal estrogen therapy is the development of endometrial cancer. The addition of a progestin appears to protect against the development of endometrial hyperplasia without having an adverse effect on bone density. The choice of progestin may overwhelm or negate the beneficial effects of estrogen on serum lipid profile. The 19-norprogestin series has the greatest negative effect and natural progesterone the least effect on HDL levels. The implications that these changes have for the risk of cardiovascular events have not been clarified, and further studies are needed to evaluate this question. It seems prudent at this time to advocate the use of the smallest dosage of progestin possible to adequately antagonize estrogen effects on the endometrium.

Chemotherapy

DES has been used to treat patients with breast cancer.

Estrogens such as DES have been used in the treatment of advanced metastatic breast cancer in postmenopausal women and in men. Those tumors that have receptors for estrogen respond best to this alteration in hormonal milieu. Other potential agents include antiestrogens. In premenopausal women, estrogen may promote rather than suppress tumor growth.

In men, estrogen treatment has been used as a palliative treatment for advanced metastic carcinoma of the prostate gland. The LH-RH agonist, however, may be a better therapeutic choice in this setting. Like estrogens, it suppresses the serum testosterone level, but with fewer side effects and less risk of adverse cardiovascular events.

Antiestrogens

Tamoxifen and clomiphene are weak estrogen agonists.

Two weak estrogen agonists, tamoxifen and clomiphene, have found wide therapeutic use as estrogen antagonists. Tamoxifen is useful in the treatment of estrogen-receptor–positive breast cancer in postmenopausal women. Clomiphene is used for the induction of ovulation in anovulatory women.

CONTRAINDICATIONS

There are no indications for the use of estrogen in pregnancy. DES was prescribed for the prevention of miscarriage from 1950 to 1963, but there is no evidence that estrogens are effective for this use.

Estrogen should not be used by any patient with an estrogen-dependent tumor such as carcinoma of the breast or endometrium. Estrogens are contraindicated in patients with known or suspected thromboembolic disease or thrombophlebitis, undiagnosed genital bleeding, or active liver disease.

Relative contraindications to estrogen treatment include a family history of estrogen-dependent neoplasia, uterine leiomyomata, a history of liver disease, diabetes mellitus, porphyria, and hypertension. Other risk factors for cardiovascular disease and thromboembolism such as obesity and heavy smoking increase the risk of estrogen use.

DRUG INTERACTIONS

Most of the drug interactions seen with estrogen treatment are associated with routes of administration (oral) that have a significant first-pass effect on the liver and thereby induce hepatic proteins. Oral anticoagulant action may be decreased by estrogen therapy, an effect that may be mediated through an increase in vitamin K levels.

The action of estrogens may be decreased when they are given with other agents that induce hepatic microsomal enzymes. This probably occurs because of an accelerated metabolism of estrogens to less active compounds. This effect is commonly seen with rifampin, phenylbutazone, phenytoin, primidone, carbamazepine, and the barbiturates.

CHOICE OF PREPARATIONS AND DOSAGES

Estrogens may be given as oral, intramuscular, and topical preparations. Oral administration is most common and its effects are best understood. Intramuscular administration has the potential advantage of improved compliance, requiring only monthly administration with certain agents, and also avoids the hepatic effects. However, the initial peak concentration of estrogen is high, and absorption may be variable. Topical routes such as transvaginal or transdermal administration may lead to a greater physiological estrone-to-estradiol ratio. Vaginal absorption may be erratic, however, and experience with the transdermal preparations is as yet limited.

The large number of estrogen preparations available may make the choice of a given preparation difficult (Table 42–1). The recommendations for specific therapeutic situations include regimens in common use as well as some of the more recent therapeutic options.

The regimen for hormonal replacement therapy in premenopausal women is generally chosen to mimic the normal cycle and avoid deleterious side effects. Oral contraceptives containing the lowest dose of estrogen (20–35 μg ethinyl estradiol) and progestin (norethindrone acetate 1 mg, or levonorgestrel in a triphasic pattern) are commonly used. This approach exceeds the replacement dosage of estrogen (about 20 μg/day of ethinyl

Oral, intramuscular, and topical administration of estrogens

Table 42–1   ESTROGEN PREPARATIONS

Type of Estrogen	Doses Available			
	Oral (mg)	Parenteral (mg/ml)	Vaginal (%)	Transdermal
Steroidal				
ESTRADIOL				
Ethinyl estradiol	0.02, 0.05, 0.5	None	None	None
Estradiol valerate	None	10, 20, 40	None	None
Estradiol cypionate	None	1, 5	None	None
Estradiol benzoate	None	0.5	None	None
Estradiol hemisuccinate	1, 2	None	None	0.6*
Polyestradiol phosphate	None	20	None	None
Micronized estradiol	1, 2	None	0.01	0.05, 0.1†
ESTRONE	None	1, 2, 5	None	None
Esterified estrogens	0.3, 0.625, 1.25, 2.5	None	None	None
Estropipate‡	0.3, 0.625, 1.25, 2.5, 5	None	0.15	None
CONJUGATED EQUINE				
Estrogens	0.3, 0.625, 0.9, 1.25, 2.5	25	0.0625	None
Nonsteroidal				
Chlorotrianisene	12, 25, 72	None	None	None
Dienestrol	None	None	0.01	None
Diethylstilbestrol	0.1, 1, 5	50	None	None
Quinestrol	0.1	None	None	None

* mg/g.
† mg/24 hours.
‡ Equivalent dose of estrone sodium sulfate.

Table 42-2 DOSE-RESPONSE EFFECTS OF COMMONLY USED ESTROGENS

Estrogen Preparation	Bone Density Improvement*	Superficial Vaginal Cell Cytology*	Induction Hepatic Proteins*
Ethinyl estradiol (μg)			
Oral	20	5-50	5
Conjugated estrogens			
Oral (mg)	0.625	1.25	0.625
Vaginal (mg)	ND†	0.3	1.25
Estradiol			
Transdermal (μg/day)	100	100	>200

* Minimal effective dose.
† ND = no data.

Hormonal replacement regimens for postmenopausal women

Synthetic progestins come from progesterone or testosterone.

estradiol) and has the disadvantages discussed under Steroidal Contraceptive Agents. The mnemonic packaging of these agents makes it a convenient approach that can be recommended for women less than 35 years of age. Other physiological regimens can be designed to mimic the menstrual cycle, using a low daily dosage of estrogen and a low dosage of progestin for the first 12 days of each calendar month. Micronized estradiol given by the transdermal, oral, or vaginal route in combination with the more recently available micronized progesterone given by mouth may best mimic normal hormone levels and physiological effects, but experience with this approach is limited (Jensen et al, 1987).

Hormonal replacement regimens for postmenopausal women should be designed to maximize effects on urogenital organs and the bones and to minimize undesirable side effects. Strong consideration should be given to the addition of a progestin in those women with an intact uterus. Table 42-2 compares the effects of some of the more commonly used estrogen preparations given by the oral and topical routes. The dose-response effects of a single preparation are different for different organs. Few studies have evaluated the dose-response effects of a combined estrogen-progestin preparation as regards gonadotropin levels, vaginal cytology, or the induction of (nonlipid) hepatic proteins. It appears that the addition of a progestin either enhances slightly or has no effect on bone density. The beneficial effect of oral estrogens on lipid metabolism may be negated or overwhelmed by the addition of progestin. This undesirable result depends on the type of progestin, with the 19-nor series having the most adverse effect, and micronized oral progesterone having the least effect (Fahraeus et al, 1983; Jensen et al, 1987; Sitruk-Ware et al, 1987). More work is needed to define the optimal type and route of administration of estrogens and progestins in the postmenopausal woman.

Progestins

CHEMISTRY

Structure

Progestins, as implied by the name, are compounds capable of sustaining pregnancy. Progesterone is the only naturally occurring progestin, but many synthetic compounds have progestin activity. The synthetic progestins derive either from progesterone or from testosterone.

The progesterone derivatives (pregnanes) have properties most like native progesterone (Fig. 42-3). These compounds were developed from 17α-hydroxyprogesterone, which has no biological activity unless it is esterified to other compounds. 10α-acetoxyprogesterone, a moderately active progestin, was one of the first agents produced in this way. Prolon-

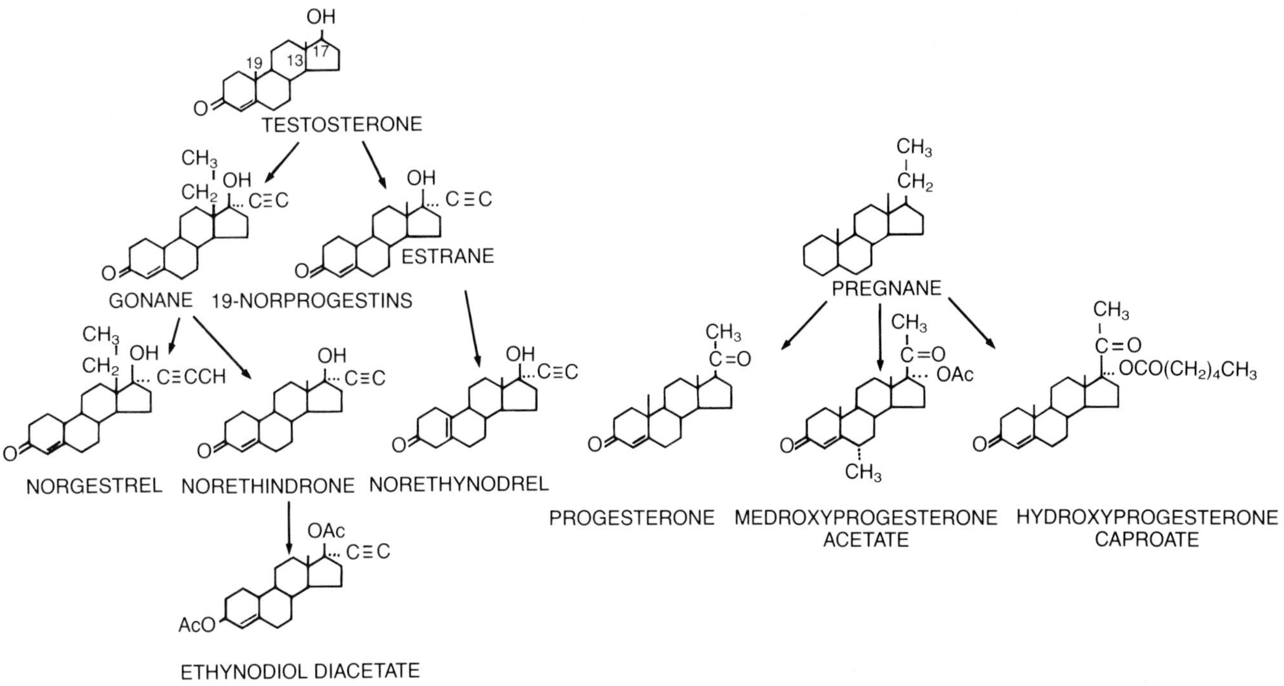

Figure 42–3

Structure of the gonane-, estrane-, and pregnane-derived progestins. The estranes are derived from testosterone by removal of the C19 methyl group and addition of an ethinyl group at C17. The gonanes share this structure with an ethyl group at C13.

gation of the alkyl α chain yields long-acting compounds such as 10α-hydroxyprogesterone caproate. Changes at the C6 position increase potency and convey oral activity, resulting in compounds such as medroxyprogesterone acetate. The insertion of a chloride atom at the C6 position or formation of a double bond at C6–C7 also increases potency.

The testosterone derivatives (estranes and gonanes) have alterations at the C19 and C17 positions (Fig. 42–3). The estranes lack the C19 methyl group and have an ethinyl group at C17. The gonanes share these structural features with the addition of an ethyl group at position 13. Removal of the C19 methyl group from testosterone yields a series of compounds, called C19-norprogestins, with enhanced progestin and decreased androgenic activity. The addition of an ethinyl group at C17 further decreases androgenic activity and allows the compound to be orally active. The first of these compounds, 17α ethinyl-19-nortestosterone (norethindrone) was synthesized by Djerassi in 1951. The addition of an ethyl group at C13 yielded one of the most active steroids parenterally, norgestrel, but at the cost of some androgenic side effects. The estrane-derived progestins are converted to norethisterone in the liver. The gonane-derived progestins do not require hepatic transformation for biological activity.

Estranes and gonanes are testosterone derivatives.

Production

Progesterone is secreted from the dominant follicle beginning just before ovulation, and from the corpus luteum once ovulation has occurred, reaching peak plasma concentrations of 10–30 ng/ml in the midluteal phase. When pregnancy does not occur, the corpus luteum regresses, progesterone levels decrease, and menses begin. In fertile cycles, human chorionic gonadotropin (hCG) secretion by the trophoblast rescues the corpus luteum, and progesterone production is maintained. The placenta begins to produce progesterone in amounts adequate to maintain pregnancy by the second or third month of gestation. After this, the corpus luteum is not essential for the maintenance of the pregnancy.

Progesterone is made also by the adrenal cortex and testis. These sources account for the low plasma concentrations (<2 ng/ml) seen in men and in anovulatory and postmenopausal women.

Circulating plasma progesterone is bound largely to CBG. The pregnane-derived progestins show little binding to CBG or SHBG. The estrane-derivatives, in contrast, bind strongly to SHBG.

Unlike the pregnanes, estranes bind strongly to SHBG.

MECHANISM OF ACTION

Unbound progesterone, like other steroids, diffuses into its target cell where it binds to an intranuclear protein receptor that is specific for the progestins. The progestin-receptor complex binds to DNA and activates specific mRNA synthesis, resulting ultimately in the production of proteins. Progesterone action is modulated by the concentration of receptors in the cell. Estrogen secreted during the follicular phase increases the amount of progesterone receptor in the endometrium. Progesterone in turn inhibits the synthesis of both its own receptor and that of estradiol.

ORGAN/SYSTEM PHARMACOLOGY

Absorption, Distribution, Elimination

The absorption of oral progesterone is inefficient and subject to first-pass hepatic hydroxylation and conjugation. Micronized progesterone (UTROGESTIN), however, is well absorbed and has significant oral activity. The oral absorption of the synthetic progestins is variable.

Oral progesterone absorption is inefficient, but micronized progesterone is well absorbed.

Progesterone is well absorbed from the vaginal, rectal, and intramuscular routes of administration. The long-acting parenteral preparations rely on the injection of a hydrophobic suspension or solution or on the incorporation of an active compound into a carrier substance. Both approaches provide long-term steady state levels of drug.

Progesterone is metabolized primarily in the liver. The metabolites are conjugated with glucuronide or sulfate and excreted. The major urinary metabolite is pregnane-3α,20α-diol-glucuronide (pregnanediol).

BIOLOGICAL EFFECTS

The primary target organs of progesterone are the uterus and the breast. Progesterone action at these tissues is dependent on prior estrogen exposure, as outlined earlier. Progesterone induces secretory changes in the uterine endometrium that prepare the uterine lining for the nidation of a fertilized egg. Progesterone withdrawal causes the breakdown and eventual shedding of the endometrium. The mass of the uterine myometrium is increased by progesterone. Cervical mucus decreases in quantity and thickens under the influence of progesterone. Progesterone decreases the contractility of the fallopian tube. Mammary alveolar tissue growth increases slightly in the luteal phase, and dramatically during pregnancy.

Progesterone increases the mass of the uterine myometrium.

Progesterone has a thermogenic effect and increases body temperature by 0.5–1°F. This effect, mediated by the hypothalamus, is seen in the luteal phase and persists in pregnancy.

Progestins also inhibit LH and FSH secretion by the pituitary gland, a property exploited in the contraceptive use of these agents.

Progesterone has natriuretic activity mediated through an antagonism of aldosterone action on the renal tubule.

Other biological effects are seen with the synthetic progestins. These compounds can bind to other steroid receptors and act as hormone agonists or antagonists. The 17-hydroxy or acetoxy compounds are the most similar to progesterone. The 19-nor derivatives, on the other hand, exhibit some estrogenic or androgenic properties, including nitrogen retention, weight gain, exacerbation of acne, and impaired glucose tolerance.

Hepatic lipid metabolism is affected also by the administration of synthetic progestins, especially the 19-nor compounds. These agents tend to decrease the concentrations of very low density lipoprotein (VLDL) triglycerides and HDL, especially HDL2. It remains unclear whether or not a dose of progestin that affects the endometrium, but not lipids, can be defined. The physiological implications of the lipid changes are unknown and require more study.

ADVERSE EFFECTS

The most common untoward effect of progestin treatment is abnormal menstrual bleeding: breakthrough bleeding, spotting, change in the amount of flow, or amenorrhea.

Use of the synthetic progestins in pregnancy has been associated with masculinization of female fetuses and feminization of male fetuses. These compounds should not be given to pregnant women.

Effects seen with combined estrogen-progestin preparation are discussed under Steroidal Contraceptive Agents.

Abnormal menstrual bleeding is an adverse effect of progestin treatment.

THERAPEUTIC USES

Dysfunctional uterine bleeding is common at the extremes of reproductive life when anovulatory cycles frequently occur. It probably results from the breakdown of an estrogen-stimulated hyperplastic endometrium that has not been exposed to progesterone, with the attendant withdrawal bleeding. Active bleeding can be treated with progestins alone (5–10 mg norethindrone every 4–6 hours for 24 hours and then 5 mg twice daily for 1–2 weeks) or with an estrogen-progestin combination (ethinyl estradiol, 100 μg or mestranol, with a progestin given daily). Once bleeding is controlled, the monthly administration of progesterone may normalize bleeding episodes.

Progesterone (megestrol acetate or medroxyprogesterone acetate) is used in the palliative treatment of recurrent metastatic endometrial carcinoma. Up to 50% of patients derive improvement from this regimen, which should be continued for a few months to achieve full efficacy. The best results are seen in younger patients whose tumor contains progesterone or estradiol receptors.

Natural progesterone has been advocated for the treatment of threatened abortion or inadequate luteal phase. Although this is a widespread practice, few controlled studies are available to evaluate its efficacy.

Progesterone can be used to evaluate the cause of amenorrhea and to test for estrogenic effects on the endometrium. For this purpose natural progesterone (75–100 mg) can be given in oil intramuscularly, or medroxyprogesterone acetate (10 mg daily for 5 days) can be given by mouth. Withdrawal bleeding will ensue as progesterone levels fall in women with previous estrogen exposure. Intramuscular medroxyprogesterone acetate should not be used for this indication to avoid the possibility of prolonged suppression of gonadotropin secretion.

Progesterone has been used alone (norethindrone, norgestrel) and in combination with estrogen for contraception as described under Steroidal Contraceptive Agents and may be used in conjunction with estrogen in the therapy of postmenopausal women (see Estrogens).

Table 42–3 PREPARATIONS AND DOSAGES OF PROGESTINS

Preparation	Dosage	
	Oral (mg)	Parenteral (mg/ml)
Progesterone	None*	50
Medoxyprogesterone acetate	2.5, 5, 10	100, 400
Hydroxyprogesterone caproate	None	125, 250
Megestrol acetate	20, 40	10
Norethindrone	0.35, 5	None
Norethindrone acetate	5	None
Norgestrel	0.075	None

* Micronized progesterone, 100 mg for oral administration, is not available in the United States at this time.

CONTRAINDICATIONS

Progesterone is contraindicated in patients with a history of thrombophlebitis, thromboembolic disease, and cancer of the breast. It should not be given to women with undiagnosed vaginal bleeding, missed abortion, or active liver disease.

DRUG INTERACTIONS, PREPARATIONS, AND DOSAGES

Rifampin can decrease progestin effectiveness when used concurrently.

Concurrent use of rifampin may decrease the effectiveness of the progestins because of accelerated metabolism.

Preparations and dosages of the progestins are shown in Table 42–3.

Steroidal Contraceptive Agents

CHEMISTRY

Estrogens and progestins, alone or in combination, are used as contraceptive agents worldwide. Progestins alone, taken in a small continuous daily dosage, have an efficacy of about 97%. This mini-pill approach avoids estrogenic side effects but is frequently associated with breakthrough bleeding. Progesterone can be administered systemically by injections or subcutaneous implants. Both approaches provide long-term reversible contraception without problems of compliance. The intrauterine device can be used as a vehicle to deliver progesterone locally to the endometrium, another effective contraceptive method. Estrogens alone have not been used as long-term contraceptive agents, but they can prevent implantation when given within 48 hours of unprotected intercourse. DES is commonly prescribed for this indication, often referred to as the *morning after pill*.

DES has been called the *morning after pill*.

The combined formulation of an estrogen and a progestin is used so commonly for contraception that it is referred to as the *birth control pill* or *oral contraceptive*. These agents are the most effective form of medical contraception for women, being about 99% effective when used as directed. They vary in terms of the type, dosage, and schedule of estrogen and progestin administration. The pills usually are taken continually for 21 out of every 28 days.

Formulations with a fixed daily dosage of both estrogen and progestin are referred to as *combination* or *monophasic* preparations. The estrogenic component is given in a fixed daily dosage considered low ($<50 \mu$g) or high ($\geq 50 \mu$g) and consists of ethinyl estradiol, a potent semisynthetic estrogen, or mestranol (the 3-methyl ester of ethinyl estradiol), a slightly less potent compound. The progestin component is usually a 19-nortestosterone derivative. Of these, levonorgestrel and norgestrel are the most, and norethynodrel the least, potent progestins. Levonorgestrel, norgestrel, and norethindrone have the greatest androgenic effects. Ethynodiol diacetate, a 17α-hydroxyprogesterone derivative, is used also.

Preparations with a variable dosage of estrogen or progesterone, or both, are designed to mimic the hormonal pattern of a normal cycle. These preparations are referred to as *sequential* or *phasic* formulations. Phasic preparations contain two (biphasic) or three (triphasic) different combinations of progestin and estrogen to be given sequentially during separate periods within the same cycle. Ethinyl estradiol, the estrogenic component, is given either at a fixed (35 μg) or variable (30–40 μg) daily dosage. L-norgestrel or norethindrone is used as the progestin component. Preparations containing other gonane-derived progestins with potentially fewer adverse metabolic effects are being evaluated but are not available yet in the United States.

Levonorgestrel and norgestrel are examples of combination preparations.

MECHANISM OF ACTION

The progestin-estrogen combination pills prevent ovulation by direct negative feedback at the hypothalamus and pituitary gland. The progestin component thickens cervical mucus, impedes sperm penetration, and alters the normal endometrial development, rendering it hostile to implantation. These properties are shared by the progestin-only mini-pills, which have a variable effect on ovulation. The progesterone-containing intrauterine device (IUD) acts locally to create a hostile endometrium. Large dosages of estrogen alter endometrial physiology and result in withdrawal bleeding.

ORGAN/SYSTEM PHARMACOLOGY

Absorption, Distribution, Elimination

The oral contraceptive formulations in widespread use are well absorbed. As discussed in the respective sections on estrogens and progestins, the compounds undergo hepatic metabolism and conjugation and then are excreted. Mestranol undergoes hepatic demethylation to ethinyl estradiol, a conversion that appears responsible for most of its biological activity. Ethinyl estradiol is metabolized and conjugated in the liver and undergoes significant enterohepatic circulation or is excreted. Most 19-norprogestins are metabolized to norethindrone. Levonorgestrel and norethindrone do not undergo significant enterohepatic circulation but are metabolized and conjugated in the liver and are eliminated in urine and feces.

BIOLOGICAL EFFECTS

The biological effects of estrogen-progestin combination pills represent, for the most part, the additive effects of each agent. The endometrium tends to regress, leading to decreased menstrual flow and, occasionally, amenorrhea. When birth control pills are discontinued, the pituitary recovers first, followed by the ovary (ovulation), and finally, the endometrium.

Oral contraceptives induce a variety of both desirable and undesirable effects. These effects have been reviewed by the FDA, and the package insert has been revised (FDA, 1988). The beneficial effects of oral contraceptive use include a decreased incidence of ovarian cysts, menorrhagia, ovarian and endometrial carcinoma, endometriosis, iron deficiency, and dysmenorrhea.

Benefits of oral contraceptive use include decreased incidences of ovarian cysts and ovarian carcinoma.

ADVERSE EFFECTS

Weight gain, nausea, and breast tenderness are frequent mild side effects attributed to estrogen. They may diminish with increased duration of use or at a smaller dosage of estrogen. Chloasma may appear with prolonged use. The estrogenic component of oral contraceptives may precipitate or exacerbate migraine headaches.

Glucose tolerance is impaired in some women using oral contraceptives. This is usually manifested by an increase in the fasting blood sugar and not by overt diabetes. The progestin component has been implicated, especially the 19-nor compounds, with norgestrel having the most deleterious effect.

The alterations in lipid metabolism associated with oral contraceptives reflect a balance between the estrogen-induced stimulation and the progestin-induced supression of HDL (Gaspard, 1987; Wahl et al, 1983). Formulations containing ethinyl estradiol (30–50 μg/day) and norethisterone (1000 μg/day) preserve the normal HDL-to-cholesterol and HDL-to-triglyceride ratios. A trend to increased HDL levels is seen at a lower dosage of norethisterone (400 μg/day). Preparations containing levonorgestrel, 150–200 μg/day, had favorable or neutral effects on lipid metabolism. The triphasic preparations appear to have minimal effects on lipid metabolism (Hale, 1987).

The liver is affected by these agents. The incidence of benign hepatic adenoma, a rare tumor, is increased, especially after prolonged use. The incidence of gallbladder disease and gallstones is increased in women who used oral contraceptives. This is caused by an estrogen-induced increase in biliary cholesterol concentration. Cholestatic jaundice, a dose-dependent phenomenon, has been reported as well.

The primary morbidity and mortality associated with the use of oral contraceptives relate to an increased risk of thrombosis (Stadel, 1981), presumably because of an estrogen-induced increase of Factors VII, VIII, IX, and X concentration and a decrease in antithrombin III (Bonnar, 1987). Pulmonary thromboembolism is increased in users fourfold. Thrombotic stroke is increased to a similar degree and is more likely in hypertensive patients and in those who smoke.

Fatal and nonfatal myocardial infarctions are increased two to five times. The risk increases with the duration of oral contraceptive use, age, smoking (especially if more than 15 cigarettes daily), and coexisting hypertension. The risk of myocardial infarction is decreased but not eliminated at the lowest dosages of estrogen. The overall mortality is increased two- to fourfold, primarily as a result of fatal myocardial infarction or cerebrovascular accident. These findings have led to the recommendation that oral contraceptive use be limited to nonsmoking women less than 35 years of age who have normal blood pressure.

Hypertension will develop in up to 5% of women using oral contraceptives. Although this is usually gradual in onset, it may be rapid and severe. The cause is unknown but may be related to stimulation of the renin-angiotensin system. It subsides when the agents are discontinued. The risk of hypertension increases with age, a family history of hypertension, history of renal disease, and increasing duration of use.

Neither short-term nor long-term use of oral contraceptives appears to increase the risk of malignancy. The incidence of breast cancer is similar in users and nonusers (The Centers for Disease Control [CDC], 1983a). Oral contraceptive use appears to convey some protection against the development of ovarian (CDC, 1983b) and uterine cancer (CDC, 1983c). In one study, women using combination agents for at least 12 months had a relative risk of developing uterine cancer of 0.5. This positive effect per-

Adverse effects include increased incidences of liver and gallbladder diseases.

Five percent of oral contraceptive users develop hypertension.

sisted for at least 10 years. Given the clear-cut risk of estrogen on the development of uterine cancer, this effect has been attributed to progesterone antagonism of estrogen effect on the endometrium. Similarly, the relative risk for development of ovarian cancer in women using oral contraceptives was 0.6.

Vitamin metabolism is changed by oral contraceptive use. Serum B_{12} levels may decrease. A relative deficiency of pyridoxine secondary to impaired tryptophan metabolism has been reported. Estrogen may interfere with the absorption of dietary folate, leading to a deficiency.

The estrogenic component of oral contraceptives stimulates hepatic synthesis of a variety of proteins, including the carrier proteins for copper (ceruloplasmin), iron (transferrin), thyroid hormone (TBG), estrogen (SHBG), and cortisol (CBG). Patients do not manifest a clinical deficiency of these compounds, however, because production or absorption increases to fill the newly available carrier sites, and the unbound fraction remains normal.

The interpretation of a number of laboratory tests is affected by oral contraceptive use. Radioimmunoassays that measure the total amount of hormone or mineral transported by carrier proteins may yield a result that is increased above the normal range and may be interpreted falsely as indicating an increase in the unbound or free fraction. The response to metyrapone is decreased in women taking oral contraceptive agents. These agents may also cause false-positive results for lupus erythematosus (LE) cells or antinuclear antibodies (ANA) titer.

THERAPEUTIC USES

These agents are prescribed for contraceptive use. Preparations containing ethinyl estradiol at a daily dosage of 30 μg or less may be used also for steroid replacement therapy in hypogonadal women.

CONTRAINDICATIONS

Women with a history of thromboembolic disease or thrombophlebitis should not receive oral contraceptive agents. These agents are contraindicated also in women with a history of cerebrovascular or coronary artery disease. Oral contraceptives are contraindicated in pregnancy and should not be started until 1 month after parturition. Similarly, they should be discontinued 1 month before and not started until 1 month after elective surgery. Women with active liver disease or a history of cholestatic jaundice should not use these agents. Oral contraceptives should not be prescribed to women with undiagnosed genital bleeding or with endocrine-dependent tumors. These include benign or malignant liver tumors that developed during prior estrogen use as well as cancer of the breast, uterus, cervix, and vagina.

Oral contraceptive agents should be used with caution in women with hypertension, diabetes mellitus, hyperlipidemia, uterine leiomyoma, or migraine headaches.

DRUG INTERACTIONS

Oral contraceptives increase the metabolic clearance of coumarin, acetaminophen, and prednisolone. The dosages of these drugs may need to be increased. Oral contraceptives increase the bioavailable amounts of imipramine and theophylline.

Barbiturates, hydantoins, griseofulvin, and rifampin increase the he-

Table 42-4 CURRENTLY AVAILABLE COMBINATION ORAL CONTRACEPTIVE AGENTS	
Estrogen (μg/day)	Progestin (mg/day)
Ethinyl estradiol	
MONOPHASIC PREPARATIONS	
20	Norethindrone acetate (1)
30	L-norgestrel (0.15)
30	Norethindrone acetate (1.5)
30	Norgestrel (0.3)
35	Ethynodiol diacetate (1)
35	Norethindrone (0.4)
35	Norethindrone (0.5)
35	Norethindrone (1)
50	Ethynodiol diacetate (1)
50	Norethindrone acetate (1)
50	Norethindrone acetate (2.5)
50	Norgestrel (0.5)
BIPHASIC PREPARATIONS	
35	Norethindrone 0.5 for 10 days then 1.0 for 11 days
TRIPHASIC PREPARATIONS	
30	L-norgestrel 0.05 for 6 days then
40	L-norgestrel 0.075 for 5 days then
30	L-norgestrel 0.125 for 10 days
35	Norethindrone 0.5 for 7 days then
35	Norethindrone 0.75 for 7 days then
35	Norethindrone 1 for 7 days
35	Norethindrone 0.5 for 7 days then
35	Norethindrone 1 for 9 days then
35	Norethindrone 0.5 for 5 days
Mestranol	
MONOPHASIC PREPARATIONS	
50	Norethindrone (1)
75	Norethynodrel (5)*
150	Norethynodrel (9.85)*

* Used to induce cyclic withdrawal bleeding for the treatment of hypermenorrhea; not recommended for contraception.

patic metabolism of estrogens by mixed function oxidases. Antibiotics decrease the plasma concentrations and efficacy of estrogens and progestins, probably by killing the gut flora responsible for hydrolysis of hepatic conjugates and thereby interrupting the enterohepatic circulation.

PREPARATIONS AND DOSAGES

The oral contraceptive chosen should contain the smallest quantity of steroid possible to minimize potential side effects. High-dose estrogens (containing more than 50 μg ethinyl estradiol) have been taken off the market by the FDA. Table 42-4 lists the preparations available currently.

The FDA has removed high-dose estrogens from the market.

References

Bonnar J: Coagulation effects of oral contraceptives. Am J Obstet Gynecol 157:1042–1048, 1987.

The Boston Collaborative Drug Surveillance Program: Surgically confirmed gallbladder disease, venous thromboembolism, and breast tumors in relation to postmenopausal estrogen therapy. N Engl J Med 290:15–19, 1974.

Bush T, Barrett-Connor E: Noncontraceptive estrogen use and cardiovascular disease. Epidemiol Rev 7:80–104, 1985.

The Centers for Disease Control: Cancer and steroid hormone study. Long-term oral contraceptive use and the risk of breast cancer. JAMA 249:1591–1595, 1983a.

The Centers for Disease Control: Cancer and steroid hormone study. Long-term oral contraceptive use and the risk of ovarian cancer. JAMA 249:1596–1599, 1983b.

The Centers for Disease Control: Cancer and steroid hormone study. Oral contraceptive use and the risk of endometrial cancer. JAMA 249:1600–1604, 1983c.

Chetkowski RJ, Meldrum DR, Steingold KA, et al: Biologic effects of transdermal estradiol. N Engl J Med 314:1615–1620, 1986.

Ettinger B, Genant HK, Cann CE: Long-term estrogen replacement therapy prevents bone loss and fractures. Ann Intern Med 102:319–324, 1985.

Fahraeus L, Larsson-Cohn U, Wallentin L: L-norgestrel and progesterone have different influences on plasma lipoproteins. Eur J Clin Invest 13:447–453, 1983.

FDA: Labeling guidance text for combination oral contraceptives. Physician labeling. Contraception 37:434–455, 1988.

Fieser LF, Fieser M: Steroids, 444–502, 539–576. New York: Reinhold, 1959.

Gambrell RD: The role of hormones in the etiology and prevention of endometrial cancer. Clin Obstet Gynecol 13:695–723, 1986.

Gaspard UJ: Metabolic effects of oral contraceptives. Am J Obstet Gynecol 157:1029–1041, 1987.

Geola FL, Frumar AM, Tataryn IV, et al: Biological effects of various doses of conjugated equine estrogens in postmenopausal women. J Clin Endocrinol Metab 51:620–625, 1980.

Gordon T, Kannel WB, Hjortland MC, et al: Menopause and coronary heart disease: The Framingham Study. Ann Intern Med 89:157–161, 1978.

Hale RW: Phasic approach to oral contraceptives. Am J Obstet Gynecol 157:1052–1058, 1987.

Henderson BE, Ross RK, Paganini-Hill A: Estrogen use and cardiovascular disease. J Reprod Med 30(Suppl):814–820, 1985.

HEW recommends follow-up on DES patients. FDA Drug Bull 8:10–11, 1978.

Hunt K: Long-term effects of postmenopausal hormone therapy. Br J Hosp Med 38:450–459, 1987.

Hutchinson TA, Polansky JM, Feinstein AR: Postmenopausal oestrogens protect against fracture of hip and distal radius. Lancet 2:705–709, 1979.

Jensen J, Riis B, Strom V, et al: Long-term effects of percutaneous estrogens and oral progesterone on serum lipoproteins in postmenopausal women. Am J Obstet Gynecol 156:66–71, 1987.

Lindsay R, Hart DM, Clark DM: The minimum effective dose of estrogen for prevention of postmenopausal bone loss. Obstet Gynecol 63:759–763, 1984.

Mandel FP, Geola FL, Lu JKH, et al: Biologic effects of various doses of ethinyl estradiol in postmenopausal women. Obstet Gynecol 59:673–679, 1982.

Mandel FP, Geola FL, Meldrum DR, et al: Biological effects of various doses of vaginally administered conjugated equine estrogens in postmenopausal women. J Clin Endocrinol Metab 57:133–139, 1983.

Peterson HB, Lee NC, Rubin GL: Genital neoplasia: *In* Mishell D. Jr (ed): Menopause: Physiology plus Pharmacology, 275–298. Chicago: Yearbook Medical Publishers Inc, 1987.

Ross JL, Cassorla FG, Skerda MC, et al: A preliminary study of the effect of estrogen dose on growth in Turner's syndrome. N Engl J Med 309:1104–1106, 1983.

Sitruk-Ware R, Bricaire C, DeLignieres B, et al: Oral micronized progesterone. Contraception 36:373–403, 1987.

Stadel BV: Oral contraceptives and cardiovascular disease. N Engl J Med 305:612–618, 672–677, 1981.

Sturdee DW, Wade-Evans T, Paterson MEL, et al: Relationships between bleeding pattern, endometrial histology, and oestrogen treatment in menopausal women. Br Med J 1:1575–1577, 1978.

Sullivan JM, Vander Zwaag R, Lemp GF, et al: Postmenopausal estrogen use and coronary atherosclerosis. Ann Intern Med 108:358–363, 1988.

Wahl P, Walden C, Knopp R, et al: Effect of estrogen/progestin potency on lipid/lipoprotein cholesterol. N Engl J Med 308:862–867, 1983.

Weiss NS, Szekely DR, Austin DF: Increasing incidence of endometrial cancer in the United States. N Engl J Med 294:1259–1262, 1976.

Weiss NS, Ure CL, Ballard JH: Decreased risk of fractures of the hip and lower forearm with postmenopausal use of estrogen. N Engl J Med 303:1195–1198, 1980.

Whitehead MI, Townsend PT, Pryse-Davies J, et al: Effects of various types and dosages of progestagens on the postmenopausal endometrium. J Reprod Med 27(Suppl):539–548, 1982.

Wingo PA, Layde PM, Lee NC, et al: The risk of breast cancer in postmenopausal women who have used estrogen replacement therapy. JAMA 257:209–215, 1987.

43

Adrenal Cortex

Paul J. Davis
Kathleen M. Tornatore
Alexander C. Brownie

The principal secretory products of the adrenal cortex in humans are the steroid hormones, cortisol, aldosterone, and androgens. The gland exhibits functional zonation with aldosterone being biosynthesized and secreted by the outer zona glomerulosa and cortisol and androgens by the zona fasciculata/reticularis.

Cholesterol, the precursor of all the adrenocortical steroid hormones, is derived from circulating low-density lipoproteins (LDL). Most of the reactions involved in cholesterol conversion to steroid hormones (Fig. 43–1) are catalyzed by a family of mixed-function oxidases that are specific cytochromes P-450. The first reaction, catalyzed by cholesterol side-chain cleavage cytochrome P-450 (P-450$_{scc}$), is the rate-limiting step in adrenal steroidogenesis (Pedersen and Brownie, 1983). Adrenocorticotropic hormone (ACTH) controls cortisol and androgen production through the activation of P-450$_{scc}$ in zona fasciculata/reticularis cells, whereas angiotensin II stimulates the same reaction, and therefore aldosterone production, in zona glomerulosa cells. Thus, the adrenal gland elaborates three types of steroids: glucocorticoids, which, among other actions, regulate hepatic gluconeogenesis; mineralocorticoids, which have important actions on sodium and potassium homeostasis; and adrenal androgens. Cortisol and aldosterone are primary examples, respectively, of glucocorticoids and mineralocorticoids.

The spontaneous syndromes of hyperfunction of the adrenal cortex (hypercortisolism and hyperaldosteronism—each associated with either adrenocortical hyperplasia or adrenal adenoma), of hypoadrenocorticism, and of defects in adrenal steroidogenesis (congenital adrenal hyperplasia) that result in excess adrenal androgen production have been important historically in defining the nature of the pituitary-adrenal hormonal feedback loop and complex steps in steroidogenesis. *Cushing's syndrome* refers to the clinical picture of hypercortisolism, regardless of pathogenesis, and includes ectopic, i.e., nonpituitary, production of ACTH by cancers and the setting of therapeutic administration of large doses of synthetic anti-inflammatory glucocorticoids; *Cushing's disease* specifically refers to hypercortisolism that results from excess pituitary release of ACTH. The risk of iatrogenic Cushing's syndrome is appreciably greater than that of endogenous hypercortisolism: the prevalence of anti-inflammatory glucocorticoid administration in our teaching general hospital inpatient population is 6.1%. *Conn's syndrome* describes the clinical pattern of spontaneous

Cholesterol is the precursor of all adrenocortical steroid hormones.

Cushing's syndrome refers to the clinical picture of hypercortisolism.

Cushing's disease describes only the hypercortisolism that results from excess pituitary ACTH.

717

Figure 43-1

Biosynthetic pathway for adrenocortical steroids in the human adrenal cortex.

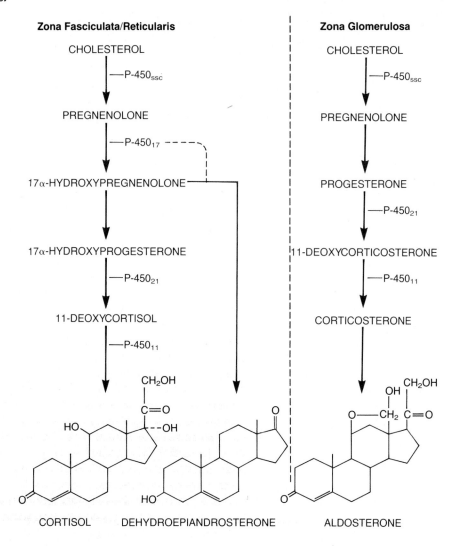

Conn's syndrome describes the clinical course of primary hyperaldosteronism.

excess of adrenal mineralocorticoid production (primary hyperaldosteronism). Although primary hyperaldosteronism is rare, clinical syndromes in which aldosterone production is increased owing to heart failure or hepatic cirrhosis (secondary hyperaldosteronism) are frequent. An aldosterone inhibitor, spironolactone, may be employed in these settings, and the prevalence of inpatient spironolactone use in our teaching hospital is 1.7%. Primary failure of the adrenal cortex was described by Addison in the mid-nineteenth century and includes loss of both glucocorticoid and mineralocorticoid secretory capacity.

Pituitary-Adrenal Cortex Physiology

ACTH controls the growth of the adrenal cortex.

The pituitary-adrenocortical axis is a classic hormonal feedback loop in which a target gland secretory product, cortisol, inhibits pituitary gland secretion of a trophic hormone, ACTH; ACTH in turn is responsible for regulation of cortisol biosynthesis and release by the adrenal cortex (Fig. 43-2). ACTH also controls the growth of the adrenal cortex and the synthesis of steroidogenic enzymes.

ACTH is part of a 26,000-dalton polypeptide, proopiomelanocortin (POMC), which is synthesized in the corticotrophs of the anterior pituitary (Smith and Funder, 1988). POMC also contains β-endorphin and melanocyte-stimulating hormone (MSH) sequences. Production and secretion of ACTH by pituitary corticotrophs involves specific processing of POMC

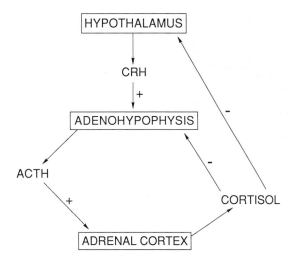

Figure 43-2

The hypothalamic-adenohypophyseal-adrenocortical axis.

under the influence of the hypothalamic hormone, corticotropin-releasing hormone (CRH) (Nieman and Loriaux, 1989). Negative feedback inhibition of pituitary ACTH secretion by cortisol, and by potent synthetic glucocorticoids such as prednisolone and dexamethasone, occurs at both the pituitary and the hypothalamic (CRH) levels.

ACTH secretion is pulsatile, with a dozen or more principal pulses through each 24 hours, conforming to a cycle that imposes a characteristic circadian (diurnal) rhythm of cortisol secretion (highest plasma concentrations at 5:00–7:00 A.M. in humans, lowest at 3:00–6:00 P.M., assuming a traditional wake-sleep cycle). The pulsatile nature of ACTH/cortisol secretion is generated by central nervous system (CNS) input to the hypothalamus. Stress on the organism, whether physical, including systemic (nonadrenal) disease, or emotional, alters importantly ACTH/cortisol secretion and metabolism. The major effects of stress on the pituitary-adrenocortical axis include (1) increased cortisol secretion, (2) enhanced degradation of cortisol (shortened $t_{1/2}$), (3) loss of circadian variation in ACTH/cortisol release, e.g., absence of the afternoon nadir, and (4) reduced susceptibility of the hypothalamus/pituitary gland to inhibition by cortisol and dexamethasone.

Body habitus may affect cortisol secretion, in that obesity is associated with enhanced secretion but the response of the hypothalamic/pituitary unit to dexamethasone is intact. Also, there is evidence for alterations in the circadian rhythm of cortisol secretion in depression, apparently related to changes in the negative feedback inhibition of ACTH by cortisol in such patients. Alteration of the wake-sleep cycle in normal subjects is associated with a change in the circadian rhythm of cortisol secretion, so that the peak anticipates the new wake period. Two weeks of an altered wake-sleep cycle is required to achieve a new, stable cortisol secretion pattern.

In contrast to cortisol and despite their secretion being increased by ACTH, aldosterone and adrenal androgens do not affect hypothalamic-pituitary control of ACTH release. Pharmacological suppression of endogenous ACTH is associated in humans with a 25% decline in circulating levels of aldosterone; the major regulators of aldosterone secretion, however, are the renin-angiotensin system and circulating levels of potassium. Adrenal androgen secretion is controlled by one or more POMC-derived peptides, the most well characterized is ACTH, and another, cortical androgen–stimulating hormone, is a product of the processing of the N-terminal portion of POMC. Interruption of normal cortisol production in the adrenal cortex, e.g., in the setting of the 11β- and 21-hydroxylase forms of congeni-

ACTH secretion is pulsatile and produced by CNS input to the hypothalamus.

Stress can cause increased cortisol secretion, enhanced degradation of cortisol secretion, loss of circadian variation in ACTH/cortisol release, and reduced susceptibility to cortisol inhibition in the hypothalamus/pituitary gland.

Aldosterone secretion is primarily regulated by the renin-angiotensin system and circulating levels of potassium.

Cortical androgen–stimulating hormone

tal adrenal hyperplasia, results in excessive ACTH secretion (release of negative feedback inhibition), increased adrenal androgen release, and virilization in affected females. Administration of ACTH-suppressive doses of dexamethasone can reduce adrenal androgen secretion in this setting.

The system-specific actions of cortisol and aldosterone are reviewed later in this chapter, under Specific Organ System Effects of Glucocorticoids and Mineralocorticoids.

Angiotensin-Aldosterone Axis

Products from angiotensinogen hydrolysis regulate aldosterone secretion.

Angiotensin-converting enzyme (ACE)

Beta-adrenergic stimulation enhances renin production.

Potassium *stimulates* aldosterone production.

Aldosterone secretion by the zona glomerulosa of the adrenal cortex is regulated primarily by the products of the hydrolysis of a liver-derived protein, angiotensinogen (renin substrate) (Bondy, 1985). Renin, an enzyme secreted by renal juxtaglomerular cells, catalyzes the production from angiotensinogen of a decapeptide (angiotensin I) that has little or no biological role and is itself hydrolyzed rapidly in lung and blood by angiotensin-converting enzyme (ACE) to an octapeptide, angiotensin II. Angiotensin II is the principal stimulator of aldosterone synthesis, but it is also a pressor substance. Enzymatic removal of the N-terminal aspartic acid residue of angiotensin II results in angiotensin III, a peptide with less pressor activity but aldosterone-stimulating ability comparable to angiotensin II (Bondy, 1985). Renin release is provoked by decreased renal artery blood pressure or intravascular volume depletion, reflecting apparent baroreceptor function of the renal juxtaglomerular apparatus. Beta-adrenergic stimulation and lowered filtered sodium load, as well as potassium depletion, also act to enhance renin production. The biochemical mechanisms involved in mediating the effects of these various factors on renin release are not entirely clear, but prostaglandins may be involved; e.g., inhibition of prostaglandin synthesis by nonsteroidal anti-inflammatory agents induces a low-renin–low-aldosterone state (hyporeninemic hypoaldosteronism) that promotes hyperkalemia. The actions of angiotensin II and III on the adrenal cortex involve enhanced conversion of cholesterol to pregnenolone and corticosterone to aldosterone (see Fig. 43–1).

In contrast to its damping effect on renin production, potassium is a potent stimulator of aldosterone production through a direct action on the adrenal cortex. Ambient plasma sodium concentration appears to have little effect on aldosterone synthesis.

ACTH Preparations

CHEMISTRY

The NH_2-terminal 24 residues of the ACTH polypeptide make up the bioactive portion of the molecule. Residues 25–39 represent the immunogenic end of ACTH. Thus, a commercially available $ACTH_{1-24}$ peptide, cosyntropin, is minimally allergenic.

MECHANISM OF ACTION

ACTH interacts with specific receptors on the surfaces of adrenocortical cells, promoting adenylate cyclase activity and cyclic 3′,5′-AMP (adenosine monophosphate) (second-messenger) generation with subsequent phosphorylation of adrenal proteins, a process related in some unknown way to the production of a polypeptide(s), which facilitates the interaction of cholesterol with $P-450_{scc}$ (Pedersen and Brownie, 1983). Another second-messenger system in adrenal plasma membranes, the phosphatidylinositol (PI) cycle, can also be activated by ACTH and appears to be the principal mechanism involved in the stimulation by angiotensin II of aldosterone secretion by adrenal zona glomerulosa cells.

ADVERSE EFFECTS

Chronic ACTH administration results in excess adrenal steroid production (hypercortisolism), the consequences of which are reviewed later.

Chronic ACTH administration causes excessive production of adrenal steroids.

USE: ACTH STIMULATION TEST

ACTH, specifically the α_{1-24} peptide (cosyntropin) is a diagnostic agent. The patient is given 0.25 mg of cosyntropin as an intravenous (IV) bolus or intramuscularly (IM) (1-hour test) or as an 8–24-hour infusion in patients with suspected adrenocortical insufficiency, with plasma cortisol determinations taken either before bolus IV or IM injection and 60 minutes after injection or before and at the conclusion of 8- or 24-hour infusion. Failure of plasma cortisol concentration to rise within 60 minutes of IV bolus or IM cosyntropin supports the diagnosis of primary adrenocortical insufficiency (Addison's disease) but does not exclude the diagnosis of secondary (hypo-pituitary) adrenocortical insufficiency. Very rarely, confirmation of the latter may require 8–24 hours of ACTH infusion. In the presence of non-endocrine illness ("stress"), the endogenous response of the adrenal cortex to exogenous ACTH may be limited in terms of adrenal androgen secretion and of renin release (see Chemistry, Distribution, and Metabolism under Adrenal Corticosteroids).

Agent	Structure	Use
Cosyntropin	α_{1-24} ACTH peptide	Diagnostic agent
ACTH	Intact 39-amino acid molecule	Diagnostic agent
ACTH gel	Intact 39-amino acid molecule in gelatin	Diagnostic agent

ACTH and ACTH gel offer no advantage as diagnostic agents over α_{1-24} ACTH.

USE: ACTH THERAPY

The therapeutic advantage of systemic ACTH administration, employing ACTH (intact 39-amino acid molecule) or ACTH gel, rather than glucocorticoid use, is not established in the treatment of clinical states described later that respond to anti-inflammatory steroids. It should be noted that ACTH administration will promote the release of biologically active steroids—such as adrenal androgens and aldosterone—in addition to glucocorticoids, but it is not clear that these agents offer therapeutic benefits in anti-inflammatory steroid–responsive conditions. It has been postulated that exogenous ACTH-related peptides mimic endogenous repair signals in nervous tissue. The utility of ACTH in other neuropathological states, such as demyelinating disorders, has not been established, but neurotoxicity associated with certain cancer chemotherapeutic agents, such as cisplatin, may be prevented by administration of an ACTH (4–9) analog.

CHEMISTRY, DISTRIBUTION, AND METABOLISM

Adrenal Corticosteroids

The ultimate pharmacological effect of glucocorticoids is dependent on dose of the agent, type of disease to be treated, clinical status of patient (patient age, gender, renal and hepatic function), and the interaction of these factors at the level of disposition of the specific steroid administered.

Cortisol and its analogs can be administered orally.

Oral administration of aldosterone is not practical.

CBG is the principal corticosteroid transport protein.

Increased ACTH secretion occurs during stress.

Glucocorticoids are absorbed through the skin and can suppress endogenous ACTH secretion.

Cortisol and its analogs are absorbed from the gastrointestinal (GI) tract to degrees that are clinically very useful, despite variability; e.g., oral cortisol absorption ranges from 45% to 80%. The absorption of cortisone acetate is similarly variable, but such agents are clinically effective in patients with adrenocortical insufficiency, indicating there is a fairly broad therapeutic range with replacement dosage. It should also be understood that cortisone and prednisone are inactive analogs; the 11-ketone must undergo reduction to an 11β-hydroxyl in order to achieve biological activity. The bioavailability of oral prednisone formulations is more consistent than those of cortisol and ranges from 75% to more than 90%. Oral administration of mineralocorticoid is more problematical. Desoxycorticosterone acetate (DOCA) is not absorbed significantly from the GI tract, and aldosterone, itself, has a very short $t_{1/2}$ (15 minutes; see later), making its oral administration impractical.

Cortisol and prednisolone are largely protein-bound (90%); the free fraction is biologically active (Mendel et al, 1989). The principal corticosteroid transport protein, cortisol-binding globulin (CBG), is a low–binding capacity, high-affinity moiety. CBG synthesis in the liver is stimulated by estrogen, and administration of the latter, or spontaneously hyperestrogenemic clinical states (e.g., pregnancy), elevate CBG and plasma cortisol levels. Albumin also binds glucocorticoids, but with low affinity, and changes in circulating levels of albumin glucocorticoids have no significant effect on cortisol kinetics. Mineralocorticoids are about 60% protein-bound, but at low-affinity sites; this largely determines the short plasma half-life of aldosterone.

Metabolism of glucocorticoids includes reductions of the 4,5 double bond and of the 3-ketone or of the 20-ketone (Fig. 43–3), usually carried out in the liver (Bondy, 1980). These reductions yield generally inactive by-products. Reductions which occur in the A ring (3 or 4–5 positions) presage hepatic sulfoconjugation or glucuronidations of the steroid at the 3-position. These water-soluble metabolites are excreted by the kidney, together with small quantities of unconjugated (designated *free*) cortisol. The GI tract is not a significant contributor to the metabolism of glucocorticoids.

The pituitary-adrenal axis has a characteristic response to major medical and psychiatric stress (Parker et al, 1985). This includes increased ACTH secretion and resultant rise in plasma cortisol concentration. Adrenal androgen response to exogenous ACTH administration in the setting of stress may be blunted. The diurnal rhythm of ACTH-cortisol secretion may be lost, and exogenous glucocorticoid, e.g., dexamethasone, may not predictably suppress endogenous ACTH and cortisol secretion. Failure of the pituitary-adrenal axis to suppress normally after dexamethasone administration to psychiatric patients has been interpreted by a few observers to have psychiatric/diagnostic significance (Berger et al, 1984). Hyporeninemic hypoaldosteronism may also occur transiently in the setting of stress.

Glucocorticoids are absorbed through the skin, particularly erythematous or denuded skin. In order to alter the steroid molecule for topical administration, glucocorticoid is conjugated with a lipophilic ester, e.g., an acetonide, that permits high topical steroid dosage but reduced systemic absorption. Applied over a large area, particularly occlusively, steroids may nonetheless be absorbed in sufficient quantities to suppress endogenous ACTH secretion. Corticosteroids are effective when applied topically to mucosal membranes, such as in the conjunctivae or airway. Mucosal administration offers the advantage of achieving high local concentrations with reduced systemic side effects and is effective in the management of asthma

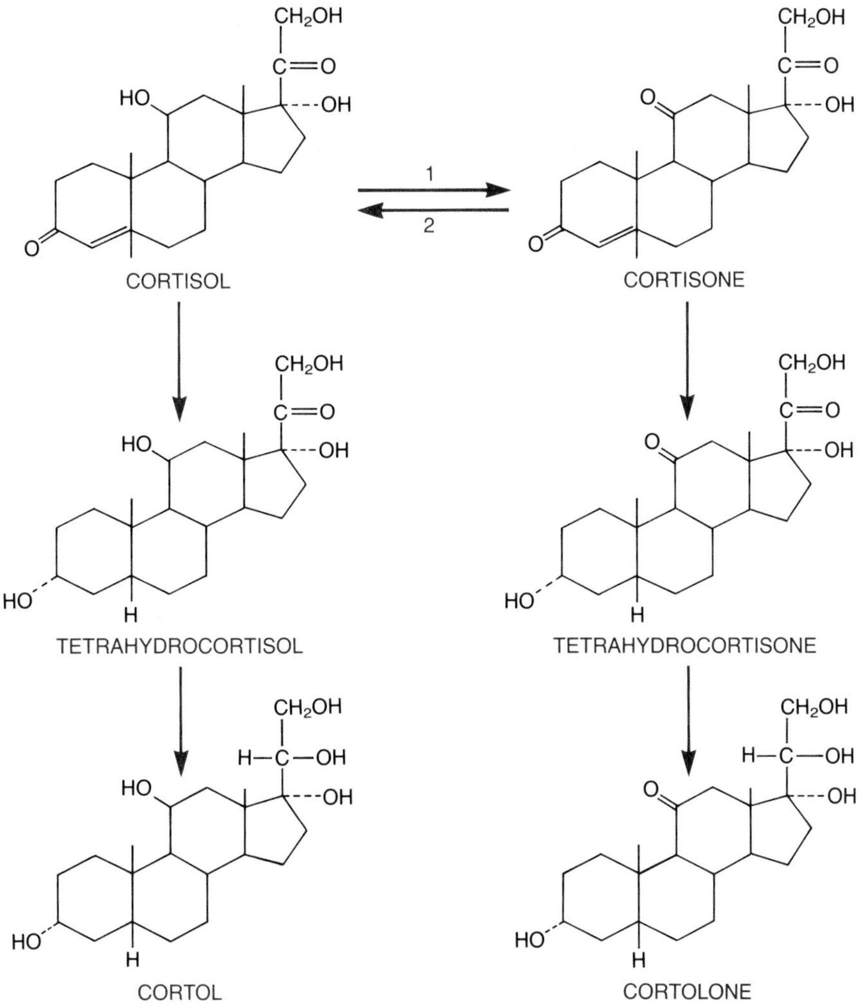

Figure 43-3

The catabolism of cortisol in the liver. Reaction 1 is catalyzed by 11β-hydroxy-steroid dehydrogenase; reaction 2 by 11-ketosteroid reductase activity.

(aerosolized steroid) and ulcerative colitis, particularly that restricted to the rectosigmoid area (steroid enema).

Intra-articular administration of glucocorticoids can deliver temporary anti-inflammatory relief in afflicted joints. The steroid molecule is manipulated with the substitution of a tert-butylacetate (prednisolone tebutate) or a hexacetonide group (triamcinolone) that decreases the water solubility of these drugs' microcrystalline suspension (Gifford, 1975; Intra-articular steroids, 1984). These microcrystalline suspensions result in delayed systemic absorption and prolonged exposure to the inflamed joint space (Gifford, 1975).

To enable the parenteral (IV, IM) administration of glucocorticoids, manipulation of the water solubility of the steroid molecule is achieved through conjugation at the 21 carbon. Steroids (hydrocortisone, methylprednisolone, prednisolone, dexamethasone) that are formulated as sodium phosphate or sodium succinate salts exhibit a rapid rate of absorption owing to increased water solubility. These formulations are appropriate for IV or IM administration when a rapid effect is desirable (Szefler, 1989; Tyrell and Baxter, 1987). The glucocorticoids that are conjugated with acetate (prednisolone, methylprednisolone, cortisone, dexamethasone, hydrocortisone) or acetonide (triamcinolone) esters demonstrate an enhanced lipid solubility resulting in a slower rate of absorption and a prolonged duration of effect. For example, a single IM injection of triamcinolone acetonide is absorbed slowly with an effect lasting a few weeks (Dluhy, 1975; Fariss et al, 1978). These lipid-soluble ester formulations are inappropriate steroid selections when a rapid clinical response is required after IM injection (Tyrell and Baxter, 1987). IM or IV administration of glucocorticoids is indicated when the oral/GI route is impractical. IV hormone is mandatory in patients with acute adrenocortical insufficiency; blood volume is reduced in such patients, making the absorption of IM (or oral) agents unpredictable.

Glucocorticoids administered through aerosolized inhalation result in minimal systemic absorption with directed application to the pulmonary vasculature. One of the most commonly utilized steroids is beclomethasone diproprionate, which has esterification of the hydroxyl group at carbons 17 and 21. Chemical modification results in a potent local effect from a weak glucocorticoid (Martin et al, 1975).

PHARMACOLOGICAL MODIFICATION OF CORTICOSTEROID STRUCTURE

Introduction of a 1,2 double bond to the glucocorticoid nucleus (prednisolone and methylprednisolone) enhances glucocorticoid (anti-inflammatory) activity (Fig. 43–4) and reduces mineralocorticoid effect. Cortisone and prednisone are inactive anti-inflammatory agents until they are converted in the body from 11-keto formulations to 11β-hydroxyl compounds (cortisol and prednisolone, respectively). The introduction of a 6α-methyl group to prednisolone modestly enhances anti-inflammatory activity, but this results in an important change in pharmacokinetic properties. Introduction of fluorine at the 9α-position in the steroid B ring very significantly improves salt-retaining qualities of the steroid (9α-fluorocortisol). 9α-fluorination also enhances anti-inflammatory properties, but in order to exploit this quality therapeutically, the salt-retaining potency of 9α-fluorination must be diminished by introductions of other modifications of the

Cortisol and prednisolone are 11β-hydroxy-corticosteroids.

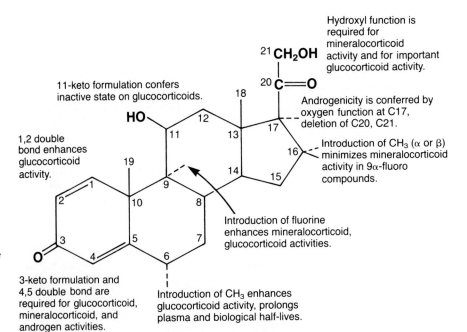

Figure 43–4

Corticosteroid structure-activity relationships. *Dotted lines* reflect projection below the plane of the ring (α configuration); side chain bonds, represented by *intact lines*, project about the plane of the ring (β configuration). (Modified from Liddle GW: Clinical pharmacology of the anti-inflammatory steroids. Clin Pharmacol Ther 2:615–635, 1961.)

Hydroxyl function is required for mineralocorticoid activity and for important glucocorticoid activity.

11-keto formulation confers inactive state on glucocorticoids.

Androgenicity is conferred by oxygen function at C17, deletion of C20, C21.

Introduction of CH₃ (α or β) minimizes mineralocorticoid activity in 9α-fluoro compounds.

1,2 double bond enhances glucocorticoid activity.

Introduction of fluorine enhances mineralocorticoid, glucocorticoid activities.

3-keto formulation and 4,5 double bond are required for glucocorticoid, mineralocorticoid, and androgen activities.

Introduction of CH₃ enhances glucocorticoid activity, prolongs plasma and biological half-lives.

steroid nucleus. For example, betamethasone and dexamethasone are potent 9α-fluorinated anti-inflammatory agents with C16 modifications (α- or β-methyl group introductions) to minimize the mineralocorticoid effect.

Although salt-retaining properties do not require an oxygen moiety at C11, aldosterone does have an 11-oxygen; the 11-oxygen in the form of the 11β-hydroxyl *is* required for glucocorticoid effects. A 21-hydroxy function is needed for both mineralocorticoid and glucocorticoid action. Adrenal steroid androgenicity is invested in the replacement of C20 and C21 with an oxygen function at C17. A potent glucocorticoid antagonist with negligible agonist activity has resulted from organic residue substitutions at the 17α-, 17β-, and 11-positions of the estrogen nucleus (17α-hydroxy-11β - (4 - dimethylaminophenyl) - 17β - (prop - 1 - ynyl) - estra - 4,9 - dien - 3-one) (RU 486) (Lahteenmaki et al, 1987). This compound is also an anti-estrogen (see Chapter 42). Potencies of various glucocorticoids and mineralocorticoids are compared in Table 43 – 2.

Glucocorticoids are also classified according to their biological half-lives in humans (see Table 43 – 2), on the basis of the duration of ACTH suppression after single-dose exposure. These data are limited in amount, but widely cited.

9α-fluorinated anti-inflammatory agents: betamethasone and dexamethasone

MECHANISMS OF ACTION

Biological effects of glucocorticoids (cortisol and its natural and synthetic analogs) occur in target cells following the interaction of the steroid with a specific glucocorticoid receptor (GR). GRs are now recognized to be members of a superfamily of ligand-responsive DNA-binding proteins having a zinc-finger structure that allows them to interact with the genome (Fig. 43 – 5). This family also includes mineralocorticoids, thyroid hormone (c-*erb*-A), 1,25-dihydroxy-vitamin D_3, retinoic acid, estrogen, progesterone, and androgen receptors (Green and Chambon, 1986; Weinberger et al, 1987). As opposed to the receptors for progesterone, estrogen, and androgen, the GR is localized in the cytoplasm and following binding of the glucocorticoid the complex moves to the nucleus. The steroid-binding domain is located at the C-terminal end of the receptor separate from the more centrally located DNA-binding domains (see Fig. 43 – 4). Occupancy of the steroid-binding sites by cortisol or dexamethasone has allosteric effects on the receptor protein that enable its interaction with specific glucocorticoid responsive elements (GRE) in nuclear DNA. The interaction of the GR complex with its DNA-binding site is abnormal in the familial syndrome of glucocorticoid resistance, associated with high serum ACTH and endogenous cortisol levels, but no clinical stigmata of Cushing's syndrome (Nawata et al, 1987).

There is some evidence for direct effects of glucocorticoids on the plasma membrane of target cells (Gelehrter, 1979), perhaps through the induction of changes in membrane phospholipid content.

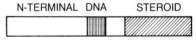

| N-TERMINAL | DNA | STEROID |

Figure 43 – 5

Schematic structure of steroid hormone receptors illustrating the steroid-binding and DNA-binding domains.

Steroid hormone – binding occurs at the C-terminal region of the receptor. This domain is preceded by two zinc-finger DNA-binding motifs. The N-terminal region is hypervariable but is thought to fine-tune the regulation of gene expression. Occupancy of the ligand-binding sites on the glucocorticoid receptor (GR) by cortisol or dexamethasone has allosteroic effects on the receptor protein that enable its interaction(s) with genes. Steroids appear critical to the nuclear action of the steroid receptor proteins *in vivo*, but they may not be necessary under certain experimental *in vitro* conditions. The nuclear effects of these steroid receptor proteins promote nucleus-directed synthesis of certain proteins and inhibit synthesis of other proteins (see later). Aldosterone action also is cell nucleus – mediated through its binding to the mineralocorticoid receptor (MR) in target tissues. There is 94% homology between the DNA-binding domains of GR and of MR and, understandably, significantly less (57%) in the hormone-binding domain. Glucocorticoids have catabolic effects (increased protein degradation) as well, the biochemical mechanisms of which are not understood.

SYSTEMIC PHARMACOLOGY OF ADRENAL CORTICOSTEROIDS

The systemic and organ-specific effects of glucocorticoids are extensive (Loriaux and Cutler, 1986) (Table 43 – 1). They promote hepatic gluconeo-

Table 43–1 PRINCIPAL EFFECTS OF GLUCOCORTICOIDS

Metabolic Effects of Physiological Concentrations of Glucocorticoids

Effect	Consequence
FUEL HOMEOSTASIS	
Increased hepatic glycogenolysis* Increased hepatic gluconeogenesis* Decreased uptake of glucose by peripheral tissues	Contribution to counterregulation (restoration of normoglycemia after hypoglycemia); promotion of hyperglycemia
Increased protein degradation in striated muscle and adipose and lymphoid tissues†‡ Decreased protein synthesis in striated muscle and adipose and lymphoid tissues‡	Provision of amino acid substrates for gluconeogenesis; catabolic state
Increased lipolysis*	Mobilization of free fatty acids and glycerol
METABOLIC ADAPTATION	
Increased myocardial contractility Increased sensitivity of myocardium to catecholamines	Increased cardiac output
Increased capacity for work of striated muscle§	

System-Specific Effects of Pharmacological Concentrations of Glucocorticoids

Host Defense/Inflammatory Response

Decreased resistance to bacterial, viral, and fungal infections‖
Decreased antibody formation
Decreased phagocytic performance of granulocytes
Decreased lymphocyte, thymocyte mass, with impairment of delayed hypersensitivity
Decreased vascular permeability

Gastrointestinal Tract

Decreased absorption of calcium

Endocrine System

Decreased peripheral, i.e., extrathyroidal, conversion of L-thyroxine to 3,5,3′-L-triiodothyronine
Decreased pituitary thyrotropin (TSH) secretion
Increased pituitary ACTH secretion

Musculoskeletal System

Myopathy of proximal (limb girdle) striated muscles§
Osteopenia
Decreased growth of bone in immature skeleton

Connective Tissue

Decreased collagen, glycosaminoglycan formation¶
Decreased wound healing

Eye

Posterior subcapsular cataract

Data from Loriaux DL, Cutler DB Jr: Diseases of the adrenal gland. *In* Kohler PO, Jordan RM (eds): Clinical Endocrinology, 167–238. New York: John Wiley & Sons, 1986. Additional details of the side-effect profile of glucocorticoids are presented in Table 43–3.
* Glucocorticoids are essential to endogenous epinephrine- and glucagon-stimulated gluconeogenesis, glycogenolysis, and lipolysis.
† Myocardium and diaphragm are spared, as may be exercise-hypertrophied striated muscle.
‡ Protein (enzyme) synthesis in liver is enhanced by glucocorticoids and supports gluconeogenesis.
§ Enhanced work capacity is a short-term effect of glucocorticoids. Long-term increases in endogenous cortisol secretion (Cushing's syndrome) or administration of pharmacological doses of glucocorticoids enhances striated muscle catabolism, chiefly of the proximal muscles.
‖ Compromised host response to infectious agents, particularly opportunistic organisms, is characteristic of clinical settings in which pharmacological doses of glucocorticoids are administered as anti-inflammatory agents, but opportunistic infections may occur occasionally in states of endogenous hypercortisolism.
¶ Physiological concentrations of glucocorticoids may also regulate glycosaminoglycan formation.

genesis and also mobilize amino acids through muscle (and other tissue) protein catabolism to support gluconeogenesis. This action underlies cortisol's classification as a counterregulatory hormone, i.e., defending the intact organism against hypoglycemia, particularly insulin-induced hypoglycemia. Glucocorticoids also support or elevate blood glucose concentration by inhibiting glucose uptake/utilization in peripheral tissues, e.g., fat cells. Supraphysiological doses of corticosteroids cause frank hyperglycemia. In addition to these effects on carbohydrate metabolism, corticosteroids importantly affect lipid metabolism by stimulating lipolysis (free fatty acid liberation from triglycerides); they also enhance the lipolytic effects of catecholamines on adipose tissue. Supraphysiological amounts of glucocorticoids, whether exogenous or endogenous (Cushing's syndrome), foster redistribution of body fat into a centripetal pattern (truncal obesity) characteristic of Cushing's syndrome.

> Glucocorticoids elevate blood glucose concentration.

The cell nucleus–dependent effects of glucocorticoids on protein metabolism have been mentioned previously; they are generally catabolic, resulting in loss of muscle mass (at least in part through enhanced proteolysis), bone mass (osteoporosis), and lymphoid tissue elements. Mineralocorticoids (aldosterone, corticosterone) are critical to body sodium and potassium homeostasis and enhance urinary potassium excretion and the reabsorption of sodium from renal tubular filtrate at Site 3 (distal tubule) (Marver and Kokko, 1983). Cortisol has modest sodium-retaining capacity, whereas certain synthetic glucocorticoids (dexamethasone) (Table 43–2) have virtually no effect on renal sodium-handling. Cortisol also facilitates the action of antidiuretic hormone (ADH; arginine vasopressin, AVP) on water reabsorption in the renal collecting tubule, perhaps in part by enhancing glomerular filtration rate (GFR). Mineralocorticoids do not directly affect GFR or water metabolism, but their effects on renal sodium reabsorption result in expanded plasma volume and normalization of GFR in subjects who were previously volume-depleted.

> Mineralocorticoids are essential to body sodium and potassium homeostasis.

Table 43–2 COMPARISON OF PHARMACOKINETICS AND POTENCIES OF CORTICOSTEROIDS

Corticosteroid	Plasma $t_{\frac{1}{2}}$ (minutes)	Tissue $t_{\frac{1}{2}}$ (hours)	Relative Potency Glucocorticoid Activity	Relative Potency Mineralocorticoid Activity	Equivalent Dose* (mg)
Cortisol (hydrocortisone)	90	8–12	1	1	20
Cortisone (11-dehydrocortisol)	30	8–12	0.8	0.8	25
Prednisone (Δ^1-cortisone)	60	12–36	4	0.8	5
Prednisolone (Δ^1-cortisol)	200	12–36	4	0.8	5
6α-methylprednisolone	180	12–36	5	0.5	4
Fludrocortisone (9α-fluorocortisol)	200	8–12	10	125	—
Triamcinolone (9α-fluoro-16α-hydroxyprednisolone)	300	12–36	5	0	4
Betamethasone (9α-fluoro-16β-methylprednisolone)	100–300	36–54	25	0	0.75
Dexamethasone (9α-fluoro-16α-methylprednisolone)	100–300	36–54	25	0	0.75

Modified from Truhan AP, Ahmed AR: Corticosteroids: A review with emphasis on complications of prolonged systemic therapy. Ann Allergy 62:375–390, 1989.
* Equivalent dosages are approximate and apply only to oral or intravenous administration. Potencies will vary importantly when agents are administered intramuscularly or into the joint space.

SPECIFIC ORGAN SYSTEM EFFECTS OF GLUCOCORTICOIDS AND MINERALOCORTICOIDS

Endocrine System

As indicated earlier, cortisol and its glucocorticoid analogs defend against hypoglycemia (counterregulation) and can, particularly when present in excess, exacerbate carbohydrate intolerance (see Table 43–1). The normal release of another counterregulatory hormone, growth hormone (GH), requires cortisol. In excess, glucocorticoids suppress endogenous thyrotropin (TSH) release.

The release of growth hormone requires cortisol.

Cardiovascular System

Glucocorticoids appear to sensitize blood vessels to the actions on vasomotor tone of catecholamines and angiotensin. Excess glucocorticoids usually provoke hypertension. Although incompletely understood, steroid-associated hypertension is thought to have a component of volume-dependence, that is, a mineralocorticoid/sodium retention component.

Hypertensive effects

Skeletal Muscle

Although muscle weakness is a hallmark of adrenocortical insufficiency, this manifestation very likely respresents decreased plasma volume and cardiac output. Administered in pharmacological doses, cortisol and the glucocorticoid analogs produce profound muscle wasting, particularly of the proximal muscles of the shoulders and hip girdle.

Muscle-wasting effects of glucocorticoids

Bone

In supraphysiological concentrations, glucocorticoids inhibit osteoblast activity or the proliferation of periosteal cells that give rise to osteoblasts. Although this contributes to the loss of bone mass associated with pharmacological use of anti-inflammatory steroids, the latter agents also affect calcium absorption (see later). The role of cortisol in physiological concentrations on bone metabolism is unclear.

Gastrointestinal Tract

Glucocorticoids decrease absorption of calcium by the GI tract. In part, this reflects glucocorticoid inhibition of vitamin D activation and removal of the stimulation by 1,25-dihydroxyvitamin-D_3 of calcium absorption. This effect is observed at supraphysiological levels of cortisol. The reduction in plasma calcium levels that results from glucocorticoid action causes a homeostatic rise in circulating concentrations of parathyroid hormone (PTH). When clinical glucocorticoid use is prolonged, a new steady state of induced hyperparathyroidism is developed, associated with PTH-induced osteoclast activation and loss of bone mass. Mineralocorticoids stimulate GI tract mucosal membrane Na,K-ATPase activity and enhance sodium absorption from the gut. This action of aldosterone occurs at physiological levels of the steroid.

Glucocorticoids decrease calcium absorption.

Bone Marrow and Lymphoid Tissues

Glucocorticoids are growth factors for cells cultured *in vitro*, and these agents may have modest trophic effects on erythroid precursors in bone marrow. Modest normochromic anemia in the setting of sustained primary adrenocortical insufficiency has been attributed to the loss of the putative trophic action of cortisol; it is likely, however, that this finding may be a nonspecific anemia of chronic disease.

Administration of pharmacological doses of anti-inflammatory corticoids results in elevated peripheral white blood cell counts, owing to recruitment of mature granulocytes into the circulation. Eosinophils are reduced in this setting, and eosinophil counts are increased in patients with primary adrenocortical insufficiency, indicating that there exists a cell-specific response of glucocorticoids of this cell line. Peripheral blood eosinophil count also is decreased in spontaneous Cushing's syndrome. The steroid effect on eosinophils appears to reflect the clinically useful application of steroids to the management of allergic conditions of various origins.

Lymphoid tissue atrophies under the influence of supraphysiological levels of anti-inflammatory glucocorticoids, and peripheral lymphocytosis develops in the face of chronic adrenocortical insufficiency. Although the action of corticoids has been described as acutely lympholytic in animal models, the lymphopenia that accompanies excessive endogenous or exogenous glucocorticoid exposure in humans relates to longer-term genomic effects on lymphoid tissue and to heightened turnover of circulating lymphocytes, without necessarily a lytic effect on the mononuclear cells.

Immune System

Glucocorticoids in supraphysiological concentrations inhibit the proliferation of macrophages and lymphocytes, as well as of antigen-presenting cells. They also block the production of interleukin-2 (IL-2), a lymphokine critical to the normal immune response. Thus, prolonged glucocorticoid use clinically induces an immunocompromised state in which opportunistic bacteria and fungi may establish tissue infections in the steroid-treated host. On the other hand, it is sometimes necessary to suppress the immune response, e.g., in the settings of rejection of a transplanted (allograft) organ or a serious systemic allergic reaction; here, systemic glucocorticoid administration may be essential.

Glucocorticoids can induce an immunocompromised state.

Inflammatory Response

Glucocorticoids suppress the features of local inflammatory response (erythema, warmth, edema) and a major systemic inflammatory response, fever. These suppressive actions are mediated by the ability of anti-inflammatory steroids to diminish cytokine production, including interleukins, prostaglandins, and leukocyte migration inhibition factor (MIF), and to inhibit the proliferation of various mononuclear cell types important to the inflammatory process. Suppression of inflammatory or immune responses may justify high-dose systemic glucocorticoid administration in the management of rheumatological disorders (collagen vascular diseases), sarcoidosis, or local edema associated with primary or metastatic tumors in closed spaces, specifically, the CNS. The ophthalmopathy of Graves' disease (diffuse toxic goiter) is a complex localized inflammatory and secretory response involving retrobulbar cellular elements, including fibroblasts, and is responsive to high-dose dexamethasone therapy (Bartalena et al, 1989).

Glucocorticoids suppress fever.

High-dose dexamethasone therapy is used to treat ophthalmopathy of Graves' disease.

Nervous System

Although the efficacy of high-dose glucocorticoid administration has been established in localized tumor–related edema within the CNS, it is not established that glucocorticoids alter the course of trauma-induced brain edema. Dexamethasone alone, or with metoclopramide, may be effective as an antiemetic in patients who receive cancer chemotherapy with cisplatin.

ADVERSE EFFECTS OF GLUCOCORTICOIDS

The side-effect profile of glucocorticoids is presented in Table 43–3. These adverse effects largely represent exaggerations of Cushing's syndrome. All glucocorticoids are capable of inducing the effects listed in Table 43–3, except that pharmacological doses of cortisol rarely induce mineralocorti-

---

Table 43–3   PRINCIPAL SIDE EFFECTS OF ANTI-INFLAMMATORY CORTICOSTEROID THERAPY

System-Specific Side Effects

Endocrine-Metabolic
Hyperglycemia, including hyperosmolar nonketotic stupor/coma and, rarely, diabetic ketoacidosis
Truncal obesity, enlargement of cervical, supraclavicular, and mediastinal fat pads
Retarded somatic growth (pediatric patient population)
Acne
Hirsutism
Negative nitrogen and calcium balances
Sodium retention (except with synthetic 16-substituted, 9α-fluorinated corticosteroids)

Cardiovascular System
Hypertension

Gastrointestinal Tract
Pancreatitis
Peptic ulcer disease*

Musculoskeletal System
Osteoporosis
Aseptic necrosis of femoral and humeral heads
Myopathy

Nervous System
Pseudotumor cerebri
Mood disorders, including both euphoria and depressive states
Psychosis

Host Defenses Against Infectious Agents
Increased susceptibility to opportunistic infections, owing to impaired cellular and humoral responses

Eye
Posterior subcapsular cataract

Incidence of Major Side Effects

Complication	Incidence Range (%)	Duration of Therapy Prior to Appearance of Complication	Minimal Daily Dose Reported to Result in Complication	Reversibility
Diabetes mellitus	2–28	Days to months	7.5 mg prednisone	Yes
Redistribution of body fat	13	<2 months	4–12 mg triamcinolone	Variable
Hypertension	4–25	2 weeks	7.5 mg prednisone	Yes
Peptic ulcer disease*	0–14	<1 month		Yes
Aseptic necrosis of bone	1–10	<6 weeks	5–20 mg prednisone	No
Myopathy	10	1 week	10 mg prednisone	Yes
Psychiatric disorders	1–18	Days	60 mg hydrocortisone	Yes
Cataract	4	2 months	5 mg prednisone	No

Adapted from Axelrod L: Glucocorticoid therapy. Medicine 55:39–65, 1976; and Truhan AP, Ahmed AR: Corticosteroids: A review with emphasis on complications of prolonged systemic therapy. Ann Allergy 62:375–390, 1989. Duration and dosage requirements cited are estimates and highly dependent on concurrent clinical factors that may, in addition to glucocorticoid administration, promote certain of the complications listed, such as diabetes mellitus, hypertension, and psychiatric disturbances.
* The risk of peptic ulcer disease during glucocorticoid administration is controversial (Conn and Blitzer, 1976).

coid side effects. It must also be emphasized that, in addition to their unfavorable side-effect profile, anti-inflammatory glucocorticoids, administered for 3 weeks or more, suppress the hypothalamic-pituitary-adrenal axis. Withdrawal of exogenous steroid may leave the pituitary-adrenal axis inadequately responsive to stress.

The incidence of each of the major adverse effects from glucocorticoid administration is difficult to define (see Table 43–3) (Truhan and Ahmed, 1989). The cumulative steroid dose and duration of steroid exposure associated with specific side effects are not clearly established in the literature, but ranges for these factors are provided in Table 43–3. The psychiatric side effects of corticosteroids are not predicted by patients' prior histories of psychopathy and may occur at any point in long-term pharmacological-dose steroid use (Ling et al, 1981). Patients develop side effects of glucocorticoids at various rates, which may reflect interpatient variability in pharmacokinetics or, possibly, altered cellular sensitivity to steroids. Whether steroids facilitate upper GI tract ulceration remains controversial. Data on this issue are biased by the severity of the disease states for which corticosteroids are indicated, that is, stress is acknowledged to promote peptide ulcer disease, regardless of steroid therapy. As indicated previously, introduction of steroid treatment locally—aerosolized for airway disease or topically for skin disease—minimizes the risks of glucocorticoid treatment, although enough agent may be absorbed into the systemic circulation to cause some degree of hypothalamic-pituitary suppression.

DIAGNOSTIC USE OF CORTICOSTEROIDS

The intactness of the normal relationship between the pituitary gland and the adrenal cortex may be assessed in the setting of suspected hyperadrenocorticism by administering an exogenous corticosteroid in amounts sufficient to suppress endogenous ACTH and measuring the latter or plasma cortisol. Dexamethasone is usually utilized for this purpose; this glucocorticoid does not cross-react with cortisol antibodies in the cortisol radioimmunoassay and permits monitoring of endogenous cortisol levels while dexamethasone is administered.

The normal pituitary gland interrupts its ACTH release after administration of 0.75 mg of dexamethasone (*overnight dexamethasone suppression test*, DST). The paradigm for further testing of the pituitary-adrenal axis is as follows: 0.5 mg of dexamethasone is administered orally every 6 hours for 48 hours ("low dose"), then 2.0 mg is administered orally every 6 hours ("high dose") for an additional 48 hours. Plasma cortisol at 8:00 A.M. or 24-hour urine excretion of cortisol, or both, is measured during this sequence. Normal response is a reduction in plasma cortisol to < 5 μg/dl with the low-dose test. Failure to suppress with the low-dose regimen usually indicates an abnormal hypothalamic-pituitary-adrenal axis. Patients who do not suppress at 2.0 mg/day, but do at 8.0 mg/day, have Cushing's disease (bilateral adrenocortical hyperplasia, owing to excess pituitary ACTH or CRF-ACTH output). Patients who fail to suppress in the high-dose paradigm have adrenocortical adenoma, adrenal carcinoma, or ectopic ACTH syndrome.

It should be noted, however, that abnormal DST may occur in patients with glucocorticoid-resistance syndrome or who are receiving phenytoin. Modified DST has been widely applied to patients with psychiatric syndromes in an effort to standardize diagnoses or predict responses to therapy. DST has not yet proved to be reliable for either purpose. The regimen has been midnight administration of 0.75 or 1.0 mg of dexamethasone, with measurement of plasma cortisol concentration at 4:00 P.M., rather than at 8:00 A.M., the following day.

Suppression of the hypothalamic-pituitary-adrenal axis

Variability of adverse effects among patients

Overnight dexamethasone suppression test

Failure to suppress at low dosage and suppression at high dosage indicates an abnormal hypothalamic-pituitary-adrenal axis.

THERAPEUTIC USES OF CORTICOSTEROIDS

Adrenocortical Insufficiency

Addison's disease is characterized by primary destruction of the adrenal gland.

Inadequate function of the adrenal cortex in humans results from (1) primary destruction of the adrenal gland (Addison's disease), usually on an autoimmune basis, (2) loss of pituitary ACTH secretory capacity or hypothalamic CRF secretory capacity (secondary adrenal insufficiency), or (3) suppression of the hypothalamic-pituitary axis by sustained administration of exogenous glucocorticoid and subsequent withdrawal of the steroid.

The principal symptoms and signs of the state relate to loss of both glucocorticoids and aldosterone—asthenia, orthostatic dizziness, weight loss, GI tract dysfunction—although certain findings are due to cortisol loss alone (hypoglycemia) or inadequate aldosterone secretion (hyperkalemia). Hyponatremia reflects primarily absence of the sodium-retaining effect of mineralocorticoid, but it is complicated by compensatory increases in central arginine vasopressin (AVP) release in response to decreased plasma volume, which results in decreased renal free-water clearance. Lack of glucocorticoid activity also decreases free-water clearance. The hyperpigmentation noted in previously fair-skinned patients who become addisonian reflects ACTH and β-lipotropin action on susceptible melanophores in skin creases, elbows, knees, mucocutaneous junctions, and mucosae. Freckling and moles also darken. Subjects with secondary adrenal insufficiency have minimal hyponatremia and lack hyperkalemia, because the renin-angiotensin-aldosterone axis is intact. Asthenia or hypoglycemia may be predominant findings, and signs of loss of other pituitary trophic hormones (hypothyroidism, hypogonadism) are frequently present. Excessive cutaneous pigmentation cannot develop.

Long-term steroid administration causes adrenocortical insufficiency.

Adrenocortical insufficiency resulting from anti-inflammatory steroid withdrawal after long-term steroid administration is usually manifested by weakness and hypotension. It may be subtle or, in the context of major physical stress (e.g., surgery or systemic infection), dramatic. Hyperpigmentation is not encountered because of the chronic suppression of the hypothalamic-pituitary axis that exogenous steroid therapy causes. Daily anti-inflammatory steroid dosage equivalent to more than 60 mg of cortisol (i.e., 15 mg of prednisone daily) is frequently sufficient to suppress the hypothalamic-pituitary axis when such therapy is continued for more than 3 weeks. High-dose steroid therapy of 40–60 mg of prednisone daily for 1 week or less has no consequence in terms of pituitary-adrenal suppression. Duration of therapy, size of dose, and periodicity of dosing are the critical factors in determining axis suppression.

Alternate-day corticosteroid administration

Daily prednisone administration is a risk for hypothalamic-pituitary suppression, whereas *alternate-day corticosteroid administration* is not; that is, a regimen of 40 mg of prednisone daily when modified to one dose of 80 mg every second day has minimal impact on the ACTH axis (Axelrod, 1976; MacGregor et al, 1968). Because of the pharmacokinetics of prednisone, ACTH secretion is restored by 36–48 hours after a dose of the agent.

Glucocorticoid Replacement Therapy

Acute adrenocortical insufficiency (adrenal crisis, addisonian crisis) may be life-threatening; its management is to be conducted in the hospital and includes

1. Restoration of intravascular volume with 0.9% saline solution, 1 or more liters over minutes to several hours, titrating against (orthostatic) blood pressure and heart rate and taking cognizance of the age and possible intrinsic heart disease of affected patients;

2. Replacement IV bolus glucocorticoid, 100 mg of hydrocortisone, then 50–100 mg of hydrocortisone every 8 hours as a continuous infusion for 24 hours or more, according to clinical state, converting to oral glucocorticoid replacement (see later) at 24–72 hours;

3. Specific management of concomitant nonendocrine illness (stress), which may have incited acute adrenocortical insufficiency.

Acute adrenocortical insufficiency is a potentially life-threatening state; when its presence is suspected, therapy, as described, should be introduced even though a definitive diagnosis has not been made. Confirmatory studies (e.g., ACTH stimulation test) may be carried out after replacement therapy has been initiated.

> ACTH stimulation test can confirm adrenocortical insufficiency.

Chronic adrenocortical insufficiency is managed by replacement corticosteroid—cortisol (hydrocortisone), 20 mg, or cortisone (acetate), 25 mg—orally each morning and 10 or 12.5 mg, respectively, of each agent in midafternoon, mimicking the diurnal variation in plasma cortisol levels that occurs in intact subjects. Some mineralocorticoid activity is obtained with these agents. A significant minority of adrenocortical insufficiency patients may require adjunctive mineralocorticoid treatment with 0.05–0.10 mg of 9α-fluorocortisol (fludrocortisone) by mouth daily or on alternate days. Indications for mineralocorticoid replacement include evidence of plasma volume depletion, impaired sense of well-being, myalgia, or modest hyperkalemia.

An alternative regimen for hypoadrenocorticism is prednisone (5.0 mg in the morning, 2.5 mg in the afternoon) with mineralocorticoid. It should be noted that excessive mineralocorticoid therapy promotes hypertension and sodium retention with edema.

The fully replaced adrenocortically insufficient patient requires increased glucocorticoid dosage when she or he is subjected to the stress of acute or intermittent systemic illness. Steroid half-lives decrease under these circumstances. The daily dose of glucocorticoid is doubled for the duration of the illness. Profound illness—e.g., acute myocardial infarction, bacteremia—should be treated with the equivalent of maximal endogenous corticoid output from the normal adrenal gland, 200–300 mg of hydrocortisone daily as an IV infusion. Mineralocorticoid is not used in this setting because, in such inpatients, volume and solute replacement are critically and selectively managed.

Mineralocorticoid Replacement Therapy: Hypoaldosteronism

Hypoaldosteronism may also occur independently of glucocorticoid insufficiency. This may be an isolated, idiopathic event; a consequence of dysfunction of the renin-angiotensin axis (hyporeninemic hypoaldosteronism); or a reversible biochemical action of high-dose IV heparin administration.

Isolated hypoaldosteronism is a very rare clinical syndrome associated with hyperkalemia. It is treated with 0.05–0.10 mg of fludrocortisone by mouth daily. Hyporeninemic hypoaldosteronism is occasionally encountered in patients with mild renal insufficiency (serum creatinine concentrations 1.5–2.5 mg/dl) and presents as hyperkalemia (Schambelan et al, 1972). The syndrome is seen with increased frequency in non–insulin-dependent diabetic patients. Hyperkalemia is sometimes alarming in these patients (>7.0 mEq/l) and may be managed with sodium polystyrene sulfonate (KAYEXALATE) chronically or with fludrocortisone. The dosage of the latter required to control serum potassium concentration ranges from 0.05 mg by mouth daily up to 1.0 mg or more. Caution is to be exercised in the use of high doses of synthetic mineralocorticoid.

> Isolated hypoaldosteronism is very rare.

> Non–insulin-dependent diabetics are susceptible to hyperkalemia.

Mineralocorticoid may also be indicated in the management of idiopathic orthostatic hypotension or in other dysautonomic states in which hypotension is symptomatic.

Chronic Use of Glucocorticoids As Anti-Inflammatory Agents

The goal of the anti-inflammatory use of glucocorticoids is acceptable control of the inflammatory, immunological, or allergic state for which it is employed, at the same time minimizing, insofar as possible, the unfavorable side-effect profile of glucocorticoids. The principles of anti-inflammatory steroid therapy include (1) continuation of steroid therapy only as long as the disease state for which steroid treatment is indicated is active; (2) use of the lowest steroid dose effective against the disease treated and tapering of the glucocorticoid as the activity of the disease permits; (3) use of local steroid where feasible (airway; skin); (4) use of *alternate-day systemic steroid administration* (Axelrod, 1976; MacGregor et al, 1968) when the disease under treatment permits such a regimen; (5) anticipation of side effects; (6) appreciation that withdrawal of chronic daily systemic steroid therapy leaves a pituitary-adrenal axis that may not be fully normal for months; (7) understanding that 1–2 weeks of high-dose daily systemic glucocorticoid administration has no clinically significant effect on the hypothalamic-pituitary-adrenal axis.

The advantages of alternate-day therapy are well-characterized (Axelrod, 1976) in terms of reduced risk of corticosteroid side effects and of suppression of the hypothalamic-pituitary axis. Steroid-responsive disease states are frequently, but not invariably (Hunder et al, 1975), controlled by alternate-day steroid administration.

When a disease process responsive to daily corticosteroid permits reduction or withdrawal of steroids, the strategy is (1) taper dosage systematically and (2) convert, whenever feasible, to an alternate-day administration regimen. A conventional program is to convert to alternate-day, e.g., for a patient receiving 40 mg prednisone daily, change to 80 mg every other day, then reduce prednisone dose by 5 mg weekly, monitoring the subject closely for appearance of activity of the underlying disease or symptoms of adrenal insufficiency. At 20 mg/dose, tapering may proceed at a reduced pace (2.5 mg/week or every other week), but the regimen should be individualized. Withdrawal of chronic anti-inflammatory corticosteroid therapy can result in adrenocortical insufficiency, in exacerbation of the disease for which steroid therapy was indicated, or in the *steroid withdrawal syndrome*, an occasional state of fever, asthenia, and myalgias. The latter appears not to be a hypocortisolemic state, but it responds to reinstitution of glucocorticoid treatment and slower tapering of dosage.

Corticosteroids As Replacement Therapy for Hypoadrenocorticism

Hydrocortisone   **Therapeutic agent**

Available for oral administration in 5, 10, 20 mg tablets for administration as 20 mg in A.M., 10 mg in P.M.

Available for IV administration as the sodium phosphate (solution), 100 mg IV every 8 hours for 24 hours or more for management of hypoadrenal (addisonian) crisis.

Cortisone   **Therapeutic agent**

Available for oral administration as the acetate in 5, 10, 25 mg tablets for administration as 25 mg in A.M., 12.5 mg in P.M.

Margin notes:

Principles of anti-inflammatory steroid therapy

Advantages of alternate-day systemic steroid administration

Available for IM administration as the acetate in 25 mg/ml and 50 mg/ml suspension in dosage comparable to oral administration.

Fludrocortisone   Therapeutic agent

Available for oral administration as the acetate in 0.1 mg tablets for administration in conjunction with glucocorticoid in hypoadrenal patients as 0.05 mg – 0.1 mg daily or every other day. Higher doses may be required to treat salt-losing forms of congenital adrenal hyperplasia or the hyperkalemia of hyporeninemic hypoaldosteronism.

Anti-Inflammatory Use

Hydrocortisone   Therapeutic agent

Available as enema, 100 mg/60 ml, for management of localized inflammatory bowel disease.

Cortisone   Therapeutic agent

Available as rectal foam, 10%, for management of localized inflammatory bowel disease.

Prednisone   Therapeutic agent

Available for oral administration as 1, 2.5, 5, 10, 20, 25, and 50 mg tablets, prescribed in dosage needed to control corticosteroid-responsive systemic illness. Initial dosage may be 5 – 80 mg/day or more. The lower-dose tablets may be useful in completing withdrawal of steroid therapy after control of systemic illness.

Prednisolone   Therapeutic agent

Available for oral administration in 5 mg tablets prescribed in dosage required to control corticosteroid-responsive systemic illness. Oral solution and syrup are also available. Initial dosage may be 5 – 80 mg/day or more.

Available as the acetate, 25 or 50 mg/ml, for intra-articular or soft tissue (*not* IV) administration.

Methylprednisolone   Therapeutic agent

Available for oral administration in 2, 8, 16, 24, and 32 mg tablets for administration in daily doses of 2 – 60 mg.

Available as the acetate in sterile suspension (20, 40, or 80 mg/ml) for intra-articular or soft tissue injection.

Triamcinolone   Therapeutic agent

Available for oral administration as 1, 2, 4, 8, 16 mg tablets and as syrups, prescribed in dosage required to control corticosteroid-responsive illness.

Available as the diacetate in suspensions, 25 or 40 mg/ml, or as acetonide, 10 and 40 mg/ml, for intra-articular or skin (*not* IV) injection.

Available in various formulations for topical administration to patients with skin diseases.

Betamethasone   Therapeutic agent

Available for oral administration as 0.6 mg tablets.

Available as the sodium phosphate/acetate suspension, 3 mg of each form/ml, for local injection (intra-articular, soft tissue).

Dexamethasone   Therapeutic agent

Available for oral administration as 0.25, 0.5, 0.75, 1, 1.5, 2, 4, 6 mg tablets to control corticosteroid-responsive illness or for diagnostic purposes (DST).

Available as acetate or sodium phosphate for systemic therapy IM (*not* IV) or for intra-articular or soft tissue administration.

Beclomethasone   Therapeutic agent

Available as dipropionate aerosol for inhalant therapy, 42 mcg delivered/ puff to patient, of bronchial asthma.

Use of Inhibitors of Steroidogenesis or Steroid Action in Adrenocortical Hyperfunction

Adrenocortical Hyperfunction. Excessive corticoid action may be the result of (1) increased pituitary secretion of ACTH, resulting in bilateral adrenocortical hyperplasia and usually a consequence of unregulated hypothalamic release of CRF into the pituitary-portal circulation, (2) unilateral disease of an adrenal gland, e.g., adenoma or carcinoma, (3) nonpituitary (ectopic) production of ACTH, usually by a lung or GI tract carcinoma, or (4) prolonged administration of therapeutic glucocorticoid.

Symptoms of hypercortisolism

The major signs and symptoms of hypothalamic-pituitary hypercortisolism (Cushing's disease) are centripetal fat distribution (truncal obesity), excess facial fat (moon facies), hypertension, muscle weakness, and osteoporosis. Changes in the skin induced by steroids result in easy bruisability, and the appearance of violaceous striae in areas of the body that are subject to stretch stress occurs frequently. When hypercortisolism is of hypothalamic-pituitary origin, it may be associated with increased skin pigmentation owing to modest elevations of circulating ACTH and β-lipotropin (β-LPH). Hypokalemia is observed in only about 20% of patients with Cushing's disease, reflecting the small effect of ACTH on the aldosterone secretory mechanism of the adrenal cortex. In hypothalamic-pituitary hypercortisolism, dexamethasone at 2 mg daily for 2 days does not suppress ACTH (or endogenous cortisol), whereas 8 mg for 2 days results in suppression.

Cushing's syndrome owing to adrenocortical adenoma produces a clinical pattern similar to that of hypothalamic-pituitary hypercortisolism. Dexamethasone administration at 2 or 8 mg daily for 2 days does not suppress circulating levels of endogenous cortisol. Hypercortisolism owing to adrenocortical carcinoma is frequently associated with excessive adrenal androgen production and is not dexamethasone-suppressible.

Ectopic ACTH syndrome presents quite differently. Systemic levels of ACTH are very high, sufficient to promote aldosterone production and cortisol levels substantial enough to manifest mineralocorticoid activity. Thus, hypokalemia results. Hyperpigmentation may also be dramatic. The lung tumors (small cell carcinoma) associated with ACTH elaboration are extraordinarily aggressive, and patients usually do not survive long enough to manifest other classic signs of hypercortisolism.

Hyperpigmentation can be dramatic in ectopic ACTH syndrome.

High-dose anti-inflammatory steroid use leads to a side-effect profile of body fat redistribution, skin changes, hypertension, osteoporosis, and diabetes mellitus. Because the potency of the synthetic steroids far exceeds that of endogenous corticoids, immunological suppression may be achieved, and increased susceptibility to infection may be apparent. This state is rarely achieved with endogenous hypercortisolism. Infections may develop with conventional or opportunistic bacteria or with fungi or myco-bacteria. Wound-healing is also impaired.

Excessive endogenous aldosterone production without hypercorti-solism results from either bilateral adrenocortical hyperplasia or an adreno-cortical adenoma. Primary aldosteronism is manifested by hypertension and hypokalemia. Other occasional findings are neuromuscular irritability and hypomagnesemia. Renin levels are suppressed in this condition.

Pharmacological Interventions in Hyperadrenocorticism. A number of pharmacological agents have actions on the adrenal cortex that are clini-cally important.

Metyrapone (METOPIRONE)	11β-hydroxylase inhibitor	Diagnostic agent Therapeutic agent

Administration of this agent inhibits cortisol production, leading to de-re-pression of endogenous ACTH production and increased circulating levels of 11-deoxycortisol. The latter has little bioactivity and does not sup-press ACTH production. Metyrapone (single dose, 2–3 gm by mouth at midnight, plasma cortisol levels at 8 A.M.) has been used to test for hypopituitary hypoadrenocorticism (failure of plasma 11-deoxycortisol levels to rise after drug administration supports hypopituitarism). Avail-ability of other diagnostic approaches for hypopituitarism (radioimmuno-assays for ACTH, thyrotropin, gonadotropins, growth hormone) minimize the diagnostic need for this agent. In addition, administration of the drug to patients with borderline (and untreated) primary adrenocortical insuffi-ciency has provoked profound adrenocortical failure ("crisis") and, rarely, death.

Metyrapone (250–500 mg by mouth three times a day) has been used to palliate the syndromes of ectopic ACTH production and of excess corti-sol production by adrenocortical carcinoma. Inhibition of 11β-hydroxyla-tion inhibits both cortisol and aldosterone biosynthesis. They may reduce the risk of potassium depletion associated with excessive aldosterone se-cretion, although desoxycorticosterone (DOC) secretion increases and pro-vides some mineralocorticoid activity. Adrenal androgen production per-sists unabated during metyrapone administration.

Aminoglutethimide	Inhibits cholesterol side-chain cleavage	Therapeutic agent

Administered as 250–500 mg by mouth four times a day, aminoglutethi-mide palliates the hypercortisolism of ectopic ACTH production and of adrenocortical carcinoma. Mineralocorticoid biosynthesis may be insuffi-cient with this agent (in contrast to metyrapone), and clinically significant hypoadrenocorticism with hyperkalemia may result.

Ketoconazole	Inhibits steroid synthesis through enzyme blockage	Therapeutic agent

Ketoconazole is an imidazole broad-spectrum antifungal agent that inter-feres with gonadal and adrenal steroid synthesis *in vivo* and *in vitro* (Pont et al, 1982) by inhibition of adrenal P-450–dependent enzymes, 11β-hydrox-ylase, and C17–20-lyase. The inhibition of cortisol synthesis is dose-de-pendent when 400 mg or greater of ketoconazole is administered as single or multiple doses. Ketoconazole causes a diminished adrenocortical response to ACTH administration with a reduction in serum and urinary cortisol concentrations and can produce acute adrenocortical insufficiency (Khosla et al, 1989). The long-term efficacy and safety of the use of ketoconazole in hyperadrenocorticism has not yet been established.

Mitotane (o,p'-DDD)   Direct adrenocortical   Therapeutic agent
cytotoxic

Mitotane can cause primary degeneration in the zonae fasciculata and reticularis. This drug may also specifically inhibit cortisol and aldosterone synthesis (Luten et al, 1979) by action at the 11β-hydroxylation step. The adrenocortical response to ACTH is of course depressed by mitotane. For treatment of Cushing's syndrome due to adrenal carcinoma, this adrenolytic agent is generally initiated as 3 – 6 mg daily in three or four divided doses with maintenance doses ranging from 500 mg biweekly to 2 gm daily. When mitotane is administered chronically, glucocorticoid (and mineralocorticoid) replacement therapy is usually necessary to avoid adrenocortical insufficiency. Side effects are relatively frequent with mitotane. GI tract disturbances occur in approximately 60% of patients, and CNS effects are observed in 40% of patients and include lethargy and, less often, vertigo and depression.

RU-486   Therapeutic agent

RU-486 is a glucocorticoid analog (17α-hydroxy-11β-(4-dimethylaminophenyl)-17β-(prop-1-ynyl)-estra-4,9-dien-3-one) with negligible agonist action and potent antiglucocorticoid, antiprogesterone, and antiestrogen activities. It has been shown to be effective in the treatment of Cushing's syndrome (Nieman et al, 1985) and may be effective in reversing the immunosuppressive actions of traditional glucocorticoids (Van Voorhis et al, 1989). The agent has not been approved by the United States Food and Drug Administration for clinical applications.

It should be noted that several other agents may interfere with adrenal steroidogenesis to clinically significant degrees, but these are not used as antiadrenal drugs. The anticoagulant *heparin* selectively interferes with aldosterone synthesis and, when it is used in high-dose IV bolus regimens, may result acutely in hypoaldosteronism and hyperkalemia. This biochemical effect is reversible with interruption of heparin therapy; heparin and coumarin anticoagulants may also, but rarely, promote bilateral adrenal gland hemorrhage and permanent hypoadrenocorticism. *Cyclosporin* is a cyclic peptide of fungal origin and has useful immunosuppressive qualities (see Chapter 59). This peptide induces hyperreninemic hypoaldosteronism in rats but can result in hypertension and hypoaldosteronism in humans. Among its adrenocortical effects are acute blockage of induction by angiotensin II of aldosterone secretion by the zona glomerulosa. *Phenytoin, rifampin,* and *barbiturates* enhance hepatic microsomal metabolism of corticosteroids. The half-life of dexamethasone may be sufficiently shortened in the setting of phenytoin administration to create, in patients with normal hypothalamic-pituitary-adrenocortical function, "nonsuppressibility" of this axis (abnormal DST). Macrolide antibiotics, e.g., erythromycin and troleandomycin, impair the elimination of methylprednisolone owing to their inhibitory action on the cytochrome P-450 system.

Heparin interferes with aldosterone synthesis.

Cyclosporine blocks aldosterone synthesis.

CONTRAINDICATIONS TO STEROID THERAPY

There are no contraindications to *replacement* glucocorticoid use in patients with adrenocortical insufficiency. Replacement therapy, including *stress dose replacement* (100–300 mg hydrocortisone, or its equivalent, daily) does not predispose patients to infection or other complications of pharmacological doses of anti-inflammatory steroids.

Relative contraindications to high-dose anti-inflammatory steroid use are the presence of systemic bacterial infection, poorly controlled diabetes mellitus, and advanced demineralizing bond disease. Mineralocorticoid use is relatively contraindicated in the setting of expanded intravascular volume, e.g., congestive heart failure.

PRECAUTIONS DURING STEROID THERAPY

Patients receiving glucocorticoids as a component of chronic immunosuppressive therapy should be monitored closely for the appearance of secondary bacterial or viral infections.

The decision to employ long-term administration of glucocorticoids in high dosage to children must be carefully weighed; close patient observation is mandatory during high-dose glucocorticoid therapy in the pediatric population, owing to the impact of steroids on growth and bone maturation (Tyrell and Baxter, 1987). It has been demonstrated that alternate-day therapy in children results in less inhibition of growth as well as decreased cushingoid effects.

> Glucocorticoid administration in high doses to children should be carefully weighed.

Administration of glucocorticoids in pharmacological doses during pregnancy may result in increased fetal deaths and congenital malformations, such as cleft palate. These drugs should be avoided, if possible, in the first trimester of pregnancy and be utilized in a discriminate manner in this patient population. However, glucocorticoids should not be withheld in conditions that are considered life-threatening to the pregnant mother.

> Fetal death and congenital malformations can result from administration of glucocorticoids to pregnant women.

References

Axelrod L: Glucocorticoid therapy. Medicine 55:39–65, 1976.

Bartalena L, Marcocci C, Bogazzi F, et al: Use of corticosteroids to prevent progression of Graves' ophthalmopathy after radioiodine therapy for hyperthyroidism. N Engl J Med 321:1349–1352, 1989.

Bondy PK: The adrenal cortex. *In* Bondy PK, Rosenberg LE (eds): Metabolic Control and Disease. 8th ed, 1427–1499. Philadelphia: WB Saunders, 1980.

Bondy PK: Disorders of the adrenal cortex. *In* Wilson JD, Foster DW: Williams Textbook of Endocrinology. 7th ed, 825–826. Philadelphia: WB Saunders, 1985.

Dluhy RG, Newmark SR, Lauler DP, Thorn GW: Pharmacology and chemistry of adrenal glucocorticoids. *In* Azarnoff DL (ed): Steroid Therapy, 1. Philadelphia: WB Saunders, 1975.

Fariss BL, Hane S, Shinsako J, Forsham PH: Comparison of absorption of cortisone acetate and hydrocortisone hemisuccinate. J Clin Endocrinol Metab 47:1137, 1978.

Gelehrter TD: Glucocorticoids and the plasma membrane. Monogr Endocrinol 12:561–574, 1979.

Gifford RH: Corticosteroid therapy for rheumatoid arthritis. *In* Azarnoff DL (ed): Steroid Therapy, 78. Philadelphia: WB Saunders, 1975.

Green S, Chambon P: A superfamily of potentially oncogenic hormone receptors. Nature 324:615–617, 1986.

Hunder GG, Sheps S, Allen GL, Joyce JW: Daily and alternate-day corticosteroid regimens in treatment of giant cell arteritis: Comparison in a prospective study. Ann Int Med 82:613–618, 1975.

Intra-articular steroids. [Editorial] Lancet 1:38, 1984.

Lahteenmaki P, Heikinheimo O, Croxatto H, et al: Pharmacokinetics and metabolism of RU 486. J Steroid Biochem 27:859–863, 1987.

Ling MHM, Perry PJ, Tsuang MT: Side effects of corticosteroid therapy. Arch Gen Psychiatry 38:471–477, 1981.

Loriaux DL, Cutler DB Jr: Diseases of the adrenal gland. *In* Kohler PO, Jordan RM (eds): Clinical Endocrinology, 167–238. New York: John Wiley & Sons, 1986.

MacGregor RR, Sheagren JN, Lipsett MB, Wolff SM: Alternate-day prednisone therapy. Evaluation of delayed hypersensitivity responses, control of disease and steroid side effects. N Engl J Med 280:1427–1431, 1969.

Martin LE, Harrison C, Tanner RJN: Metabolism of beclomethasone dipropionate by animals and man. Postgrad Med J 51(Suppl 4):11–20, 1975.

Marver D, Kokko JP: Renal target sites and the mechanism of action of aldosterone. Miner Electrolyte Metab 9:1–18, 1983.

Mendel CM, Kuhn RW, Weisiger RA, et al: Uptake of cortisol by the perfused rat liver: Validity of the free hormone hypothesis applied to cortisol. Endocrinology 124:468–476, 1989.

Nieman LK, Loriaux DL: Corticotropin-releasing hormone: Clinical applications. Annu Rev Med 40:331–339, 1989.

Parker LN, Levin ER, Lifrak ET: Evidence for adrenocortical adaptation to severe illness. J Clin Endocrinol Metab 60:947–952, 1985.

Pedersen RC, Brownie AC: Cholesterol side-chain cleavage in the rat adrenal cortex: Isolation of a cycloheximide-sensitive activator peptide. Proc Natl Acad Sci USA 80:1882–1886, 1983.

Smith AI, Funder JW: Proopiomelanocortin processing in the pituitary, central nervous system, and periphral tissues. Endocr Rev 9:159–179, 1988.

Szefler SJ: General pharmacology of glucocorticoids. *In* Schleimer RP, Claman HN, Oronsky A (eds): Anti-inflammatory Steroid Action: Basic and Clinical Action, 354–376. Toronto: Academic Press, 1989.

Truhan AP, Ahmed AR: Corticosteroids: A review with emphasis on complications of prolonged systemic therapy. Ann Allergy 62:375–391, 1989.

Tyrell JB, Baxter JD: Glucocorticoid therapy. *In* Felig P, Baxter JD, Broadus AE, Frohman LA (eds): Endocrinology and Metabolism. 2nd ed, 788–817. New York: McGraw-Hill, 1987.

Van Voorhis BJ, Anderson DJ, Hill JA: The effects of RU 486 on immune function and steroid-induced immunosuppression *in vitro.* J Clin Endocrinol Metab 69:1195–1199, 1989.

Weinberger C, Giguere V, Hollenberg SM, et al: Human steroid receptors and erb-A gene products form a superfamily of enhancer-binding proteins. Clin Physiol Biochem 5:179–189, 1987.

Carbohydrate Metabolism

44

K. S. Nair
Shyam D. Karki

Therapeutics of the disorders involving carbohydrate metabolism are discussed in this chapter. In humans the most important of these disorders is diabetes mellitus. Diabetes mellitus involves not only carbohydrate metabolism but also other substrates, especially lipids and proteins. Therefore, the treatment of diabetes involves changes in the metabolism of the entire range of substrates in the body. However, the effects of diabetes and insulin treatment on carbohydrate metabolism can be measured more easily by clinical features and biochemical tests than the metabolism of other substrates.

Carbohydrate constitutes 40 – 45% of the normal caloric intake in the Western diet and a much higher portion in the non-Western diet. The sources of the dietary carbohydrate vary from complex carbohydrates, such as starch, to refined sugars, such as sucrose. Irrespective of the sources of carbohydrate, the end products of the digestion of carbohydrates that are absorbed in the intestine are the hexoses glucose, fructose, and galactose. Of these simple sugars, glucose is by far the largest constituent.

Maintenance of blood glucose within certain limits is vital for the survival of humans. Blood glucose is regulated precisely by the concerted actions of insulin and the counterregulatory hormones, such as glucagon, epinephrine, norepinephrine, cortisol, and growth hormone. Figure 44 – 1 summarizes the mechanisms of maintenance of blood glucose in humans. Blood glucose concentration is determined by the difference between glucose appearance and disappearance. Glucose appearance depends on the amount of exogenous glucose ingestion and on the endogenous glucose appearance (or glucose production). The endogenous glucose appearance depends on glycogenolysis and gluconeogenesis. The glucose disappearance involves both glucose catabolism for producing energy (aerobic and anaerobic oxidation) and glucose storage as glycogen and fat. Immediately after ingestion, the glucose that is not oxidized is stored mostly as glycogen. Because the glycogen store in the liver is small, the major portion of the glycogen is stored in muscle. The glycogen store in the liver is available for systemic use, unlike muscle glycogen, which is only available for local consumption. The storage of glucose is relevant only in the fed state. The control of these metabolic processes by hormones is shown in Table 44 – 1.

The source of glucose in the postabsorptive state is exclusively from hepatic glucose production (75% from glycogenolysis and 25% from gluconeogenesis) after an overnight fast. All animal cells can metabolize glucose

Carbohydrate Metabolism

Unused glucose is stored as glycogen and fat.

Figure 44-1

The mechanism of maintenance of blood glucose in humans.

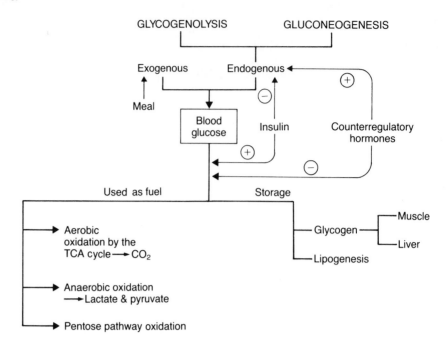

Glucose is the sole source of energy for the brain.

in some way. However, brain, blood cells (erythrocytes and white blood cells), and muscles are the major consumers of glucose. The brain, even though it accounts for less than 2% of body weight, consumes about 20% of the basal calories. Glucose is the sole source of energy for the brain in humans except during prolonged states of starvation. About 60–70% of endogenous glucose production is used exclusively for the energy requirement of the brain. In a prolonged state of starvation (when blood levels of ketones increase), ketones become an alternate source of energy for the brain. The brain requires an uninterrupted supply of fuels during sleep or activities. Diminished supply of glucose to the brain results in various degrees of intellectual dysfunction, including coma and ultimately death. Therefore, it is imperative that a continuous supply of glucose is maintained as a fuel for the brain. Blood cells depend on glucose for their energy requirements in fed or starved states. Some other tissues, such as eye and renal medulla, also rely on glucose as a fuel.

Hypoglycemia is acutely life-threatening, whereas hyperglycemia has more chronic effects. Acute hyperglycemia is life-threatening when it causes hyperosmolar coma. If free water loss that occurs with hyperglycemia is not compensated by increased water intake, it results in hyperos-

Table 44-1 EFFECTS OF INSULIN AND GLUCOSE COUNTERREGULATORY HORMONES ON GLUCOSE METABOLISM		
Hormones	**Liver**	**Muscle**
Insulin	Glycogen synthesis ↑ Glycogenolysis ↓ Gluconeogenesis ↓	Glycogen synthesis ↑ Glycogenolysis ↓
Glucagon	Glycogenolysis ↑ Gluconeogenesis ↑	
Catecholamines	Glycogenolysis ↑ Gluconeogenesis ↑	Glucose uptake ↓ Glycogenolysis ↑
Cortisol	Gluconeogenesis ↑	Glucose uptake ↓
Growth hormone		Glucose uptake ↓

molarity in the blood and hyperosmolar coma. Hyperglycemia is believed also to cause many chronic complications in diabetes.

HISTORICAL PERSPECTIVE

Diabetes was a disease known to ancient civilizations (Chinese, Egyptian, Indian, and Greeks). As far back as 600 BC the Hindu physician Susruta described "honey urine disease" of two different types—one associated with emaciation and another with obesity. The latter group was recognized to be related to gluttony and inactivity. The Greek physician Aretaeus in AD 130 referred to the "melting down of the flesh into urine," implying muscle wasting and polyuria. In 1889 Minkowski and von Mering demonstrated that extirpation of the pancreas produced diabetes. During the early part of this century, several investigators were close to the discovery of the pancreatic substance that reduces blood glucose. It was the discovery of insulin by Banting and Best in 1921 that resulted in the most remarkable advance in our knowledge about diabetes and its treatment.

Following the extraction of the active principle from pancreas, Banting and Best treated a 14-year-old diabetic patient at the Toronto General Hospital. This patient's blood glucose was 500 mg/dl while on a strict diet of 450 kcal/day. The patient would likely not have lived for more than a few weeks on this preinsulin diet. Insulin treatment reduced his urinary glucose excretion from 100 to 7.5 g per day, and the patient made dramatic improvement. The impressive change in body composition in this patient is the best possible demonstration of insulin action on human metabolism. Soon after the discovery of insulin, Collip developed improved isolation procedures. Thereafter, the isolation and commercial production of insulin from beef and pork pancreas began. Description of the amino acid sequence of insulin by Sanger, of proinsulin by Steiner and associates, and of pre-proinsulin by Chan and colleagues were important landmarks in our understanding of this important pancreatic hormone. Even though various types of bioassays were available for measuring insulin, it was the development of the radioimmunoassay by Bersen and Yallow that made a precise measurement of insulin concentrations in blood possible. Discovery of insulin receptors by Roth and coworkers, use of the glucose clamp technique, and tracer kinetic studies substantially improved our understanding of insulin action.

DEFINITION

Diabetes mellitus refers to a spectrum of related disorders characterized by a common factor: relative or absolute deficiency of insulin or its metabolic action. A comprehensive and complete definition of diabetes eludes every author. It is essentially a metabolic disorder resulting in diseases involving multiple organ systems of the body. The complications of this disorder can be acute but are usually secondary to metabolic disturbances, e.g., diabetic ketoacidosis and hyperosmolar coma. The chronic complications of diabetes are believed to be secondary to the chronic effect of metabolic disturbances. These chronic complications include microvascular disease and atherosclerosis involving medium and large vessels. Renal complications in diabetes are a major cause of morbidity and mortality. Renal disease in diabetes ranges from microalbuminuria to chronic renal failure. Diabetes also predisposes patients to infection and accelerates the effects of other diseases (e.g., atherosclerosis). In a pathological sense it is correct to describe one of the main effects of diabetes as the acceleration of the aging process, which is true for most organs but especially for vessels and connective tissues. For details of these complications and other clinical features readers are advised to read textbooks of medicine or endocrinology.

Diabetes Mellitus

Banting and Best's discovery of insulin in 1921 greatly advanced our understanding of diabetes.

Sanger described the amino acid sequence of insulin in 1960.

Renal complications in diabetes are a major cause of death.

CLASSIFICATION

A classification of diabetes and related disorders by an international workgroup sponsored by the National Diabetes Data Group and the National Institutes of Health is given. The therapeutic options differ for these groups. With advances in our knowledge about diabetes, a new look at the classification of diabetes mellitus is warranted. The criteria for diagnosis of diabetes mellitus in the adult (nonpregnant) human include (1) a random plasma glucose of 200 mg/dl or above plus classic symptoms and signs of diabetes, such as polyuria, polydypsia, polyphagia, and weight loss; (2) a fasting plasma glucose of 140 mg/dl or greater on at least two occasions; and (3) a fasting plasma glucose level of less than 140 mg/dl plus a sustained elevated plasma glucose level during at least two oral glucose tolerance tests (75 g glucose level). In the third criterion, both the 2-hour plasma glucose level and at least one other between 0 and 2 hours after the 75 g glucose dose must be 200 mg/dl or greater.

In children the criteria for diagnosing diabetes differs from adults. The quantity of glucose administered is based on ideal body weight (1.75 g/kg, up to a maximum of 100 g). A fasting glucose of above 100 mg/dl, a 1-hour glucose of above 160 mg/dl, and a 2-hour glucose of more than 140 mg/dl are diagnostic of diabetes.

For diagnosing diabetes in pregnant women, the criteria are different from children and nonpregnant adults, because plasma glucose levels tend to fall during pregnancy. A diagnosis of gestational diabetes may be made if two plasma glucose values during a glucose tolerance test (100 g glucose load) equal or exceed the following: fasting = 105 mg/dl; 1 hour = 190 mg/dl; 2 hour = 165 mg/dl; 3 hour = 145 mg/dl. For diagnosing impaired glucose tolerance in nonpregnant adults all of the following criteria are essential: (1) a fasting plasma glucose of less than 140 mg/dl; (2) a 2-hour glucose tolerance test plasma glucose level between 140 and 200 mg/dl; and (3) an intervening oral glucose-tolerance test plasma glucose value of 200 mg/dl or greater.

Type I diabetes is marked by abrupt onset of symptoms with insulinopenia before the age of 40.

Type I Diabetes Mellitus or Insulin-Dependent Diabetes Mellitus. Insulin-dependent diabetes mellitus (IDDM) was formerly known as juvenile diabetes. About 10–20% of known cases of diabetes in the United States are Type I. Type I diabetic patients are usually thin. This type of diabetes is characterized by a rather abrupt onset of symptoms and signs with insulinopenia before the age of 40 years. These patients are dependent on injected insulin to prevent ketosis and preserve life. Even though the genetic and etiological factors are heterogeneous, certain histocompatibility antigens (HLA) on chromosome 6 are increased or decreased in frequency in these patients. Islet cell antibodies are frequently present at diagnosis.

Eighty to 90% of all diabetics are Type II; 60–90% of Type II diabetics are obese.

Type II Diabetes Mellitus or Non-Insulin-Dependent Diabetes Mellitus. Non-insulin-dependent diabetes mellitus (NIDDM) was formerly known as adult or maturity-onset diabetes, about 80–90% of all cases of diabetes in the United States are this Type II. About 60–90% of all Type II diabetic patients are obese (weight/height^2 > 25 kg/sq m). The onset of the disease, unlike that of Type I diabetes, is insidious and is diagnosed often when patients present with complications such as infections or vascular disorders. Patients are frequently diagnosed on blood glucose or urine sugar measurements during routine physical examination. Weight reduction often corrects their hyperglycemia.

Secondary Diabetes. Secondary diabetes results from the following:

1. pancreatic diseases such as chronic pancreatitis or pancreatomy;

2. hormonal abnormalities, e.g., acromegaly, pheochromocytoma, Cushing's syndrome, primary aldosteronism, glucagonoma;

3. drug- or chemical-induced reactions, e.g., thiazide, glucocorticoids, some psychoactive agents, anticancer treatment such as streptozocin or diasoxide;

4. insulin receptor abnormalities, e.g., acanthosis nigricans;

5. certain genetic syndromes, e.g., hyperlipidemia and muscular dystrophy;

6. malnutrition-related reasons—this is a poorly defined group of diabetic patients with no detailed information available on the etiopathophysiology of the disorder.

These categories of patients are relatively rare in the United States. Certain disorders, such as chronic pancreatitis, constitute a major cause of diabetes in certain geographical locations, such as South India (Kerala), some Southeast Asian countries, and African countries such as Uganda and Nigeria.

> Secondary diabetes is rarely observed in the United States.

Impaired Glucose Tolerance Test. Impaired glucose tolerance (IGT) was previously known as *chemical diabetes* or *subclinical diabetes*. The criteria for impaired glucose tolerance are (1) a fasting plasma glucose of less than 140 mg/dl; (2) a 2-hour oral glucose tolerance test plasma glucose level between 140 and 200 mg/dl; and (3) an intervening oral glucose tolerance test plasma glucose value of 200 mg/dl or greater. There is an age-related deterioration of glucose tolerance. Obesity also impairs glucose tolerance. About 25% of patients with IGT eventually become diabetic.

> One fourth of patients with IGT develop diabetes.

Gestational Diabetes Mellitus. Patients with gestational diabetes mellitus (GDM) have onset or discovery of glucose intolerance during pregnancy, usually in the second or third trimester. The criteria for diagnosis is discussed earlier. Because of the effectiveness of meticulous blood glucose control in preventing maternal and fetal complications, an early diagnosis and effective therapy are important.

CHEMISTRY AND BIOSYNTHESIS

Insulin

Insulin is a hormone secreted by the β cells of the pancreatic islet of Langerhans. It is a small protein with a molecular weight of 5734. It contains 51 amino acids arranged in two peptide chains (A and B) connected by three disulfide linkages. Proinsulin is the precursor of insulin. The structure and amino acid sequence of human proinsulin is given in Figure 44–2. The

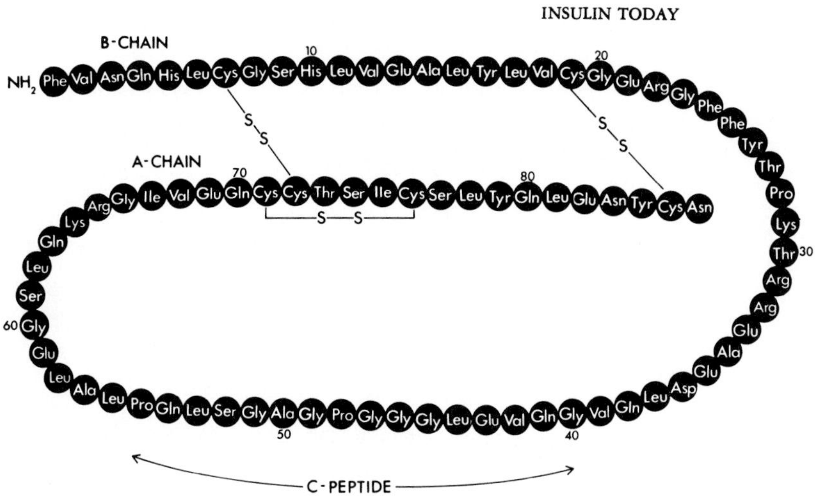

INSULIN TODAY

Figure 44–2

The structure and amino acid sequence of human proinsulin. (From DR Steiner, Diabetes, Vol 26, 1976. Copyright © 1976 by the American Diabetes Association. Reprinted with permission.)

sequence of amino acids in the insulin molecule varies with the animal species. The major sites of differences between porcine, bovine, and human insulin are Positions 8, 9, and 10 of the A chain. Porcine insulin is most similar to that of humans, differing only by the substitution of an alanine residue for threonine at the carboxy terminus of the A chain whereas bovine insulin also has different amino acids in Positions 8 and 10 of the A chain.

Proinsulin is a single polypeptide chain with a molecular weight of approximately 9000. It has an extended peptide sequence connecting the amino terminus of the insulin A chain with the carboxyl terminus of the insulin B chain. The segment that connects the A and B chains in proinsulin is called the C-peptide.

Investigations into the cellular mechanisms of insulin biosynthesis indicate that the biosynthetic process involves a cascade of increasingly smaller molecules before the formation of the active hormone is finally achieved. Figure 44–3 shows schematically the steps in the biosynthesis of insulin. Proinsulin is synthesized in the rough endoplasmic reticulum. Translation of insulin mRNA results first in a molecule larger than proinsulin (pre-proinsulin). Conversion of pre-proinsulin to proinsulin takes place in the membrane-associated polyribosome of the rough endoplasmic reticulum. Proinsulin from the cisternae of the reticulum is transferred to the Golgi complex through microvesicles. Proinsulin is concentrated within the

> Proinsulin, the precursor of insulin, is synthesized in the rough endoplasmic reticulum.

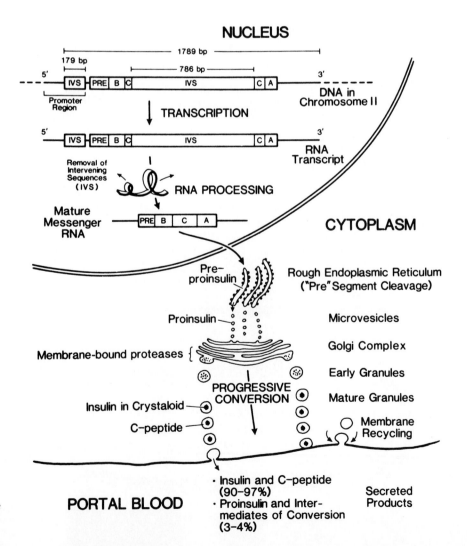

Figure 44–3

The mechanism of the biosynthesis of insulin in the pancreatic β cell. (From Robbins DC, Tager HS, Rubenstein AH: Biologic and clinical importance of proinsulin. Reprinted, by permission of the New England Journal of Medicine 310:1165–1175, 1984.)

immature granules of the Golgi complex. After passage through the Golgi complex, proinsulin is packaged in membrane-enclosed secretory granules that contain proteases that cleave the precursor at the paired dibasic amino acid residues linking the C-peptide (26-31 amino acid residues, according to species) and insulin. As a result of this posttransitional processing of proinsulin, both C-peptide and insulin are secreted in equimolar proportions into the blood. Peripheral blood concentrations of C-peptide are higher than insulin because of greater catabolism of insulin by the liver.

Granules within the β cells store insulin in the form of crystals consisting of two atoms of zinc and six molecules of insulin. The biologically active form is thought to be the monomer. Release of the contents of the mature secretory granules involves exocytosis, the progressive migration of granules toward the plasma membrane, where the granule membrane, and plasma membrane fuse together. This fusion is followed by extrusions of insulin and C-peptide from the granule.

An increase in serum glucose is the most important stimulus for insulin secretion. The insulin secretion is initiated at a serum glucose concentration of about 90 mg/dl (5 mmol/1) and the overall insulin response to serum glucose is sigmoidal, reaching a plateau at about 360 mg/dl (20 mmol/1). Other stimuli for insulin secretion include amino acids (especially leucine and arginine), ketones, and fatty acids. If amino acids are given along with glucose, insulin secretion is accelerated. Potentiators of insulin secretion include secretin, pancreozymin, glucose-dependent insulinotropic peptide (GIP), and acetylcholine. Inhibitors of insulin secretion include epinephrine, norepinephrine, and somatostatin.

> Insulin secretion is stimulated by an increase in serum glucose.

Epinephrine and norepinephrine inhibit insulin secretion. This inhibitory effect is mediated by α stimulation. Beta$_2$ stimulation, as by isoproteronol, stimulates insulin release, possibly via cyclic adenosine monophosphate (cAMP). Vagal stimulation releases insulin also. Hypothalamic control of insulin secretion through inhibition of insulin by the ventromedial and stimulation by the ventrolateral hypothalamus has been recognized also.

Peptide hormones, such as pancreozymin-cholecystokinin, secretin, glucagon, vasointestinal peptide, and gastric inhibitory polypeptide, may all augment insulin secretion.

A paracrine relationship between insulin-secreting B cells, glucagon-secreting A cells, and somatostatin-secreting D cells, has been suggested. The anatomical proximity of these cells along with the *in vitro* demonstration of interactions strongly support this paracrine relationship, although it has never been demonstrated *in vivo*. Blood, plasma, or other biological fluid concentrations of insulin, C-peptide, and proinsulin may be measured by radioenzymatic technique.

INSULIN ACTION

Effects of Insulin Action

No other hormone's metabolic effects and mechanism of action have been as extensively investigated as that of insulin. Insulin can be rightly described as the most important hormone, not only because of its influence on the fuel metabolism and growth processes but also because it is indispensable for life. Insulin action involves a complex response that ultimately affects carbohydrate, lipid, and protein metabolism. The action of insulin occurs in three principal tissues: liver, muscle, and adipose tissue. Glucose metabolism of the brain is unaffected by insulin, and the function of the nervous system is not affected by insulin *per se*. Insulin has both metabolic and growth-promoting effects. The metabolic effects are on carbohydrate, lipid, and protein metabolism. Insulin increases glycogen synthesis in liver

> Insulin action occurs primarily in the liver, muscle, and adipose tissue.

and muscle, and decreases glycogenolysis and gluconeogenesis. Insulin exerts a moment-to-moment effect on blood glucose concentration by virtue of rapid changes in glycogen synthase and phosphorylase. Insulin's effect on lipid metabolism is through inhibition of lipolysis and stimulation of lipogenesis. In the liver, insulin stimulates the synthesis of free fatty acids (FFA) from glucose as well as their esterification to form triglycerides. Insulin also accelerates the removal of circulating triglycerides and the uptake of FFA by adipose tissue by its stimulating effect on lipoprotein lipase. Insulin stimulates glucose uptake by adipose cells to provide the α-glycerophosphate necessary for esterification of FFA. Insulin inhibits tissue lipase within the adipose cell. Insulin also inhibits ketogenesis in liver.

Most of insulin's effects on protein metabolism are related to its growth-promoting effects. The growth-promoting effects of insulin are stimulation of DNA synthesis and stimulation of cell growth and differentiation. Insulin has some mixed metabolic and growth effects, such as the transport of amino acid across membranes, the inhibition of oxidation of branched-chain amino acids, stimulation of protein synthesis, the inhibition of protein degradation, and the stimulation of RNA synthesis. More recent studies in humans using amino acid tracers indicate that once the genetic potential for growth is achieved, insulin's role in maintaining protein mass in the postabsorptive state depends on its inhibition of proteolysis. Based on human studies, it can be said that insulin promotes protein synthesis when amino acids are supplied.

Insulin plays an important role in the maintenance and regulation of energy stores in humans. Insulin's physiological effect *in vivo* is modulated by the availability of substrates and the effects of other hormones. In an insulin-deprived state, energy expenditure increases because of the unopposed action of catabolic hormones, such as glucagon, epinephrine, norepinephrine, and cortisol. Insulin administration normalizes energy expenditure, presumably by decreasing the accelerated rates of gluconeogenesis, protein turnover, and substrate cycles. Insulin is also a thermogenic hormone, because it promotes energy-requiring substrate storage (e.g., glycogen synthesis, lipid synthesis, and protein synthesis). The thermogenic effect of insulin is manifested usually after meal ingestion.

Energy expenditure is normalized by insulin.

It must be stressed that the growth-promoting effects of insulin are intimately related to insulin-like growth factors (IGFs). Two different IGFs have been identified: IGF-I and IGF-II. IGFs act like insulin; insulin is more potent in producing metabolic effects, whereas the IGFs have greater growth-promoting effects.

IGFs (insulin-like growth factors) have greater growth-promoting effects than insulin.

Mechanism of Insulin Action

Insulin binds to specific receptors on the plasma membrane of the cell and thus initiates a cascade of events leading to its metabolic and growth-promoting effects. The receptor recognizes the hormone among all other substances in the blood and binds it with high affinity and specificity. This binding of hormone to receptor transmits a transmembrane signal, resulting in alterations in intracellular metabolic pathways (Fig. 44–4).

The structure of the insulin receptor has been elucidated (Fig. 44–5). The insulin receptor is a glycoprotein with complex carbohydrate side chains and consists of two distinct subunits: α (molecular weight 135,000) and β (molecular weight 95,000). The α subunit is considered to be the insulin-binding site, whereas the β subunit appears to be an insulin-sensitive protein kinase. It is believed that the β subunit is involved in signal transduction across the membrane.

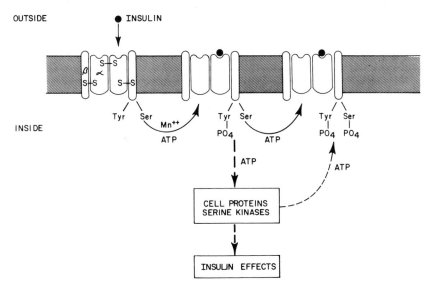

Figure 44-4

Proposed mechanism of insulin action. Insulin binds to the extracellular α unit of the receptor and activates tyrosine kinase (part of β unit) by autophosphorylation. The cascade of phosphorylation reactions initiated by insulin binding to the α unit is essential for insulin actions. (See text and Kahn, 1985, for details.) (From Kahn CR: The molecular mechanism of insulin action. Reproduced, with permission, from the Annual Review of Medicine, Vol. 36, © 1985 by Annual Reviews Inc.)

Evidence indicates that the insulin receptor itself is an insulin-sensitive enzyme, namely a tyrosine-specific protein kinase. This protein kinase enzyme is involved in autophosphorylation reactions. Insulin binds to an external α subunit of the receptor, which activates the tyrosine activity of the β subunit, and the insulin receptor undergoes autophosphorylation. Alterations in intracellular activities may be mediated through a cAMP-independent phosphorylation cascade subsequent to autophosphorylation at the membrane site. The activity of tyrosine kinase is affected by (1) receptor-bound insulin; (2) Mn^{2+}; and (3) the state of receptor phosphorylation, which sustains the activity after removal of insulin. It is likely that the activated receptor kinase continues to phosphorylate other intracellular proteins and enzymes with regulatory function, thereby propagating the insulin message. The serine residues on the receptor are also phosphorylated in the basal state, thereby increasing the course of signal transmissions.

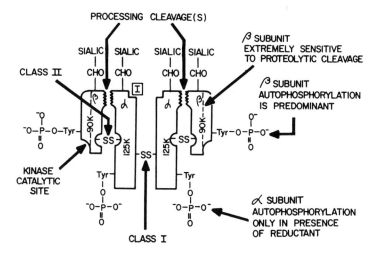

Figure 44-5

Schematic representation of several major features of the insulin receptor structure as currently understood. The major form of the mature insulin receptor appears to be a heterotetrameric, disulfide-linked configuration of α and β subunits. The disulfide linkages are of two classes (class I and class II) that can be distinguished experimentally by their differential sensitivity to reduction by dithiothreitol and other reductants. Both α and β subunits contain oligosaccharide and sialic acid. The mature α and β subunits appear to be derived from a single precursor polypeptide chain by a proteolytic cleavage or cleavages. The β subunit exhibits a site at about the center of its amino acid sequence that is exquisitely sensitive to elastase-like proteases. Tyrosine-kinase catalytic sites are associated with the β subunits that are autophosphorylated *in vitro* in the presence or absence of reductant. Alpha subunits, which appear to bind insulin, are also autophosphorylated on tyrosine residues *in vitro*, but only in the presence of millimolar concentrations of reductants. The insulin receptor tyrosine-kinase activity is markedly activated upon binding insulin. (See text for further details.) (From Czeck MP: The nature and regulation of the insulin receptor: Structure and function. Reproduced, with permission, from the Annual Review of Psychology, Vol. 47, © 1985 by Annual Reviews Inc.)

Figure 44-6

Hypothetical model of insulin's stimulatory action on glucose transport. According to this hypothesis, insulin binds to its specific cell surface receptor, inducing a signal. In response to this signal, intracellular vesicles containing the glucose transporter are translocated by an exocytic-like mechanism to the plasma membrane. Following fusion of these vesicles with the plasma membrane, glucose transporters are then exposed to the extracellular medium, giving rise to the increase in glucose transport activity. On removal of insulin from its receptor, glucose transporters are retranslocated back to the intracellular fluid by an endocytic-like mechanism similar to receptor-mediated endocytosis. (For details of this mechanism, see Simpson and Cushman, 1986, and Karnieli et al, 1981.) (From Karnieli E, Zarnowski MJ, Hissin PJ, et al: Insulin-stimulated translocation of glucose transport systems in the isolated rat adipose cell: Time course, reversal, insulin concentration, dependency and relationship of glucose transport activity. J Biol Chem 256:4772–4777, 1981.)

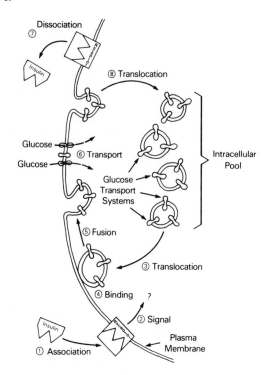

Membrane vesicles are responsible for intracellular transport of glucose and are called *glucose tansporters.*

The internalization of insulin-bound receptors and the entry of insulin into the cell nucleus stimulate mRNA synthesis. Chronic hyperinsulinization results in the reduction of the number and the sensitivity of insulin receptors, which in turn inhibits the biosynthesis of mRNA. This down-regulation of insulin receptors by hyperinsulinism is reversible on correction of hyperinsulinism.

Investigations demonstrated that intracellular transport of glucose is carried out by membrane vesicles, termed *glucose transporters.* Generation of a family of cytoplasmic mediators of insulin action has been considered also. Figure 44–6 shows the suggested mechanism for insulin stimulatory action on glucose transport. Similar transport systems have not been identified so far for other substrates.

Insulin Resistance

Decreased insulin action may result from insulin resistance. Insulin resistance can be due to pre-receptor causes, such as increased degradation of insulin or the binding of insulin by anti-insulin antibodies. Abnormal β cell secretory products, such as abnormal insulin molecules or the incomplete conversion of proinsulin to insulin, can cause insulin resistance also in some patients. Such patients have normal sensitivity to exogenously administered insulin. Circulating insulin antagonists include elevated levels of counterregulatory hormones, anti-insulin antibodies, and anti-insulin receptor antibodies. The possible causes of insulin resistance at the receptor level include alterations in insulin binding, decreased receptor number, decreased receptor affinity, and alterations in signal transduction. The postreceptor causes of insulin resistance may be due to alterations in intracellular pathways of insulin action, alterations in common pathways, and alterations of a specific pathway. A defect in receptor binding, described as decreased sensitivity and decreased responsiveness, is represented as a postreceptor defect. A classification of insulin-resistant states by a dose-response curve of insulin action is given in Figure 44–7.

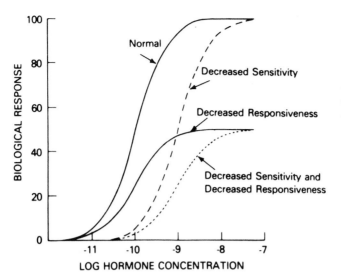

Figure 44-7

Classification of insulin-resistant states by the dose-response curve for insulin action. Decreased insulin sensitivity usually represents a receptor binding defect, whereas decreased responsiveness usually represents a postbinding defect. (From Kahn CR: The molecular mechanism of insulin action. Reproduced, with permission, from the Annual Review of Medicine, Vol. 36, © 1985 by Annual Reviews Inc.)

PHARMACOKINETICS

Insulin is destroyed in the gastrointestinal (GI) tract and therefore must be given parenterally. When injected subcutaneously or intramuscularly (IM), it is well absorbed in the blood. The rate of absorption, serum insulin concentrations, and bioavailability of injected insulin are determined by many factors, including the site of injection, exercise of the limb, depth of injection, ambient temperature, circulating insulin antibodies, volume, concentration, and type of insulin. Different insulin preparations differ in onset, peak, and duration of action as shown in Table 44-2. The three major characteristics distinguishing insulin preparations are (1) degree of purity, (2) time course of action, and (3) species of origin.

The intraindividual variation in insulin absorption from day to day is about 25% and between patients is up to 50%. This may be attributed to blood flow variations. For example, in conditions with peripheral vasoconstriction (e.g., shock) subcutaneous and IM injections have an uncertain absorption rate. Its absorption is highly influenced by the site of injection. Absorption is most rapid from the abdomen, followed by the arm, buttocks, and thigh. The deeper insulin is injected, the quicker and higher is its peak. Other factors, like ambient temperature, exercise of injected limb, local massage, and smoking, affect the rate of absorption also. Local degradation of insulin seems of less importance, but in rare cases, may be the cause of high insulin requirements.

Insulin is destroyed in the GI tract; therefore, it must be administered parenterally.

Table 44-2 PHARMACOKINETICS OF THE INSULINS

Types	Onset (hours)	Peak (hours)	Duration (hours)	Appearance
Rapid				
Regular	1/2-1	2-3	5-7	Clear
Semilente	1/2-1	4-6	12-16	Cloudy
Intermediate				
Lente	1-2	8-12	18-24	Cloudy
Isophane (NPH)	1-2	8-12	18-24	Cloudy
Long-acting				
Ultralente	4-8	16-18	36	Cloudy
PZI	4-8	14-20	36	Cloudy

Insulin seems to be absorbed directly into the blood stream rather than by way of the lymphatics, irrespective of the preparation of insulin. Once absorbed, it is distributed rapidly throughout the extracellular fluids. The plasma half-life of insulin is less than 9 minutes, and there does not appear to be any difference in half-life between normal healthy subjects and diabetic subjects. However, binding of insulins by antibodies in diabetic patients may prolong its half-life. Antibody-bound insulin is in equilibrium with the free insulin. It clearly prolongs the biological half-life and thus causes hypoglycemia at unexpected times. It may also protect against rapid development of ketosis in situations of insulin deprivation.

About 50% of the insulin that reaches the liver through the portal vein is metabolized by the liver and never reaches the general circulation. Insulin is filtered at the glomerulus and is reabsorbed (80%) in the proximal tubules. About 60% of the reabsorbed insulin is metabolized in the cells lining the proximal convoluted tubules. Renal impairment affects the clearance of insulins, and therefore, the dosage has to be adjusted. Peripheral tissues such as muscle and fat bind and inactivate insulin, but this is of minor significance.

Insulin Preparations

Zinc and protamine are added to insulin preparations to delay absorption.

Insulin is available in many forms. The different forms are made by the addition of zinc, protamine, or both in the presence of a suitable buffer, and these modifications delay the absorption of insulin from a subcutaneous or IM depot, resulting in extended duration of action. Short-acting insulin is a crystalline zinc-insulin complex provided in soluble form. All other insulins have been modified to prolong action and are dispensed as cloudy suspensions. They are mixed either with protamine in phosphate buffer (protamine zinc and neutral protamine Hagedorn [NPH] insulin) or with varying concentrations of zinc in acetate buffer (ultralente, lente, and semilente insulins). Various insulins differ in time of onset, peak, and duration of action. Broadly, they can be classified as rapid, intermediate, or prolonged acting. The characteristics of these different types of insulin, their sources, and manufacturers are given in Table 44–3. All types of insulin are effective. Selection of a particular type depends on the individual patient, the type of diabetes, and the nature of glucose control desired. Regular insulin is the only preparation that can be administered intravenously (IV).

Potency of Insulin Preparations

Potency of insulin is expressed as USP (United States Pharmacopeia) units. The potency is determined by a bioassay based on the capacity of samples to lower blood glucose concentrations. The standard of unit is the USP Insulin Reference standard. All types of insulin are prepared in solutions of two different strengths, designated U-40 and U-100. The number after the U indicates the number of units in 1 ml. U-40 insulin bottles are marked with a red top; U-100 with orange. Most insulin currently in clinical use is U-100.

Purity of Insulin

The first insulin preparations contained contaminating proteins greater than 10,000 ppm. These included proinsulin and partially cleaved proinsulin that were metabolically inactive but capable of inducing anti-insulin antibodies. Increased technological advancements, such as gel filtration chromatography and ion-exchange chromatography, have enabled the production of insulin with less than 10 ppm contaminating proteins. When

Table 44–3 INSULINS AVAILABLE IN THE UNITED STATES

Type/Duration of Action	Animal Source	Brand Name	Manufacturer	Proinsulin Content	Comment
Short-acting					
Regular					
Standard	Beef/pork	Regular Iletin I	Lilly	<10	
	Pork	Regular insulin	Squibb/Novo	<10	
Purified	Beef	Beef regular Iletin II	Lilly	<1	
	Pork	Regular purified pork Iletin II	Lilly	<1	
	Pork	Velosulin	Nordisk-USA	<1	Phosphate buffer
Human	Recombinant DNA	Humulin R	Lilly	0	
		Humulin BR	Lilly	0	"Buffered regular." Phosphate buffered for pump use
	Semisynthetic	Novolin R	Squibb-Novo	<1	Also available in cartridge for Novopen use
		Velosulin human	Nordisk	<1	
Semilente (Insulin zinc suspension, prompt)					
Standard	Beef/pork	Semilente Iletin I	Lilly	<10	
	Pork	Semilente insulin	Squibb-Novo	<10	
Purified	Pork	Semilente purified pork	Squibb-Novo	<1	
Intermediate-acting					
NPH (Isophane insulin suspension)					
Standard	Beef/pork	NPH Iletin I	Lilly	<10	
	Beef	NPH insulin	Squibb-Novo	<10	
Purified	Beef	Beef NPH Iletin II	Lilly	<1	
	Pork	Pork NPH Iletin II	Lilly	<1	
		NPH purified pork	Squibb-Novo	<1	
		Insulatard NPH	Nordisk	<1	Phosphate buffer
Human	Recombinant DNA	Humulin N	Lilly	0	
	Semisynthetic	Novolin N	Squibb-Novo	<1	
		Insulatard NPH	Nordisk-USA	<1	
Lente (Insulin Zn suspension)					
Standard	Beef/pork	Lente Iletin I	Lilly	<10	
	Beef	Lente insulin	Squibb-Novo	<10	
Purified	Beef	Lente Iletin II	Lilly	<1	
	Pork	Lente Iletin II	Lilly	<1	
	Pork	Lente purified pork insulin	Squibb-Novo	<1	
Human	Recombinant DNA	Humulin L	Lilly	<1	
	Semisynthetic	Novolin L	Squibb-Novo	<1	
NPH/Regular Mixtures (70%/30%)					
Purified	Pork	Mixtard	Nordisk-USA	<1	
Human	Recombinant DNA	Mixtard human 70/30	Lilly	0	
	Semisynthetic	Novolin 70/30	Squibb-Novo	<1	
Long-acting					
PZI (Protamine Zn insulin)					
Standard	Beef/pork	Protamine, zinc, and Iletin I	Lilly	<10	
Purified	Beef	Protamine, zinc, and Iletin II (pork)	Lilly	<1	
Ultralente (Insulin Zn suspension, extended)					
Standard	Beef/pork	Ultralente Iletin I	Lilly	<10	
	Beef	Ultralente insulin	Squibb-Novo	<10	
Purified	Beef	Ultralente purified beef	Squibb-Novo	<1	
Human	Biosynthetic	Humulin U	Lilly	0	

Reproduced by permission from Applied Therapeutics: The Clinical Use of Drugs, fourth edition edited by Lloyd Yee Young and Mary Anne Koda-Kimble published by Applied Therapeutics, Inc., Vancouver, Washington © 1988.

Human insulin has been biosynthesized using recombinant DNA technology.

the proinsulin content is less than 10 ppm, the manufacturers are allowed by the United States Food and Drug Administration (FDA) to label their products as "purified."

A number of modifications in the insulin production procedures have resulted in preparations of superior purity and various action profiles. A semisynthetic human insulin has been produced by the chemical modification of pork insulin, whereby threonine is substituted for the alanine residue at Position 30 of the B chain. Advances in genetic engineering enabled the biosynthesis of human insulin by *Escherichia coli,* using recombinant DNA technology.

Storage of Insulin

All insulin preparations should be stored in a refrigerator. However, they do maintain their potency at room temperature for a long period of time. The convenient practice is to store extra insulin vials in the refrigerator and store the open vial at room temperature. Insulin should not be kept in the freezer compartment of a refrigerator.

Indications of Insulin Treatment

Insulin therapy is indicated for the following reasons:

1. all patients with Type I diabetes mellitus regardless of age;
2. patients who have ketoacidosis or hyperosmolar coma;
3. patients with non–insulin-dependent diabetes when diet restriction, exercise, and oral hypoglycemic agents have failed to maintain satisfactory blood glucose concentrations;
4. patients with non–insulin-dependent diabetes in the presence of surgery, fever, infections, serious renal or hepatic dysfunction, pregnancy, and other metabolic disturbances;
5. pregnant diabetic women.

Methods of Insulin Delivery

Insulin is usually injected subcutaneously. In nondiabetic humans, insulin secreted from the pancreas goes directly into the hepatic portal vein and thus to the liver, where approximately 50% of it is metabolized. Therefore, the circulating level of insulin in the nondiabetic human is much lower than in diabetic patients receiving insulin by subcutaneous injection. The biological effects of these differences in circulating insulin is not fully understood. Figure 44–8 shows the pattern of blood glucose and insulin levels in a nondiabetic person. Figure 44–9 shows blood glucose and insulin levels in a diabetic patient receiving two NPH-insulin injections and two regular insulin dosages daily. It is clear from these figures that the blood insulin pattern resulting from subcutaneous insulin injections (given as two or more injections) does not match that seen in normal human subjects.

Continuous subcutaneous insulin infusion (CSII), with bolus dosages of insulin given before each meal, most closely resembles the insulin pattern in normal subjects (see Fig. 44–8). The CSII technique, using an open loop system, has been used more recently for treating Type I diabetic patients. The insulin infuser in this system consists of a syringe containing a small amount of regular insulin, a small electronic pump, an infusion rate selector (to adjust the rate of insulin release), a small rechargeable battery, and a small plastic catheter with a needle. Improvements and refinements are constantly being made on this basic unit to make it smaller and programmable with respect to time and rate of delivery of insulin, both continuously and in bolus.

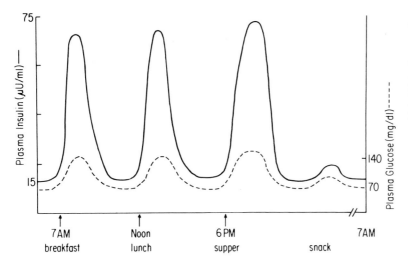

Figure 44–8

The insulin-glucose relationship in a normal human, showing the fine regulatory role of insulin in blood glucose. (From Kahn CB: Advances in insulin therapy of diabetes mellitus. *In* Brownlee M [ed]: Handbook of Diabetes Mellitus. Vol 5, Current and Future Therapies, 75–94. New York: John Wiley & Sons, 1981.)

Insulin can be delivered IV. In acute conditions, such as diabetic ketoacidosis, hyperosmolar coma, or conditions with peripheral vasoconstriction that require insulin treatment, IV administration of insulin is recommended. The uncertainties of insulin absorption are excluded by IV administrations. IM injections have been used in the treatment of diabetic ketoacidosis. Small-dose, multiple IM injections may be used for treating diabetic ketoacidosis when an IV infusion facility is not available.

Insulin can be administered by jet injections also. Although extensive experience using jet injections for insulin administration is not available, some reports document favorable results by this technique. However, many diabetologists believe that it is expensive and inconvenient, and that blood glucose is not consistently reduced. Others find it useful, especially in children.

Intranasal delivery of insulin has been tried. When insulin was administered as an aerosol after mixing it with 1% deoxycholate, reproducible effects have been reported. Serum insulin levels peaked 10 minutes after spraying. Nasal sniffing has the same intraindividual variability of absorption as injected insulin and causes nasal irritation.

IV administration of insulin is recommended in acute conditions.

Administration of Insulin

Disposable plastic syringes with needles attached are available with three different calibrations: 30 units, 50 units, and 100 units. These disposable syringes may be reused several times if proper sterile precautions are taken.

With the current concept of split dosing of insulins, different types of insulin preparations are given at the same time. When ultralente, NPH, lente, or semilente insulin are used, it is important to gently invert the bottle several times until the sediment in the bottom is suspended in the solution. For convenience, they can be mixed together in a syringe. The more rapid-acting insulin (clear) should be drawn first into the syringe, and then the less rapid-acting insulin (cloudy) can be drawn up.

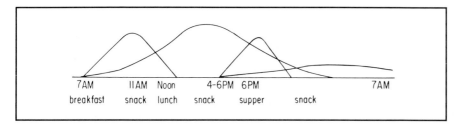

Figure 44–9

The insulin action-pattern in a type I diabetic patient receiving regimen II. (See also Table 44–4.) (From Kahn CB: Advances in insulin therapy of diabetes mellitus. *In* Brownlee M [ed]: Handbook of Diabetes Mellitus. Vol 5, Current and Future Therapies, 75–94. New York: John Wiley & Sons, 1981.)

Types of Insulin Treatment

The objective of insulin treatment is to prevent the chronic complications of diabetes by monitoring and adjusting blood glucose levels.

The objective of treatment of diabetic patients is to correct the metabolic abnormalities that result from insulin deficiency, with hopes of preventing the acute and chronic complications of diabetes. Because blood glucose monitoring is easy and universally available, blood glucose levels or glycosylated hemoglobin (an index of 3–6 weeks of blood glucose) is widely used as a measure of metabolic control in diabetic patients. The short-term benefits of meticulous blood glucose control are well established. Such benefits include subjective well-being, less frequent catabolic crises resulting from underinsulinization, normal growth in children, and decreased frequency of infections. It is also well established that meticulous blood glucose control prevents many maternal-fetal complications of diabetic pregnancy. Even though most of the evidence strongly indicates that meticulous blood glucose control prevents or delays chronic complications of diabetes, unequivocal evidence of such a hope is still lacking. Such evidence is desired from the multicenter study sponsored by the National Institutes of Health (NIH) National Institute of Diabetes and Digestive and Kidney Diseases (NIDDK), known as *DCCT study.*

However, meticulous glucose control has potential serious short-term risks, such as frequent hypoglycemic episodes, possibly resulting in severe neuroglycopenia and increased retinopathy in patients previously in a poor state of control. More recent clinical studies demonstrated that many insulin-dependent diabetic patients, especially those with long-term disease, have delayed recovery from hypoglycemia because of a defective glucagon response to hypoglycemia. Glucagon response is critical for recovery from hypoglycemia in these patients because of the common occurrence of autonomic neuropathy. Studies in normal human subjects have demonstrated that in the absence of epinephrine and norepinephrine action, glucagon is essential for recovery from hypoglycemia in the first several minutes after its onset. A delayed recovery could cause irreversible brain damage and even death. Meticulous glucose control has been reported also to reduce the awareness of diabetic patients to early symptoms of hypoglycemia. Such a lack of awareness could result in unarrested progression to severe hypoglycemia.

Hypoglycemic episodes are a major side effect of insulin treatment.

It is clear from the available evidence that even though meticulous glucose control is desirable, such an objective is not reasonable in every diabetic patient because of the risks involved. Physicians have to exercise their clinical judgment in each patient regarding the type of insulin treatment. Based on current knowledge, it is prudent to achieve as meticulous control as possible in pregnant diabetic mothers, even prior to conception; in diabetic patients following renal transplantation irrespective of their general health; and in other diabetic patients in otherwise good health without hypoglycemic risk factors or advanced diabetic complications. Meticulous glucose control is not always desirable in elderly patients, in patients with autonomic neuropathy, and in patients with other hypoglycemia risk factors.

The type of insulin treatment varies from patient to patient. CSII therapy needs to be more widely tested before it can be recommended universally for diabetic patients. Table 44–4 gives the different combinations of insulin that can be administered to a Type I diabetic patient.

Insulin regimens depend upon the preference of the patient as well as the clinical status. In patients in whom tight diabetic control is desired, multiple injections are preferred. Regimen I is well suited for most patients. The choice of an intermediate-acting insulin at bedtime is due to its peak action (8–12 hours) and the usual early morning increase of blood glucose in diabetic patients (dawn phenomenon). If NPH/lente insulin is taken

Table 44–4 CHOICES OF INSULIN REGIMENS

Regimen	Combination/Insulins	Time of Administration			
		Before Breakfast	**Before Lunch**	**Before Supper**	**Before Bedtime**
I.	Lente/NPH	Yes	No	No	Yes
	Regular	Yes	No	Yes	No
II.	Lente/NPH	Yes	No	Yes	No
	Regular	Yes	No	Yes	No
III.	Lente/NPH	No	No	No	Yes
	Regular	Yes	Yes	Yes	No
IV.	Lente/NPH	Yes	No	No	Yes
V.	Ultralente	No	No	No	Yes
	Regular	Yes	Yes	Yes	No
VI.	Lente/NPH	Yes	No	No	No
	Regular	Yes	No	No	No
VII.	Ultralente	Yes	No	No	No
	Regular	No	No	No	No

before supper (between 5–6 P.M.), its peak action occurs in the early morning (about 2 A.M.), whereas a bedtime (9 P.M.–10 P.M.) injection tends to peak when the patient is awake (about 6 A.M.). Hypoglycemia during sleep is particularly worrisome for elderly patients and in patients with a compromised glucose regulatory mechanism. In general, regular insulin injection has to be avoided at bedtime because of possible hypoglycemia during sleep. These optimal regimens may not be applicable, because there are individual variabilities.

In general, regular insulin injections should not be administered before sleep.

For patients whose meticulous blood glucose control is not desired and who refuse multiple injections, a single injection of long-acting insulin may prevent very high blood glucose levels.

Blood glucose measurements are superior to urine sugar tests for monitoring diabetic control. Blood glucose measurement as an index at a particular time and glycosylated hemoglobin as an index of long-term control continue to be the gold standards. With different types of glucose monitoring equipment and finger-stick techniques, it is possible to monitor blood glucose with little effort but with reasonable accuracy. Use of BG chemstrips with color comparison is also adequate if the person performing the blood glucose measurement uses the proper technique and has good vision. Four separate blood glucose measurements are recommended initially for adjusting insulin dosage. An example of adjusted insulin dosage according to blood glucose is given in Table 44–5. It is to be emphasized that the diet and exercise of patients must be considered in any readjustments of insulin dosage.

Blood glucose measurements are more effective than urine sugar tests for monitoring diabetic control.

Table 44–5 INSULIN DOSE ADJUSTMENT IN A PATIENT ON REGIMEN I

Blood Glucose	NPH/Lente	Regular
Before breakfast High	Increase at bedtime	No change
Before breakfast Low	Decrease at bedtime	No change
Before lunch High	No change	Increase before breakfast
Before lunch Low	No change	Decrease before breakfast
Before supper High	Increase before lunch	
Before bedtime Low	No change	Increase before dinner

Once an insulin regimen is achieved with stable blood glucose control, the frequency of blood glucose monitoring can be reduced.

The criteria for meticulous blood glucose control are still widely debated. A blood glucose level of less than 125 mg/dl is considered to be excellent by most diabetologists. In patients over 65 years old at the time of diagnosis, acceptable blood glucose control is a premeal blood glucose of less than 150 mg/dl.

Measurement of glycosylated hemoglobin provides the physician with a retrospective view of the prevailing time-integrated elevation of blood glucose levels over the previous 10–14 weeks. It also helps physicians to determine whether self-monitoring is being performed accurately and consistently.

COMPLICATIONS OF INSULIN TREATMENT

Hypoglycemic reactions are the most common complications of insulin therapy. When normal or near-normal blood glucose is attained, it is difficult to avoid occasional hypoglycemic episodes. They are seen frequently in patients with brittle diabetes, which is characterized by unpredictable spontaneous reductions in insulin requirement. They may also result from an excessively large dose of insulin. With current practice of tight glucose control, its incidence is likely to increase. Symptoms of hypoglycemia include sweating, weakness, hunger, tachycardia, tremor, headache, blurred vision, mental confusion, incoherent speech, coma, and convulsions. If left untreated, it may result in irreversible brain damage. Mild recurrent hypoglycemia can be debilitating to many patients performing skilled work. Even asymptomatic mild hypoglycemia may cause subtle permanent neuropsychopathology in very young children.

The symptoms of mild hypoglycemia are relieved by the oral administration of carbohydrates, whereas severe hypoglycemia may require IV administration of 50% dextrose. Administration of glucagon is recommended in patients who are stuporous or unconscious because oral administration of glucose may cause aspiration to lungs. Beta blockers mask many of the signs and symptoms of hypoglycemia and also may delay recovery from hypoglycemic episodes. Beta-1-blockers are more selective and do not delay recovery from hypoglycemia or mask its signs and symptoms to the same degree as nonselective β blockers.

Local allergic reactions, such as itching, redness, or swelling, may develop in patients receiving insulin for the first time or when insulin therapy is restarted. Usually they disappear within a few weeks. These reactions generally appear within 15–60 minutes after the injection. With the availability of purer forms of insulin, the incidence of allergy has decreased. Systemic allergic reactions characterized by generalized urticaria, lymphadenopathy, angioedema, and anaphylaxis are rare.

Rapid desensitization may be achieved by subcutaneous or intradermal administration of 0.001 units of insulin and doubling each subsequent dosage every 30 minutes.

Atrophy of subcutaneous fat at the site of injection may lead to scarring, but its incidence has decreased with the introduction of purer forms of insulin. Resistance to insulin may occur in some patients and is manifested by requirements of a very high insulin dosage of usually more than 200 units daily. All patients on insulin therapy develop a low titer of circulating IgG anti-insulin antibodies that neutralize the action of insulin. In some patients, a high titer of IgG anti-insulin antibodies develops and results in insulin resistance. Switching to a less antigenic insulin may help decrease the insulin dosage requirement. It is also important to initiate insulin treat-

Tighter glucose control can increase the incidence of hypoglycemic reactions.

Oral administration of carbohydrates can relieve the symptoms of mild hypoglycemia.

Table 44-6 INTERACTION OF INSULIN WITH OTHER DRUGS

Drug Name	Effect	Mechanism of Action
Alcohol metabolism	Hypoglycemia	Ethanol alters glucose
Beta-adrenergic blockers (nonselective)	Prolonged hypoglycemic effect and masking of certain symptoms of hypoglycemia	Retard blood glucose rebound following insulin
Fenfluramine	Increased hypoglycemic effect	Increases skeletal muscle uptake of glucose
Monoamine oxidase inhibitor	Increased hypoglycemic effect	Possible direct effect on insulin release and interference with sympathetic response to hypoglycemia

ment with one of the pure insulin preparations in order to reduce the chances of antibody formations.

Hyperglycemic rebound (Somogyi effect) may develop when a patient chronically receives overdoses of insulin. Morning hyperglycemia may result from hypoglycemia in the early morning. Symptoms of hypoglycemia in the early morning may not be evident in all diabetic patients, especially in patients with autonomic neuropathy. Morning headache should raise the threshold for checking blood glucose in the early morning (3 A.M.) The importance of the Somogyi effect has been questioned by more recent clinical research. There is little doubt that the primary cause of rebound hyperglycemia is overeating in response to low blood glucose. Weight gain is a clue in some patients. Its treatment involves lowering the insulin dosage, with close monitoring of glucose.

A summary of insulin's interactions with other drugs is given in Table 44-6.

Insulin Treatment in Special Situations

In certain special situations, such as diabetic ketoacidosis, diabetic hyperosmolar coma, surgery, and infections, insulin administration requires special care.

Diabetic Ketoacidosis. In diabetic ketoacidosis, insulin deficiency, dehydration, acidosis, and electrolyte imbalance have to be corrected. Meticulous professional supervision is needed, not only to correct the named abnormalities but also to determine the precipitating factors and to treat them.

Insulin replacement is an essential part of the treatment in diabetic ketoacidosis. Diabetic ketoacidosis is associated with insulin resistance, and therefore the rule in the past was to treat with large dosages of insulin. Clinical investigations in the early 1970s clearly demonstrated the therapeutic efficiency of small dosages of insulin administered either by continuous IV infusions or intramuscularly in diabetic ketoacidosis. It has been documented in several studies that 2–10 units per hour of regular insulin results in a predictable fall, averaging a 75–100 mg/dl/hour decline in blood glucose. In most patients, blood glucose reaches 200–300 mg/dl in approximately 4–6 hours. The response of blood glucose to insulin varies from patient to patient and is affected also by many other factors, such as infections or trauma and other stress factors, and blood pH.

Both IV infusions and repeated IM injections have been reported to be equally effective. However, it is prudent not to use IM and subcutaneous administration of low dose insulin in patients with severe dehydration and

Diabetic ketoacidosis is associated with insulin resistance.

Fluid replacement is an important measure in treating diabetic ketoacidosis.

Serum potassium levels should be monitored in patients with diabetic ketoacidosis.

Hyperosmolar nonketotic coma in Type II patients is life-threatening.

acidosis, because initial absorption may be irregular because of vasoconstriction.

In the treatment of diabetic ketoacidosis, replacement of fluids and correction of electrolytes and acidosis are equally important. Water deficits may be as high as 100 ml/kg body weight, and sodium deficits of 7–10 mg/kg body weight may be expected. Usually water and sodium deficits are corrected by normal saline infusion. In conditions with high serum osmolarity hypo-osmolar saline is indicated initially. Correction of fluid deficit and insulin is adequate usually to correct pH, but in severe cases of metabolic acidosis (pH <7.0), bicarbonate replacement may be indicated expecially if there is fall in blood pressure or deterioration of hemodynamic parameters. However, it must be emphasized that rapid correction of blood osmolality or pH may cause deterioration of brain function due to the delayed correction of these abnormalities in the brain. It may contribute to cerebral edema if blood osmolality is lower than that of cerebrospinal fluid (CSF). The exact cause of cerebral edema remains unknown. Hyperinsulinism is considered to be a cause also. An increased CSF acidity in comparison with blood could cause hyperventilation and respiratory alkalosis when metabolic acidosis is improving. Diabetic ketoacidosis is invariably associated with total body potassium deficit of the magnitude of 3–10 mEq/kg body weight. When these patients are acidotic, they have a normal serum potassium. Once the fluid is replaced and insulin is given, acidosis is corrected, and there is marked shift of potassium from the extracellular to the intracellular compartment resulting in a rather dangerous fall in serum potassium. Such hypokalemia can precipitate cardiac arrhythmias. Therefore, it is prudent to start on potassium replacement early, and to monitor serum potassium frequently during the course of treatment.

Replacement of deficiencies of phosphorus and magnesium is considered important also on a theoretical basis. However, no control studies have been done to prove that phosphorus replacement is essential. Potassium can be given as potassium phosphate.

Hyperosmolar Nonketotic Coma in Type II Diabetic Patients. A plasma glucose concentration that exceeds 600 mg/dl and a serum osmolarity of above 350/mosm/l is necessary to make the diagnosis. It is a life-threatening situation. Insulin is only one part of the therapeutic program in these patients. An integral part of the therapy is the search for correctable precipitating factors, such as infection, and prompt treatment of these.

Replacing water loss is the highest priority. If hypotension or shock exists, large volumes of a volume expander must be administered. To replace water loss initially, hypotonic saline is preferred. Isotonic solutions should be started when hyperosmolarity is partially corrected. The amount of fluid replacement required varies from patient to patient. A water loss of between 4–12 l has been reported to occur. The rate of fluid replacement is determined on the basis of age and cardiovascular status of the patient. Hypernatremia and coma without hypotension suggest severe intracellular water depletion and warrants water replacement preferably as one half normal saline. If hypotension is present, volume expanders must be given. Replacements of electrolytes, such as potassium, phosphorus, and in some cases magnesium, must be monitored carefully.

Low-dose insulin treatment, as in diabetic ketoacidosis, is effective. After a bolus dose (10-20 units), regular insulin can be given as a continuous IV infusion at a rate of 4–6 units per hour. IM injections are also sufficient in many patients, although the IV route is preferred in patients with shock and hypotension. It must be remembered that administration of insulin can suddenly shift the fluids owing to a fall in blood glucose, causing hypotension. Therefore, it is important to start the fluid replacement before insulin administration.

Insulin Treatment During Surgery

The objective of management of diabetes during surgery is to avoid either sustained hyperglycemia or hypoglycemia. It is also important to maintain fluid and electrolyte balance. An ambient blood glucose level between 120–200 mg/dl is generally desired.

A preferred technique is to administer regular insulin IV with a glucose solution. In this case no subcutaneous insulin should be given preoperatively. About 35% of the usual daily insulin dosage is given in a 5% dextrose solution (2–4 l) throughout the day of the operation. The infusion rate of the solution is to be adjusted to maintain blood glucose between 120–200 mg/dl. Another common way to administer insulin is to divide the usual insulin dosage, giving one third to one half of the total subcutaneously on the morning of operation. The morning meal is replaced by a 5% dextrose infusion, adjusting the infusion rate to maintain blood glucose between 120–200 mg/dl. Postoperatively, a similar dosage of insulin can be given subcutaneously.

Oral Hypoglycemic Agents

The oral medications currently available in the United States for treating hyperglycemia in NIDDM are the sulfonylureas. The biguanides (metformin) are currently not approved for use in the United States, but they are used extensively in Europe and many other parts of the world.

In contrast to Type I diabetic patients, whose insulin deficiency is the major defect, Type II diabetic patients have insulin resistance as the major defect. Most of the Type II diabetic patients have a compensatory increase in insulin secretion, resulting in hyperinsulinism. Diabetes in these patients represents the failure of the pancreas to compensate sufficiently for the degree of insulin resistance. Defective first-phase insulin secretion during an IV glucose tolerance test has been recognized also. The physiological relevance of first-phase insulin release has been questioned, because first-phase release is not desired after an oral glucose load. However, studies with closed-loop insulin infusion devices indicate that first-phase insulin release is required in the algorithms to prime the insulin-target tissues and to prevent overinsulinization and secondary hypoglycemia. First-phase release of insulin has been found to be important also in regulating hepatic glucose output.

It is well established that obesity is associated with insulin resistance or diminished sensitivity to insulin in human tissues. It is generally agreed that the diabetogenic effect of obesity is mediated through insulin resistance. Defects at the major sites of insulin action—hormone binding, glucose transport, and intracellular glucose metabolism—have all been recognized.

About 85% of Type II diabetic patients are obese. Obesity not only precipitates diabetes in predisposed individuals, but also causes deterioration in mild diabetes. Weight reduction by dietary restriction has been shown to improve diabetic control. Substantial weight reduction in some obese diabetic patients may result in discontinuation of oral hypoglycemic agents or insulin.

A subpopulation of Type II diabetic patients is reported to have reduced insulin secretions and normal insulin sensitivity. This group of Type II patients has not been clearly defined; thus, the approach to treatment of these patients remains incompletely defined. However, it is reasonable to

Type II patients have insulin resistance, not insulin deficiency, as the major defect.

Obesity is associated with insulin resistance.

assume that a symptomatic nonobese Type II diabetic patient with high fasting blood glucose (more than 250 mg/dl) is likely to need a treatment similar to that of Type I diabetic patients.

Inactivity decreases insulin sensitivity. Exercise acutely enhances insulin sensitivity and glucose disposal. Exercise training also improves glucose tolerance. Cessation of exercise reverses the results from exercise that had been achieved.

A logical approach to diabetic patients is to correct their abnormality. In Type I diabetic patients with β cell failure and insulin deficiency, there is no alternative to insulin replacement. In Type II diabetic patients with obesity and insulin resistance, the primary objective is to achieve weight reduction and to improve insulin sensitivity. Exercise, specifically a program of physical training, is an important and valuable adjunct to caloric restriction. Oral hypoglycemic agents or insulin is indicated only when dietary restrictions and exercise programs fail to achieve adequate diabetic control.

Often, it is the failure of patients to change or modify their beliefs, attitudes, and habits with respect to eating and physical activity that results in the failure of nondrug treatment. In some patients with severe diabetes, dietary restriction alone is not sufficient to control the diabetes. In addition, such patients require oral hypoglycemic agents or insulin.

HISTORICAL PERSPECTIVE

In 1926 Frank and coworkers altered the guanidine molecule to prepare synthalin. Synthalin was used for several years in Germany to treat diabetes, but its use was discontinued because of its severe side effects. Synthalin was a forerunner of the later biguanides (phenformin and metformin). In 1942 Janbon, in France, accidentally discovered the hypoglycemic effect of a sulfonamide derivative (2254RP) during the treatment of typhoid fever. Following this discovery, extensive research on this sulfonylurea derivative resulted in the following information: the sulfonylurea derivative did not act in pancreatectomized animals; following its administration there was a progressive fall in blood glucose; and the appearance of a substance with insulin-like activity was detected in the blood of treated animals. These investigations led to the discovery of tolbutamide and, subsequently, other sulfonylureas, such as acetohexamide, tolazamide, and chlorpropamide. These drugs are widely known as the first-generation sulfonylureas.

There are several second-generation sulfonylureas undergoing clinical trials. Two second-generation sulfonylureas that are available for use in the United States are glyburide and glipizide. Glyburide was previously used extensively in Europe and Asia under the name glybenclamide.

Phenformin was used widely in the 1960s and 1970s but was later discontinued in view of its side effects, especially lactic acidosis. Currently, metformin is a widely used biguanide in many parts of the world. Its use has not been approved yet by the FDA for use in the United States.

SULFONYLUREAS

All the sulfonylureas have the same basic molecular structure.

R₁—⟨○⟩—SO₂—NH—CO—NH—R₂

Sulfonylureas   Basic structure

Chemistry

The structural formulas of the first-generation sulfonylurea compounds available for use as oral hypoglycemics—tolbutamide, acetohexamide, tolazamide, and chlorpropamide—are shown in the margin.

CH₃—⟨○⟩—SO₂—NH—CO—NH—(CH₂)₃CH₃

Tolbutamide

CH₃CO—⟨○⟩—SO₂—NH—CO—NH—⟨○⟩

Acetohexamide

Many members of the second-generation sulfonylureas are in different stages of clinical trial, and two of these, glyburide and glipizide, are already in use. Their structural formulas are also shown.

CH_3—◯—SO_2—NH—CO—NH—N◯

Tolazamide

Mechanism of Action

The sulfonylureas lower blood glucose mainly by stimulating insulin release from the islet cells of the pancreas and are thus effective in NIDDM patients in whom the islets retain the capacity to secrete insulin. They are ineffective in completely pancreatectomized patients and in IDDM patients. Sulfonylureas cause degranulation of β cells of the islets and thus cause increased insulin secretion. It is believed that the sulfonylureas act by depolarization of the cell membrane and reduction of the movement of K^+ through an adenosine triphosphate-sensitive K^+ channel, producing a secondary increase in intracellular calcium. This results in the activation of microfilaments involved in the insulin secretory process. The mediator of this activation is calmodulin.

After prolonged sulfonylurea therapy, serum insulin levels no longer are increased by the drug and may return to baseline values. The sulfonylureas continue to exert beneficial hypoglycemic effects even after this effect on enhancing insulin secretion is no longer present. To account for this, extrapancreatic effects have been proposed.

The extrapancreatic effects of the sulfonylureas appear to be a combination of an increase in the absolute number of insulin receptors and the increased sensitivity of the insulin receptors.

Sulfonylureas lower blood glucose levels by stimulating insulin release from the islet cells of the pancreas.

Cl—◯—SO_2—NH—$\overset{\overset{\displaystyle O}{\|}}{C}$—NH—$(CH_2)_2CH_3$

Chlorpropamide

Glyburide (or glibenclamide)

Glipizide

Pharmacokinetics (Table 44–7)

Sulfonylureas are readily absorbed from the GI tract. Differences in chemical structure and in metabolic fate when ingested result in functional differences between these agents, affecting their potency and duration of action. The duration of hypoglycemic activity is related to the half-life of these drugs only in general terms and may correlate poorly in some cases. All of these compounds are highly protein bound (92–99%).

Tolbutamide (ORAMIDE, ORINASE) is about 95% bound to plasma pro-

Table 44–7 PHARMACOKINETICS OF SULFONYLUREAS

Drug	Duration of Biological Action (hours)	Mode of Metabolism	Renal Excretion (%/24 hours)	Activity of Metabolites	Therapeutic Equivalent Doses (mg)	Comments
First-Generation						
Acetohexamide	12–18	Hepatic reduction to 1-hydrohexamide	60	++++	500	Contraindicated in renal failure
Chlorpropamide	24–72	Hepatic hydroxylation of side-chain cleavage	60	±	250	ADH action; alcohol flushing
Tolazamide	2–18	Hepatic metabolites	85	+	250	Safe in patients with impaired renal function
Tolbutamide	6–8	Hepatic carboxylation	100	Inactive	1000	Safe in patients with impaired renal function
Second-Generation						
Glyburide	16–24	Hepatic metabolites	65	Inactive	5.0	Affects insulin secretions on long-term basis
Glipizide	12–18	Hepatic metabolites	75	Inactive	7.5	Less secondary failure than first-generation drugs

teins. Peak concentrations are reached in 3–5 hours. It is carboxylated in the liver, rapidly metabolized, and almost entirely excreted in the urine. The half-life is approximately 7 hours, but great individual variations have been reported. The hypoglycemic action lasts about 6–12 hours and, therefore, it should be dosed two to three times a day. It is supplied in tablets of 250 and 500 mg. The usual starting dosage is 500 mg three times a day, and it must be adjusted in patients with renal impairment.

Chlorpropamide (DIABINASE) is about 90% bound to plasma proteins. Peak plasma concentrations are reached in 2–4 hours. It was formerly believed that chlorpropamide was not significantly metabolized, but new data indicate that it is extensively metabolized in the liver, and both the metabolites and unchanged drug are excreted in the urine. According to the manufacturer, 6–60% of the drug is excreted renally; within 96 hours, 80–90% of a single oral dose of chlorpropamide is excreted in urine as unchanged drug and metabolite. It has a half-life of 36 hours and can be much higher in patients with renal impairment. The hypoglycemic action lasts for more than 40 hours, and it is dosed once a day. It is supplied in tablets of 100 and 250 mg, and the usual dosage is 250 mg daily.

Peak concentrations of acetohexamide (DYMELOR) are reached in about 2 hours, and that of its metabolite in about 4 hours. It is metabolized in the liver to hydroxyhexamide, which has more than twice the hypoglycemic action of the parent drug. The half-life of the drug is about 1.5 hours, and that of the active metabolite 6 hours. Approximately 80% of an oral dose of acetohexamide is excreted in urine as unchanged drug and its metabolite. The duration of hypoglycemic action is about 12–18 hours, and it is dosed once or twice a day. It is supplied in tablets of 250 and 500 mg. The usual dosage is 500 mg to 1 g daily, and it must be adjusted in patients with renal impairment.

Tolazamide (TOLINASE) is absorbed much more slowly than the other sulfonylureas. Peak concentrations occur within 4–8 hours. It is metabolized in the liver to six compounds, three of which are inactive, whereas the other three retain partial activity. Most of the drug is excreted in urine as metabolites. It has a half-life of about 7 hours. The duration of hypoglycemic action is about 20 hours. It is usually dosed once a day. It is supplied in tablets of 100, 250, and 500 mg, and the usual dosage is 250 mg a day.

Glipizide (GLUCOTROL) is rapidly and completely absorbed from the GI tract. Food delays the absorption of the drug but does not affect the peak serum concentrations or the extent of absorption. Peak concentrations occur in 1–3 hours. It is completely metabolized, and the metabolites are excreted mainly in the urine. The drug and its metabolites are fecally excreted. The metabolites are not pharmacologically active. It is extensively (95%) bound to plasma proteins. The protein binding of glipizide seems to be nonionic, and hence the drug is less likely to be displaced from binding sites and less likely to displace other highly bound drugs from their binding sites. It has a half-life of about 4 hours. The hypoglycemic effects persist for about 10–16 hours. The discrepancy between the half-life and its duration of action has not been explained. It is usually dosed twice a day. Glipizide is supplied in tablets of 5 and 10 mg, and the usual dosage is 5–20 mg daily.

Glyburide (DIABETA, MICRONASE) is absorbed rapidly from the GI tract. Peak concentrations occur in about 2–4 hours. Food does not affect the rate or extent of absorption. It is more than 99% bound to plasma proteins. The protein binding is nonionic, and thus it does not displace other highly protein bound drugs. It is completely metabolized. The metabolites are excreted almost equally in urine and feces. Fecal excretion appears to occur almost completely through biliary eliminations. It has a half-life of about 10 hours. The duration of hypoglycemic action is about 24 hours, and it is

Tolbutamide, chlorpropamide, and acetohexamide are readily absorbed from the GI tract.

Peak concentrations of glipizide (GLUCO-TROL) occur in 1–3 hours.

usually dosed once a day. Glyburide is supplied in tablets of 1.25, 2.5, and 5 mg. The usual daily dosage is 5–10 mg.

Adverse Effects

Hypoglycemia is the major adverse effect of sulfonylureas. This can lead to permanent neurological damage and even death. More than 6% of patients receiving chlorpropamide have been reported to have had hypoglycemia as an adverse reaction. Chlorpropamide is more likely to promote long-lasting hypoglycemia probably because it is eliminated slowly—its half-life is 36 hours—so significant accumulations can occur. Generally, the more prolonged the activity of the agent, the more common is hypoglycemia. Most reactions are observed in patients over 50 years of age. Patients with impaired renal or hepatic functions are more likely to have hypoglycemic episodes, because the liver and kidney are important in metabolism and excretion of sulfonylureas.

Chlorpropamide potentiates the action of antidiuretic hormone and may precipitate the syndrome of inappropriate antidiuretic hormone (SIADH) manifested as symptoms and signs of water intoxication. Geriatric patients are at high risk of chlorpropamide-induced SIADH, which can be managed by discontinuing the drug along with water restriction.

Chlorpropamide causes a disulfiram-like reaction in patients ingesting alcohol. It is believed that the plasma acetaldehyde level is increased when alcohol is concomitantly ingested.

Nausea, vomiting, and epigastric pain have occurred in patients receiving sulfonylurea drugs. Allergic skin reactions have been reported also.

> Hypoglycemia is the primary adverse effect of sulfonylurea administration.

> Other adverse effects include nausea, epigastric pain, and allergic skin reactions.

Drug Interactions

Sulfonylureas are highly protein bound. They may displace other protein-bound drugs or may be displaced by other protein-bound drugs, such as oral anticoagulants, hydantoins, salicylates and other nonsteroidal anti-inflammatory agents, and sulfonamides. This type of interaction does not occur with second-generation sulfonylureas, because their protein binding is nonionic. Phenylbutazone enhances the hypoglycemic action of the sulfonylureas by a combination of protein-binding displacement, an inhibitory effect on hepatic enzyme activity, and decreased renal excretion.

Beta-adrenergic blocking agents may cause several problems for patients on sulfonylurea therapy. These include impairment of glucose tolerance, blockage of hypoglycemia-induced tachycardia, and alteration of the hemodynamic response to hypoglycemia. It is best to avoid the concomitant use of sulfonylureas and β-adrenergic blockers.

Drugs such as chloramphenicol, monoaminase oxidase inhibitors, and probenecid enhance the hypoglycemic effect of the sulfonylureas, whereas corticosteroids, contraceptives, phenytoin, rifampin, isoniazid, calcium channel-blocking agents, and phenothiazines decrease the hypoglycemic effect. When these drugs are initiated or discontinued in patients receiving sulfonylureas, the patients should be monitored carefully. A summary of interactions of sulfonylureas with other drugs is provided in Table 44–8.

In summary, sulfonylureas are effective drugs for control of hyperglycemia. The individual drugs and dosages should be chosen carefully, and patients must be closely monitored in the initial stage. After initial stabilization, patients should be educated about the signs and symptoms of hypoglycemia as well as hyperglycemia, so that these can be reported

> The combined use of sulfonylureas and β blockers should be avoided.

Table 44-8 INTERACTIONS OF SULFONYLUREAS WITH OTHER DRUGS

Drug Name	Effect	Mechanism of Action
Anticoagulant (Dicumarol)	Increased hypoglycemic effect	Inhibition of metabolism of sulfonylureas
Ethanol	Both hypoglycemia and hyperglycemia; acute alcohol intolerance may occur	Inhibition of hepatic gluconeogenesis and increased metabolism of drug
Monoamine oxidase	Increased hypoglycemic effect	Probably direct effect on insulin release and interference with symptomatic response
Phenylbutazone	Increased hypoglycemic effect	Impaired metabolism
β blockers (nonspecific)	Possible increased hypoglycemic effect; blunting of symptoms of hypoglycemia	

immediately to the physician for necessary dosage adjustments. Home blood glucose monitoring is desirable initially to determine the appropriate dosage of the medication. After the initial period, less frequent blood glucose monitoring than advised in Type I diabetic patients is required.

Drugs with a longer duration of action afford the advantage of fewer dosages per day while at the same time carrying a greater risk of prolonged hypoglycemia. First-generation sulfonylureas, because of their ionic type of protein binding, displace or are displaced by many highly protein-bound drugs. Second-generation sulfonylureas, because of their nonionic type of binding, do not undergo displacement interactions. Furthermore, second-generation sulfonylureas are efficacious in cases of secondary failure to first-generation sulfonylureas.

BIGUANIDES

Biguanides (metformin and phenformin) were available from the 1950s until 1977. The University Group of Diabetes Project (UGDP) studies included phenformin to test its efficacy in the prevention of complications of NIDDM. Experiences with lactic acidosis resulted in the withdrawal of both biguanides from the United States market. In most other parts of the world metformin continues to be used in view of its low risk of causing lactic acidosis. Phenformin also remains available in many countries. In the United States, the biguanides are not currently available for clinical use.

Chemistry

Metformin (meltrylbiguamide) is a compound of two guanidine groups in which there is a monopolar linkage of two methyl groups. It can be assayed in serum by high-performance liquid chromatography using an ultraviolet absorbance detector.

Mechanism of Action

The precise mechanism of action of the biguanides is incompletely understood. *In vitro* experiments indicated that metformin stimulates anaerobic glycolysis and inhibits hepatic and renal gluconeogenesis. It must be remembered that the dosages used to produce these effects *in vitro* generally exceeded those used in patients.

Metformin does not stimulate insulin secretion. It is ineffective in pancreatectomized humans, but it reduces insulin requirements of persons

Second-generation sulfonylureas do not undergo displacement interactions.

$$CH_3 \diagdown \atop CH_3 \diagup N - \underset{\underset{NH}{\|}}{C} - NH - \underset{\underset{NH}{\|}}{C} - NH_2$$

Metformin

with insulin-dependent diabetes and improves glucose tolerance in NIDDM patients. It does not cause hypoglycemia in normal humans even in very high dosages. It is believed that metformin enhances the peripheral action of insulin. Metformin has been shown to enhance the insulin-induced peripheral glucose uptake in obese NIDDM patients. Metformin has been shown also to reduce the elevated splanchanic glucose output in NIDDM patients.

Metformin has been reported to inhibit GI absorption of glucose, as well as to have an anorexigenic effect. These two properties may be major contributors to its hypoglycemic effect.

Metformin has been reported also to increase high-density lipoprotein (HDL) cholesterol and to reduce triglycerides. It has been reported to reduce blood pressure also. A diminution in platelet aggregation, apparently independent of the cyclooxygenase-prostaglandin pathway, has been described. It is unclear whether these effects are primary or secondary to improved diabetic control.

Metformin does not stimulate insulin secretion.

Metformin can reduce HDL cholesterol.

Pharmacokinetics

Unlike most other drugs, metformin is not bound to serum proteins and thus is not displaced by competitive binding of other drugs. It is excreted primarily by the kidney (80–100%). The plasma half-life of metformin varies from 1.5 to 4.5 hours (2½ hour average). However, kinetic studies indicate two compartments, with a slow turning-over compartment with a metformin half-life of 12–14 hours. The bioavailability of metformin is about 50% of the ingested dose.

Metformin's bioavailability is about 50% of the ingested dose.

Therapeutic Use

The therapeutic indications are similar to those for sulfonylureas. Metformin, like the sulfonylureas, is indicated in NIDDM patients after diet and exercise fail to control diabetes.

Because the hypoglycemic effect of metformin does not depend on insulin secretion, there is a strong case for administering it to obese, hyperinsulinemic NIDDM patients. Metformin alone or in combination with a second-generation sulfonylurea is another combination widely used in Europe. Metformin has been used also in certain insulin-resistant patients to reduce the insulin requirement.

The therapeutic dosage ranges between 0.5 and 2.5 g daily. It is recommended that metformin be administered before breakfast, lunch, and supper with a 500 mg tablet each time. This dosage has to be gradually increased, in order to avoid the unpleasant side effects, until the therapeutic target is achieved or the maximal recommended dosage is reached.

Side Effects

Lactic Acidosis. Lactic acidosis is a problem when phenformin is used, especially in patients with renal or hepatic insufficiency. This has rarely been encountered during metformin use. GI upsets tend to occur frequently. Metformin use is frequently associated with the occurrence of severe diarrhea. Unlike sulfonylureas, hypoglycemia is not a complication for the use of biguanides.

HISTORICAL PERSPECTIVE

The discovery of glucagon and the perfection of its radioimmunoassay closely followed that of its sister hormone insulin. In contrast to the glu-

Glucagon

Glucagon is the major hormone involved in ketoacidosis.

cose-lowering hormone secreted by the β cell of the pancreas, the glucogenic hormone secreted by the α cell received less attention for a long time. Unger, who developed the radioimmunoassay of this hormone along with Orci, proposed diabetes as a bihormonal disease. This was disputed by many other workers. More recently it has become clear that glucagon is the major hormone involved in ketoacidosis, and it is increasingly recognized as the primary defense against severe hypoglycemia. It is recognized also that a high glucagon level in insulin deficiency state accelerates protein catabolism and energy expenditure.

CHEMISTRY

Glucagon is a single chain polypeptide with a molecular weight of 3485 daltons. There is a striking structural analogy between glucagon and secretin, which implies a common embryological origin. All mammalian glucagon, with the exception of the guinea pig, appears to have an identical amino acid sequence. The terminal amino group of glucagon is active in both binding and cellular action of the hormone. However, the terminal carboxyl group confers high affinity for its receptors, which allows the hormone binding, thereby facilitating its action.

BIOSYNTHESIS AND SECRETION OF GLUCAGON

The α cells of the islets of Langerhans are the cells that synthesize glucagon. Figure 44–10 gives a schematic representation of a rat islet cell, demonstrating the topographical relationships of the major cell types. The insulin-secreting cells and glucagon-secreting cells share close topographical

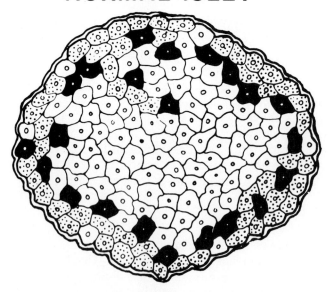

NORMAL ISLET

A CELLS	Glucagon
D CELLS	Somatostatin
B CELLS	Insulin

Figure 44–10

Schematic representation of a rat islet showing the topographical relationships of the major cell types. (Reprinted by permission of the publisher from Unger RH, Orci L: Glucagon. *In* Ellenberg M, Rifkin H [eds]: Diabetes Mellitus: Theory and Practice, 3rd ed, 203–224. New York: Medical Examination Publishing Co., 1983. Copyright 1983 by Elsevier Science Publishing Co., Inc.)

relationship with the somatostatin-secreting cells. Somatostatin is known to inhibit insulin and growth hormone secretion. It is not clear whether the topographical proximity of somatostatin-secreting cells to those secreting insulin and glucagon is related to its regulatory role on the secretion of insulin and glucagon. Glucagon-producing α cells are usually preserved when the β cells are destroyed by the autoimmune process of Type I diabetes.

The primary translation product of α cells is preproglucagon with 180 amino acids. Pre-proglucagon is converted to proglucagon with 69 amino acids. Proglucagon has glucagon-like immunoreactivity and is known as glycentin. The conversion of proglucagon to glucagon requires two enzyme activities—one trypsin-like and the other carboxypeptidase-B-like. The secretory granules of α cells contain glucagon as the central core with proglucagon in the outer rim. Analogous to insulin secretion, glucagon from the granules is excreted by the process of exocytosis.

Glucagon secretion is primarily governed by the prevailing arterial glucose concentration. Hypoglycemia is a major stimulant of glucagon secretion, and hyperglycemia inhibits glucagon secretion. Glucose secretagogues are more effective when hyperglycemia is not present. A mixture of amino acids or a protein meal stimulates glucagon secretion. Most amino acids stimulate both insulin and glucagon secretions. There are certain amino acids, such as alanine and arginine, which are potent stimulants of glucagon. Arginine stimulates insulin secretions as well, whereas alanine is only a weak stimulant of insulin secretion. Leucine stimulates insulin secretion but is an ineffective α cell stimulant. Fatty acids also have been reported to reduce glucagon secretion. The physiological significance of the fatty acid effect on glucagon secretion is incompletely understood.

Mechanism of Action and Effects

Glucagon binds to its receptor and activates adenylate cyclase through a cascade of reactions, resulting in cAMP. This further activates cAMP-dependent protein kinase, leading to phosphorylation of key enzymes, leading to glycogenolysis and increasing glycogenesis. Glucagon also stimulates ketogenesis. Glucagon action is modulated by insulin. Therefore, it is believed that the glucagon action depends on the relative concentrations of glucagon to insulin.

Glucagon action is modulated by insulin.

Plasma glucagon levels are elevated in insulin-deficient Type I diabetic patients and in a variety of stress conditions, such as trauma, burns, surgery, and bacterial infections. Glucagon-producing tumors in the pancreas are associated with the highest plasma concentrations of glucagon.

Pharmacokinetics, Therapeutic Uses, and Undesirable Side Effects

Glucagon is available in 1 or 10 ml vials as a dry powder. It is dissolved easily in water. It is an unstable peptide hormone and, therefore, has to be used immediately after it is made into a solution. It circulates in the body fluids bound to protein. If infusion of glucagon is desired, glucagon has to be dissolved in a solution containing albumin.

Glucagon's main therapeutic use is in the emergency treatment of hypoglycemic coma in insulin-treated diabatic patients. It can be given IV for rapid action, but it may also be given IM or subcutaneously. Because prolonged hypoglycemia is life-threatening and glucagon is a powerful glucose stimulant, prudent use of glucagon can be life-saving.

Glucagon's main therapeutic use is emergency treatment of hypoglycemic coma in insulin-treated diabetics.

Glucagon causes nausea and vomiting in some patients and, therefore, carries the risk of aspiration in unconscious patients.

References

Banerge MA, Lebowitz HE: Insulin-sensitive and insulin resistant variants in NIDDM. Diabetes 38:84–92, 1989.

Binder C, Lauritzen T, Faber O, Pramming S: Insulin pharmacokinetics. Diabetes Care 7:188–199, 1984.

Cryer PE, Gerich JE: Glucose counterregulation during intensive insulin therapy in diabetes mellitus. N Eng J Med 312:232–241, 1985.

Czeck MP: The nature and regulation of the insulin receptor: Structure and function. Annu Rev Physiol 47:357–381, 1985.

Felig P: Physiologic action of insulin. In Ellenberg M, Riflan H (eds): Diabetes Mellitus, Theory and Practice. 3rd ed, 77–96. New York: Medical Examination Publishing, 1983.

Foster D, McGarry JD: The metabolic derangements and treatment of diabetes keto-acidosis. N Engl J Med 309:159–169, 1983.

Gerich JE: Somatostatin and Diabetes. Am J Med 70:619–626, 1981.

Geyelin HR, Harrop G, Murray MF, et al: The use of insulin in juvenile diabetes. J Metab Res 2:767–791, 1922.

Kahn CB: Advances in insulin therapy of diabetes mellitus. In Brownlee M (ed): Handbook of Diabetes Mellitus, Current and Future Therapies, Vol 5, 75–94. New York: John Wiley & Sons, 1981.

Kahn CR: The molecular mechanism of insulin action. Annu Rev Med 36:429–451, 1985.

Karnieli E, Zarnowski MJ, Hissin PJ, et al: Insulin-stimulated translocation of glucose transport systems in the isolated rat adipose cell: Time course, reversal, insulin concentration-dependency and relationship to glucose transport activity. J Biol Chem 256:4772–4777, 1981.

Khardori R, Soler NG: Hyperosmolar hyperglycemic nonketotic syndrome. Am J Med 77:899–904, 1984.

Kitabchi AE: Pro-insulin and C-peptide: A review. Metabolism 26:547–587, 1977.

Lockwood DH, Ferick JE, Goldfine I: Effects of oral hypoglycemic agents on receptor and post receptor actions of insulin. Diabetes Care (Suppl) 7:1–2, 1984.

Melander A: Clinical pharmacology of sulfonylureas. Metabolism 36:12–16, 1987.

Nair KS, Halliday D: Energy and protein metabolism in diabetes and obesity. In Garrow JS, Halliday D (eds): Substrate and Energy Metabolism in Man, 195–202. London: John Libbey, 1985.

Nair KS, Halliday D, Matthews DE, Welle SL: Hyperglucagonemia during insulin deficiency accelerates protein catabolism. Am J Physiol 253:E208–213, 1987.

National Diabetes Data Group: Classification and diagnosis of diabetes mellitus and other categories of glucose intolerance. Diabetes 28:1039–1057, 1979.

Osei K: Concomitant insulin and sulfonylurea therapy in patients with type II diabetes —Effects on glucoregulation and lipid metabolism. Am J Med 77:1002–1009, 1984.

Owen OE, Den G: Insulin and sufonylurea agents in noninsulin dependent diabetes mellitus. Arch Intern Med 146:673, 1986.

Reaven GM: Role of insulin resistance in human disease. Diabetes 37:1595–1607, 1988.

Rizza RA, Greene DA: Diabetes mellitus. Med Clin North Am 72:1–1576, 1988.

Robbins DC, Tager HS, Rubenstein AH: Biologic and clinical importance of proinsulin. N Engl J Med 310:1165–1175, 1984.

Simpson IA, Cushman SW: Hormonal regulation of mammalian glucose transport. Annu Rev Biochem 55:1059–1089, 1986.

Sims DF, Sims EAH (eds): Motivation, adherence and the therapeutic alliance. Diabetes spectrum: From research to practice. Am Diabetes Assoc Jan/Feb: 17–52, 1989.

Skyler JS: Insulin pharmacology. Med Clin North Am 72:1337–1354, 1988.

Steiner DR: Insulin today. Diabetes 26:322–340, 1976.

Tamborlane WV, Sherwin RS, Genel M, et al: Restoration of normal lipid and amino acid metabolism in diabetic patients with a portable insulin infusion pump. Lancet 1:1258–1261, 1979.

Unger RH: Meticulous control of diabetes: Benefits, risks and precautions. Diabetes 3:479–483, 1982.

Unger RH, Orci L: Glucagon. *In* Ellenberg M, Riflan H (eds): Diabetes Mellitus, Theory and Practice. 3rd ed, 203–224. New York: Medical Examination Publishing, 1983.

Wrenshall GA, Hetenyi G, Feaby WR (eds): The Story of Insulin: Forty Years of Success Against Diabetes 767–792. Toronto: Max Reinhardt, 1962.

Young L, Koda-Kible MN: Applied Therapeutics: The Clinical Use of Drugs, 1674–1675. Spokane, WA: Applied Therapeutics, 1988.

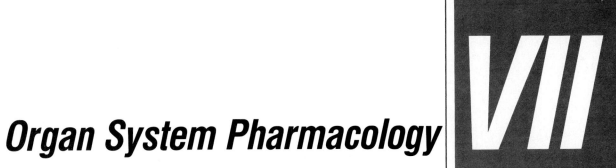

Organan System Pharmacology

VII

Gastrointestinal Drugs

Daniel S. Camara

45

The treatment of peptic ulcer disease (PUD) was formerly limited to the neutralization of acid by antacid preparations and the modest inhibition of acid production by anticholinergics. With the advent of H_2 receptor antagonists, namely cimetidine, a resurgence of interest took place in the development of new compounds for PUD. In this section, antacids, H_2 receptor antagonists, sucralfate, and other new modalities for the treatment of PUD are presented.

Peptic Ulcer Disease

SHORT REVIEW OF GASTRIC PHYSIOLOGY

Hydrochloric acid is produced by the parietal cells (oxyntic cells) in the gastric glands. These cells also secrete intrinsic factor for the absorption of vitamin B_{12}. Other cellular components of the gastric glands include the chief cell, the G cell, and the mucus cells. These cells are primarily responsible for the production of pepsinogen, gastrin, and mucus, respectively.

The regulation of acid secretion is the subject of complex orchestration of neuroendocrine influences. The parietal cell has three receptors in its surface: H_2 receptors for histamine, receptors for acetylcholine, and receptors for gastrin (Fig. 45–1). When histamine interacts with its receptor, it induces stimulation of adenylcyclase, resulting in an increased concentration of cellular cyclic adenosine monophosphate (AMP). This, in turn, activates a protein kinase that catalyzes the transfer of a high-energy phosphate from adenosine triphosphate (ATP) to a protein. This protein interacts with the enzyme H^+/K^+ ATPase (adenosine triphosphatase, the proton pump), resulting in secretion of hydrogen ion.

The other two receptors, when activated, increase the permeability of the cellular membrane to calcium, resulting in an increased secretion of hydrochloric acid (HCl) mediated by activation of the proton pump.

Mucus produced by the gastric gland adheres to the surface of the epithelium, immobilizing bicarbonate secreted by the surface cells. Mucus is composed of 95% water and 5% glycoprotein. The diffusion of a hydrogen ion through mucus is only one quarter of the diffusion rate through the gastric mucosa. Therefore, a pH gradient is generated by the mucus lining the surface of the gastric epithelium. The ability of the stomach to secrete acid and pepsin is dependent upon the maintenance of the cellular integrity of the gastric mucosa by the gastric mucosal barrier.

Acid secretion is initiated by the anticipation of eating (cephalic phase) with excitation of the vagus nerve liberating acetylcholine and gastrin, resulting in the activation of the parietal cell. Once the food reaches the stomach, distention of the antrum occurs with mucosal exposure to protein products. The exposure of the mucosa to protein products results in the release of gastrin (gastric phase) with the secretion of more HCl. With the

H^+/K^+ ATPase is also known as the *proton pump*.

Cephalic and gastric phases of acid secretion

Figure 45-1

Diagram of the parietal cell of the gastric mucosa illustrating the three types of membrane receptors and some of the bio-chemical pathways involved in the secretion of acid into the lumen of the stomach. (H_2=histamine receptor; ACh = acetylcholine receptor; G = gastrin receptor.)

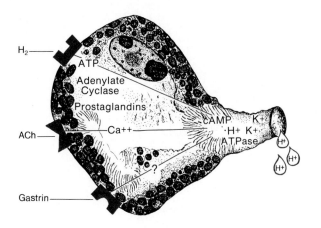

progression of the gastric digestive process a decrease in antral pH inhibits further release of gastrin. As the products of digestion and acid leave the stomach, duodenal acidification triggers the release of hormonal peptides, including secretin, which inhibits the gastric acid secretion.

ANTACIDS

Antacids have been the cornerstone of the treatment of peptic ulcer disease for many decades despite a paucity of controlled trials documenting their efficacy. Most of the popular preparations are mixtures of magnesium and aluminum hydroxide. The mechanism of action of these compounds involves the neutralization of acid by the following chemical reaction:

$$Al(OH)_3 + 3\ HCl \longrightarrow AlCl_3 + 3\ H_2O$$

$$Mg(OH)_2 + 2\ HCl \longrightarrow MgCl_2 + 2\ H_2O$$

$$NaHCO_3 + HCl \longrightarrow NaCl + H_2O + CO_2$$

Of note is the variability in the acid-neutralizing capacity (number of milliequivalents of 1 N HCl that can be brought to a pH of 3.5 in 15 minutes) and cost of the different preparations. Sodium bicarbonate (baking soda), although an effective antacid, should be avoided because of its rapid absorption, resulting in alkalosis and sodium overload. Calcium carbonate (the active ingredient of TUMS) in excess is associated with increased absorption of calcium, resulting in hypercalcemia, particularly in patients who consume an excessive amount of milk (milk alkali syndrome). Calcium carbonate preparations are associated also with rebound gastric hypersecretion due to the stimulation of gastrin release by the gastrin-producing cells in the stomach and upper small bowel.

Antacids are used primarily in the treatment of peptic diseases of the upper gastrointestinal (GI) tract. These include reflux esophagitis and gastric and duodenal ulcers. The value of antacids in the treatment of common dyspepsia has never been proved. In patients with chronic renal failure, aluminum hydroxide preparations are used to increase the absorption of calcium by reacting with phosphate.

Milk alkali syndrome represents the combination of peptic ulcer disease, hypercalcemia, and renal failure owing to excessive consumption of calcium salts.

Efficacy of antacids for dyspepsia has never been proved.

DOSAGE AND SIDE EFFECTS

Correct administration of antacids has been a subject of controversy for many years. There is a consensus that antacids should be given after meals,

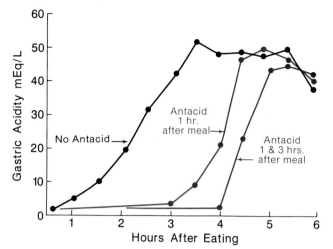

Figure 45-2

Effect of timing of antacid administration in relation to a meal on gastric acidity. Ordinate is gastric acidity expressed as milliequivalents per liter. The abscissa is hours after eating a meal. The *curve in black* on the left was obtained with no antacid, showing a maximal acid secretion within 3 hours following eating. Administration of antacid 1 hour after eating results *(curve in color, on left)* in a delay in the appearance of acid for more than 2 hours, with a peak after 4 hours. Administration of antacid at both 1 and 3 hours *(curve in color, on right)* further delays and reduces acid secretion.

ideally 1 and 3 hours after meals, so that the elevation of gastric pH can be maintained for a longer period of time. In an empty stomach the increase of gastric pH is transient; therefore, to effectively neutralize HCl, hourly dosages would be needed. Figure 45-2 illustrates the differences in the duration of effective gastric alkalization provided by different schedules of administration of the same amount of antacid. The recommended total dose of acid-neutralizing capacity in an antacid preparation ranges from 207 mM to 1008 mM. More recently antacid tablets have been shown to be effective in healing duodenal ulcers.

The primary factor limiting the use of high-dose antacid therapy is the frequent occurrence of diarrhea, decreasing patient compliance. Owing to both the inconvenience of taking liquid antacids and the associated side effects with poor compliance, antacids are rarely employed at the present time as the sole treatment for PUD. Other regimens are just as effective and associated with a higher patient compliance.

H_2 RECEPTOR ANTAGONISTS

The development of agents that selectively antagonize histamine at the level of its receptor in the parietal cell (H_2 blocker) emphasizes the importance of endogenous histamine in the control of acid secretion. Although H_2 receptors have been described in other organs and tissues, their main role is the histaminic modulation of acid secretion. Thus, the H_2 receptor blockers produce little interference with any other physiological mechanisms and are a remarkably safe family of drugs. Cimetidine became available in the United States in 1977, and since then more than 10 million patients have been treated with this drug worldwide, making it one of the most widely prescribed drugs in the world.

The chemical structure of H_2 receptor blockers bears some close resemblances to the structure of histamine and H_1 histamine antagonists (Chapter 65). Currently there are four H_2 receptor antagonists available on the market for the treatment of peptic ulcer disease: cimetidine, ranitidine, famotidine, and nizatidine. Ranitidine is 10 times more potent than cimetidine, whereas famotidine is 30 times more potent than cimetidine and 8 times more than ranitidine. Nizatidine is similar to ranitidine in potency and dosage. H_2 antagonists inhibit all aspects of gastric secretion (fasting, nocturnal, stimulated by meals, or pentagastrin). These agents are absorbed rapidly from the GI tract, with peak plasma concentration achieved 45-90 minutes after oral administration. These H_2 antagonists exhibit half-lives of approximately 1–2 hours. They are eliminated primarily by the kidneys and appear in the urine more than 60% unchanged.

Indications

Numerous studies have demonstrated the efficacy of H_2 antagonists in the treatment of duodenal and gastric ulcers. Approximately 80% of the ulcers are healed after 4–6 weeks of treatment. Other indications for H_2 antagonists include the treatment of hypersecretory syndromes (Zollinger-Ellison syndrome), systemic mastocytosis, basophilic leukemia, preoperative prevention of aspiration pneumonia, coadjuvant treatment of pancreatic insufficiency, prevention of stress gastritis, and treatment of reflux esophagitis.

Side Effects

These drugs have a remarkable safety record, and the great majority of patients have no side effects. Cimetidine, owing to its inhibition of P-450 cytochrome oxidase system of the liver, can induce a prolongation of the action of many drugs that are metabolized by this system. Attention to signs of toxicity and monitoring of serum levels should be obtained when cimetidine is used concomitantly with warfarin, phenytoin, diazepam, chlordiazepoxide, theophylline, and lidocaine. Other H_2 blockers do not appear to interfere with the P-450 system and, therefore, are associated with less potential for drug interactions. Rare cases of thrombocytopenia, hepatitis, and bone marrow suppression have been described. Changes in mental status characterized by confusion, disorientation, and coma have been described in patients using high dosages of the parenteral form of cimetidine, usually in intensive care patients with liver and renal failure. These symptoms usually subside upon discontinuation of drug administration.

Although H_2 antagonists suppress all types of acid stimuli, several studies have demonstrated the important role played by nocturnal acid secretion in the pathogenesis of PUD. Figure 45–3 depicts the gastric pH over 24-hour periods in subjects taking placebo or different dosages of cimetidine. These profiles demonstrate that the major deviation from pla-

Figure 45–3

Temporal pattern of the acid secretion as modified by different regimens and dosages of the H_2 blocker, cimetidine. Ordinate is the mean hydrogen ion secretion per hour. The abscissa is time plotted as a 24-hour clock divided into the periods over which the acid secretion was measured: morning from 0730 to 1230; afternoon from 1230 to 1630; night from 0030 to 1730. In the placebo condition *(black circles)*, acid secretion was high during all three periods. Cimetidine given twice a day (400 mg b.i.d. *[colored circles]*) reduced acid production at all three time periods. Administration of single daily doses of cimetidine at bedtime (800 mg and 1600 mg h.s. *[colored squares and colored triangles, respectively]*) was effective in reducing nocturnal acid secretion to almost zero. Total acid secretion over 24 hours was approximately the same for all three of the cimetidine dosage regimens.

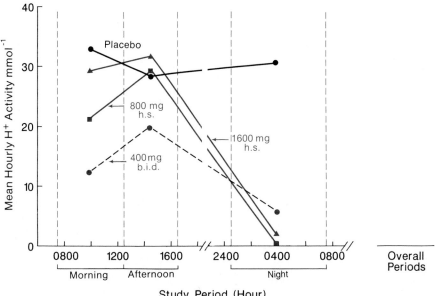

cebo treatment is the acid secretion occurring at night. Based on these observations a number of studies have established the effectiveness of different doses of H_2 antagonists given as a single nightly dose (cimetidine 800 mg; ranitidine 300 mg; famotidine 40 mg). This effectiveness highlights the importance of the suppression of nocturnal acid secretion, because the healing rates were similar to the traditional multiple daily doses. Furthermore, a single nightly dose improves patient compliance.

Once-a-day pills result in better compliance than that achieved with multiple doses each day.

ANTICHOLINERGICS

Anticholinergics have been available for many years for the treatment of gastric and duodenal disorders. These drugs are described in more detail in Chapter 11. Their mechanism of action involves the competitive antagonism of acetylcholine with a resultant decrease in acid secretion. The high incidence of side effects such as dry mouth, precipitation of glaucoma, and urinary retention limits their use for the treatment of peptic ulcer disease. Propantheline is used occasionally with H_2 receptor antagonists in the treatment of hypersecretory syndromes.

SUCRALFATE

Sucralfate (CARAFATE) is a basic aluminum salt of sucrose substituted with eight sulfate groups. In an acid environment some of the $Al_2(OH)_5$ ions dissociate, forming the polymer sucrose octosulfate. This polymeric viscous substance is thought to adhere to denatured proteins in the base of the ulcer. A barrier is thus formed protecting the ulcer from further aggression by pepsin and HCl. Sucralfate has six to seven times more affinity for the ulcerated mucosa than the normal mucosa. However, this mechanism of action has been recently challenged by experimental evidence showing that sucralfate has cytoprotective properties. The use of sucralfate is associated also with increased production in the gastric mucosa of prostaglandins, bicarbonate, and increased thickening of the mucus covering the gastric epithelium. Numerous studies have demonstrated that this drug is superior to placebo and is as effective as H_2 antagonists in the treatment of PUD. Sucralfate is not absorbed by the GI tract, and side effects such as constipation occur in less than 5% of the patients studied.

DRUGS AND TREATMENTS OF THE FUTURE

The substituted benzimidazoles represent a new approach for the control of gastric acid secretion. These compounds irreversibly inactivate the enzyme H^+/K^+ ATPase (proton pump) in the secretory membrane of the parietal cell, which represents the final step in the secretion of hydrogen ion. A single dose of omeprazole (the first substituted benzimidazole to undergo clinical trials) can suppress the production of HCl for 24–48 hours. These drugs may have an important role in the treatment of hypersecretory states and gastroesophageal reflux disease.

Zollinger-Ellison syndrome is produced by a tumor of the gastrin-producing cells resulting in extremely high serum concentration of gastrin (over 1000 pg/ml). This results in gastric acid hypersecretion and severe PUD, frequently associated with complications (e.g., perforation, bleeding).

A new anticholinergic (pirenzepine) that selectively blocks the gastric muscarinic receptors will soon become available in the United States for the treatment of PUD. The incidence of traditional anticholinergic side effects is reported to be less.

Several derivatives of natural-occurring prostaglandins have been developed for the treatment of PUD. Prostaglandins are derived from the metabolism of arachidonic acid catalyzed by the enzyme cyclooxygenase. These products participate in a variety of biological activities affecting many organs and organ systems. In the gastric mucosa they inhibit produc-

Cytoprotection is defined as the ability of certain drugs (prostaglandin, sucralfate, and others) to protect the mucosa under the surface epithelium from the damaging effects of a variety of noxious agents (100% alcohol, 25% NaCl, and even boiling water).

tion of HCl when given in pharmacological dosages. PGE_2 has been shown to be as effective as the H_2 antagonists in the treatment of PUD. Furthermore, prostaglandins appear to be the primary compounds responsible for cytoprotective action.

These prostaglandin derivatives have a potential use for the treatment of lesions in the upper GI tract produced by aspirin and other nonsteroidal anti-inflammatory drugs inasmuch as prostaglandin deficiency appears to be an important pathophysiological factor in their development. Prostaglandin and sucralfate represent new approaches in the treatment of PUD, e.g., they enhance mucosal defense.

Laxatives

Rarely in medicine is there an absolute indication for the use of laxatives. A high-fiber, well-balanced diet rich in fruits and vegetables supplemented by bran should be enough to normalize bowel function. The fear of autointoxication and the constant concern of many patients regarding the frequency and quality of bowel movements make laxatives one of the most popular over-the-counter drugs on the market with serious potential for user abuse. Accepted indications for laxatives and stool softeners include preparation for diagnostic colonic examination (barium enema, colonoscopy); treatment of anorectal disorders (anal fissures, hemorrhoids); and prevention of hepatic encephalopathy. Laxatives can be divided into bulk, osmotic, and irritant (or stimulant).

IRRITANT LAXATIVES

Castor Oil. The irritant laxative mode of action usually involves interference with normal function of the small bowel and colon, usually reversing the primary absorptive function into a secretory function. Castor oil's active moiety is ricinoleic acid (a hydroxy fatty acid) that evokes the secretion of water and electrolytes in the colon and small bowel. It also increases small bowel peristaltic activity. Castor oil is commonly used for preparation of patients to undergo diagnostic colonic examination such as barium enema and colonoscopy.

Bile Salts. Bile salts in general have laxative properties, although they are not commercially available as such. One of the major side effects of the use of chenodeoxycholic acid used for the dissolution of cholesterol gallstones is diarrhea. The diarrhea is due to the following mechanisms:

- unconjugated bile salts induce active electrolyte secretion, stimulating adenylate cyclase activities, and increase intestinal cyclic AMP;
- increase in intestinal motility;
- increase in intestinal permeability.

In the colon, unconjugated bile acid reduces absorptive capacity and induces water and electrolyte secretion.

Bisacodyl. Bisacodyl, the active ingredient of DULCOLAX, is an effective laxative. It has different modes of action that include decreased water and glucose absorption in the colon and small bowel, and a stimulatory effect on small bowel peristalsis.

Phenolphthalein. Structurally similar to bisacodyl, phenolphthalein is present in a variety of commonly available laxatives. Its mode of action involves the interference with absorption at different levels of the GI tract. In experimental animals it decreases the sodium and glucose absorption in the small bowel. This drug affects intestinal motility also.

As indicated earlier none of the irritant laxatives has absolute indications in medicine. Moreover, chronic use may be responsible for colonic atonia and inability to have spontaneous bowel movements (cathartic colon).

OSMOTIC LAXATIVES

The mode of action of these agents is based on the increase in stool osmolarity, thus water is trapped in the stool resulting in its reduced consistency. A combination of polyethylene glycol and electrolytes (COLYTE or GOLYTELY) is used now for the preparation of diagnostic procedures of the colon (barium enema or endoscopy). The advantage of colonic lavage is the reduction of the time needed for preparation of the patients. Instead of 2 days of clear liquids and administration of castor oil or bisacodyl, patients ingest 1 gallon of this solution the evening before or a few hours before the procedure, resulting in an outstanding preparation.

BULK LAXATIVES

Bulk laxatives, such as the derivatives of psyllium seeds (e.g., METAMUCIL, KONSYL), natural bran, semisynthetic cellulose, or gum, are substances poorly absorbed through the GI tract, thus causing a retention of water in the lumen, increasing the volume and decreasing the consistency of the fecal bolus. If clinically required, these are the drugs of choice for the treatment of chronic constipation.

MINERAL OIL

Mineral oil has been used extensively as an over-the-counter preparation, most commonly in children with chronic constipation. It is composed of a mixture of aliphatic hydrocarbons derived from petroleum. It is not absorbed from the GI tract, and after 2 – 3 days it softens the stools and may interfere with colonic absorption of water. It also interferes with the absorption of fat-soluble vitamins, and its administration presents the risk of aspiration.

Antidiarrheal Drugs

Acute diarrhea of infectious etiology is a common clinical problem, particularly in underdeveloped countries, where it is a major cause of mortality in children. Diarrhea should be approached as a symptom rather than a disease. There is a long list of causes of diarrhea, ranging from a self-limited viral gastroenteritis lasting 2 – 3 days, to a severe malabsorptive state such as that secondary to pancreatic insufficiency, or celiac disease characterized by a prolonged, protracted diarrhea lasting several months or years. Acute diarrhea of an infectious etiology (viral or bacterial) lasts no more than 3 – 5 days. Most of the patients affected do not require any therapy and do not seek medical help. Occasionally in elderly patients or in young children excessive fluid losses induce dehydration requiring parenteral fluids.

Whenever one approaches a patient with diarrhea it is important to find out if the process is acute (less than 2 weeks) or chronic; if there is a recent travel history (ameba, *Giardia lamblia*, or traveler's diarrhea secondary to enterotoxigenic *Escherichia coli* [ETEC] should be considered); if there are associated symptoms such as fever and malaise, features suggestive of an infectious process. It is also important to examine the stools, particularly for the presence of blood (acute infection or idiopathic colitis) and fecal leukocytes. The initial work-up includes examination of the stools

All diseases associated with reactive mucosal inflammation are associated with the leukocytes in stool.

for ova and parasites, routine cultures (including *Salmonella, Shigella, Campylobacter jejuni,* and *Yersinia enterocolitica*), and stools for fecal leukocytes.

The presence of fecal leukocytes is helpful in distinguishing patients with infectious diarrhea (with the exception of viral and traveler's diarrhea) from patients with irritable bowel. In the latter, no fecal leukocytes will be observed. Sigmoidoscopy and biopsy are performed occasionally. The typical bacteria responsible for acute diarrhea are *C. jejuni, Shigella, Salmonella,* and *Y. enterocolitica*. These organisms invade the GI mucosa producing an inflammatory reaction that interferes with normal absorption of fluids and nutrients with stimulation of peristalsis, resulting in an excessive number of bowel movements. Other bacteria are not directly cytopathic but elaborate enterotoxins, resulting in diarrhea devoid of intestinal mucosal inflammation. Typical organisms include ETEC (traveler's diarrhea), *Vibrio cholerae, Clostridium perfringens,* and others.

PHARMACOTHERAPY

Most of the acute infectious diarrheas do not require specific therapy because they are usually self-limited. The general approach should be prevention and treatment of dehydration (patients should be on a low-fiber diet, avoiding salads, fruits, and milk products); occasionally nonspecific and antimicrobial treatment may be necessary due to severe symptoms.

Antimotility Drugs

Derivatives of opiates (paregoric, codeine, diphenoxylate plus atropine [LOMOTIL] or loperamide [IMODIUM]) are used for the treatment of diarrhea. The mechanisms of action of these agents involve decreased peristalsis, increased bowel capacity secondary to a reduction in smooth muscle tone, and possibly antisecretory action resulting from interaction with intestinal opiate receptors. Loperamide has a particular advantage over the other agents owing to its inability to cross the blood-brain barrier; therefore, it has less potential for abuse when compared with codeine or paregoric (see Chapter 18). These agents should be avoided in patients with acute *Salmonella, Shigella,* or *Campylobacter* infections because they may prolong the febrile state, malaise, and passage of bloody stools.

Bismuth Subsalicylate

This drug is used in the prevention and treatment of traveler's diarrhea secondary to ETEC. Bismuth subsalicylate (the active ingredient in PEPTO-BISMOL) appears to inhibit the effects of the ETEC toxin in the gut in addition to a possible direct antibacterial effect. Liquid PEPTO-BISMOL can be used for the prevention and treatment of traveler's diarrhea.

Inert Compounds

Kaolin (hydrated aluminum silicate) is claimed to absorb water and toxins and decrease the amount of free water in the GI tract and, therefore, reduce the number of stools in a diarrheal state. Other aluminum salts such as aluminum hydroxide (AMPHOJEL) are known to have a constipating effect directly related to the aluminum component. Other products derived of plants and their fruits include polygacturonic acid and pectins. These products are not absorbed in the small bowel but are degraded by the colonic bacteria, producing short-chain fatty acids. These short-chain fatty acids (propionate, acetic, and butyrate) facilitate the absorption of sodium and water from the colon. KAOPECTATE (kaolin plus pectin) is a common over-the-counter preparation used in diarrheal illnesses; however, studies definitively documenting its efficacy are lacking.

Specific Therapy—Antibiotics

Only rarely are antibiotics used for the treatment of diarrhea. Again, children and elderly patients with severe diarrhea associated with systemic manifestations such as fever, dehydration, and occasionally bacteremia are exceptions to this statement. In these cases the antibiotics should be specific to the bacterial pathogen (see Part VIII).

Metoclopramide

Metoclopramide (REGLAN) is a dopamine antagonist that sensitizes the intestinal smooth muscle to the effects of acetylcholine. The combination of the central nervous system dopamine antagonism resulting in increasing the vomiting threshold and the acceleration of gastric emptying makes this drug a unique antiemetic. As a smooth muscle stimulant it raises the lower esophageal sphincter pressure and decreases gastric transit time. Because of these properties metoclopramide has been used with success in the treatment of reflux esophagitis and gastric stasis syndromes. The drug is rapidly absorbed, achieving peak plasma concentrations within 40–120 minutes. The usual dosage is 10 mg orally three to four times a day. Side effects can be relatively common, particularly when used in high doses for prolonged periods of time; these include somnolence, nervousness, and dystonic extrapyramidal reactions.

References

Banwell JG: Non-specific therapy. *In* Gorbach SL (ed): Infectious Diarrhea, 219–225. Cambridge, MA: Blackwell Scientific Publications, 1986.

Bongiovanni GL, Giannella RA: Acute infectious diarrhea. *In* Bayless TM (ed): Current Therapy in Gastroenterology and Liver Disease, Vol 2, 253–257. St Louis: CV Mosby, 1986.

Danowitz M: Current concepts of laxative action. J Clin Gastroenterol 1:77–84, 1979.

Farley A, Levesque P, Pare ABN, et al: Comparative trial of ranitidine 300 mg at night with ranitidine 150 mg twice a day in the treatment of duodenal and gastric ulcer. Am J Gastroenterol 80:665–668, 1985.

Fordtran JS, Morawski SF, Richardson CT: *In vivo* and *in vitro* evaluation of liquid antacids. N Engl J Med 288:923–928, 1973.

Freston JW: Cimetidine. I. Development, pharmacology and efficacy. Ann Intern Med 97:573–580, 1982.

Freston JW: Cimetidine. II. Adverse reactions and patterns of use. Ann Intern Med 97:728–734, 1982.

Kumar N, Vij JC, Karol A, et al: Controlled therapeutic trial to determine the optimum dose of antacids in duodenal ulcer. Gut 25:1199–1202, 1984.

Peterson WL, Sturdevant RAL, Frankl HD, et al: Healing of duodenal ulcer with an antacid regimen. N Engl J Med 297:341–345, 1977.

Sack RB: The treatment of diarrhea with antibiotics. *In* Gorbach SL (ed): Infectious Diarrhea, 227–236. Cambridge, MA: Blackwell Scientific Publications, 1986.

Schulze-Delrieu K: Metoclopramide. N Engl J Med 305:28–33, 1981.

Shuster MM: Evaluation and treatment of chronic constipation. Practical Gastroenterol 10:15–18, 1986.

Tytgat GNJ, Hameetma W, Van Olffen GH: Sucralfate, bismuth compounds and substituted benzimidazoles, tripramine and pirenzepine in the short and long term treatment of duodenal ulcer. Clin Gastroenterol 13:543–566, 1984.

46

Drugs Acting on the Blood and Blood-Forming Organs

Richard E. Bettigole

Substances absorbed or injected into our bodies are transported usually in the blood. Thus, they and their metabolites easily can affect the red cells, white cells, platelets and plasma, as well as all the tissues to which the blood circulates. This chapter concentrates on drugs used to treat anemia and on drugs affecting the hemostatic system.

Anemia

Anemia defined

Anemia is defined as a hemoglobin level or hematocrit (packed red cell volume) more than two standard deviations below the mean for healthy individuals the same age and sex as the patient. By this definition, assuming a normal distribution, 2.5% of healthy individuals are anemic (and 2.5% are polycythemic).

MECHANISMS OF ANEMIA

Causes

Anemia almost always results from blood loss, decreased red cell production, decreased red cell survival, or some combination of these. A rare cause is a rapid expansion of the blood volume (intravascular volume) as may be seen in young children with sickle cell anemia whose spleens can enlarge rapidly in what is called a sequestration crisis. Average red cell survival is about 120 days (with variation from person to person).

Red cell production

Red cells are produced normally in bone marrow. The otherwise healthy person's response to chronic tissue hypoxia is to increase the production of erythropoietin by the kidneys. This glycoprotein stimulates stem cells in the bone marrow to differentiate into red cell precursors, which as they divide and mature eventually extrude their nuclei, leave the bone marrow, and enter the blood circulation.

There is a stimulus to red cell production also simply as a result of increased red cell destruction or even chronic blood loss without anemia or oxygen lack in the tissues of the body. The physiological mechanism for this is unknown. For example, a nonhypoxemic person with a compensated hemolytic anemia (normal hemoglobin and hematocrit, increased red cell production, and increased red cell destruction) clearly has increased erythropoiesis but no tissue hypoxia. Similarly, a healthy person who donates blood frequently but whose iron stores are maintained will have reticulocytosis without anemia.

Iron Deficiency

Iron is an essential component not only of hemoglobin but also of myoglobin and of numerous enzymes essential for human metabolism. However, iron deficiency, even when it is severe, does not seem to show itself clinically except as anemia. Iron has been used for the treatment of anemia for over 2000 years.

Total body iron in adults is 3–5 g of which 0.5 g or less is in myoglobin and iron-containing enzymes. Depending on the blood volume and the hematocrit, about 1.5–3 g of iron exist as hemoglobin in red cells. Iron stores average about 0.5–1.5 g. Iron deficiency causes a hypochromic, microcytic anemia with a mean red cell volume (MCV) usually well below normal.

Iron stores

Humans have no known excretory system for iron. Healthy people have about 0.5 mg iron/ml blood (depending on the hemoglobin level in the blood). Blood loss is the main cause of iron deficiency in older children and adults. Menstruating women lose, and therefore require, about 1–2 mg iron daily, whereas men and nonmenstruating women need only half that amount. The amount of menstrual blood loss varies widely, however, even in women who consider their menstrual cycles entirely normal. Absent iron stores and anemia due to iron deficiency are rather frequent among menstruating women.

Iron requirements

In infancy and childhood when body growth is rapid, the need to fill the expanding blood volume can easily lead to iron deficiency despite the absence of blood loss unless foods other than milk are started in a timely fashion. In adults, nutritional iron deficiency for practical purposes is never seen and *iron deficiency means blood loss.* It cannot be stressed too often that in adults *iron deficiency anemia is not a disease; it is a sign of blood loss.*

Iron-containing compounds are useful in the treatment of anemia due to iron deficiency and as a dietary supplement for pregnant women.

Absorption. Over one third of ingested heme iron is absorbed, compared with only about one twentieth or less of nonheme iron in adults with normal iron stores. Vitamin C and meat increase the absorption of nonheme iron. Thus, diets vary in the bioavailability of iron. In addition, with increasing iron stores, the absorption of dietary iron is increasingly inhibited. With adequate iron stores, iron absorption is less than 5% whether the bioavailability of nonheme iron in the diet is low, average, or high. But when iron stores are absent, absorption of nonheme dietary iron is less than 5% from a diet with low iron bioavailability but 15% or more when bioavailability is high. This variable block in active transport of ferrous iron by the mucosal cells of the duodenum and the first portion of the jejunum is known as the *mucosal block.*

Iron absorption

Iron Transport. Absorbed ferrous iron is bound to transferrin, a plasma protein produced by hepatic cells. Transferrin is measured in the clinical laboratory by its ability to bind iron and is reported as total iron-binding capacity (TIBC). Iron deficiency in otherwise healthy individuals leads to a fall in serum iron and a rise in transferrin (TIBC), so that the percent of plasma iron saturation, which normally is about 30–35%, falls to less than 13% in iron deficiency. (In acute and chronic illnesses, serum iron *and* TIBC fall, so despite the low serum iron, the percent of iron saturation usually exceeds 13%.)

Iron transport

Iron from transferrin is used either in heme synthesis (one atom of iron in each heme group, four of which, combined with four globin chains, form the tetramer called a hemoglobin molecule) or is stored in the reticuloendothelial system, hepatocytes, and elsewhere in the protein *ferritin* as single molecules or as microscopically visible aggregates known as *hemosiderin.*

Iron storage

Over 80% of the iron used to produce red cells normally comes from heme iron derived from the roughly 1% of those red cells that, having lived out their life span, are destroyed daily. Much of the rest comes from transferrin-bound, newly absorbed dietary iron. Therefore, the iron stores normally lie relatively undisturbed unless there is a deficiency in iron. The rate of clearance of iron from plasma is high in iron deficiency and low when iron stores are ample.

In iron deficiency serum ferritin levels are low; in iron overload levels are quite high. However, serum ferritin is a *reactive protein* (like fibrinogen, haptoglobin, Factor VIII) and tends to rise with acute or chronic illness; therefore, although a low serum level of ferritin is good evidence of iron deficiency, a normal ferritin may not rule it out.

Iron deficiency is present in many millions of people all over the world. Even in prosperous nations with good nutrition and medical care, many infants and many women in the years between menarche and menopause are iron-deficient. *Iron deficiency always should be suspected* when there is microcytosis (small red cells), even without overt anemia. The other common causes of microcytosis are the thalassemia syndromes. Even with an obvious possible cause of iron deficiency such as excessive menstrual blood loss, gastrointestinal (GI) blood loss may be a factor also. *One possible cause of iron deficiency does not relieve one of the responsibility to search for other causes.*

IRON PREPARATIONS

Oral. Ferrous salts are better absorbed than ferric salts. *Ferrous sulfate* has about the same bioavailability as other ferrous compounds when calculated as milligrams of iron. The usual therapeutic dosage is $2-3$ mg/kg of iron. For ferrous sulfate ($FeSO_4 7H_2O$) iron is about 20% by weight, so for a 50 kg woman the $FeSO_4$ dosage would be $50 \times 5 \times 2 - 50 \times 5 \times 3 = 500 - 750$ mg/day. In actual practice 300 mg three times a day (900 mg) is a widely used dosage regardless of the adult patient's size. Dosage probably should be adjusted more often for the weight of adult patients, as of course it always must be for children. *As the dosage of iron is increased, the percent that is absorbed decreases.* At the usual adult dosage of about 180 mg/day of iron (300 mg three times a day of $FeSO_4$), about $15-20\%$ is absorbed ($27-36$ mg). At a dosage of 60 mg (one 300 mg $FeSO_4$ tablet), probably $25-30\%$ is absorbed ($15-18$ mg). Thus, cutting the dosage to one third only cuts the absorbed amount by about one half.

Duration of Treatment With Oral Iron

Correction of anemia caused by iron deficiency by the use of oral iron in an otherwise healthy adult can take up to 2 months, assuming iron absorption is normal and there is no continuing loss of blood. If blood loss continues or if there are additional illnesses, return to a normal hemoglobin level may take longer or may not take place at all. Assuming that blood loss due to abnormal conditions is not continuing, *the oral therapy is continued usually from 3 to 6 months after the hemoglobin has returned to normal in order to replenish iron stores.* Because the rate of iron absorption decreases as iron stores increase, this kind of prolonged therapy is needed in order to replace iron stores.

Side Effects of Oral Preparations of Iron

Intolerance to oral preparations of iron is mainly a function of the iron content of the particular medication. Some studies have shown relatively few side effects of oral iron compared to placebo. Side effects relate mainly

Iron turnover

Serum ferritin

Iron deficiency

Oral iron therapy

to the abdomen and GI tract and include abdominal distress, constipation, diarrhea, and nausea. If there has been a history of intolerance to oral iron, or if the anemia is not severe, therapy can be started with a small dosage, gradually increasing the dosage to the desired level. Symptoms are reported by about one fourth of treated individuals compared with about one seventh of controls receiving placebos. However, this is at a dosage delivering approximately 200 mg of iron per day (300 mg of ferrous sulfate taken three times a day delivers approximately 180 mg of iron/day).

Iatrogenic Iron Overload. Long-term toxicity may result from continued administration of oral iron in therapeutic amounts to patients who are not iron deficient, with the gradual production of an overload of iron. This has resulted, in general, either from the careless notion that all anemia should be treated with iron, or that all microcytic anemia should be treated with iron. Thalassemia minor affects millions of people on every continent. Although it is seen most often in the United States in black people and Italian Americans, it is widespread in people from Greece, India, Southeast Asia, and China and occurs also in many other populations. These people with α or β thalassemia syndromes have microcytic (small) red cells and usually have little or no anemia. Unless they are iron deficient also, oral iron therapy is inappropriate and can lead over a period of years to iron overload. This form of iron toxicity can never be justified.

It is vital to establish whether or not an anemia is due to iron deficiency, for a diagnosis of iron deficiency means an obligation to seek the source of the blood loss, except in growing infants who are known to lack the usual dietary sources of iron.

IRON POISONING

Iron poisoning due to the ingestion of large amounts of ferrous salts of iron is a fairly common cause of childhood poisoning in infants in some parts of the world, although not particularly common in the United States. Iron pills are dispensed often in bottles of 100. The availability of oral iron preparations in many households, whether for the treatment of iron deficiency or as an iron supplement during pregnancy, makes the problem a difficult one. The use of childproof containers has helped greatly in preventing this form of poisoning.

Ferrous salts are directly toxic to the upper GI tract, and signs of a toxic overdose occur often within an hour or less, although they may be delayed for several hours longer. Nausea and vomiting (often of grayish black or bloody stomach contents) may occur, with abdominal pain and diarrhea. In patients who die, there is hepatocellular damage with a diffuse hemorrhagic lesion of the GI tract.

Treatment of Iron Poisoning

Iron pills are opaque to x-rays and may be seen in x-rays of the abdomen. If the serum iron is less than 500 μg/dl, there should not be immediate danger. However, often emergency measurement of serum iron is not available.

The iron-chelating agent *deferoxamine* is available as 500 mg vials of deferoxamine mesylate. It can be given intravenously (IV) if the patient is hypotensive but usually is given intramuscularly (IM) at an initial dose of 1 g followed by 500 mg 4 hours and 8 hours after the initial dose. Depending on the clinical response, injections may be continued, but it has been recommended that the dosage not exceed 6 g/day. The IV route is used only for patients in shock with an infusion rate that *does not exceed*

Side effects

Avoid iron overload.

Iron toxicity

Deferoxamine

15 mg/kg/hour, with return to the IM route as soon as hypotension is no longer a problem.

Deferoxamine is used also in subcutaneous infusions with a battery-powered pump worn on the forearm of the patient. This has been useful in preventing and treating iron accumulation in patients such as those with thalassemia major who receive transfusions throughout their lives. Remembering that each blood transfusion contains about 250 mg of iron, it is easy to see that an adult getting 40 or 50 units a year is getting around 10–12 g of iron per year. Because the maximal excretion of iron, even in the iron-loaded adult, is only about 10 mg a day, maximum iron excretion is less than 4 g per year. In patients requiring continuing transfusions, phlebotomy obviously is not an available means of decreasing body iron. Subcutaneous infusion of deferoxamine is currently extending the lives and preserving the health of many patients with thalassemia major, but its chronic use is not without problems, including allergic reactions, abdominal pain, and cataracts.

PARENTERAL IRON THERAPY

Parenteral iron therapy

Iron dextran injection has been available in the United States for many years. During most of this time, it was available only in a preparation recommended for IM use. Despite this, the IM preparation was used IV, particularly in the Third World, as a means of rapid replacement of the total iron deficit in iron deficient individuals. It is available now both as an IM preparation containing 0.5% phenol and in 2 ml ampules containing 50 mg/ml of iron for IM or IV administration. The iron from iron dextran must be processed by the body before it becomes available for hematopoiesis. The compound is taken in by reticuloendothelial cells where the sugar portion of the complex is removed and the iron becomes available. The iron gradually leaves the reticuloendothelial cells then, becoming bound to transferrin, but the availability of the administered iron dextran takes weeks to months to become complete. IM injection is usually in the buttock, using a *Z track injection* to prevent leakage of the material to the skin where it can discolor the skin surface. At 2 ml/injection, which is the usual dose, it takes 20 injections to give the patient 2 g of iron if that is the goal in replacing iron stores.

There may be severe reactions to parenteral iron dextran.

Severe reactions to parenteral iron dextran have been recorded, including a few fatal anaphylactic reactions. Other reported reactions include joint pain, hives, headache, and fever. Thus there must be specific indications for the parenteral administration of iron.

Intravenous Iron Dextran

IV iron dextran is an option if oral administration is to be avoided.

When the physician believes an iron-deficient patient is likely neither to take oral iron nor to return for follow-up, IV iron dextran may be a suitable option despite its small but real risks. The same is true when continuing blood loss requires an amount of iron replacement with which only IV iron dextran can keep up, as in some patients with hereditary hemorrhagic telangiectasia. To try to avoid anaphylactic reactions, the injection of IV iron dextran is started usually with 0.1 or 0.2 ml over a period of 5 minutes and then the remaining amount is given over 5–10 minutes if there is no sign of a reaction. The total dosage may be calculated in a fairly simple fashion by estimating what proportion of the roughly 2 g of iron in hemoglobin in an average-sized adult is missing and adding to that an additional 1–2 g of iron for replenishment of iron stores. For larger or smaller adults, and especially for children, obviously the dosage has to be adjusted in proportion to size. It is probably better to figure out this total dosage using common sense rather than to apply a formula blindly, because if it is known that probably the maximum for any iron deficient adult is 3 g of iron replacement, then it can be estimated how the results should come out in smaller adults and children, and arithmetic errors cannot be made without recognizing them.

Failure to Respond to Iron Therapy

The only common causes for an iron-deficient patient not to respond to oral iron (if the patient is not otherwise ill) are not taking the medication or continued bleeding. Good rapport with the patient should enable one to deal with this. Starting therapy with lower dosages makes it more likely that the patient will comply with the physician's recommendation. *It cannot be stressed too much that because there is really no life-threatening toxicity from the use of oral iron in the usually prescribed dosages, the even small risk of a fatal anaphylactic reaction to parenteral iron cannot be justified if a little bit more time and attention can achieve the same objective using oral therapy. Parenteral iron should be used when only parenteral iron would be useful.*

Vitamin B$_{12}$

Human *dietary sources of vitamin B$_{12}$* are largely animal protein, including dairy products and eggs. Total body content is about 1–10 mg. The daily requirement for an average adult is probably no more than 1 μg. About 3 μg daily are secreted in the bile and reabsorbed in the ileum. This secretion and reabsorption accelerates the development of vitamin B$_{12}$ deficiency when intestinal vitamin B$_{12}$ absorption is defective.

> The sources of vitamin B$_{12}$ are dairy products, eggs, and other animal proteins.

Normal individuals have plasma vitamin B$_{12}$ concentrations between 200 and 900 pg/ml. Values of less than 100 are definitely abnormal; those between 100 and 200 raise a suspicion of vitamin B$_{12}$ deficiency. Cobalamin deficiency, including neuropsychiatric manifestations, can exist, albeit infrequently, in the face of normal serum cobalamin levels and in the absence of anemia. Vitamin B$_{12}$ is mainly bound in the plasma to a β globulin called transcobalamin II, by which it is transported to the tissues. Vitamin B$_{12}$ bound to transcobalamin II is rapidly cleared from the plasma, being taken up by hepatic parenchymal cells. Urine or serum levels of methyl malonic acid have been used as a sign of the metabolic effects of vitamin B$_{12}$ deficiency.

FUNCTION OF VITAMIN B$_{12}$

The active vitamin B$_{12}$ coenzymes are thought to be methylcobalamin and 5-deoxyadenosylcobalamin. These are essential for the growth of cells and for mitosis. Methylcobalamin is necessary for the formation of methionine from homocysteine. Also, folic acid cannot be used properly in the presence of vitamin B$_{12}$ deficiency, so there is a functional deficiency of folic acid metabolites in the presence of vitamin B$_{12}$ deficiency. Changes analogous to those in the bone marrow in red cell precursors occur also in the GI mucosa in vitamin B$_{12}$ deficiency and in folic acid deficiency. These changes in the GI mucosa may lead to decreased absorption of vitamin B$_{12}$. Thus, folic acid deficiency can lead to decreased absorption of vitamin B$_{12}$, which becomes normal after folic acid repletion. Even with vitamin B$_{12}$ deficiency that is not due to lack of Intrinsic Factor but instead is a result of some cause such as a blind loop syndrome, vitamin B$_{12}$ absorption may in part be decreased because of the mucosal changes caused by the deficiency.

> Vitamin B$_{12}$ deficiency can cause a functional deficiency in folic acid. True folic acid deficiency can lead to vitamin B$_{12}$ deficiency.

5-deoxyadenosylcobalamin is used for the conversion of L-methyl-malonyl CoA to succinyl CoA and therefore is the mechanism for the methylmalonic acidemia and methylmalonic aciduria seen in vitamin B_{12} deficiency.

ABSORPTION

Intrinsic factor is necessary for vitamin B_{12} absorption.

Vitamin B_{12} is absorbed in the terminal ileum only if it is bound by a material known as *intrinsic factor* (IF), which is synthesized by gastric parietal cells. Addisonian pernicious anemia is an autoimmune disorder in which there is atrophic gastritis and decreased-to-absent synthesis of IF with consequent decreased-to-absent absorption of vitamin B_{12}-IF complex. Pancreatic enzymes help release vitamin B_{12} from proteins so that it can be bound by IF, and this explains the B_{12} malabsorption that may be seen in some forms of pancreatic disease. Vitamin B_{12} absorption obviously may be decreased by ileal disease and certainly is prevented by surgical removal of the stomach or of the terminal ileum. Bacterial overgrowth in blind-loop syndromes prevents an adequate supply of vitamin B_{12} from reaching the ileum. The fish tapeworm *Diphyllobothrium latum* is thought to use vitamin B_{12} as it passes through the upper small intestine and prevents it from reaching the terminal ileum. Congenital absence of B_{12}–binding protein results in megaloblastic anemia, which responds to large dosages of parenteral vitamin B_{12}, apparently by permitting unbound vitamin B_{12} in the plasma to gain access to the cells where it is needed. A functional deficiency of vitamin B_{12} has been reported also in individuals with large increases in transcobalamin I and III as a result of hepatic disease or myeloproliferative disorders.

VITAMIN B_{12} DEFICIENCY

Megaloblastic anemia

Vitamin B_{12} deficiency causes ineffective red cell production with megaloblastic changes in the bone marrow. The peripheral blood shows macrocytosis, hypersegmented polys, and often thrombocytopenia. Red cell survival tends to be decreased. Usually the MCV is increased and the hemoglobin level is decreased. It is vital to remember that the neurological and psychiatrical results of vitamin B_{12} deficiency can occur without anemia, without macrocytosis, or without both. In contrast to the neurological changes, the *hematological* changes due to B_{12} deficiency are all reversible. *Neurological* damage due to vitamin B_{12} deficiency is not always completely reversible. The classic neurological disorder of vitamin B_{12} deficiency is *subacute combined degeneration.* It is associated with degeneration of axons in the posterior and lateral columns of the spinal cord. Vitamin B_{12} deficiency causes demyelination and cell death both in the spinal column and the cerebral cortex. Paresthesias of the hands, feet, and tongue occur in 5–10% of patients, along with the more common decreases in vibratory and position senses and motor disturbances. Psychological changes can occur in the presence or absence of anemia; these include hallucinations, emotional lability, and dementia. There may be more subtle personality changes also. In general, the changes reversible with treatment are milder and recent, whereas those most likely to be incompletely reversible are more severe and of longer duration.

Vitamin B_{12} deficiency due to a lack of B_{12} in the diet occurs only in strict vegetarians (vegans) who avoid all animal-derived food including eggs and dairy products; vitamin B_{12}–deficient babies may be born to women who are vegans.

Therapy

Vitamin B_{12} is given IM, usually in 100 μg dosages. Initially, it usually is given daily for a few days, then weekly three or four times, and then monthly.

Even though therapy for vitamin B_{12} deficiency is given only once a month after repletion of stores, it is an injection once a month for the remainder of the life of the patient. For this reason, it is important that the physician be sure that the treatment is justified, and that the patient understands the importance of continued treatment. It is important to suspect, diagnose, and treat vitamin B_{12} deficiency. Without adequate sustained treatment the patient can be damaged permanently by a condition that is completely treatable once the need is known.

Vitamin B_{12} has no known toxicity. (How many other medications come to mind for which this can be said?)

OTHER USES OF VITAMIN B_{12}

The only proven indication for the use of parenteral vitamin B_{12} is B_{12} deficiency. The standard work-up for dementia, especially in the elderly, includes a search for hypothyroidism, intracranial abnormalities and vitamin B_{12} deficiency, possibly including a therapeutic trial of vitamin B_{12} for suspected deficiency because, in rare instances, laboratory levels can be normal in the presence of actual B_{12} deficiency.

Vitamin B_{12} has been widely used also for an assortment of neurological and psychiatrical disorders and as a tonic for a wide variety of patients, some of whom are certain the injections help them. None of these uses has been shown to be effective.

Folic Acid Deficiency

Folic acid or pteroylglutamic acid is the usual pharmaceutical form of this vitamin. The daily requirement in a normal adult is approximately 25–50 μg. During pregnancy or when nursing their babies, women may require as much as 100–200 μg or more daily. Folic acid is used up in the synthesis of hemoglobin and, therefore, patients with high rates of red cell turnover may also require increased amounts of folic acid. The standard American diet provides between 50 and 500 μg or more, the main sources being fresh green vegetables. Cooking can destroy up to 90% of the folic acid content of food if the cooking is prolonged. In addition to fresh green vegetables, most foods contain some folates. Folate in food occurs mainly in the form of polyglutamates. Most dietary folate is absorbed in the upper portion of the jejunum and in the duodenum. Small intestinal disease in these areas may result in decreased absorption of folate and therefore in its deficiency. Various forms of the coenzyme have different functions: conversion of serine to glycine, synthesis of thymidylate, conversion of homocysteine to methionine, and synthesis of purines. The folates present in food are transported as methyl tetrahydrofolate to tissues where they are stored as polyglutamates.

Folate deficiency is most common where small intestinal disease is most common. Because tropical sprue is widespread in tropical areas, folate deficiency is widespread there too. In temperate climates, folate deficiency is seen commonly in alcoholics, who can become deficient in folic acid in 2 or 3 weeks if, as often is the case, their diet lacks folic acid and they are drinking heavily. It is seen also in people with small intestinal diseases such as regional enteritis (Crohn's disease). Folic acid deficiency due to increased

Folate needs and sources

There are a number of possible causes of folate deficiency.

need for folic acid may occur in hemolytic anemias. The cause of the rapid onset of folate deficiency in acute and chronic alcoholism probably is interference with the enterohepatic cycle of the vitamin due to the damage to hepatic cells seen in alcoholism. Some anticonvulsants, and occasionally oral contraceptives, are believed to interfere with the absorption and storage of folates and, of course, cancer chemotherapeutic drugs such as methotrexate, which inhibit dihydrofolate reductase, were designed to have antifolate activity. Folate deficiency, like deficiency of vitamin B_{12}, causes a macrocytic, megaloblastic anemia. The hematological findings in folate deficiency and in vitamin B_{12} deficiency are indistinguishable. *Folic acid cures the hematological abnormalities, but not the neurological abnormalities seen in vitamin B_{12} deficiency. Vitamin B_{12} does not cure the hematological abnormalities seen in folic acid deficiencies. Because administration of therapeutic dosages of folic acid can cure the hematological manifestations of vitamin B_{12} deficiency, it can obscure the presence of vitamin B_{12} deficiency and lead to neurological damage that can be severe and, at least in part, irreversible.* For this reason, folic acid was removed some years ago from most multivitamin preparations. It is present in the multivitamin preparations prescribed for pregnant women; therefore, those preparations should not be used except during pregnancy.

SIDE EFFECTS

Unlike vitamin B_{12}, there are rare reports of systemic reaction to parenteral injections of folic acid or its relative folinic acid (leucovorin). Oral folic acid is not toxic. However, large dosages of oral folic acid may decrease the effect of antiepileptic medications.

THERAPEUTIC USE

Folate deficiency in adults usually is treated with oral folic acid: 1 mg tablets given up to two or three times daily. When folid acid is given prophylactically (as for patients with chronic hemolytic anemias) 1 mg daily is the usual adult dosage. Patients receiving pharmacological dosages of folic acid should be examined periodically for any sign of development of the neurological manifestations of vitamin B_{12} deficiency; although there is no known association of vitamin B_{12} deficiency with the usual causes of folate deficiency, there is also no reason to think that individuals with disorders leading to folate deficiency are immune to deficiency in vitamin B_{12}.

Other Agents for Treating Anemia

There are several agents for treating anemia. The agent to be used depends on the cause of the anemia.

Recombinant erythropoietin was released by the Food and Drug Administration (FDA) in 1989. It is a glycoprotein normally produced by the kidney that stimulates marrow erythroid progenitors to produce red cells. Its therapeutic indications already include the anemia of renal failure and the anemia of acquired immunodeficiency syndrome (AIDS). Response requires adequate iron, folic acid, and vitamin B_{12}. The rise in hematocrit in patients with renal failure may be complicated by hypertension, seizures, and clotting of the vascular access or of the dialysis apparatus. Headache, arthralgia, vomiting, and diarrhea also occur more often in treated patients than controls. It is given IV or subcutaneously with a target hematocrit of 30–33%. Other uses of erythropoietin are being studied.

Anemia resulting from *copper* deficiency has been reported after surgical therapy for obesity (intestinal bypass) and also in people receiving total parenteral nutrition. Daily dosages (0.1 mg/kg) of copper sulfate have been given by mouth in such patients and have resulted in clinical responses. A portion of this amount might be added to the material given for total parenteral nutrition. *Cobalt* has been used in the treatment of anemia. It is thought that it tends to raise the hemoglobin level by increasing erythropoietin production as a response to cobalt-induced tissue hypoxia. It has never been shown that anemic patients are clinically benefited by cobalt.

Pyridoxine (vitamin B_6) has produced clinical improvement in up to half of patients both with hereditary and acquired sideroblastic anemias. In these patients, pyridoxine is given orally, 50 mg–100 mg daily. These are amounts far above the usual requirement (pharmacological rather than physiological doses). Hence, these are called *pyridoxine-responsive* (not pyridoxine deficiency) anemias. These are anemias characterized by a mixed red cell population in the peripheral blood, some of which are hypochromic, and by marrow iron stains showing a ring of intramitochondrial iron surrounding the nuclei of red cell precursors. Pyridoxine, administered in order to prevent the occurrence of isoniazid-induced peripheral neuropathy, has also corrected the sideroblastic anemia associated occasionally with the use of isoniazid.

Anticoagulant, Antithrombotic, and Thrombolytic Agents

Thrombosis is merely the obverse of normal hemostasis. We need our circulating blood to stay liquid so that it can perform its numerous vital functions. But we need a mechanism by which bleeding can be stopped, so that a hole in the plumbing does not result in excessive loss of fluid. The same mechanism that seals a leaking small blood vessel can cause a thrombosis at the site of an area of abnormal endothelium, such as an atherosclerotic plaque.

When a vessel is injured or the endothelium is damaged, blood *platelets adhere* to the exposed basement membrane or collagen. These platelets then normally *release* a number of substances including serotonin and adenosine diphosphate (ADP). The released ADP causes other passing platelets to agglutinate and stick to the area of damage. This is the mechanism called primary hemostasis, and at the same time it is a mechanism by which an atherosclerotic plaque in a coronary artery can lead to a coronary artery occlusion. This is also the origin of the so-called white thrombus seen in the arterial system when there is an abnormal suface to which the circulating blood is being exposed.

In the laboratory the agglutination of platelets has been studied by examining the reactivity of platelets in citrated plasma when ADP, collagen, and other materials are added, using light transmission through a cuvette containing stirred platelet-rich plasma as the method of measurement.

In normal hemostasis, if flow from a cut vessel is stopped by a platelet plug, the platelets serve also as the nidus for the formation of fibrin strands when fibrinogen is clotted by thrombin. On the venous side, thromboses in this low flow, low pressure system are clots usually rather than platelet thrombi; these are the red thrombi of the venous system as opposed to the white thrombi of the arterial system. Platelet plugs tend to be unstable and to disaggregate unless they are reinforced by fibrin formation within and around the platelet plug.

Because both platelet plug formation and clot formation are normal adaptive activities leading to protection of the organism, interference with platelet plug formation, interference with blood clot formation, and the use of agents to accelerate the disappearance of clots all affect both normal and pathological platelet plugs and clots. The "magic bullet" that affects only clots and platelet agglutinates that are not wanted, while leaving intact those that are, has not been developed.

HEPARIN

Heparin was found accidentally by a medical student in 1916 while he was investigating ether-soluble materials that accelerated blood clotting. Heparin was purified further in the 1920s and used *in vitro* to prevent the clotting of blood. It seemed logical that such an agent might be used also to treat venous thrombosis, and clinical trials with large dosages took place in the late 1930s. However, studies of the efficacy of low dosages of heparin did not begin until the 1960s and 1970s.

Chemistry

Heparin is not a single substance. It is a group of straight chain, anionic mucopolysaccharides or glycosaminoglycans. Heparin has a low pH because of its covalently linked carboxylic acid groups and sulfate groups. Commercially available heparins consist of polymers of two disaccharides. They are prepared from the intestinal mucosa of pigs and the lungs of cattle. However, the incidence of heparin-induced thrombocytopenia is said to be lower with the porcine product. Semisynthetic heparins have been prepared also from sulfated polymers of the disaccharides, D-glucosamine and D-glucuronic acid. The physiological function of the heparin normally present in mammalian mast cells is unknown.

Actions of Heparin

Heparin itself is not an anticoagulant. The anticoagulant effect of heparin requires the presence of a plasma factor known as antithrombin III, and it occurs *in vivo* as well as *in vitro*. Heparin vastly potentiates the activity of antithrombin III in neutralizing activated Factors II, IX, X, XI, XII, and XIII. Activated Factor II, of course, is thrombin, the proteolytic enzyme that acts on fibrinogen resulting in the formation of a fibrin clot. Even low concentrations of heparin considerably increase the activity of antithrombin III, especially against activated Factor X and thrombin, which is the rationale for the experimental administration of low dosages of heparin that has proven to be therapeutically useful.

> Heparin potentiates the activity of antithrombin III.

The injection of heparin results also in the disappearance of turbidity from lipemic plasma due to the release, under the influence of heparin, of lipid-hydrolyzing enzymes, especially lipoprotein lipase. Lipoprotein lipase acts on chylomicrons and low density lipoproteins bound to capillary endothelial cells.

Absorption

Heparin is a polar molecule with an average weight of 15,000 daltons. Probably for this reason it is not absorbed through the GI tract or the skin, nor does it pass the placenta. It is given subcutaneously or IV, but *IM heparin is not used because of reports of large IM hematomas* at the sites of injection. IV use can be either intermittent or continuous. The higher the dosage, the longer the half-life. Hepatic cells metabolize heparin by means of the enzyme heparinase. Its inactive byproducts are excreted in the urine. Both renal and hepatic insufficiency result in a prolongation of the half-life of heparin. The larger heparin dosages recommended for patients with pulmonary embolism are thought to be required because of rapid heparin clearance in such patients.

Therapeutic Use

Heparin has been standardized at various times, both as units and as milligrams. However, because of considerable variations in activity per milligram, only units are now used. One unit of heparin is the amount that prevents 1 ml of recalcified citrated plasma from clotting. *Low-dose heparin* is given by deep subcutaneous injection for prophylaxis of venous thrombosis. If done in connection with surgery, it is begun usually several hours before the surgery with a dosage of 5000 units in an average-sized adult patient, repeated two or three times daily for a week. Therapy is stopped sooner if the patient is ambulatory earlier, and continued longer if not.

Patients receiving heparin should not receive medications that interfere with platelet function, because interfering with two hemostatic systems at the same time is more likely to produce bleeding. Heparin used for therapy rather than prophylaxis *(standard-dose heparin)* is given usually by continuous IV infusion. For continuous IV therapy, 6000 units of heparin are added to 100 ml of 5% dextrose, normal saline or similar solution, and infused at a rate of 1000 units/hour. The rate of infusion is adjusted to keep the partial thromboplastic time at about 1½–2 times the patient's pretreatment value. This infusion follows an *IV loading dose* of 5000 units in an average-sized adult for deep venous thrombosis and 10,000 units for an average-sized adult in the event that one is treating a pulmonary embolism. Some use intermittent IV therapy through heparin locks, giving 5000–10,000 units initially, followed by 5000–10,000 units every 4 to 6 hours, adjusting the dosage so that the partial thromboplastin time shortly before the next dose is 1½–2 times the patient's control value. Heparin also can be given by deep subcutaneous injection at a dose in adults of 5000–10,000 units every 6 hours, adjusting the dose according to the partial thromboplastin time (PTT) as with intermittent IV therapy.

Side Effects

Allergy to heparin is unusual but can occur, with fever, urticaria, or anaphylactic shock. For this reason, a trial dosage of 1000 units is given ordinarily before the usual therapeutic dosages. The most common long-term side effect of heparin, aside from bleeding, is osteoporosis in patients treated for over 3 months with over 15,000 units of heparin/day.

Hemorrhage is the most common and most dangerous complication of the use of heparin. All aspirin-containing medications should be avoided when this agent is being used. Any bleeding in the patient receiving heparin should be viewed also as a sign of a significant lesion. There are many reports of GI hemorrhage while on anticoagulants as the first sign of a GI malignancy.

Thrombocytopenia of a mild and transient nature probably occurs in a significant minority of people receiving heparin. This is of no clinical significance. On the other hand, a severe thrombocytopenia may occur, usually in the second week of heparin therapy. This is characterized by *severe thrombocytopenia and multiple episodes of thromboembolism.* An IgG/antibody directed against a heparin antigen has been detected in the plasma of some patients with this reaction. This is a life-threatening complication,

Severe heparin-induced thrombocytopenia

both because of the severe thrombocytopenia and because of the possibility of severe disease and death from thrombotic complications. If this form of heparin-induced thrombocytopenia is present, heparin should be stopped immediately. If another agent to inhibit thrombosis is needed, either oral anticoagulants, antiplatelet agents, or both should be used. This form of severe heparin-induced thrombocytopenia with thromboembolism has been seen also in patients on low-dose heparin. Tests of serum antiheparin antibodies are being developed and may be able to provide a definitive diagnosis of heparin-induced thrombocytopenia. Perhaps this will provide a means of monitoring patients so that the heparin can be stopped before the development of the severe thrombocytopenia and thrombosis.

Contraindications

Because patients who are bleeding actively have holes in their blood vessels, it is obvious that heparin is contraindicated in such patients unless the bleeding can be controlled by other means, such as pressure. Heparin is generally contraindicated also in patients with thrombocytopenic purpura, congenital or acquired coagulation disorders, intracranial hemorrhage, acute or subacute bacterial endocarditis, and should be avoided after surgery on the eye, central nervous system, or other critical areas.

Therapy of Heparin-Associated Bleeding

Protamine sulfate can be used to combat heparin-induced bleeding.

If time is not of the essence, the dosage of heparin should be lowered or discontinued. If the bleeding is more severe, *protamine sulfate* may be used. This is available as a solution for IV use containing 10 mg/ml. One milligram of protamine sulfate blocks the anticoagulant effect of 100 units of heparin. Protamine sulfate should not be given at a rate of more than 20 mg/minute nor more than 50 mg in a 10-minute period. Rapid injection of protamine has been reported to cause flushing, hypertension and other symptoms, possibly as a result of histamine release.

ORAL ANTICOAGULANTS: WARFARIN

A number of medications can affect the activity of warfarin.

Warfarin sodium is the only oral anticoagulant in common use in the United States at this time, although several other agents are available. Its anticoagulant properties were discovered in 1924 as a result of the observation of cattle with a hemorrhagic disorder traced to eating spoiled sweet clover. The effect of warfarin is to cause the synthesis of inactive forms of the vitamin K–requiring clotting Factors II, VII, IX, X, and protein C, and protein S. Note that whereas lack of Factors II, VII, IX, and X would be expected to have an anticoagulant activity, lack of protein C or S leads to a thrombotic tendency. Warfarin is the active agent also in commonly used rat poisons that cause the animals to bleed to death internally. Warfarin can be used as an example of many of the things that affect the biological activity of a medication. Some medications, such as phenobarbital by enzyme induction, increase the rate of disappearance of warfarin and thus decrease its anticoagulant effect. Other agents, such as aspirin, potentiate the effect. As a general rule, it is not safe to add or withdraw any medication in a patient on warfarin without checking to see whether there is an effect on the amount of warfarin needed to maintain therapeutic anticoagulation. Warfarin, like heparin, is not itself an anticoagulant. However, its action is different from that of heparin, which immediately becomes an anticoagulant when linked to antithrombin III.

Factors That Affect the Activity of Warfarin

There are reports of congenital resistance to warfarin in rare families. More common factors that increase the effect of warfarin include any conditions that might lead to vitamin K deficiency, including the use of antimicrobial agents that produce vitamin K deficiency in as little as 10 days to 2 weeks without the use of oral anticoagulants. This effect of antibiotics on the vitamin K synthesized by intestinal bacteria is sometimes overlooked as a possible cause of prolonged coagulation tests and postoperative bleeding. Patients with damaged livers and already impaired hepatic synthesis of coagulation factors are likely also to have a greater effect from warfarin. (All the clotting factors, with the exception of Factor VIII, are thought to be synthesized by hepatocytes.) It is thought that older people in general are more sensitive to warfarin as are those with fever or hyperthyroidism. Aspirin should not be used in association with oral anticoagulant therapy because it interferes with platelet function, leads to increased blood loss from the GI mucosa even without anticoagulation, and also potentiates the effect of oral anticoagulants.

Absorption and Dosage

Warfarin is rapidly and uniformly absorbed after oral administration. It is given once daily. Peak plasma concentrations are reached within 1 hour. Ingestion of food with warfarin decreases the rate but not the extent of absorption. Because warfarin is essentially totally bound to plasma albumin, it does not enter breast milk. However, it is teratogenic. Because small amounts cross the placenta, warfarin should not be given to pregnant women. Warfarin usually is started at a dose of 5 mg daily, adjusting the dose after 3–5 days and thereafter so as to maintain the prothrombin time (PT) at 1.2–1.5 times control.

Side Effects

Hemorrhage is by far the greatest and most frequent risk in patients receiving oral anticoagulants. It can occur even when the prothrombin time is well within the expected therapeutic range. In Europe less hemorrhage seems to occur with warfarin than had been the American experience. Apparently this is due to the different thromboplastin used in the monitoring of oral anticoagulant therapy in the United States as opposed to Western Europe. It is now recommended that the patient/control ratio of the prothrombin time, using the standard United States commercial rabbit brain thromboplastin, should be in the range of 1.2–1.5, going up to a ratio of 1.5–2.0 only for the prophylaxis of thrombosis in patients with recurrent systemic embolism on lower dosages and those with prosthetic heart valves.

Treatment of hemorrhage caused by oral anticoagulants depends on the severity of the hemorrhage. One can smply stop the drug and wait for the coagulation abnormality to disappear. If bleeding is not an active problem, 10–20 mg of vitamin K1 (phytonadione) can be given orally, which should return the prothrombin time to normal within 24 hours. For serious or life-threatening bleeding, IV vitamin K1 should be used with dosages usually of 5–10 mg, although up to 50 mg can be used. The effect of vitamin K is not a coagulant one, however, and correction of the hemorrhagic tendency must await hepatic synthesis of normal Factors II, VII, IX, and X. For this reason, the only rapidly effective means to correct the hemorrhagic tendency due to warfarin is by the use of plasma. This can be either

Warfarin skin necrosis

Anticoagulation regimen: heparin and warfarin

fresh-frozen plasma or cryoprecipitate-depleted plasma (which has less fibrinogen and Factor VIII than normal plasma, but should have normal amounts of Factors II, VI, IX, and X).

Rare patients may show a complication known as *skin necrosis* or other thrombotic tendencies. It is thought that the reason for this is that protein C (an inhibitor of activated Factors V and VIII) falls to low levels more rapidly than Factor IX at the beginning of a course of warfarin. For this reason, it is recommended that when a patient is anticoagulated for venous thrombosis, heparin should be started and then *warfarin,* usually at a dosage of 5 mg/day in adults, and the dosage adjusted as the prothrombin time gradually prolongs. Using this more gradual approach to oral anticoagulation heparin should protect the individual if the protein C gets particularly low before Factor IX falls, and the incidence of skin necrosis also should be lower or absent. In the event of what is thought to be warfarin skin necrosis, heparin should be reinstituted (or instituted if not given before) and consideration should be given to the administration of thawed frozen plasma as a source of protein C.

The warfarin-related purple toes syndrome is another rare complication of oral anticoagulant therapy. It presents several weeks after the start of oral anticoagulation and gradually improves after oral anticoagulants are stopped. This syndrome appears to be due to cholesterol microembolization.

THROMBOLYTIC DRUGS

Streptokinase, urokinase, and tissue plasminogen activator cause the dissolution of clots.

Thrombolytic agents are enzymes that cause the dissolution of clots. *Streptokinase* is a protein derived from Group C β-hemolytic streptococci. It binds to plasminogen and the streptokinase-plasminogen complex activates uncomplexed plasminogen to the proteolytic enzyme plasmin. Streptokinase is an effective fibrinolytic agent for reasonably fresh clots even up to 4 days old. It also induces bleeding from surgical wounds, sites of arterial puncture, and so forth. Fever is a common side effect. Perhaps because it is derived from streptococci, allergic reactions are not uncommon. *Urokinase* probably is at least as effective as streptokinase, is not antigenic (no allergic reactions), but costs several times as much. It directly converts plasminogen to plasmin. The incidence of bleeding complications is probably about the same with urokinase as it is with streptokinase.

Tissue plasminogen activators (TPA) are much-heralded agents about which a great deal of enthusiastic expectation had been generated. This was based on the idea that these agents would have a greater effect on clots and cause less bleeding because they are not fibrinogenolytic but only fibrinolytic. However, in reports of their clinical use bleeding complications seem to be about as common. It remains to be seen whether these agents are superior to streptokinase and urokinase. It would be expected that *recombinant urokinase,* if it becomes available and is inexpensive enough, will replace streptokinase as a therapeutic agent because it is not antigenic. The role of tissue plasminogen activators remains incompletely defined, although they are increasingly widely used. The hope was that these agents, by acting largely on fibrin, would not induce a systemic lytic state and that bleeding complications would be few. But the hope of avoiding a systemic lytic state has not been realized. Because bleeding complications of fibrinolytic agents presumably must involve blood vessels with defects in their walls or blood vessels that have been severed, it probably was wishful thinking to think that the action of lytic agents on fibrinogen contributes much to the incidence of bleeding due to these agents.

Regimens for Fibrinolytic Therapy

The usual loading dose of *streptokinase* is 250,000 International Units (IU) given over a 30-minute period. Thereafter, 100,000 units/hour is a common dosage, with therapy continued for 1–3 days. Therapy can be monitored by any coagulation test, which shows that there is a therapeutic effect of the lytic agent. Because prothrombin times and PTTs are influenced by low levels of fibrinogen, these are adequate. The most sensitive test is a thrombin time, but it is not available at all times of the day in all hospitals. The prothrombin time is a perfectly adequate way of telling whether the desired effect has been achieved. For *urokinase* the usual loading dose is 4400 IU/kg given IV over 10 minutes followed by a continuous IV infusion at 4400 IU/kg/hour for 12 hours. Because urokinase does not bind to plasminogen, it is not possible (as it is with streptokinase) to give a dosage such that all of the plasminogen is bound and none is available for conversion to plasmin. Therefore, it is not necessary to monitor the lytic effect of urokinase. Urokinase should work unless there is a grossly low level of plasminogen.

Regimens for tissue plasminogen activators still are evolving rapidly. Bleeding complications are the main untoward effects: especially GI and intracranial bleeding. Reperfusion arrhythmias often occur when these drugs are used in patients with recent myocardial infarction. Arterial and venous punctures should be minimized. Check for current regimens and precautions.

ANTIPLATELET-AGGREGATION AGENTS

Use of these agents is aimed at the arterial system. There is scanty evidence that antiplatelet agents have any effect on venous thrombosis.

Platelet aggregation seems not only to be involved in thromboembolic disorders, but also in the formation of atherosclerotic plaques. Clearly, this is an area of vast clinical and research interest.

Different prostaglandins have opposing effects on platelet function. Thromboxane, a platelet product, potentiates platelet aggregation. Prostacyclin (PGI$_2$) is synthesized by vascular endothelium and inhibits aggregation of platelets by ADP. *Aspirin* inhibits synthesis both of prostacyclin and of thromboxane. Its effects on platelets last for the 8–9-day life span of the platelets affected. Low dosages of aspirin (60–75 mg/day) have been shown to inhibit thromboxane synthesis more than prostacyclin synthesis. Thus, platelet aggregation is inhibited but there is no significant decrease in the antiaggregatory effect of the prostacyclin at the vessel wall. Essentially, all the studies of the antithrombotic effects of aspirin, however, have used larger dosages (usually at least 300 mg/day), which effectively inhibit both thromboxane and prostacyclin synthesis. For this reason, it is not now possible to know what dosage of aspirin proves to be best. Clotting of Silastic arteriovenous shunts for hemodialysis can be prevented by the use of aspirin. This presumably is related to the fact that thromboxane synthesis in the blood passing through these shunts is effectively inhibited by the aspirin, but Silastic catheters do not synthesize prostacyclin.

Aspirin probably is useful in preventing transient ischemic attacks (TIAs) and strokes. It reduces the risk of myocardial infarction and of reinfarction after myocardial infarction. In a widely publicized study of middle-aged male American physicians, aspirin reduced acute cardiac deaths but had no effect on overall mortality.

Aspirin inhibits synthesis of prostacyclin and thromboxane.

Sulfinpyrazone has been used as a uricosuric agent in the treatment of hyperuricemia in the past but has been largely supplanted for this indication by allopurinol. Sulfinpyrazone inhibits the platelet-release reaction as well as inhibiting the adherence of platelets to subendothelial structures; it also inhibits the synthesis of prostaglandins. Reports have indicated a reduction in the incidence of sudden death after myocardial infarction, but there has been criticism of the methodology of the studies and sulfinpyrazone is not approved presently by the FDA as an antithrombotic agent.

Dipyridamole has been in use for some years as a vasodilator. It probably interferes with platelet function by inhibiting phosphodiesterase. The only present official recommended use of dipyridamole as an antithrombotic agent is in conjunction with warfarin for the prevention of thromboemboli in patients who have had prosthetic heart valves implanted.

REFLECTIONS ON THE FUTURE

The *appropriate use of anticoagulant, antithrombotic, and thrombolytic drugs* remains an area of active research. The risk of severe thrombocytopenia and thromboembolism with heparin was totally unsuspected in the mid-1970s. The risk to patients of the presence of lupus inhibitors and what should be done about them in each patient is not well defined. The risk of bleeding with these agents is probably greatest with the thrombolytic drug regimens, intermediate with anticoagulants, and least with antiplatelet agents. If these agents are given in combination, risks as well as benefits can be expected to increase. *Low-molecular-weight heparins* are being studied with the hope that equivalent antithrombotic efficacy can be obtained with less risk of bleeding. More recent reports suggest this is probably the case.

Platelet aggregation and fibrin clot formation are involved not only in thromboembolism but also in arteriosclerosis and the spread of cancer. Fish oils as well as some ingredients of traditional Chinese cooking have inhibitory effects on laboratory tests of platelet function. Therapeutic effects are less well established, but Eskimos' diet does seem to give them a mild bleeding disorder. Cancer cells grow better in a fibrin mesh than without one; anticoagulation in experimental animals slows the growth of experimental metastases and decreases their numbers. Anticoagulation inhibits formation of a positive tuberculin test in tuberculin-sensitized animals, although other aspects of cellular immunity can be demonstrated in these animals. Clearly these are areas with immense potential for benefit to human health.

Use of Drugs to Reduce Surgical Blood Loss

Blood transfusion is well known to carry a risk of disease transmission. It is the risk of human immunodeficiency virus (HIV-I) transmission that has created truly widespread concern, and some would say hysteria, although there are more frequent risks of transfusion.

The intuitive response to the problem of limiting surgical blood loss is to tie off or cauterize more bleeders. However, normal hemostatic mechanisms clearly are required to limit surgical blood loss from capillaries, venules, and arterioles.

Prostacyclin (PGI_2) inhibits platelet aggregation. Given IV just before cardiopulmonary bypass in patients having coronary artery bypass grafting procedures, it results in higher intraoperative and postoperative platelet counts but has no significant effect on total blood loss.

Several agents are being explored for ability to reduce surgical blood loss.

DDAVP (desmopressin, a synthetic analog of arginine vasopressin) shortens the bleeding time and the partial thromboplastin time in normal people and people with uremia, platelet function defects, von Willebrand's disease, and hemophilia A (Factor VIII deficiency). It increases plasma levels of high molecular weight multimers of von Willebrand Factor. DDAVP has been shown in several studies to decrease blood loss in cardiac and noncardiac surgery.

Aprotinin inhibits trypsin, plasmin, and kallikrein. Its use has been reported to produce impressive decreases in blood loss in both cardiac and noncardiac surgery.

Adverse effects of these drugs include hypotension with prostacyclin and DDAVP, and water retention and hyponatremia with DDAVP. The obvious possibility of increasing the risk of thromboembolism with DDAVP and aprotinin is also a major concern.

The appropriate use and proper dosage (if any) of these agents remains to be established.

General References

Clouse LH, Comp PC: The regulation of hemostasis: The protein C system. N Engl J Med 314:1298–1304, 1986.

Hirsh J: Drug therapy: Heparin. N Engl J Med 324:1565–1574, 1991.

Hirsh J: Is the dose of warfarin prescribed by American physicians unnecessarily high? Arch Intern Med 147:769–771, 1987.

Hirsh J: Oral anticoagulant drugs. N Engl J Med 324:1865–1875, 1991.

National Conference on Antithrombotic Therapy. Chest 89:1S–106S, 1986.

Samama MM: Thrombolytic agents and treatments. Semin Thromb Hemost 13:131–227, 1987.

Antimicrobial Chemotherapy

VIII

Principles of Anti-Infective Use*

Thomas R. Beam, Jr.

47

Anti-infective drug products may be used in three different ways: first, as prophylactic agents; second, for presumptive therapy of a suspected infection; and third, as therapy of a defined infectious process. Antibiotics employed as prophylactic agents are used to eliminate or reduce the amount of bacterial contamination to a degree that host defenses can successfully prevent an infection from becoming established. Prophylactic antibiotic use may be divided into surgical and medical applications.

The rationale for surgical prophylaxis was established by Burke. He created a standardized incision of known depth and length on the abdominal surface of guinea pigs. A predetermined number of bacteria with known antimicrobial susceptibilities were applied to the freshly created wound, allowed to dwell for 3 minutes, then lavaged away with sterile saline. The wound was closed with clips.

Positive (heat-killed bacteria) and negative (sterile saline) wound controls were included on the abdominal surface of each animal. An antibiotic was administered before, during, or at varying times after surgery. Intravenous (IV) saline was administered as an antibiotic control. The results are summarized in Figure 47–1.

Induration was measured 24–30 hours after completion of surgery; infection was verified, by biopsy and culture of the wound and surrounding tissue, to cause the induration. Antimicrobial efficacy was greatest when the drug was administered 1 hour prior to surgery. Efficacy lessened progressively when the drug was administered simultaneously or within 1, 2, or 3 hours after completion of surgery. No benefit was conferred 4 or more hours after creation of the wound.

Subsequent studies have shown that it is important to maintain serum concentrations of an effective antibiotic throughout the course of surgery, and that tissue concentrations should exceed the minimal inhibitory concentration (MIC) of anticipated pathogens that might contaminate the wound.

Numerous additional factors contribute to the risk of postoperative infection. Antibiotics help to reduce, but do not eliminate, this risk. Patient risk factors include age over 60 years; malnutrition; obesity; diabetes mellitus; malignancy; immunosuppressive chemotherapy or radiotherapy; corticosteroids at dosages of 20 mg or more of prednisone per day; and underlying chronic cardiac, pulmonary, hepatic, or renal disease.

The circumstances under which surgery is performed also influence postoperative wound infection rates. These factors include duration of preoperative hospitalization, the use of antiseptic soaps for preoperative showering or bathing, the performance of elective rather than emergency

Prophylaxis

Antimicrobials may be used to prevent or treat defined infections or may be employed for presumptive infection.

Prophylaxis is best administered immediately prior to surgery.

Patient characteristics, the circumstances of the surgical procedure, and the type of surgery define the risk for infection.

* The work was supported by the Veterans Administration.

Figure 47–1

Active control (infected) lesions showed about 10-mm induration in the absence of antibiotic. Negative control (killed staphylococci) showed about 3-mm induration. The effect of antibiotic is progressively reduced after surgery begins, reaching control values at 4 hours. The most effective time of administration is 1 hour before surgery begins. (From Burke JF: The effective period of preventive antibiotic action in experimental incisions and dermal lesions. Surgery 50:162, 1961.)

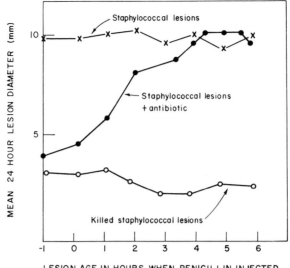

surgical procedures, timing and type of hair removal, use of drains, insertion of foreign bodies or implants, presence of pre-existing foreign bodies or implants, reoperation — particularly during the same hospitalization — duration of the surgical procedure, and presence of hematoma.

However, the most important variable in determining the risk of postoperative infection is the classification of the wound. Five categories have been described and are summarized in Table 47–1. Two caveats are applied to the use of prophylactic antibiotics. First, prophylaxis has been convincingly demonstrated to be of value for clean-contaminated surgery. Second, prophylactic use of antibiotics has not been reproducibly demonstrated to be of value for most clean surgeries. But with clean surgery and insertion of a prosthesis, the severe morbidity or mortality associated with a single infection is believed to justify the risk of exposing a large number of patients to antibiotics, even though they will not necessarily benefit from the drug.

Prophylactic antibiotics cannot be given to patients with contaminated or dirty wounds. For contaminated wounds, early, anticipatory, or preventive treatment is employed. For dirty wounds, infection is established, and treatment must be given. The responsibility for defining the category of the

> Wounds are classified as clean, clean-contaminated, contaminated, and dirty.

> Antimicrobial prophylaxis can be given only for clean or clean-contaminated surgery.

Table 47–1   CLASSIFICATION OF SURGICAL WOUNDS*

Category	Antibiotic Prophylaxis/Therapy	Proportion of Surgical Procedures (%)	Wound Infection Rates (%)	Examples
Clean	No/No	70	≤5	Thyroidectomy Mastectomy
Clean with prosthesis	Yes/No	5	≤2	Insertion of heart valve, prosthetic joint
Clean-contaminated	Yes/No	15	≤10	Elective colon surgery
Contaminated	No/Yes	5	≤20	Biliary or urological surgery in presence of bacteria
Dirty	No/Yes	5	≤40	Drainage of intraabdominal abscess

* Most hospitals achieve rates of ≤2% without use of prophylactic antibiotics.

wound belongs to the surgeon and should be established during the operative procedure. Proper classification is essential for assuring quality care.

Common surgical procedures and the recommended prophylactic antibiotic for each are listed in Table 47–2. The antibiotic of choice is difficult to identify for several reasons. Clean surgical procedures require evaluation of thousands of patients before a legitimate distinction between drugs can be made. These studies have generally not been done. For clean-contaminated surgery, the best available information is derived often from

It is difficult to define optimal antimicrobial prophylaxis.

Table 47–2 COMMON SURGICAL PROCEDURES AND RECOMMENDED PROPHYLACTIC ANTIBIOTICS

Type of Surgery	Documented Need	Drug of Choice	Alternative(s)
Clean Surgery			
CARDIAC			
Prosthetic valve	No	Cefazolin or vanocomycin	Nafcillin
Coronary artery bypass	Equivocal	Cefazolin	Vancomycin
Pacemaker implantation	No	None	None
ORTHOPEDIC			
With prosthesis	No	Cefazolin	Vancomycin
Without prosthesis	No	None	None
VASCULAR			
Involving groin	Yes	Cefazolin	Cefuroxime
Abdominal aorta	Equivocal	Cefazolin	Cefuroxime
Other vascular	No	None	None
UROLOGICAL			
Orchiectomy	No	None	None
Anterior cystourethropexy	No	None	None
Varicocelectomy	No	None	None
Insertion of prosthesis	Equivocal	Cefazolin	TMP/SMZ*
Clean-Contaminated Surgery			
HEAD AND NECK WITH TRANSECTION OF OROPHARYNX	Yes	Cefazolin	Cefotaxime or cefoperazone
THORACIC (NONCARDIAC)	Equivocal	Cefazolin	
GASTROINTESTINAL			
Gastric, small intestine	Yes	Cefazolin	Cefoxitin or cefotetan
Biliary tract	High risk†	Cefazolin	Cefoxitin or Cefotetan
Appendix	Equivocal	Cefoxitin or cefotetan	Clindamycin and gentamicin
Colorectal	Yes	Oral erythromycin and neomycin	Cefoxitin or cefotetan
GYNECOLOGICAL			
Vaginal hysterectomy	Yes	Cefazolin	Cefoxitin or cefotetan
Abdominal hysterectomy	Yes	Cefazolin	Cefoxitin or cefotetan
Cesarean section	Yes	Cefazolin	Cefoxitin or cefotetan
UROLOGICAL			
Ureterolithotomy	High risk‡	Cefazolin	TMP/SMZ
Pyelolithotomy	High risk	Cefazolin	TMP/SMZ
Nephrectomy	High risk	Cefazolin	TMP/SMZ
Partial cystectomy	High risk	Cefazolin	TMP/SMZ
Cystotomy	High risk	Cefazolin	TMP/SMZ

* TMP/SMZ—trimethoprim/sulfamethoxazole.
† High risk (biliary tract)—age over 70, past or present jaundice, previous biliary surgery, sepsis within 1 week, common bile duct pathology, diabetes, obesity.
‡ High risk (urological)—elderly, malnourished, debilitated, diabetic, immunosuppressed, prosthetic device.

Medical prophylaxis may be primary (to
prevent acquisition of infection) or
secondary (to prevent clinical manifestations of infection).

premarketing trials of new antibiotics. The structure of these studies is not necessarily developed to address the issue of defining the optimal antimicrobial agent. Finally, pharmacokinetics of antimicrobial agents may be critically important in determining efficacy. The ability of many older antimicrobial agents to effectively penetrate into the tissues surrounding the surgical wound has generally not been evaluated.

Prophylaxis for medical reasons is employed in a wide variety of clinical circumstances. It is usually targeted at specific pathogens and usually prescribed only during a period of high-likelihood of exposure. The infections to be prevented range in severity from spontaneously resolving (travelers' diarrhea) to life-threatening (infective endocarditis). Applying the same standards as for surgical prophylaxis, medical conditions warranting prophylactic use of antibiotics are listed in Table 47–3.

One situation commonly described as prophylactic use of an antimicrobial agent is isoniazid prescription for an individual who has recently converted from purified protein derivative (PPD) negative to positive. This actually represents early or presumptive therapy, because infection of the host by mycobacteria has already occurred. The number of organisms present is relatively small, and the rate of growth is slow. Therefore, treatment with isoniazid for 1 year significantly reduces the number of viable mycobacteria and minimizes the risk of developing clinically apparent disease. However, infection has already occurred prior to the institution of prophylaxis.

In general, exposure to infectious agents that are most highly commu-

Table 47–3 PROPHYLAXIS AGAINST INFECTION FOR MEDICAL DISEASES

Condition	Proven Efficacy	Agent of Choice	Alternative(s)
Childhood Illnesses			
Ophthalmia neonatorum —standard	Yes	Erythromycin or tetracycline ointment	Silver nitrate
Ophthalmia neonatorum —high risk	Yes	Penicillin G	Cefotaxime
Pertussis	Equivocal	Erythromycin	TMP/SMZ*
Recurrent otitis media	Equivocal	Sulfisoxazole	Amoxicillin, TMP/SMZ
Haemophilus influenzae	Equivocal	Rifampin*	None
Splenectomy; pneumococcal infection	Equivocal	Penicillin V	Amoxicillin*
Rheumatic fever	Yes	Benzathine penicillin G	Sulfadiazine, penicillin V
Children and Adults			
Meningococcal disease	Yes	Rifampin	Sulfadiazine, minocycline
Recurrent urinary tract infections in females	Yes	TMP/SMZ	Nitrofurantoin, trimethoprim
Influenza A	Yes	Amantadine*	None
Bacterial endocarditis	No	Amoxicillin, ampicillin plus gentamicin, or vancomycin ± gentamicin†	Erythromycin, clindamycin
Adults			
Traveler's diarrhea	Equivocal	TMP/SMZ	Ciprofloxacin, doxycycline, Pepto-Bismol
Malaria	Yes	Chloroquine or mefloguine	Primaquine, fansidar
Contact of person with STD	Equivocal	Variable—depends on STD	Variable

* Vaccination recommended when clinically appropriate.
† Drug depends on type of procedure to be performed.

nicable occurs in situations of intimate contact. Examples are sexual activities and family dwellings. Risk diminishes in the work environment (including the hospital setting). Risk is also highest from those microorganisms that can function as colonizing strains (*Streptococcus pneumoniae, Haemophilus influenzae,* and *Neisseria meningitidis*), or organisms that are part of the normal flora of an individual but gain access to deep tissue because of disruption of the anatomic barrier that usually limits spread (*S. viridans* from the oropharynx, *Enterococcus faecalis* from the gastrointestinal or genitourinary tract). Dissemination through foodstuffs or vectors such as the mosquito is a relatively low risk, unless the duration of exposure is prolonged or the degree of exposure is intense.

All medical conditions listed in Table 47–3 require detailed explanation for determining appropriate use of antibiotics. Primary reference source material is cited and should be reviewed to support clinical decision making.

Exposure to infectious agents occurs in situations of close (intimate) contact.

Dosing

Many of the basic principles of clinical pharmacokinetics have been derived from the use of antibiotics to treat infectious diseases. Clinical pharmacokinetics is the study of drug absorption, distribution, metabolism, and excretion over time in an individual patient. Of greater importance is the concept of pharmacodynamics, i.e., the relationship between drug concentration at the target receptor site and the pharmacological response it produces. Many infections occur at sites inaccessible to easy recovery of tissue. Fortunately, there generally is a strong correlation between concentrations of drug in the blood and clinical or microbiological outcome.

Pharmacokinetics is what the body does to a drug. Pharmacodynamics is what the drug does to the body.

When penicillin became available in the 1940s, dosing of the drug was limited by scarce supply. Low dosages (almost immeasurable by today's standards) administered for a brief period of time produced cure of serious infections such as pneumococcal pneumonia (for example, 30,000 units/day for 3 days). Clinical observation determined that this treatment schedule was inadequate for pneumococcal meningitis, so "massive" dosages (1.2 million units/day) were employed with favorable results.

These observations led to a dosing routine that has persisted to the present. That is, mild infections (as judged by the physician) require relatively small dosages of antibiotics administered infrequently; moderate infections require more; and serious infections require the largest dosages tolerable administered at the briefest intervals. Although toxicity may be produced by extremely large quantities of penicillin (40 million units/day), the therapeutic index (toxic/therapeutic ratio) is large and allows for this kind of approach.

Dosing is often proportioned to the severity of illness.

Cephalosporin antibiotics possess this same degree of safety over a wide dosing range. But aminoglycoside antibiotics provide a ready example that dose-dependent toxicity is an important consideration for certain antibiotic prescriptions, and that the therapeutic index of some antibiotics limits their clinical utility. Many pharmacokinetic dosing principles evolved during the time that accurate gentamicin dosing became an important clinical concern.

Gentamicin is a polar, water-soluble antibiotic. Therefore, it is poorly absorbed from the gastrointestinal (GI) tract. Intramuscular (IM) or IV administration is best described by the one compartment model with a small volume of distribution. The drug is not metabolized, and almost all is recovered unchanged from the urine by first-order elimination. However, this drug does accumulate in the kidney, and the major toxicity of gentamicin is nephrotoxicity.

No clinical parameters accurately predict vulnerability to gentamicin nephrotoxicity. Routine laboratory testing through urinalysis or serum cre-

Pharmacokinetic modeling is the preferred dosing method.

atinine can only define toxicity after it has occurred. Therefore, dosing is best determined by pharmacokinetic modeling. The most commonly employed formula was described by Cockcroft and Gault. The formula incorporates the important features of ideal body weight, sex, and age-associated decline in renal function. Because gentamicin is poorly lipid-soluble, administration of a dose based upon a simple mg/kg calculation is inappropriate for the obese person. Women have a different calculation for ideal body weight than that of men. Furthermore, elderly individuals lose muscle mass over time. This is approximately matched by a decline in glomerular filtration. The result is a serum creatinine in the normal range that does not accurately reflect renal function. Therefore, the elderly are also vulnerable to excessive dosing unless a correction is made.

Despite the general applicability of the formula, confounding variables limit the accuracy of dosing. Examples include dehydration and concurrent administration of nephrotoxic drugs, such as furosemide, cephalosporin antibiotics, and cisplatin. On the other hand, underdosing may occur with children and burn patients, because the drug is cleared more rapidly than predicted.

Measurement of serum peak and trough concentrations maximizes efficacy and minimizes toxicity.

In order to adjust dosing, serum peak and trough determinations must be made periodically. The peak value is assayed on a serum sample obtained 30 minutes after administration of an IV dose or 1 hour after an IM dose of drug. The trough is measured on a serum sample obtained 30 minutes prior to administration of the subsequent dose. Based on these results, the serum half-life can be calculated and the dosing interval adjusted. By following serum peak and trough values during a course of therapy, the risk of nephrotoxicity can be minimized.

However, efficacy is also critically important. It has been well established that clinical efficacy is most closely associated with the serum peak achieved by the first dose. In order to achieve a rapid serum peak concentration and to keep drug concentration within the therapeutic window, a

---

Table 47-4 AMINOGLYCOSIDE DOSING

Determination of Loading Dose

Aminoglycoside	Loading dose*	Expected serum peak
Gentamicin	1.5–2.0 mg/kg	4.0–10.0 μg/ml
Tobramycin	1.5–2.0 mg/kg	4.0–10.0 μg/ml
Amikacin	5.0–7.5 mg/kg	15.0–30.0 μg/ml
Kanamycin	5.0–7.5 mg/kg	15.0–30.0 μg/ml
Netilmicin	1.3–3.3 mg/kg	4.0–12.0 μg/ml

Determination of Interval Dose
Administer 50% of loading dose at estimated serum half-life or calculate creatinine clearance.

$$C_{cr} \text{ male} = \frac{140 - \text{age}}{\text{serum creatinine}}$$

$$C_{cr} \text{ female} = 0.85 \times C_{cr} \text{ male}$$

Choose the preferred dosing interval and percentage at loading dose interval.

C_{cr} (ml/mm)	Half-life (hours)	8 hours (%)	12 hours (%)	24 hours (%)
90	3.1	84	—	—
60	4.5	71	84	—
30	8.4	48	63	86
20	11.9	37	50	75
10	20.4	24	34	56

Adapted from Cockcroft DW, Gault MH: Prediction of creatinine clearance from serum creatinine. Nephron 16:31, 1976. By permission of S. Karger AG, Basel.
* Based on ideal body weight: male—50 kg + 2.3 kg for every inch over 5 feet; female—45.5 kg + 2.3 kg for every inch over 5 feet.

loading dose should be administered (Table 47–4). The loading dose is calculated based on ideal body weight and does *not* require consideration of renal function. A 70 kg man with a serum creatinine of 0.7 mg/dl and a 70 kg man with a serum creatinine of 5.0 mg/dl should receive the same loading dose. However, the dosing interval will differ markedly for these two individuals.

What is most important therapeutically is the concentration of drug at the site of infection. Most organs are perfused by porous capillary beds that permit antibiotics to penetrate the extravascular interstitial space. The concentration of drug achieved within such tissues depends upon the amount of free drug in serum and the distance the drug has to travel to reach the site of infection. If the distance traveled is short, tissue concentrations approximate unbound serum concentrations. If the distance is long, the tissue concentration may be approximated by the logarithmic mean of the peak and trough determinations.

Certain body sites are perfused by capillaries with tight membrane junctions. Examples include the central nervous system (CNS), vitreous humor, and prostate gland. Lipid-soluble antibiotics, such as chloramphenicol, penetrate much more effectively than water-soluble gentamicin. Even though the prostate is bathed in urine that may contain 1000–2000 μg/ml of gentamicin, less than 0.1% may reach the gland unless there is significant inflammation, producing disruption of the barrier.

Having learned these lessons about aminoglycosides, pharmacokinetic and pharmacodynamic studies are now performed routinely in the

Certain body sites are "restricted access" sites. Lipid solubility determines penetrability.

Table 47–5 DOSE INTERVAL ADJUSTMENTS FOR COMMONLY PRESCRIBED β-LACTAM ANTIBIOTICS IN RENAL FAILURE (ADULTS)*

Drug	Dose	Interval for C_{cr} (ml/minute)			
		>90	60–90	10–60	<10
Amoxicillin	0.25–0.50 g	8	8	12	12–24
Ampicillin	0.5–2.0 g	4–6	6	8	12
Cloxacillin	0.5–1.0 g	6	6	6	6
Dicloxacillin	0.25–0.5 g	6	6	6	6
Mezlocillin	3–4 g	4–6	4–6	6–8	8–12
Nafcillin	0.5–1.5 g	4–6	4–6	4–6	4–6
Oxacillin	0.5–2.0 g	4–6	4–6	4–6	4–6
Penicillin G	0.3–2.4 × 10⁶ U	2–12	2–12	2–12	⅓–½ dose
Penicillin V	0.25–0.5 g	6	6	8	12
Piperacillin	3–4 g	4–6	4–6	6–12	12
Ticarcillin	3 g	4–6	4–6	8	2 g q 12
Cefazolin	0.5–1 g	8	8	12	24
Cefalexin	0.25–1 g	6	6	8–12	24–48
Cephalothin	0.5–2 g	4–6	6	8	12
Cefaclor	0.25–0.5 g	8	8	8	8
Cefamandole	0.5–2 g	4–6	6	8	0.5–1 g q 12
Cefonicid	0.5–2 g	24	0.5–1.5 g q 24	0.5–1 g q 24	0.5–1 g q 3–5 days
Cefoxitin	1–3 g	4–6	1–2 g q 8	1–2 g q 12	0.8–1 g q 12–24
Cefuroxime	0.75–1.5 g	8	8	12	24
Cefoperazone	1–4 g	6–8	6–8	6–8	6–8
Cefotaxime	1–2 g	4–6	4–6	6–12	12
Cefotetan	1–2 g	12	12	24	48
Ceftazidime	0.5–2 g	8–12	8–12	1 g q 12–24	0.5 g q 24–48
Ceftizoxime	1–4 g	8–12	0.25–1 g	0.25–1 g q 12	0.25–1 g q 24–48
Ceftriaxone	0.5–1 g	12–24	12–24	12–24	12–24

* All intervals expressed in hours.

analysis and development of new drugs. For certain older drugs, careful monitoring of serum levels is considered the standard of care. These include vancomycin and chloramphenicol, in addition to aminoglycosides. Because most β-lactams are excreted by the kidney, dose adjustment is required in renal failure. Adjustment recommendations are summarized in Table 47–5.

Certain newly developed cephalosporins have bimodal routes of excretion, including cefotaxime and ceftriaxone. Cefotaxime is metabolized to a desacetyl derivative, which enters the enterohepatic circulation. The parent compound and metabolite are excreted also in the urine. Ceftriaxone is excreted unchanged through the biliary tract and kidney. With both drugs, dose modification is generally unnecessary except for treatment of patients with simultaneous end-stage hepatic and renal disease.

Antibiotics cleared primarily by hepatic metabolism, such as chloramphenicol, have no reliable mechanism for predicting dosing adjustments. The premature infant and neonate lack a mature glucuronyl transferase enzyme system and, therefore, accumulate the active drug. Patients with cirrhosis or active hepatic dysfunction conjugate chloramphenicol at a slower rate. The only practical way to determine appropriate dosing is to frequently monitor drug concentrations in serum. The consequence of chloramphenicol accumulation is inhibition of mitochondrial transport in the liver, heart, and skeletal muscle. This produces clinical manifestations of vomiting, tachypnea, cyanosis, and an ashen color identified as the *gray syndrome.* If unrecognized, it can progress to vascular collapse and death.

Thus, dosing has progressed from standard quantities (250 mg, 500 mg, 1000 mg) administered to patients of various size, and weights, based solely on their degree of illness, to pharmacokinetic analysis and dosing based on weight, sex, renal function, and measured concentrations of drugs. With the development of a wide variety of new antimicrobial agents, sufficient choices exist often to provide an alternative therapeutic agent of equal efficacy but lesser toxicity.

The next consideration for dosing of antibiotics is pharmacodynamics. What is the most effective method to deliver high concentrations of an antibiotic to the site of infection—continuous infusion; large dosages achieving high serum concentrations at infrequent intervals; or smaller dosages at more frequent intervals? Is it more important to achieve a high initial concentration or a sustained lower concentration at the site of infection? These issues are only more recently being explored, and responses to the questions may depend on the drug, the causative organism, the site of infection, and the status of host defenses.

Finally, certain antibiotics, most notably the aminoglycosides, produce a postantibiotic effect. In animal and *in vitro* models of infection, an aminoglycoside antibiotic continues to inhibit bacterial growth several hours after it has declined below inhibitory concentration. Bacteria are most vulnerable to killing only after they initiate growth again. Therefore, there may be therapeutic value to allowing serum trough concentrations to remain subinhibitory for several hours. The exact number of hours is species- and drug-dependent. Thus, there remain additional areas to explore in order to define optimal dosing and dose modifications for antimicrobial agents.

Resistance

Resistance to antimicrobial agents arises generally through one of three mechanisms: (1) intrinsic; (2) mutation; and (3) plasmid-mediated. Intrinsic resistance is a naturally occurring form of resistance that antedates the development or marketing of an antimicrobial agent. It has been identified in remote tribes of Indians not previously exposed to antibiotics. Because

Certain antibiotics have bimodal excretion.

Antibiotics cleared by the liver require monitoring of serum concentrations to maximize safety.

Pharmacodynamics of antibiotics are just now being analyzed.

Postantibiotic effect is persistent suppression of bacterial growth below inhibitory concentrations.

Resistance occurs by intrinsic, mutation, or plasmid-mediated mechanisms.

most antimicrobials are natural products or derivatives thereof, intrinsic resistance is believed to represent a survival mechanism possessed by strains of microorganisms to give them selective advantage in population dynamics.

A second form of intrinsic resistance is inducible β-lactamase production. This has been best described among certain *Enterobacteriaceae,* such as *Enterobacter, Klebsiella,* and *Serratia* species. Original isolates from clinical sources appear susceptible upon initial *in vitro* testing. However, treatment with an antimicrobial agent that induces β-lactamase production, such as cefoxitin, stimulates production of an enzyme that may destroy the therapeutic agent, other β-lactam antibiotics, or both. Although this may give the appearance of acquired resistance, testing of the original isolate (prior to antibiotic exposure) shows the resistance to be intrinsic.

The third form of intrinsic resistance exists in the construct of the bacterial cell wall. Channels known as porins are used by bacteria to transport materials in and out of the cell. *Escherichia coli* have a choice in porin structure. In the absence of antimicrobials, the OmpF porin is incorporated into the cell wall; this has a large pore diameter and allows more entry by charged and hydrophilic molecules. In the presence of antibiotics, the OmpC protein is incorporated, a smaller, more restrictive channel.

Mutational events include change in penicillin-binding proteins (PBPs), ribosomal proteins, DNA gyrase, RNA polymerase, and bacterial energy-generation systems. All bacteria possess target proteins in their cystoplasmic membranes for β-lactam antibiotics. Multiple mutational steps are required to change the PBP target, and it is presumed that widespread use of β-lactam antibiotics contributes to the selective pressure that promotes this change. Resistance among *S. pneumoniae* to penicillin is an excellent example. An alternative form of this resistance is change of the PBP-binding capacity, requiring greater and greater concentrations of the β-lactam antibiotic to saturate the target site and exert a lethal effect. Methicillin-resistant staphylococci employ this mechanism.

Mutational resistance in ribosomal proteins involves alteration of one or two amino acids in the protein content of the 30S subunit. The result is a single-step, high level of resistance to streptomycin. This form of resistance has been seen also for spectinomycin and gentamicin, but remains rare for these antibiotics at this time.

The newly developed fluoroquinolone antibiotics have a broad spectrum of activity and represent a significant therapeutic advance. However, alteration of their DNA gyrase target by a single mutation can render a strain of bacteria resistant. Thus far, the occurrence of such events remains infrequent (1 in 10^{11}).

A one-step mutational event can result in an altered protein component of the bacterial 30S ribosomal subunit and decreased binding affinity for both macrolides and lincosamides. It has been described in *S. pyogenes, Staphylococcus aureus,* and *E. coli.* It is particularly common among bacteria exposed to subinhibitory concentrations of antibiotic.

The logic behind the combination of trimethoprim-sulfamethoxazole was to attack bacterial tetrahydrofolic acid synthesis at two distinct steps, minimizing the likelihood that a mutational event could circumvent the lethal effect. The *in vitro* killing by the combination was synergistic rather than additive. Intrinsic susceptibility to trimethoprim was the major factor in determining efficacy of the combination. But certain strains of bacteria have developed an alternative tetrahydrofolic acid synthesis pathway, circumventing the theoretical advantage of the combination drug.

Plasmid-mediated resistance can take multiple forms. The most common is production of an enzyme that inactivates the antimicrobial mole-

Intrinsic resistance is naturally occurring, inducible (enzyme production), or mediated by structural changes.

Mutations generally modify target sites.

cule. Plasmid activity may be constitutive or inducible. Antibiotics vulnerable to plasmid-mediated resistance include penicillins, cephalosporins, aminoglycosides, macrolides, lincosamides, trimethoprim, sulfonamides, chloramphenicol, and tetracycline. Macrolides and lincosamides have reduced target affinity through plasmid-mediated resistance; trimethoprim and sulfamethoxazole activity is bypassed by new dihydrofolate reductase and dihydropteroate synthetase production; chloramphenicol has reduced uptake; and tetracycline has enhanced efflux from the cell through production of the tetracycline energy-dependent transfer (TET) protein.

Resistance mechanisms may be combined.

Finally, bacteria may combine certain of the mechanisms of resistance. A more recent common problem among clinical isolates has been reduced permeability combined with enzymatic induction. In this case the enzyme is given a longer time period to exert a destructive action; the enzyme may compete with the antibiotic for the target site; or the enzyme may act like a sponge, preventing the antibiotic from reaching its target. Both β-lactam and aminoglycoside molecules are vulnerable to these mechanisms.

Appropriate antibiotic prescriptions decrease the likelihood for resistant strains to emerge.

Knowledge of these various mechanisms reinforces the concept that antibiotics must be prescribed appropriately in order to maintain the therapeutic usefulness of these drugs as long as possible. It must be realized also that antibiotics are incorporated into animal feeds in order to reduce illness among herds in the food chain. This adds to the environmental burden of drug-induced resistance. Also, many countries around the world allow over-the-counter purchase of antibiotics, again exerting a significant impact on resistance.

On a global perspective, bacterial resistance is widespread. Sulfonamides were the first systemic antibacterial agents. Sulfa-resistant gonococci were widespread 10 years after their introduction; meningococcal resistance has become so widespread that prophylaxis with sulfonamides can no longer be recommended; and sulfa resistance among *E. coli* is more common than for any other class of antibacterial agents.

Penicillin was introduced in the 1940s. Although originally highly susceptible, *S. aureus* quickly developed β-lactamase–mediated resistance and caused epidemics of infection among hospitalized patients in the 1950s. The current prevalence of penicillin resistance among both community and nosocomial isolates approaches 90%. A similar phenomenon mediated by a different mechanism of resistance (altered target) is currently occurring among staphylococci and their susceptibility to methicillin. All indications are that methicillin resistance is headed toward epidemic proportions.

Ampicillin was the first semisynthetic penicillin with activity against gram-negative bacteria. For many years it was the most widely prescribed antibiotic in the United States. Amoxicillin currently occupies this position. From 20 to 70% of *E. coli* are ampicillin-resistant, depending on the community in which resistance is evaluated.

Resistance is most common in hospitals.

The most intense pressure for selection of resistant strains occurs in the hospital setting. This is also the most common test site for newly developed antibiotics. Prevalence studies conducted for 3–6 months generally indicate no resistance among hospital strains for new antibiotics prior to marketing. The subsequent likelihood of resistant strains emerging during the therapeutic prescription of a new antimicrobial agent varies with the class of drug. A survey of published studies showed that rates of resistance during clinical trial of a new drug were 9.2% for broad-spectrum penicillins, 8.6% for second- and third-generation cephalosporins, 4.7% for imipenem, 11.8% for ciprofloxacin, and 13.4% for aminoglycosides. Not all these resistant strains caused significant infections during the course of therapy, and most strains reverted to susceptible when therapy was completed.

However, the focus of appropriate antibiotic prescriptions must be the individual patient. Often, careful tracking can identify the source of an epidemic of resistant bacteria as an individual patient who has received multiple courses of antibiotics. Resistant strains are transmitted then to other vulnerable patients by the hands of hospital personnel. These patients are vulnerable because of their underlying disease, receipt of immunosuppressive drugs, invasion by devices, or receipt of antibiotics. The epidemic may be contained by infection control practices, such as contact isolation, or the resistant strain may become part of the nosocomial flora. In the latter circumstance, antibiotic prescriptions must be tailored to take this resistance into account, prompting selective pressure toward a different pattern of resistance.

Thus, every antibiotic prescription must be written carefully. Factors favoring resistance include excessive dose and duration of therapy, use in unwarranted circumstances, and broad-spectrum coverage when organism-targeted therapy would suffice. The responsibility for maintaining therapeutic viability of antimicrobial agents rests with every practitioner.

Transfer of resistant organisms from patient to patient through personnel is a hazard of hospitalization.

General References

Prophylaxis

Altemeier WA, Burke JP, Pruitt BA Jr, Sandersky WR (eds): Definitions and classifications of surgical infections. *In* Altemeier WA (ed): Manual on Control of Infection in Surgical Patients, 2nd ed, 1. Philadelphia: JB Lippincott CO, 1984.

Antimicrobial therapy and chemprophylaxis of infectious diseases. *In* Drug Evaluations, 6th ed, 1225. Chicago: American Medical Association, 1986.

Beam TR Jr: First-generation cephalosporins in surgical prophylaxis. Infect Med 10:275, 1988.

Burke JF: The effective period of preventive antibiotic action in experimental incisions and dermal lesions. Surgery 50:161, 1961.

Conte JE Jr, Jacob LS, Polk HC Jr: Antibiotic Prophylaxis in Surgery. Philadelpha: JB Lippincott Co, 1984.

Morsgard F, Lykkegaard-Nielsen MC, Justesen T, Scheibel JM: Wound infection rate following preoperative versus intraoperative commencement of antibiotic prophylaxis. Eur J Clin Microbiol 3:199, 1984.

VanScoy RE, Wilkowski CJ: Prophylactic use of antimicrobial agents in adult patients. Mayo Clin Proc 62:1137, 1987.

Dosing and Dose Modification

Barza M: Principles of tissue penetration antibiotics. J Antimicrob Chemother 8(Suppl C): 7, 1981.

Bennett WM, Aronoff GR, Morrison G, et al: Drug prescribing in renal failure: Dosing guidelines for adults. Am J Kidney Dis 3:155, 1983.

Bundzten RW, Gerber AU, Cohn DL, et al: Postantibiotic suppression of bacterial growth. Rev Infect Dis 3:28, 1981.

Cockcroft DW, Gault MH: Prediction of creatinine clearance from serum creatinine. Nephron 16:31, 1976.

DiPiro JT, Blouin RA, Pruemer JM: Concepts in Clinical Pharmacokinetics. Bethesda, MD: American Society of Hospital Pharmacists, 1988.

Moore RD, Smith CR, Leitman PS: The association of aminoglycoside plasma levels with mortality in patients wth gram-negative sepsis. J Infect Dis 149:443, 1984.

Spyker DA, Guerrant RL: Dosage nomograms for aminoglycoside antibiotics. Hosp Formulary 16:132, 1981.

Resistance

Bryan LE: General mechanisms of resistance to antibiotics. J Antimicrob Chemother 22(Suppl A): 1, 1988.

Eliopoulos GM: Induction of beta-lactamase. J Antimicrob Chemother 22(Suppl A):37, 1988.

Kozarsky PE, Terry PM, Romland D: Development of antibiotic resistance by *Staphylococcus aureus* in a single patient. Am J Med 80:1208, 1986.

Levy SB: Microbial resistance to antibiotics. An evolving and persistent problem. Lancet 2:83, 1982.

Milatovic D. Braverny I: Development of resistance during antibiotic therapy. Eur J Clin Microbiol 6:234, 1987.

Nikaido H: Bacterial resistance to antibiotics as a function of outer membrane permeability. J Antimicrob Chemother 22(Suppl A):17, 1988.

O'Brien TF, Members of Task Force 2: Resistance of bacteria to antibacterial agents: Report of task force 2. Rev Infect Dis 9(Suppl 3):S244, 1987.

48

The Penicillins, Vancomycin, and Bacitracin

Alan M. Reynard

The discovery of penicillin G marks the real beginning of the antibiotic era. There had been earlier discoveries of antibiotics such as salvarsan by Paul Ehrlich and the sulfonamides by Gerhard Dogmak. However, salvarsan was a very toxic drug that would never be considered for clinical use now, and the sulfonamides, although effective and still in use, were completely overshadowed by the extremely effective and less toxic penicillin G.

Penicillin G was discovered in 1929 by Alexander Fleming. He left a culture plate containing staphylococci on a work table while he went on vacation. On his return he noticed that a mold growing on the plate had stopped the growth of the colonies of staphylococci, especially those that were growing near the mold. He isolated the mold and used it to produce more of the inhibitory substance, which he named *penicillin*.

Fleming uncovered many of the properties of penicillin, such as its spectrum of action and that resistance to it could occur. He treated several patients with it, but because he was unable to purify the penicillin he could only use it topically and the treatments were unsuccessful.

In 1939 England was at war with Germany, and Howard Flory, Professor of Pathology at Oxford, was searching for substances with antibacterial properties for use in treating wounds inflicted during bombing raids and later in the field. He had the advantage of having a well-trained chemist on his staff, Abraham Chain, who partially purified penicillin, thereby enabling Flory to treat a series of patients parenterally. The first patient was a policeman from the town of Oxford who was suffering from a severe, mixed staphylococcal/streptococcal infection. The improvement that penicillin G initially made in the policeman's condition was dramatic. However, the supply of penicillin G was limited, and when the supply was exhausted the patient died. The results were so encouraging that eight other patients were later treated with extremely good results.

The penicillin discovered by Fleming was penicillin G. Shortly afterward an analog was discovered, penicillin V, also produced by a mold, but with the property of being resistant to degradation by acid, thereby permitting it to be administered orally. Since that time, numerous other analogs have been discovered with a variety of special properties.

Fleming and Chain were knighted, Flory was made a lord, and all three shared the Nobel Prize.

The importance of penicillin at that time was that it was the first antibiotic with extremely good activity against the then most serious organisms, staphylococci, streptococci, pneumococci, and neisseria, and it had very few adverse effects. Here is an example of how profound the effects of penicillin G were. Puerperal fever (a streptococcal infection of mothers at

The Penicillins

Penicillin G is discovered by Alexander Fleming.

Abraham Chain and Howard Flory purify penicillin G and demonstrate that it is useful to treat infection in humans.

Penicillin V is discovered. It can be administered orally.

Penicillin G has profound effects on whole populations of bacteria.

the time of childbirth) was a frequent, serious, reportable disease in the 1930s. The sulfonamides, used initially in 1936, were able to reduce the number of deaths due to puerperal fever by a factor of ten. In contrast, penicillin, introduced into civilian hospitals in 1945, not only could be used to treat the disease but also actually reduced the incidence of the disease to nearly zero. The sulfonamides were able to treat the disease, but penicillin all but eradicated it.

CHEMISTRY

The penicillins have two rings.

The penicillins are compounds that share a common double-ring system and are differentiated only by a single side chain that is unique for each penicillin. The two rings are a β-lactam ring and a thiazolidene ring. The β-lactam ring is the more important because it plays a role in all the actions of the penicillins. The thiazolidene ring plays a role in specifying the potential for allergic reactions to the drug. It can be noted that the cephalosporins (see Chapter 49) also have a β-lactam ring but have a dihydrothiazine ring instead of a thiazolidene ring. Many people who are allergic to penicillin are not allergic to the cephalosporins.

The thiazolidine ring plays a role in allergic reactions.

The β-lactam ring is involved in (1) antibacterial activity, (2) instability to acid, (3) bacterial resistance, and (4) allergic reactions.

The β-lactam ring is involved in most of the activities of the penicillins.

An additional feature of the penicillins is a carboxyl group attached to the thiazolidene ring. Penicillins are never administered as the free acid; they are administered as either the sodium or the potassium salt. Because the penicillins have relatively few dose-related adverse effects, and because they are sometimes used in situations in which a dramatic effect is required, they may be administered in enormous doses. This poses a problem for patients with heart conditions, for whom the potassium administered as part of a large dose of penicillin may be sufficient to adversely affect heart muscle.

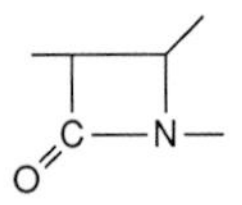

Penicillins are administered as salts.

β-lactam ring

The β-lactam ring is very reactive.

The β-lactam ring is a four-member ring and, therefore, is inherently unstable. It tends to hydrolyze, but it will react with other ligands, and this property provides the penicillins with their antibacterial activity. When penicillin is hydrolyzed, the bond between the nitrogen and the carbonyl in the β-lactam ring opens and the carbonyl becomes a carboxyl. The ensuing product is called *penicilloic acid* (Fig. 48–1). When the penicillin reacts with something other than water, such as the bacterial transpeptidase, it acylates the target molecule, thereby forming a covalent bond.

The common moiety in the penicillins is 6-aminopenicillanic acid (6-APA).

The side chain of the penicillins can be removed by hydrolysis with or without enzyme catalysis, and the product is 6-aminopenicillanic acid (6-APA). 6-APA is used as the base material to produce most of the penicillin analogs. Because of this, penicillins G and V, the only ones produced solely by fermentation, are called the *natural penicillins*, and the others,

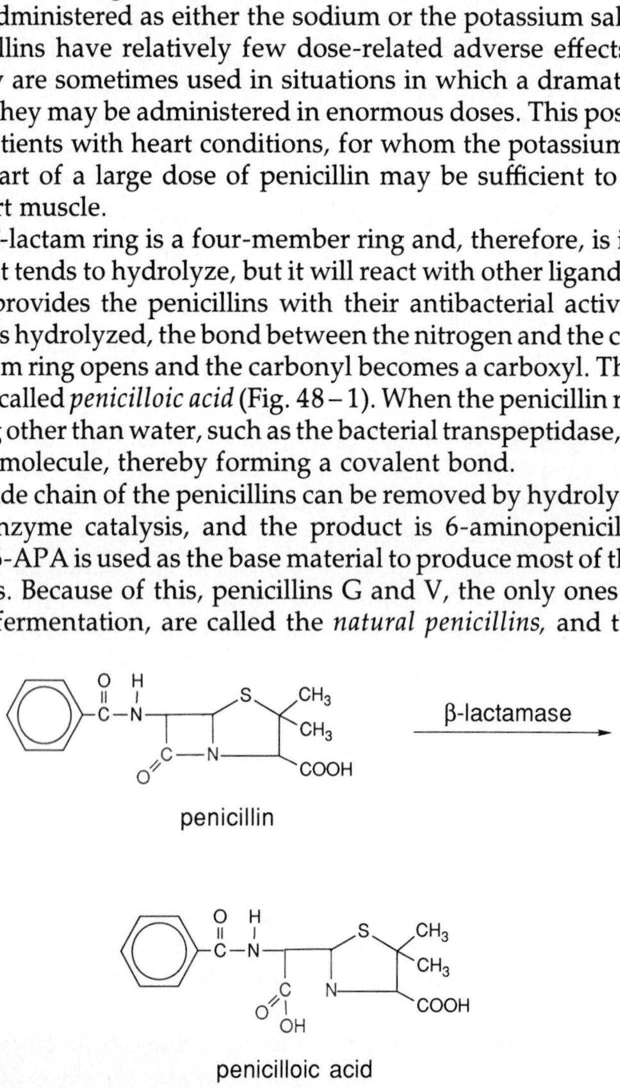

penicillin

Figure 48–1

Hydrolysis of penicillin to penicilloic acid is catalyzed by the β-lactamase enzyme.

penicilloic acid

The penicillins
Side chain (R)

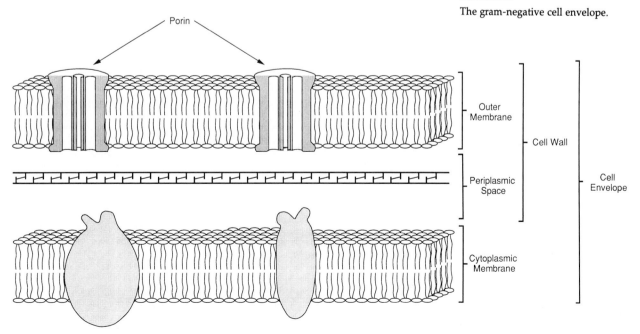

Penicillin G (benzyl)

Penicillin V (phenoxymethyl)

Methicillin

Oxacillin

Ampicillin (α-aminobenzyl)

Amoxicillin

Carbenicillin

Ticarillin

such as ampicillin, which are produced by chemically adding a side chain to 6-APA, are called the *semisynthetic penicillins*.

When penicillin G was first used clinically, it was so impure that weight was not a good determinant of dose. Instead, each batch of penicillin G was calibrated against a standard strain of *Staphylococcus aureus*, and penicillin was administered by unitage. It is now known that 1 unit of penicillin G contains 0.6 μg of pure sodium penicillin G (1 mg = 1667 units). All other penicillins are administered by weight.

Penicillin G is administered as units. The other penicillins are administered by weight.

MECHANISM OF ACTION

The Bacterial Cell Envelope. The cell envelope of a bacterial cell (Fig. 48–2) consists of several structures. A *cytoplasmic membrane*, similar to the

Figure 48–2

The gram-negative cell envelope.

Porin

Outer Membrane

Periplasmic Space

Cytoplasmic Membrane

Cell Wall

Cell Envelope

The envelope of a gram-positive bacterial cell consists of a cytoplasmic membrane and a cell wall.

The envelope of a gram-negative cell consists of the two structures found in a gram-positive cell and an outer membrane.

Completion of the bacterial cell wall occurs outside the cytoplasmid membrane where the usual energy sources are not available.

Peptidoglycan is composed of a polymer of alternating *N*-acetylglucosamine and *N*-acetylmuramic acid with short peptide chains attached to the muramic acid moieties.

membrane of a mammalian cell, is the cell's principle permeability barrier and contains a number of enzyme systems. The bacterial transpeptidase resides near the outer surface of the cytoplasmic membrane. Covering the cytoplasmic membrane is the *cell wall*, a relatively rigid structure that provides shape and stability to the cell. Gram-negative cells have an additional membrane, the *outer membrane*, that acts as a partial permeability barrier. The outer membrane is composed largely of lipid but has a number of proteins. Some of the proteins stretch through the entire membrane and provide cross-membrane channels called *porins*. In gram-negative cells, the space between the cytoplasmic and the outer membranes is called the *periplasmic space*.

Because the cell wall is located outside the cytoplasmic membrane, the bacterial cell is faced with completing synthesis of its cell wall essentially on its exterior surface. Thus, completion of the cell wall requires the making of chemical bonds at a place where there is no natural energy supply; the natural sources of cellular energy, such as adenosine triphosphate (ATP), are confined by the cytoplasmic membrane to the interior of the cell. This problem is overcome by the strategy of breaking one bond so that another can be made.

The Bacterial Cell Wall. It is necessary to know the structure of the bacterial cell wall to understand how it is synthesized. It consists of a polymer, called *glycan*, made of repeating units of *N*-acetylglucosamine moieties. Every other *N*-acetylglucosamine molecule has a molecule of lactic acid attached, and the *N*-acetylglucosamine–lactic acid molecule is called *N*-acetylmuramic acid. Another way to view the structure of glycan is as alternating units of *N*-acetylglucosamine and *N*-acetyl muramic acid. Attached to each *N*-acetylmuramic acid is a small chain of amino acids (a small peptide). The amino acid composition of the peptide is different for the different species of bacteria. For example, it is ala-glu-lys-ala-ala for *Escherichia coli* and

$$\begin{array}{c} \text{gly-gly-gly-gly-gly} \\ | \\ \text{ala-glu-lys-ala-ala} \end{array}$$

Staphylococcal cell walls are thick, and the *E. coli* cell wall is thin.

for *S. aureus*. However, the two terminal amino acids are ala-ala in each case. The entire polymer is referred to as *peptidoglycan*. The bacterial cell wall is composed of peptidoglycan molecules bridged together by the peptide side chains of the peptidoglycan. In *S. aureus* the cell wall is quite thick and rigid and gives the cell its spheroid shape. Correspondingly, *S. aureus* cells are relatively difficult to break with methods such as sonic oscillators. In contrast *E. coli* cells have thin cell walls, are rod-shaped, and are relatively easy to break.

Synthesis of the cell wall is completed by making cross-links between peptide side chains of adjacent peptidoglycan polymers.

Removal of an amino acid from the end of one of the chains provides the energy to make the new peptide bond.

The Synthesis of Cell Wall. The site of action of the penicillins is the last step in synthesis of the bacterial cell wall. In this step, the peptide side chains of two adjacent peptidoglycan molecules are covalently linked, i.e., a new peptide bond is formed. This step is facilitated by a transpeptidase, an enzyme that resides on the outer surface of the cytoplasmic membrane. The transpeptidase accomplishes its task in two steps (Fig. 48–3). In the first, it catalyzes the removal of the terminal (ultimate) amino acid (alanine) from the peptide side chain. This step produces energy that is coupled into the formation of a bond in the second step. If the enzyme were not to accomplish the second step, the energy would be dissipated as heat. In the second step, the energy produced by the breaking of the bond in the first

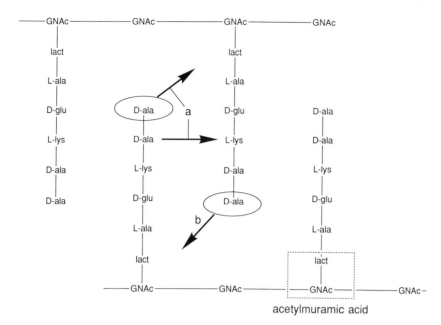

acetylmuramic acid

Figure 48-3

Sites of action of two enzymes on the bacterial cell wall. Letter a represents the action of the transpeptidase as it makes a cross-link between two peptide side chains of the *E. coli* cell wall. Letter b represents the cleavage of a terminal amino acid by the carboxypeptidase.

step is used to make a covalent bond between the penultimate amino acid and an amino acid on a neighboring chain. In the case of *E. coli* it is the remaining alanine (the penultimate amino acid) in the chain from which the ultimate alanine was removed that binds to a lysine on an adjacent chain. In the case of *S. aureus* the penultimate alanine binds to a glycine on the glycine side chain.

The cross-linking is catalyzed by an enzyme, the transpeptidase, residing at the outer surface of the cytoplasmic membrane.

Penicillins Inhibit the Transpeptidase. The penicillins inhibit the action of the transpeptidase in two stages. First, a penicillin molecule binds to the transpeptidase and acts as a competitive inhibitor of the enzyme. Second, the β-lactam ring of the penicillin acylates the transpeptidase and forms a covalent bond, thereby becoming an irreversible inhibitor.

Penicillins inhibit the transpeptidase.

Recall that the natural substrate of the enzyme is the ala-ala dipeptide that is the end of the peptide side chain of the peptidoglycan. The 6-APA portion of the penicillins, although composed of a double-ring system, resembles two amino acids. It is thought that the rigid, double ring of 6-APA is in a proper configuration for fitting the active site of the enzyme. As such, the rigid penicillin molecule has a thermodynamic advantage in attaching to the active site over the natural substrate, which is free to rotate in solution. This explains why the penicillins are such effective inhibitors of the transpeptidase.

Penicillins bind well to the transpeptidase because their rigid, two-ring system mimics the natural substrate of the enzyme, ala-ala.

Cells contain enzymes called *autolysins* that catalyze hydrolysis of cell wall material. When penicillin stops the growth of the bacterial cell wall and when autolysins are active, the cells undergo lysis. The lysis of cells subsequent to treatment with penicillin causes the cells to die. For this reason the penicillins are classified as *bactericidal*. Cells deficient in autolysins are inhibited in growth by penicillins, but they do not lyse and the cells survive.

Autolysins play a role in the killing of penicillin-inhibited cells.

The transpeptidase is only one of several penicillin-binding proteins (PBPs) involved in the mechanism of action of the penicillins. These other PBPs are responsible for septum formation in dividing bacteria, for their shape, and other effects. The PBPs are bound by penicillin and other penicillin-like compounds, such as the monobactams. The strength of binding varies with the type of antibiotic, but binding can result in effects such as filament formation or oval shape as well as cell death. There is also a

Penicillin-binding proteins (PBPs) play a role in the actions of the penicillins and other compounds.

carboxypeptidase enzyme that is an exopeptidase. It functions in bacteria to catalyze removal of terminal alanine molecule from peptide side chains of the peptidoglycan (see Fig. 48–3). This results in a reduction in the number of side chains available for linking to other side chains and in the amount of cross-linking of the peptidoglycan molecules. In *E. coli* there is considerable carboxypeptidase activity, the cell wall is thin, and only about 50% of the side chains are cross-linked. As noted earlier, the *E. coli* cell wall is easily broken by mechanical means. In *S. aureus* there is little carboxypeptidase activity, the cell wall is thick, and the peptidoglycan is nearly 100% cross-linked. The cell wall is broken by mechanical means only with comparative difficulty. Penicillin inhibits the activity of the caboxypeptidase, but there is probably no significance to this in regard to cell lysis.

> The carboxypeptidase is also inhibited by the penicillins.

An additional characteristic of the penicillins is that they are active against growing, but not resting, cells. This is a result of their mechanism of action. If the cell is not growing, it does not need additional cell wall material, and consequently, inhibition of the transpeptidase has no effect. There is some clinical significance to this observation. In general, penicillins are not used in conjunction with a bacteriostatic antibiotic because the growth inhibition by the bacteriostatic antibiotic results in diminished effectiveness of the penicillin. This was unfortunately demonstrated in the mid-1950s during an epidemic of pneumococcal pneumonia when tetracycline (bacteriostatic) was administered with penicillin in an attempt to provide more antibacterial activity.

> Penicillins are active against growing, but not resting, cells.

The relative insensitivity of the gram-negative rods to penicillin G and several of the other penicillins is probably due to the permeability barrier function of the outer membrane of these species. The penicillin molecules are not able to reach their target, the transpeptidase, located on the outer edge of the cytoplasmic membrane. Ampicillin, carbenicillin, and others are active against gram-negative cells because they can breach the outer membrane. They enter the periplasmic space by penetrating through channels (porins).

> The outer membrane of gram-negative cells provides a permeability barrier that prevents penicillin G and others from reaching the transpeptidase. Analogs such as ampicillin can penetrate the outer membrane.

BACTERIAL RESISTANCE

Almost all bacterial resistance to the penicillins comes from the effects of an enzyme that catalyzes the hydrolysis of the β-lactam ring (Fig. 48–3). This enzyme is often referred to as the *penicillinase* but is more appropriately called the *β-lactamase*. The emergence of this enzyme in the bacterial population has been tracked in a number of hospitals with similar findings. The percentage of strains bearing the enzyme and, consequently, resistant to the penicillins rose over a few years, from a few percent to about 80%, where it stands now. This high level of resistance is apparently due to the large amount of penicillin used in hospitals. When use of antibiotics in general, and penicillins in particular, has been reduced in hospitals, the number of strains resistant to the antibiotics correspondingly decreases.

> Bacteria become resistant to the penicillins by production of the enzyme β-lactamase.

The function of the β-lactamase is to destroy, by hydrolysis, the bond between the amino and the carbonyl groups in the β-lactam ring of the penicillin. When this bond is destroyed, the β-lactam ring is no longer active as an acylating agent and the penicillin molecule is not able to participate in its usual β-lactam–mediated actions.

> The β-lactamase catalyzes the hydrolysis of the β-lactam ring of the penicillins.

There are a number of β-lactamase enzymes, with specificities for the various β-lactam–containing antibiotics, including the cephalosporins. In *E. coli*, the β-lactamase is produced continually at low levels and is confined in the periplasmic space where it waits for the intrusion of a β-lactam antibiotic. In *S. aureus* there is no periplasmic space, and consequently the enzyme is elaborated directly into the medium. Here, enzyme is produced at a higher rate but production of the enzyme is under repressor control, so that enzyme is produced only after contact with the antibiotic. In this way, staphylococci do not consume resources by producing large amounts of enzyme unless it is necessary.

Several of the penicillins are not affected by the β-lactamase of staphylococci, i.e., they are resistant to it. Although it is confusing, they are occasionally referred to as the β-lactam–resistant penicillins. These include methicillin, oxacillin, cloxacillin, dicloxacillin, and nafcillin. These antibiotics are useful against most β-lactamase–producing strains of *Staphylococcus*. However, in a small percentage of strains there is a different mechanism of resistance, long known as *intrinsic resistance*, that provides resistance to all penicillins including the β-lactamase–resistant analogs. This latter resistance is probably due to a lack of binding to the PBPs.

> Several penicillins are not affected by β-lactamase.

Clavulanic acid is a β-lactamase inhibitor that covalently binds to the enzyme (a suicide inhibitor) and prevents it from further catalyzing hydrolysis of β-lactam antibiotics. It is produced by the mold *Streptomyces clavuligerus*, but it does not have significant antimicrobial activity. It is marketed in combination with amoxicillin (AUGMENTIN) for oral use and with ticarcillin (TIMENTIN) for parenteral use. These combinations are used to provide antimicrobial activity against certain β-lactamase–producing bacteria. Clinically, amoxicillin–clavulanic acid is used to treat bronchitis, lower respiratory tract infections, and otitis media. Ticarcillin–clavulanic acid is used for osteomyelitis as well as for skin, respiratory, and intra-abdominal infections. Clavulanic acid contains a β-lactam ring but has little antimicrobial activity. Another inhibitor, sulbactam, is marketed in combination with ampicillin (UNASYN) for parenteral use.

> Clavulanic acid is an inhibitor of β-lactamase. When combined with a penicillin, it prevents the β-lactamase from destroying the penicillin.

ABSORPTION, DISTRIBUTION, METABOLISM, AND EXCRETION

Some of the penicillins can be administered orally. Because food interferes with absorption, orally administered penicillins should be given at least 1 hour before or 2 hours after meals.

> Some penicillins can be administered orally. Others should be given parenterally.

Some of the penicillins should be given parenterally because of their instability in gastric acid. The instability manifests as an acid-catalyzed hydrolysis of the β-lactam ring. This results in uncertainty in the amount of active agent that can be absorbed by the gastrointestinal tract. Intramuscular injection is irritating and painful. For this reason, in treatment of diseases such as gonorrhea, the clinician will attempt to achieve a cure with one treatment only (a "one-shot cure").

The penicillins are widely distributed in the body, but they do not enter cells. They do not accumulate in cerebrospinal fluid in normal individuals. However, in diseases in which the meninges are inflamed the decrease in the blood-brain barrier permits therapeutic amounts of drug to enter. This precludes the necessity for intrathecal injection when treating pneumococcal or meningococcal meningitis. Therapeutic concentrations of penicillins are achieved in pleural, joint, and pericardial fluids, and at least some penicillin can be found in gingival crevicular fluid. Indanyl carbenicillin is excreted so rapidly that therapeutic levels are not achieved in the blood stream and high concentrations are seen in the urinary tract.

Penicillins are excreted largely by tubular secretion, with a small amount by glomerular filtration. Probenecid, an inhibitor of secretion of organic acids (see Chapters 30 and 34), can raise blood levels and prolong the half-life of penicillins in the body. It has been used in treatment of gonorrhea and in various prophylactic regimens. Penicillins are generally not lipid-soluble. However, the more lipid-soluble penicillins such as nafcillin are excreted largely through the biliary tract.

> Probenecid can elevate the level of some penicillins in the blood stream by blocking their tubular excretion.

There are two forms of penicillin that are excreted very slowly, pro-

Procaine and benzathine penicillin G are used for prophylaxis.

Procaine penicillin G and benzathine penicillin G are marketed as microcrystals that dissolve slowly from an intramuscular site of injection. They are depot preparations.

caine penicillin G and benzathine penicillin G. They are used in prophylactic regimens. Procaine penicillin G has been used for prophylaxis against bacterial endocarditis in conjunction with certain types of surgery, especially dental surgery, but its use in this instance has been reduced and other drugs have replaced it. Benzathine penicillin G is still used for prophylaxis against recurrences of rheumatic fever. A single injection of benzathine penicillin G produces a useful prophylactic blood level for 1 month. Both procaine and benzathine penicillin G have very low solubility and are administered in a microcrystalline form. An intramuscular injection results in the deposit of the crystals as a bolus in the muscle tissue. As the drug is absorbed into the blood stream, the crystals slowly dissolve, providing more drug in molecular form suitable for absorption. Procaine penicillin G is occasionally used for therapy as well as for prophylaxis.

SPECIAL PROPERTIES

The penicillins are a group of drugs with a common ring structure. However, the various side chains attached to the ring system provide the penicillins with a variety of properties. Table 48 – 1 illustrates this point. It also shows that penicillin G, probably the most important of the penicillins, has none of the special properties of the other members of the group, except for its superior activity against certain organisms.

INDICATIONS AND CONTRAINDICATIONS

Meningococci. Meningococcal meningitis is still uniquely susceptible to penicillin G. It is treated by intravenous injection of 20 – 24 million units of penicillin G.

Pneumococci. Infections caused by *Streptococcus pneumoniae* are regularly treated with penicillin G, although several occurrences of resistance to

---

Table 48 – 1   PROPERTIES OF THE PENCILLINS

Agent	Oral Administration*	Beta-Lactamase Resistance†	Gram-Negative Activity‡	Gram-Positive Activity§
Penicillin G				+++
Penicillin V	+			++
Nafcillin‖		+		+
Oxacillin¶	+	+		+
Ampicillin	+		+	+
Carbenicillin**			+	+
Ticarcillin††			+	+

* Resistance to gastric acidity is required for oral administration.
† Nafcillin and oxacillin are resistant to the β-lactamase enzymes that are elaborated by *Staphylococci*. These agents are never used against gram-negative bacteria.
‡ Ampicillin has good activity against gram-negative bacteria except for *Pseudomonas aeruginosa* and some strains of *Proteus*. Amoxicillin has similar activity, but absorption from gastrointestinal tract is better.
§ Penicillin G is by far the most active agent for many gram-positive species, including *Staphylococcus aureus* and *Streptococcus pyogenes*.
‖ Methicillin, with properties similar to those of nafcillin, has less activity and is little used.
¶ Two other very similar agents are cloxacillin and dicloxacillin.
** Carbenicillin has activity against *Pseudomonas* and *Proteus*, but it has to be injected. Indanyl carbenicillin is administered orally. It is hydrolyzed to carbenicillin in the blood but is cleared so rapidly that it achieves useful concentrations only in the urine.
†† Ticarcillin has two to four times as much activity against *Pseudomonas* as that of carbenicillin. Drugs similar to ticarcillin but even more active are azlocillin, mezlocillin, and piperacillin.

penicillin G have been noted. The dose depends on the disease; pneumo-coccal pneumonia may be treated with 600,000 units of procaine penicillin G twice a day, whereas pneumococcal meningitis requires 20–24 million units every 2–3 hours. Oral administration in cases of serious infections such as these is not recommended.

Streptococci. In general, *S. pyogenes* is very susceptible to penicillin, *S. viridans* is more variable with most strains susceptible but a few relatively resistant, and *S. faecalis* is least susceptible and is usually treated with a combination of penicillin and an aminoglycoside.

Strep throat, usually caused by *S. pyogenes,* may be treated with oral penicillin V, intramuscular procaine penicillin G, or intramuscular ben-zathine penicillin G. Other infections with *S. pyogenes* are regularly treated with penicillin G, the dose depending on the type of infection. Such infec-tions include otitis media, pneumonia, meningitis, and endocarditis.

Endocarditis is most often caused by *S. viridans,* and treatment with penicillin alone is usually adequate. In diseases such as this it is important to determine the susceptibility of the offending strain to penicillin G and other antibiotics. In the event that the organism is not susceptible to penicillin G, usually the combination of penicillin G and an aminoglycoside will suffice. However, some cases may be caused by a strain resistant to penicillin or the aminoglycoside, or both.

Staphylococci. Whereas approximately 20% of strains of staphylococcus found in the community are resistant to penicillin G, approximately 80% of strains found in hospital are resistant. Treatment of localized infection by a penicillin-resistant strain is usually accomplished with one of the β-lactamase–resistant penicillins: oxacillin, cloxacillin, dicloxacillin, or naf-cillin. Nafcillin is usually used for systemic infection.

Staphylococci that exhibit intrinsic resistance will be resistant to all the penicillins, and an alternative class of drug will have to be used. A common choice is an aminoglycoside.

Gonococci. *Neisseria gonorrhoeae* once was extremely susceptible to peni-cillin G. In the 1950s most cases of uncomplicated gonorrhoea could be cured with a single intramuscular injection of 200,000 units of penicillin G. By the 1960s, because of a gradual change in the susceptibility of the organism to penicillin G, the amount required had risen to 4.8 million units. By the 1970s, probenecid had to be added to the regimen to achieve a cure. In the late 1970s, a strain was discovered that produced very large amounts of β-lactamase, thereby completely frustrating treatment with penicillin G. In the 1980s, there were so many cases due to these high-level-penicillin-ase–producing (HLPP) strains that initial treatment in epidemic areas was no longer with penicillin G but with alternative drugs. In nonepidemic areas initial treatment is 4.8 million units procaine penicillin G combined with probenecid, ampicillin plus probenecid, or amoxicillin plus probene-cid. In epidemic areas (greater than 15% of strains are HLPP), initial treat-ment is the cephalosporin ceftriaxone.

Treponema. *Treponema pallidum* is susceptible to penicillin G; both pri-mary and secondary syphilis are treatable with procaine penicillin G plus probenecid.

Other diseases for which penicillin G is the agent of choice include anthrax, clostridial infections (gas gangrene, tetanus, rabbit-bite fever), erysipelas, rat-bite fever, listerial infection, trench mouth, and actinomy-cosis.

ADVERSE EFFECTS

The penicillins produce relatively few dose-related adverse effects. The broad-spectrum penicillins may produce superinfection.

The penicillins cause relatively few dose-related adverse effects—that is, they have very good selective toxicity because their target site on the bacterial cell (the cell wall/transpeptidase) has no counterpart in mammalian cells. Intramuscular injection is painful, and penicillin is irritating to tissues. Oral doses may cause nausea and vomiting. Toxicity of the potassium ions administered with large doses of potassium penicillin G or penicillin V may adversely affect already damaged heart muscle. Granulocytopenia and bone marrow depression have been reported.

Superinfection has been known to occur after administration of the penicillins. It is more frequent with oral administration and is seen with broad-spectrum penicillins, such as ampicillin, more frequently than with narrow-spectrum agents, such as penicillin G or V or methicillin. The superinfection may be serious, however, and pseudomembranous colitis has been observed.

The penicillins produce allergic reactions in a large number of patients. Some of the allergic reactions are very serious.

More important are the allergic reactions. About 5% of individuals in the United States are allergic to the penicillins. All penicillins are implicated, and when an individual is allergic to one penicillin, she or he is allergic to all penicillins; this is termed a *cross-reaction*. A history designed to discover possible allergic reactions is necessary when a penicillin is administered. A second reaction to a penicillin is often more serious than the first. If the patient appears to have had an allergic reaction to penicillin, an alternative drug ought to be considered, and a cephalosporin is often used. Even though the cephalosporins have a β-lactam ring, the substitution of a dihydrothiazine ring for the thiazolidene ring in the penicillins appears to introduce a sufficient difference to markedly reduce the possibility of a cross-reaction.

The allergic reactions are categorized as immediate, accelerated, and delayed.

There are several types of allergic reaction that are seen infrequently. These are thrombocytopenia, hemolytic anemia, drug fever, and serum sickness. More frequent are allergic reactions that can be classified as (1) immediate, (2) accelerated, and (3) delayed. The *immediate reaction* usually occurs within 30 minutes following a dose of penicillin. It is characterized by intense urticaria and other skin reactions, local inflammatory reactions, angioedema, and laryngeal edema sometimes leading to anaphylaxis and culminating in death. The *accelerated reaction* occurs within a day of receiving the drug and involves most of the same manifestations as the immediate reaction, but not the acute anaphylactic reaction. The *delayed reaction* may occur weeks after a dose of penicillin. It consists of a mild fever and rash. It is usually not treated, and it subsides spontaneously. The accelerated and immediate reactions should be treated with a glucocorticosteroid or an antihistamine, or both. In addition, the immediate reaction will probably have to be treated with epinephrine.

The incidence of skin reactions following administration of ampicillin is reported to be especially high. There are fewer allergic reactions following oral administration than parenteral administration.

It is possible to test for allergy with a skin test.

The major determinant contributing to the acute allergic reaction is a plasma protein (acting as the carrier) and penicillin acylating the protein (acting as a hapten). The plasma protein appears to be rich in lysine residues at the site of acylation. Minor determinants of the acute reaction appear to be penicillin degradation products. Skin testing with penicillin can be done but results in a high number of false-positive and false-negative responses. In addition, anaphylactic reactions have been reported following skin testing with very small doses of penicillin. A mixture of the minor determinants can be prepared and used for skin testing. The most reliable test is with penicilloyl-polylysine (PRE-PEN), a preparation containing a synthetic polypeptide consisting of about 18 lysine residues acylated with penicillin. Penicilloyl-polylysine does not appear to invoke anaphylactic reactions.

Desensitization of individuals with a prior history of penicillin allergy can be accomplished by intradermal injection of increasingly larger doses of penicillin, followed by subcutaneous injection of even larger doses. It may also be accomplished by oral administration. The procedure continues until full doses can be administered. Desensitization is obviously a dangerous procedure and should only be attempted when absolutely required, and it should be done under conditions in which an anaphylactic reaction can be dealt with. Several theories have been proposed that describe what occurs during the desensitization procedure. One is that IgG antibodies are discharged and block access of the allergy-producing IgE antibodies to their target sites, and another is that IgE antibodies are discharged at subclinical levels and are fully discharged by the time the desensitization period is finished.

Desensitization of a patient to penicillin is possible but difficult.

Imipenem

Imipenem is the *N*-formimidoyl derivative of a mold-produced antibiotic, thienamycin. It contains a β-lactam ring and closely resembles the penicillins, but its 5-member ring lacks the sulfur atom that is part of the penicillin's dihydrothiazine ring. In addition, imipenem has a -CH group in the location where the penicillins have the -NH group that is used to attach the various side chains.

Imipenem has very good activity against a wide variety of organisms. It has a β-lactam ring but is not a penicillin.

It has excellent activity against both gram-positive and gram-negative organisms, including anaerobic organisms such as *Bacteroides* species. It is resistant to most types of β-lactamase, although not to those from *Pseudomonas* species. It has been used to treat a wide variety of infections, particularly those in which the organism is resistant to most other drugs. Because of the possibility of resistance it should be used with an aminoglycoside when treating infection caused by *Pseudomonas*.

It is marketed in combination with cilastatin to reduce inactivation of the imipenem in the kidney by renal dihydropeptidase. Use of cilastin increases the concentration of imipenem in urine, although it does not affect concentration in the blood.

The most common adverse reactions are nausea and vomiting, and seizures have been noted. Patients allergic to the penicillins may be allergic to imipenem.

Aztreonam

Aztreonam is the first of a group of antibiotics referred to as the *monobactams*. The name derives from the fact that these agents have a β-lactam ring but lack the second ring characteristic of the penicillins and cephalosporins. Aztreonam has activity only against aerobic gram-negative bacteria. It is susceptible to inactivation by certain β-lactamases.

Aztreonam has a β-lactam ring but no other ring. It is a monobactam.

Aztreonam has been used in treatment of urinary and respiratory tract infections, as well as bacteremia and osteomyelitis. It acts by binding to PBPs to produce long, filamentous bacterial shapes that eventually lyse. Aztreonam has few adverse effects, and many patients allergic to the penicillins do not appear to be allergic to it.

Vancomycin

Vancomycin is a glycopeptide, molecular weight about 1500, produced by mold culture. It is marketed as the hydrochloride, which is soluble in water and very stable.

Vancomycin has good activity against gram-positive cocci but has almost no activity against gram-negative bacteria and mycobacteria. Specifically, it is bactericidal against *Staphylococcus aureus*, *Streptococcus pyo-*

Vancomycin has good activity against gram-positive cocci. It is more toxic than the penicillins.

genes, and *Strep. viridans*. It is less effective against *Strep. faecalis*, but in combination with gentamicin it is bactericidal. A few strains of *Staph. hemolyticus* and *Strep. faecalis* exhibit plasmid-mediated resistance. In practice, vancomycin is used to treat serious infections due to the gram-positive cocci when penicillin G is not able to be used because of resistance or allergy to the penicillins. Such infections include disseminated staphylococcal infection and endocarditis. When the causitive agent is *Strep. faecalis*, an aminoglycoside should be used in combination. Vancomycin has been used to treat meningitis. Because of irregular penetration of the central nervous system, intravenous administration has not always been effective, and intraventricular administration has also been used. When the infection is less serious, other, less toxic drugs may be used, such as erythromycin.

Vancomycin inhibits one of the final steps in the synthesis of the peptidoglycan-pentapeptide-pentaglycine moiety of the bacterial cell wall. Like the penicillins, it is effective only against growing organisms.

Vancomycin is poorly absorbed from the gastrointestinal tract, and the usual route of administration is intravenous. The drug is excreted mainly by glomerular filtration; the dose should be adjusted in the case of renal failure. Oral administration may be used to treat infection in the lower bowel, such as a superinfection, especially when due to *Clostridium difficile*.

The two major adverse effects are ototoxicity and nephrotoxicity. Hearing loss may be permanent. Both hearing loss and kidney damage can be minimized by careful attention to dose and by monitoring blood levels of the drug. Hearing loss and kidney damage can be potentiated by concurrent administration of another drug that causes the same adverse reactions, such as gentamicin.

Bacitracin

Bacitracin is used only topically.

Bacitracin was first obtained from a strain of *Bacillus subtilis* obtained from the broken leg of a young girl named Tracy. It is an inhibitor of one of the last steps in the synthesis of peptidoglycan and is active against gram-positive cocci. Bacitracin is extremely nephrotoxic. At one time it was administered parenterally, but currently it is used only topically.

Bacitracin is available in ophthalmic and dermatological ointments. Over-the-counter preparations are available that contain bacitracin either alone or in combination with other antibiotics such as neomycin and polymixin.

Bacitracin has been shown to be of benefit in infections of the eye, but its benefit in other infections, such as occur with mild skin abrasions, has not been proved.

Bacitracin has almost no adverse effects when administered topically. Hypersensitivity reactions occur but are rare.

General References

Cooper GL, Given DB: Vancomycin: A Comprehensive Review of 30 Years of Clinical Experience. New York: John Wiley & Sons, 1986.

Erffmeyer JE: Adverse reactions to penicillin. I. Ann Allergy 47:288–293, 1981.

Erffmeyer JE: Adverse reactions to penicillin. II. Ann Allergy 47:294–300, 1981.

Pratt WB, Fekerty R: The Antimicrobial Drugs, 85–112. New York: Oxford University Press, 1986.

Weiss ME, Adkinson NF: β-lactam allergy. *In* Mandell GL, Douglas RG Jr, Bennett JE (eds): Principles and Practice in Infectious Diseases, 3rd ed, 264–269. New York: Churchill Livingstone, 1990.

Wendel GD Jr, Stark BJ, Jamison RB, et al: Penicillin allergy and desensitization in serious infections during pregnancy. N Engl J Med 312:1229–1232, 1985.

Cephalosporins*

Thomas R. Beam, Jr.

49

Cephalosporin antibiotics proliferated in number, spectrum of activity, prescriptions by physicians, and cost to the health care system during the 1970s and 1980s. Development of new drugs was spurred by the recognition that gram-negative bacilli were responsible for most nosocomial infections, and cephalosporin antibiotics were generally safe and effective in the treatment of these infections. Biochemical manipulation of the cephalosporin molecule could affect spectrum of antibacterial activity, the serum half-life, or both. These observations led to intense investigational activity in the pharmaceutical industry and to a profusion of new antibiotics.

For purposes of convenience and in an attempt to categorize the large number of similar-sounding compounds, cephalosporins have been classified in generations. The classification is arbitrary and based on chemical structure, pharmacokinetic properties, antimicrobial spectrum, and time of entry into the marketplace. First-generation cephalosporins have excellent gram-positive activity except for enterococci and methicillin-resistant staphylococci. Gram-negative coverage is modest in spectrum. Second-generation cephalosporins lose some gram-positive activity (by weight) and gain limited gram-negative coverage (*Haemophilus influenzae* or *Bacteroides fragilis*, for example). Third-generation cephalosporins generally sacrifice further gram-positive activity by weight but gain substantial gram-negative coverage against Enterobacteriaceae (by weight and spectrum) and sometimes include coverage against Pseudomonadaceae. Classification and generic and trade names are summarized in Table 49–1.

Cephalosporins were first identified as antibacterial compounds toward the end of World War II. Giuseppe Brotzu hypothesized that the cleanliness of water might be related to products of microorganisms. In 1945 he isolated a fungus, *Cephalosporium acremonium*, from seawater near a sewage outlet in Sardinia. He found that a filtrate of the organism had antibacterial activity in animals and humans. He sent the organism to Edward P. Abraham at Oxford University, who isolated cephalosporins C, N, and P from the filtrate. Cephalosporin C showed the most activity; it currently provides the molecular structure from which other cephalosporins have been derived.

Cephalosporin C contains a β-lactam ring and an adjacent dihydrothiazine ring. Acid treatment of cephalosporin C hydrolyzes the compound to 7-aminocephalosporanic acid (7-ACA). Substitutions at position 7 of the 7-ACA nucleus alter antibacterial activity. Insertion of a 7-methoxy group yields compounds called *cephamycins*; cefoxitin is an example. Substitutions at position 3 of the dihydrothiazine ring affect the metabolism and

---

*The work was supported by the Veterans Administration.

General Characteristics

Many cephalosporins were developed in response to the increased number of hospital-acquired infections caused by gram-negative bacilli.

Table 49–1 CEPHALOSPORIN ANTIBIOTICS

Generic Name	Trade Name
First Generation	
Cephalothin	Generic
	Keflin
	Seffin
Cephapirin	Cefadyl
Cefazolin	Generic
	Ancef
	Kefzol
Cephalexin	Generic
	Keflex
Cephradine	Generic
	Velosef
	Anspor
Cefadroxil	Duricef
	Ultracef
Second Generation	
Cefamandole	Mandol
Cefoxitin	Mefoxin
Cefonaride	Precef
Cefuroxime	Zinacef
	Kefurox
Cefuroxime axetil	Ceftin
Cefaclor	Ceclor
Cefonicid	Monocid
Cefotetan	Cefotan
Third Generation	
Cefotaxime	Claforan
Moxalactam	Moxam
Ceftizoxime	Cefizox
Ceftriaxone	Rocephin
Cefoperazone	Cefobid
Ceftazidime	Fortaz
	Tazicef
	Tazidime

Figure 49-1

The basic cephalosporin structure.

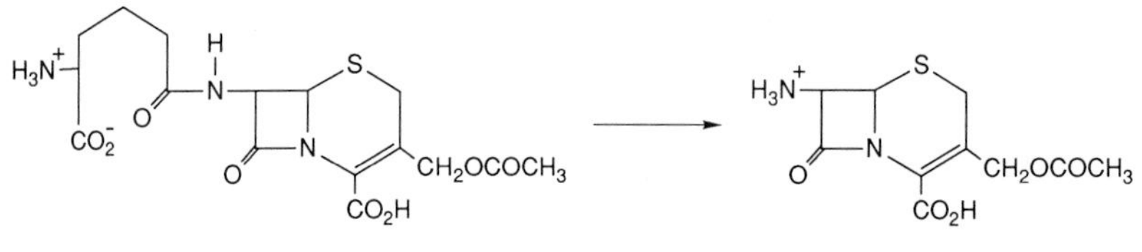

cephalosporin C   7-ACA

The cephalosporin molecule is amenable to multiple biochemical manipulations yielding a wide diversity of antimicrobials.

Cephalosporins are divided into first-, second-, and third-generation products.

elimination (serum half-life) of the compound. Insertion of a methylthio-tetrazole group at this position is associated with certain adverse reactions, including a disulfiram-like response when alcohol is ingested, and bleeding diathesis particularly among the malnourished and the elderly. The basic cephalosporin structure is shown in Figure 49–1. Substituent groups and resulting compounds are shown in Figure 49–2.

Figure 49-2

Cephalosporins: Constituent groups and resulting compounds.

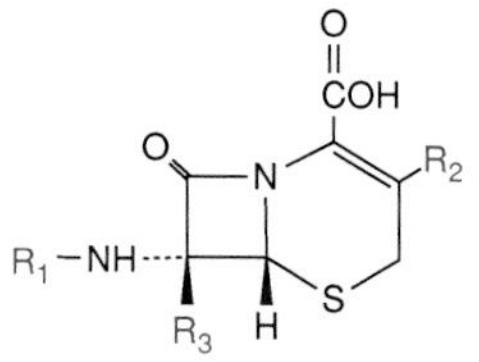

cephalosporin nucleus

First Generation	R_1	R_2	R_3
cefadroxil	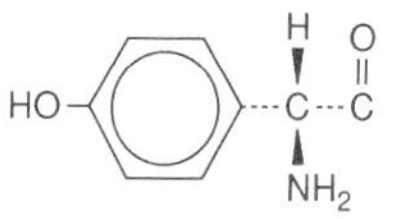	CH_3	H
cefazolin	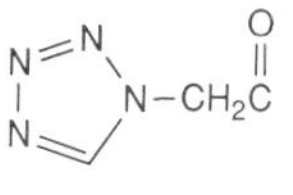	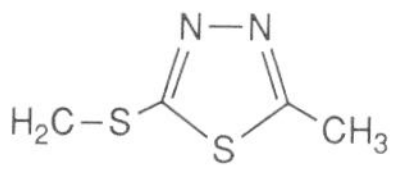	H
cephalexin	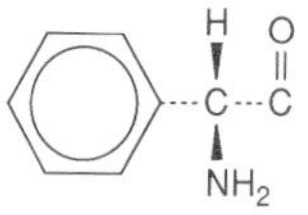	CH_3	H
cephalothin	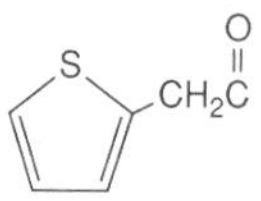	CH_2OCCH_3	H
cephapirin	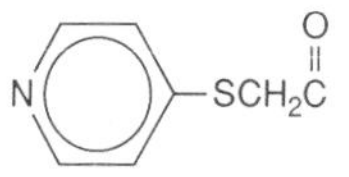	CH_2OCCH_3	H
cephradine	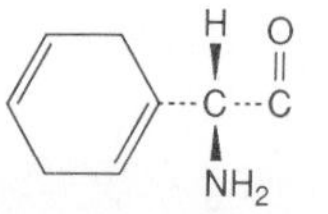	CH_3	H

Second Generation	R_1	R_2	R_3
cefaclor	phenyl–CH(NH₂)–CO–	Cl	H
cefamandole nafate	phenyl–CH(OCHO)–CO–	CH₃-tetrazole-CH₂S–	H
cefonicid	phenyl–CH(OH)–CO–	(CH₂SO₃H)-tetrazole-CH₂S–	H
ceforanide	(o-CH₂NH₂-phenyl)–CH₂C(O)–	(CH₂COOH)-tetrazole-CH₂S–	H
cefoxitin	thiophene–CH₂C(O)–	CH₂OC(O)CH₃	OCH₃
cefuroxime	furan–C(=NOCH₃)–C(O)–	CH₂OC(O)CH₃	H

Third Generation	R_1	R_2	R_3
cefmenoxime	(2-amino-thiazol-4-yl)–C(=NOCH₃)–C(O)–	CH₃-tetrazole-CH₂S–	H
cefoperazone	(4-ethyl-2,3-dioxopiperazine)-N-C(O)NH–CH(p-OH-phenyl)–C(O)–	CH₃-tetrazole-CH₂S–	H
cefotaxime	(2-amino-thiazol-4-yl)–C(=NOCH₃)–C(O)–	CH₂OC(O)CH₃	H
cefsulodin	phenyl–CH(SO₃H)–C(O)–	H₂C–N⁺(pyridinium-CONH₂)	H

Illustration continued on following page

Figure 49-2 Continued

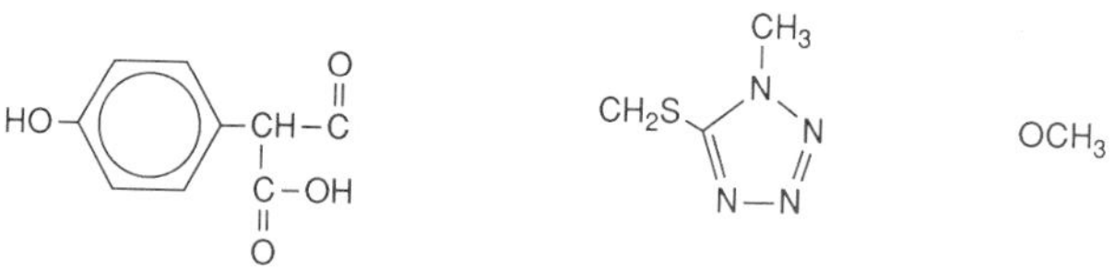

Cephalosporins generally bind to penicillin-binding proteins and exert a lethal action against bacteria.

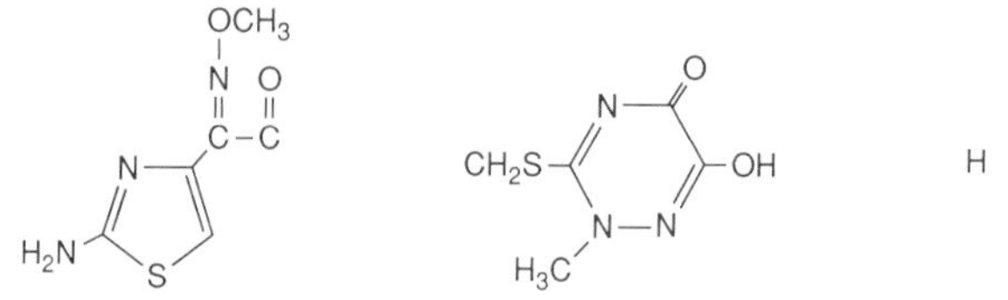

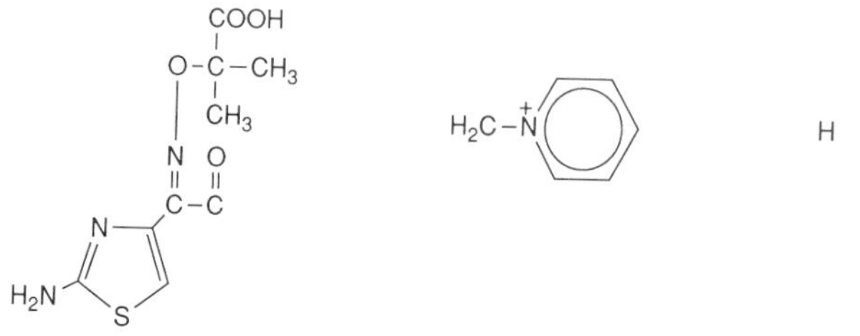

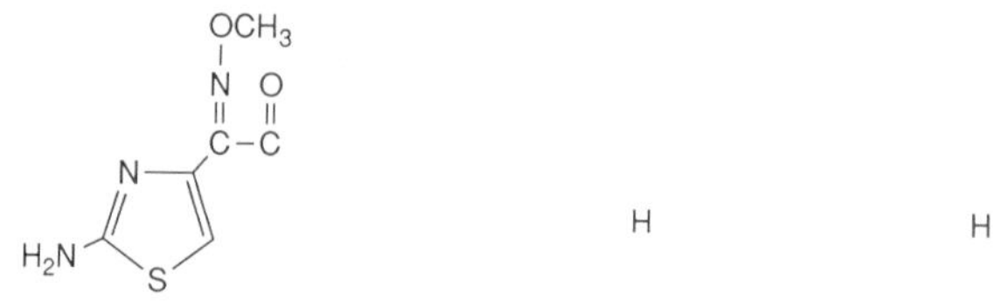

Cephalosporins are generally safe.

Cephalosporins bind to penicillin-binding proteins (PBPs) with varying affinity. The pattern of binding produces the various morphological changes observed during bacterial growth and, ultimately, the bactericidal effect. Once binding to PBPs occurs, protein synthesis is inhibited and an autolysin no longer develops. If bacterial cells do not contain an autolysin, cephalosporins may still be effective through exertion of a bacteriostatic effect. If cephalosporins have different PBP target sites, then combinations of different cephalosporins or cephalosporins plus penicillins may have some therapeutic logic.

A summary of basic pharmacokinetic parameters is presented in Table 49-2. Specific comments are provided in the text under each drug name.

Cephalosporins, like other β-lactam antibiotics, have certain general toxicities. However, they are usually very well tolerated. Hypersensitivity reactions include maculopapular rash with or without drug fever and eosinophilia. Type I anaphylactic reactions are rare. Immune-mediated suppression of bone marrow cell lines is also distinctly uncommon. Coombs' test may become positive but rarely is associated with a hemolytic anemia.

Cross-allergenicity is generally not a problem with penicillin and does not occur with the monobactam aztreonam. However, it is prudent not to administer a cephalosporin antibiotic to a patient with a known type I hypersensitivity to penicillin products.

Gastrointestinal side effects include nausea, vomiting, diarrhea, anorexia, and pseudomembranous colitis. Hepatic enzymes may be transiently and reversibly elevated during therapy, but true hepatotoxicity is rare. Cephalosporins are generally not nephrotoxic, although cephalothin has been reported to cause tubular necrosis. Cephalosporins may interact with nephrotoxic drugs (particularly aminoglycosides) to increase the amount of toxicity.

Cephalosporins can cause pain at the injection site when administered

Table 49–2 PHARMACOKINETIC PARAMETERS OF CEPHALOSPORIN ANTIBIOTICS

Name	Route of Administration*	Protein Binding (%)	Serum Half-Life (hours)	Metabolized (%)	Secreted	Urine Recovery (%)
First Generation						
Cephalothin	IV/IM	70	0.5–0.9	20–30	Yes	50–80
Cephapirin	IV/IM	45–50	0.6–0.8	40	Yes	50–90
Cefazolin	IV/IM	85	1.5–1.8	None	Yes	95
Cephalexin	PO	10–15	0.9–1.3	None	Yes	90
Cephradine	IV/IM/PO	10–20	0.8–1.3	None	Yes	90
Cefadroxil	PO	15–20	1.4–1.5	None	Yes	90
Second Generation						
Cefamandole	IV/IM	70–80	0.6–1.0	None	Yes	80–95
Cefoxitin	IV/IM	70–80	0.75–1.0	<2	Yes	80–95
Ceforanide	IV/IM	80	2.7–3.0	None	Yes	80–95
Cefuroxime	IV/IM	33	1.3–1.7	None	Yes	90–95
Cefuroxime axetil	PO	50	1.2	None	Yes	90–95
Cefaclor	PO	25	0.6–0.9	None	No	60–85
Cefonicid	IV/IM	95–98	3.5–4.5	None	Yes	90
Cefotetan	IV/IM	88	3.5	7	Yes	80
Third Generation						
Cefotaxime	IV/IM	38	1.0–1.1	30–50	Yes	85
Moxalactam	IV/IM	50	2.0–2.3	None	No	70–95
Ceftizoxime	IV/IM	30	1.4–1.8	None	Yes	80–90
Ceftriaxone	IV/IM	83–96	6.0–9.0	None	No	40–65
Cefoperazone	IV/IM	87–93	1.9–2.1	None	No	25
Ceftazidime	IV/IM	17	1.6–1.9	None	No	75–90

*IV = intravenously; IM = intramuscularly; PO = *per os* (by mouth).

intramuscularly. They also are associated with phlebitis at an intravenous site of delivery. Both reactions are uncommon and somewhat drug-specific. For example, intramuscular cephalothin is significantly more painful than cefazolin.

Therapy with cephalosporins is associated with colonization and sometimes superinfection by resistant bacteria or various fungi. Risk depends on dose and duration of therapy, as well as on the medical status of the patient being treated.

Because of their broad spectrum of activity, superinfections are possible adverse effects of cephalosporin therapy.

Despite their overall safety profile, cephalosporins are not well studied in pregnant women. There is no evidence of teratogenicity in humans for any cephalosporin preparation.

Drug interactions are limited in scope and number. Cephalosporins and aminoglycosides, when coadministered, may yield enhanced nephrotoxicity. Cephalosporins containing a methylthiotetrazole ring can cause a disulfiram-like reaction when alcohol is ingested. A false-positive test for urine glucose may be seen with Benedict's or Fehling's solution or Clinitest tablets. False elevation of serum creatinine has also been reported with cefoxitin, ceforanide, and cephalothin.

CEPHALOTHIN

Cephalothin is the prototype cephalosporin. After a 2-g intravenous dose, peak serum concentrations are 100 μg/ml and decline rapidly. The drug is widely distributed throughout body water, but it does not reliably penetrate the central nervous system. A pump in the choroid plexus metabolizes cephalothin prior to its entry into cerebrospinal fluid and renders it inactive. About 65% of cephalothin is excreted unchanged in the urine and the

First-Generation Cephalosporins

Cephalothin is indicated for treatment of serious infections due to susceptible organisms. Its use has declined because of its short half-life.

remainder as the desacetyl metabolite. Small amounts of drug are also excreted in the bile. Minor dose modifications are required in patients with severe renal failure. Cephalothin is removed by peritoneal and hemodialysis.

For therapeutic use cephalothin may be perceived as an alternative to penicillin or penicillin derivatives for treatment of streptococcal or pneumococcal infections (outside the central nervous system), staphylococcal infections, urinary tract infections, and gram-negative bacteremia caused by susceptible organisms. However, because of its short half-life, cephalothin has generally been replaced by cefazolin for all these indications. The drug is contraindicated only in patients known to be hypersensitive to cephalosporin antibiotics.

CEPHAPIRIN

The differences between cephapirin and cephalothin are clinically insignificant. See Cephalothin.

CEFAZOLIN

Cefazolin does not reliably penetrate into the central nervous system.

After an intravenous infusion of 500 mg over 20 minutes, the peak serum concentration of this drug is 118 μg/ml. Almost all of the drug is recovered unchanged in the urine. Because of the high degree of protein binding, the volume of distribution is the smallest among all cephalosporins. The drug does not reliably penetrate into the central nervous system or other restricted sites. The drug accumulates in renal failure, and dose adjustment is required. No unique toxicity has been ascribed to this agent.

Cefazolin is the most widely prescribed parenteral first-generation cephalosporin, particularly for prophylaxis against infection in surgery.

Cefazolin is indicated for treatment of respiratory tract, urinary tract, skin and skin structure, biliary tract, bone and joint, genital, bacteremic, and endocarditic infections caused by susceptible organisms. It is generally perceived as an alternative to some other antibiotic for most of these indications. However, it is the drug of choice as prophylaxis against infection for most clean and clean-contaminated surgeries.

CEPHALEXIN

Cephalexin is relatively well absorbed and distributes widely.

Cephalexin is almost completely absorbed after oral administration. Food delays but minimally affects total drug absorbed. The serum peak of 15 μg/ml is achieved 1 hour after a 500-mg dose. The drug is excreted unchanged in the urine, but small amounts do enter the bile. Tissue distribution is good in most body fluids except restricted-access sites (eye, central nervous system, and prostate).

Cephalexin is indicated for outpatient therapy of mild to moderate infections caused by susceptible organisms.

No unique toxicities have been noted with cephalexin. The drug has been administered safely during pregnancy without evidence of fetal damage. However, its use in pregnancy is incompletely studied. It is indicated for treatment of respiratory tract, skin and soft tissue, bone and joint, and urinary tract infections caused by susceptible organisms. It is generally perceived as an alternative drug to other antibiotics.

CEPHRADINE

The oral form of this drug is clinically similar to cephalexin. Indications for the oral preparation are the same as those for cephalexin. For the intravenous preparation, a serum peak of 60 μg/ml is attained 15 minutes after a 1-g dose infused over 5 minutes. The drug is widely distributed except for the central nervous system. Some cephradine is excreted into the bile. The antibiotic has no unique toxicities, but there are no clear indications for use of the parenteral form of the drug. Cefazolin and cephalothin have greater *in vitro* activity and should be employed in preference to cephradine.

CEFADROXIL

Cefadroxil differs from cephalexin and cephradine because of its longer serum half-life. The serum peak is achieved 1 hour after administration of a 1-g oral dose and is slightly lower than that achieved with cephalexin. After a peak of 15 μg/ml at 1 hour, the serum concentration declines to 12.5, 4.5, 1.8, 1.1, and 0.6 μg/ml at 2, 4, 6, 8, and 12 hours, respectively. The delayed elimination is attributed to saturated binding sites for secretion in the renal tubules. Absorption is not impaired by food, and the drug distributes in a pattern analogous to that of cephalexin. Excretion is through glomerular filtration, tubular secretion, and biliary excretion.

The only unique side effect is that mild elevation of blood urea nitrogen may occur during therapy but is not believed to indicate nephrotoxicity. The drug is indicated for treatment of urinary tract infections, skin and skin structure infections, and tonsillopharyngitis caused by susceptible organisms. There are no adequate studies in pregnant women.

Cefadroxil is often chosen for outpatient prescriptions because of its once-a-day dosing convenience.

CEFAMANDOLE

Cefamandole can only be given parenterally. A serum peak of 88 μg/ml is reached immediately after completion of infusion of a 1-g dose. The drug distributes widely except for the central nervous system, even in the presence of inflammation. The drug is not metabolized, and nearly all of the drug is excreted by the kidney in unchanged form. Some drug is excreted through the bile but is undetectable in patients with complete biliary obstruction. Dose adjustment is required in renal failure.

Cefamandole has been widely prescribed for multiple indications among patients with a variety of disease and nutritional states. It has infrequently been reported to cause hypoprothrombinemia and bleeding, but the condition is rapidly reversible by administration of vitamin K. Cefamandole can also impair platelet function, but only at very high serum concentrations of 300–400 μg/ml. Because it contains a methylthiotetrazole side chain, disulfiram-like adverse reactions have been seen when alcohol is ingested during therapy.

Cefamandole is indicated for treatment of urinary tract, skin and skin structure, bone and joint, and respiratory tract infections caused by susceptible organisms. Its designation as a second-generation cephalosporin relates to its *in vitro* activity against *H. influenzae*. Because of distribution problems of the drug, cefamandole should only be used for treatment of infections outside the central nervous system. In fact, meningitis caused by susceptible organisms has developed among patients receiving cefamandole therapy. Cefamandole has been used for surgical prophylaxis in biliary tract, cardiac, and orthopedic procedures. Alternative, less expensive drugs such as cefazolin are generally preferred.

Second-Generation Cephalosporins

Cefamandole is available only for parenteral therapy. It is cleared through the kidney.

Caution is advised in treating seriously ill patients. Cefamandole does not reliably penetrate into the central nervous system.

CEFOXITIN

Cefoxitin is only suitable for parenteral administration. A serum peak of 222 μg/ml is reached 3 minutes after infusion of 1 g of drug over 5 minutes. The drug distributes well to most tissues and body fluids except the central nervous system. Even in the presence of inflammation, penetration into

Cefoxitin has clinically relevant activity against *B. fragilis*. Therefore, it has frequently been used for prevention and treatment of intra-abdominal and pelvic infections.

cerebrospinal fluid is unreliable. Excretion in unchanged form by the kidney is essentially the only mode of elimination. A very small amount (2%) is desacetylated, and this occurs only in a limited proportion of the population. Less than 1% of the drug appears in bile. Careful dose modification is therefore required for patients who have renal failure.

Cefoxitin is indicated for urinary tract, respiratory tract, skin and soft tissue, and bone and joint infections caused by susceptible organisms. It is considered a second-generation cephalosporin because of its activity against *B. fragilis*. Therefore, it is indicated for treatment of intra-abdominal and pelvic infections probably caused by this organism. It also is indicated for anaerobic pleuropulmonary infections, decubitus ulcers, and sepsis caused by organisms (including *Bacteroides)* that are susceptible to the drug.

The drug is considered the agent of choice for prophylaxis in emergency bowel surgery. It is also a frequent choice as prophylaxis against infection for female pelvic surgery, although it has not been proved superior to alternative, less expensive agents such as cefazolin.

CEFORANIDE

Ceforanide has a serum half-life of 3 hours.

The distinguishing feature of ceforanide is its serum half-life of 3 hours. Following a 1-g dose administered intravenously over 30 minutes, the serum peak is 135 μg/ml. Twelve hours later the serum concentration is 5 μg/ml. The drug is approximately 80% bound to serum protein but distributes well through tissue and body fluids outside the central nervous system. It is not metabolized but is cleared by glomerular filtration and tubular secretion. Some drug is also eliminated in the bile.

There have been no unique toxicities identified with this drug. Ceforanide is indicated for treatment of bone and joint infections, endocarditis, lower respiratory tract infections, bacterial septicemia, skin and skin structure infections, and urinary tract infections caused by susceptible organisms. It also is approved for use as a prophylactic agent for open heart (coronary artery bypass graft), biliary tract (high-risk patients), and female genital tract surgery. Because its spectrum of *in vitro* activity is minimally different from first-generation cephalosporins, the drug has not been widely used.

Because ceforanide has a spectrum of activity that differs little from first-generation cephalosporins, it has infrequently been used.

CEFUROXIME

Cefuroxime is available in both parenteral and oral formulations.

Cefuroxime may be given intravenously, intramuscularly, or by mouth. Following a 1-g dose given intramuscularly, the serum peak of 40 μg/ml is reached 45–60 minutes later. Following a rapid intravenous infusion of 1 g, the serum peak is 80 μg/ml at the end of the infusion. Following a 1-g dose by mouth, cefuroxime axetil is rapidly hydrolyzed to cefuroxime by esterases in the intestinal mucosa; the serum peak concentration of 13.6 μg/ml is achieved about 2 hours later.

Cefuroxime distributes throughout body tissues and fluids. It enters cerebrospinal fluid reliably in the presence of inflammation and may be used to treat bacterial meningitis caused by certain susceptible strains. Most cefuroxime is eliminated unchanged in the urine. Small amounts enter the bile.

Cefuroxime is indicated for treatment of respiratory tract, urinary tract, skin and skin structure, and bone and joint infections caused by susceptible organisms. It is also indicated for treatment of bacterial septicemia and both mucous membrane and disseminated gonococcal infections. It is not a drug of choice for the latter. Cefuroxime has been successfully used for the treatment of meningitis caused by *Streptococcus pneumoniae, H.*

influenzae, and *Neisseria meningitidis.* Its use for central nervous system infections should be confined to these three organisms. Cefuroxime has also been used to prevent infection in gynecological, vascular, and cardiac surgery procedures. It should be perceived as an alternative to cefazolin for these prophylaxis indications.

If cefuroxime is used to treat serious infections, such as meningitis, it should be limited to therapy of *S. pneumoniae, H. influenzae,* and *N. meningitidis.*

CEFACLOR

Cefaclor is an orally administered, second-generation cephalosporin. Food delays absorption and reduces the serum peak concentration but does not reduce the total amount of drug absorbed. Following a 1-g dose, the serum peak concentration of 23 μg/ml is achieved in 30–60 minutes. The drug distributes into soft tissue and interstitial fluid; it is 50% protein-bound. About 70% of a dose is recovered unchanged in the urine. The rest is metabolized, although the nature of the metabolites is unknown.

One unique reaction of this drug is a serum sickness–like reaction, which has been infrequently reported. It is characterized by erythema multiforme or a morbilliform rash, arthritis/arthralgia, and fever. It has been seen more commonly in children than adults and more often after a second rather than a first therapeutic course. The syndrome generally resolves several days after therapy is discontinued.

A unique adverse reaction to cefaclor is a serum sickness–like illness.

Cefaclor is indicated for the treatment of otitis media, upper and lower respiratory tract infections, urinary tract infections, and skin and skin structure infections due to susceptible organisms. Care must be taken in the treatment of infections that may spread to the central nervous system, such as orbital cellulitis or epiglottitis. Cefaclor does not adequately penetrate the central nervous system to be therapeutic.

Cefaclor is widely prescribed for treatment of infections in pediatric patients.

CEFONICID

Cefonicid is suitable for intramuscular or intravenous administration. The serum peak concentration of 100 μg/ml is achieved 1–2 hours after intramuscular administration, and 220 μg/ml is reached 5 minutes after intravenous infusion of a 1-g dose. Protein binding is extremely high (95–98%), but distribution into tissue and interstitial fluids is reasonable. The drug does not achieve therapeutic concentrations in the central nervous system.

Cefonicid has a long serum half-life and may be dosed once per day.

The serum half-life of approximately 4 hours allows for once-daily dosing. The drug is excreted unchanged in the urine. Small amounts appear in the bile. Dose modification is required for patients with renal failure. Cefonicid is well tolerated by intramuscular administration.

Cefonicid is indicated for treatment of lower respiratory tract, urinary tract, skin and skin structure, and bone and joint infections caused by susceptible organisms. Its spectrum of activity is very similar to that of cefamandole. Cefonicid may be particularly useful for outpatient treatment of chronic, non–life-threatening infections such as osteomyelitis. Cefonicid has also proved useful for prophylaxis against infection in certain surgeries, such as colorectal (in conjunction with an oral bowel preparation), gynecological, high-risk biliary tract, prosthetic joint, or open heart procedures. It is useful because single-dose prophylaxis is appropriate for these procedures.

Cefonicid has been employed for outpatient parenteral therapy of chronic infections such as osteomyelitis.

CEFOTETAN

Cefotetan is a semisynthetic cephalosporin suitable for parenteral administration. The serum peak of 160 μg/ml is achieved 30 minutes after intravenous infusion, and 70 μg/ml is achieved 1–2 hours after intramuscular

Cefotetan may be regarded as an alternative to cefoxitin with a longer half-life but slightly less *in vitro* activity.

injection of a 1-g dose. The drug is highly protein-bound (88%) and has a serum half-life of 3 – 4 hours. It distributes well into body fluids and tissues other than the central nervous system and has a spectrum of activity similar to cefoxitin, although it is less active against *B. fragilis*. A small portion of drug is metabolized to a tautomer that has activity similar to the parent compound. The majority is excreted unchanged in the urine, and therefore dose modification is required for patients in renal failure.

Because of the methylthiotetrazole side chain present in cefotetan, caution must be advised when the drug is administered to patients who may be deficient in vitamin K. Caution is also advised because of the potential for disulfiram-like adverse reaction among patients who may ingest alcohol. Other adverse effects are those typical of cephalosporin antibiotics.

Cefotetan is indicated for the treatment of urinary tract, lower respiratory tract, skin and skin structure, gynecological, intra-abdominal, and bone and joint infections caused by susceptible organisms. Cefotetan is also indicated for prophylaxis against infection in surgeries such as colorectal, female genital tract, and high-risk biliary tract procedures. It may be generally perceived as an alternative to cefoxitin, with a longer half-life but slightly less *in vitro* activity.

Third-Generation Cephalosporins

Cefotaxime was the first third-generation cephalosporin marketed in the United States.

Cefotaxime possesses an exceptional safety record.

Cefotaxime treats many serious gram-negative bacillary infections, including meningitis. It is not effective against Pseudomonadaceae.

CEFOTAXIME

Cefotaxime may be administered intramuscularly or intravenously. Following a 1-g dose intramuscularly, the peak serum concentration of 20 μg/ml is reached 30 minutes later; following rapid infusion of 1 g intravenously, the serum peak of 86 μg/ml is achieved 5 minutes later. Serum protein binding is low and averages 35 – 40%. The drug distributes well into most tissues and body fluids. It does not penetrate the central nervous system in the absence of inflammation. In the presence of inflammation, drug entry is sufficient to provide adequate concentrations for effective therapy of many meningeal pathogens. The parent compound is partially desacetylated by the choroid plexus during transport, and the metabolite retains about 10% of the antimicrobial activity.

Cefotaxime is excreted through the urine unchanged by glomerular filtration and tubular secretion. About 30% of the drug is converted by the liver into desacetyl cefotaxime, which also is cleared by the kidney. Two other inactive metabolites are renally eliminated. Biliary clearance is negligible. There are no unique toxicities for this compound. The drug has had a remarkable safety profile since its approval for marketing in the United States as the first third-generation cephalosporin to be made available.

Cefotaxime is indicated for treatment of lower respiratory tract, urinary tract, gynecological, skin and skin structure, intra-abdominal, bone and joint, and central nervous system infections caused by susceptible organisms. It is also indicated for treatment of bacteremia and septicemia, particularly gram-negative aerobic bacteria other than Pseudomonadaceae. The drug retains good gram-positive coverage. A combination of exquisite susceptibility of meningeal pathogens plus adequate central nervous system penetration allow for treatment of bacterial meningitis. Cefotaxime has also proved useful as prophylaxis against infection in gynecological, urological, and colon surgery. Cefotaxime should be administered as a supplement to an oral bowel preparation for colon surgery.

MOXALACTAM (LATAMOXEF)

Moxalactam may be administered intramuscularly or intravenously. Approximately 1 hour after an intramuscular injection of 1 g, a serum peak concentration of 38 μg/ml is achieved; following rapid intravenous infusion of 2 g, a serum peak concentration of 210 μg/ml is achieved 10 minutes later. Moxalactam penetrates well into body tissues and fluids. Measurable amounts are detected in cerebrospinal fluid in the absence of inflammation, and therapeutic amounts in the presence of inflammation. Protein binding averages 50%. Most of the drug is excreted unchanged in the urine. A lesser amount is excreted in bile, but this quantity is sufficient to have an impact on fecal flora. A small amount may be metabolized, but no metabolites have been identified.

Moxalactam is an excellent antimicrobial agent that distributes widely throughout the body.

The side effect profile of moxalactam is distinctive. It has been associated with severe bleeding diathesis. In seriously ill, elderly, and undernourished patients, moxalactam causes vitamin K deficiency and hypoprothrombinemia. These are reversible by parenteral administration of vitamin K. The adverse reaction occurs with sufficient frequency to advise that all patients given moxalactam should receive prophylactic vitamin K. Moxalactam also inhibits adenosine diphosphate (ADP)–induced platelet aggregation, resulting in a prolonged bleeding time. Moxalactam seems to be associated with this adverse effect more than any other cephalosporin.

Moxalactam's side-effect profile, especially hemorrhage and superinfection, has limited its use.

Because of its impact on fecal flora, moxalactam has been associated with colonization and infection by resistant organisms. These particularly include enterococci, *Pseudomonas* species, and *Candida albicans*. The rate of enterococcal colonization or superinfection has been established at 2% and enterococcal bacteremia at 0.3% of moxalactam recipients.

Additional third-generation cephalosporins with a better safety profile have been developed. Because the bleeding diathesis or enterococcal bacteremia can be life-threatening, moxalactam has become infrequently prescribed. The drug remains available in the United States but is not listed in the 1990 Physicians' Desk Reference.

Moxalactam has a United States Food and Drug Administration (FDA)–approved indication for the treatment of meningitis caused by gram-negative bacteria. It is not indicated for treatment of pneumococcal, group B streptococcal, or the rare case of *P. aeruginosa* meningitis. Moxalactam has been successfully used to treat lower respiratory tract, urinary tract, gynecological, skin and skin structure, bone and joint, and intra-abdominal infections due to susceptible organisms. It also is effective in septicemia/bacteremia. However, for all these indications, an alternative cephalosporin or a combination of antimicrobials is preferred because of the excessive risk of adverse reactions. Furthermore, any drug that affects coagulation may interact with moxalactam to produce an accelerated bleeding disorder.

CEFTIZOXIME

Ceftizoxime is very similar to cefotaxime except that it is not metabolized *in vivo*. After administration of 1 g intramuscularly, the serum peak of 20 μg/ml is reached 30 minutes later. Following a 1-g bolus delivered intravenously over 3 minutes, the serum peak concentration of 86 μg/ml is reached 5 minutes later. The elimination half-life is about 1.4 hours.

This drug distributes in a fashion analogous to cefotaxime. It does not penetrate the central nervous system except in the presence of inflammation. Protein binding is about 30%. No metabolites have been identified in humans. There is negligible biliary excretion, and unchanged drug is excreted by glomerular filtration and tubular secretion in the kidney.

The antimicrobial spectrum is very similar to that of cefotaxime. The drug is indicated for treatment of lower respiratory tract, urinary tract, uncomplicated gonococcal, intra-abdominal, skin and skin structure, bone and joint, and meningeal infections caused by susceptible organisms. It is

Ceftizoxime is essentially the same as cefotaxime except that it is cleared exclusively through the kidney.

also indicated for treatment of septicemia/bacteremia. Ceftizoxime retains good coverage against gram-positive cocci, possesses excellent activity against most Enterobacteriaceae, and lacks anti-*Pseudomonas* coverage. It is more active *in vitro* against *B. fragilis* than other third-generation cephalosporins except moxalactam.

CEFTRIAXONE

Ceftriaxone must be delivered parenterally. Following a 1-g intramuscular injection, a peak serum concentration of 76 μg/ml is achieved 2 hours later. Lidocaine must be added to the injection to reduce pain at the site but does not affect kinetic parameters. Following infusion of 1 g intravenously over 30 minutes, a peak serum concentration of 150 μg/ml is achieved 30 minutes later. The serum half-life in children with meningitis averages 4.5 hours; it is 6–8 hours in healthy adults. Single daily dosing is strongly recommended.

Ceftriaxone is 98% protein-bound at a serum concentration of 25 μg/ml or less, and 85% bound at serum concentrations of 300 or more μg/ml. Dose modification is generally not required in the elderly or in patients with either renal or hepatic dysfunction. Combined excretory organ dysfunction does lead to drug accumulation and potential toxicity. The drug distributes well to body tissues and fluids except the central nervous system. However, in the presence of meningeal inflammation, therapeutic concentrations of drug are achieved in cerebrospinal fluid. Although absolute concentrations of drug are lower than those of moxalactam, the cerebrospinal fluid half-life and duration of bactericidal activity are longer.

Ceftriaxone is not metabolized. About one half is eliminated unchanged in the urine by glomerular filtration. The remainder is eliminated through the bile. Stool samples do not yield active drug, and it is assumed that intestinal bacteria or enzymes break down the drug into an inert compound.

Only one side effect and one interaction warrant mention. The rate of diarrhea associated with ceftriaxone therapy may be higher than that occurring with renally excreted third-generation cephalosporins (cefotaxime, ceftizoxime), but this remains unproved in a direct comparative trial. Ceftriaxone can displace bilirubin from its protein-binding sites. Care should be employed if the drug is used in premature infants or neonates with hyperbilirubinemia. Ceftriaxone is indicated for the treatment of lower respiratory tract, skin and skin structure, urinary tract, gonococcal, bone and joint, intra-abdominal, and central nervous system infections caused by susceptible organisms. It also is indicated for treatment of septicemia/bacteremia, and pelvic inflammatory disease caused by *N. gonorrhoeae*. Ceftriaxone has also been used as prophylaxis against infection in female genital and coronary artery bypass graft surgeries. It is not the drug of choice for either of these procedures.

CEFOPERAZONE

Cefoperazone is suitable for intramuscular or intravenous administration. After intramuscular injection of 1 g, a serum peak concentration of 65 μg/ml is reached 1 hour later; after 2 g administered by intravenous infusion over 3 minutes, the peak serum concentration is 256 μg/ml at the end of the infusion. Protein binding is relatively high at 90%, and cefoperazone has a smaller volume of distribution than that of less highly bound cephalosporins. Despite the protein binding, therapeutic concentrations of cefo-

Ceftriaxone distributes well to infected body sites, including the central nervous system, despite its high degree of protein binding.

Ceftriaxone has a large number of approved indications and is the most widely prescribed injectable cephalosporin antibiotic in the United States.

Cefoperazone differs from other third-generation cephalosporins because of its hepatic excretion and anti-*Pseudomonas* activity.

perazone are reached in tissues and body fluids other than the central nervous system. Even in the presence of inflammation, central nervous system penetration is not reliable.

Only 20–30% of a dose is recovered unchanged in the urine. Renal excretion is primarily by glomerular filtration. A very small amount of metabolite, cefoperazone A, is formed. This has minor antimicrobial activity. The main route of excretion of drug is in the bile in unchanged form. This degree of biliary elimination is unique among cephalosporin antibiotics.

Because of cefoperazone's biliary excretion, diarrhea is a relatively common adverse effect. Cefoperazone also causes major changes in fecal flora. Enterococci, *Candida* species, and *Clostridium difficile* all may overgrow. Cefoperazone contains a methylthiotetrazole side chain. Therefore, vulnerable patients may sustain bleeding complications. Both vitamin K deficiency producing hypoprothrombinemia and inhibition of ADP-induced platelet aggregation have been reported. The frequency seems much less than that associated with moxalactam and about the same as that occurring with cefamandole. Patients likely to be vitamin K deficient should receive parenteral vitamin K supplements if cefoperazone therapy is instituted. A disulfiram-like adverse reaction has also been sustained by patients who have ingested alcohol while receiving cefoperazone therapy. Other adverse reactions are those characteristic of cephalosporin antibiotics.

The rate of bleeding diathesis or superinfection with cefoperazone therapy is far less than that seen with moxalactam. The reason for this is obscure.

Cefoperazone is indicated for treatment of respiratory tract infections, peritonitis and intra-abdominal infections, bacterial septicemia, urinary tract infections, skin and skin structure infections, pelvic inflammatory disease, endometritis, and other infections of the female genital tract caused by susceptible organisms. Cefoperazone is distinguished from other third-generation cephalosporins by its activity against *P. aeruginosa* and its vulnerability to degradation by β-lactamase. Susceptibility testing of clinical isolates is particularly important because *in vitro* results may be less predictable than those achieved with more β-lactamase–stable cephalosporins.

CEFTAZIDIME

Ceftazidime is suitable for intravenous and intramuscular administration. However, the intramuscular route is limited by the large amount of diluent required to solubilize the drug, therefore yielding a volume that is difficult to administer. Following intramuscular injection of 1 g, the peak serum concentration of 40 μg/ml is achieved 1 hour later; following intravenous infusion of 1 g over 5 minutes, the peak serum concentration of 107 μg/ml is achieved 10 minutes later. The serum half-life ranges from 1 to 2 hours in normal volunteers.

Ceftazidime is a renally excreted third-generation cephalosporin with a relatively short half-life.

Protein binding is 20% or less. The drug distributes well into tissues and body fluids except for the central nervous system. Drug concentrations reach therapeutic values in the presence of meningeal irritation, but studies of efficacy in meningitis have been limited. The major route of excretion is by glomerular filtration in unchanged form through the kidneys. No active metabolites have been identified. Dose modification is required in renal failure.

Pain at the site of intramuscular injection is commonly reported, in part related to volume. No unique toxicities have been identified.

Ceftazidime is indicated for the treatment of lower respiratory tract, skin and skin structure, bone and joint, urinary tract, gynecological, intra-abdominal, and central nervous system infections caused by susceptible

Ceftazidime is the most potent cephalo-sporin against *Pseudomonas aeruginosa.*

organisms. Ceftazidime has more potent anti-*Pseudomonas* activity *in vitro* than any other cephalosporin antibiotic. It therefore has been used to treat patients with cystic fibrosis and patients with malignancy and granulocy-topenia, in anticipation of *Pseudomonas* infections. Ceftazidime is also indi-cated for treatment of septicemia/bacteremia.

New Developments

The enthusiasm for development of new cephalosporin antibiotics has diminished. In part this is related to the large number of compounds al-ready available, in part the increasing prevalence of gram-positive nosoco-mial infections, and in part the inability to develop a unique niche for new products. Orally administered third-generation cephalosporins continue to be pursued. The logic for these drugs would be to provide a formulation that could be employed following parenteral therapy, could be adminis-tered on an outpatient basis, and could be used in selected circumstances to avoid hospitalization. The fluoroquinolones are also being pursued for these very same reasons.

Drugs in development include (1) cefsulodin, with primarily anti-*Pseudomonas* and anti-*Staphylococcus* activity; the drug is administered parenterally; (2) cefmenoxime, with similar activity to cefotaxime, a re-quirement for parenteral administration, and the presence of a methylthio-tetrazole side chain; this drug is unlikely to be marketed in the United States; (3) cefmetazole, with activity similar to cefoxitin, a requirement for parenteral administration, and the presence of a methylthiotetrazole side chain; this drug is also unlikely to become available in the United States; (4) cefoticin, with susceptibility to β-lactamase degradation and a requirement for parenteral administration; development of this drug will not be pur-sued; (5) cefpimizole, with no advantages over current third-generation cephalosporins, will not be pursued; (6) cefpiramide, with no apparent advantages, will probably not be pursued; (7) cefpirome (HR 810)—with better *in vitro* activity than currently available third-generation cephalo-sporins, and equivalent activity against *Pseudomonas* compared with cef-tazidime, plus better gram-positive activity—is undergoing clinical trials. Several additional drugs are too early in their evaluation to determine whether they will offer significant advantage. These include BMY 28142 (parenteral), cefbuperazone [BMY 25182] (parenteral), cefetamet [R015 8074] (oral), and ceftetrame [RO 19–5247] (oral).

General References

First-Generation Cephalosporins

Griffith RS, Black HR: Cephalothin—A new antibiotic. JAMA 189:823, 1964.

Jones RN, Preston DA: Antimicrobial activity of cephalexin against old and new patho-gens. Postgrad Med J 57(Suppl 5):9, 1983.

Moellering RC Jr, Swartz M: Drug therapy: The newer cephalosporins. New Engl J Med 294:24, 1976.

Nightingale CH, Greene DS, Quintiliani R: Pharmacokinetics and clinical use of cepha-losporin antibiotics. J Pharm Sci 64:1899, 1975.

Perkins RL, Saslow S: Experience with cephalothin. Ann Intern Med 64:13, 1966.

Phillips J, Ward ER (eds): Role of cefadroxil in oral antibiotic therapy. J Antimicrob Chemother 10(Suppl B):1, 1982.

Quintiliani R, Nightingale CH: Cefazolin. Ann Intern Med 89 (Part 1):650, 1978.

Second-Generation Cephalosporins

Kammer RB, Short LJ: Cefaclor—Summary of clinical experience. Postgrad Med J 55(Suppl 4):93, 1979.

Kass EH, Evans DA (eds): Future prospects and past problems in antimicrobial therapy: The role of cefoxitin. Rev Infect Dis 1:1, 1979.

Long M, Anderson PO: Serum sickness with cefaclor. Drug Intell Clin Pharmacol 19:186, 1985.

Sanders CV, Greenberg RN, Marier RL: Cefamandole and cefoxitin. Ann Intern Med 103:70, 1985.

Tartaglione TA, Polk RF: Review of the new second-generation cephalosporins: Cefonicid, ceforanide and cefuroxime. Drug Intell Clin Pharm 19:188, 1985.

Ward A, Richards DM: Cefotetan: Review of its antibacterial activity, pharmacokinetic properties and therapeutic use. Drugs 30:382, 1985.

Third-Generation Cephalosporins

Beam TR Jr: Ceftriaxone: Beta-lactamase stable, broad-spectrum cephalosporin with an extended half-life. Pharmacotherapy 5:237, 1985.

Carmine AA, Brogden RN, Heel RC, et al: Cefotaxime: A review of its antimicrobial activity, pharmacological properties and therapeutic use. Drugs 25:223, 1983.

Fitzpatrick BJ, Standiford HC: Comparative evaluation of moxalactam: Antimicrobial activity, pharmacokinetics, adverse reactions, and clinical efficacy. Pharmacotherapy 2:197, 1982.

Funk EA, Strausbaugh LJ: Antimicrobial activity, pharmacokinetics, adverse reactions, and therapeutic indications of cefoperazone. Pharmacotherapy 2:185, 1982.

Neu HC: Ceftizoxime: Beta-lactamase stable, broad-spectrum cephalosporin: pharmacokinetics, adverse effects and clinical use. Pharmacotherapy 4:47, 1984.

Yost RL, Ramphal R: Ceftazidime review. Drug Intell Clin Pharm 19:509, 1985.

50

Aminoglycosides

Alan M. Reynard

After the 1939 demonstration that penicillin, a mold-derived substance, was a highly effective, clinically useful antimicrobial agent, Selman Waksman initiated a program to find other mold exudates that had antimicrobial properties. His search culminated in 1943 in the discovery of streptomycin, for which he was subsequently awarded the Nobel Prize. The introduction of streptomycin had considerable significance because its activity against gram-negative rods was considerably higher than that of the sulfonamides, the only other type of agent with gram-negative activity available at that time. In the following years, a number of other antibiotics similar to streptomycin were discovered. In addition to streptomycin, the aminoglycosides currently available are amikacin, gentamicin, kanamycin, neomycin, netilmicin, paromomycin, and tobramycin.

The aminoglycosides have many features in common. All contain one or more sugar molecules, and the sugar moieties have one or more amino groups. The sugar moieties are joined to each other or to other moieties by glycosidic links. Hence, these antibiotics are known as the *aminoglycosides*. They are also sometimes referred to as *aminocyclitols*.

Aminoglycosides are similar in many properties.

In addition to structure, the aminoglycosides are similar in mechanism of action and a variety of other properties. However, differences in some of these properties have led to a decrease in use of some of the aminoglycosides and an increase in use of others. Most of the aminoglycosides are still used at least in some circumstances. Over the years since the discovery of streptomycin, kanamycin replaced streptomycin for general use because of a slightly lower toxicity and a slightly broader spectrum of action; gentamicin replaced kanamycin because of a broader spectrum of action and a lower susceptibility to bacterial resistance; and amikacin replaced gentamicin because of a lower susceptibility to bacterial resistance.

The aminoglycosides, although differing slightly in spectrum of action, have activity against both gram-positive and gram-negative organisms.

Chemistry

Aminoglycosides are more active in alkaline media.

The aminoglycosides have several structural features in common. They each contain one or more sugar moieties and a streptidine ring. In addition they have one or more amino or guanidino groups. The aminoglycosides are very soluble in water, are stable in solution, and are more active in alkaline than in acid media. This latter property is of importance in treatment of urinary tract infections because the relatively low pH of the urine (5.5) must be raised so that the aminoglycoside will be effective.

Mechanism of Action

The aminoglycosides all act by the same mechanism. They bind to proteins on the 30S ribosome of bacteria thereby inhibiting protein synthesis, particularly the initiation step. Inhibition of protein synthesis is not a lethal event in bacteria in the same sense as destruction of the cell envelope. Nevertheless, the aminoglycosides bind so strongly to their receptors that the binding is essentially irreversible and the end result is death of the bacterial cell. Thus, the aminoglycosides are considered to be bactericidal. This is in contrast to other inhibitors of protein synthesis such as chloramphenicol and the tetracyclines in which binding to the ribosome is weaker and the agents are bacteriostatic.

Aminoglycosides inhibit protein synthesis.

The aminoglycosides also cause misreading of the genetic code, so that incorrect amino acids are incorporated into proteins of the bacterial cell. This mechanism is probably less important than inhibition of protein synthesis in killing cells.

At high concentrations, aminoglycosides cause disruption of membranes of both bacterial and mammalian cells. The concentration required for this is higher than that usually achieved in the blood during therapy. However, aminoglycosides accumulate in the fluids of the ear and the kidney in high concentration, and this high concentration is probably responsible for the adverse effects seen in these two organs.

Aminoglycosides, at high concentration, disrupt cell membranes.

Mechanism of Resistance

There are several ways bacteria can become resistant to the aminoglycosides. The most important, clinically, is the plasmid-mediated production of drug-inactivating enzymes by resistant cells. Three different enzyme reactions have been identified

Plasmid-mediated resistance is effected by three different types of enzyme.

$$AcCoA + AG \longrightarrow Ac\text{-}AG + CoA$$

$$ATP + AG \longrightarrow P\text{-}Ag + ADP$$

$$ATP + AG \longrightarrow AMP\text{-}AG + PP_i$$

In the first reaction, an amino group on the aminoglycoside (AG) is acetylated (AcCoA = acetylcoenzyme A). In the second, a hydroxyl group on the aminoglycoside is phosphorylated (ATP = adenosine triphosphate; ADP = adenosine diphosphate). In the third, a hydroxyl group on the aminoglycoside receives the adenosine monophosphate (AMP) portion of ATP (the aminoglycoside is adenylylated) (PPi = inorganic pyrophosphate.) In all cases conjugation of the aminoglycoside inactivates it.

The phosphorylation reaction was discovered soon after the discovery of plasmid-mediated resistance and caused inactivation of the first two aminoglycosides, streptomycin and kanamycin. Gentamicin, lacking the hydroxyl group that was the target of that reaction, was free of inactivation for a number of years. Eventually, a plasmid appeared that specified the enzyme that catalyzed the third reaction (adenylylation), a reaction to which gentamicin is susceptible. At about the same time a derivative of kanamycin, amikacin, was produced that was not susceptible to either phosphorylation or adenylylation. Amikacin is essentially kanamycin B with an α-amino-γ-hydroxybutaryl moiety attached. The complete formula is α-amino-γ-hydroxybutaryl kanamycin B. This group protects the molecule from the inactivating enzymes by steric hindrance.

In general, plasmid-mediated resistance results in low-level resistance where minimal inhibitory concentrations range from 25 to 200 μg/ml.

Another mechanism of resistance is a mutation that results in the

Chromosomal mutation results in high-level resistance.

production of a 30S ribosomal subunit that contains an altered protein, such that the ribosome still functions in protein synthesis but no longer binds an aminoglycoside. This mechanism results in an organism with very high levels of resistance (1000–3000 μg/ml), but this mechanism has less clinical significance than enzyme-mediated resistance.

A third mechanism derives from the fact that aminoglycosides are transported to the interior of a cell, where they bind to ribosomes by an oxygen-dependent transport mechanism. Some organisms can live in anaerobic conditions, where the oxygen-dependent transport is lacking. In this circumstance, aminoglycosides are not transported into the cells of the bacteria, and the cells survive despite the presence of aminoglycoside in the environment.

Facultative anaerobes are not susceptible to aminoglycosides in anaerobic conditions.

Absorption, Distribution, Metabolism, Excretion

Administration is usually intramuscular.

The most common route of administration of the aminoglycosides is intramuscular with good absorption; peak plasma levels are achieved in 30–90 minutes. Administration is rarely oral or intravenous. The drugs are not absorbed from the gastrointestinal tract. The aminoglycosides, when administered orally, affect only the microbes in the gastrointestinal tract and do not exhibit their usual adverse effects.

Less than 20% of absorbed drug is bound to plasma protein. The drugs are highly charged and do not enter mammalian cells readily. There is little metabolism of the drugs. Excretion is largely by glomerular filtration and is reduced in renal damage. In patients with reduced kidney function the dose of an aminoglycoside must be reduced. There are a number of nomograms available to calculate dose on the basis of creatinine clearance and weight of patient.

Adverse Effects

Adverse effects include hearing loss and vertigo.

The principal dangers associated with the use of aminoglycosides are ototoxicity and nephrotoxicity. In both types of toxicity the high concentration of drug that accumulates in the fluids of these tissues probably plays a role.

The ototoxicity is associated with either hearing loss (cochlear damage) or vertigo (vestibular damage), or both. An early sign is tinnitus accompanied by loss of high-frequency hearing. The hearing loss, if detected early, can be reversed, but it will become permanent after prolonged treatment with aminoglycosides. Patients receiving an aminoglycoside should have periodic hearing tests. The various aminoglycosides differ in the relative proportion of hearing loss and vertigo that they produce. The high amount of hearing loss produced by neomycin precludes its systemic use.

The nephrotoxicity caused by the aminoglycosides is dose-related and reversible if not too severe.

Other drugs may potentiate the adverse effects.

The concomitant administration of other drugs that cause similar adverse effects will potentiate the adverse effects caused by the aminoglycosides. Drugs that cause ototoxicity include ethacrynic acid and furosemide. Drugs that cause nephrotoxicity include ethacrynic acid, furosemide and cisplatin, and polymixin.

A third adverse reaction caused by the aminoglycosides is a curare-like neuromuscular blockade resulting in respiratory paralysis. This occurs mainly after intraperitoneal administration.

Allergic reactions in the form of fever and rash may occasionally occur. These usually appear only after prolonged contact with the drug, as in the treatment of tuberculosis.

Clinical Uses

The aminoglycosides are usually reserved for the more serious microbial infections because they have very severe adverse effects.

Streptomycin is currently used mainly in the treatment of tuberculosis, usually in conjunction with another agent such as isoniazid. Streptomycin is also used in the therapy of plague and tularemia.

Gentamicin may be used for treatment of many aerobic Gram-negative infections such as by *Escherichia coli, Klebsiella, Enterobacter, Proteus,* and *Serratia.* Another use for gentamicin is in treatment of infection by methicillin-resistant staphylococci. Gentamicin and the penicillins act synergistically in the treatment of *Pseudomonas aeruginosa.* However, gentamicin is inactivated by the penicillins when they are in the same solution, and consequently, they are administered separately to the patient.

Aminoglycosides and penicillins act synergistically in treatment of *Pseudomonas.*

There is a narrow window of plasma concentration of gentamicin between the minimum needed to produce a therapeutic effect (8 μg/ml) and a toxic effect (12 μg/ml). In addition, there is considerable variability in achievable plasma levels between individuals. Therefore, the plasma concentration of gentamicin is often monitored.

Amikacin has essentially the same spectrum of action as gentamicin and is largely replacing it for general use because of the increased occurrence of resistance to gentamicin by gram-negative organisms.

Tobramycin and netilmicin have essentially the same spectrum of action as gentamicin. Netilmicin, because of its structure, is protected from inactivation by the phosphorylating enzyme and, therefore, exhibits less frequency of resistance than gentamicin.

Neomycin, because of its high toxicity, is never administered parenterally, but it is available in a variety of over-the-counter preparations for topical administration. Neomycin is administered orally for preparation of the lower bowel for surgery. It is not absorbed from the gastrointestinal tract, thereby not exhibiting its toxic properties. It is excreted in the feces. Paromomycin may also be used similarly.

References

Neu HC: New antibiotics: Areas of appropriate use. J Infect Dis 134 (Suppl):S3, 1987.
Meyer RD: Drugs five years later. Ann Intern Med 95, 1981.
Phillips I: Aminoglycosides. Lancet 2:311, 1982.

51

Sulfonamides, Trimethoprim, and Their Combination*

Thomas R. Beam, Jr.

Sulfonamides

Sulfanilamide was synthesized as a potential coloring dye.

Sulfanilamide was synthesized in the German dye industry in 1908. Its antimicrobial properties were unrecognized for more than 20 years. In 1932 Gerhard Domagk noted a protective effect of prontosil against murine streptococcal infections. It was later learned that this therapeutic effect could be attributed to its metabolic product para-aminobenzenesulfonamide (sulfanilamide). The first therapeutic use in humans occurred when a 10-year-old girl with *Haemophilus influenzae* meningitis was treated in the United States. It was unsuccessful. However, major efforts were then made to synthesize new derivatives that might be less toxic and more efficacious.

CHEMISTRY AND MECHANISM

Clinically useful sulfonamides have all been derived from sulfanilamide (Fig. 51–1). This compound is similar in structure to para-aminobenzoic acid (PABA) an essential precursor for bacterial synthesis of folic acid. The amino group at Position 4 of sulfanilamide expands antibacterial activity, as does addition of a sulfonyl radical at Position 1. Substitutions at the 4 amino group can block systemic absorption.

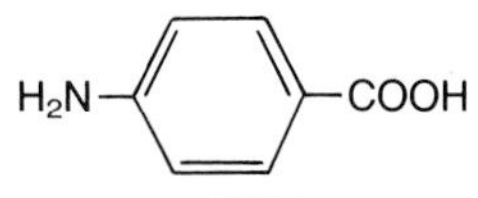

Sulfonamides inhibit folic acid synthesis.

For bacteria, tetrahydrofolic acid is a required cofactor in the synthesis of thymidine, purines, and DNA; bacteria are unable to use external sources of folic acid because of impermeability of the cell wall. On the other hand, humans require preformed folic acid, largely obtained through dietary sources, and are unable to synthesize it. These distinctions lend a relatively high therapeutic index to sulfonamides. Sulfonamides competitively inhibit the incorporation of PABA into tetrahydropteroic acid and are incorporated into dihydropteroate. Sulfonamides have a higher affinity for microbial tetrahydropteroic acid synthetase than the natural substrate PABA. The result is generally a bacteriostatic inhibition of growth.

H_2N—⬡—COOH

PABA

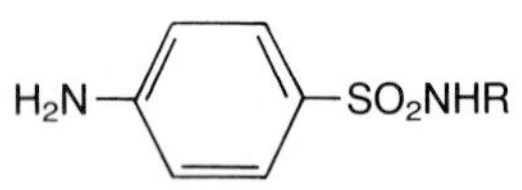

H_2N—⬡—SO_2NHR

Sulfonamide nucleus

ABSORPTION, DISTRIBUTION, METABOLISM, AND EXCRETION

For use as antimicrobial agents most sulfonamides are administered orally. Absorption is almost complete, except for certain preparations substituted at the N-1 position. Topical preparations are absorbed also and can result in measurable serum levels.

Serum peak concentrations are variable from 30 to 100 μg/ml, de-

* This work was supported by the Veterans Administration.

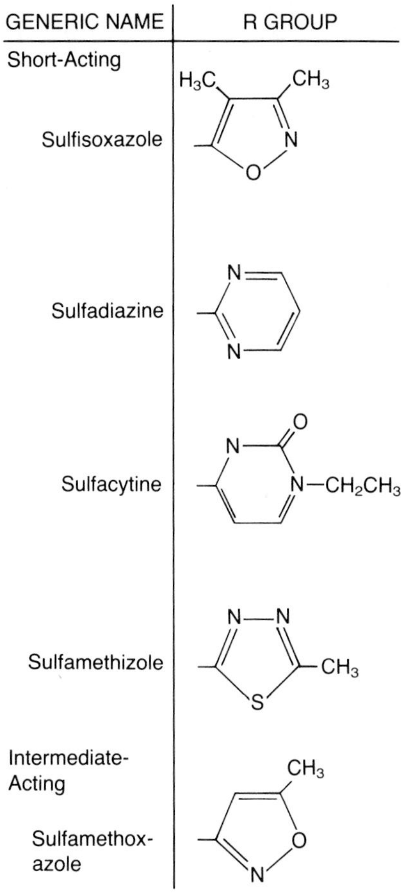

GENERIC NAME	R GROUP
Short-Acting	
Sulfisoxazole	
Sulfadiazine	
Sulfacytine	
Sulfamethizole	
Intermediate-Acting	
Sulfamethox-azole	

Figure 51–1

Chemical structures of various sulfonamides.

pending on the preparation. Protein binding, plasma half-life, and penetration into the cerebrospinal fluid (CSF) are summarized in Table 51–1. The sulfonamides distribute widely, generally reaching 70–80% of simultaneous serum values in extravascular body fluids. Sulfonamides readily cross the placenta and are present in fetal blood and amniotic fluid.

To clear sulfonamides from the body, these drugs are generally acetylated or conjugated with glucuronic acid in the liver. Most metabolites are inactive and excreted through the urine. Excretion is mainly by glomerular filtration, but tubular resorption and secretion have been described also. Alkalization usually enhances urinary excretion. Dosing schedules for pa-

Sulfa drugs are mostly administered orally, well absorbed, and distributed widely through body tissues.

Table 51–1 LEVELS IN BLOOD, CEREBROSPINAL FLUID, PLASMA HALF-LIFE, AND PROTEIN BINDING OF SOME SULFONAMIDES

Drug	Peak Blood Level* (μg/ml)	Serum Level in CSF (%)	Plasma Half-Life (hours)	Protein Binding (%)
Sulfadiazine	30–60	40–80	17	45
Sulfisoxazole	40–50	30–50	5–6	92
Sulfamethoxazole	80–100	25–30	11	70
Sulfadoxine	50–75	20–30	100–230	80–98

From Zinner SH, Mayer KH: Sulfonamides and trimethoprim. *In* Mandell GL, Douglas RG, Bennett JE (eds): Principles and Practice of Infectious Diseases, 3rd ed, 327. New York: Churchill Livingstone, 1990.
* Approximate free sulfonamide level after a 2-g oral dose.

Table 51-2 PREPARATIONS AND DOSAGES: SULFONAMIDES		
Preparation	**Manufacturer**	**Dosage Forms**
Sulfacytine (Renoquid)	Glenwood	250 mg tablets
Sulfadiazine	Generic	500 mg tablets
Sulfadiazine sodium	Generic	Powder for IV use
Sulfamethizole (Thiosulfil forte)	Ayerst	500 mg tablets
Sulfisoxazole (Gantrisin)	Roche; Generic	500 mg tablets
Sulfisoxazole acetyl (Gantrisin)	Roche	500 mg/5 ml suspension 500 mg/5 ml syrup 1 g/5 ml liquid
Sulfisoxazole diolamine (Gantrisin)	Roche	IV discontinued in United States Ophthalmic ointment and suspension, 4%
Sulfamethoxazole (Gantanol)	Roche; Generic	500 mg and 1 g tablets 500 mg/5 ml suspension
Sulfonamide and Phenazopyridine		
Azo Gantanol	Roche	500 mg sulfamethoxazole plus 100 mg phenazopyridine
Azo Gantrisin	Roche	500 mg sulfisoxazole plus 50 mg phenazopyridine
Thiosulfil A	Ayerst	250 mg sulfamethizole plus 50 mg phenazopyridine
Thiosulfil A Forte	Ayerst	500 mg sulfamethizole plus 50 mg phenazopyridine
Urobiotic	Roerig	250 mg sulfamethizole plus 250 mg oxytetracycline plus 50 mg phenazopyridine
Erythromycin ethylsuccinate plus sulfisoxazole acetyl (Pediazole)	Ross	200 mg erythromycin plus 600 mg sulfisoxazole/5 ml suspension
Sulfabenzamide		
Sultrin	Ortho	Sulfathiazole plus sulfa cefamide plus sulfabenzamide cream
Sultrin	Ortho	Vaginal tablets
Sulfacetamide sodium		
Sulamyd	Schering	10% ophthalmic ointment and solution; 30% ophthalmic solution
Sulfanilamide		
AVC	Merrell Dow	15% cream 1.05 g suppositories

tients with compromised renal function have not been studied. Because of reduced renal clearance, inadequate concentration of the sulfonamide may be achieved in the urine. Therefore, alternative agents are generally preferred for treatment of patients who have serious infections and renal failure.

There are several parenteral preparations available for clinical use (see Table 51–2). Sulfisoxazole diolamine may be given subcutaneously or intravenously (IV). Sulfadiazine sodium may also be given IV. However, because of poor water solubility, the drugs must be diluted in large volumes of 5% dextrose in water and, therefore, require prolonged infusion times.

ADVERSE EFFECTS

Despite modifcations of the molecular structure to improve solubility and decrease adverse reactions, side effects still occur with sulfonamide therapy. The major adverse effects of currently available preparations are hypersensitivity phenomena and hematological toxicity. Cutaneous hypersensitivity is most commonly manifested by photosensitivity, erythema nodosum, exfoliative dermatitis, or Stevens-Johnson syndrome. Rashes may be accompanied by a serum-sickness–type illness.

Stevens-Johnson syndrome is the most serious cutaneous toxicity and includes erythema multiforme and mucosal ulcerations. It can be fatal.

The most common side effects are different types of skin rash.

Stevens-Johnson syndrome is a potentially lethal adverse reaction to this class of drugs.

Because of the frequency and severity of this adverse reaction, the long-acting sulfonamide preparations are no longer available in the United States. The estimated risk is 1–2/10 million therapeutic courses of any sulfa preparation.

Adverse reactions, particularly rash, seem to occur more commonly among acquired immune deficiency syndrome (AIDS) patients who are prescribed a sulfa preparation than among the population at large. Because there is no standard mechanism for testing sulfonamide hypersensitivity, allergy to one preparation should be construed to represent allergy to all preparations.

Hematological toxicity may result in agranulocytosis, aplastic anemia, megaloblastic anemia, and thrombocytopenia. All of these are rare occurrences with currently available sulfa preparations. Fortunately, the agranulocytosis, megaloblastic anemia, and thrombocytopenia are generally reversible with discontinuation of the drug.

Nephrotoxicity was common with older preparations but is rarely seen today. Sulfadiazine may cause crystalluria, pain, hematuria, and anuria. Hydration and alkalization of the urine minimize the likelihood of crystal precipitation. Sufonamides also may cause tubular necrosis in the absence of crystal precipitation. Therefore, these drugs should be used with caution in patients with impaired renal function, if at all.

> Newly developed sulfa preparations have little nephrotoxicity.

Hepatotoxicity manifested by focal or diffuse necrosis and cholestatic jaundice is also rare with newer preparations of sulfonamides. Sulfonamides can displace bilirubin from albumin-binding sites and can lead to kernicterus in newborns. Gastrointestinal (GI) side effects of anorexia, nausea, vomiting, and diarrhea are also less common than in the past.

A wide variety of neurotoxicities have been rarely reported. These include headache, lethargy, dizziness, and mental depression. IV delivery is associated infrequently with pain at the infusion site.

INDICATIONS AND CONTRAINDICATIONS

The uses of sulfonamide preparations are limited by a high prevalence of resistance that has developed among previously susceptible microorganisms, safer alternatives, and lack of systemic efficacy (oral preparations). Current indications are for treatment of uncomplicated urinary tract infections, nocardiosis, and respiratory tract infections caused by susceptible pathogens. But even these uses have been supplanted by sulfa combined with trimethoprim or erythromycin.

> Sulfa antimicrobials are most commonly used to treat urinary tract infections.

Sulfadiazine is recommended as an alternative to penicillin for prophylaxis against rheumatic fever in the penicillin-allergic patient. Sulfadiazine or sulfadoxime in combination with pyrimethamine is indicated for treatment or prophylaxis of cholorquine-resistant malaria and treatment of toxoplasmosis. Preparations and dosages are shown in Table 51–2.

The drug is contraindicated for those patients known to be hypersensitive to it, in children less than 12 years of age, and in pregnancy at term or during breast feeding. Besides bilirubin, as noted earlier, sulfonamides may displace drugs from albumin or decrease metabolism of these drugs, thus enhancing activity of the compounds. These effects may occur with oral hypoglycemics, coumarin anticoagulants, phenytoin, and methotrexate. Sulfonamides may interact with thiazide diuretics, particularly in elderly individuals, yielding an increased risk of thrombocytopenia and purpura.

> Caution is warranted when prescribing sulfa drugs simultaneously with oral hypoglycemics, anticoagulants, phenytoin, and methotrexate.

In contrast to bilirubin, sulfa drugs may be displaced by agents with higher avidity for albumin-binding sites, including phenylbutazone, salicylates, and probenecid. The increase in free drug results in increased sulfonamide activity.

Sulfimethazole and sulfathiozole may form insoluble precipitates with formaldehyde. Therefore, coadministration of methenamine should be avoided. PABA-containing compounds, including local anesthetics, may inhibit sulfonamide activity. They also should not be concurrently administered.

Finally, interference with laboratory tests may be caused by the sulfonamides. Included are false-positive Benedict's test for glucose, false-positive sulfosalicylic acid test for urine protein, false-negative Urobilistix for urobilinogen, and 10% increase in serum creatinine performed by the Jaffe alkaline picrate test for creatinine.

Trimethoprim

Trimethoprim is a dihydrofolate reductase inhibitor that was synthesized by Hitchings at the Wellcome Research Laboratories in the United States in 1956. It was available only in combination with sulfamethoxazole until 1980, when it was released for use as a single (uncombined) anti-infective agent.

CHEMISTRY AND MECHANISM

The chemical structure of this drug is 2,4-diamino-5-(3'-4'-5'-trimethoxybenzyl) pyrimidine. Trimethoprim inhibits bacterial dihydrofolate reductase, which converts dihydrofolic to tetrahydrofolic acid. The latter is used for bacterial purine and DNA synthesis. Trimethoprim selectively inhibits the bacterial enzyme at 50,000- to 100,000-fold lower concentration than the human enzyme. It is also 2000-fold more active against the malarial enzyme than the human form. This represents high specificity against pathogenic microorganisms.

ABSORPTION, DISTRIBUTION, METABOLISM, AND EXCRETION

Trimethoprim is essentially 100% absorbed following an oral dose. The serum peak concentration of 0.8–1.0 mcg/ml is reached 1–4 hours after a 100 mg dose. The drug is widely distributed into tissues and body fluids, including CSF in the absence of inflammation. Particularly high concentrations are found in kidney and liver. Equal concentrations are found in serum and within erythrocytes. Thus, cell membranes do not act as restrictive barriers to drug distribution.

Trimethoprim is 42–46% protein-bound and has a serum half-life of 9–11 hours. Between 60 and 80% of a dose is excreted unchanged in the urine. Trimethoprim is metabolized in the liver but also may be metabolized in peripheral tissues. Inactive oxide or hydroxyl metabolites are cleared through the kidney. The rate of renal excretion of parent drug plus metabolites is increased by an acid urine. Therapeutic dosages need to be adjusted only for the patient with a creatinine clearance less than 30 ml/minute.

ADVERSE EFFECTS

The most common adverse reaction to trimethoprim is rash, including maculopapular, morbilliform, and occasionally exfoliative dermatitis. GI intolerance is common also and is evidenced by epigastric distress, nausea, vomiting, and glossitis. Hematological toxicities may include thrombocytopenia, leukopenia, and megaloblastic anemia. These are indicators that the high specificity against microbial enzymes is not without effect on

Trimethoprim inhibits microbial folic acid production.

Trimethoprim

(2,4-diamino-5-(3',4',5'-trimethoxy-benzyl)pyrimidine)

Trimethoprim is almost completely absorbed, distributes throughout the body without restriction, and has a long (9–11 hour) serum half-life.

The most common side effect is rash.

human folate use. Therefore, trimethoprim should be used with caution among individuals with possible folate deficiency. Folinic acid can be provided for human folic acid needs without impeding the antibacterial effectiveness of the drug.

Fever, elevated hepatocellular enzymes, and increased blood urea nitrogen (BUN) or creatinine have been reported also. Because of lack of information about safety in humans, this drug should not be prescribed during pregnancy. It should be avoided also in nursing mothers and infants less than 2 months of age.

Trimethoprim should not be used in persons with folate deficiency or in newborns.

INDICATIONS AND CONTRAINDICATIONS

Trimethoprim is indicated for treatment of acute, uncomplicated urinary tract infections, prophylaxis against recurrent urinary tract infections, and treatment of chronic prostatitis caused by susceptible organisms. It may be used also to treat traveler's diarrhea caused by bacterial pathogens (particularly *Escherichia coli*).

Trimethoprim is used to treat urinary tract infections, including prostatitis.

The drug is contraindicated for patients known to be hypersensitive to it and those with documented folate deficiency.

There are few problems with drug interactions. Trimethoprim may inhibit hepatic metabolism of phenytoin and increase serum concentrations of the latter to toxic levels. Therefore, serum concentrations should be monitored. Trimethoprim can interfere also with serum methotrexate determinations performed by the competitive protein-binding technique, but not by radioimmunoassay. It also may falsely elevate serum creatinine values determined by the Jaffe alkaline picrate method. Preparations and dosages are shown in Table 51–3.

Table 51–3 PREPARATIONS AND DOSAGES: TRIMETHOPRIM

Preparation	Manufacturer	Dosage Forms
Trimethoprim	Generic	100 mg tablets
Trimpex	Roche	100 mg tablets
Proloprim	Burroughs Wellcome	100 and 200 mg tablets

Trimethoprim-sulfamethoxazole (TMP-SMZ) was developed and marketed for two main reasons: the absorption and serum half-lives of the two drugs were similar, and the sequential inhibition of bacterial folic acid synthesis produced synergistic bacterial killing. The drugs were combined in a fixed ratio of 1:5 trimethoprim/sulfamethoxazole, and the drug mixture was first introduced into the United States in 1974.

Whereas a single enzymatic block of bacterial folic acid production usually results in a bacteriostatic effect, the two-step block is usually bactericidal. In addition, the likelihood of emerging resistance is theoretically less because of the use of two antimicrobials with different sites of action.

Trimethoprim-Sulfamethoxazole Combinations

The sequential enzyme inhibition provided by the combination of trimethoprim and sulfamethoxazole produces bacterial killing and lessens bacterial resistance.

ADVERSE EFFECTS

As is generally true for drug combinations, any adverse reaction reported for either agent may be seen with the combination. Skin rash is the most common and is usually attributed to hypersensitivity to the sulfa component. Although generally mild and reversible on discontinuation, toxic epidermyl necrolysis, erythema multiforme, exfoliative dermatitis, and the Stevens-Johnson syndrome may occur. Allergic or toxic suppression of bone marrow cells has been reported also. Chills, fever, allergic vasculitis, and a systemic lupus erythematosus syndrome may be seen.

Skin rash is the most common adverse reaction and may be severe or life-threatening.

Nephrotoxicity and hepatotoxicity are rare, but anorexia, nausea, and vomiting are relatively common GI complaints. Central nervous system (CNS) toxicity has been reported but is unusual. The combination should not be used during pregnancy, at term, or for nursing mothers up to 2 months following delivery. It should be restricted in use for those patients likely to have a folate deficiency.

Patients with HIV infections are particularly vulnerable to skin rash, fever, and marrow suppression.

AIDS patients are particularly vulnerable to adverse reactions characterized by recurrent fever, maculopapular skin rash, and peripheral cytopenias. These are believed to represent hypersensitivity phenomena and recur upon rechallenge. Discontinuation of the drug combination is often necessary.

INDICATIONS AND CONTRAINDICATIONS

The drug combination has broad-spectrum activity against many different types of pathogens. Therefore, the drug may be used to treat or prevent a large number of clinical conditions. TMP-SMZ is indicated for the treatment of both upper and lower urinary tract infections. It may be used also as prophylaxis against recurrent urinary tract infections.

The spectrum of indications for the drug combination far exceeds the indications for the component parts.

TMP-SMZ is the drug of choice for acute and chronic bacterial prostatitis, in part because of trimethoprim's ability to penetrate tissue. It is also useful for treatment of respiratory tract infections such as otitis media, sinusitis, acute exacerbations of chronic bronchitis, and pneumonia caused by susceptible organisms. It may be useful for prophylaxis against recurrent otitis and is an alternative to erythromycin for eradication of the *Bordetella pertussis* carrier state.

TMP-SMZ is the treatment of choice for infections caused by *Shigella flexneri* and *S. sonnei;* for typhoid fever and serious infections caused by *Salmonella;* traveler's diarrhea caused by enterotoxigenic *E. coli;* and as an alternative to tetracycline for treatment of cholera. TMP-SMZ is an alternative therapy for treatment of chancroid, *Chlamydia trachomatis,* and granuloma inguinale. It may be useful also for therapy of melioidosis, nocardiosis, and brucellosis. It is an alternative to minocycline for treatment of *Mycobacterium marinum* infections.

A common use of this drug combination has been treatment of *P. carinii* pneumonia.

TMP-SMZ is the treatment of choice for *Pneumocystis carinii* pneumonia, particularly among patients with cancer or transplantation. It is also useful for treatment of *P. carinii* pneumonia in AIDS patients, recognizing that toxicity often limits completion of a full therapeutic course. It may be employed also to prevent recurrence of *Pneumocystis* in the same population. Finally, TMP-SMZ has been used as prophylaxis against gram-nega-

Table 51-4 PREPARATIONS AND DOSAGES: TRIMETHOPRIM-SULFAMETHOXAZOLE COMBINATIONS		
Preparation	**Manufacturer**	**Dosage Forms**
TMP-SMZ	Generic	200 mg SMZ + 40 mg TMP/5 ml suspension
		400 mg SMZ + 80 mg TMP/tablet
Bactrim	Roche	200 mg SMZ + 40 mg TMP/5 ml suspension
		400 mg SMZ + 80 mg TMP/tablet
Septra	Burroughs Wellcome	200 mg SMZ + 40 mg TMP/5 ml suspension
		400 mg SMZ + 80 mg TMP/tablet
Bactrim DS	Roche	800 mg SMZ + 160 mg TMP/tablet
Septra DS	Burroughs Wellcome	
Bactrim IV	Roche	16 mg/ml SMZ + 80 mg/ml TMP solution in 5, 10, and 30 ml containers
Septra IV	Burroughs Wellcome	16 mg/ml SMZ + 80 mg/ml TMP solution in 5, 10, and 20 ml containers
TMP-SMZ IV	Generic	16 mg/ml SMZ + 80 mg/ml TMP solution in 5 and 10 ml containers

tive sepsis in neutropenic patients. Efficacy in this setting is controversial.

All drug interactions previously noted for each single agent, and all interference with laboratory tests, can be seen with the combination product. Preparations and dosages are shown in Table 51–4.

General References

Brogden RN, Carmine AA, Heel RC, et al: Trimethoprim: A review of its antibacterial activity, pharmacokinetics and therapeutic use in urinary tract infections. Drugs 23:405, 1982.

Cockerill FR, Edson RS: Trimethoprim-sulfamethoxazole. Mayo Clin Proc 58:147, 1983.

Kucers A, Bennett NM: Sulfonamides. *In* Kucers A, Bennett NM (eds): The Use of Antibiotics, 4th ed, 1075. Philadelphia: JB Lippincott Co, 1987.

Rubin RH, Swartz MN: Trimethoprim-sulfamethoxazole. N Engl J Med 303:426, 1980.

52

Tetracyclines and Chloramphenicol

Alan M. Reynard

The tetracyclines and chloramphenicol are known as the *broad-spectrum antibiotics,* because of their affects on gram-positive and gram-negative bacteria as well as a few nonbacterial species. These drugs are still used to a certain extent, but other, less toxic and more effective agents have supplanted them. In addition, there has been a change in therapeutic philosophy, from using one drug for many things to using drugs with very specific indications.

Tetracyclines

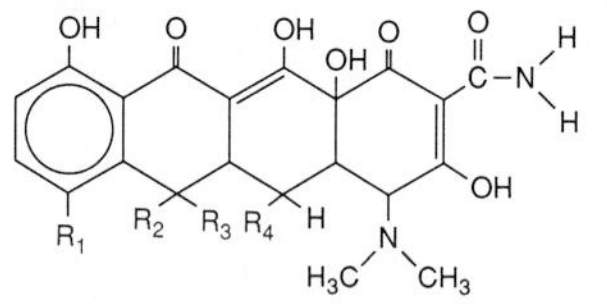

	R_1	R_2	R_3	R_4
chlortetracycline	Cl	CH_3	OH	H
demeclocycline	Cl	H	OH	H
doxycycline	H	CH_3	H	OH
methacycline	H	CH_2	—	OH
minocycline	N(CH_3)_2	H	H	H
oxytetracycline	H	CH_3	OH	OH
tetracycline	H	CH_3	OH	H

Tetracycline

Tetracyclines chelate divalent and trivalent cations.

Tetracyclines inhibit protein synthesis. They are bacteriostatic.

The tetracyclines are a group of drugs with a common 4-ring structure, hence the name. The first of these, chlortetracycline, was introduced in 1948. The most recent, minocycline, was introduced in 1972. The available tetracyclines are shown in the margin.

CHEMISTRY

The tetracyclines are bright-yellow compounds, poorly soluble in water as the free base but soluble as the hydrochloride. The hydrochloride is the form available for use. With the exception of chlortetracycline, they are moderately stable in solution. However, breakdown products form over a period of several years even in solid form, and these products can be toxic. The tetracyclines chelate divalent and trivalent metal ions. This chelation is responsible for their incorporation into tooth and bone material and for poor absorption from the gastrointestinal tract in the presence of food and other substances.

MECHANISM OF ACTION

The tetracyclines bind to the 30S subunit of microbial ribosomes. This results in inhibition of protein synthesis by interference with attachment of aminoacyl-tRNA. Tetracyclines are actively transported into microbial cells but not into mammalian cells, which is the basis for their selective toxicity. Tetracyclines are bacteriostatic drugs.

Plasmid-mediated resistance to the tetracyclines is extremely common among the gram-negative rods. It results from an increased efflux of drug from the resistant cells, thereby reducing intracellular concentration. There is no known chromosomally mediated resistance to the tetracyclines.

ABSORPTION, DISTRIBUTION, METABOLISM, AND EXCRETION

Absorption of the tetracyclines following oral administration is somewhat variable. In general, chlortetracycline is least well absorbed, and doxycycline and minocycline are almost completely absorbed. Absorption is poor in the presence of food, so the drugs should be taken at least 1 hour before or 2 hours after a meal. Absorption is reduced by the presence of divalent and trivalent cations, such as are found in milk and in many antacid products.

The tetracyclines are bound in various amounts to plasma proteins and are distributed to most tissues. Unlike chloramphenicol, the tetracyclines do not reach useful concentrations in cerebrospinal fluid.

A considerable portion of an oral dose of a tetracycline is excreted in the feces. This varies among the tetracyclines. Tetracyclines that are not absorbed in the intestine are excreted in the feces. Tetracyclines are relatively lipophilic and therefore appear in the enterohepatic circulation, which also contributes to fecal excretion. Absorbed tetracyclines are excreted largely by glomerular filtration, making their plasma levels very dependent on kidney function. Exceptions are minocycline and doxycycline; for these agents glomerular filtration appears to have little role in excretion.

Absorption of tetracyclines is reduced by divalent and trivalent cations and food.

ADVERSE EFFECTS

The tetracyclines produce a variety of dose-related gastrointestinal effects, including nausea, vomiting, and epigastric distress. Diarrhea may also result and should be distinguished from the pseudomembraneous colitis associated with growth of *Clostridium difficile.*

Tetracyclines, like other broad-spectrum antibiotics, have a relatively high potential to produce superinfection. This is caused by the suppression of certain body flora with subsequent appearance of other organisms, particularly staphylococci, clostridia, and *Candida*. Drugs with narrow spectra of action, such as penicillin, produce superinfection much less frequently. When the appearance of superinfection is determined, administration of the causative drug, in this case tetracycline, is stopped and treatment of the offending organism is started.

Broad-spectrum antibiotics are more likely to cause superinfection.

Hepatic toxicity can occur with administration of large doses (usually 2 g/day or more) of drug. The symptoms include jaundice, azotemia, acidosis, and possibly, shock. Biopsy reveals a diffuse, fatty infiltrate.

Kidney toxicity in the form of azotemia has been observed in some patients, especially in the presence of kidney failure. The shelf life of tetracycline is limited, and ingestion of outdated tetracycline has been the cause of a clinical picture similar to that of the Fanconi syndrome, presumably due to the effects of degradation products. The symptoms include nausea, vomiting, and kidney failure.

Outdated tetracycline can cause kidney damage.

Treatment with tetracyclines, especially demeclocycline and doxycycline, may cause sensitivity to sunlight, leading to mild to severe skin reactions.

Tetracycline, because it chelates to divalent metals, binds strongly to bone and tooth material. The binding can cause depression of bone growth. Because tetracycline is a bright-yellow compound, it can cause a discoloration of teeth that changes from yellow to grayish brown over time. Because of these effects, tetracyclines are contraindicated in children of tooth-formation age and also in women from midpregnancy onward.

Administration of minocycline has been associated with vestibular reactions such as dizziness and nausea.

Intravenous administration of a tetracycline can lead to thrombophlebitis.

Various hypersensitivity reactions to the tetracyclines have been described including rash, fever, glossitis, angioedema, and anaphylaxis. However, these reactions, especially the more serious ones, are quite rare.

In contrast to the great benefit derived from the use of tetracyclines, the enormous amounts of tetracycline used have contributed to greatly increased numbers of resistant organisms. This comes not only from use of tetracycline in medical practice but also from the inclusion of tetracycline in animal feeds for the purpose of growth promotion.

INDICATIONS AND CONTRAINDICATIONS

The tetracyclines are the drugs of choice for treatment of

Tetracyclines are the drugs of choice for a limited number of infections.

- rickettsial infections such as Rocky Mountain spotted fever, rickettsialpox, Q fever, Brill's disease, murine typhus, and scrub typhus;
- chlamydial infections such as lymphogranuloma venereum, pneumonia, psittacosis, inclusion conjunctivitis, and trachoma;
- mycoplasma infections such as pneumonia.

Rickettsial and mycoplasma infections are usually treated with tetracycline, whereas chlamydial infections are often treated with doxycycline.

Neisseria gonorrhoeae is susceptible to the tetracyclines, and treatment of gonorrhea in areas in which there is a high prevalence of penicillinase-producing *N. gonorrhoeae* can be accomplished with tetracycline or doxycycline. However, resistance to the tetracyclines has also increased, reducing effectiveness of these agents, and ceftriaxone (see Chapter 49) has become the treatment of choice. Tetracyclines have the advantage of being effective against chlamydia, which often accompanies gonorrhea, and they may be administered along with ceftriaxone.

The tetracyclines can be useful in cases of syphilis for which it is not possible to use a penicillin or a cephalosporin.

Minocycline has been used to eradicate the meningococcal carrier state, but its serious toxicity (vertigo) limits its usefulness.

Tetracycline is often used in treatment of acne when it occurs in young people and in adults as acne rosacea. It is thought that inhibition of propionibacteria results in a decrease in the amount of fatty acids occurring in sebaceous follicles. The low dose of tetracycline used seems to produce few adverse effects, but there is the possibility, because of the long term of treatment, of developing tetracycline-resistant organisms.

Tetracyclines may be used for a number of infections for which they are no longer the drug of choice when the drug of choice is not useful because of hypersensitivity, resistance, or some other reason. These infections include cholera, brucellosis, tularemia, urinary tract infection by some gram-negative strains, actinomycosis, Lyme disease, yaws, relapsing fever, tetanus, and plague.

Tetracyclines are contraindicated in children whose teeth are still developing and in pregnant women.

Tetracyclines are contraindicated in children up to about 10 years of age, in whom long bones or tooth enamel is being formed, and are contraindicated in pregnant women.

Chloramphenicol

When chloramphenicol appeared on the market it was hailed as the wonder drug of the century. It was a broad-spectrum antibiotic with activity against gram-positive and gram-negative bacteria as well as some nonbacterial species. It could be produced by synthetic processes, which made it relatively inexpensive to market. It could be administered by mouth, and it was virtually nontoxic. However, it was shortly discovered that some patients treated with chloramphenicol were dying of aplastic anemia. Although the percentage of patients affected was small, the large number of people receiving the drug resulted in upward of 300 deaths/year for several years. Chloramphenicol was taken off the market in the United States while a Senate committee reviewed it and other drugs. It was returned to the market with much sterner warnings of toxicity on the package insert. In addition, the Food and Drug Administration was given new powers to regulate the marketing of drugs.

CHEMISTRY

Chloramphenicol has a relatively simple structure. It is produced by chemical synthesis, in contrast to most other antibiotics that are produced as a by-product of mold growth. It is a colorless compound, relatively insoluble in water.

Chloramphenicol

MECHANISM OF ACTION

Chloramphenicol binds to the 50S ribosomal subunit of susceptible species and inhibits the peptidyl transferase enzyme that is part of the subunit. The result is inhibition of protein synthesis. It is a bacteriostatic drug.

Chloramphenicol inhibits protein synthesis. It is bacteriostatic.

As with the tetracyclines, plasmid-mediated resistance is very common in gram-negative rods. This resistance is especially troublesome in *Hemophilus influenzae* because chloramphenicol and ampicillin were the drugs of choice before the prevalence of resistant strains became too high. The mechanism of resistance is production of an intracellular enzyme that catalyzes the acetylation of chloramphenicol, thereby inactivating it.

ABSORPTION, DISTRIBUTION, METABOLISM, AND EXCRETION

Chloramphenicol is administered orally either as chloramphenicol or as chloramphenicol palmitate. The palmitate ester is hydrolyzed to free drug in the intestine from which the chloramphenicol is absorbed. Chloramphenicol is not very soluble in water and is marketed for injection as the more soluble succinate ester. The inactive ester is hydrolyzed to free drug in various tissues in the body.

The drug is distributed well to most tissues of the body, including the cerebrospinal fluid, whether or not there is meningitis. It can be found in bile and in maternal milk and crosses the placenta. It is bound to plasma proteins.

Chloramphenicol penetrates into the cerebrospinal fluid.

Chloramphenicol is inactivated in the liver by glucuronide formation, and therefore its concentration in plasma is dependent on liver function. Patients with liver disease may have abnormally high concentrations of the drug if the dose is not adjusted. Similarly, infants with immature liver development are subject to abnormally high concentrations of the drug.

Excretion of chloramphenicol and the glucuronide is mainly in the urine, but the dose does not have to be altered in the presence of renal failure.

ADVERSE EFFECTS

The most important adverse effect of chloramphenicol is a rare (about 1 in 30,000 courses) but often fatal aplasia of the bone marrow, leading to pancytopenia. The mechanism is not yet understood. In patients who survive there is an abnormally high incidence of leukemia. There seems to be no correlation between outcome following aplastic anemia and dose, but the incidence of the malady increases with increased length of treatment with chloramphenicol.

Chloramphenicol can cause aplastic anemia, which is usually fatal.

Chloramphenicol also causes a dose-related anemia characterized by a defect in red cell maturation. This probably results from an inhibition by chloramphenicol of mitochondrial protein synthesis. This may be fatal but usually reverses after the drug is discontinued.

Chloramphenicol is contraindicated in infants.

Administration of chloramphenicol has had fatal results in infants owing to the gray syndrome. As mentioned earlier, infants under approximately 4 weeks of age have immature liver function and are not able to inactivate chloramphenicol by glucuronidation. In addition, such infants have immature kidneys and cannot excrete the drug at the same rate as older children or adults. In this circumstance chloramphenicol can accumulate and cause vomiting, hypothermia, and shock. The infants die with a cyanotic gray color.

Chloramphenicol, like the tetracyclines, has a propensity to cause superinfection.

Hypersensitivity reactions are relatively rare.

INDICATIONS AND CONTRAINDICATIONS

Chloramphenicol is used in the treatment of serious infections, especially those in cerebrospinal fluid and brain tissue.

Chloramphenicol is effective against a large number of microorganisms but is used for only a limited number of infections because of its adverse effects. The infections for which it is used tend to be the more serious types such as meningitis.

Chloramphenicol is sometimes used for treatment of typhoid fever due to *Salmonella typhi*, but ampicillin is also highly effective. Resistance may occur to one or both of these agents. In this case trimethoprim-sulfamethoxazole and several of the cephalosporins may be used. Meningitis due to *H. influenzae* usually responds well to chloramphenicol. Again, ampicillin is also effective, but resistance to ampicillin has increased to over 25% of strains. Meningitis due to *N. meningitidis* or *Streptococcus pneumoniae* is usually treated with penicillin, but when the patient is allergic to ampicillin, chloramphenicol is an alternative. It is often stated that a static drug should not be used in combination with a penicillin antibiotic. Nevertheless, chloramphenicol has been used, with good results, in conjunction with ampicillin for treatment of meningitis, especially in children between 3 months and 10 years of age, in which *H. influenzae* may be the causative organism.

Chloramphenicol is effective in treatment of infection by several anaerobic organisms, particularly *Bacteroides fragilis* and is used for some of the more serious forms such as infection of the central nervous system or brain abscess. Metronidazole is also effective against bacteroides and is often used with penicillin for these infections. Clindamycin has activity against bacteroides but, unlike chloramphenicol and metronidazole, does not penetrate the blood-brain barrier.

Chloramphenicol is used as an alternative drug for treatment of infection due to rickettsiae and brucella when tetracycline cannot be used.

INTERACTIONS

Chloramphenicol has been reported to increase the toxicity of phenytoin and to decrease the effects of iron salts and vitamin B_{12}.

General References

Gump DW: Chloramphenicol: A 1981 view. [Editorial] Arch Intern Med 141:573, 1981.

Kucers A, Bennett N: Chloramphenicol and thiamphenicol. *In* The Uses of Antibiotics, 4th ed, 757–807. Philadelphia: JB Lippincott Co, 1987.

Neu HC: A symposium on tetracyclines: A major appraisal. Introduction. Bull NY Acad Med 54:141–155, 1978.

Standiford HC: Tetracyclines and chloramphenicol. *In* Mandell GL, Douglas RG Jr, Bennett JE (eds): Principles and Practice of Infectious Diseases, 3rd ed, 284–295. New York: John Wiley & Sons, 1990.

53

Drugs Used in the Treatment of Tuberculosis: Antimycobacterial Agents*

Thomas R. Beam, Jr.

Antimycobacterial agents may be directed at treatment of *Mycobacterium tuberculosis,* atypical mycobacterial infection, or *M. leprae.* The objectives of therapy are to cure the individual patient of infection, render the patient noncontagious as soon as possible, and avoid relapse or failure following therapy. Acceptable relapse rates are 5% or less.

In general, therapy must consist of two or more agents. The number of drugs employed depends on the organism load and the susceptibility pattern of the patient's infecting strain. Antimycobacterials exert their therapeutic effect only on actively growing organisms. These organisms may exist in cavitary lesions; closed, caseous lesions; and macrophages. Pharmacokinetic information (and particularly distribution properties of the drug) is critical to predict efficacy for treatment of susceptible organisms. In addition, mycobacterial resistance is always a concern. This may exist as primary resistance (original isolate before chemotherapy) or acquired resistance (usually seen in noncompliant patients who erratically take the prescribed drug). Mutational resistance to two drugs is rare; therefore, therapy usually consists of two or more drugs.

Duration of therapy is divided into conventional and short-course. Conventional therapy lasts for 18 months, short-course therapy for 9 months or less. At issue is the rate of relapse. Studies have confirmed equal efficacy for as little as 6 months of treatment if therapy is initiated with four drugs for 2 months, followed by two drugs for 4 months. Another equally efficacious option is treatment twice or three times per week rather than daily.

Corticosteroids have been used as adjuncts for treatment of tuberculous meningitis, peritonitis, and pericarditis. The objectives are to reduce scarring and late complications of the infection such as neurologic dysfunction or constrictive pericarditis. Corticosteroids also have been administered to patients with fulminant disease.

Isoniazid (INH) is the cornerstone of most therapeutic regimens and the only drug used for prophylaxis against early infection. Isonicotinic acid hydrazide was discovered in 1952 at Squibb and Roche Laboratories. Animal and human studies quickly demonstrated its efficacy against *M. tuberculosis.* INH is a totally synthetic molecule. Preparations and dosage forms are given in Table 53–1.

Therapy of mycobacterial disease usually consists of two or more drugs.

The pharmacokinetic profile of the drug and *in vitro* susceptibility accurately predict clinical response.

Short-course therapy (6 months) has become widely accepted.

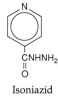

Isoniazid

Isoniazid

INH is bactericidal against growing organisms.

* The work was supported by the Veterans Administration.

Table 53-1 ISONIAZID PREPARATIONS AND DOSAGES		
Preparation	Manufacturer	Dosage Forms
Isoniazid	Generic	50, 100, and 300 mg tablets
Dow-Isoniazid	Merrell Dow	300 mg tablets
Nydrazid	Squibb	100 mg tablets
		100 mg/ml in 10 ml solution containers for injection
Laniazid Syrup	Lannett	10 mg/ml syrup
Combination Products With Rifampin		
Rimactine/INH	CIBA	30 × 300 mg isonizid tablets plus 60 × 300 mg rifampin capsules
Rifamate	Merrell Dow	150 mg isoniazid plus 300 mg rifampin capsules

INH is bactericidal against growing organisms and bacteriostatic against dormant strains. It can penetrate human cell membranes and is active against intracellular organisms. It has been proposed that the drug interferes with cell wall mycolic acid biosynthesis.

INH is readily absorbed following oral or intramuscular administration. The drug has a large volume of distribution in the central nervous system (CNS), including cerebrospinal fluid (CSF), even in the absence of inflamed meninges. CSF concentrations average 20% of simultaneous serum values. When given orally, the drug is vulnerable to significant first-pass metabolism by the liver. Protein binding is negligible. The time to peak following an oral dose is 1–2 hours.

INH penetrates into the CNS, even in the absence of inflammation.

INH is metabolized in the liver by acetylation and hydroxylation and the rate of acetylation is bimodal in the population. Approximately half the population of the United States is estimated to acetylate this drug rapidly. Certain other populations have widely divergent rates (Eskimos 95%, Egyptians 17% rapid acetylators). This phenomenon does not have therapeutic implications if the drug is dosed daily, but it may if intermittent dosing is employed. The large majority of metabolites are excreted in the urine. A small fraction of unchanged drug is also cleared by the kidney. Dose modification may be required for patients with severe liver dysfunction, kidney failure, or a combination of hepatic and renal insufficiency.

There are a wide variety of adverse reactions to INH. Gastrointestinal and hypersensitivity adverse effects are rare, but include nausea, vomiting, diarrhea, fever, and maculopapular rash. If hypersensitivity appears during administration of several antimycobacterial agents, all drugs should be stopped and allowed to clear. Therapy should be reinstituted with INH first because of its chemotherapeutic importance and excellent safety profile. Long-term administration may be associated with a positive antinuclear antibody (ANA) test or full-blown lupus erythematosus syndrome.

Patients with poor dietary habits should receive pyridoxine with their INH therapy.

Neurotoxicity can be seen with INH. The drug can cause pyridoxine (vitamin B_6) deficiency by forming hydrazones that inhibit conversion of pyridoxine to pyridoxyl phosphate or inactivate it. Because pyridoxine is a cofactor for production of neurotransmitters, neuropathy results. Clinical manifestations include paresthesias and peripheral neuropathy but may extend to sensory or motor dysfunction if unrecognized. The peripheral neuropathy is more common in slow acetylators. Small-dose dietary supplementation with pyridoxine can avoid this complication. However, large doses may block the effectiveness of INH. CNS toxicity is most commonly seen with excessive dosing or suicide attempts. Manifestations include altered personality, psychosis, and coma. Niacin deficiency (pellagra) is also an uncommon adverse reaction.

INH also produces hepatocellular dysfunction in approximately 15% of recipients. Enzyme elevations are usually asymptomatic and resolve with discontinuation of the drug. Clinically significant toxicity is rare. Evidence suggests that the elderly are not more prone to this adverse reaction than the young. The mechanism of hepatotoxicity is not known.

Treatment for all forms of *M. tuberculosis* infection should include INH, except when the infecting strain is resistant to the drug. In the latter circumstances most authorities still advocate use of INH. The logic is that in the large pool of organisms causing infection, some will be susceptible to INH and are best treated with this drug.

INH is also used in combination therapy of disease caused by atypical mycobacteria, irrespective of susceptibility results. Treatment of pulmonary tuberculosis with INH may be standard, intermittent, or short-course. INH is also indicated for treatment of tuberculosis in children and pregnant women. INH should be routinely employed for therapy of extrapulmonary tuberculosis, including CNS infection.

Preventive treatment with INH is indicated for purified protein derivative (PPD) convertors within the past 2 years, household contacts of patients, persons with positive PPD tests plus abnormal chest x-rays who have not received previous adequate chemotherapy, or patients at excess risk for developing disease (silicosis, diabetes mellitus, receipt of adrenocorticosteroids, hematological malignancy). INH has been safely employed in the nursing home setting to prevent development of an epidemic of disease.

INH is contraindicated in patients who develop severe hypersensitivity reactions, including drug-induced hepatitis. It is also contraindicated for patients with previous INH-induced hepatic injury; for people who sustain severe adverse reactions during therapy including drug fever, chills, and arthritis; and for people with acute liver disease of any etiology.

INH inhibits microsomal inactivation of carbamazepine, producing toxicity. In turn, carbamazepine is an enzyme inducer and can increase the formation of toxic INH metabolites. INH may also interfere with the metabolism of primidone and barbiturates and reduce serum concentrations of ketoconazole. INH may also inhibit hepatic monoamine oxidase (MAO). Drug interactions could occur among patients taking MAO inhibitors or could follow ingestion of foodstuffs rich in monoamines, such as cheese and port wine.

A second antimycobacterial drug less commonly used than INH is ethambutol. This drug was discovered at Lederle Laboratories in a program to randomly screen chemical compounds for antimycobacterial activity. It has activity only against mycobacteria. Ethambutol is dextro-2,2'-(ethylenedi-imino)-di-1-butanol dihydrochloride. A preparation and its dosage form are given in Table 53–2.

Ethambutol inhibits the transfer of mycolic acids into the cell wall of the tubercle bacillus. It may also inhibit the synthesis of spermidine in mycobacteria. The action is usually bactericidal, and the drug can penetrate human cell membranes to exert its lethal effect.

Hepatocellular dysfunction is relatively common but infrequently clinically significant.

Most therapeutic regimens for typical or atypical mycobacterial infection include INH.

INH can prevent development of disease among vulnerable individuals.

Drug interactions occur with carbamazepine, primidone, and barbiturates.

Ethambutol

Ethambutol hydrochloride

Table 53–2 ETHAMBUTOL: PREPARATION AND DOSAGE FORM

Preparation	Manufacturer	Dosage Form
Myambutol	Lederle	100 and 400 mg tablets

Human pharmacokinetics have not been extensively studied. The drug is administered orally, and 75–80% is absorbed. Peak serum concentrations average 5 μg/ml. Based on animal data and therapeutic results, the volume of distribution is large. However, the drug does not effectively penetrate into the CNS in the absence of inflammation and does so only erratically with inflammation. Up to 15% of drug is converted to inactive metabolites. Approximately 80% is excreted unchanged in the urine. Thus, dose modification is required in the presence of renal failure. Unabsorbed drug is excreted unchanged in the stool. Protein binding averages 40%.

> A special toxic effect of ethambutol is retrobulbar neuritis; it is usually reversible.

The chief toxicity of ethambutol is retrobulbar neuritis. Symptoms may include blurred vision, blind spots, and colorblindness. All effects are usually reversible with discontinuation of the drug. Toxicity seems to be dose-related. Visual acuity and visual fields may be tested every 4–6 weeks during therapy. Rarely, a peripheral neuritis may develop or nephrotoxicity may occur. The drug is nonteratogenic in animals and may be safely administered to pregnant women.

> Ethambutol may be used in place of or in combination with INH.

The main current indication for ethambutol is as an alternative for the patient unable to tolerate INH or rifampin in the treatment of tuberculosis. It is also employed when there is primary or acquired resistance to one of these agents. Ethambutol is also recommended as one component of combination therapy of mycobacterial infections due to *M. kansasii, M. avium-intracellulare,* and granulomas caused by *Nocardia brasiliensis,* if the isolated pathogen is susceptible to the drug.

> Ethambutol has activity against atypical mycobacteria and *Nocardia.*

It is contraindicated in patients known to be hypersensitive to the drug and relatively contraindicated among patients with optic neuritis. No clinically significant interactions have been identified.

Rifampin

> Rifampin is a semisynthetic drug.

The rifamycin complex is a different class of antimycobacterial drugs. The rifamycins were isolated from *Nocardia (Streptomyces) mediterranei* in 1957 at Lepetit Laboratories in Italy. Chemical modifications were made to one of the original isolates, rifamycin B, which showed antimycobacterial activity. However, most were metabolized and excreted rapidly. Rifampin avoids rapid degradation by entering the enterohepatic circulation. It was first synthesized in 1965 and became available for clinical use in 1968. The drug is called *rifampicin* in the United Kingdom, Europe, and Australia. Preparations and dosage forms are given in Table 53–3.

Rifampin

Rifampin has the chemical formula 3–4 (4 methyl-piperazinyl-imino-methylidine) rifamycin. It is a semisynthetic derivative of rifamycin B. Rifampin inhibits the B subunit of DNA-dependent RNA-polymerase of bacteria. The drug does not exert significant effect on the human enzyme. The action is bactericidal against growing microorganisms, but there is also some effect on resting cells.

> Rifampin is mycobactericidal and kills intracellular bacteria.

> The drug is highly lipid soluble and diffuses into most body compartments.

Rifampin is well absorbed after an oral dose. Peak serum concentrations reach 7–8 μg/ml after 600 mg is ingested. The drug is widely distributed throughout the body because of its high degree of lipid solubility. Penetration into the CSF of normal people is erratic, but CSF concentra-

Table 53–3 RIFAMPIN: PREPARATIONS AND DOSAGE FORMS		
Preparation	**Manufacturer**	**Dosage Forms**
Rimactane	CIBA	300 mg capsules
Rifadin	Merrell Dow	150 and 300 mg capsules
Rifadin IV	Merrell Dow	600 mg vials

tions approach 50% of simultaneous serum values in the presence of inflammation. The high degree of lipid solubility facilitates entry into polymorphonuclear leukocytes and macrophages, where a chemotherapeutic effect can be exerted.

Protein binding is 80%. The drug is metabolized (desacetylated) in the liver and excreted in the bile; it reenters the portal venous circulation and participates in an enterohepatic cycle. The functional mass of the liver and hepatic blood flow affect the transfer of drug into the bile. Dose modification is required for persons with severe hepatic dysfunction. Desacetylrifampin exerts antimicrobial activity, but less than the parent compound. Eventually 60% of an administered dose is excreted in the stool, 15% is glucuronidated, and the balance is cleared through the kidneys.

Rifampin enters the enterohepatic circulation.

The major toxicity is hepatic. Mild disturbances in liver enzymes are common but resolve without need for discontinuation of the drug. Bilirubin and alkaline phosphatase are most commonly affected. Alcoholics with preexisting liver disease are most prone to serious hepatotoxicity. Children may also be at increased risk. Combination INH/rifampin therapy is associated with a 40% risk of hepatocellular dysfunction, but this is usually not sufficiently severe to warrant discontinuation of drug therapy.

Rifampin's main toxicity is hepatic. In treating a patient for tuberculosis, other commonly used drugs have overlapping toxicity.

Hypersensitivity reactions are rare. But intermittent therapy is associated with a "cutaneous syndrome" of facial flushing, pruritus, and conjunctivitis; rash may or may not occur. Anorexia, nausea, vomiting and diarrhea, and pseudomembranous colitis have all been infrequently reported. *Clostridium difficile* that develops rifampin resistance during therapy has been identified as the responsible pathogen for the latter.

Hematological toxicities include thrombocytopenia, mediated through IgG and IgM antibodies among patients on intermittent therapy. Hemolysis and neutropenia rarely occur. Sudden oliguria or anuric renal failure can be seen. Acute tubular necrosis, interstitial nephritis, and cortical necrosis have all been observed on microscopic examination of kidney biopsy specimens. The time course of these effects on renal function is unpredictable.

A "flu syndrome" is reported with intermittent therapy. Symptoms and signs include fever, headache, malaise, arthralgias, and myalgias. The syndrome occurs 1–2 hours after a dose is taken; onset is delayed 3–6 months into therapy. Symptoms generally resolve spontaneously. This syndrome is particularly common among patients receiving high-dose (1200 mg) once-weekly therapy. A change in regimen to lower-dose or daily therapy, or both, aborts the syndrome, which appears to be immunologically mediated. A respiratory syndrome of dyspnea and wheezing has a similar etiological mechanism.

A unique adverse reaction is the "flu syndrome," believed to be most common among patients receiving the drug intermittently.

Although *in vitro* studies have suggested an immunosuppressive effect of rifampin on both T and B lymphocytes, clear-cut *in vivo* documentation is lacking. Finally, experiments in rats and mice have indicated fetal abnormalities. But no evidence of human fetal toxicity is known, and the drug has been administered safely to pregnant women.

Rifampin in combination with INH is considered the therapy of choice for treatment of tuberculosis. Rifampin should not be used as the sole therapeutic agent for treatment of any infectious disease because of the rapid emergence of resistance. Rifampin has been recommended for preventive therapy of the PPD convertor among patients who are intolerant of INH, but its efficacy in this circumstance is unproved.

Many physicians consider INH plus rifampin to represent optimal chemotherapy for pulmonary tuberculosis.

Rifampin is indicated for treatment of atypical mycobacterial infections if *in vitro* susceptibility is documented. Such therapy usually consists of four or more drugs. Rifampin is also used as adjunctive therapy to dapsone for treatment of leprosy.

Rifampin also has significant *in vitro* activity against aerobic gram-

Table 53–4 DRUG INTERACTIONS WITH RIFAMPIN AND THERAPEUTIC IMPLICATIONS

Drug	Rate of Metabolism	Therapeutic Impact
Tolbutamide	Increased	Adjust according to serum glucose
Oral contraceptives	Increased	Alternative contraceptive measures should be employed
Corticosteroids	Increased	Increase dose as required clinically
Cyclosporine	Increased	Increase dose according to blood levels
Warfarin	Increased	Adjust according to prothrombin time
Methadone	Increased	Increase dose to control narcotic withdrawal
Theophylline	Increased	Monitor blood levels
Digoxin/digitoxin	Increased	Monitor blood levels
Quinidine	Increased	Monitor blood levels
Propranolol	Increased	Monitor according to clinical response
Dapsone	Increased	Not clinically significant
Ketoconazole	Increased	Alter dosing schedule to administer each drug 12 hours after the other
Chloramphenicol	Increased	Monitor blood levels

Rifampin may be used to treat nonmycobacterial infections.

Rifampin may be used to prevent acquisition of H. influenzae and N. meningitidis.

Rifampin interacts with most drugs cleared by the liver.

positive cocci and certain aerobic gram-negative cocci and bacilli. In combination with other antistaphylococcal antibiotics, the drug has been used to treat staphylococcal infections in essentially all body sites. Its use for this indication remains controversial.

Rifampin has also been recommended as the drug of choice for prophylaxis against *Neisseria meningitidis* and *Haemophilus influenzae* in a dose of 600 mg twice a day for 2 days. It has been successfully employed to eradicate the carrier state with *Staphylococcus aureus* when combined with topical or additional oral antistaphylococcal agents.

Rifampin plus trimethoprim-sulfamethoxazole has been used to treat urinary tract infections caused by Enterobacteriaceae. Better agents are available, and this combination is no longer advocated. Rifampin has also been employed as single-dose therapy for gonococcal urethritis, with a success rate of 89%. Alternative agents consistently achieve better than 95% cure; therefore, rifampin should not be used for this indication.

Rifampin has been used in the treatment of chancroid, brucellosis, Q fever, leishmaniasis, fungal infections, meningoencophalitis caused by *Naegleria,* and a variety of other uncommon infectious diseases. Its true value as a therapeutic agent for treatment of these infections is undefined; *in vitro* data generally indicate susceptibility of the infecting organism.

Rifampin is contraindicated in patients with a previous history of hypersensitivity to any rifamycin. It interacts with a multitude of chemicals normally excreted or metabolized by the liver. It competes with bilirubin for excretion, causing elevated serum bilirubin concentrations, then induces glucuronidation of bilirubin, causing levels to return to normal. Rifampin also induces a proliferation of hepatic cell smooth endoplasmic reticulum and microsomal enzymes responsible for drug metabolism. The effects of increased enzyme activity are summarized in Table 53–4.

Ansamycin (LM 427) is a derivative of rifamycin S. It possesses excellent *in vitro* activity against *M. tuberculosis, M. avium-intracellurae* (MAI), and *M. fortuitum.* It is currently in clinical trials, particularly for treatment of MAI infection among AIDS patients. Other investigational compounds include rifamycin DL-473 and FCE 22250.

Streptomycin

The first drug possessing antimycobacterial activity to become available for clinical use was streptomycin; however, it is infrequently prescribed today because of its ototoxicity. It was isolated from *Streptomyces griseus* by Waksman and colleagues in 1943 (cited in Leitman, 1990). The drug is an aminoglycosidic aminocyclitol. Many salts can be prepared, but the sulfate salt is best tolerated on intramuscular injection.

Streptomycin remains a commonly used drug for treatment of pulmonary tuberculosis in combination with other antimycobacterials. It may be administered daily in early therapy and two or three times per week on an outpatient basis. (See Chapter 50 for more details about streptomycin.)

> Streptomycin is an aminoglycoside antimicrobial with good activity against mycobacteria.

A number of antimycobacterial agents are classified as second-line, because of either lack of activity or high rates of toxicity, or both. These drugs are most often employed for treatment of resistant strains of mycobacterial species. Each is briefly described.

Second-Line Antimycobacterial Agents

PARA-AMINOSALICYLIC ACID

Para-aminosalicylic acid (PAS) was discovered as part of a deliberate search for antimycobacterial agents. In 1941 Bernheim showed that salicylic acid increased oxygen consumption of tubercle bacilli, and in 1946 Lehmann discovered PAS. It is a synthetic derivative. PAS probably inhibits bacterial folic acid synthesis by falsely being incorporated (instead of para-aminobenzoic acid) during cell growth. Preparations and dosage forms are given in Table 53–5.

Para-aminosalicylic acid

PAS is well absorbed following oral ingestion; a serum peak of 7–8 μg/ml, following a 4-g dose, is reached in 1–2 hours. Up to one third of the drug is excreted unchanged in the urine. The balance is metabolized in the liver and excreted in the urine. The drug is distributed well to tissues and interstitial fluid but not the CNS. Serum protein binding is 60–70%.

> PAS is a folic acid antagonist.

Gastrointestinal intolerance is the most common side effect. Symptoms include nausea, vomiting, anorexia, abdominal cramps, and diarrhea, and many patients refuse to take the drug because of these. Hypersensitivity occurs in 5–10% of patients. Less common adverse reactions include neutropenia, agranulocytosis, renal failure, hypokalemia, and sodium retention.

> Use of PAS is most often limited by gastrointestinal intolerance.

PAS may be used for treatment of tuberculosis, particularly in children less than 2 years of age as a substitute for ethambutol. Because it is inexpensive, PAS is commonly used in underdeveloped countries for treatment of tuberculosis occurring in all ages.

PAS is contraindicated for patients who have shown previous hypersensitivity to the drug. Furthermore, hypersensitivity to INH and rifampin may be cross-induced by PAS when administered concurrently.

> In the United States, PAS may substitute for ethambutol in the treatment of children.

PYRAZINAMIDE

One of the older antimycobacterial drugs originally perceived as too toxic for routine use is pyrazinamide. Pyrazinamide was synthesized from nico-

---

Table 53–5 PARA-AMINOSALICYLIC ACID: PREPARATIONS AND DOSAGE FORMS

Preparation	Manufacturer	Dosage Forms
Aminosalicylic acid	Generic	Powder
Aminosalicylate sodium	Generic	500 mg and 1 g tablets Powder
Aminosalicylic resin	Generic	4 g resin pack

Table 53-6 PYRAZINAMIDE: PREPARATION AND DOSAGE FORM		
Preparation	Manufacturer	Dosage Form
Pyrazinamide	Lederle	500 mg tablets

Pyrazinamide is a derivative of nicotinamide and is highly active against *M. tuberculosis.*

Pyrazinamide

tinamide in 1952. It has assumed increased importance in the treatment of tuberculosis because it is highly active and has tolerable toxicity in short-course chemotherapy. Pyrazinamide, an analog of nicotinamide, is not water-soluble and exerts its greatest antimycobacterial effect in an acid medium. A preparation and its dosage form are given in Table 53–6.

Pyrazinamide is bactericidal, but its mechanism of action is unknown. Organisms must be actively growing for the drug to exert its effect.

Pyrazinamide distributes widely throughout the body, including the CNS when inflammation is present.

Pyrazinamide is well absorbed after an oral dose and reaches peak serum concentration in 2 hours. The recommended dose is 20–35 mg/kg/day in two equally divided doses. For adults, this is usually 750–1000 mg twice a day. Because of its lipid solubility it is widely distributed throughout the body, including the CNS in the presence of inflammation. It penetrates leukocyte membranes and is capable of killing intracellular organisms.

The serum half-life ranges from 10 to 16 hours. It is metabolized in the liver to hydrolyzed and hydroxylated products. The major metabolite is 5-hydroxyprazinoic acid which is eliminated by glomerular filtration. High concentrations of the drug are achieved in the liver, lung, and kidneys, but lesser concentrations are reached in other organs.

The most important adverse reactions are hepatotoxicity and hyperuricemia.

Pyrazinamide causes dose-related hepatotoxicity manifested by hepatocellular dysfunction. Baseline transaminase determinations and follow-up samples every 2–4 weeks are advised. Hepatocellular dysfunction is generally reversible upon withdrawal of the drug. The second major adverse effect is hyperuricemia that may lead to gout. Nongouty arthralgias also commonly occur. Shoulders, knees, and fingers are most often affected. The hyperuricemia is attributable to blocked tubular secretion of uric acid mediated by the metabolite pyrazinoic acid. Concurrent administration of rifampin may reduce the rate of both hyperuricemia and joint complaints. Finally, pyrazinamide has infrequently been associated with gastrointestinal intolerance and hypersensitivity reactions.

This drug is used only for treatment of mycobacterial infections. Pyrazinamide is commonly prescribed in combination with INH and rifampin until susceptibility study results become available. It also is a frequent component of the early phase (2 months) of short-course (6 months) chemotherapy for pulmonary tuberculosis.

Toxicity is tolerable when the drug is used for 2 months of therapy.

Pyrazinamide is contraindicated only in patients with a known hypersensitivity to the drug. The drug has a complex interaction with probenecid. Pretreatment with pyrazinamide prolongs the serum half-life of probenecid, which prolongs the latter drug's uricosuric effect and lessens the effect of pyrazinamide. These interactions may be modified by adjusting the dosing schedule.

ETHIONAMIDE

Ethionamide

Ethionamide is another second-line agent. It was synthesized from isonicotinic acid in France in 1956. Prothionamide is another derivative with similar activity against *M. tuberculosis.* The drug inhibits mycolic acid synthesis in a fashion analogous to INH and ethambutol. A preparation and its dosage form are given in Table 53–7.

Ethionamide inhibits mycobacterial mycolic acid synthesis.

Ethionamide is well absorbed after oral ingestion and distributes throughout the body (including the CNS) in the absence of inflammation.

Table 53-7	ETHIONAMIDE: PREPARATION AND DOSAGE FORM	
Preparation	**Manufacturer**	**Dosage Form**
Trecator SC	Wyeth-Ayerst	250 mg tablets

The drug is metabolized to sulfoxides, which retain antimycobacterial activity. Metabolites are excreted in the urine.

Gastrointestinal side effects are most common and include metallic taste, nausea, vomiting, anorexia, abdominal pain, and diarrhea. Hepatocellular dysfunction occurs infrequently. Neurotoxicity and altered mental status may occur. A wide variety of other adverse reactions have rarely been reported. The drug is teratogenic in animals.

> Gastrointestinal side effects may compromise patient compliance.

Ethionamide is indicated for treatment of tuberculosis caused by organisms resistant to more commonly employed agents. It also may be used for treatment of leprosy. There are no drug interactions of clinical significance.

> Ethionamide should be used to treat infections caused by organisms resistant to primary agents.

CYCLOSERINE

Cycloserine was isolated from cultures of *Streptomyces orchidaceus* by Harned and associates and *Streptomyces garyphalus* by Harris and co-workers in 1955. It was originally produced as a fermentation product but now is synthesized. The structure is D-4-amino-s-isoxizolidone. It is unrelated to aminoglycosides or polypeptides and shows no cross-resistance with them. Cycloserine interferes with cell wall synthesis, acting as a competitive antagonist of the enzymes that link D-alanine molecules in the bacterial cell wall. A preparation and its dosage form are given in Table 53-8.

Cycloserine

Cycloserine is administered orally. Serum concentrations reach a peak of 10 μg/ml following a dose of 250 mg. About 60–70% is excreted unchanged in the urine, and the remainder is metabolized. The drug is distributed well through all tissues and fluids including the CNS, even in the absence of inflammation. Neurotoxicity is the most common and serious adverse reaction. Headache, tumor, drowsiness, and convulsions may occur. Psychotic disturbances are also commonplace. Hypersensitivity reactions are rare.

> Cycloserine distributes to the CNS but also has serious nervous system toxicity.

Cycloserine is employed for treatment of tuberculosis caused by organisms resistant to the more commonly prescribed drugs and may also be useful in the treatment of MAI infections.

> Cycloserine should be used to treat infections caused by resistant mycobacteria.

Isoniazid and ethionamide should not be administered simultaneously because of additive CNS toxicity. Alcohol should not be ingested when taking cycloserine because of the drug's ability to reduce the seizure threshold. Renal dysfunction and previous history of seizures are relative contraindications to use of the drug.

VIOMYCIN

Viomycin is a rarely used polypeptide antimycobacterial with relatively low activity against *M. tuberculosis,* but it usually is active against strains

Table 53-8	CYCLOSERINE: PREPARATION AND DOSAGE FORM	
Preparation	**Manufacturer**	**Dosage Form**
Seromycin	Lilly	250 mg capsules

Table 53-9 CAPREOMYCIN: PREPARATION AND DOSAGE FORM

Preparation	Manufacturer	Dosage Form
Capastat Sulfate	Lilly	1 g/10 ml vials

Viomycin is sometimes useful for treatment of streptomycin-resistant mycobacteria.

	R	
capreomycin 1A	OH	$C_{25}H_{44}N_{14}O_8$
capreomycin 1B	H	$C_{25}H_{44}N_{14}O_7$

Capreomycin is a mixture of four components and is bactericidal.

Capreomycin should be avoided in patients with renal dysfunction.

resistant to streptomycin. It shows complete cross-resistance with capreomycin. It is administered intramuscularly and pharmacokinetics mimic those of streptomycin. Toxicity is analogous to capreomycin but occurs to a greater degree. The drug is available in 1-g and 5-g vials. It should not be used in combination with other ototoxic or nephrotoxic drugs.

CAPREOMYCIN

Capreomycin was isolated from *Streptomyces capreolus* in 1960 and it consists of four microbiologically active components. The drug is bactericidal by an unknown mechanism. A preparation and its dosage form are given in Table 53-9.

Capreomycin is well absorbed following intramuscular administration. Serum peaks of 30 μg/ml are reached 1-2 hours after administration of 1 g. Half the dose is excreted unchanged by the kidneys and the other half is assumed to be metabolized. Drug distribution has not been studied. Nephrotoxicity is the most common adverse reaction, with tubular damage the most common manifestation. Ototoxicity causing vertigo or hearing loss is uncommon. Other side effects are rare.

In combination with at least one other active agent, capreomycin is indicated for the treatment of drug-resistant tuberculosis. Capreomycin is contraindicated in patients hypersensitive to the drug and relatively contraindicated in patients with renal dysfunction. Neuromuscular blockade may be enhanced when capreomycin is administered simultaneously with other drugs exerting this reaction.

References

Alford RH: Antimycobacterial agents. *In* Mandell GL, Douglas RG Jr, Bennett JE (eds): Anti-Infective Therapy, 280. New York: John Wiley & Sons, 1985.

Antimycobacterial agents. *In* Drug Evaluations, 6th ed, 1531. Chicago: American Medical Association, 1986.

Girling DJ: Adverse effects of antituberculous drugs. Drugs 23:56, 1982.

Leitman PS: Aminoglycosides and spectromycin: Aminocyclitols. *In* Mandell GL, Douglas RG, Bennett JE (eds): Principles and Practice of Infectious Diseases, 3rd ed, 269. New York: Churchill Livingstone, 1989.

Rifampicin: A review. Drugs 1:353, 1971.

Sanders WE Jr: Rifampin. Ann Intern Med 85:82, 1976.

VanScoy RE, Wilkowski CJ: Antituberculous agenst. Mayo Clin Proc 58:233, 1983.

54

Miscellaneous Antimicrobial Drugs*

Thomas R. Beam, Jr.

There are several compounds that have been developed for clinical use but exert their only antibacterial effect in the urinary tract. These include methenamine, nitrofurantoin, and nalidixic acid. Derivatives of the latter, the fluoroquinolones, represent such a new and exciting therapeutic array, that they are addressed separately.

METHENAMINE

The potential value of methenamine was recognized in the late 1800s; it was introduced in 1895 by Nicolaier specifically for the treatment of urinary tract infections.

Chemistry and Mechanism

Methenamine has been combined with either mandelic acid or hippuric acid in an attempt to acidify the urine (Table 54-1). Acidification is necessary to convert mandelamine to formaldehyde, the active antibacterial agent. In order to have antibacterial effect, the following chemical reaction must take place in the urine:

$$N_4(CH_2)_6 + 6H_2O \rightarrow 4\,NH_4^+ + 6HCHO$$

At urine pH 6, only 6% of methenamine is converted to formaldehyde, whereas at urine pH 5, this conversion approximates 20%. Formaldehyde is equally active at acidic or basic pH but cannot be generated from methenamine under basic conditions. A second limitation to antimicrobial efficacy is time. At urine pH 5, it takes 3 hours to reach 90% of the final equilibrium of the formaldehyde generation. Therefore, current opinion is that addition of weak acids (mandelic, hippuric, ascorbic) or dietary supplements (cranberry juice) confers no benefit in generating additional formaldehyde from methenamine. The formaldehyde produced is bacteriostatic by denaturing bacterial proteins.

Absorption, Distribution, Metabolism, and Excretion

Once ingested, rapid absorption occurs from the gastrointestinal (GI) tract, and the peak serum concentration of 35.2 μg/ml is achieved 1 hour after a 1-g dose. The elimination half-life is 4.3 hours with about 85–90% of the

Urinary Tract Antiseptics

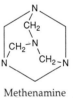

Methenamine

Formaldehyde is the antibacterial agent.

* The work was supported by the Veterans Administration.

Table 54–1 PREPARATIONS AND DOSAGES: METHENAMINE

Preparation	Manufacturer	Dosage Forms
Methenamine	Generic	500 mg tablets
Methenamine mandelate	Generic	500 mg/ml suspension 500 mg and 1 g tablets 250 mg, 500 mg, and 1 g enteric-coated tablets
Mendelamine	Parke-Davis	500 mg and 1 g granules 250 and 500 mg/5 ml suspension 500 mg and 1 g plain and enteric-coated tablets
Methenamine hippurate	Generic Merrill Dow	1 g tablets 1 g tablets

absorbed drug being recovered from the urine. Renal clearance approximates creatinine clearance, although there is some tubular secretion of drug as well.

Adverse Effects

Side effects are few.

Side effects are generally minor in nature. Some patients develop nausea, vomiting, or diarrhea. Formaldehyde may exert a local irritative effect, yielding urgency, frequency, dysuria, hematuria, and proteinuria. These symptoms mimic infection and, therefore, suggest drug failure. Microscopic evaluation of the urine should clarify the cause. Finally, skin rash is rarely observed.

Indications and Contraindications

Methenamine is indicated only for UTI.

Methenamine should be avoided in patients with gout or renal failure, or taking sulfa drugs.

The only indications for using methenamine are to treat acute urinary tract infections (UTI) or suppress recurrent ones. The drug's efficacy in this latter circumstance is debated.

Methenamine should not be prescribed for patients with gout, because it may cause precipitation of urate crystals. It is also contraindicated for patients who have renal failure or those who have shown previous hypersensitivity to it.

Methenamine should not be prescribed in combination with sulfa antimicrobials, because it chemically combines with the sulfa preparation resulting in mutual antagonism. The active breakdown product, formaldehyde, may cause a number of laboratory test abnormalities, such as increased catecholamines and vanillylmandelic acid (VMA), decreased estriol, increased 17-hydroxycorticosteroid, and decreased 5-hydroxyindoleacetic acid (5HIAA).

NITROFURANTOIN

Nitrofurantoin is a second urinary antiseptic. It became available for clinical use in 1953, and a macrocrystal formulation was developed in 1967 in an attempt to reduce GI side effects (Table 54–2).

Nitrofurantoin

Chemistry and Mechanism

Nitrofurantoin is 0-(5-nitrofurfurylideneamino)-hydantoin. It is a synthetic nitrofuran compound belonging to a class of organic chemicals characterized by a ring containing one oxygen and four carbon atoms. The drug

Table 54-2 PREPARATIONS AND DOSAGES: NITROFURANTOIN		
Preparation	**Manufacturer**	**Dosage Forms**
Nitrofurantoin macrocrystals	Generic	50 and 100 mg capsules
Furadantin	Norwich-Eaton	50 and 100 mg tablets 5 mg/ml oral suspension
Macrodantin capsules	Norwich-Eaton	25, 50, and 100 mg capsules

may inhibit bacterial enzymes or directly damage bacterial DNA, but the precise mechanism of action is unknown.

Absorption, Distribution, Metabolism, and Excretion

Following oral administration, absorption occurs from the small intestine and, in contrast to many antimicrobials, it is enhanced by food. Therapeutic serum concentrations are never achieved, and the drug is rapidly broken down in tissues and excreted in the urine. The serum half-life is only 20 minutes, and 90% of the absorbed drug is protein bound.

Once reaching the kidney, the drug is excreted in the urine in its active form. About one third of the amount absorbed actually reaches the urine, in which concentrations average 50–250 μg/ml. Acidification of urine increases renal parenchymal concentrations. Patients with compromised renal function do not obtain therapeutic urine concentrations of the drug.

Absorption is enhanced by food.

Adverse Effects

Anorexia, nausea, and vomiting are the most common side effects and are dose-related. The macrocrystalline form of the drug may reduce the incidence of these reactions by slowing absorption. Parotitis, a truly unique adverse effect, has been described. Hypersensitivity reactions, including skin rash, eosinophilia, and fever, are uncommon. A wide variety of central nervous system (CNS) toxicities have also been reported. Examples include headache, dizziness, depression, confusion, slurred speech, and blurred vision. Peripheral neuritis occurs at a rate of 7/10,000 and seems to be dose-related. This toxicity is reversible if the diagnosis is made early and the drug withdrawn.

Pulmonary toxicity should cause the greatest concern for physicians who prescribe the drug. It may be divided into acute, subacute, and chronic. The acute reaction is characterized by cough, fever, and dyspnea, sometimes with infiltrates on chest x-ray. This is probably a hypersensitivity reaction and usually is associated with eosinophilia. The subacute form of toxicity is associated with respiratory complaints such as shortness of breath or diminished exercise tolerance. Infiltrates are present on x-ray but reversible. These usually develop about 1 year after initiating therapy or prophylaxis. Chronic pulmonary reactions are characterized by irreversible interstitial fibrosis associated with bilateral pulmonary infiltrates on chest x-ray. Although clinical and radiographic manifestations may improve upon withdrawal of the drug, the fibrosis persists. Hepatotoxicity and blood dyscrasias are rare adverse effects.

Toxicities (GI, CNS, pulmonary) limit the usefulness of this drug.

Indications and Contraindications

The only indication for use of nitrofurantoin is treatment of UTI caused by susceptible organisms. This includes urethritis, prostatitis, cystitis, and pyelonephritis (in the absence of septicemia or bacteremia). The drug may

Nitrofurantoin is indicated only for treatment of UTIs.

also be used to suppress recurrent UTIs. However, the toxic potential of the drug must be carefully considered. Most physicians do not use the drug for chronic suppression of UTIs.

The drug is contraindicated for patients known to be hypersensitive to it and for patients with renal dysfunction. In the latter circumstance, therapeutically inadequate concentrations of drug are achieved in the urinary tract, whereas toxic amounts may accumulate in serum. Nitrofurantoin is also contraindicated in pregnant patients at term and for use in infants less than 1 month of age (because of hemolytic anemia attributed to immature erythrocyte enzyme systems).

The number and type of drug interactions are limited. Magnesium trisilicate reduces the rate and extent of absorption and should not be coadministered. Probenicid and sulfinpyrazone inhibit tubular secretion of the drug and may cause toxic accumulation; they also may decrease efficacy and should not be coadministered.

In sum, the two urinary antiseptics are well absorbed but reach therapeutic concentrations only in the urinary tract. They should never be prescribed for a septic patient. Chemical and physical properties limit the usefulness of methenamine. Toxicity is the major concern with nitrofurantoin.

NALIDIXIC ACID

Nalidixic acid is the original compound of this class.

Nalidixic acid

Nalidixic acid and its derivatives inhibit DNA supercoiling and produce bacterial cell death.

Nalidixic acid is a naphthyridine derivative described by Lesher and colleagues in 1962 at the Sterling-Winthrop Research Institute in the United States and introduced into clinical use in 1964 (Table 54–3). It is the progenitor of a class of drugs, the fluoroquinolones, which are discussed later in the chapter.

Chemistry and Mechanism

The 1,8-naphthyridine compounds are totally synthetic and unrelated to any other antimicrobial agents. Nalidixic acid is 1-ethyl-1, 4 dihydro-7 methyl-4-oxo-1, 8 naphthyridine-3 carboxylic acid. Two other early derivatives, oxolonic acid and cinoxacin, were marketed in the United States but rarely used because of GI intolerance.

Nalidixic acid and its derivatives bind to DNA and interfere with the A subunit of DNA gyrase, leading to impaired DNA replication and eventual bacterial cell lysis. DNA gyrase (topoisomerase II) catalyzes negative supercoiling of double-standard DNA. Quinolones block reactions that require breakage and reunion of DNA, including supercoiling, relaxation, catenation, and decatenation. RNA-mediated protein synthesis continues, causing cells to filament and ultimately die.

Absorption, Distribution, Metabolism, and Excretion

Nalidixic acid is almost completely absorbed from the GI tract. Two hours following a 1-g dose, serum peak concentrations reach 20–50 μg/ml.

Table 54–3 PREPARATIONS AND DOSAGES: NALIDIXIC ACID		
Preparation	**Manufacturer**	**Dosage Forms**
Nalidixic acid	Generic	250, 500, and 1000 mg tablets
Neg Gram Caplets	Winthrop Pharmaceuticals	250, 500, and 1000 mg caplets
Neg Gram Suspension	Winthrop Pharmaceuticals	250 mg/5 ml suspension
Cinobac Pulvules	Dista	250 and 500 mg capsules
Utibid	Warner/Chilcott	No longer available

Individual serum peak concentrations are reproducible, but person-to-person variability is substantial. Nalidixic acid is 93% protein bound and rapidly metabolized. About one third of the parent compound is converted to the active metabolite hydroxynalidixic acid. It does not accumulate in tissues other than the kidney. The drug is excreted in breast milk.

Nalidixic acid metabolites are also cleared by the kidney. About 15% is hydroxynalidixic acid; the remainder is inactive metabolites. The drug continues to be cleared in potentially therapeutic concentrations during mild to moderate renal failure.

In contrast to other urinary antiseptics, nalidixic acid continues to be cleared through the kidney in mild to moderate renal failure.

Adverse Effects

Side effects are generally mild in degree and few in number. The most common adverse reactions are GI, including nausea, vomiting, abdominal pain, and diarrhea. Occasionally, these are sufficiently severe to warrant discontinuation of therapy. An allergic rash, usually concurrent with eosinophilia, is infrequently seen; photosensitivity is more common. All patients who are prescribed this class of drugs should be warned to avoid excessive exposure to the sun or to use sunscreens. A hemolytic anemia may develop, most often in patients with glucose 6 phosphate dehydrogenase (G6PD) deficiency. Leukopenia and thrombocytopenia are extremely rare.

Patients should be warned about photosensitivity reactions.

CNS side effects include visual disturbances, excitement, depression, confusion, and hallucinations. Caution is advised when this drug is used to treat patients who have an underlying seizure disorder or psychiatric illness, because these conditions may worsen. Intracranial hypertension and pseudotumor cerebri are also rare complications.

CNS side effects can be sufficiently severe to warrant discontinuation of the drug.

No teratogenic effects have been reported in animals, and pregnant women have taken nalidixic acid without adverse effect on the fetus. However, there are no data about safety during the first trimester of pregnancy, and fluoroquinolones do not share this safety profile.

Indications and Contraindications

Nalidixic acid, like other urinary tract antiseptics, should only be used for the treatment of lower urinary tract infections caused by susceptible organisms. It may be employed as a prophylactic agent against recurrent lower urinary tract infections. The drug is contraindicated for persons known to be hypersensitive to it, or those who have a convulsive disorder. Nalidixic acid can displace warfarin-like anticoagulants from protein-binding sites resulting in increased warfarin activity. Nalidixic acid and nitrofurantoin interact and directly impede the antimicrobial activity of each other. They should never be coadministered.

Caution is advised for monitoring interaction with warfarin.

In the laboratory, nalidixic acid metabolites give a false-positive test for urine glucose if Benedict's solution or Clinitest tablets are employed. Clinistix and Tes-tape are not affected. Nalidixic acid also interferes with the determination of urinary keto- and ketogenic steroids in the M-dinitrobenzene reaction. The Porter-Silber method should be used instead.

Nalidixic acid can interfere with urine glucose test systems giving false-positive results.

Fluoroquinolones

The fluoroquinolones are currently the most actively investigated group of antimicrobial agents. The reasons are several:

1. broad spectrum of antimicrobial activity, including species other than bacteria;
2. good absorption following oral administration with serum concentrations approaching those achieved by intravenous (IV) infusion;
3. wide distribution through extravascular tissue sites;
4. long serum half-life, resulting in infrequent administration;

The fluoroquinolones offer significant advantages in pharmacokinetics, spectrum of activity, and reduced cost.

5. potential of substituting for parenteral therapy, resulting in avoidance of hospitalization or early discharge from hospital;
6. significant financial savings compared with parenteral therapy;
7. relatively low incidence of adverse reactions, most of which are minor in nature.

Three fluoroquinolone antimicrobials have been marketed in the United States. The first was norfloxacin, synthesized at the Kyorin Central Research Laboratory in Japan. The key change in molecular structure made by the chemists was the addition of a fluoride to the ring structure of nalidixic acid. The compound was developed by Merck in the United States.

The first quinolone to become available in the United States was norfloxacin.

NORFLOXACIN

Chemistry and Mechanism

Norfloxacin is 1-ethyl-6-fluoro-1,4-dihydro-4-oxo-7-(1-piperazinyl)-3-quinolone carboxylic acid. In contrast to nalidixic acid, it is water-soluble through the pH range 2.9–7.6. At physiological pH, norfloxacin is a zwitterion. Other biochemical changes include conversion of the naphthyridine ring to the quinolone ring (increased potency) and substitution of the piperazinyl ring for the methyl group at position 7 (antipseudomonal activity). Despite these changes, the mechanism of action is the same as nalidixic acid.

Biochemical manipulation of the nalidixic acid molecule increased its spectrum of activity and reduced its toxicity.

Norfloxacin

Absorption, Distribution, Metabolism, and Excretion

Norfloxacin is rapidly absorbed following oral administration. Serum peak concentrations average 1.3–1.6 μg/ml following a 400-mg dose, and there is a linear relationship between dose and serum peak up to 800 mg per dose. The serum half-life is 3–4 hours. Food both delays and inhibits absorption.

About 30% of norfloxacin is metabolized into six different compounds, which possess minimal antimicrobial activity. Metabolites are excreted through both urine and bile. Approximately 30% of the drug is excreted unchanged through the kidneys, where both filtration and active tubular secretion occur. The remainder of the drug is not absorbed but rather excreted unchanged in the stool. This provides colonic concentrations sufficient to kill many enteric pathogens.

Therapeutic concentrations of norfloxacin are achieved in the urogenital and GI tracts.

Protein binding is estimated at 5–15%, but tissue distribution is poor, with therapeutic concentrations only achieved in the urinary tract. However, urine concentrations remain high even in the presence of renal failure. Dose modification is required for patients who have a creatinine clearance less than 30 ml/minute.

Adverse Effects

In their brief history of widespread clinical use, fluoroquinolones have been well tolerated. Severe adverse reactions are extremely uncommon. Nausea (2.8%), headache (2.7%), and dizziness (1.8%) were the most common side effects reported during clinical trials of norfloxacin. Cartilage erosion has developed in juvenile animals given this agent, and tendonitis has been reported in a small number of patients.

The most important toxicity is cartilage erosion documented in animals. Norfloxacin should not be used in pregnant women or growing children.

Indications and Contraindications

Norfloxacin has proved to be of significant value in the treatment of uncomplicated and complicated infections of the urinary tract. Clinical trials

Table 54-4 PREPARATIONS AND DOSAGES: NORFLOXACIN		
Preparation	**Manufacturer**	**Dosage Forms**
Noroxin	Merck, Sharp and Dohme	400 mg tablets

also support its use in the treatment of prostatitis, gonococcal urethritis or cervicitis, traveler's diarrhea caused by susceptible strains of bacteria, and prophylaxis against infection in neutropenic patients.

The drug is contraindicated in pregnant patients, persons whose skeletal growth is incomplete, or those who have a history of hypersensitivity to nalidixic acid or quinolone antibiotics.

Concurrent administration of probenecid diminishes urinary excretion of norfloxacin. Coadministration of nitrofurantoin results in inactivation of the antimicrobial activity of both compounds. Antacids may delay or inhibit absorption of the drug and should be avoided (Table 54-4).

Antacids delay or inhibit absorption.

CIPROFLOXACIN

The second fluoroquinolone marketed in the United States is ciprofloxacin. This drug was developed at Bayer Pharmaceuticals in Germany. An oral preparation is currently marketed in the United States, and a parenteral preparation has just been approved for marketing by the Food and Drug Administration (FDA).

Chemistry and Mechanism

Ciprofloxacin is 1-cyclopropyl-6-fluoro-1,4-dihydro-4-oxo-7-(1-piperazinyl) 3-quinolone carboxylic acid hydrochloride (Table 54-5). Its mechanism of action is also inhibition of supercoiling of DNA.

Ciprofloxacin

Absorption, Distribution, Metabolism, and Excretion

About 70% of an oral dose of the drug is absorbed. Peak serum concentrations are achieved 1-2 hours later; these are 1.3-1.4 $\mu g/ml$ (250 mg), 2.6-2.9 $\mu g/ml$ (500 mg), and 3.4-4.2 $\mu g/ml$ (750 mg). Like norfloxacin, aluminum- and magnesium-containing antacids both delay and inhibit absorption.

Ciprofloxacin differs from nalidixic acid and norfloxacin because of its pharmacokinetic properties. The volume of distribution of ciprofloxacin far exceeds total body water. Therapeutic concentrations are achieved in most tissues, including the prostate, but penetration into the CNS is unpredictable. Of interest particularly for treatment of diseases such as Legionnaire's pneumonia, ciprofloxacin penetrates into both leukocytes and macrophages and can kill intraphagocytic organisms.

The drug is eliminated through multiple routes. Like norfloxacin, about 30% is not absorbed and excreted unchanged in the stool. An additional 30-45% of active drug can be recovered from the urine. Small amounts of drug are excreted through the bile. There are at least four

Table 54-5 PREPARATIONS AND DOSAGES: CIPROFLOXACIN		
Preparation	**Manufacturer**	**Dosage Forms**
Ciprofloxacin	Miles Pharmaceutical Division	250, 500, and 750 mg tablets

metabolites, each of which has some antimicrobial activity. There seems to be decreased metabolism and increased renal clearance of the parent compound following repeated dosages of drug. Administration of ciprofloxacin with food delays absorption but does not affect the total amount of drug absorbed.

Adverse Effects

Nausea, vomiting, diarrhea, and abdominal pain are the most common side effects noted with ciprofloxacin. Administration with food may reduce the intensity of these reactions but also will give a lower serum peak concentration. Like nalidixic acid, ciprofloxacin has certain CNS toxicities. These include headache, tremors, dizziness, restlessness, and confusion and are more common among the elderly. Ciprofloxacin is an inhibitor of γ aminobutyric acid and may increase the risk of seizures in seizure-prone individuals. Rash and photosensitivity have been infrequently reported. The drug has caused arthropathy and cartilage damage in young animals and some humans.

Indications and Contraindications

Because of its wide distribution throughout most of the body, ciprofloxacin is indicated for the treatment of respiratory tract, skin and skin structure, bone and joint, and UTIs caused by susceptible organisms. It is also indicated for the treatment of infectious diarrhea. In clinical trials the drug has proven useful for treatment of endophthalmitis, prophylaxis against infection in neutropenic patients, and treatment of gonorrhea.

Ciprofloxacin is contraindicated in patients who are pregnant or children under the age of 17 years. It is contraindicated also in patients who have a known hypersensitivity to quinolone antibiotics. Ciprofloxacin may increase serum concentrations of theophylline; either the drugs should not be administered concurrently or serum concentrations of theophylline should be carefully monitored. Drug interactions also occur with other therapeutic agents. Antacids containing magnesium/aluminum hydroxide should not be concurrently administered, because they block absorption. Probenicid sufficiently blocks tubular secretion so that it increases serum concentrations of ciprofloxacin and may result in a need for dose adjustment. Ciprofloxacin increases the stimulant properties of caffeine. Therefore, patients should be cautioned regarding intake of caffeinated beverages. Ciprofloxacin may also increase warfarin concentrations by displacing this drug from its albumin-binding sites. Prothrombin time should be carefully monitored in patients receiving both drugs.

New Developments

In addition to the IV formulation of ciprofloxacin, there are at least 25 other quinolones in development. Some have undergone evaluation in clinical trials and are under review at the FDA. Others are still early in clinical trials. Ofloxacin was approved in December 1990 for marketing in the United States by the FDA. Drugs that may soon become available to practicing physicians include pefloxacin and flexroxacin.

Ofloxacin

Pefloxacin

Enoxacin

Erythromycin

Erythromycin belongs to a class of drugs known as macrolides. In 1952, erythromycin was derived from *Streptomyces erythreus* found in a soil sample in the Philippines by McGuire and associates (Table 54–6).

Table 54–6 PREPARATIONS AND DOSAGES: ERYTHROMYCIN

Product	Manufacturer	Dosages
Erythromycin		
Generic	—	250 and 500 mg powder, tablets
Base Filmtab	Abbott	250 and 500 mg tablets
E-Mycin	Upjohn	250 and 333 mg tablets
ERYC	Parke Davis	250 mg capsules
Ery-Tab	Abbott	250, 333, and 500 mg tablets
Ilotycin	Dista	250 mg tablets
Robimycin	Robins	250 mg tablets
RP Mycin	Reid-Provident	250 mg tablets
Erythromycin estolate		
Generic	—	250 mg tablets
Ilosone	Dista	125 and 250 mg/5 ml suspension
		125 and 250 mg tablets
		125 and 250 mg chewable tablets
		100 mg/ml drops
		125 and 250 mg/5 ml suspension
		500 mg tablets
Erythromycin ethylsuccinate		
Generic	—	200 mg/5 ml powder for suspension
		200 mg and 400 mg/5 ml suspension
		400 mg tablets
EES	Abbott	100 mg/2.5 ml powder for suspension
		200 mg/5 ml granules for suspension
		200 and 400 mg/5 ml suspension
		200 mg chewable tablets
		400 mg tablets
E-Mycin E	Upjohn	200 and 400 mg/5 ml suspension
Wyapamycin E	Whett	200 and 400 mg/5 ml suspension
Ery Ped	Abbott	400 mg/5 ml powder for suspension
Pediamycin	Ross	100 mg/2.5 ml powder for suspension
		200 mg/5 ml granules for suspension
		200 and 400 mg/5 ml suspension
Erythromycin stearate		
Generic	—	250 and 500 mg tablets
Ery Par	Parke Davis	250 and 500 mg tablets
Erythrocin Stearate	Abbott	250 and 500 mg tablets
Ethril	Squibb	250 and 500 mg tablets
SK-Erythromycin	SK + F	250 and 500 mg tablets
Wyamycin S	Whett	250 and 500 mg tablets
Pfizer-E	Pfipharmes	250 mg tablets
Erythromycin gluceptate		
Ilotycin gluceptate	Dista	200, 500, and 1000 mg powder
Erythromycin lactobionate		
Generic	—	500 and 1000 mg powder
Erythrocin lactobionate IV	Abbott	500 and 1000 mg powder

Chemistry and Mechanism

Erythromycin base is a bitter-tasting crystalline substance that is poorly water-soluble. It is a weak base (with a pK of 8.8), and susceptible to inactivation by acid. *In vitro* activity of the drug progressively increases from pH 5.5 to 8.5. It is a stable compound in isotonic saline and 5% dextrose in water, with preservation of activity for 21 days at 25°C.

Because of its vulnerability to acid inactivation, two mechanisms have been employed to avoid acid degradation in the stomach. The first is to apply an enteric coating; unfortunately, this also tends to diminish absorption. The second is to alter the chemical structure specifically to lessen acid inactivation. This has been accomplished by formation of a salt (stearate), ester (ethyl succinate or propionate), or lauryl sulfate salt of an ester (estolate). Chemical formulas are shown in Figure 54–1.

Erythromycin is a weak base and is vulnerable to acid degradation in the stomach.

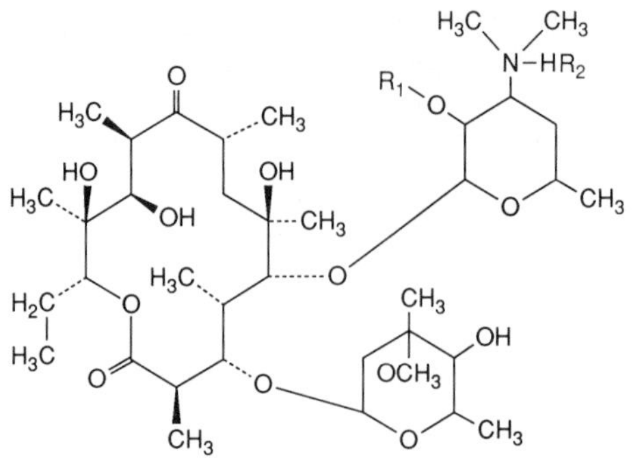

Figure 54-1

Erythromycin. *(Top)* The basic chemical structure. *(Bottom)* Structural formulas of erythromycin and some of its derivatives.

	R₁	R₂
Erythromycin base	H	
Erythromycin stearate	H	$C_{17}H_{35}COO$
Erythromycin estolate	CH_2CH_2CO	$C_{12}H_{25}OSO_3$
Erythromycin ethylsuccinate	$CH_2CH_2OOCCH_2$	CH_2COO

Erythromycin may exert a bacteriostatic or bactericidal effect.

The spectrum of activity includes nonbacterial pathogens such as mycoplasma, chlamydia, and mycobacteria.

None of the available oral formulations differs significantly in pharmacokinetic properties from the others.

Erythromycin is a bacteriostatic antibiotic against most susceptible strains. It binds to the 50S subunit of 70S ribosomes, resulting in inhibition of protein synthesis. Erythromycin antagonizes chloramphenicol action by binding to the 50S subunit. But erythromycin differs by inhibiting a translocation reaction, whereas chloramphenicol inhibits a peptidyl transferase reaction.

Erythromycin has a broad spectrum of activity against gram-positive and gram-negative aerobic and anaerobic bacteria, plus mycobacteria *Mycoplasma* species, and chlamydia. It may be bacteriostatic or bactericidal, depending on the concentration achieved at tissue sites of infection. It possesses bactericidal activity against Enterobacteriaceae and Pseudomonadaceae in stringently alkaline conditions that can only be achieved by systemic alkalization.

Absorption, Distribution, Metabolism, and Excretion

Erythromycin base or stearate is absorbed from the upper small intestine. Food reduces absorption of these preparations. Peak serum concentrations are reached approximately 4 hours after ingestion of enteric-coated tablets and range from 0.3–0.5 μg/ml for a 250-mg tablet to 0.3–2.0 μg/ml for a 500-mg tablet.

The estolate is less susceptible to acid degradation, and absorption is minimally inhibited by food. Peak serum concentrations are reached in 2 hours and are approximately 1.5 μg/ml following a 250-mg dose and 4.0 μg/ml following a 500-mg dose. However, the estolate must be hydrolyzed to the base, and only the base interacts with bacterial ribosomes. Actual concentrations of base are similar to those achieved by giving the base preparation of drug, as noted earlier.

Erythromycin ethylsuccinate is less acid-vulnerable, and absorption is less inhibited by food. However, serum concentrations also approximate those of the base. Thus, none of the preparations has unique pharmacokinetic advantage.

Erythromycin gluceptate and lactobionate are IV formulations of the drug. Peak serum concentrations average 8 μg/ml 1 hour following a 500-mg dose and 12 μg/ml 1 hour following a 1-g dose.

Protein binding of different erythromycin formulations varies from 40 to 90%. The drug persists in tissues longer than blood, therefore allowing some accumulation over time. Erythromycin distributes throughout the total body water. It achieves therapeutic concentrations for susceptible organisms in most body sites, including aqueous humor, ascitic fluid, bile, middle ear fluid, pleural fluid, prostatic fluid, sinus fluid, and tonsils—all in the presence of inflammation.

Limited data are available about penetration into the CNS, and they are insufficient to warrant recommending the drug for treatment of CNS infections except when there is no alternative. Erythromycin is transferred across the placenta, and the drug is excreted in breast milk.

Erythromycin also penetrates through host and bacterial cell membranes. Therefore, it has proved useful in the treatment of intraphagocytic infections such as *Legionella* and infections caused by organisms lacking a true cell wall, such as chlamydia and mycoplasma. Four mechanisms may contribute to intracellular concentration of erythromycin:

1. engulfment of surrounding fluid by phagocytic vacuoles;
2. pH gradients;
3. lipid solubility;
4. active transport using an energy-dependent process.

Only lipid solubility seems not to play a role in erythromycin's intraphagocytic concentration.

About 5% of an oral dose and 15% of a parenteral dose of erythromycin are recoverable in the urine. Erythromycin is concentrated in the liver and excreted into the bile, but only a small portion reaches the intestine. Most drug is found unchanged in the stool, presumably reflecting nonabsorption. The remainder is probably inactivated by demethylation in the liver. The serum half-life is approximately 1.4 hours. Dose adjustment is not required in renal failure. The drug is not removed by peritoneal dialysis or hemodialysis.

Erythromycin is poorly absorbed but distributes widely in body fluids.

Erythromycin penetrates human cell membranes and can kill intraphagocytic organisms.

Adverse Effects

The most common adverse effect associated with oral administration of erythromycin is GI distress. This may include epigastric pain or discomfort, nausea, vomiting, and diarrhea. The effect is often dose related. Relief may sometimes be obtained by switching from one preparation to another, or by administering the drug with food. However, it should be remembered that food inhibits the absorption of certain preparations.

Hypersensitivity reactions are unusual. Type I allergic manifestations are rare. The most serious side effect is cholestatic hepatitis, which is most commonly associated with the estolate preparation. All cases reported have occurred in patients older than 12 years. The reaction characteristically begins 10 or more days after initiation of therapy and progresses rapidly. Rare adverse effects include sensorineural hearing loss and pseudomembranous colitis. Safety in pregnancy has not been established; the estolate ester should probably be avoided in the pregnant woman.

The major adverse reaction associated with IV delivery is pain at the infusion site associated with phlebitis. Slow infusion rate, dilute solutions, and use of a large-caliber vein such as the subclavian may minimize this side effect.

Erythromycin is sometimes toxic to the GI tract. This may compromise patient compliance with therapy.

Erythromycin is phlebitogenic. Patients learn to fear administration of the drug.

Indications and Contraindications

Erythromycin is the drug of choice for treatment, prophylaxis, or reduction of risk of dissemination of pathogens by eliminating the carrier state of

Erythromycin may be used to prevent, treat, or avoid dissemination of a wide spectrum of pathogens.

several infectious diseases. It is considered optimal therapy for *Mycoplasma pneumoniae* respiratory tract infections, *Legionella pneumophila* pneumonia, *Chlamydia trachomatis* pneumonia or conjunctivitis, chlamydia pelvic infection during pregnancy (even though safety is not fully established), and *Campylobacter jejuni* gastroenteritis. It has been used in combination with neomycin as oral prophylaxis for elective colorectal surgery, oral prophylaxis against dissemination of pertussis, and topical prophylaxis to prevent neonatal ophthalmia caused by chlamydia. It is also used to eradicate the carrier state of *Corynebacterium diphtheriae.* Most infectious disease specialists consider it the drug of choice for these conditions.

Erythromycin is the most commonly prescribed alternative for penicillin-allergic patients.

Erythromycin is an important alternative, particularly in the penicillin-allergic patient, for treatment of Group A, B, C, or G streptococcal infection, pneumococcal infections, and disseminated gonococcal disease. Nongonococcal urethritis, usually treated with tetracycline, may be treated successfully with erythromycin as an alternative. Erythromycin is also recommended as an alternative therapy for early and late syphilis, although its efficacy is unproven. It is recommended for treatment of syphilis in pregnancy for the penicillin-allergic patient. Erythromycin has been employed in the treatment of anaerobic bronchopulmonary infections with success, Q fever pneumonitis among patients unable to tolerate tetracycline, and pneumonitis caused by *Nocardia* or *Actinomyces israelii.* Acne vulgaris may be treated with oral or topical erythromycin. Lymphogranuloma venereum, granuloma inguinale, and chancroid may be treated with this drug also.

As a prophylactic agent, erythromycin represents a valuable alternative to penicillin for the prevention of rheumatic fever. It may also be used for prophylaxis against bacteremia among patients undergoing dental procedures who are at risk for endocarditis. Erythromycin is only contraindicated in patients with a known hypersensitivity to the drug.

Drug Interactions

Caution must be used when administering other drugs simultaneously with erythromycin IV.

IV erythromycin is incompatible with a variety of other medications that might be administered through the same infusion. These include vitamins B and C; antibiotics: cephalothin, tetracycline, chloramphenicol, and colistin; and other drugs: heparin, metaminol, and diphenylhydantoin. Simultaneous administration of oral erythromycin and theophylline results in elevated theophylline concentrations and potential toxicity. A similar phenomenon has been observed with cyclosporine, carbamazepine, warfarin, and methylprednisolone. All are assumed to be due to erythromycin-induced inhibition of hepatic metabolism of these drugs.

New Developments

Clarithromycin (Abbott 56268 or 6-0 methylerythromycin) and azithromycin (Pfizer) are under active investigation in the United States. They are administered less frequently than other erythromycin formulations because of a longer serum half-life. Spiramycin, josamycin, and rosaramicin are older investigational agents that are being extensively studied but may or may not be pursued for marketing. Their spectrum of activity is similar to that of erythromycin; rosaramicin seems most active by weight.

Spectinomycin

Spectinomycin is an aminocyclitol antibiotic that was originally called actinospecticin. It was isolated in 1960 from *Streptomyces spectabilis* during the fermentation of beer. Spectinomycin contains neither an amino sugar

Table 54–7 PREPARATIONS AND DOSAGES: SPECTINOMYCIN		
Compound	**Manufacturer**	**Dosages**
Trobicin	Upjohn	2 and 4 g of powder with 3.2 and 6.4 ml of diluent (400 mg/ml)

Spectinomycin

nor a glycosidic bond. Therefore, it is not an aminoglycosidic aminocyclitol (such as gentamicin) (Table 54–7).

Spectinomycin binds to the bacterial 30S ribosomal subunit to inhibit protein synthesis. However, there is no misreading of the genetic code, and the effect actually may be an alteration in membrane permeability. Spectinomycin exerts an inhibitory effect for most susceptible strains but is bactericidal against *Neisseria gonorrhoeae*.

Spectinomycin is poorly absorbed by the oral route. It is available as a hydrochloride salt and administered intramuscularly (IM). Although an IV preparation was developed, it has not been marketed. Following IM administration of a 2-g dose, the serum peak of 100 μg/ml is achieved 1 hour later. There is little tendency for accumulation following repeated dosages over time. Approximately 75% of the dose is excreted unchanged in the urine. Tissue distribution has not been studied except in uterus and fallopian tube; concentrations averaged 25–33% of simultaneous serum values and were subinhibitory for most pathogens. The serum half-life is 1 hour, and protein binding is minimal. No metabolites of the drug have been identified.

Spectinomycin has neither ototoxicity nor nephrotoxicity. It is well tolerated at dosages up to 2 g given at a single IM site, even with repeated administration up to 21 days. Rarely reported side effects include chills, fever, dizziness, nausea and vomiting, and urticaria. Single-dose therapy accounts for the excellent safety profile, in part. Repeated dose therapy has been associated with minor abnormalities in hemoglobin, alkaline phosphatase, serum glutamic-oxaloacetic transaminase (SGOT), blood urea nitrogen (BUN), and creatinine clearance.

Spectinomycin is an alternative therapy for urogenital or disseminated gonorrhea, and is especially useful for penicillin-allergic patients or in areas where penicillinase-producing *N. gonorrhoeae* are prevalent. It is not indicated for treatment of pharyngeal gonorrhea or anorectal gonorrhea in men. It may be safely administered to pregnant women who are allergic to penicillin. It has been replaced by ceftriaxone, however, at most centers providing treatment for gonococcal infections.

Because *Chlamydia trachomatis* or *Mycoplasma urealyticum* may coexist with gonococcal infection, spectinomycin has been evaluated *in vitro* and *in vivo* against these pathogens. It is not reliably effective, and supplemental tetracycline therapy should be prescribed if these pathogens are suspected or proven to be present. Spectinomycin has no useful activity against *Treponema pallidum*.

Spectinomycin is contraindicated in patients with a known hypersensitivity to the drug. There are no known drug interactions of concern.

Lincomycin and clindamycin are lincosamide antimicrobials. Lincomycin was isolated as a product of *Streptomyces lincolnesis* in 1962 from soil samples screened near Lincoln, Nebraska. Clindamycin is a semisynthetic derivative of lincomycin. Lincosamides consist of an amino acid linked to an amino sugar (Fig. 54–2). Chemically, clindamycin is 7-chloro-7-deoxy-

Spectinomycin is bactericidal against gonococci.

Spectinomycin is only administered intramuscularly.

The drug is well tolerated.

The main use of spectinomycin is to treat gonococcal infections resistant to penicillin.

Spectinomycin therapy should be supplemented with tetracycline to treat *Chlamydia trachomatis* or *Mycoplasma urealyticum*.

Lincomycin and Clindamycin

Figure 54-2

The lincosamide antibiotics: lincomycin, R = OH; clindamycin, R = Cl. (From Steigbigel NH: Erythromycin, lincomycin, and clindamycin. *In* Mandell GL, Douglas RG, Bennett JE: Principles and Practice of Infectious Diseases. 3rd ed, 312. Churchill Livingstone, New York, 1990.)

trans-L-4-n-propyl hygrinic acid

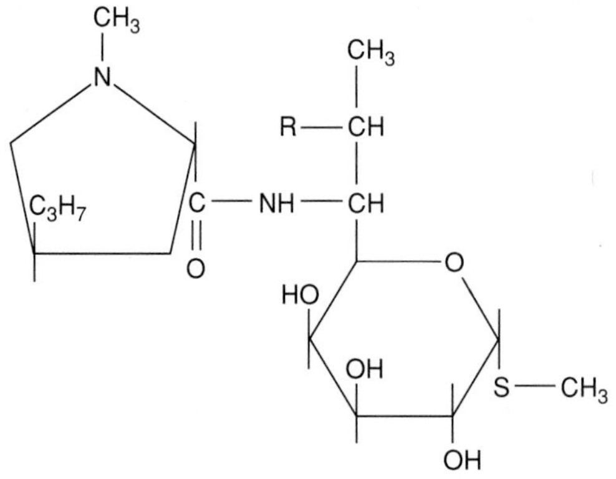

methyl-α-thiol lincosaminide

Figure 54-2

The lincosamide antibiotics: lincomycin, R = OH; clindamycin, R = Cl. (From Steigbigel NH: Erythromycin, lincomycin, and clindamycin. *In* Mandell GL, Douglas RG, Bennett JE: Principles and Practice of Infectious Diseases. 3rd ed, 312. Churchill Livingstone, New York, 1990.)

lincomycin. Both drugs are weak bases and water-soluble as salts (Table 54-8).

Both lincomycin and clindamycin inhibit bacterial protein synthesis by binding to the 50S ribosomal subunit. They compete with erythromycin and chloramphenicol for the same binding site, but in an overlapping rather than matching fashion. Both lincomycin and clindamycin may be bacteriostatic or bactericidal, depending on concentration, relative susceptibility of the organism, and inoculum size.

Clindamycin and lincomycin may be bacteriostatic or bactericidal.

Clindamycin has better absorption following an oral dose and has a broader spectrum of activity than lincomycin. Lincomycin is infrequently prescribed. Therefore, the pharmacokinetics of clindamycin are emphasized.

Lincomycin is rarely prescribed because it is poorly absorbed following an oral dose and has a narrower spectrum of activity than clindamycin.

Up to 90% of an oral dose of clindamycin hydrochloric acid (HCl) is absorbed. Peak serum concentrations measured 45-60 minutes after administration average 2.5 and 3.6 μg/ml following ingestion of 150 and 300 mg, respectively. Food does not significantly affect the rate or amount of drug absorbed. The palmitate salt yields lower serum peaks.

Clindamycin phosphate may be administered IM or IV. Peak concentrations are reached 3 hours after an IM dose. Peak concentrations following IV administration increase linearly but not in proportion to the increase in dose.

Clindamycin is 90% protein bound. However, it diffuses well into most tissues and body fluids except the CNS. It readily crosses the placenta. Like erythromycin, it concentrates in polymorphonuclear leukocytes and macrophages. The mechanism of penetration is believed to be active transport into the cell. Therefore, clindamycin is particularly useful in treatment of abscesses.

Clindamycin penetrates cell membranes and is particularly useful for treating the anaerobic component of abscesses.

The drug is metabolized in the liver; metabolites are excreted in both

Table 54-8   PREPARATIONS AND DOSAGES: CLINDAMYCIN AND LINCOMYCIN

Formulation	Manufacturer	Dosages
Clindamycin HCl	Upjohn	75 and 150 mg capsules
Clindamycin palmitate	Upjohn	75 mg/5 ml granules for suspension
Clindamycin phosphate	Generic	150 mg/ml in 2, 4, and 6 ml vials
	Upjohn	150 mg/ml in 2, 4, and 6 ml containers
Lincocin	Upjohn	250 and 500 mg capsules
	Upjohn	300 mg/ml in 2 and 10 ml containers
Cleocin T Topical Solution	Upjohn	10 mg/ml in 30 and 60 ml bottles

urine and bile. Approximately 10% is excreted unchanged through the urine. Clindamycin metabolites (active and inactive) continue to be excreted through the stool at least 5 days after administration is stopped. Its antimicrobial effect on GI flora may persist for 2 or more weeks.

The serum half-life of clindamycin ranges from 2.4 to 3.0 hours in healthy volunteers. The standard dosing may be reduced by 50% in patients with end-stage renal disease. Dosing should be reduced in patients with liver disease, but dose modification is unstandardized. Neither hemodialysis nor peritoneal dialysis removes clindamycin.

Diarrhea is the most common adverse reaction observed following therapy with clindamycin or lincomycin; the estimated incidence is 8%. A unique form of diarrhea was described in the mid-1970s and associated with clindamycin use. However, it now has been reported with essentially all antimicrobials and is most commonly seen in association with ampicillin, clindamycin, and cephalosporin use, in that order of frequency. This adverse reaction is antibiotic-associated pseudomembranous colitis (AAPMC).

Patients most vulnerable are hospitalized, elderly, chronically debilitated, and recipients of previous antibiotic therapy. The disease is caused by a toxin produced by *Clostridium difficile,* an anaerobic bacterium normally found in the GI tract. The disease usually occurs between days 4 and 9 of treatment with an antibiotic, but may occur as late as 2–6 weeks after the provocative agent has been discontinued. Patients often present with watery diarrhea, crampy abdominal pain, fever, and leukocytosis. In its worst form the clinical manifestations mimic an acute abdominal event, and surgery may be contemplated. Surgery should be avoided, because if performed, patient death often ensues.

The diagnosis of AAPMC is most often made by performance of a toxin assay on a stool sample. The organism may also be cultured, but its presence on culture does not confirm the diagnosis. Another diagnostic modality is sigmoidoscopy and visual or histopathological confirmation of the presence of pseudomembranes. Treatment depends on severity of illness and ranges from discontinuation of the provocative antibiotic, to cholestyramine, to oral antimicrobial therapy with vancomycin, metronidazole or bacitracin, or a combination of these therapies.

AAPMC may also occur in epidemic form among vulnerable individuals, such as nursing home residents or hospitalized patients. In this circumstance health care professionals are believed to acquire the organism in their provision of care and transmit it to other high-risk patients through hand carriage. Proper hand-washing is the best way to avoid such outbreaks.

Other adverse reactions associated with clindamycin and lincomycin include nausea and vomiting, cutaneous hypersensitivity manifested by a morbilliform rash, transient abnormalities in blood counts (leukopenia, eosinophilia, thrombocytopenia), and minor elevations of hepatic enzymes. Rapid infusion has been reported to rarely cause cardiovascular collapse; a medicinal taste is observed as a less serious manifestation of rapid infusion. The drug is well tolerated by IM injection.

Therapeutic Uses

Clindamycin is often the drug of choice for infections caused by anaerobic bacteria, particularly *Bacteroides* species, or mixed aerobic/anaerobic infection in combination with other antimicrobials. Clindamycin is usually considered an alternative for treatment of infections caused by susceptible strains of aerobic gram-positive cocci, such as pneumococci or staphylococci, but not enterococci.

Clindamycin exhibits delayed clearance from the GI tract. This may explain the occurrence of diarrhea after the drug is stopped.

Pseudomembranous colitis is not unique to clindamycin. It may occur subsequent to use of any antimicrobial or sometimes without any antimicrobial therapy.

Treatment of pseudomembranous colitis depends on the severity of illness provoked by the responsible toxin.

Clindamycin is effective against many aerobic and anaerobic gram-positive cocci, and anaerobic gram-positive bacilli.

Clindamycin is a therapeutic alternative (for susceptible pathogens) to penicillin for penicillin-allergic patients.

Examples of infections caused by anaerobic bacteria include intra-abdominal abscess associated with a ruptured bowel wall (appendicitis, diverticulitis, trauma, intraoperative spillage of colon content) and gynecological infections (postoperative myometritis, tubo-ovarian abscess). A third example is infection or sepsis associated with pressure sores.

Clindamycin represents a therapeutic alternative to penicillin treatment of anaerobic infections above the diaphragm. Periodontal infections, including actinomycosis, pharyngeal infections such as peritonsillar abscess, aspiration pneumonitis, lung abscess, and empyema all may be effectively treated with clindamycin.

Clindamycin is also alternative therapy for certain staphylococcal infections, such as skin and soft-tissue infections, septic arthritis, and osteomyelitis. The pharmacokinetic properties of the drug plus its availability as an oral agent make it a common choice for staphylococcal osteomyelitis. However, because it is not reliably bactericidal against *Staphylococcus aureus*, it should not be used for life-threatening infections such as infective endocarditis. Clindamycin is also a useful alternative for treatment of staphylococcal or streptococcal pyoderma, streptococcal pharyngitis, and pneumococcal infections of the upper and lower respiratory tract. Clindamycin has no clinically useful activity against enterococci.

Clindamycin in combination with an aminoglycoside may be used for prophylaxis against wound infection in colon surgery. Topical clindamycin is a valuable therapeutic agent for treatment of acne.

Contraindications

Clindamycin is contraindicated in patients with a known hypersensitivity to clindamycin or lincomycin.

Both clindamycin and lincomycin possess slight activity that may provoke neuromuscular blockade. More importantly, either may enhance the activity of a drug that causes neuromuscular blockade. Clindamycin is incompatible in IV solutions with ampicillin, aminophylline, barbiturates, calcium gluconate, magnesium sulfate, and phenytoin. Clindamycin may be combined and infused simultaneously with aminoglycosides, assuming the dosing schedule of the aminoglycoside is appropriately matched.

General References

Arcieri G, Griffith E, Gruenwaldt CT, et al: A survey of clinical experience with ciprofloxacin, a new quinolone antimicrobial. J Clin Pharmacol 28:179, 1988.

Chu DT, Fernandes PB: Structure-activity relationships of the fluoroquinolones. Antimicrob Agents Chemother 33:136, 1989.

D'Aray PF: Nitrofurantoin. Drug Intell Clin Pharmacol 19:540, 1985.

Derrick CW Jr, Reilly KM: Erythromycin, lincomycin and clindamycin. Pediatr Clin North Am 30:63, 1983.

Dhawan VK, Thadepalli H: Clindamycin: A review of fifteen years of experience. Rev Infect Dis 4:1133, 1982.

Fernandes PB: Mode of action and *in vitro* and *in vivo* activities of the fluoroquinolones. J Clin Pharmacol 28:156, 1988.

Holloway WJ: Spectinomycin. Med Clin North Am 66:169, 1982.

Hooper DG, Wolfson JS: The fluoroquinolones: Pharmacology, clinical uses and toxicities in humans. Antimicrob Agents Chemother 28:716, 1985.

LeFrock JL, Molavi, A, Prince RA: Clindamycin. Med Clin North Am 66:103, 1982.

Mayrer AR, Andriole VT: Urinary tract antiseptics. Med Clin North Am 66:199, 1982.

McCormick WM, Finland M: Spectinomycin. Ann Intern Med 84:712, 1976.

Moellering RC Jr (ed): Norfloxacin: A fluoroquinolone carboxylic acid antimicrobial agent. Am J Med 82(6B):1, 1987.

Nelson JD (ed): Evolving role of erythromycin in medicine. Proceedings of a symposium. Pediatr Infect Dis J 5:118, 1986.

Neu HC, Percival A, Lode H: Ciprofloxacin: A major advance in quinolone chemotherapy. Am J Med 82(4A):1, 1987.

Nix DE, Schentag JJ: The quinolones: An overview and comparative appraisal of their pharmacokinetics and pharmacodynamics. J Clin Pharmacol 28:169, 1988.

Phillips I: Past and current use of clindamycin and lincomycin. J Antimicrob Chemother 7(Suppl A):11, 1981.

Ronald AR, Turck M, Petersdorf RG: A critical evaluation of nalidixic acid in urinary tract infections. N Engl J Med 275:1081, 1966.

Rowen RC, Michel DJ, Thompson JC: Norfloxacin: Pharmacology and clinical use. Pharmacotheray 7:92, 1987.

Rubenstein E, Adam D, Moellering RC Jr, Woldvogel F: International symposium in new quinolones. Rev Infect Dis 10(Suppl 1):1, 1988.

Stein GE: The 4-quinolone antibiotics: Past, present and future. Pharmacotherapy 8:301, 1988.

Tedesco FJ: Pseudomembranous colitis. Pathogenesis and therapy. Med Clin North Am 66:655, 1982.

Washington JA, Wilson WR: Erythromycin: A microbial and clinical perspective after 30 years of clinical use. Mayo Clin Proc 60:189, 271, 1985.

Wolfson JS, Hooper DC: Norfloxacin: A new targeted fluoroquinolone antimicrobial agent. Ann Intern Med 108:238, 1988.

55

Antifungal Agents

Thomas R. Beam, Jr.

Polyene Antifungal Agents

Amphotericin is a polyene antifungal that is poorly water-soluble.

AMPHOTERICIN B

There are a limited number of antifungal agents available for treatment of fungal diseases. The foremost is amphotericin B, a drug produced by *Streptomyces nodosus*, an organism first isolated in the Orinoco River Valley of Venezuela.

Amphotericin B is a polyene antifungal agent characterized by a macrocyclic lactone ring and a series of conjugated double bonds, a free carboxyl, and a glycosidic side chain (Fig. 55–1). Amphotericin is amphoteric,

Figure 55–1

Structure of amphotericin B.

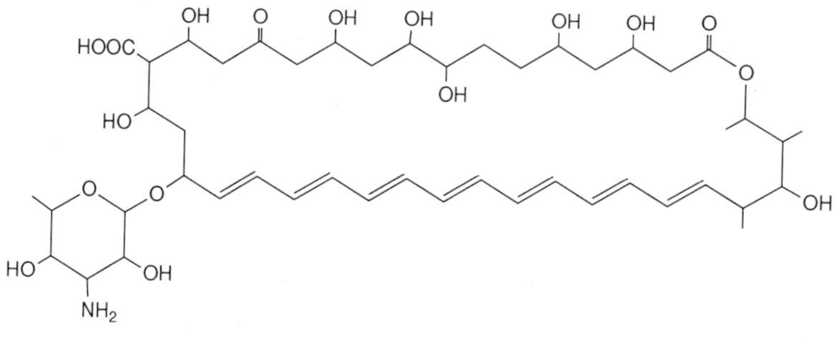

forming soluble salts in both acidic and basic media. It is highly insoluble in aqueous solutions at physiological pH. Thus, the intravenous (IV) form of the drug is a colloidal suspension using sodium desoxycholate as a dispersing agent. There are two forms of amphotericin, labelled A and B. The latter is more active against fungi and is the major form used clinically.

Amphotericin B binds to a sterol component of the fungal membrane of susceptible species, increases membrane permeability, and causes leakage of intracellular components, leading to cell death. The binding occurs in two stages. At low concentrations the binding is reversible and the effect is fungistatic. At high concentrations the binding is irreversible and leads to cell death. This two-stage binding seems to be related to the molecular size of the polyene; smaller polyenes are only fungicidal.

Because of its poor water solubility, amphotericin B is not well absorbed when administered orally or intramuscularly and has no therapeutic effect. When administered IV, a 50-mg vial should be reconstituted with 10 ml of sterile water. This mixture is then diluted at least 1:50 in 5%

Amphotericin is incorporated into the fungal cell wall and causes leakage and cell death.

The drug must be administered IV.

dextrose with a pH of 4.2. No other salts or antibiotics should be administered through the same vascular access line because of the likelihood of causing a precipitation reaction. A preparation and its dosage form are given in Table 55–1.

Most physicians administer a test dose of 1.0 mg before beginning therapeutic infusions. The test dose is administered over 6 hours, while the patient is carefully monitored for adverse reactions. If none occurs, the dosing schedule may be advanced rapidly (0.3 mg/kg on day 1, then 0.6 mg/kg on day 2 and subsequent days) or slowly (5–10 mg increments per day) depending on personal preference. In life-threatening disease, a full therapeutic dose may be given as the first drug administration.

Following delivery of a 0.65 mg/kg dose over 4–6 hours, a serum peak of 1.8–3.5 μg/ml is reached 1 hour later, maintained for 6–8 hours, and declines to 50% of peak 20 hours later. The drug distributes into a central and a peripheral compartment. It has a serum half-life of 24–48 hours but does not accumulate in the presence of normal renal function. The peripheral compartment has two components, one equilibrating rapidly and one slowly. The latter component has a half-life of approximately 6 days. Following administration of a full therapeutic course of 1.0–2.0 g, measurable drug persists in serum and urine for 3–7 weeks.

Only 3% of active drug is excreted unchanged in the urine. More than 95% is bound to serum proteins, primarily to cholesterol on β lipoprotein. It is presumed that the remainder of the drug is bound to cholesterol in human cell membranes. A small amount of drug is excreted through the bile, and the remainder is probably degraded *in situ*. Blood levels are not influenced by renal or hepatic failure, and the drug is not effectively removed by dialysis.

In the presence of inflammation the drug distributes into pleural, peritoneal, synovial, and vitreal fluids. It does not reliably penetrate into the central nervous system (CNS).

Adverse effects are common and often severe. During infusion, headache, fever and chills, malaise, arthralgias and myalgias, nausea, vomiting, and hypotension can occur. Because there often is no therapeutic alternative to amphotericin B, a number of agents have been tried to block these side effects, including antihistamines, antipyretics, antiemetics, and narcotic analgesics. Thrombophlebitis is also a common complication at the infusion site. Heparin has been added to the infusate to reduce the likelihood of this adverse reaction. Finally, low-dose corticosteroids (25–50 mg of hydrocortisone) have been added to block or diminish all these effects. Unfortunately, there is no proof that any of these maneuvers is efficacious.

All patients who receive amphotericin B sustain nephrotoxicity. The toxic effect may be reduced by providing sodium to the salt-depleted patient, but otherwise there is no effective intervention to lessen this concomitant of therapy. If the patient's serum creatinine exceeds 2.5–3.0 mg/dl, either a rest period of 2–5 days or a delay of therapy until serum creatinine declines below the threshold of intolerance (3.0 mg/dl) is advised. The nephrotoxic effects are of two types: (1) cortical ischemia, and (2) diminished glomerular filtration plus renal tubular damage leading to altered potassium-, magnesium-, and acid-handling capabilities.

Dosing schedules are unique and subject to physician preference.

The route of elimination of the drug is uncertain.

Toxicities may warrant immediate discontinuation of drug infusion.

Renal toxicity is universal among drug recipients.

Table 55–1	AMPHOTERICIN B: PREPARATION AND DOSAGE FORM		
	Preparation	**Manufacturer**	**Dosage Form**
	Fungizone	Squibb	50 mg powder

Hematological toxicity is manifested by a normocytic, normochromic anemia attributed to inhibition of erythropoietin by amphotericin B. Leukopenia and thrombocytopenia are less common. CNS toxicity is unusual, even with intrathecal injection of the drug. Cardiac arrest has been reported with rapid infusion; otherwise, direct cardiac toxicity is rare. Pulmonary and hepatic toxicity are also uncommon.

The drug has been safely administered to pregnant women, without toxic effects on the fetus; the drug does cross the placenta. Safety in the first trimester is not established.

True allergic reactions are rare, and although amphotericin has been shown to suppress immune responses *in vitro,* there is no known clinical correlate of these observations. In sum, this is one of the most toxic antimicrobials prescribed by physicians. Therapeutic alternatives would be welcomed.

Amphotericin B effectively treats almost all geographical and opportunistic fungal pathogens.

The spectrum of activity is broad, and the therapeutic uses of amphotericin B are many. Blastomycosis; candidiasis involving bone and joint, lung, heart, CNS, urinary tract, esophagus, peritoneum, and disseminated disease; histoplasmosis; cryptococcosis; paracoccidioidomycosis; coccidioidomycosis; aspergillosis; mucormycosis; and extracutaneous sporotrichosis have all been successfully treated with amphotericin B.

Granulocytopenic patients with persistent fever often receive amphotericin B empirically as presumptive therapy for suspected but unproven candidiasis. In that same patient population, amphotericin B appears effective in the treatment of infections caused by *Torulopsis glabrata* and also may be effective for treatment of invasive or disseminated aspergillosis.

Total dose and duration for treatment of most fungal infections is poorly defined.

The appropriate dose and duration of therapy for treatment of fungal infections are not well established. Most diseases seem to be effectively treated by a total of 1.5–3.0 g. Smaller amounts may be effective for catheter-related candidiasis (500 mg or less). Duration of therapy typically averages 6–12 weeks.

Local injection or instillation of drug has been employed for treatment of septic arthritis caused by sporotrichosis or coccidioidomycosis and CNS infection caused by coccidioidomycosis. A dose of 5–15 mg may be injected into the joint and 0.2–0.5 mg into cerebrospinal fluid. Hydrocortisone, 5–15 mg, is often added to the latter to diminish fever and other adverse effects.

Amphotericin B has been combined with flucytosine, rifampin, and tetracycline to treat selected infections. Flucytosine is discussed in the next section. Rifampin may exert an amphotericin B–sparing effect but does not seem to enhance its antifungal activity. It has been used in conjunction with amphotericin B for treatment of *Candida, Histoplasma, Cryptococcus,* and *Aspergillus* infections. Tetracycline has proved effective in animal experiments but has not been tested in humans because of toxic interactions with amphotericin B.

The only contraindication to amphotericin B use occurs in patients who are hypersensitive to the drug, unless there is no therapeutic alternative for treatment of the disease. No desensitization scheme has been adequately studied.

Many of the drugs commonly employed to treat other diseases (e.g., cancer chemotherapy) have toxicities similar to those of amphotericin B.

Besides the large number of toxicities associated with the drug, drug interactions are also common. Renal toxicity may be enhanced when amphotericin is concurrently administered with antineoplastic agents. Amphotericin B–induced hypokalemia may be exacerbated by coadministration of corticosteroids or corticotropin. Synergistic toxicity has been reported with flucytosine and is caused by increased cellular uptake and impaired renal excretion of amphotericin. The potential for renal toxicity of other drugs (aminoglycosides) may be enhanced, and skeletal muscle relaxants may be promoted because of amphotericin-induced hypokalemia.

Table 55-2   NYSTATIN: PREPARATIONS AND DOSAGE FORMS

Preparation	Manufacturer	Dosage Forms
Oral		
Nystatin	Generic	Oral suspension, 100,000 U
Mycostatin	Squibb	and
Nilstat	Lederle	Tablets, 500,000 U
Vaginal		
Nystatin	Generic	Vaginal tablets, 100,000 U
Mycostatin	Squibb	Vaginal tablets, 100,000 U
Nilstat	Lederle	Vaginal tablets, 100,000 U
Combination		
O-V Statin	Squibb	42 × 500,000 U oral tablets plus 14 × 100,000 U vaginal tablets
Cream/Ointment		
Nystatin	Generic	100,000 U/g of cream or ointment
Mycostatin	Squibb	100,000 U/g of cream or ointment
Nilstat	Lederle	100,000 U/g of cream or ointment
Pastilles		
Mycostatin	Squibb	200,000 U/troche

New Developments

A methyl ester salt of amphotericin B was developed that was more water-soluble. It produced higher serum levels and lesser toxicity in animals. In humans the drug has been associated with a leukoencephalopathy and progressive neurological dysfunction. Clinical trials have been terminated.

Amphotericin B has also been encapsulated in liposomes. Theoretical advantages include more selective targeting of therapy (liposomes are concentrated in reticuloendothelial organs), reduced toxicity, and higher concentrations of drug at infected sites. Studies of this formulation are ongoing.

NYSTATIN

The only other clinically useful polyene antifungal agent is nystatin. This drug was isolated from *Streptomyces noursei* in 1950. It was originally called *fungicidin*. It is a mixture of chemically related substances that were developed and refined by Squibb Research Laboratories, and the name was changed to *nystatin* because the work was done in New York state. Preparations and dosage forms are given in Table 55-2. The major component of nystatin is shown in Figure 55-2.

A second polyene antifungal is nystatin.

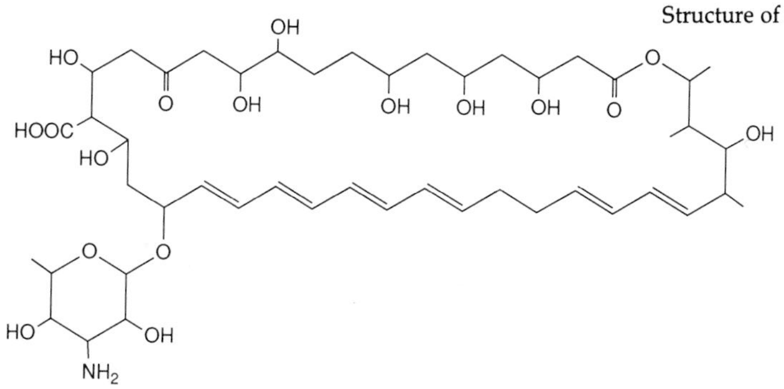

Figure 55-2

Structure of nystatin.

Its use is limited to treatment of superficial mycoses but not dermatophytes.

Nystatin acts in a manner analogous to that of amphotericin B. There is no systemic absorption following oral ingestion, topical application, or mucous membrane application, and there is no parenteral formulation.

The topical drug is generally benign. There are no local irritative or allergy-producing effects. Nausea or diarrhea may follow inadvertent oral ingestion of large doses. No adverse effects have been noted on children born to mothers treated with vaginal tablets during pregnancy.

The drug is indicated for treatment of superficial mycoses caused by susceptible organisms. *Candida* infection of the skin (but not infections caused by dermatophytes) and oral, gastrointestinal, and vaginal candidiasis are commonly treated with this drug. Although other fungi are susceptible, they do not cause superficial infections amenable to topical therapy.

The drug should not be used in patients known to be hypersensitive to it. There are no known drug interactions.

Fluorinated Pyrimidine Antifungal Agents

FLUCYTOSINE

A second class of antifungal agents is the fluorinated pyrimidine molecules. Only one clinically useful product has been developed; that is 5-fluorocytosine (flucytosine). This drug was synthesized in 1957 at Roche Laboratories as part of a screening program for antitumor agents in the treatment of leukemia. It is relatively noncytotoxic but does exert antifungal activity. A preparation and its dosage form are given in Table 55–3.

5-fluorocytosine is a fluorinated pyrimidine antifungal agent.

5-fluorocytosine

The drug may be given orally or IV, depending on the severity of patient illness.

Flucytosine is the fluorinated analog of cytosine. It acts by entering the yeast cell through a permease system. The intracellular drug is deaminated to 5-fluorouracil, which is then incorporated into fungal RNA instead of uracil. The genetic code is misread and growth desists. A second mechanism of action occurs through another metabolite, 5-fluorodeoxyuridine monophosphate, which inhibits thymidylate synthetase and blocks DNA synthesis. These effects may result in fungistatic or fungicidal activity, depending on drug concentration and time of exposure.

The drug may be administered orally or IV. Oral absorption is almost complete. The peak serum concentration of 45 μg/ml is reached 2–6 hours after ingestion of 2 g, and serum half-life is 3–5 hours. It distributes widely throughout body water, and protein binding is insignificant. Cerebrospinal fluid concentrations are approximately 75% of simultaneous serum values. The drug is cleared by both hemodialysis and peritoneal dialysis.

After IV infusion of 2 g over 15 minutes, a serum peak of 45–50 μg/ml is achieved at the end of the infusion.

The half-life is prolonged in patients with renal dysfunction. Nearly 100% of drug is excreted unchanged by glomerular filtration. A small amount is metabolized to 5-fluorouracil. As a compensatory mechanism, metabolic degradation increases with worsening renal function. The compensation is generally inadequate, however.

Toxicities are common and often may be related to concurrently administered drugs or underlying disease.

The major toxicity is hematological, although quantitating this toxicity has been difficult because patients treated with flucytosine often receive concurrent drugs with hematological toxicity or have diseases of the hematopoietic system. Suppression of red cells, white cells, and platelets is dose-dependent.

Table 55–3 FLUCYTOSINE: PREPARATION AND DOSAGE FORM

Preparation	Manufacturer	Dosage Form
Ancobon	Roche Laboratories	250 and 500 mg capsules

Other adverse effects include hypersensitivity manifested by rash; this is infrequent. Nausea, vomiting, and diarrhea are also uncommon. Hepatotoxicity may be manifested by elevation of hepatocellular enzymes. Finally, the drug is not nephrotoxic, but it accumulates rapidly, with the nephrotoxicity caused by concurrent treatment with amphotericin B. The safety of the drug in pregnancy is not established.

Flucytosine is most often combined with amphotericin B to treat deep-seated mycoses. It is not the drug of choice for treatment of any infection other than chromomycosis. Either the amphotericin B is more active or the relatively high likelihood of resistant strains emerging precludes flucytosine use as a single agent. Infections commonly treated include cryptococcosis, candidiasis, and *T. glabrata.* Response by *Aspergillus* species has been variable at best.

> The main therapeutic use has been treatment of cryptococcal meningitis (in conjunction with amphotericin B therapy).

The drug is contraindicated in patients known to be hypersensitive to it. Drug interactions are limited in scope. Cytosine arabinoside inactivates the antifungal activity of flucytosine by competitive inhibition. Any nephrotoxic drug can prolong the serum half-life of flucytosine and enhance its toxicity. Finally, flucytosine may cause false elevation of the serum creatinine level when determined by the slide enzymatic method.

Griseofulvin

A third class of antifungal agents is illustrated by griseofulvin, a drug that was isolated from *Penicillium griseofulvium* in 1939 but not pursued because it lacked antibacterial activity. Although its potential as an antifungal for botanical purposes was recognized in 1947, it was not evaluated in animals or humans until 1957–1959. Preparations and dosage forms are given in Table 55–4.

> Griseofulvin was discovered in the 1930s, but its clinical potential went unrecognized for two decades.

Griseofulvin binds to fungal RNA and interferes with microtubules of the mitotic spindle and cytoplasm. These microtubules transport material through the cytoplasm to the cell wall. Damage to the tubules impairs cell wall synthesis at the growing tips of hyphae; therefore, griseofulvin is effective only against growing organisms.

The drug is administered orally. The rate and amount of absorption are enhanced by a high-fat meal. After a 1.0-g dose the serum peak of 1–2 μg/ml is reached within 4 hours; 50% elimination occurs 12 hours later. Administration with milk is to be encouraged.

> Griseofulvin should be administered in conjunction with high-fat foods.

Griseofulvin is widely distributed throughout the internal organs, particularly liver, fat, and muscle. It distributes to skin, hair, and nails and is actively secreted from eccrine sweat glands. Griseofulvin is concentrated in keratin precursor cells. New keratin formed during treatment is thus resistant to infection, but the drug does not affect already formed keratin layers. These must be shed, and therapy must therefore be prolonged.

> The drug is distributed preferentially to skin, hair, and nails.

Most griseofulvin is dealkylated in the liver, and metabolites are cleared through the kidney. Less than 1% is cleared unchanged. A considerable portion of the drug is excreted unchanged in the stool.

Griseofulvin

Table 55–4 GRISEOFULVIN: PREPARATIONS AND DOSAGE FORMS

Preparation	Manufacturer	Dosage Forms
Griseofulvin	Generic	125 and 250 mg tablets
Fulvicin P/G	Schering	125 and 250 mg tablets, ultramicrosize crystals
Fulvicin P/G 165 and 330	Schering	165 and 330 mg tablets
Fulvicin-U/F	Schering	250 and 500 mg tablets, microsize crystals
Grifulvin V	Ortho Pharmaceuticals	250 and 500 mg tablets; 125 mg/5 ml suspension
Grisactin	Wyeth-Ayerst	125, 250, and 500 mg tablets, microsize crystals
Grisactin Ultra	Wyeth-Ayerst	125, 250, and 330 mg tablets, ultramicrosize crystals

Side effects are uncommon, but therapy must be prolonged in order to be effective.

Griseofulvin should be used to treat dermatophytic infections except tinea versicolor.

Because griseofulvin induces hepatic enzymes, drug interactions are common.

The most common side effect is headache, which generally resolves even with continuation of therapy. Serious adverse reactions are rare, but include leukopenia, fixed drug eruption, and hepatotoxicity. Other uncommon reactions include dysgenesis, dry mouth, nausea, vomiting or diarrhea, arthralgias, peripheral neuritis, and fever. Griseofulvin rarely may affect mentation and induce forgetfulness or memory loss. The drug is teratogenic in animals and contraindicated during pregnancy.

Griseofulvin is indicated for dermatophytic infections (tinea) except tinea versicolor. It is the drug of choice for tinea barbae and tinea capitis. Duration of therapy depends on rapidity of keratin turnover at the site of infection and may range from 1 (scalp) to 15 months (toenails).

Griseofulvin induces hepatic enzymes; drug interactions with agents metabolized in the liver are common. Coumarin-type anticoagulants may have diminished efficacy owing to increased turnover. Barbiturates decrease systemic absorption of griseofulvin, and increased doses of the latter drug may be necessary to achieve therapeutic effect. The effects of alcohol, including tachycardia and flushing, may be potentiated by griseofulvin. Finally, reduced efficacy of oral contraceptives is possible because of stimulated hepatic metabolism.

Potassium Iodide

Another chemical that possesses interesting antifungal activity is potassium iodide. Its mechanism of action is unknown. A saturated solution of potassium iodide is the drug of choice for treatment of cutaneous sporotrichosis. Local heat is applied to the lesions as adjunctive therapy. Amphotericin B is the treatment of choice for extracutaneous and disseminated disease. Side effects of potassium iodide include brassy taste, heartburn, and nausea; rhinitis coryza, salivation, lacrimation, sneezing, and burning of the mouth or throat; ocular irritation; sialoadenitis; and pustular acne over the chest. Use of the drug is contraindicated during pregnancy. A preparation and its dosage form are given in Table 55–5.

Imidazole Derivatives

Clotrimazole

Imidazoles inhibit fungal cell wall synthesis.

CLOTRIMAZOLE

The fifth class of antifungal agents is the imidazole derivatives. These drugs are being actively pursued as alternatives to amphotericin B but have not fulfilled that expectation. Clotrimazole was synthesized at the Bayer Research Laboratories in Germany in 1967. It was originally hoped that systemic fungal infections could be treated, but the drug is indicated for superficial mycoses only. The drug is closely related to miconazole (see later). Preparations and dosage forms are given in Table 55–6.

Clotrimazole is fungistatic at low concentrations and fungicidal at high concentrations. At low concentrations, all imidazoles (clotrimazole, econazole, miconazole, and ketoconazole) inhibit *de novo* synthesis of sterols required for cell membrane formation in actively growing organisms. The biochemical blockade occurs at the conversion of lanosterol to ergosterol. At high concentrations, imidazoles cause direct damage and increased permeability of the fungal cell membranes, producing a lethal effect. Unfortunately, these concentrations are generally not achievable in clinical medicine.

Table 55–5   POTASSIUM IODIDE: PREPARATION AND DOSAGE FORM

Preparation	Manufacturer	Dosage Form
SSKI	Generic	1 g/ml in 30 ml bottles

Table 55-6 CLOTRIMAZOLE: PREPARATIONS AND DOSAGE FORMS

Preparation	Manufacturer	Dosage Forms
Topical		
Lotrimin	Schering	1% cream in 15, 30, 45, and 90 g tubes
Mycelex	Miles	1% cream in 15, 30, and 45 g tubes
Lotrimin	Schering	1% solution in 15 and 30 ml bottles
Mycelex	Miles	1% solution in 15 and 30 ml bottles
Lotrimin	Schering	1% lotion in 30 ml bottles
Vaginal		
Gyne-Lotrimin	Schering	1% cream in 45 g tube
Mycelex-G	Miles	1% cream in 45 and 90 g tubes
Gyne-Lotrimin	Schering	100 and 500 mg tablets
Mycelex-G	Miles	100 and 500 mg tablets

Clotrimazole is poorly water-soluble and poorly absorbed after oral administration. The drug is a potent inducer of its own hepatic microsomal enzymes, resulting in progressively less drug being available during a course of therapy. Little drug is excreted through the kidney, and metabolites do not have antifungal activity. Therefore, the oral formulation is no longer available in the United States.

Side effects of topical preparations are generally minor. Minor local irritative phenomena, including burning, erythema, or urticaria, are associated with application of the cream. Contact allergy has rarely been reported. Small amounts are absorbed systemically following application to mucous membranes. Although there have been no reports of fetal toxicity, use of the drug during pregnancy is not indicated. The troche may be associated with nausea, vomiting, and reversible elevation of hepatocellular enzymes.

Clotrimazole is indicated for treatment of tinea infections, including tinea versicolor, cutaneous candidiasis, and *Candida* infections of mucous membranes or mucocutaneous junctions. The troche form has also been employed to reduce the risk of colonization or infection of the oropharynx and esophagus in immunosuppressed patients.

> Imidazoles (systemics) induce hepatic microsomal enzymes and can produce significant drug interactions.

> Clotrimazole is indicated for treatment of cutaneous and mucous membrane fungal infections.

ECONAZOLE

Econazole was developed at Janssen Pharmaceutical Research Laboratories in Belgium in 1969. A preparation and its dosage form are given in Table 55-7.

This drug is only available as a topical preparation. There is no systemic toxicity. Local reactions are infrequent and minor, including pruritus, burning, and erythema. The drug does not cause fetotoxic or embryotoxic effects in animals. During the first trimester of pregnancy, it should be used only when considered essential.

Econazole is indicated for treatment of dermatophyte infections and cutaneous and mucous membrane candidiasis. Because of its excellent activity against *Aspergillus* it has been used as local infusion to treat *Aspergillus* sinus infections.

Econazole nitrate

> Econazole is also indicated for treatment of dermatophytic infections.

Table 55-7 ECONAZOLE: PREPARATION AND DOSAGE FORM

Preparation	Manufacturer	Dosage Form
Spectazole	Ortho Pharmaceuticals	1% cream in 15, 30, and 85 g tubes

Miconazole nitrate

Miconazole must be administered IV to treat systemic mycoses.

Side effects associated with drug delivery can be life-threatening.

Miconazole is not the drug of choice for treatment of any systemic mycosis.

Drug interactions are common and must be carefully monitored.

MICONAZOLE

The next imidazole developed was miconazole. This drug was also synthesized at Janssen Pharmaceutical Research Laboratories in Belgium. It has a broad spectrum of antifungal activity and may be applied topically or administered parenterally. It is only slightly water-soluble. A preparation and its dosage form are given in Table 55–8.

Oral absorption is unreliable; therefore, systemic mycoses must be treated with the IV form of the drug. A serum peak concentration of 1.6 μg/ml is achieved at the completion of the infusion of 200 mg of miconazole IV over 1 hour. There is a rapid, early decline in serum levels, and the half-life is 30 minutes. There is slow elimination from a peripheral compartment, with a half-life of 20 hours. Serum protein binding is approximately 90%. Distribution into extravascular body fluids is poor. Cerebrospinal fluid penetration is unreliable.

About 1% of the drug is excreted unchanged in the urine. Ten percent of the total dose is excreted by renal clearance of metabolites. The remainder of the drug is metabolized in the liver by O-dealkylation and N-dealkylation to inactive metabolites, which are excreted in the stool.

Special precautions are necessary when administering miconazole IV. Nausea and vomiting may be induced by rapid infusion. So may cardiac arrest, and a delivery period of no less than 60 minutes is advised. CNS toxicity occurs in a significant proportion of patients; it includes tremors, hallucinations, confusion, dizziness, and rarely, seizures. Miconazole can also cause hemolysis, a hypoplastic bone marrow, and normochromic, normocytic anemia. The drug is phlebitogenic, and administration through a central venous access device is advocated. Pruritus and rash may occur and occasionally are sufficiently severe to warrant discontinuation of the drug. Finally, the vehicle for soluble miconazole is cremaphor EL. This may induce elevated cholesterol, elevated triglycerides, and rouleaux formation by red blood cells. Thus, the hope that this drug would be less toxic than amphotericin B has not been realized.

Miconazole may be effective for treatment of cryptococcosis that fails to respond to amphotericin B plus flucytosine therapy. But it is not the drug of first choice for this indication. It plays a similar back-up role in the treatment of systemic candidiasis, nonmeningeal coccidioidomycosis, and histoplasmosis. The total number of patients treated for each of these indications is small. Amphotericin B remains the drug of choice, and ketoconazole (see next section) has replaced miconazole for treatment of most infections caused by susceptible organisms. The IV solution may be injected intrathecally in a dose of 20 mg to supplement IV administration. Superficial mycoses of the skin and mucous membranes, including tinea versicolor, can be treated by local application of the drug.

As a systemically administered product and because of its high degree of protein binding, miconazole can displace warfarin into serum and result in an increased anticoagulant effect. Miconazole has also been reported to inhibit hepatic enzymes responsible for phenytoin and carbamazepine metabolism, producing toxic levels of these drugs. An interaction between miconazole and oral hypoglycemics has been reported to produce severe hypoglycemia.

Table 55–8 MICONAZOLE: PREPARATION AND DOSAGE FORM

Preparation	Manufacturer	Dosage Form
Monistat I.V.	Janssen	10 mg/ml in 20 ml solutions

KETOCONAZOLE

Ketoconazole was developed at Janssen Pharmaceutical Research Laboratory in Belgium in the 1970s; clinical trials began in 1977. Ketoconazole is unique among imidazoles because it is soluble in acidic aqueous solutions owing to a piperazine ring in its structure. Unfortunately, absorption is inadequate to produce serum concentrations necessary to exert a fungicidal effect. Ketoconazole is also unique in its capability to inhibit pseudomycelium formation of *Candida albicans,* because it is 100 times more potent than miconazole. Preparations and dosage forms are given in Table 55–9.

Ketoconazole is administered by the oral route. Sufficient gastric acidity is required to transform it into a hydrochloride salt. Antacids, anticholinergics, and H_2 blockers should be avoided for at least 2 hours following ingestion of the drug. There is large person-to-person variability in pharmacokinetic parameters. There is also a variable effect of combining the drug with a high fat meal. In general a serum peak of 3.0–4.5 μg/ml is achieved 2 hours after ingestion of a 200-mg oral dose. After an initial period of stabilization, individual patient serum peak concentrations are highly reproducible. Up to a dose of 800 mg, the pharmacokinetics seem to be dose-dependent.

After absorption, the drug is widely distributed through saliva, sebum, cerumen, and eccrine sweat. Ketoconazole is found in pleural, peritoneal, and ophthalmic fluids. It does not penetrate into the CNS reliably. A small fraction (2–4%) is excreted unchanged in the urine. Lesser quantities are found in bile. The drug is primarily metabolized by the liver to inactive forms and excreted either unchanged or as metabolites in the stool.

The most frequent side effects are gastrointestinal, including nausea and vomiting, abdominal pain, anorexia, diarrhea, and flatulence. These may be relieved by ingestion of the drug with food. Transient elevations of hepatocellular enzymes, which resolve without discontinuation of the drug, are seen in a small percentage of patients. On rare occasions the drug may have significant hepatotoxicity.

In doses of 400 mg or more, there can be suppression of testosterone formation in males, leading to breast tenderness, gynecomastia, decreased libido, oligospermia, and hair loss. The hair loss may also occur in women. These effects are reversible upon withdrawal of the drug. Ketoconazole in doses of 800–1200 mg/day can block cortisol production and suppress adrenal response to corticotropin. Ketoconazole also may reduce serum cholesterol (but elevate triglycerides), cause transient leukopenia, and interact with host defenses synergistically against fungi *(in vitro).*

Ketoconazole is indicated for treatment of serious dermatophyte infections; cutaneous, oral, and vaginal *Candida* infections; chronic mucocutaneous candidiasis; paracoccidioidomycosis; histoplasmosis in persons with normal host defenses; and blastomycosis. In certain cases of candidiasis and coccidioidomycosis, it may be a useful adjunctive therapy when combined with amphotericin B. It also has been employed as prophylaxis against *Candida* colonization among granulocytopenic immunocompromised hosts.

Ketoconazole interferes with cyclosporine metabolism in the liver,

Ketoconazole

Ketoconazole is well absorbed after oral administration but does not achieve fungicidal concentrations in infected tissues.

Antacids and H_2 blockers inhibit ketoconazole absorption.

The drug is widely distributed through most body systems but does not reliably penetrate into the CNS.

A unique toxicity is suppression of testosterone; this is reversible.

Ketoconazole is indicated for treatment of superficial and systemic mycoses, especially in patients with normal host defenses.

Table 55–9 KETOCONAZOLE: PREPARATIONS AND DOSAGE FORMS		
Preparation	**Manufacturer**	**Dosage Forms**
Nizoral	Janssen	200 mg tablets
Nizoral	Janssen	2% cream in 15, 30, and 60 g tubes

Drug interactions are common with those agents metabolized in the liver.

producing elevated serum concentrations that may be nephrotoxic. Reduced renal elimination of ketoconazole exacerbates its toxicity. Rifampin may induce more rapid metabolism of ketoconazole, yielding therapeutically inadequate concentrations. Ketoconazole may enhance the anticoagulant effect of coumarin-like drugs. Concurrent administration with diphenylhydantoin may affect the metabolism of one or both drugs. Levels of both should be monitored. Caution should be used when ketoconazole is administered concurrently with oral hypoglycemic agents. The hypoglycemic effect may be enhanced.

Fluconazole

Pharmacokinetic properties for the oral and the IV preparations of fluconazole are similar.

Fluconazole reliably penetrates into the CNS.

The adverse reaction profile is similar to that of other imidazoles, as are drug interactions.

Drug levels of phenytoin (DILANTIN) should be monitored when this drug is coadministered with fluconazole.

FLUCONAZOLE

The most recent imidazole to be developed and marketed is fluconazole. This drug is a white, crystalline solid that is slightly soluble in water and saline solution. It is available for oral or IV administration. Like other imidazoles, fluconazole inhibits sterol incorporation into fungal cell walls and exerts a fungistatic effect. A preparation and its dosage forms are given in Table 55–10.

The pharmacokinetics of orally and IV administered drug are similar. A serum peak of 6.7 μg/ml is reached 1–2 hours after administration of a single 400-mg dose. Plasma concentrations and area under the curve calculations are dose-proportional; steady state is achieved in 5–10 days.

Protein binding averages 12%. Fluconazole distributes into all body fluids, including cerebrospinal fluid, and therefore is unique among imidazoles. Approximately 80% of an administered dose of drug appears unchanged in the urine. Another 10% of drug is excreted by the kidney as inactive metabolites. There is an inverse relationship between serum half-life and renal function, and dose adjustment must be made for patients with renal failure. The drug is removed by hemodialysis.

Nausea, headache, skin rash, vomiting, abdominal pain, and diarrhea are the most common adverse reactions, occurring in 1–4% of recipients. Hepatocellular dysfunction manifested by elevated liver function tests is the most common laboratory abnormality.

Drug interactions with agents metabolized in the liver must be carefully monitored. Minimal effect on oral contraceptive metabolism has been reported. Hydrochlorothiazide increases serum concentrations of fluconazole; rifampin has the opposite effect. Fluconazole increases the effect of warfarin, sulfonylureas, phenytoin, and cyclosporine. Its greatest effect is on phenytoin (DILANTIN).

Fluconazole is indicated for the treatment of oropharyngeal and esophageal candidiasis; serious systemic *Candida* infections including urinary tract infections, peritonitis, and pneumonia; and cryptococcal meningitis. It has been particularly useful for therapy of cryptococcal disease among patients with acquired immunodeficiency syndrome (AIDS). After treatment of the acute infection with amphotericin B, maintenance therapy with fluconazole prevents relapse of the infection.

Table 55–10 FLUCONAZOLE: PREPARATION AND DOSAGE FORMS

Preparation	Manufacturer	Dosage Forms
Diflucan	Pfizer/Roerig	50, 100, and 200 mg tablets; 2 mg/ml in 100 ml and 200 ml containers

NEW DEVELOPMENTS

A number of imidazoles are being evaluated in clinical trials. Systemic drugs include triazole and itraconazole; topical preparations include terconazole and bifonazole.

General References

Antifungal agents for systemic mycoses. *In* Drug Evaluations, 6th ed, 1553. Chicago: American Medical Association, 1986.

Bennett JE: Flucytosine. Ann Intern Med 86:319, 1977.

Berestein GL: Liposomal amphotericin B in the treatment of fungal infections. Ann Intern Med 105:130, 1986.

Cohen J: Antifungal chemotherapy. Lancet 2:532, 1982.

Drueg DJ (ed): Systemic fungal infections: Diagnosis and treatment II. Infect Dis Clin North Am 3(1):1, 1989.

Drugs for treatment of systemic fungal infections. Med Letter 28:41, 1986.

Graybill JR (ed): Proceedings of a symposium on new developments in therapy for the mycoses. Am J Med 74(1B):1, 1983.

Graybill JR, Craven PC: Antifungal agents used in systemic mycoses. Activity and therapeutic uses. Drugs 25:41, 1983.

Hermans PF, Keys TF: Antifungal agents used for deep-seated mycotic infections. Mayo Clin Proc 58:223, 1983.

Medoff G, Kobayashi GS: Strategies in the treatment of systemic fungal infections. N Engl J Med 302:145, 1980.

Stevens DA: Current perspectives on miconazole. Drug Therapy 12:85, 1982.

VanTyle JH: Ketoconazole: Mechanism of action, spectrum of activity, pharmacokinetics, drug interactions, adverse reactions and therapeutic use. Pharmacotherapy 4:343, 1984.

56

Antiviral Drugs

Ann M. Arvin

The replication of both RNA and DNA viruses is an intracellular process that is difficult to inhibit without disrupting the metabolism of the host cell. The analysis of the biochemistry of viral synthesis has led to the development of effective antiviral therapy for infections caused by some herpesviruses, some respiratory viruses, and human immunodeficiency virus (HIV).

Nucleoside Analogs

The antiviral activity of nucleoside analogs, many of which were identified originally as antitumor agents, was established during the 1950s and 1960s (Elion, 1986). 5-iododeoxyuridine (IUDR) and cytosine arabinoside were used in early clinical investigations of the antiviral efficacy of compounds that inhibited DNA replication. The systemic administration of these drugs was associated with significant toxicity because of damage to rapidly dividing host cells, e.g., granulocytes and lymphocytes. The effect of cytosine arabinoside upon host cell DNA synthesis was such that patients with herpes zoster who received the drug had a more severe infection than placebo recipients. IUDR continues to be used as a topical antiviral agent for herpes simplex virus (HSV) keratitis. Otherwise, these original nucleoside analogs have been replaced by related antiviral agents with enhanced antiviral activity and limited interference with host cell DNA metabolism.

VIDARABINE

History. The antiviral activity of vidarabine (adenine arabinoside, ara-A) *in vivo* was described in murine models of vaccinia and herpes simplex virus infections. It was one of the first nucleoside analogs evaluated extensively for the antiviral therapy of human herpesviral infections because it was much less toxic than IUDR and cytosine arabinoside.

Chemistry. Vidarabine, 9-β-D-arabinofuranosyladenine monohydrate, is a fermentation product of *Streptomyces antiboticus* and has been synthesized also. Its chemical structure is identical to that of adenosine except for the substitution of arabinose for ribose.

Mechanism of Action. The drug is taken up by mammalian cells in its intact form and as arabinosylhypoxanthine, an inactive metabolite produced by deamination. The intact form of the drug is phosphorylated intracellularly by cellular enzymes. The triphosphate form, ara-ATP, inhibits the DNA polymerase of HSV and other herpesviruses and also acts as chain terminator when incorporated into HSV DNA. The drug binds to

The triphosphate form is the active compound.

cellular DNA polymerases but its specificity is several-fold greater for the viral DNA polymerases. Vidarabine inhibits many DNA viruses *in vitro* but not most RNA viruses.

Organ System Pharmacology. Vidarabine is distributed into all tissues but undergoes rapid deamination into arabinosylhypoxanthine extracellularly as well as after its uptake by cells. Cerebrospinal fluid concentrations are proportional to plasma concentrations, with a ratio of approximately 1:3. Both the native and the metabolized forms of the drug are eliminated primarily by renal excretion.

Adverse Effects. Common side effects of vidarabine that do not require the interruption of therapy include nausea, vomiting, and diarrhea. Its most serious adverse effect is encephalopathy associated with headache, dizziness, confusion, hallucinations, ataxia, and tremors, which can progress to coma. Patients with impaired renal function are at particular risk of this adverse effect. At dosages above 20 mg/kg/day, hematological suppression can occur causing a decrease in hemoglobin and in granulocyte and platelet counts. Liver function tests, e.g., serum glutamic-oxaloacetic transaminase (SGOT), may become elevated. Vidarabine administration occasionally causes rash and pruritus or malaise. The clinical use of the drug is complicated by its relative insolubility, requiring its administration in large volumes of intravenous (IV) fluid.

Therapeutic Uses (Indications/Contraindications). The clinical efficacy of vidarabine has been demonstrated in patients with HSV-1 encephalitis, infants with neonatal HSV infections, and immunocompromised patients with varicella (chickenpox) or herpes zoster, both of which are caused by varicella-zoster virus (VZV) (Whitley et al, 1983). It is effective as a topical antiviral agent for acute keratoconjunctivitis due to HSV. Vidarabine has no clinical efficacy against cytomegalovirus (CMV) infections.

Drug Interactions. Allopurinol may interfere with vidarabine metabolism.

Preparations and Dosages. The IV preparation is given at 10 mg/kg/day as a 12-hour infusion for 5 days to immunocompromised patients with VZV infections. It is given to patients with HSV encephalitis at 15 mg/kg/day for 7 days and to infants with neonatal herpes at 30 mg/kg/day for 10 days. The ophthalmic ointment is a 3% concentration of the drug in a petrolatum base and is applied five times/day.

New Developments. Vidarabine has been replaced by acyclovir as the drug of choice for the treatment of HSV encephalitis (Whitley et al, 1986). Preliminary data indicate that the efficacy of vidarabine is comparable to acyclovir in neonatal HSV infections, but acyclovir therapy avoids the problem of IV fluid volume required for vidarabine administration. Acyclovir was more effective for the treatment of herpes zoster in bone marrow transplant recipients than vidarabine (Shepp et al, 1986).

Summary. Vidarabine provided significant clinical benefit to patients with life-threatening HSV and VZV infections during the 1970s, but it has been replaced by acyclovir for most of its original indications.

ACYCLOVIR

History. Acyclovir was identified in the course of screening acyclic derivatives of adenine for antitumor and antiviral activity (Elion, 1986).

Chemistry. Acyclovir is a synthetic acyclic purine nucleoside, 9-[(2-hydroxyethoxy)methyl] guanine.

Mechanism of Action. Acyclovir is taken up selectively by cells infected with herpesviruses. Like vidarabine, its activity depends upon conversion to the triphosphate form. However, the antiviral specificity of acyclovir for HSV and VZV is enhanced relative to vidarabine because its phosphorylation is mediated selectively by the viral thymidine kinase of these viruses. The consequence of this is that phosphorylation of acyclovir occurs mainly in virus-infected cells, thereby sparing cells not infected with the virus. The triphosphate form of acyclovir interferes with HSV DNA polymerase; incorporation of the compound into viral DNA results in chain termination. The initial conversion of acyclovir to the monophosphate form does not occur in uninfected cells, so that drug toxicity for host cells is minimal. The triphosphate form does have some inhibitory effect on the cellular a-DNA polymerase. Natural resistance of HSV and VZV strains to acyclovir is rare but can occur if the strain is a thymidine kinase–deficient mutant. Other viruses, including herpesviruses like CMV and Epstein-Barr virus (EBV), do not require viral thymidine kinase for replication, so that their inhibition by acyclovir is limited. EBV replication is reduced by the drug because the viral DNA polymerase of EBV is highly sensitive to acyclovir triphosphate.

Selective activity in virus-infected cells is due to the requirement of viral thymidine kinase for metabolism.

Organ System Pharmacology. The pharmacokinetics of acyclovir is consistent with a two-compartment model with the distribution at steady state being approximately equal to the body fluid volume (deMiranda and Blum, 1983). Plasma concentrations at steady state after oral administration to adults are 0.5 μg/ml (200-mg dose) and 1.3 μg/ml (600-mg dose). The plasma half-life of acyclovir given orally to adults is 3–4 hours. Drug levels are measurable in saliva, lesion fluid, and vaginal secretions; cerebrospinal fluid levels are approximately half the plasma concentration. More than 80% of a drug dose is eliminated by renal excretion through glomerular filtration and, to a lesser extent, by tubular secretion. Renal tissue levels are substantially higher than plasma concentrations.

Adverse Effects. Clinical symptoms reported by some patients include nausea, vomiting, and headache, but these side effects rarely interfere with drug treatment. Acyclovir is soluble at 2.5 mg/ml. The drug can precipitate in the renal tubules with excessive dosages or when the therapeutic dosage is given by rapid infusion or to patients who are dehydrated. Impaired renal function as reflected by an increase in serum creatinine and decreased creatinine clearance may result. A few cases of encephalopathy, with signs including lethargy, tremors, hallucinations, seizures, and coma have been reported in patients with deficient renal clearance. Extravasation of the drug into soft tissues can produce severe cutaneous lesions. Theoretically, the selection of drug-resistant mutants of HSV and VZV could occur during acyclovir therapy, but the emergence of resistance has been quite unusual in clinical experience with the drug (Lehrman et al, 1986).

Acyclovir toxicity is primarily renal.

Therapeutic Uses (Indications/Contraindications). Acyclovir is most active against HSV-1 and HSV-2. *In vitro* replication of HSV-1 is reduced by 90% with drug concentrations less than 1.0 μg/ml, and by 50% with less than 0.2 μg/ml; HSV-2 is only slightly less sensitive than HSV-1. IV acyclovir is indicated for HSV encephalitis, neonatal HSV, and life-threatening HSV and VZV infections in immunocompromised patients (Whitley et al, 1986). Oral acyclovir is indicated for the treatment of primary and recurrent genital herpes (Reichman et al, 1984). Topical acyclovir reduces the duration of primary genital herpes but is not effective for recurrences. Treatment of primary HSV infections with acyclovir does not prevent recurrent disease, indicating that the drug does not prevent the establishment of latent neural cell infection. Acyclovir ophthalmic ointment is effective for herpes simplex keratitis. Acyclovir is not effective for CMV infection. The safety of acyclovir administration during pregnancy has not been established.

Drug Interactions. Concurrent administration of other drugs that reduce renal clearance, e.g., amphotericin, would be expected to raise the plasma and renal concentrations of acyclovir. Some patients given acyclovir and interferon or intrathecal methotrexate have had severe neurological complications, but these reactions were not clearly related to acyclovir. Probenecid reduces its renal excretion.

Preparations and Dosages. Acyclovir capsules contain 200 mg of drug. The bioavailability of the oral dose is 15–20%. The oral regimens for HSV infections are (1) 200-mg capsule five times a day for 10 days for initial episodes or for 5 days for recurrences, and (2) 200-mg capsule three times a day for up to 6 months for suppression of recurrent genital herpes. Topical acyclovir ointment (5%) is prescribed for initial genital herpes in otherwise healthy patients and for recurrent mucocutaneous herpes in immunocompromised patients. The ointment is used to cover the lesions every 3 hours, six times a day for 7 days. IV acyclovir (500 mg/vial) is given as 750 mg/sq m/day divided into three dosages and given every 8 hours for HSV infections in immunocompromised patients and as 1500 mg/sq m or 30 mg/kg/day (500 mg/sq m or 10 mg/kg every 8 hours) for VZV infections in high-risk patients. The dosage for neonatal HSV and HSV encephalitis is 30 mg/kg/day (10 mg/kg every 8 hours). The IV drug must be given as a 1-hour infusion. The dosage is adjusted for impaired clearance if the creatinine clearance is less than 50 ml/minute/1.73 sq m.

New Developments. The prodrug of acyclovir, 6-deoxyacyclovir, which is converted to acyclovir *in vivo* by xanthine oxidase, provides much higher plasma concentrations after oral administration and may be more effective for oral therapy of VZV infections. The current preparation, given orally as 800 mg per dose five times a day, has been effective for the treatment of herpes zoster in nonimmunocompromised patients in clinical trials and will probably be licensed for this indication. The experience to date with acyclovir for treatment of infectious mononucleosis caused by EBV does not suggest significant clinical efficacy. Oral acyclovir prophylaxis has been useful for the suppression of recurrent HSV infections in organ and bone marrow transplant recipients.

Summary. Acyclovir is the drug of choice for HSV infections and has proven clinical value for the treatment of VZV infections in immunocompromised patients. The possible emergence of drug resistance in clinical strains of HSV and VZV has not yet created a major therapeutic problem but will require careful monitoring as the drug is used widely. Drug resistance has been encountered in severely immunocompromised patients given prolonged acyclovir therapy.

GANCICLOVIR

History. Ganciclovir was synthesized as an acyclic nucleoside analog of guanine in the course of a search for an antiviral drug with activity against CMV.

Chemistry. Ganciclovir is 9-(1,3 dihydroxy-2-propoxymethyl) guanine; the drug is sometimes referred to as DHPG.

Mechanism of Action. Like acyclovir, ganciclovir is phosphorylated by the viral thymidine kinase of HSV-1 or HSV-2 to its monophosphate form within infected cells; the triphosphate form, which is generated by the activity of cellular enzymes, interferes with viral replication by insertion into the viral DNA. DNA replication is inhibited by chain termination and competitive inhibition of viral DNA polymerase. Ganciclovir also inhibits VZV replication *in vitro*, probably by the same pathway. The drug has antiviral effects on CMV and EBV as well. However, because these viruses do not have viral thymidine kinases, the mechanism by which ganciclovir inhibits CMV and EBV replication is less certain. The initial phosphorylation of ganciclovir is presumed to occur by the action of viral or cellular deoxyguanosine kinases, allowing its incorporation into replicating CMV or EBV DNA. The triphosphate form of the drug is known to accumulate in significantly higher concentrations in CMV- or EBV-infected cells, compared with uninfected cells. Viral infection is then restricted by the phosphorylated drug because of chain termination and inhibition of the viral polymerase.

Organ System Pharmacology. Animal studies have demonstrated that ganciclovir is excreted by the kidneys without undergoing any metabolic change, in concentrations equaling 90% of the dose given by IV administration. The drug is widely distributed in tissues, including brain, and concentrations can be maintained in plasma that are above the mean inhibitory concentration for CMV isolates, which is 0.02–3.0 μg/ml.

Adverse Effects. Ganciclovir has bone marrow suppressive effects in animals and also reduces spermatogenesis. The drug has been shown to have tumorigenic potential in mice. Therefore, the use of ganciclovir has been restricted to life-threatening or sight-threatening infections in immunocompromised patients. The severity of the underlying illnesses in these patient populations has complicated assessments of ganciclovir toxicity in clinical use. However, patients can develop neutropenia, thrombocytopenia or anemia, gastrointestinal symptoms, rashes, and abnormal hepatic and renal function; neurological syndromes including altered mental status, seizures, hallucinations, and psychosis have also been described during ganciclovir therapy. Suppression of the bone marrow is dose related and occurred within 10 days after initiating ganciclovir treatment of CMV infection in transplant recipients. Approximately 40% of patients given the drug can be expected to have neutrophil counts less than 1000 cells/cu mm. Adverse effects on reproductive function and carcinogenicity are also possible, based on observations in animals. Phlebitis is common with ganciclovir administration.

Therapeutic Uses (Indications/Contraindications). Because of its potential for causing serious adverse effects, ganciclovir is indicated only for life-threatening or sight-threatening infections caused by CMV. The patients who are most likely to experience such infections include bone marrow and organ transplant recipients and patients with the acquired immunodeficiency syndrome (AIDS) caused by HIV. The licensed indication for ganciclovir is limited to CMV retinitis. Ganciclovir has antiviral activity in severely immunocompromised patients with CMV pneumonia, when measured as a reduction in the quantity of infectious virus in urine, blood, and respiratory secretions. However, the impact of drug treatment on the survival rate of severely immunosuppressed patients with CMV pneumonitis has been variable in clinical trials. Although it has the capacity to inhibit HSV and VZV, its potential toxicity is a contraindication to the clinical use of ganciclovir for HSV and VZV infections, even in severely immunocompromised patients.

Drug Interactions. Because of the potential of both ganciclovir and azidothymidine to cause severe bone marrow suppresson, the concomitant administration of these drugs is not recommended. Theoretically, other drugs, such as chemotherapeutic agents, that inhibit rapidly dividing cells may have additive toxicity in patients receiving ganciclovir. As in the case of acyclovir, probenecid is likely to reduce the renal clearance of ganciclovir. Seizures have been reported in some patients who were receiving ganciclovir and imipenem-cilastin.

Preparations and Dosages. Ganciclovir is available as an IV preparation. The use of ganciclovir for CMV retinitis is based on an induction phase, in which the drug is given at a dose of 5 mg/kg, as a 1-hour IV infusion, administered every 12 hours for 14–21 days. Maintenance therapy consists of 5 mg/kg, given once a day, as a 1-hour infusion, or 6 mg/kg for 5 of every 7 days. Excretion of the drug by the kidneys requires adequate hydration; dosage reductions are essential if renal function is impaired.

New Developments. CMV isolates that are resistant to ganciclovir have been recovered from AIDS patients following ganciclovir treatment.

Summary. Ganciclovir is the only antiviral agent that is currently licensed for the treatment of CMV infection in high-risk patients.

AZIDOTHYMIDINE

History. Azidothymidine (zidovudine) was originally synthesized as a compound with potential antitumor activity. Its specific therapeutic value remained undefined until its substantial *in vitro* activity against HIV was demonstrated in the search for agents to treat AIDS (Mitsuya et al, 1985).

Chemistry. Azidothymidine is 3'-azido-3'deoxythymidine.

Mechanism of Action. The conversion of azidothymidine to its triphosphate form by cellular enzymes produces a compound that is very active as a competitive inhibitor of the reverse transcriptase of HIV and other retroviruses. This effect is manifest at low intracellular concentrations of the drug ($<1 \mu g/ml$) whereas the cellular a-DNA polymerase is much less sensitive to the agent, so that host cell toxicity is minimal (Hirsch and Kaplan, 1987). Incorporation of the drug also acts to terminate DNA synthesis.

Organ System Pharmacology. Azidothymidine is absorbed at more than 50% of the oral dose, and the plasma and body fluid concentrations produced are well above the 1–5 μm required to inhibit HIV *in vitro*. The drug is detected in cerebrospinal fluid after oral or IV administration.

Adverse Effects. Patients treated with azidothymidine for 4–6 weeks can be expected to develop anemia severe enough to require intermittent blood transfusions (Richman et al, 1987). Most patients also have granulocytopenia. Patients receiving the drug should have a complete blood count every 1–2 weeks. Clinical data are lacking, but like vidarabine and acyclovir, the toxicity of azidothymidine is probably increased in patients with impaired renal or hepatic function.

Therapeutic Uses (Indications/Contraindications). Azidothymidine is indicated for the treatment of HIV infection in patients who have symptomatic HIV infection with past *Pneumocystis carinii* pneumonia or an absolute CD4 T lymphocyte count less than 200/cu mm (Fischl et al, 1987). It also has value for the treatment of HIV infection, which is asymptomatic, by prolonging the interval until the development of symptomatic disease.

Drug Interactions. Any drugs that have adverse effects upon bone marrow or renal function may enhance the toxicity of azidothymidine, e.g., dapsone, pentamidine, amphotericin B, flucytosine, interferon, and cancer chemotherapeutic agents. Probenecid reduces the renal excretion of the drug and may inhibit glucuronidation; it has been recommended that patients receiving azidothymidine should not be given acetaminophen, aspirin, or indomethacin. Neurological symptoms have been described in a few patients given azidothymidine and acyclovir.

Preparations and Dosages. Azidothymidine is formulated as a 250-mg capsule and as an IV preparation. The dosage in the multicenter treatment trials for patients with AIDS and AIDS-related complex was 250 mg of oral drug every 4 hours.

New Developments. Clinical trials are in progress to determine the value of combinations of azidothymidine with other drugs or lymphokines, such as interferons, in symptomatic HIV infection.

Summary. Azidothymidine is the first drug with proven efficacy against HIV infection, but the initial clinical experience does not indicate that HIV infection can be eradicated by the drug.

RIBAVIRIN

History. Like the other nucleoside analogs, ribavirin was synthesized originally in a program designed to screen this class of compounds for antiviral activity.

Chemistry. Ribavirin is 1-β-D-ribofuranosyl-11-1,2-triazole-3-carboxamide and is most closely related to guanosine by x-ray crystallography studies.

Mechanism of Action. Ribavirin is phosphorylated intracellularly by cellular enzymes with the triphosphate form being the most active antiviral form. In contrast to vidarabine and acyclovir, ribavirin has broad activity against both RNA and DNA viruses. Its mode of action is best understood for respiratory viruses (Wray et al, 1985). *In vitro* studies of activity against influenza A infection of mammalian cells demonstrated a decrease in the intracellular nucleoside pool, inhibition of 5'-cap formation of cellular mRNAs, and viral RNA polymerase inhibition. RNA viruses are generally more susceptible to ribavirin, but the replication of HSV, CMV, and many other viruses is inhibited by this agent. Ribavirin reduces HIV replication in T lymphocyte cultures (McCormick et al, 1984).

Organ System Pharmacology. Information about the tissue distribution of ribavirin in human subjects is limited (Connor et al, 1984). Ribavirin is actively taken up by erythrocytes when given orally or IV with the half-life in these cells being 40 days. Penetration of the drug into cerebrospinal fluid has been documented. Most of the drug is excreted by the kidneys without undergoing metabolism. The drug is detected in plasma after 3 or more days of aerosol administration at concentrations of $3-6\,\mu m$; these concentrations are 1000-fold lower than concentrations in respiratory secretions.

Adverse Effects. Oral ribavirin administration causes a transient, dose-related anemia. Its administration by aerosol has produced serious mechanical interference with assisted ventilation because of drug precipitation in mechanical ventilators. Deterioration of respiratory function has been documented in some infants and adults treated with aerosolized ribavirin, but the role of the drug in causing such clinical events is not certain.

Therapeutic Uses (Indications/Contraindications). Ribavirin given by aerosol into an infant oxygen hood has been effective for the treatment of respiratory syncytical virus (RSV) pneumonia (Hall et al, 1983; Taber et al, 1983). It is not approved for use in infants with RSV pneumonia who require assisted ventilation. Ribavirin, given systemically, is highly effective for the treatment of Lassa fever, a rare arenavirus infection. The oral drug is not useful for the treatment of respiratory viral infections (Smith et al, 1980).

Drug Interactions. No specific drug interactions have been identified, but clinical experience with the systemic administration of ribavirin is limited.

Preparations and Dosages. Ribavirin is prepared as both oral and IV formulations. Only the aerosol formulation is available in the United States. The drug is aerosolized by putting 20 mg/ml of drug in the reservoir of a small particle Collison generator and administering it along with humidified air and oxygen for 12–18 hours/24 hours. The usual duration of treatment is 3–7 days.

New Developments. Ribavirin is one of the antiviral agents being investigated for clinical efficacy in patients with HIV infection. Further experience with its aerosol administration to infants who require mechanical ventilation for RSV pneumonia is needed to determine the safety and efficacy of the drug in these patients. Although oral ribavirin has been used for hepatitis A and measles infections elsewhere, these indications for the drug have not been established definitely.

Summary. Ribavirin is the first antiviral agent licensed for the treatment of RSV, which is the most common cause of severe pneumonia in infants and has been lifesaving for patients with lassa fever. Its efficacy for respiratory and other viral infections in adults remains to be established, although

The primary clinical indication is for treatment of RSV.

initial studies indicate some benefit from aerosol therapy of influenza A and B infections (Gilbert et al, 1985).

Interferons

History. The inhibition of vaccina virus replication in patients with measles, as described by Erasmus Darwin in 1803, probably represents the first description of the effect of interferon *in vivo*. Isaacs and Lindemann (1957) first reported the *in vitro* effects of interferon upon viral replication.

Chemistry. The interferons constitute a family of glycoproteins that are made by mammalian cells exposed to viruses, double-stranded RNAs, and other compounds. The interferons are classified as α, β, and γ-IFN. Alpha-IFN and β-IFN exhibit a significant degree of homology in amino acid sequences whereas γ-IFN differs substantially. Alpha-IFN is produced primarily by leukocytes, β-IFN by fibroblasts and epithelial cells, and γ-IFN by T lymphocytes. Genetic engineering methods have been used to prepare recombinant IFNs of each class.

Mechanism of Action. IFNs have diverse effects upon viral replication, including interference with viral uncoating, viral RNA transcription, viral protein synthesis, and the assembly of whole virions. The antiviral efficacy of IFNs is probably enhanced by their natural activities as immunomodulating lymphokines *in vivo*.

Organ System Pharmacology. The tissue distribution and metabolism of IFNs is incompletely understood. IFN activity is detected in serum after intramuscular administration but diminishes rapidly, probably because of the catabolism of IFN protein by the liver. Topical and intralesional administration does not produce detectable serum concentrations of IFN.

Adverse Effects. IFN therapy has been associated with fever, malaise, and fatigue; prolonged administration produces hair loss. A dose-related leukopenia occurs with natural and recombinant IFNs. The topical intranasal application of α-IFN was associated with punctate hemorrhages of the nasal mucosa in some patients.

Therapeutic Uses (Indications/Contraindications). IFNs have been effective against several viral infections in clinical trials, but licensure for a specific indication has not been made. Clinical benefit has been demonstrated with α-IFN used as in placebo-controlled trials as treatment of primary and recurrent VZV infections in immunocompromised patients, prophylaxis of recurrent HSV-1 infections, CMV prophylaxis in renal transplant recipients, prophylaxis and treatment of respiratory viral infections, and systemic and intralesional therapy for papillomavirus infections (Merigan et al, 1978; Douglas et al, 1986).

Drug Interactions. Concurrent therapy using α-IFN and vidarabine or acyclovir can cause neurological toxicity.

Preparations and Dosages. Most clinical trials have been carried out with human leukocyte α-IFN in dosages of $1-3 \times 10^6$ U per dose given once or twice daily by intramuscular injection.

New Developments. The evaluation of the antiviral efficacy of IFNs against human viral infections has been limited by the difficulty of producing sufficient quantities of the protein. The preparation of IFNs using recombinant DNA technology will allow much broader investigation of their value as antiviral agents alone and in combination with other compounds.

Summary. Although IFNs and IFN inducers were considered promising early in the effort to identify antiviral agents of clinical value, widespread use has been limited by short supply and by the concomitant development of other drugs, e.g., acyclovir, that have met the need for treatment of some herpesviral infections. However, better understanding of these natural antiviral substances is likely to generate new approaches to their clinical application.

History. Amantadine hydrochloride was synthesized in the 1960s in a program to identify antiviral agents effective against respiratory and other viruses.

Amantadine

Chemistry. 1-adamantanamine hydrochloride is a tricyclic amine derived from a 10-carbon alicyclic compound, adamantane (Couch and Six, 1986).

Mechanism of Action. The mechanism of the antiviral activity of amantadine is not fully defined. Its action appears to occur early in the course of viral infection of the mammalian cell with effects upon uncoating and fusion as well as assembly of progeny virions.

Organ System Pharmacology. Amantadine hydrochloride is not metabolized, and more than 90% of the dose is excreted by the kidneys (Dolin, 1986). Plasma and tissue fluid concentrations of $0.5-1\,\mu g/ml$ are observed with the usual dosage, whereas concentrations in respiratory secretions are about two thirds of the plasma levels. Higher plasma concentrations occur in patients with impaired glomerular filtration.

Adverse Effects. Amantadine causes mild adverse effects including dizziness, anxiety, and insomnia; some patients have had ataxia and confusion. In some controlled clinical trials of amantadine as an antiviral agent, such symptoms were reported as commonly by participants receiving aspirin or acetaminophen only. Urinary retention is another potential side effect. Serious adverse effects in patients treated for Parkinson's disease have included hypotension, congestive failure, altered mental status including psychosis and depression, seizures, and leukopenia.

Therapeutic Uses (Indications/Contraindications). Amantadine is indicated for the prophylaxis and treatment of influenza A virus infections. Low concentrations of the drug, achievable after its oral administration, inhibit clinical isolates of all types of influenza A, i.e., H_1N_1, H_2N_2, and H_3N_2 strains. Amantadine is considered an adjunct to the primary management of patients who are at risk for severe influenza A infection, which consists of annual influenza immunization. Those who may develop severe influenza A infection include the elderly, patients with chronic pulmonary or cardiac disease, and immunocompromised patients. Those who have not received vaccine prophylaxis can benefit from amantadine prophylaxis given for at least 10 days after a known exposure to influenza A or up to 90 days during a community epidemic. The early treatment of influenza A pneumonia with amantadine, continuing for $24-48$ hours after the resolution of symptoms, also reduces the severity of the illness in high-risk patients. Amantadine is contraindicated during pregnancy.

Drug Interactions. Amantadine hydrochloride interacts with anticholinergic drugs to produce atropine-like effects unless the dosage of the anticholinergic drug is reduced. Alterations of mental status may occur if patients are receiving central nervous system stimulants. Decreased excretion of the drug has been reported after concomitant administration with hydrochlorthiazide and triamterene. Amantadine prophylaxis or treatment does not interfere with the immune response to influenza vaccination given concurrently.

Preparations and Dosages. Amantadine is available as a capsule (100 mg) and as a pediatric suspension (50 mg/5 ml). The dosage for adults and children above 9 years of age is 200 mg given once or twice (100 mg/dose) a day; children from 1–9 years should receive 4.4–8.8 mg/kg/day with a maximal dosage of 150 mg/kg/day.

New Developments. Rimantadine is a compound that is closely related to amantadine but that produces higher concentrations in respiratory secretions. Rimantadine appears to cause fewer side effects and is now being evaluated for the therapy of influenza A infections. This compound has been used extensively in the Soviet Union and was comparable to amantadine in initial clinical trials in the United States.

Amantadine is underutilized in clinical practice.

Summary. Amantadine is an antiviral agent that is underutilized currently in clinical practice, given its demonstrated efficacy for the prophylaxis and treatment of influenza A infections. This circumstance is due to the difficulty of making a specific diagnosis of influenza A and should be alleviated as rapid viral diagnostic methods become available for this purpose.

References

Nucleoside Analogs

Elion GB: History, mechanism of action, spectrum and selectivity of nucleoside analogs. *In* Mills J, Corey L (eds): Antiviral Chemotherapy: New Directions for Clinical Application and Research, 118–137. New York: Elsevier, 1986.

Vidarabine

Shepp D, Dandliker P, Myers J: Treatment of varicella-zoster infection in severely immunocompromised patients: A randomized comparison of acyclovir and vidarabine. N Engl J Med 314:208–212, 1986.
Whitley RJ, Alford CA, Hirsch MS, et al: Vidarabine versus acyclovir therapy in herpes simplex encephalitis. N Engl J Med 314:144–149, 1986.
Whitley RJ, Yeager A, Kartus P, et al: Neonatal herpes simplex infection: Follow-up evaluation of vidarabine therapy. Pediatrics 72:778–785, 1983.

Acyclovir

de Miranda P, Blum MR: Pharmacokinetics of acyclovir after intravenous and oral administration. J Antimicrob Chemother 12(Suppl B):29–37, 1983.
Elion GB: History, mechanism of action, spectrum and selectivity of nucleoside analogs. *In* Mills J, Corey L (eds): Antiviral Chemotherapy: New Directions for Clinical Application and Research, 118–137. New York: Elsevier, 1986.
Lehrman SN, Douglas JM, Corey L, Barry DW: Recurrent genital herpes and suppressive oral acyclovir therapy. Relation between clinical outcome and *in vitro* drug sensitivity. Ann Intern Med 104:786–790, 1986.
Reichman RC, Badger GJ, Mertz GJ, et al: Treatment of recurrent genital herpes simplex infections with oral acyclovir. A controlled trial. JAMA 251:2103–2107, 1984.

Ganciclovir

Bach MC, Bagwell SP, Knapp NP, et al: 9-(1,3 dihydroxy-2-propoxymethyl) guanine for cytomegalovirus infections in patients with the acquired immunodeficiency syndrome. Ann Intern Med 103:381–384, 1985.

Collaboratory DHPG Treatment Study Group: Treatment of serious cytomegalovirus infections using 9-(1,3 dihydroxy-2-propoxymethyl) guanine in patients with AIDS and other immunodeficiencies. N Engl J Med 314:801–805, 1986.

Field AK, Davies ME, DeWitt C, et al: 9-([2-hydroxyl-1-(hydroxymethyl)ethoxyl] methyl) guanine: A selective inhibitor of herpes group virus replication. Proc Natl Acad Sci USA 80:4139–4143, 1983.

Laskin OL, Stahl-Bayliss CM, Kalman CM, Rosecan LR: Use of ganciclovir to treat serious cytomegalovirus infections in patients with AIDS. J Infect Dis 155:323–327, 1987.

Mar EC, Cheng YC, Huang ES: Effect of 9-(1,3 dihydroxy-2-propoxymethyl) guanine on human cytomegalovirus replication in vitro. Antimicrob Agents Chemother 24:518–521, 1983.

Martin JC, Dvorak CA, Smee DE, et al: 9-[(1,3 dihydroxy-2-propoxy)methyl] guanine: A new potent and selective antiherpes agent. J Med Chem 26:759–761, 1983.

Shepp DH, Dandliker PS, de Miranda P, et al: Activity of 9-[2-hydroxy-1-(hydroxymethyl)ethoxymethyl] guanine in the treatment of cytomegalovirus pneumonia. Ann Inter Med 103:368–373, 1985.

Azidothymidine

Fischl FA, Richman DD, Grieco MH, et al: The efficacy of azidothymidine (AZT) in the treatment of patients with AIDS and AIDS-related complex. A double-blind placebo-controlled trial. N Engl J Med 317:185–191, 1987.

Hirsch MS, Kaplan JC: Treatment of human immunodeficiency virus infections. Antimicrob Agents Chemother 31:839–843, 1987.

Mitsuya H, Weingold KJ, Furman PA, et al: 3'azido 3'deoxythymidine: An antiviral agent that inhibits the infectivity and cytopathic effect of human T-lymphotropic virus type III/lymphadenopathy associated virus *in vitro.* Proc Natl Acad Sci USA 82:7096–7100, 1985.

Richman DD, Fischl MA, Grieco MH, et al: The toxicity of azidothymidine (AZT) in the treatment of patients with AIDS and AIDS-related complex. N Engl J Med 317:192–197, 1987.

Ribavirin

Connor JD, Hintz M, VanDyke R, et al: Ribavirin pharmacokinetics in children and adults during therapeutic trials. *In* Smith RA, Knight V, Smith SAD (eds): Clinical Applications of Ribavirin, 107–123. New York: Academic Press, 1984.

Gilbert BE, Wilson SZ, Knight V, et al: Ribavirin small-particle aerosol treatment of infections caused by influenza virus strains A/Victoria/7/83 (H_1N_1) and B/Texas/1/84. Antimicrob Agents Chemother 27:309–313, 1985.

Hall CB, McBride JT, Walsh EE, et al: Aerosolized ribavirin treatment of infants with respiratory syncytial virus infection: A randomized doubleblind study. N Engl J Med 308:1443–1447, 1983.

McCormick JB, Mitchell SW, Getchell JP, Hicks D: Ribavirin suppresses replication of lymphadenopathy associated virus in cultures of human adult T lymphocytes. Lancet 2:1367–1369, 1984.

Smith CB, Charette RP, Fox JP, et al: Lack of effect of oral ribavirin in naturally occuring influenza A (H_1N_1) infection. J Infect Dis 141:548–554, 1980.

Taber LH, Knight V, Gilbert BE, et al: Ribavirin aerosol treatment of bronchiolitis associated with respiratory syncytial virus infection in infants. Pediatrics 72:613–618, 1983.

Wray SK, Gilbert BE, Noall NW, Knight V: Mode of action of ribavirin: Effect of nucleoside pool alterations on influenza virus ribonucleoprotein synthesis. Antiviral Res 5:29–37, 1985.

Interferons

Douglas RM, Moore BW, Miles HB, et al: Prophylactic efficacy of intranasal alpha$_2$-interferon against rhinovirus infections in the family setting. N Engl J Med 314:65–70, 1986.

Issacs A, Lindemann J: Virus interference. I. The interferon. Proc R Soc Lond [Biol] 147:258–267, 1957.

Merigan TC, Rand KH, Pollard RB, et al: Human leukocyte interferon for the treatment of herpes zoster in patients with cancer. N Engl J Med 298:891–897, 1978.

Amantadine

Couch RB, Six HR: The antiviral spectrum and mechanism of action of amantadine and rimantadine. *In* Mills J, Corey L (eds): Antiviral Chemotherapy: New Directions for Clinical Application and Research, 50–57. New York: Elsevier, 1986.

Dolin R: Antiviral chemotherapy and chemoprophylaxis. Science 227:1296–1303, 1986.

Dolin R: Clinical efficacy, pharmacology and toxicity of amantadine and derivatives. *In* Mills J, Corey L (eds): Antiviral Chemotherapy: New Directions for Clinical Application and Research, 58–62. New York: Elsevier, 1986.

Antiparasitic Agents

57

Elizabeth A. Vande Waa
James W. Tracy

Throughout the world, particularly in less developed countries, parasitic diseases are among the most pressing and serious, yet most neglected, public health problems. A majority of the world's population harbors one or more protozoan or metazoan parasites. These infections are associated with a high degree of morbidity and have a profound impact on the economic development of endemic regions. The prevalence of parasitic infections is increasing dramatically.

In the past, such "tropical" or "exotic" diseases were of little concern to physicians practicing in the Unites States (U.S.). The advent of jet aircraft and extensive worldwide travel for both business and pleasure has made these endemic regions readily accessible, and with that accessibility comes increased risk of infection. Furthermore, many parasitic diseases are not restricted to the tropics. It has been estimated that over 60 million Americans are infested with helminths, including pinworms, ascarids, whipworms, and hookworms.

ADVICE TO TRAVELERS

For a physician in the U.S., one of the best ways to deal with "travelers' diseases" is prevention. Appropriate counseling of patients prior to overseas travel and follow-up examinations on their return can greatly reduce their chances of acquiring such infections. Which travelers are at risk depends on such things as the purpose of their trip, their destination, and the duration of their visit. Low-risk travelers include business people who stay in international hotels in major cities for short periods of time. At the other end of the spectrum might be a Peace Corps volunteer who will live in a rural area in indigenous housing for a year or more.

Advice Prior to Travel. The patient should be advised against drinking untreated water, including ice prepared from the water. Fresh milk should be avoided, but bottled beverages such as beer and wine are usually acceptable. Hot coffee or tea made from boiled water is reasonably safe. It is very dangerous to eat raw or undercooked meat of any kind; raw or undercooked fresh-water fish frequently contains flukes or tapeworms. Peelable raw fruits and vegetables are relatively safe, if peeled by the eater. Salads are particularly dangerous because the vegetables are often washed in local water that has not been treated.

It is very important to advise travelers to take precautions to minimize the number of insect bites they receive. An unprotected individual in the

Parasitic Diseases and Their Management

Over 60 million Americans are infested with helminths.

Business people residing in international hotels are at low risk for parasitic infections; Peace Corps volunteers living in rural indigenous housing for more than a year are at a much higher risk of infection.

913

tropics can suffer over 270 mosquito bites per day! The use of mosquito netting, long-sleeved garments, and insect repellents is necessary. Bites from tsetse flies, black flies, and reduviid bugs should be avoided, as these also are parasite vectors.

Travelers should be warned of special hazards. For example, wading or swimming in fresh-water streams, lakes, or rivers may well lead to a schistosome infection. Chlorinated swimming pools, found at many hotels, and sea water are safe for schistosomiasis.

Follow-up After Travel. It is important to advise the traveler to be alert for symptoms that may be indicative of a parasitic infection. In particular, travelers to regions endemic for malaria should be alert for signs of febrile illness and should seek medical attention immediately. A follow-up visit after returning to the U.S. should be recommended.

PARASITIC DISEASE MANAGEMENT

Improved hygiene, vector and intermediate host control, vaccines, and chemotherapy are four approaches to the management of parasitic disease.

In terms of dealing with parasitic infections, there are four approaches to consider: (1) improved hygiene, (2) vector and intermediate host control, (3) vaccines, and (4) chemotherapy. Programs for improving sanitation and hygiene in developing countries have been somewhat successful, but many nations do not have the fiscal resources to modernize public water, sewage treatment, and housing. There have been many programs worldwide to eradicate the vectors and intermediate hosts of parasites. After World War II, the use of insecticides such as DDT was successful in lowering mosquito populations in a number of countries. However, resistance to such compounds has developed, and as a result, the vector population is increasing. The use of chemical molluscicides to kill the intermediate snail host of schistosomiasis has proved effective in limited regions where the water volume and flow are not too great. However, these chemicals are both expensive and toxic to other organisms, including fish and mammals. They also need to be reapplied frequently. Despite extensive research, there are at present no vaccines available against any human parasite. A malaria vaccine showed some promise in experimental animals but has proved to be of no clinical utility. It is likely to be many decades, if not centuries, before useful vaccines against helminths such as schistosomes are available.

There are no vaccines available against any human parasite.

Essentially this leaves only chemotherapy as the primary weapon against parasitic infections. Although there have been some advances in new drugs against some parasites, the number of drugs available is still limited. Of great concern is the fact that drug resistance is appearing. The emergence of chloroquine-resistant strains of falciparum malaria has reduced the list of available effective drugs for both treatment and prophylaxis. Table 57–1 summarizes the drugs used to treat parasitic infection.

PURPOSE OF CHEMOTHERAPY

Why undertake chemotherapy? When dealing with an infected individual, particularly in this country, chemotherapy is obviously undertaken to eradicate or control the infection and thus reduce the risk of disease. In such situations it is possible and desirable to individualize therapy and closely monitor clinical progress. This represents the case most often seen by U.S. physicians. However, in endemic regions chemotherapy takes on a twofold aim: The first is to treat the infected individual to eliminate the infection; the second is for public health reasons, to reduce the transmission of the parasitic infection in the community. By decreasing the number of infected

Chemotherapy can control the infection and reduce the rate of transmission of the parasitic infection inside the community.

Table 57–1　DRUGS USED TO TREAT PARASITIC INFECTIONS

Parasitic Infection	Drug of Choice	Alternative Drugs	Comments
Helminth Infections			
INTESTINAL NEMATODE INFECTIONS			
Ascariasis			
Ascaris lumbricoides	Mebendazole	Albendazole,*† pyrantel, Piperazine, ivermectin*	
Hookworm infection			
Necator americanus	Mebendazole	Albendazole,*† pyrantel	
Ancylostoma duodenale	Mebendazole	Albendazole,*† pyrantel	
A. braziliense (cutaneous larval migrans)	Thiabendazole	Albendazole*†	
Trichuriasis			
Trichuris trichiura	Mebendazole	Albendazole,*† Oxantel	
Enterobiasis			
Enterobius vermicularis	Mebendazole	Albendazole,*† pyrantel, invermectin*‡	
Strongyloides stercoralis	Thiabendazole	Albendazole,*† ivermectin*	
Trichinosis			
Trichinella spiralis	Albendazole*†	Thiabendazole	Thiabendzole efficacy limited to intestinal phase
BLOOD AND TISSUE NEMATODES			
Filariasis			
Wuchereria bancrofti	Diethylcarbamazine‡	Ivermectin*	
Brugia malayi	Diethylcarbamazine†	Ivermectin*	
Onchocerca volvulus	Ivermectin	Diethylcarbamazine‡	
TREMATODES			
Schistosomiasis			
Schistosoma mansoni	Praziquantel	Oxamniquine	
S. hematobium	Praziquantel	Metrifonate‡	
S. japonicum	Praziquantel	—	
S. mekongi	Praziquantel	—	
Liver and lung flukes			
Clonorchis sinensis, Opisthorchis spp.			
Paragonimus spp.	Praziquantel*		
Fasciola hepatica	—	—	
CESTODES			
Taeniasis			
Taenia saginata	Praziquantel*	Niclosamide	
T. solium	Praziquantel*	—	Use of niclosamide not recommended owing to risk of cysticercosis
Neurocysticercosis due to *T. solium*	Albendazole*		
Diphyllobothriasis			
Diphyllobothrium latum	Praziquantel*	Niclosamide	
Hymenolepiasis			
Hymenolepis nana	Praziquantel*	Niclosamide	
Echinococcosis			
Echinococcus granulosus	Albendazole*†	Mebendazole*	Mebendazole may be only partially effective
Protozoan Infections			
Trichomoniasis			
Trichomonas vaginalis	Metronidazole	—	
Amebiasis			
Entamoeba histolytica			
Asymptomatic cyst passers	Diloxanide furoate†	—	
Noninvastive intestinal form	Diloxanide furoate†	Paramomycin	
Invasive forms; amebic abscess	Metronidazole	Chloroquine, dehydroemetine	Alternative drugs are generally not recommended
Giardiasis			
Giardia lamblia	Metronidazole*	Quiacrine	
Leishmaniasis			
Leishmania tropica	Sodium stibogluconate†		
L. mexicana, L. braziliensis	Sodium stibogluconate†	Amphotericin B	
L. donovani	Sodium stibogluconate†	Pentamidine	

Table continued on following page.

Table 57-1   RUGS USED TO TREAT PARASITIC INFECTIONS Continued

Parasitic Infection	Drug of Choice	Alternative Drugs	Comments
Trypanosomiasis			
Trypanosoma brucei rhodesiense	Suramin	Eflornithine, pentamidine	Acute infection
T. brucei gambiense	Eflornithine	Suramin, pentamidine	No central nervous system involvement
T. brucei gambiense	Eflornithine	Suramin, then melarsoprol	Chronic infection, with central nervous system involvement
T. cruzi	Nifurtimox†		
Malaria			
Plasmodium vivax, P. oval, P. malariae	Chloroquine	—	For chemoprophylaxis and treatment of clinical attack
P. vivax, P. ovale	Primaquine	—	Radical cure agent
P. falciparum			
Chloroquine-sensitive	Chloroquine	—	For chemoprophylaxis and treatment of clinical attacks
Chloroquine-resistant or multidrug-resistant			
Chemoprophylaxis	Chloroquine, proguanil, or pyramethamine-sulfadoxine	Mefloquine	Dependent on geographical location
Treatment	Mefloquine	Quinine with or without pyramethamine-sulfadoxine	

* Accepted therapy in some countries. Use is either not approved or considered investigational in the United States.
† Contact the Parasitic Disease Drug Service, Centers for Disease Control, for availability.
‡ Recommendation based on limited clinical trials.

individuals, transmission of parasitic life stages to vectors and intermediate hosts is reduced. In some situations, it has been possible to significantly reduce both the prevalence and the incidence of infection through such community-based chemotherapy.

DRUG AVAILABILITY

Many of the drugs discussed are not routinely available in the U.S. and must be obtained from the Parasitic Disease Drug Service, Center for Infectious Disease, Centers for Disease Control, Atlanta, Georgia 30333. Telephone: (404) 329–3670 (days) or (404) 329–2888 (emergencies on evenings, weekends, and holidays). Be prepared to give detailed clinical signs and a definitive parasitological diagnosis. It is important for the physician to accurately diagnose the particular type and species of parasite infection, as drugs are effective against only a single parasite species. One should seek expert advice if there is any question about the diagnosis.

Helminth Infections

Anthelmintics combat parasitic worm infections.

The World Health Organization estimates that worldwide over 2 billion people are infected with one or more parasitic worms (helminths). Many individuals also suffer from disease manifestations of these infections. Despite the prevalence of helminthiases, only a handful of drugs, anthelmintics, are currently available for clinical use. Most anthelmintics are effective against a limited number of organisms; only a few (notably mebendazole, albendazole, and praziquantel) can be thought of as *broad-spectrum agents*. Because of the wide variety of nematodes, cestodes, and trematodes for which humans are a host, an accurate parasitological diagnosis is important to determining the drug of choice.

INTESTINAL NEMATODE INFECTIONS

Ascariasis

About one fourth of the world's population is infected with the intestinal nematode *Ascaris lumbricoides.* In the U.S., ascariasis is seen most frequently in the humid southern regions, where it is particularly prevalent among poor, rural children who have extensive contact with soil contaminated with embryonated ascarid eggs. The adult worms inhabit the lumen of the small bowel, where they can grow to 30 cm in length and live for up to 5 years.

Hookworm Infection

In the Americas the major species of hookworm is *Necator americanus,* whereas the predominant species in other parts of the world is *Ancylostoma duodenale.* The adult worms inhabit the small intestine and ingest blood, which may lead to anemia in malnourished or very heavily infected individuals. Treatment of hookworm infections has two objectives: (1) to restore the blood to normal with oral iron therapy; and (2) to expel the parasites. A zoonotic infection known as *cutaneous larval migrans* is due to the larvae of the dog hookworm, *Ancylostoma braziliense,* which penetrate and migrate through subcutaneous tissues.

Hookworm infections can lead to anemia in malnourished individuals.

Trichuriasis

Whipworm *(Trichuris trichiura)* is distributed worldwide, particularly in warm, humid climates. It normally is an innocuous infection, although penetration of the bowel can occur, leading to peritonitis.

Enterobiasis

Pinworm *(Enterobius vermicularis)* is a cosmopolitan nematode infection and is the most common cause of helminthiasis in the U.S. This parasite seldom causes appreciable clinical disease, but severe itching in the perianal region is often the impetus for seeking medical attention. In treating pinworm, it is important to recognize that autoinfection is common (rectal-oral contact resulting from scratching), so that more than one course of therapy is often required. Similarly, because the infection is easily transmitted among family members, it may be advisable to treat an entire family. Rigorous personal hygiene is also an essential adjunct to successful therapy.

Pinworm is the most common helminthiasis in the United States.

Strongyloidiasis

Infection with *Strongyloides stercoralis* is found in the tropics and subtropical regions of the world. In the U.S. it is most commonly encountered in humid southern states. This infection is the most difficult of the intestinal nematodes to treat successfully because it is prone to autoinfection. This results when rhabditiform larvae undergo two molts into filariform larvae that can penetrate intestinal mucosa, enter the circulation, and continue development into adult worms without leaving the human host.

Trichinosis

This infection, caused by *Trichinella spiralis,* is acquired only be eating raw or undercooked meat, particularly pork, that contains the infective muscle

Trichinosis is acquired by eating raw or undercooked meat, particularly pork.

stage larvae. The easiest way to prevent trichinosis is to thoroughly cook all pork products before eating. The adult worms, which inhabit the gastrointestinal tract, are susceptible to benzimidazoles; but unfortunately, the infection is seldom diagnosed during the intestinal phase. Once the larvae have migrated to muscle of the host, it is more difficult to treat.

Drugs Used to Treat Intestinal Nematode Infections

Mebendazole. Mebendazole, a 5-substituted benzimidazole, is the prototype for a large group of benzimidazole carbamates, including albendazole and flubendazole. Mebendazole is always administered orally, and because it is not unpleasant tasting, it is conveniently given as chewable tablets. The drug is poorly absorbed from the gastrointestinal tract. Bioavailability ranges from 10 to 20%. Peak plasma concentrations are achieved in 1–2 hours, and the average elimination half-life is about 1 hour. The fraction of drug absorbed undergoes extensive first-pass metabolism in the liver to a number of metabolites, about 48% of which appear in urine. Biliary excretion of mebendazole metabolites is an important route of elimination.

As a result of its poor absorption, mebendazole rarely causes systemic toxicity. Transient abdominal pain and diarrhea are sometimes seen in cases of heavy worm burden. A few patients experience allergic reactions, but these may relate to death of the parasites rather than being a direct drug-mediated effect. However, tests in laboratory animals have shown that a single dose of mebendazole is both teratogenic and embryotoxic. Thus, this drug is contraindicated for use in pregnancy. Another benzimidazole, flubendazole, which is not teratogenic, may eventually be an alternative, but it is not yet approved for use.

Mebendazole binds to the β subunit of tubulin, preventing its polymerization into microtubules (Lacey, 1990). However, the exact biochemical mechanism of action has not yet been fully explained. Although mebendazole binds avidly to parasite β tubulin, it also has significant affinity for mammalian tubulin. Mebendazole, like other members of the benzimidazole class, causes numerous other effects in parasites, such as decreased glucose transport and glycogen depletion, that are not seen in mammalian cells. Further evidence that inhibition of microtubule formation is essential for the mechanism of drug action comes from observations that benzimidazole-resistant nematodes have altered β tubulin structure and rate of subunit synthesis (Roos, 1990).

Mebendazole is the drug of choice for ascariasis. It also is highly effective against other intestinal nematodes, including hookworm, trichuriasis, and enterobiasis. It is particularly useful because two or more of these parasites often occur as mixed infections. Mebendazole has little activity toward *Strongyloides stercoralis* (strongyloidiasis). That parasite is susceptible to albendazole (see later in this chapter). Mebendazole has also shown variable activity toward several systemic nematodes, including *Trichinella spiralis* and cutaneous larval migrans. Along with albendazole, it has shown some promise for treatment of cystic hydatid disease.

Albendazole. Another benzimidazole carbamate derivative, albendazole, has been tested around the world since its introduction in 1979, but is not yet routinely available in the U.S. (Cook, 1990). Unlike mebendazole, albendazole is well absorbed after oral administration. It is primarily metabolized in the liver by a flavin-containing monooxygenase to the sulfoxide and sulfone metabolites, which are excreted in urine. The compound displays a plasma half-life of 8–9 hours.

Mebendazole

Mebendazole is the drug of choice for ascariasis.

Albendazole

Although albendazole shows higher bioavailability than mebendazole, it is relatively free of side effects. A few individuals experience transient epigastric pain, diarrhea, headaches, nausea, dizziness, and lassitude. In a few patients treated over 30 days for cystic hydatid disease, fever, reversible leukopenia, alopecia, and elevated serum enzymes were noted. The drug has not been tested for use in children. Like mebendazole, albendazole has shown teratogenic activity in some animal species and is thus contraindicated in pregnancy. It should be used with caution in patients suffering from hepatic cirrhosis.

Albendazole should be used with caution in patients suffering from hepatic cirrhosis.

In most clinical trials, albendazole consistently proved more efficacious than mebendazole against intestinal nematodes. Unlike mebendazole, albendazole shows significant activity against *Strongyloides stercoralis*, although results are variable owing to the ease with which autoinfection occurs. Albendazole has proved more effective against systemic nematode infections such as *Trichinella spiralis* and zoonotic cutaneous larval migrans (caused by dog hookworm, *Ancylostoma braziliensis*). In limited trials prolonged courses of albendazole have shown promise for treatment of systemic cestode infections (cystic hydatid disease and taeniad neurocysticercosis). This is significant because these diseases have generally been refractory to chemotherapy.

Albendazole is more efficacious than mebendazole against intestinal nematodes.

Thiabendazole. Thiabendazole is a 2-substituted benzimidazole first introduced in 1961. Like other benzimidazoles it is active against a variety of nematodes. It most cases it is administered as an oral suspension or as a chewable tablet. Unlike mebendazole, thiabendazole is rapidly absorbed from the gastrointestinal tract. Peak plasma concentrations occur after about 1 hour. The drug is extensively metabolized through aromatic ring hydroxylation to the 5-hydroxy metabolite, which is eliminated in urine either in its free form or as the corresponding O-glucuronide or sulfate conjugates.

Thiabendazole

Because a substantial fraction of the dose is bioavailable, side effects are more frequently seen with thiabendazole than with mebendazole. These are primarily central nervous system effects and include anorexia, nausea, vomiting, dizziness, and drowsiness. The drug does have hepatotoxic potential and should be used with caution in patients with compromised liver function.

As with other benzimidazole anthelmintics, the primary mechanism of action results from drug binding to β tubulin to inhibit microtubule formation (see Mebendazole).

Thiabendazole is currently the drug of choice for treating strongyloidiasis. For uncomplicated cases, a 2-day regimen is sufficient, but in cases of disseminated strongyloidiasis, a 5-day course is required. Thiabendazole is also used for treatment of cutaneous larval migrans, reducing the symptoms associated with "creeping eruptions" due to parasite migration in subcutaneous tissues. This drug is also effective for eliminating the adult stage of *Trichinella spiralis* during the intestinal phase of the infection, but it is of questionable value against the larval stage found in tissues.

Thiabendazole is the drug of choice for strongyloidiasis.

Evidence from animal studies indicates that thiabendazole will kill muscle stage larvae, but results of human trials have been mixed. Albendazole appears to represent a major advance in the treatment of trichinosis, although its use is still experimental. The administration of corticosteroids as anti-inflammatory agents seems to be of value in helping to control acute symptoms of muscle stage infection.

Pyrantel/Oxantel. Pyrantel pamoate was originally developed for use in veterinary medicine, but it has been approved for use in humans for treat-

Pyrantel

Pyrantel is well tolerated in adults and in children over 2 years old because of its poor absorption.

Piperazine

Piperazine produces a flaccid paralysis on the nematodes, thus allowing them to be expelled from the host by normal gut motility.

Bancroftian filariasis is transmitted by mosquito vectors.

ment of intestinal nematode infections. Used as the pamoate salt, it is a white, tasteless crystalline substance that is insoluble in water. The drug is administered as an oral suspension from which it is poorly absorbed from the gastrointestinal tract. Its action against intestinal nematodes is independent of its systemic bioavailability. Only about 15% of the administered dose is recovered in urine as a mixture of parent drug and metabolites.

Because of its poor absorption, the drug is well tolerated in both adults and children over 2 years of age. Side effects of pyrantel are limited to transient gastrointestinal pain, headache, fever, and dizziness, although these have not been substantiated through controlled placebo trials. No information is available regarding the safety of pyrantel in pregnancy.

The drug acts as a depolarizing neuromuscular-blocking agent, causing persistent nicotinic activation resulting in spastic paralysis of susceptible nematodes. Pyrantel and piperazine are mutually antagonistic because the latter agent causes hyperpolarization (see later). Thus, these two agents should not be given together. In laboratory animals, intravenously given pyrantel causes complete neuromuscular blockade; thus, this drug cannot be given systemically.

Pyrantel is a drug of second choice after benzimidazoles for treatment of ascariasis, hookworm, and pinworm infections, being effective after a single dose. Notably, however, pyrantel has no activity toward whipworm (trichuriasis). A single dose of oxantel, the *m*-oxyphenol analog of pyrantel, is effective against whipworm. In cases of mixed intestinal nematode infections, the two drugs can be administered simultaneously.

Piperazine. Piperazine is a simple nitrogen heterocyclic compound that is highly effective against both ascariasis and enterobiasis. With the advent of pyrantel and mebendazole, use of piperazine is declining. This is due in part to the fact that piperazine is readily absorbed from the gastrointestinal tract and is thus associated with a greater frequency of mild side effects (nausea, vomiting, diarrhea, headache, and urticaria). Because piperazine has a wide therapeutic range, serious neurotoxicity and hypersensitivity are rarely noted, except at very high doses or in patients with seriously impaired renal function. However, because of its potential for neurotoxicity piperazine is contraindicated in epileptic patients. Piperazine is an acceptable alternative to mebendazole for use in pregnancy.

The major effect of piperazine on nematodes is to produce a flaccid paralysis resulting from hyperpolarization of parasite membranes. The parasites are not killed by the drug but are expelled from the host by normal gut motility. Significantly, expelled parasites are still alive and can recover if incubated in culture medium. The drug appears to block the ability of parasite muscle to respond to acetylcholine.

BLOOD AND TISSUE NEMATODES

Filariasis

There are two type of filarial infections to be considered, both of which are among the more serious and debilitating helminthiases. The first type includes bancroftian filariasis, caused by *Wuchereria bancrofti*, which is transmitted by a mosquito vector. The adult worms live in the lymphatic system, where they cause lymphadenopathy, resulting in swelling of the extremities. It is from this pathology that the common name *elephantiasis* is derived. The parasite offspring or microfilariae circulate in the blood, where they are ingested by the mosquito vector. Brugian filariasis, caused by *Brugia malayi*, is generally similar to bancroftian filariasis in that it is transmitted by mosquito vectors. Adult *B. malayi* parasites also reside in the lymphatic system and produce microfilariae that circulate in the bloodstream. Chemotherapy of these two infections is the same. The second type of filariasis, onchocerciasis, is caused by *Onchocerca volvulus*. It is transmitted by the bite of the *Simulium* black fly that breeds near rapidly moving rivers particularly in West and Central Africa and in South America. The adult worms live in subcutaneous nodules, from which the microfilariae migrate through subcutaneous tissues. Migration of microfilariae to the eye frequently results in ocular lesions and eventual loss of vision; hence, the common name *river blindness.*

Onchocerciasis is transmitted by the bite of the *Simulium* black fly.

Drugs Used to Treat Blood and Tissue Nematodes

Diethylcarbamazine. Diethylcarbamazine, a piperazine derivative, is used as the water-soluble dicitrate salt. The drug is rapidly absorbed after oral administration, with peak plasma concentrations being attained in 1–2 hours. Diethylcarbamazine is a weak organic base. Its renal clearance is dependent on urinary pH. Under acidic conditions (pH 5), greater than 50% of the unchanged drug appears in urine, with an apparent plasma half-life of 2–3 hours. However, alkalinization of urine to pH 8 prolongs the plasma half-life (10–12 hours) and decreases renal clearance of the parent drug such that only about 10% is recovered in urine. The drug does not accumulate in tissues following multiple dosing.

Two types of side effects are associated with diethylcarbamazine administration. The first type is directly related to the drug and is dose-dependent. This includes transient nausea, anorexia, headache, joint pain, and vomiting. Although these are common, they are not too severe and usually do not limit therapy. The other type of side effect results from allergic reactions to dead and dying microfilariae. These reactions (Mazzotti reaction) often appear to be related to the intensity of microfilaremia and can be quite severe in patients harboring *O. volvulus* infections. They consist of papular rash, severe itching, tachycardia, and intense headache. Rapid drug-induced death of *O. volvulus* microfilariae in the eye can result in permanent loss of vision.

Diethylcarbamazine has two principal effects on microfilariae. It leads to decreased muscular activity and eventual paralysis. It also leads to alterations in the parasite surface, rendering microfilariae susceptible to the host's immune system. The molecular sequence of events is unknown.

It is the only agent currently used for both suppression and cure of bancroftian and brugian filariasis. The drug causes the rapid disappearance of microfilariae from peripheral blood, and there is presumptive evidence that it slowly kills the adult worms. The drug has been used extensively for the treatment of onchocerciasis, but owing to the potential severity of Mazzotti reactions and the advent of ivermectin (see later), its use for that disease is declining. Diethylcarbamazine has no activity against adult *O. volvulus.*

Diethylcarbamazine is the only agent currently used for suppression and cure of bancroftian and brugian filariasis.

Ivermectin. Avermectins are complex 16-membered macrocyclic lactones that are fermentation products of the actinomycete *Streptomyces avermitilis* that have proved to be extremely potent, broad-spectrum nematicides (Campbell, 1989). Ivermectin (Fig. 57–1), the 22, 23-dihydro derivative of avermectin B_6, was developed for use in veterinary medicine. It has become the single most widely prescribed veterinary nematicide in the U.S. Several years after its use began, ivermectin was evaluated for treatment of nematode infestations in humans.

Some pharmacokinetic data are available from studies on human vol-

Ivermectin is the most widely prescribed veterinary nematicide in the United States.

Diethylcarbamazine

Figure 57-1

Ivermectin

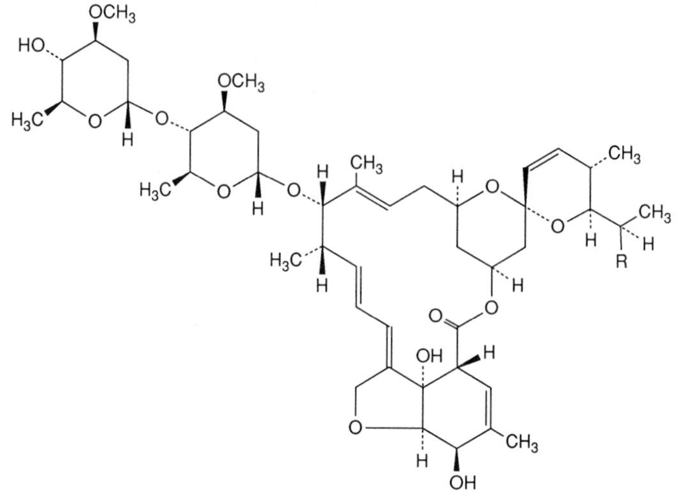

Ivermectin's success can be attributed to its potency and selective toxicity.

Ivermectin is now the drug of choice for treating onchocerciasis.

unteers administered [^{3}H]ivermectin. After oral administration, peak plasma concentration of ivermectin is reached in about 4 hours, but there appears to be some evidence for enterohepatic circulation of the drug. About 50% bioavailability was observed. The plasma half-life of ivermectin was estimated to be about 12 hours. The majority of the drug appears in the feces.

The success of ivermectin as a broad-spectrum anthelmintic is due largely to its potency and selective toxicity. Although the mechanism of action has not been fully elucidated, it is clear that ivermectin produces different effects in nematodes and vertebrates. In target organisms, ivermectin potentiates the release of γ-aminobutyric acid (GABA) from presynaptic inhibitory terminals. There is also a dose-dependent increase in chloride ion permeability. The current model of ivermectin action indicates that the drug affects the GABA receptor–chloride ion channel complex. Although various pharmacological effects can be demonstrated in vertebrate tissues *in vitro*, the concentrations of ivermectin required to produce toxicity in mammals *in vivo* are far in excess of those attained under therapeutic conditions. In addition, because ivermectin does not normally penetrate the blood-brain barrier, it does not affect mammalian GABA-mediated neurotransmission.

After extensive clinical trials, ivermectin was registered for human use in 1986, and it is now the drug of choice for treatment of onchocerciasis. A single oral dose (150 μg/kg) suppresses microfilariae in the skin and eyes and usually prevents disease progression. Ivermectin is not active against adult *O. volvulus*, but it destroys microfilariae in the uterus of the female parasite. Microfilariae eventually reappear, so treatment is optimally repeated at yearly intervals. Dramatic reductions in microfilarial burdens in infected humans also reduce the pool of parasites available to the black fly vector. Thus, it has been predicted by some that the use of ivermectin in endemic areas will eventually reduce transmission of onchocerciasis. In addition to its efficacy against *O. volvulus*, ivermectin is effective against other human nematode infections, including bancroftian filariasis, ascariasis, and trichuriasis. It may soon replace thiabendazole as the drug of choice for treating strongyloidiasis. Paradoxically, the drug displays no efficacy against hookworm infections.

TREMATODE INFECTIONS

Schistosomiasis

Of the various parasitic disease, schistosomiasis, second only to malaria in global importance as a cause of morbidity and mortality, is essentially an infection of rural and agricultural areas in tropical countries where poor sanitation and poor hygiene practices exist. Currently, 73 countries are considered endemic for schistosomiasis. Its life cycle is complicated and involves a specific snail intermediate host. The three major species of schistosome, *Schistosoma mansoni*, *S. japonicum*, and *S. haematobium*, are epidemiologically distinct, with adult worms localized in different anatomical sites in the human host and producing distinct clinical symptoms. The adult female worms produce eggs, some of which pass out of the body in the feces or urine to enter the environment and perpetuate the life cycle. Other eggs become trapped in host tissues, where they elicit a granulomatous response that results in pathology characteristic of this disease.

Schistosomiasis is second to malaria as a cause of morbidity and mortality.

Drugs Used to Treat Trematode Infections

Praziquantel. Praziquantel is a pyrazinoisoquinoline derivative discovered in 1972 and originally developed as a veterinary drug. It has since proved to be one of the primary broad-spectrum anthelmintics for therapy of cestode and trematode infections in humans. The drug is rapidly absorbed after oral administration. Peak plasma concentrations are attained after 1–2 hours. The drug undergoes extensive first-pass clearance in the liver where it is metabolized to a large number of hydroxylated and conjugated products, over 90% of which are excreted in urine. Owing to this first-pass clearance, only traces of the parent drug are detectable in plasma.

Praziquantel was discovered in 1972 and used originally as a veterinary drug.

Praziquantel

Side effects of praziquantel are generally transient and are dose-dependent. Abdominal pain, nausea, headache, and dizziness are the most common symptoms. Occasionally fever and macular eruptions are noted, but nearly half of all patients show no drug-related symptoms. Praziquantel has not been found to be mutagenic, carcinogenic, or teratogenic in extensive animal trials.

Praziquantel has two dose-related effects on susceptible parasites. At low concentrations, it causes increased muscular activity, followed by paralysis. This presumably causes parasites to release their attachment to host tissue. At higher concentrations, the drug causes irreversible vacuolization of the tegument ("blebbing"). This effect seems to make the worms susceptible to the host's immune system. The drug is not directly toxic to the parasite, and it is not metabolized by the target organism. The host's immune system seems to play a crucial role in the ultimate destruction of the parasites. The exact biochemical basis for tegumental vacuolization is still under investigation. The drug does cause increased membrane permeability to Ca^{2+}, and those divalent metal ions are essential for observing drug-induced effects *in vitro*.

Praziquantel is the drug of choice for treatment of all species of human schistosomiasis, and it is approved for that indication in the U.S. It is effective in a single oral dose or in divided doses given on a single day. Because of its broad spectrum of anthelmintic activity, it is also effective against many other trematode and cestode infections, although such indications are considered investigational. Susceptible parasites include the liver flukes *Clonorchis sinensis* and *Opisthorchis* spp. and lung fluke infections caused by *Paragonimus* spp. The drug may not be effective against *Fasciola hepatica*. The basis for this lack of activity is not understood. Prazi-

Praziquantel possesses a broad spectrum of anthelmintic activity.

quantel also is the drug of choice for treatment of the tapeworm infections taeniasis, diphyllobothriasis, and hymenolepsis.

Metrifonate. Metrifonate is an organophosphorus insecticide that is effective against *Schistosoma haematobium* infections only. It has no significant activity against other schistosome species, although the reason for this species specificity is unresolved. Metrifonate is a second choice drug in cases for which praziquantel cannot be obtained. *In vivo,* the drug is hydrolyzed to dichlorvos, a potent organophosphorus inhibitor of acetylcholinesterase. It has been postulated that schistosomal acetylcholinesterase is the target enzyme, but this is inconsistent with the drug's species specificity.

Metrifonate is given orally, and peak plasma concentrations are reached in less than 1 hour. The plasma half-life of metrifonate and dichlorvos is about 1.5 hours. Both compounds are rapidly inactivated by host esterases. The drug does inhibit both plasma and erythrocyte cholinesterases, but activity returns to normal within a few weeks. The drug is well tolerated; side effects include vertigo, nausea, and colic. Patients should not have received depolarizing neuromuscular blockers for at least 2 days before treatment. Metrifonate is contraindicated in pregnant patients and in those who have been recently exposed to organophosphorus insecticides.

Oxamniquine. Oxamniquine is a tetrahydroquinoline derivative that is effective against *Schistosoma mansoni* infections. It is ineffective against *S. japonicum* and *S. haematobium,* but it can be used in combination with metrifonate in cases of mixed *S. mansoni* and *S. haematobium* infections. The reason for oxamniquine's species specificity is unknown. Like metrifonate, it is a second-choice drug after praziquantel. The mechanism of action is thought to involve metabolic activation of the drug within the target organism to an unstable ester metabolite that spontaneously decomposes to give a reactive carbonium ion that in turn alkylates parasite macromolecules. Definitive proof for this mechanism is still lacking. There have been reports of differences in susceptibility between South American and East African strains of *S. mansoni.* There have been at least two confirmed cases of drug-resistant *S. mansoni* in South America, but there is as yet no evidence of widespread drug resistance.

Oxamniquine is given orally and is readily absorbed from the gastrointestinal tract. Absorption is slowed by the presence of food, but the drug is better tolerated after a meal. Most of the administered dose is recovered in the urine as metabolites, which color the urine orange to dark red. A major site of metabolism is the intestine. The product formed is absorbed into the systemic circulation, but this has no antischistosomal activity. Dizziness, drowsiness, nausea, and diarrhea are the most common side effects, but these are transient. Convulsions have been noted in a few individuals with a history of epilepsy. Oxamniquine is contraindicated in pregnancy.

Metrifonate is effective against *S. haematobium* infections only.

Metrifonate

Oxamniquine is effective against *S. mansoni* infections.

Oxamniquine

Oxamniquine is readily absorbed from the GI tract.

DRUGS USED TO TREAT CESTODE INFECTIONS

Taeniasis, Diphyllobothriasis, Hymenolepiasis

Several types of tapeworm infect humans: two species of *Taenia, T. saginata,* the beef tapeworm, and *T. solium,* the pork tapeworm; *Diphyllobothrium latum,* a fish tapeworm; and *Hymenolepis nana,* the dwarf tapeworm that requires no intermediate host. There are essentially two drugs currently available for the treatment of infection with these organisms: niclosamide and praziquantel. One major point needs to be made regarding the choice of drug. In the case of *T. solium* infection, the patient is at risk of developing cysticercosis, the passage of larvae (cysticerci) into the tissue, particularly the brain, orbit, muscle, liver, and lungs. This is a concern only when niclosamide is used, because it kills the adult parasite but not the ova released from gravid proglotids. For this reason, praziquantel is the drug of choice when a definitive parasitological diagnosis cannot be made.

Niclosamide. Niclosamide is a halogenated salicylanilide derivative. It is tasteless and is supplied as chewable tablets. The drug is not appreciably absorbed from the gastrointestinal tract, so it is generally free of significant side effects except for transient and mild gastrointestinal discomfort and nausea. It is safe for use in pregnant women.

The primary action of niclosamide appears to involve inhibition of energy production in parasite mitochondria through inhibition of anaerobic phosphorylation of adenosine diphosphate (ADP). Notably the drug is effective against adult tapeworms, but not against ova.

Niclosamide is indicated for all human tapeworm infections except those caused by *T. solium*, where the risk of cysticercosis exists.

The prevalence of diseases caused by parasitic protozoa is sobering. Over half of the world's population is at risk for malaria; over 150 million new cases occur annually, and at least 1 million infants and young children die from malaria each year in Africa alone. Additionally, the incidence from sexually transmitted parasitic diseases, including vaginal trichomoniasis, amebiasis, and opportunistic protozoans as a consequence of immunosuppression resulting from human immunodeficiency virus (HIV) infection, has increased dramatically since the early 1970s. Although several drugs exist for the treatment of diseases caused by these organisms, the emergence of drug resistance has presented new challenges to chemotherapeutic approaches.

Trichomoniasis

Trichomoniasis, caused by flagellated trophozoites of *Trichomonas vaginalis,* is a sexually transmitted parasitic infection often seen in the U.S. The disease presents as vaginitis in females; male partners are usually asymptomatic but can act as reservoirs for reinfection. Thus, both partners are commonly treated.

Metronidazole. Metronidazole, a 5-nitroimidazole derivative, is the sole drug of choice for treatment of trichomoniasis. The drug is rapidly and completely absorbed after oral administration. The drug is well distributed to various tissues, reaching therapeutic concentrations in vaginal secretions, semen, saliva, breast milk, and the cerebrospinal fluid. There is negligible binding to plasma proteins. Metronidazole is principally cleared in the liver by oxidative metabolism. Both the parent drug and its metabolites are excreted in urine, which may become reddish-brown.

In contrast to its oxidative metabolism in host liver, metronidazole appears to undergo enzymatic reduction of the essential nitro group within susceptible organisms, resulting in formation of chemically reactive metabolites (e.g., nitro radical anions, nitroso- and hydroxylamino- products) that produce secondary biochemical perturbations resulting in cytotoxicity.

Praziquantel is the drug of choice to treat tapeworms if a definitive diagnosis cannot be obtained.

Niclosamide

Niclosamide is effective against adult tapeworms but not against ova.

Protozoan Infections

Trichomoniasis is a sexually transmitted parasitic infection often found in the United States.

Metronidazole is the drug of choice for trichomoniasis.

Metronidazole

One putative target of such reactive intermediates is parasite DNA. There have been some confirmed reports of metronidazole-resistant organisms, but as yet the clinical utility of the drug has not been compromised. The mechanism of drug resistance is unknown, but it may involve mutation of the parasite nitroreductase.

Side effects of metronidazole, which are usually mild, include nausea, anorexia, diarrhea, epigastric pain, and cramping. More serious side effects (numbness in extremities and neurotoxicity) have been reported, but these are rare. Because the drug causes an adverse reaction when ethanol is consumed (disulfiram-like effects), patients should be cautioned to avoid alcohol consumption during treatment. Chronic administration of phenobarbital, which appears to induce enzymes responsible metabolic clearance of metronidazole, can result in subtherapeutic plasma drug concentrations.

Metronidazole, like many nitroheterocyclic drugs, is mutagenic in the Ames test. It also has been reported to be carcinogenic to rats when fed at high doses over many months. Although there is no evidence that metronidazole poses any increased risk to humans when administered at normal therapeutic doses, current wisdom dictates that the drug should not be used indiscriminately. Therefore, the presence of *T. vaginalis* in asymptomatic male partners of symptomatic females should be positively demonstrated before treatment is instituted. Metronidazole has been used during pregnancy, but its use is not recommended during the first trimester.

In addition to its activity against *T. vaginalis*, metronidazole is clinically effective against amebiasis, giardiasis, and a variety of bacterial infections caused by obligate anaerobes.

Amebiasis

Amebiasis is transmitted through fecal-oral contact with *Entamoeba histolytica*.

Amebiasis, caused by *Entamoeba histolytica*, is most prevalent in tropical regions but is also a cosmopolitan infection. Its prevalence in the U.S. is about 2–4% of the general population, and transmission is due to fecal-oral contact with the organism.

Drugs used to treat amebiasis can be classified according to the parasite stage affected. Luminal amebicides are active against intestinal forms (trophozoites) and are used to treat asymptomatic or mild intestinal infections. Diloxanide furoate is the prototypic luminal amebicide. Systemic amebicides are effective against only the pathogenic (invasive) forms of the parasite and are rarely used except for treatment of amebic dysentery or hepatic abscesses. Chloroquine and dehydroemetine are examples of systemic amebicides. Mixed amebicides are active against both intestinal and invasive stages. Metronidazole is the prototype mixed amebicide and has become the drug of choice for treating amebiasis.

Metronidazole is effective against both intestinal and invasive stages of amebiasis.

Diloxanide Furoate. Diloxanide is a dichloroacetamide derivative that is used as the furoate ester to improve efficacy. It is always given orally. The ester is hydrolyzed in the intestine and only diloxanide appears in plasma, from which it is rapidly cleared. The drug is metabolized to the corresponding glucuronide, which is cleared in urine. The drug is well tolerated. Side effects, principally flatulence, vomiting, and diarrhea, are usually mild and transient. Its safety in pregnancy has not been documented.

Diloxanide is directly toxic to *E. histolytica in vitro*, but the mechanism of its amebicidal action is unknown.

Diloxanide furoate is the drug of choice for asymptomatic patients passing trophozoites or cysts. It is ineffective against extraluminal amebiasis, but it can be used in combination with a systemic amebicide or

Diloxanide furoate

metronidazole. In the U.S., the drug is available only from the Parasitic Disease Drug Service, Centers for Disease Control.

Chloroquine. Because chloroquine is highly concentrated in liver, it has been successfully used to treat hepatic amebiasis. Its general lack of efficacy against luminal amebiasis can be attributed to its low concentration in the bowel. A combination of chloroquine and a luminal amebicide has been used successfully to treat both invasive and intestinal amebiasis. With the advent of metronidazole as a mixed amebicide, chloroquine's use has been limited to cases in which metronidazole is contraindicated. Chloroquine is discussed in detail later (see the section on antimalarial drugs).

Chloroquine is successful against hepatic amebiasis.

Dehydroemetine. Dehydroemetine is a less toxic derivative of emetine, an alkaloid derived from ipecac. Both drugs are classic examples of systemic amebicides, but they have largely been replaced by metronidazole.

Metronidazole. Metronidazole has become the drug of choice for all symptomatic cases of amebiasis. It is more effective against systemic than intestinal forms, so it is not used for cases of asymptomatic cyst passers. In those cases, diloxanide furoate is generally recommended. Metronidazole is discussed under Trichomoniasis.

Paromomycin. This aminoglycoside antibiotic is directly amebicidal. Its properties are similar to other aminoglycosides. It is given orally, but it is poorly absorbed from the gastrointestinal tract. Thus, it is effective only against intestinal forms of amebiasis and is classified as a luminal amebicide.

Paromomycin, an aminoglycoside antibiotic, is effective against intestinal forms of amebiasis.

Giardiasis

Giardiasis is the most common intestinal protozoan infection in the U.S. It is caused by *Giardia lamblia*, a flagellate. Infection occurs upon ingestion of cysts from contaminated food or water. No vector or intermediate host is involved, but animals such as dogs and beavers probably act as reservoirs of the infection. Direct transmission also may occur through fecal-oral contact. Although most individuals are asymptomatic, some experience transient or chronic diarrhea with malabsorption.

Giardiasis is the most common intestinal protozoan infection in the United States.

Quinacrine. Quinacrine is an acridine derivative originally developed as an antimalarial agent. It is readily absorbed after oral administration, even in cases of profound diarrhea. The drug accumulates in tissues and is slowly excreted over days to weeks. Its metabolic fate is poorly understood.

The side effects of quinacrine are well known. It often causes vomiting, dizziness, and headaches. Urticaria and exfoliative dermatitis are also common. Other side effects include intense yellow staining of the skin and black staining of the nails. Although quinacrine is the drug of choice for giardiasis in the U.S., its visible side effects make its use less desirable.

Quinacrine

Metronidazole. In other countries, metronidazole is more frequently used for treatment of giardiasis, but use of this drug is considered investigational in the U.S.

Leishmaniasis

Leishmaniasis is caused by four species of *Leishmania* that produce three distinct types of clinical disease. Cutaneous leishmaniasis (Oriental sore) is

There are three types of leishmaniasis: cutaneous, mucocutaneous, and visceral.

due to infection with *L. tropica* or *L. mexicana* and is the least severe form of leishmaniasis. It is usually a self-limiting infection. Mucocutaneous leishmaniasis (espundia), due to infection with *L. braziliensis*, often results in gross disfigurement of the face caused by erosion of the mucocutaneous borders of the mouth, nose, and nasal septum. Visceral leishmaniasis (kala azar) results from infection with *L. donovani* and affects all internal organs, but especially the liver, spleen (with hepatosplenomegaly), and bone marrow. It is the most severe form of leishmaniasis and is usually fatal if not treated. Sandflies (genus *Phlebotomus* or *Lutzomyia*) are the insect vectors of leishmaniasis.

Treatment of leishmaniasis is difficult because few drugs are available and those that are effective are quite toxic. Historically, chemotherapy of leishmaniasis has revolved around the use of heavy-metal poisons, specifically antimony compounds, beginning with antimony potassium tartrate (tartar emetic) and later with trivalent antimonials. Many instances of death have been observed, and the cure was often worse than the disease.

Sodium stibogluconate is a pentavalent antimonial used to treat leishmaniasis.

Sodium stibogluconate

Sodium Stibogluconate. Pentavalent antimonials, although toxic, are safer and more effective and thus have replaced trivalent antimonials as the drugs of choice. Sodium stibogluconate is the most widely used today. In the U.S., it is available through the Parasitic Disease Drug Service, Centers for Disease Control. It is a water-soluble powder that contains 30–40% antimony by weight. The drug is given by either slow intravenous or intramuscular injection. When given intravenously, about 80% of the dose is excreted in the kidneys over the first 6 hours. Another 10–12% of the dose is sequestered in an extravascular compartment from which antimony is very slowly excreted.

Stibogluconate has been incorporated into liposomes from which it is selectively taken up into infected mononuclear cells by phagocytosis. This approach of targeting the drug to the cells of the reticuloendothelial system has proved to be about 300-fold more effective in animal models than the equivalent amount of free drug. Such a formulation allows for a reduction in the severity of toxic side effects, which are of course dose-dependent. Liposome-encapsulated stibogluconate is undergoing phase I clinical trials.

The mechanism of action of sodium stibogluconate is unknown, but antimonials may act by inhibiting parasite enzymes with essential sulfhydryl groups (cysteine residues). Major side effects include pain at the injection site, joint stiffness, and gastrointestinal distress. Renal and hepatic failure have been noted. As with other antimonials, sodium stibogluconate causes other symptoms characteristic of heavy-metal poisons.

Amphotericin B. Amphotericin B, an antifungal polyene antibiotic, has been found to be somewhat effective as an alternative to pentavalent antimonials. However, this drug is likewise associated with a number of untoward effects, including impaired renal function in about 80% of treated individuals (see Chapter 55).

Allopurinol, imipramine, and primaquine are among the drugs currently being tested against leishmaniasis.

Drugs Under Investigation. Several antileishmanial drugs are now being investigated, although it may be several years before any are available for general use (Croft, 1988). They include allopurinol, which is also used for treatment of gout; liposome-encapsulated antidepressants, imipramine and 3-chloroimipramine; and the 8-aminoquinolines (primaquine), which also have antimalarial activity. The Walter Reed Army Institute of Research has examined the structure-activity relationships of a number of 8-aminoquinolines. One compound, WR6062 (an 8-*N*-alkyl derivative), is 400–700-fold more effective against *L. donovani* in a hamster model than the pentavalent antimonials. Like other 8-aminoquinolines, WR6062 causes reversible methemoglobinemia. It has a low therapeutic index, but high potency. WR6062 shows little or no activity *in vitro,* suggesting that it may require biotransformation within the mammalian host. Initial results of phase I clinical trials appear promising.

To avoid systemic drug toxicity, topical formulations are being developed for use against cutaneous leishmaniasis. An ointment containing paromomycin, an aminoglycoside antibiotic, plus methyl benzethionium chloride, a quaternary ammonium compound, given for a period of 10–30 days was used to achieve a >95% cure rate in a cohort of 100 patients. The quaternary ammonium compound acts as a penetration enhancer.

Trypanosomiasis

Two forms of trypanosomiasis affect humans: (1) African trypanosomiasis is transmitted by the tsetse fly and is caused by two subspecies of *Trypanosoma brucei: T. brucei rhodesiense* causes a rapidly progressing and usually fatal form of the disease; *T. brucei gambiense* causes a more chronic form known as *sleeping sickness.* Treatment with several toxic drugs over prolonged times is effective in treating African trypanosomiasis. A major advancement in the treatment of African trypanosomiasis has been approved. (2) American trypanosomiasis, also known as Chagas' disease, is caused by intracellular amastigotes of *T. cruzi.* This disease, which is actually a zoonosis, is transmitted by the bloodfeeding reduviid bugs that live in the mud walls of houses in several countries of South America. Chronic Chagas' disease involves destruction of myocardial cells and neurons of the myenteric plexus. There is no established treatment for *T. cruzi* infections. The circulating forms of the parasite found in acute infection can be suppressed with nitroheterocyclic drugs, notably nifurtimox.

Melarsoprol. Melarsoprol, a trivalent arsenical, is a heavy-metal poison used for treatment of African trypanosomiasis. The drug is administered by slow intravenous injection as a sterile solution in a propylene glycol vehicle. It is crucial that the drug not be allowed to leak into surrounding tissues because irritation and necrosis will result. A low but effective concentration crosses the blood-brain barrier and is thus useful for cases of cerebral infection. Because it is quickly excreted in urine, multiple injections must be given over several days. Cure rates range from 80 to 90%. Melarsoprol has no chemoprophylactic utility.

Arsenicals are nonspecific inhibitors of enzymes with essential sulfhydryl groups (cysteine residues). Thus, the basis for their antiparasitic efficacy is the same as their toxicity to the host. Side effects of melarsoprol therapy are common and frequently severe. They include fever, encephalopathy, and hypersensitivity during repeated courses of therapy. Hemolytic anemia is seen in patients with glucose-6-phosphate dehydrogenase deficiency. Because of its toxicity, melarsoprol should be administered only to hospitalized patients who have individualized therapy. It is available through the Parasitic Disease Drug Service, Centers for Disease Control.

Pentamidine. Pentamidine is an aromatic diamidine derivative that is used as the isethionate salt. It is well absorbed after intramuscular injection. The drug is sequestered in the liver and kidney and is excreted unchanged in the urine over a period of months. Binding to tissues with subsequent slow

African trypanosomiasis is transmitted by the tsetse fly.

Melarsoprol

Melarsoprol has an 80–90% cure rate against African trypanosomiasis.

Pentamidine

release is the basis for its use as a prophylactic agent in African trypanosomiasis. Doses are repeated about every 6 months. Pentamidine does not cross the blood-brain barrier. Consequently, it is of no therapeutic value against cerebral forms of trypanosomiasis.

Use of pentamidine is associated with a number of untoward effects. Intramuscular injection is often accompanied by pain at the injection site. Sterile abscesses can develop. Rapid intravenous administration results in profound hypotension, tachycardia, dizziness, vomiting, and headache that may be the result of drug-induced autacoid release from mast cells. These reactions can be minimized by administering pentamidine by intravenous infusion. Other adverse reactions to pentamidine include rash, abnormal liver function, hypoglycemia that may be fatal, and renal dysfunction. Pentamidine is contraindicated in pregnancy, as it may induce abortion.

> Pentamidine has a number of side effects, including rash, abnormal liver function, and hypoglycemia.

The mechanism of pentamidine's antiprotozoal action is unclear. The parasites accumulate the drug in an energy-dependent process, and drug transport appears reduced in pentamidine-resistant organisms. Intracellularly, it binds to parasite DNA, but a clear link between DNA binding and efficacy has not been established.

Pentamidine is effective for the treatment of several protozoan infections, including African trypanosomiasis caused by *T. brucei gambiense* and pneumonia caused by *Pneumocystis carinii*. Prolonged courses of therapy also have utility for treatment of visceral leishmaniasis caused by *L. donovani*, particularly in cases that are nonresponsive to pentavalent antimonials. Notably, it has no activity against *T. cruzi*.

Suramin. Suramin sodium (Fig. 57–2) was developed in Germany as a derivative of a series of dyes that had antitrypanosomal activity. It is sup-

Figure 57–2

Suramin

plied as a water-soluble, microcrystalline powder that must be freshly prepared and administered parenterally by slow intravenous injection. The plasma concentration of suramin falls rapidly for several hours and then is maintained at a low but therapeutically effective level for up to 3 months. The drug is extensively bound to plasma proteins, which act as a drug reservoir. Thus, suramin has proved to be an effective prophylactic agent against African trypanosomiasis for individuals residing in endemic areas for prolonged periods. The drug is cleared in the kidneys with a renal clearance rate of 0.3 ml/min. It does not undergo appreciable metabolism. Because suramin does not distribute into the central nervous system, it is of little value in treating chronic trypanosomiasis.

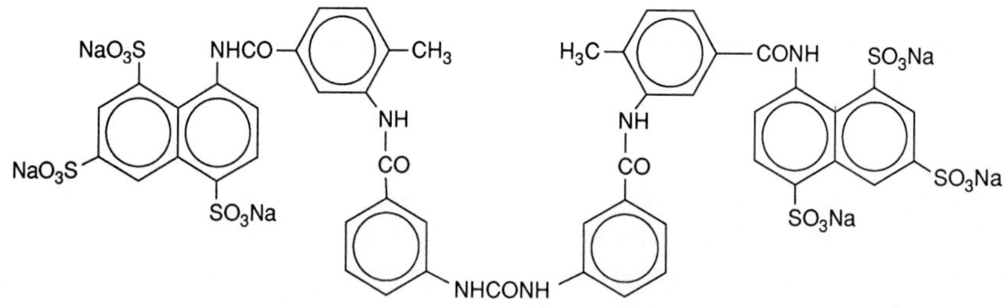

> Suramin does not distribute into the central nervous system; thus it is ineffective in treating chronic trypanosomiasis.

Administration of suramin is associated with a variety of side effects that are exacerbated in debilitated or malnourished patients. Serious immediate reactions include nausea and vomiting, shock, and unconsciousness, although the most commonly observed side effects include malaise and fatigue. Other common symptoms include fever, skin rashes, and neurotoxicity. Albuminuria that may result from drug retention in the kidneys is sometimes seen. The incidence of side effects appears greater in acquired immunodeficiency syndrome (AIDS) patients. Because some patients cannot tolerate suramin, small test doses with attention to untoward effects are given before a full course of therapy.

Suramin is most effective as a prophylactic agent against African trypanosomiasis. However, it is not recommended for short-term travel to endemic areas because of the risk of drug toxicity. Because suramin does not distribute into the central nervous system, it is of little value against cerebral infection. This limits its utility against *T. brucei rhodesiense* because these organisms migrate quickly into the central nervous system. Notably, suramin has no activity against American trypanosomiasis caused by *T. cruzi*. Suramin is the only macrofilaricidal drug available that is effective against adult *Onchocerca volvulus*.

Nifurtimox. Nifurtimox is an example of a nitroheterocyclic drug with antiparasitic efficacy against *T. cruzi*. Specifically, it is a nitrofuran derivative. The drug is given orally and is well absorbed from the gastrointestinal tract. Only small amounts of unchanged drug can be found in plasma and little if any appears in urine. However, high concentrations of metabolites are found, indicating that the drug undergoes high first-pass clearance. It is unclear whether one or more of these metabolites may also be active forms of the drug.

Nifurtimox administration is usually associated with the appearance of side effects that can be numerous. Most are dose-dependent and include nausea, vomiting, and malaise. Long-term therapy increases the incidence of gastrointestinal symptoms and is associated with an increased incidence of peripheral neuropathy. Weight loss is common and sometimes requires cessation of therapy. Hypersensitivity appears in some individuals and ranges from dermatitis to anaphylaxis. The compound also appears to be immunosuppressive. Side effects of nifurtimox are more frequent in adults than in children. Although nifurtimox is clearly a toxic drug, the lack of therapeutic alternatives and the seriousness of Chagas' disease warrant its use.

The mechanism of action of nifurtimox seems to be due to its ability to form free radical intermediates inside the parasite that results from nitroreduction catalyzed by a parasite enzyme. Such intermediates are chemically reactive and also may lead to generation of toxic forms of oxygen such as superoxide radical anion and hydrogen peroxide. *T. cruzi* appears to be deficient in antioxidant enzymes such as catalase and peroxidase.

The only indication for nifurtimox is *T. cruzi* infection. The drug is active against both the trypomastigote and the amastigote forms of *T. cruzi*. Acute Chagas' disease requires daily doses for 75 days. Although nifurtimox is more effective against the acute infection, it does show efficacy against chronic forms, for which therapy must be continued for at least 120 days.

Eflornithine. The most recent advance in the chemotherapy of African trypanosomiasis involves the use of eflorinthine, D,L-α-difluoromethylornithine (DFMO), a structural analog of the amino acid ornithine. Oral administration is associated with diarrhea, nausea, and vomiting plus a significant relapse rate and is not recommended by the World Health

Nifurtimox is a nitrofuran derivative with antiparasitic efficacy against *T. cruzi*.

Nifurtimox

Side effects of nifurtimox occur more frequently in adults than in children.

Eflornithine

Eflornithine is an irreversible inhibitor of ornithine decarboxylase.

Organization. However, these effects are not noted when the drug is administered intravenously in four doses per day over a 2-week period. The drug was registered by the U.S. Food and Drug Administration in late 1990 (World Health Organization, 1990).

Eflornithine is a highly selective, irreversible (suicide) inhibitor of ornithine decarboxylase, the enzyme that catalyzes the metabolism of ornithine to putrescine, the first step of polyamine biosynthesis. Although the physiological role of polyamines has not been entirely elucidated, they appear to function in biosynthesis of DNA, RNA, and proteins. Their concentrations increase markedly in rapidly growing tissues. In trypanosomes, polyamines are also important for formation of a unique cellular nucleophile, trypanothione, which protects the organisms against reactive oxygen species. Thus trypanothione appears to serve the same function as glutathione in other organisms. The basis for the selective toxicity of eflornithine appears to relate to the rate of ornithine decarboxylase turnover in mammalian cells compared with that in trypanosomes. In mammalian cells, the enzyme has a half-life of 20–30 minutes, whereas the half-life is on the order of several days in *T. brucei.* Rapid enzyme synthesis in the host results in a "rescue" from the drug's inhibitory effect on polyamine biosynthesis.

Eflornithine is effective in arousing comatose sleeping sickness patients; hence it has been called the "resurrection drug."

Eflornithine is more effective against *T. brucei gambiense* than against *T. brucei rhodesiense.* Research is being done on a combination of eflornithine with suramin as a more effective treatment for rhodesiense trypanosomiasis. The drug has been found to be particularly effective in arousing comatose sleeping sickness patients who have not responded to conventional therapy. It has thus been called the *resurrection drug* for its ability to help previously doomed patients. In addition to its efficacy against African trypanosomiasis, eflornithine is being used on an experimental basis in AIDS patients with opportunistic *Pneumocystis carinii* infections.

Malaria

Malaria is the most prevalent parasitic infection of humans.

Malaria, the single most prevalent parasitic infection of humans, is caused by four species of *Plasmodium: P. falciparum, P. vivax, P. ovale,* and *P. malariae.* The parasites are transmitted to humans during a blood meal by an infected mosquito vector. The parasites rapidly leave the circulation and localize in hepatic parenchymal tissue, where they multiply to form tissue schizonts. This is the *exoerythrocytic stage* of the infection and is asymptomatic. After a period of 5–16 days depending on the *Plasmodium* species, the tissue schizonts rupture, releasing merozoites into the circulation where they invade red blood cells. Within erythrocytes the asexual reproduction of merozoites takes place, resulting in rupture of infected cells and release of a new phase of infective merozoites, which then infect other red blood cells. This is referred to as the *erythrocytic stage.* The pathology and symptoms of clinical disease are due to the asexual blood forms of malaria parasites, and with the typical cyclical febrile episodes corresponding to bursting of infected erythrocytes. One feature that distinguishes infection with *P. falciparum* or *P. malariae* is that tissue schizonts rupture synchronously, leaving no latent forms in liver. In contrast, *P. vivax* and *P. ovale* schizonts can persist in tissues as hypnozoites, which can result in relapses of clinical attack months or even years after exposure.

Because antimalarial drugs are classified according to the parasite stage affected, an understanding of the life cycles of the various species is important to selecting the appropriate therapy.

Tissue schizonticides include two groups of drugs: (1) Drugs that prevent relapse: These drugs act on the latent form (hypnozoites) in the liver to prevent emergence of merozoites and thus prevent a relapse of clinical disease (erythrocytic stage). Primaquine is a good example of this class. (2) Drugs that are causal prophylactics: Such drugs act on primary tissue schizonts of *P. falciparum* and *P. malariae* to prevent initiation of the erythrocytic stage. Pyrimethamine is used for causal prophylaxis of falciparum malaria.

Blood schizonticides act on the asexual erythrocytic stage to interrupt schizogony and thus terminate clinical attacks. Quinine, chloroquine, and mefloquine are rapid-acting blood schizontocides; slow-acting ones include sulfonamides and pyrimethamine.

Gametocytocides kill sexual erythrocytic stages of the parasite to prevent transmission to the mosquito vector. Quinine and chloroquine are gametocytocidal against *P. vivax* and *P. malariae* but are inactive against *P. falciparum* gametocytes. Primaquine is active against the sexual stages of *P. falciparum*.

Sporonticides interrupt transmission by inhibiting formation of sporozoites within oocysts in the infected mosquito vector. Primaquine, which is primarily active against tissue schizonts, also has activity against the sporozoite stages.

Chloroquine. Chloroquine is the prototype of a class of antimalarial aminoquinoline derivatives. It was developed during World War II and has become the main weapon against human malaria. It is dispensed as chloroquine diphosphate, a water-soluble powder with a bitter taste. A sterile preparation of the hydrochloride salt is available for intramuscular injection. Chloroquine displays high oral bioavailability. Just over 50% of the drug is bound to plasma proteins. Significantly, it is extensively concentrated several hundredfold in tissues, including the liver, spleen, and kidney. As a result of such sequestration, the apparent volume of distribution of chloroquine is very large (100–200 l/kg body weight). About half of the absorbed drug is excreted unchanged in urine. The principal metabolite, the *N*-deethylated product, also may be pharmacologically active. Chloroquine and its major metabolite are slowly excreted in urine. Because chloroquine is a weak base, its renal clearance can be accelerated by acidification of urine.

Chloroquine is generally well tolerated. At therapeutic dosages for acute malarial attacks (25 mg base/kg body weight), gastrointestinal upset, pruritus, transient headaches, and visual disturbances are noted. At the lower dosages used for prophylaxis (5 mg base/kg), few side effects are seen in most individuals. Acute chloroquine toxicity at high doses can manifest as hypotension, lowered myocardial function, vasodilatation, and abnormal electrocardiogram pattern. Long-term high-dose administration (over 250 mg/day) can cause retinopathy. Because chloroquine is so highly concentrated in the liver and kidneys, it should be used with caution in individuals with impaired hepatic or renal function. Patients with neurological disorders usually suffer a greater incidence and intensity of side effects. Chloroquine is safe for use at normal dosages during pregnancy. Its use certainly outweighs the danger of malaria to the mother.

The mechanism of action of chloroquine and its congeners has not been fully elucidated. Because such compounds intercalate with DNA, it was suggested that they interfere with replication. However, such a mechanism is inconsistent with the rapid blood schizonticidal action of chloroquine. More recently, two other mechanisms have gained favor. It has been proposed that the drugs bind to ferriprotoporphyrin IX, a breakdown product of hemoglobin digestion by the malaria parasite. Free ferriprotoporphyrin IX is toxic to cells, causing lysis of both the erythrocyte and the

Tissue schizonticides include drugs that prevent relapse and drugs that cause prophylaxis.

Quinine, chloroquine, and mefloquine are fast-acting blood schizonticides.

Chloroquine has become the main weapon used against human malaria.

Chloroquine

intracellular parasites. The parasite is able to complex this heme product to endogenous binding sites to prevent lysis. Chloroquine binds to ferriprotoporphyrin IX, preventing its sequestration but retaining lytic activity. Another possible mechanism relates to the fact that chloroquine is a weak base. As such it is though to partition into and accumulate within acidic lysosomal compartments within the malaria parasite, where it is thought to inhibit the proteases involved in hemoglobin breakdown. Digestion of hemoglobin by the parasite is essential for its viability.

Chloroquine is not a causal prophylactic and has no effect on tissue schizonts. However, it is a rapid-acting blood schizonticide that is toxic to the asexual blood stage of all *Plasmodium* species. Because it has no action against the latent tissue forms (hypnozoites), it will not produce a radical cure of vivax or ovale malaria. It is effective in terminating acute clinical attacks of malaria. The drug lowers fever within 24–48 hours, and by 48–72 hours after treatment parasites can no longer be found in blood. Chloroquine is used as a suppressive agent against all malarias, except those strains of *P. falciparum* that are chloroquine-resistant. This suppressive use is often, and inaccurately termed, *chloroquine prophylaxis.* Note that chloroquine will not prevent infection by malaria parasites, but it does suppress clinical disease.

In addition to its use against malaria, chloroquine is one agent useful for systemic therapy of amebic liver abscesses (see earlier).

Chloroquine does not prevent infection by malaria parasites, but it suppresses the clinical disease.

Quinine. Quinine, an alkaloid derived from the bark of the cinchona tree found in South America, was the first known antimalarial drug. As early as 1633, the Spanish reported that an extract of the "fever tree" would cure the tertians (malaria). The active agent of this extract was not isolated until 1820. Extensive structure-activity relationship studies have shown that the secondary alcohol group is essential for antimalarial activity. Of the many derivatives of quinine examined, only mefloquine (see later) has proved to be therapeutically useful.

Quinine is the first known antimalarial drug.

Quinine

Quinine and its congeners are normally administered orally and are well absorbed even in patients with severe diarrhea. The drug can be given by intravenous infusion in critical cases of drug-resistant falciparum malaria. Peak plasma concentrations are seen within 1–3 hours. The plasma half-life is about 12 hours. About 70% of the drug is bound to plasma proteins. Only small amounts reach the cerebrospinal fluid, but the drug rapidly passes across the placenta. It is extensively metabolized in liver. Consequently, only 5% of the unchanged drug appears in urine. Renal clearance rate can be doubled by acidification of urine. Unlike chloroquine, quinine does not accumulate in tissues.

Quinine is significantly more toxic than chloroquine. At therapeutic dosage, it produces a spectrum of side effects called *cinchonism,* reminiscent of effects noted when extracts of cinchona bark were used for therapy. These symptoms include tinnitus, vertigo, headache, nausea, and vision impairment that includes blurred vision, photophobia, diplopia, reduce vision fields, and altered color perception. Rare cases of quinine-induced blindness have been reported. The visual and auditory symptoms appear to be manifestations of direct neurotoxicity. At higher doses, a number of organ systems, including the cardiovascular system, skeletal muscle, gastrointestinal tract, and the pancreas, are affected. Some individuals are hypersensitive to quinine and can suffer from drug-induced asthma. Overdoses of quinine can be fatal.

Quinine is more toxic than chloroquine; it produces a variety of side effects.

Despite its pharmacological use for over 170 years, the molecular mechanism of quinine action on malaria parasites remains unclear. Currently, it is assumed that its action is similar to that of chloroquine.

As an antimalarial, quinine is chiefly a blood schizonticide. It has no efficacy against exoerythrocytic forms of plasmodium. It is gametocytocidal for *P. vivax* and *P. malariae*, but not for *P. falciparum.* Because it is substantially more toxic than chloroquine, quinine is not used for suppressive cure but is reserved for treatment of drug-resistant falciparum infections. It is seldom used alone, but it is given in combination with the slower-acting pyrimethamine-sulfadoxine or with a tetracycline.

Mefloquine. Mefloquine, which is structurally related to quinine, is the only new antimalarial agent to be introduced since the 1960s. It is well absorbed after oral administration and is extensively (>70%) bound to plasma proteins. Peak plasma concentrations are reached after a few hours, but the drug has an apparent plasma half-life of 17 days. Mefloquine, like chloroquine, is concentrated in liver and in lungs. Although the drug undergoes some biotransformation, its major route of elimination seems to be in the bile. There is pharmacokinetic evidence to show that mefloquine undergoes extensive enterohepatic and enterogastric circulation. This probably explains its long half-life. Ultimately the drug is excreted in the feces. Only small amounts are recovered in urine.

Unlike quinine, mefloquine is well tolerated. Even after weekly doses of 500 mg for 1 year, no overt toxicity has been observed in adults. Dose-related (>1g) side effects include mild nausea, vomiting, and dizziness. Some instances of depression and disorientation have been noted, but these respond to symptomatic therapy. The drug does not appear to be mutagenic, carcinogenic, or teratogenic. Because of a lack of clinical experience, it is not yet recommended for pregnant women, infants, or children.

Mefloquine has been reported to produce effects in *Plasmodium* parasites that are similar to those of quinine, and it is concentrated within parasites like chloroquine. However, its precise mechanism of action has not been determined.

The only indication for mefloquine is for the treatment and prevention of chloroquine-resistant falciparum malaria. For treatment of acute clinical attacks, it is often given in combination with pyrimethamine-sulfadoxine, but this combination is not recommended for prophylaxis. In the U.S., mefloquine can be obtained from the Parasitic Disease Drug Service, Centers for Disease Control. Unfortunately, isolated instances of mefloquine-resistant falciparum malaria have already been reported.

Primaquine. Primaquine, an 8-aminoquinoline derivative, is reasonably well absorbed after oral administration. It cannot be given parenterally. It is extensively metabolized, so that only a small fraction of the absorbed drug is excreted unchanged. Three major oxidative metabolites of primaquine have been identified that may have some antimalarial activity. The plasma half-life of the parent compound is 3–6 hours, and its apparent volume of distribution is greater than total body water, suggesting some concentration in tissues. Pharmacokinetic studies have shown marked individual variability.

The major side effects of primaquine administration are methemoglobinemia, abdominal pain, and hemolysis in patients with glucose-6-phosphate dehydrogenase deficiency. Methemoglobinemia appears to be due to one or more metabolites of the drug. The possible occurrence of hemolysis must be considered when the drug is administered to blacks and to certain other ethnic groups of the Eastern Mediterranean region where the incidence of genetically inherited glucose-6-phosphate dehydrogenase deficiency is most prevalent.

Primaquine is the only tissue schizonticide currently available for the

Mefloquine

Mefloquine is well tolerated, but because of its limited clinical experience, it is not yet recommended for pregnant women and infants.

Primaquine

Primaquine is the only tissue schizonticide currently available for the cure of *P. vivax* and *P. ovale* infections.

Proguanil

Proguanil, a blood schizonticide, has been advocated by WHO for suppressive cure in areas where chloroquine resistance is prevalent.

Pyrimethamine

Pyrimethamine is an inhibitor of dihydrofolate reductase.

radical cure of *P. vivax* and *P. ovale* infections. It also is highly active against the primary tissue schizonts of *P. falciparum,* although this activity is of little therapeutic value owing to the rapidity with which falciparum progresses to clinical (erythrocytic) disease. The drug also is gametocytocidal toward all four *Plasmodium* species. Its usefulness it offset by its toxicity and the need for treatment over several days. The mechanism of antimalarial action is unknown.

Proguanil. Proguanil, also called chloroguanide, is a biguanide compound developed as an antimalarial agent during World War II. It can be administered orally as the hydrochloride salt. Proguanil is slowly absorbed from the gastrointestinal tract. Peak plasma concentrations are attained in about 4–6 hours. The apparent plasma half-life is about 18 hours. The drug is moderately bound (75%) to plasma proteins. As its name implies, proguanil is a prodrug. It is metabolized to *p*-chlorophenylbiguanide (10–25%), which is inactive, and undergoes cyclization to form a triazine ring compound (cycloguanil, 30–35%), which is the active drug form. Cycloguanil acts as an inhibitor of plasmodial dihydrofolate reductase. Dihydrofolate reductase catalyzes the reduction of dihydrofolate to tetrahydrofolate, an essential precursor for the synthesis of purines, pyrimidines, and certain amino acids.

Proguanil is classified as a blood schizonticide. Its use was suspended some time ago with the advent of more effective antifolates and because of appearance of drug resistance. More recently, however, its use has been advocated by the World Health Organization for suppressive cure (chemoprophylaxis) in areas where chloroquine resistance is prevalent. The drug is well tolerated at the recommended dose (200 mg/day). Transient nausea and diarrhea are sometimes observed. It has been used safely in infants and children at reduced doses (e.g., 100 mg/day for children 1–5 years old). Proguanil is considered safe for use during pregnancy.

Pyrimethamine. Pyrimethamine is a 2,4-diaminopyrimidine derivative. The drug is slowly but completely absorbed after oral administration. It displays an apparent elimination half-life of about 4 days because it accumulates in several tissues, most notably the kidneys, liver, and spleen. The drug is metabolized to a number of unidentified metabolites, which are excreted in urine.

Toxicity at therapeutic dosages of pyrimethamine usually presents as a mild skin rash and depression of hematopoiesis. Prolonged administration can produce a reversible megaloblastic anemia, similar to that resulting from folic acid deficiency. Although the use of antifolates is generally contraindicated during pregnancy, the combination of pyrimethamine-sulfadoxine (FANSIDAR) has been used for chemoprophylaxis over long periods of time with no apparent effect on the fetus. The danger of contracting malaria during pregnancy usually outweighs any possible drug risk.

Like other 2,4-diaminopyrimidines (trimethoprim), pyrimethamine is an inhibitor of dihydrofolate reductase. Its selective toxicity toward *Plasmodium* parasites relates to the fact that the plasmodium dihydrofolate reductase is much more sensitive to inhibition than is the mammalian enzyme. Because of the synergism between 2,4-diaminopyrimidines and sulfonamides or sulfones, structural analogs of *p*-aminobenzoic acid that inhibit the biosynthesis of dihydropteroic acid, pyrimethamine is always used in combination with sulfadoxine, a sulfonamide with a long plasma half-life (7–9 days). This combination preparation is known as FANSIDAR. Pyrimethamine also has been combined with sulfadiazine. In addition to reducing the dose of each drug required, the emergence of drug resistance is greatly reduced by the use of this combination of drugs.

The major uses of pyrimethamine-sulfadoxine are in chemoprophylaxis, for suppressive cure of vivax malaria, and in combined chemotherapy with quinine for treatment of clinical attacks of chloroquine-resistant falciparum malaria. The suppressive cure of vivax malaria requires treatment for at least 10 weeks after a patient leaves the endemic area. Such therapy is not always successful.

Resistance to Antimalarial Drugs. The first case of chloroquine-resistant falciparum malaria was reported in 1959. Since then, there has been a dramatic increase in both the incidence and the geographical distribution of drug-resistant strains of *P. falciparum.* Acquired drug resistance has been reported in virtually every area in which falciparum malaria is endemic. Drug resistance has become the most important threat to effective control of this deadly form of malaria. It has arisen largely through a combination of massive antimalarial drug use (especially chloroquine for prophylaxis and suppression) and a failure to successfully block transmission of the infection, which is due in part to extensive migration of populations. The widespread use of antifolate drugs, especially pyrimethamine-sulfadoxine combination (FANSIDAR), in areas of chloroquine resistance has resulted in the emergence of multidrug-resistant strains. These infections must now be treated with the older, more toxic drug, quinine. However, because quinine and chloroquine are similar in action, resistance is now developing to quinine as well. The biochemical basis of drug resistance may relate to the parasite's ability to rapidly excrete chloroquine, preventing its accumulation (Krogstad et al, 1987).

> Drug resistance is a major threat to controlling falciparum malaria.

Therapy of Malaria. For treatment of an acute attack of malaria, chloroquine is the drug of choice, except for chloroquine-resistant strains of *P. falciparum.* In those cases, quinine is used in combination with the slower-acting pyrimethamine-sulfadoxine combination. Recrudescence of a falciparum attack after treatment with chloroquine is indicative of drug resistance; quinine should be given immediately. Similarly, quinine should be given to a traveler returning from a region of chloroquine resistance if malaria is suspected. In endemic areas, chloroquine remains the drug of choice for prophylaxis and control of malaria other than falciparum (especially *P. vivax*). In areas of chloroquine resistance, pyrimethamine-sulfadoxine is the recommended prophylaxis. Be aware that resistance to these antifolates is increasing quickly. Radical cure of vivax malaria with primaquine can be achieved after the patient has left the endemic area. Recurrent attacks of vivax and ovale malaria are usually controlled with chloroquine combined with primaquine. The new antimalarial drug mefloquine is available for treatment of chloroquine- and multidrug-resistant falciparum malaria. Because it is the only drug available for treatment of multidrug-resistant falciparum malaria, its use should be restricted to drug-resistant strains. There have been alarming reports that resistance to mefloquine is already developing. A single tablet, triple combination (250 mg mefloquine, 25 mg pyrimethamine, and 500 mg sulfadoxine) has been tested as well, but the combination has proved to be too toxic for prophylactic use. Its use will be limited to cases of falciparum malaria that are both chloroquine- and quinine-resistant. Because the recommended therapy for malaria may change dramatically in the near future, physicians should contact the Malaria Branch, Center for Infectious Disease, Centers for Disease Control, for current information.

> Reports indicating resistance to mefloquine have been recorded.

References

Campbell WC (ed): Ivermectin and Abamectin. New York: Springer-Verlag, 1989.

Cook GC: Use of benzimidazole chemotherapy in human helminthiases: Indications and efficacy. Parasitol Today 6:133–136, 1990.

Croft SL: (1988). Recent development in the chemotherapy of leishmaniasis. Trends Pharmacol Sci 9:376–381, 1988.

Krogstad DJ, Gluzman IY, Kyle DE, et al: Efflux of chloroquine from Plasmodium falciparum: Mechanism of chloroquine resistance. Science 238:1283–1285, 1987.

Lacey E: Mode of action of benzimidazoles. Parasitol Today 6:112–115, 1990.

Roos MH: The molecular nature of benzimidazole resistance in helminths. Parasitol Today 6:125–127, 1990.

World Health Organization: "Resurrection" drug approved. TDR News 34:1–2, 1990.

Cancer Chemotherapy

Antineoplastic Drugs

58

Joseph R. Bertino

The modern era of cancer chemotherapy began after World War II with the introduction of nitrogen mustard, an alkylating agent developed for clinical use as a consequence of the hematopoietic toxicity encountered with sulfur mustard (a war gas) and aminopterin, a folate antagonist. These compounds produced dramatic remissions in patients with lymphoma and in children with acute lymphocytic leukemia. Unfortunately, cures were not obtained because of the rapid development of drug resistance, a problem that has been noted with single agent treatment of each new drug introduced into the clinic.

These encouraging results were followed by a vigorous anticancer drug development program, especially in the United States, and were fostered by support and screening facilities provided by the National Cancer Institute for academic and industrial researchers. Since this time, over 30 drugs have been approved for use for the treatment of patients with malignancies. Based on principles derived mainly from treatment of rodent tumors, combination regimens have been devised that cure a majority of patients with choriocarcinoma; testicular cancer; acute lymphocytic leukemia; certain childhood solid tumors; and several types of lymphoma that include Hodgkin's disease, large cell lymphoma, and Burkitt's lymphoma.

Cure is also obtained with combination treatment in patients with other tumors, e.g., ovarian cancer and acute myelocytic leukemia, but these cure rates are only in the range of 10–20%. Other diseases are less susceptible to treatment with chemotherapeutic drugs, although effective palliation and prolongation of survival may be obtained in some.

Another important use of chemotherapy that has evolved over the past 20 years is in the adjuvant situation. In this circumstance drugs are administered either before (neoadjuvant) definitive treatment (surgery or x-ray treatment) or following definitive treatment. Encouraging results have been obtained in patients with breast cancer and, more recently, in patients with colon cancer treated in this manner.

Dose Is Important. Studies in experimental tumors have clearly established that optimal antitumor effects occur when dosages used are the highest achievable, consistent with host tolerance. In more recent years the term *dose intensity* has been employed to define the amount of drug delivered per unit time, usually in milligrams per square meter per week. For certain drugs, such as alkylating agents that are not very schedule dependent, dose intensity delivered directly relates to treatment outcome. In most

Sulfur mustard and aminopterin were found to kill human white blood cells.

A number of tumors can now be cured.

Principles of Chemotherapy

High dosages of drug are most effective.

941

tumors in which cure is possible, this issue becomes a critical one, and less than optimal dosing may result in treatment failure.

In most human tumors that are curable by combination chemotherapy, there is a certain subset of patients, usually with advanced, bulky tumors, that are not effectively treated by these programs. The possibility of curing even this subset of patients by increasing dose intensity using autologous marrow rescue or hemotopoietic growth factors (G-CSF, GM-CSF, IL3, and so forth) is under active investigation in many centers. Preliminary results in chemotherapy-sensitive tumors (lymphoma, acute leukemia, testicular cancer) are encouraging. This approach is also being attempted for patients with other malignancies not usually cured by chemotherapy (e.g., breast cancer, low grade lymphoma). It is too early to tell if this aggressive treatment policy will benefit these patients.

Combination chemotherapy avoids drug resistance.

Combination Chemotherapy Is Necessary for Optimal Results. As mentioned earlier, drug resistance occurs rapidly when treatment with a single drug is used. The introduction of combination chemotherapy for acute lymphocytic leukemia (ALL) and Hodgkin's disease in the 1960s was an outgrowth of experimental studies that showed that combination of effective drugs gave additive cell kill and delayed or prevented drug resistance. Drugs are used in combination when the dose-limiting toxicity of one drug is nonoverlapping with the other, and if evidence has been obtained in experimental tumors that the combination gives additive or synergistic antitumor effects. When two drugs are combined that both have bone marrow suppression as the limiting toxicity, it is usually possible to use each drug at two thirds of the optimal dose without increasing toxicity. If both drugs are equally effective, then the combination increases dose intensity by 1.5 times. There may also be important reasons to sequence the use of drugs in combination, especially if one drug is used to modulate or increase the activity of a second drug. An example is the methotrexate-5-fluorouracil sequence used to treat colorectal carcinoma. An increase in the response rate was noted when methotrexate administration preceded fluorouracil treatment by 24 hours, as compared to the results obtained when both drugs were administered together.

Sequence of administration of drugs in combination can be important.

The disadvantage of combination chemotherapy is that the assumption is that both (or more than two) drugs are equally effective. If they are not, less tumor cell kill may result, because the dose of the most effective drug is decreased. When toxicity occurs, it may be difficult to adjust subsequent drug doses, because the major offending agent may not be known.

During more recent years, the idea of using alternating cycles of chemotherapy of two or more drug combinations has been tested in the clinic. This concept derived from theoretical modeling that showed that drug-resistant cells were less likely to survive alternating drug combinations as compared with repeated dosing with a fixed drug combination. Another approach now under investigation is the sequential use of combinations: the first combination is used until a maximal response is obtained (usually several months), followed by treatment with several courses of the second combination. The second combination is used at the time when there are theoretically only few drug-resistant cells remaining. If there is no cross-resistance to the drugs of the first combination, the second combination treatment may eradicate cells surviving the treatment with the first combination.

DRUG RESISTANCE

As mentioned, the major obstacle to cure with chemotherapeutic agents is survival and proliferation of cells that are resistant to further treatment. A great deal has been learned in the past 15 years of the genetic mechanisms that cause cells to become resistant to various drugs. There is often more than one resistant mechanism that may allow a cell to survive increasing concentrations of a drug. When resistance occurs after a tumor population has been initially susceptible, this is called *acquired resistance.* Some tumors may not be responsive initially to a drug, i.e., they are intrinsically resistant. Presumably, this difference reflects the number of cells in the population that are resistant. When there is good tumor regression (i.e., complete responses) to treatment, the frequency of mutant cells that have a resistant phenotype may be low (1 in 10^6). In tumor populations naturally resistant to a drug (i.e., no or minimal tumor regression), a substantial number of tumor cells may have a resistant phenotype ($> 10\%$).

An important new development in the understanding of drug resistance has been the elucidation of a type of resistance called *multidrug resistance (MDR).* MDR may be acquired or intrinsic in tumors; its importance derives from the finding that resistance to any one of several drugs (usually alkaloids — vinca alkaloids, anthracyclines, etoposide, actinomycin D) results in cross-resistance to all of the other drugs that share this phenotype. The basis of this form of resistance is the presence of a protein (P-glycoprotein, gP-170) that is capable of causing rapid efflux of MDR-type drugs, thus protecting the cells from damage by preventing these drugs from reaching their intracellular targets.

Resistance to drugs allows cancer cells to survive.

Tumors can become resistant to more than one drug—multidrug resistance.

CYCLE-ACTIVE AGENTS AND NONCYCLE-ACTIVE AGENTS

Cycle-active agents are drugs that require a cell to be "in cycle," i.e., actively going through the cell cycle preparatory to cell division to be cytotoxic. Some of these drugs are effective primarily against cells in one of the phases of the cell cycle (e.g., G_1, S, G_2, or M). The importance of this designation is that cell cycle-active agents are usually schedule-dependent, and that duration of exposure is as important and usually more important than dose. In contrast, noncell cycle–active agents are usually not schedule-dependent, and effects depend on the total dose administered, regardless of the schedule. Alkylating agents are generally considered to be noncycle active, whereas antimetabolites are prototypes of cycle-active compounds.

THE FUTURE OF CHEMOTHERAPY

Optimal use of these agents requires a thorough knowledge of chemotherapy principles, the mechanism of action, pharmacology (pharmacokinetics and risk/benefit). Many of these drugs have both acute and long-term toxicities. Efforts to reduce these toxicities have followed two major avenues: developing analogs that have less of these toxicities, or decreasing toxicity by the use of other agents. Progress has been made in both directions, and less toxic analogs of cisplatin (carboplatin) and doxorubicin (mitoxantrone) are examples of the first approach, whereas development of antinausea medication (e.g., metoclopramide) and protective agents (e.g., mesna for ifosfamide toxicity) are examples of the second approach.

Our knowledge of the role of oncogenes (growth factors) in normal and abnormal growth, as well as the role of the immune system in controlling abnormal cell growth, has markedly increased, and the 1990s will see the introduction into the clinic of new types of treatment that may be more selective and possibly less toxic. Because this field is investigational, and except for α interferon, no products have been approved for use yet, they are not discussed further in this chapter.

Antineoplastic Agents

Methotrexate is useful for choriocarcinoma and other tumors.

Methotrexate inhibits dihydrofolate reductase.

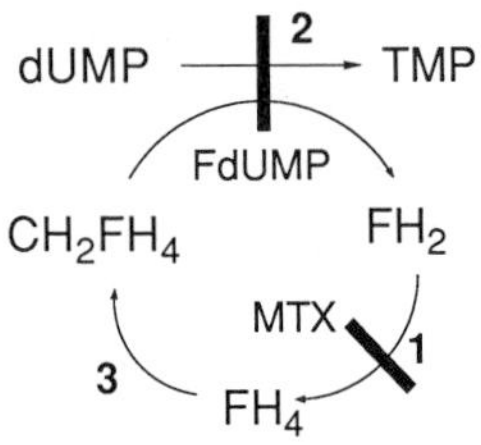

Figure 58–1

Sites of action of methotrexate (MTX) and the fluoropyrimidine antimetabolite, fluorodeoxyuridylate (FdUMP): (1) DHFR, dihydrofolate reductase; (2) TS, thymidylate synthase; (3) SHM, serine hydroxymethylate; FH_2, dihydrofolate; FH_4, tetrahydrofolate; CH_2FH_4, N^5, N^{10}-methylene-tetrahydrofolate.

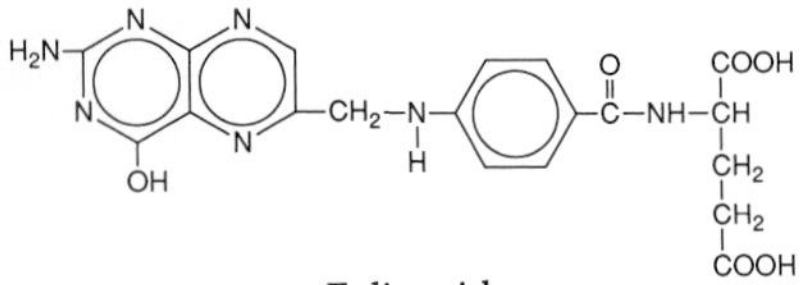

Folic acid

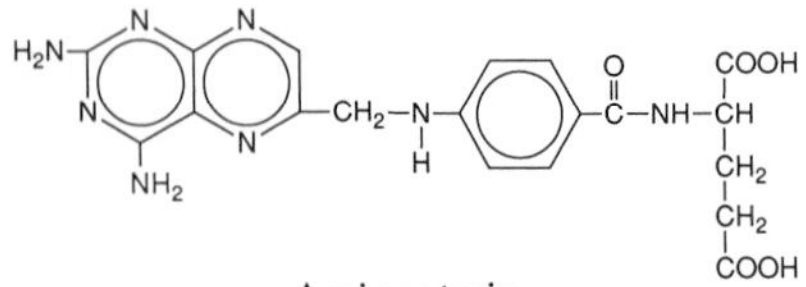

Aminopterin

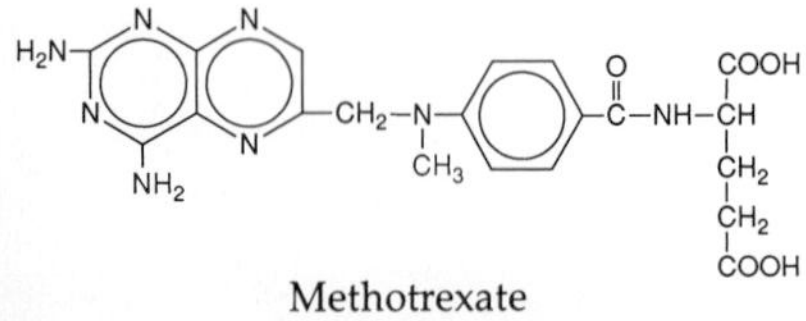

Methotrexate

CELL CYCLE–ACTIVE AGENTS

Methotrexate

The folate antagonist aminopterin was the first antimetabolite shown to induce complete remissions in children with ALL. Unfortunately, it was soon appreciated by Farber and his associates that these remissions were short-lived, and the patients' leukemia became resistant to subsequent courses of this drug. In the 1950s, methotrexate (amethopterin, MTX) supplanted aminopterin in the clinic, based on experimental studies showing that it had an improved therapeutic index as compared with aminopterin. MTX continues to be a key drug in the treatment of choriocarcinoma and in combination therapy of intermediate-grade and high-grade lymphomas, breast cancer, head and neck cancer, and bladder cancer.

MECHANISM OF ACTION. Methotrexate and aminopterin are analogs of the vitamin folic acid. The major mechanism of action of MTX is to powerfully inhibit the enzyme dihydrofolate reductase (DHFR) (Fig. 58–1). As a consequence of this inhibition, intracellular folate coenzymes are rapidly depleted (by blocking uptake of reduced folates, restoration of folate stores is also impaired). Because folate coenzymes are required for thymidylate biosynthesis as well as purine biosynthesis, DNA synthesis is blocked, and cell replication stops. More recent work has shown that MTX is retained in certain cells for long periods of time, as a consequence of an enzymatic process that adds additional glutamates (up to 5) to the antifolate. This may be an important determinant of MTX selectively, because cells capable of this conversion (e.g., lymphoblasts) may be expected to be more susceptible to cell kill by this drug.

Acquired resistance to MTX in patients with leukemia has been shown to be due to increased levels of dihydrofolate reductase as a consequence of gene amplification, defective polyglutamylation, and possibly impaired uptake of this drug. Alterations of DHFR enzyme leading to decreased binding of MTX have also been reported.

CLINICAL PHARMACOLOGY. MTX is reasonably well absorbed by mouth when administered in low dosages (5–10 mg), but when doses exceed 30 mg, progressively less of the drug is absorbed, with significant interpatient variation. Therefore, doses of MTX of 30 mg or greater should be administered intravenously (IV), intramuscularly (IM), or subcutaneously.

MTX is excreted primarily unchanged by the kidney (half-life for the β phase is 3–4 hours), although with larger doses, a significant amount of the drug (7–30%) is inactivated by hydroxylation at the 7 position (7-OH MTX). Thus, patients with renal impairment should not be treated with MTX, because the prolonged blood levels that may result may lead to increased hematological and gastrointestinal (GI) toxicity. When renal toxicity occurs following MTX treatment, leucovorin should be administered until blood levels of MTX decrease to nontoxic levels. High dose MTX (>0.5 g/sq m) is used to treat patients with osteosarcoma, diffuse lymphoma, or ALL with folinic acid (N^5-formyltetrahydrofolate leucovorin) rescue. In this circumstance, renal toxicity, which may result from precipitation of this drug (or its metabolite 7-OH MTX) in the renal tubules, may be prevented by alkalization of the urine and diuresis. Both MTX and 7-OH MTX are organic acids, which, like uric acid, are much more soluble in alkaline urine.

ADVERSE EFFECTS. The dose-limiting toxicities to MTX are myelosuppression and GI toxicity. Both thrombocytopoenia and leukopenia may be produced by methotrexate in toxic doses; the latter is more common. An early sign of MTX toxicity to the GI tract is mucositis, involving the oral mucosa. Severe toxicity may be manifested by diarrhea, which is due to small bowel damage that can progress to ulceration and bleeding.

Less common toxic effects caused by MTX are skin rash (10%), pleuritis, and chemical hepatitis. The latter is reversible in most patients, but low-dose chronic administration may lead to fibrosis and cirrhosis of the liver in a small percentage of patients. Renal toxicity is uncommon with conventional doses or more, but it has been a problem with high-dose regimens in adults. As noted earlier, alkalization and hydration, as well as monitoring MTX serum levels, are important prophylactic measures to avoid and detect this potential problem.

Methotrexate causes myelosuppression and GI toxicity.

Fluoropyrimidines (5-fluorouracil and 5-fluorodeoxyuridine)

HISTORY. 5-fluorouracil (5-FU) was developed by Heidelberger and others as a consequence of the observation that uracil was salvaged more efficiently by certain malignant cells than by normal tissues.

5-FU is metabolized to 5-FdUMP, the active molecule.

MECHANISM OF ACTION. 5-FU exerts its cytotoxic effects by inhibition of DNA synthesis, or by incorporation into RNA, thus inhibiting RNA processing and function. The active metabolite of 5-FU that inhibits DNA synthesis through potent inhibition of thymidylate synthase is 5-fluoro-deoxyuridylate (5-FdUMP) (see Fig. 58–1).

5-FdUMP inhibits thymidylate synthase.

In rapidly growing tumors, inhibition of thymidylate synthetase appears to be the key mechanism of cell death caused by 5-FU; however, in other tumors, cell death is better correlated with incorporation of 5-FU into RNA. Incorporation of 5-FU into DNA can occur also and may contribute to 5-FU cytotoxicity.

MODULATION OF 5-FU ACTION. The ternary complex formed by FdUMP and the folate coenzyme, N^5, N^{10}-methylene tetrahydrofolate with thymidylate synthase has been noted to dissociate slowly, with a half-life of several hours. The presence of excess folate coenzyme ensures maximal ternary complex formation and, in addition, retards the dissociation of FdUMP from the complex. Based on this understanding, clinical trials have employed high doses of leucovorin, a stable reduced folate precursor of N^5, N^{10}-methyltetrahydrofolate, followed by 5-FU treatment, in the hope of maximizing ternary complex formation in malignant cells, and subsequent cell death. MTX pretreatment may also increase 5-FU cytotoxicity by increasing phosphoribosylpyrophosphate (PRPP) levels in cells, thus increasing 5-FU nucleotide formation. Increased PRPP levels are a consequence of the ability of MTX to inhibit purine biosynthesis. In addition, inhibition of dihydrofolate reductase by MTX leads to an increase in dihydrofolate polyglutamates in cells, a folate that also enhances FdUMP binding to thymidylate synthetase. Sequential MTX–5-FU treatment has led to an increase in response rate in certain solid tumors, notably colon cancer.

Other strategies to modulate 5-FU cytotoxicity are also being tested in the clinic; these include pretreatment with the *de novo* pyrimidine synthesis inhibitor phosphonacetyl-L-aspartate (PALA), the use of dipyridamole, an inhibitor of nucleoside salvage, and uridine "rescue."

CLINICAL PHARMACOLOGY. 5-FU is absorbed erratically after oral administration and, therefore, is administered IV. The drug has a short plasma

Uracil

5-fluorouracil

5-fluorodeoxyuridine

half-life (10–15 minutes), and after a pulse dose with conventional doses (600 mg/sq m), cytotoxic levels ($> 1~\mu M$) are maintained in blood for only 6 hours or less. Various dosage schedules of 5-FU have been investigated, including bolus treatment daily for 5 days once a month, weekly bolus treatment, and infusions of FU lasting 24, 48, and 120 hours or longer. When infusions of 5-FU are administered, the major toxicity is GI, whereas bolus treatment usually produces leukopenia and thrombocytopenia as limiting toxicity. The drug distributes freely into third spaces (e.g., cerebrospinal fluid, ascites). Metabolism occurs mainly in the liver to dihydrofluorouracil, and further breakdown products fluoroureidoproprionic acid and CO_2. Because of its metabolism by liver, 5-FU has been infused also into the hepatic artery or administered intraperitoneally; this method achieves high local concentrations, with decreased systemic toxicity. 5-FUdR is even more rapidly metabolized by the liver than is 5-FU, and intrahepatic artery administration of this drug is used to treat isolated hepatic metastases from colon cancer.

ADVERSE EFFECTS. The major limiting toxicities of 5-FU and 5-FUdR are marrow toxicity and GI toxicity. Stomatitis and diarrhea usually occur 4–7 days after treatment. Further treatment should be withheld until recovery occurs. The nadir of leukopenia and of thrombocytopenia usually occurs 7–10 days after a single dose of a 5-day course of the drug, and recovery usually takes place by day 21. The dose-limiting toxicity to infusions of 5-FUdR through the hepatic artery is transient liver toxicity, occasionally resulting in biliary sclerosis.

Less common toxicities noted with 5-FU after systemic administration are skin rash, cerebellar symptoms (with single pulse dosages greater than 800 mg/sq m), and conjunctivitis and tearing. Myocardial infarction has been reported also in association with 5-FU administration.

THERAPEUTIC USES. 5-FU and 5-FUdR have antitumor activity against several solid tumors, most notably colon cancer, breast cancer, and head and neck cancer. A preparation containing 5-FU is used topically to treat skin hyperkeratosis and superficial basal cell carcinomas.

Cytosine Arabinoside

Cytosine arabinoside (ara-C) is an antimetabolite analog of deoxycytidine. In the analog, the OH group is in the β configuration at the 2' position. This compound was first isolated from the sponge *Cryptothethya crypta*. Ara-C is the drug of choice for the treatment of acute myelocytic leukemia (AML). When used together with an anthracycline, remissions may be achieved in 60–80% of patients with this disease.

There is some evidence that high dosages (1–3 g/sq m) of cytosine arabinoside given at 12-hour intervals for 6–12 dosages may be more effective alone or in a combination with anthracyclines than conventional doses (100–300 mg/sq m) in the treatment of AML; these high dose regimens are currently being evaluated. This drug has also been used to treat ALL, lymphoma, and the blast crisis of CML, but its exact role in the treatment of these malignancies is less well defined.

MECHANISM OF ACTION. Cytosine arabinoside is converted intracellularly to the nucleotide triphosphate (ara-CTP); this latter compound is both an inhibitor of DNA polymerase and incorporated into DNA. The latter event is considered to cause the lethal action of ara-C, because incorporation results in a defect in ligation of newly synthesized fragments of DNA.

5-FU exhibits marrow and GI toxicity.

Deoxycytidine   Cytosine arabinoside
(1-β-D-arabinosylcytosine)

Ara-C is used for acute myelocytic leukemia.

Ara-C is metabolized to ara-CTP, the active molecule.

Ara-CTP inhibits DNA polymerase and is incorporated into DNA.

Ara-C and its mononucleotide are inactivated by two intracellular enzymes, cytidine deaminase and deoxycytidylate deaminase.

Although several mechanisms for acquired resistance to ara-C have been elucidated in experimental tumor systems, an explanation for acquired resistance in leukemia cells of patients is still not clear. Deletion of deoxycytidine kinase, an increased pool size of CTP, and increased activity of cytidine deaminase have been described to occur in ara-C resistant cell lines. The level of intracellular ara-CTP formation after dosing has been reported to be useful in monitoring drug efficiency.

CLINICAL PHARMACOLOGY. Ara-C is administered IV as a pulse dose or a continuous infusion. It is not active by mouth because of degradation by cytidine deaminase present in GI epithelium and in the liver. The drug distributes rapidly into body water, and unlike many drugs, a high concentration (50% of the plasma level) may be reached in the cerebrospinal fluid (CSF) 2 hours after IV administration. Most of the drug is excreted in the urine in the form of the inactive metabolite, ara-U. As in the case of MTX, single bolus infusions (over 0.5–1 hour) of dosages as high as 5 g/sq m produce little marrow toxicity because of its rapid clearance, whereas dosages of 1 g/sq m over 48 hours produce severe marrow toxicity.

Ara-C disappears rapidly from plasma with a half-life of 7–20 minutes. With higher dosages, a longer half-life is found, presumably because of ara-U inhibition of metabolism of ara-C. Ara-U formation occurs in plasma, liver, granulocytes, and other tissues of the body.

ADVERSE REACTIONS. In conventional dosages (100–200 mg/sq m day for 5–10 days), the dose-limiting toxicity of ara-C is myelosuppression. Some nausea and vomiting are seen with this dosage, which increases markedly when high dosages are employed, although repeated administration of the drug results in some tolerance. Leukopenia and thrombocytopenia nadirs occur at about day 10, and marrow injury is rapidly reversible. In addition to increased nausea and vomiting noted with high dosages of ara-C, neurological, GI, and liver toxicity has been observed when high dose regimens are used. The severity of these effects increases with increasing duration of therapy. High dosages (2–3 g/sq m) given every 12 hours for a total of 6 dosages may be as effective as 12 dosages, and lower dosages of ara-C (0.5–1 g/sq m) given over 2 hours every 12 hours may be as effective as higher dosages.

Intrathecal ara-C is usually well tolerated, but neurological side effects have been reported (seizures, alterations in mental status).

Ara-C causes myelosuppression.

Purine Analogs (6-mercaptopurine and 6-thioguanine)

The purine analogs, 6-mercaptopurine (6-MP) and 6-thioguanine (6-TG), introduced into the clinic soon after methotrexate, are also key drugs in the curability of ALL. Other important purine analogs have also found a use in the clinic, including azathioprine, a 6-mercaptopurine "pro drug" that is a potent immunosuppressive agent; allopurinol, an inhibitor of xanthine oxidase, useful in the prevention of uric acid nephropathy; and antiviral compounds such as ara-adenine. Deoxycoformycin, a potent inhibitor of adenosine deaminase, has also been found to be a useful agent in the treatment of T-cell malignancies. This compound, as well as 2-chlorodeoxyadenosine, has impressive activity in the treatment of a rare type of chronic leukemia (hairy cell leukemia).

6-mercaptopurine

6-thioguanine

Azathioprine

2'-deoxycoformycin

6-MP and 6-TG are converted to their nucleotides, the active molecules.

MECHANISM OF ACTION OF 6-THIOPURINES. Both 6-MP and 6-TG have a thiol group substitution for the 6 oxo or hydroxyl group found in hypoxanthine or guanine, respectively. Both compounds are converted to nucleotides by the enzyme hypoxanthine-guanine phosphoribosyl transferase (HPRT). Despite considerable investigation, the exact mechanism whereby these analogs exert their cytotoxic effects is not known. *De novo* purine synthesis is blocked by the 6-thiopurine nucleotide (phosphoribosyl transferase), as well as the conversion of purine analogs. The nucleotides of both these drugs are also incorporated into DNA after conversion to the triphosphates. This incorporation may also contribute to the cytotoxic effects of the thiopurines.

In experimental tumor cells, resistance is most commonly found to be a consequence of markedly decreased activity of the activating enzyme HPRT. In human ALL, resistance was found to be associated with an increase in activity of alkaline phosphatase, found in membranes, and capable of degrading the nucleotides of the 6-thiopurines. Absence of HPRT activity was a rare cause of resistance in AML; an alteration of this enzyme leading to decreased thiopurine binding to the enzyme was found in the blast cells of some patients.

CLINICAL PHARMACOLOGY. Both 6-TG and 6-MP are administered orally, although absorption may be erratic. These drugs differ in their catabolism, and as a consequence, metabolism of 6-MP, but not 6-TG, is inhibited by allopurinol. 6-MP is metabolized primarily by xanthine oxidase to 6-thiouric acid, which is inhibited by allopurinol, whereas 6-TG is principally methylated, followed eventually by oxidation and elimination of the sulfur moiety. Therefore, a dosage reduction of 6-MP of 75% is recommended when allopurinol is used with this drug; no dose reduction is necessary when 6-TG and allopurinol are administered together. Another difference between these two drugs is GI toxicity; 6-TG causes less nausea and vomiting than 6-MP, presumably because of metabolism of this latter drug by the GI mucosa.

6-MP and 6-TG cause myelosuppression.

ADVERSE REACTIONS. Except for less GI toxicity to 6-TG as compared with 6-MP, both drugs have equivalent toxicity to the bone marrow, the dose-limiting toxicity. Mild hepatotoxicity may be noted after treatment with either of these compounds but is rapidly reversible. Long-term treatment with 6-MP has been implicated as a cause of cirrhosis in some children with leukemia on long-term therapy with this drug.

Hydroxyurea

Hydroxyurea inhibits ribonucleotide reductase.

Hydroxyurea is an inhibitor of ribonucleotide reductase, the enzyme that converts ribonucleotides at the diphosphate level to deoxyribonucleotides. Although not an antimetabolite in the true sense, i.e., it is not a substrate analog, it is a cell-cycle agent that acts in S phase. Hydroxyurea has resurfaced as an excellent drug for the treatment of chronic myelocytic leukemia (CML) and appears to be equally effective as busulfan, with potentially less toxicity. Hydroxyurea has also been used to lower the blast count rapidly during the blast crisis of CML and in patients with ALL.

Hydroxyurea is used for CML and ALL.

Resistance to hydroxyurea occurs in experimental tumors as a consequence of an increase in ribonucleotide reductase activity or an alteration of this activity leading to decreased binding to the active site of the enzyme.

CLINICAL PHARMACOLOGY. Hydroxyurea is administered orally, because it is well absorbed, even in large doses. After oral administration, plasma levels reach a maximum after 1 hour. Plasma levels fall rapidly subsequently, with renal excretion the major route of elimination.

ADVERSE REACTIONS. The major toxicity of hydroxyurea is bone marrow suppression, primarily leukopenia. Little other toxicity has been observed with this drug, even when large doses are administered. Hydroxyurea, like cytosine arabinoside, is an S-phase specific drug, and single large doses have little toxicity. The white blood cell count (WBC) nadir occurs 6–7 days after a single dose of drug, and the WBC recovers rapidly.

The Vinca Alkaloids

Of the three vinca alkaloids tested extensively in the 1970s and 1980s—vinblastine, vincristine, and vindesine—only the former two are now available for use in the United States. These drugs are used widely in the treatment of hematological neoplasms: vinblastine because of its excellent activity in the treatment of Hodgkin's disease, and vincristine for its broad spectrum of activity in non-Hodgkin's as well as Hodgkin's disease.

Vinca alkaloids are used for treatment of Hodgkin's disease and non-Hodgkin's lymphoma.

MECHANISM OF ACTION. The vinca alkaloids exert their cytotoxic action through binding to tubulin, a dimeric protein found in the cytoplasm of cells. Microtubules are essential for forming the spindle along which the chromosomes migrate during mitosis, and for maintaining cell structure. Binding of the vinca alkaloids to tubulin leads to inhibition of the process of assembly and dissolution of the mitotic spindle. As a consequence, cells are arrested in metaphase, although some studies indicate that cell kill also occurs in late S phase.

Vinca alkaloids cause metaphase arrest by binding to tubulin.

As mentioned, resistance to the vinca alkaloids has been shown in experimental cells to be associated with other drugs sharing the MDR phenotype and related to increased efflux of these drugs. Studies in progress in several laboratories may answer the question regarding the importance of this resistance mechanism in human tumor cells.

CLINICAL PHARMACOLOGY. Both vincristine and vinblastine are administered IV. The average dosage of vincristine is 1.4 mg/sq m compared with 8–9 mg/sq m of vinblastine, usually repeated at weekly or biweekly intervals. At these doses, peak plasma concentrations of approximately 1.4 μM are achieved. After a rapid distribution phase, vincristine disappears from the plasma with half-lives of 7.4 and 164 minutes. Vinblastine half-lives are 4.5 and 53 minutes, with a terminal half-life of 20 hours. Almost 70% of a dose of vincristine is metabolized by the liver and excreted in the feces. Metabolism of vinblastine is also the major route of inactivation of this drug, but details of the site of metabolism and metabolic products are lacking. Most investigators reduce the dose of vincristine or vinblastine in patients with hepatic impairment, although information on this subject is not complete. A 50% decrease in dose is recommended for patients with a bilirubin greater than 3 mg/dl, whereas no decrease in dose is advocated for impaired renal function.

	R
Vincristine	HC=O
Vinblastine	CH₃

ADVERSE REACTIONS. The dose-limiting toxicity to vincristine is neurotoxicity, which usually begins when the total dose exceeds 6 mg/sq m. The initial signs of neurotoxicity are parasthesia of the fingers and lower extremities, and loss of deep tendon reflexes. Continued use may lead to more advanced neurotoxicity, which includes profound weakness of motor strength, in particular of dorsiflexing the foot, and extensors of the wrists. Occasionally, cranial nerve palsies and severe jaw pain are noted with

Vincristine causes neurotoxicity.

vincristine administration. At high dosages of vincristine (>3 mg total single dose), autonomic neuropathy may be noted, leading to obstipation and paralytic ileus. Sensory changes and reflex abnormalities slowly improve off treatment; however, motor impairment improves less rapidly and may be irreversible. In addition to these commonly observed toxicities, inappropriate antidiuretic hormone (ADH) release is seen occasionally, resulting in symptomatic dilutional hyponatremia.

Although marrow suppression is not commonly noted with vincristine, some marrow toxicity may be noted in patients with marrow hypoplasia as a consequence of treatment with other drugs. The primary toxicity of vinblastine is leukopenia, which reaches a nadir at day 6–7 and is rapidly reversible. Therefore, the major site of action of vinblastine appears to be on a committed myeloid progenitor cell. Mucositis is occasionally observed with vinblastine at higher dosages (>8 mg/sq m) or when used in combination with drugs that also have the potential for this toxic effect. Neurotoxicity is rarely observed at conventional doses with vinblastine. Both drugs will cause severe pain and local toxicity if extravasated. Neither drug should be given intrathecally, because deaths have been reported from vincristine administered inadvertently into the CSF.

Epipodophyllotoxins

Two glycosidic semisynthetic derivatives of podophyllotoxin have received extensive clinical trials, and one of these, etoposide (VP-16), is now available in the pharmacy. This drug has significant clinical activity in Hodgkin's disease, diffuse aggressive lymphomas, leukemias, testicular cancer, and in small cell lung cancer. VM-26, the other podophyllotoxin in clinical use, but still experimental, has been used primarily to treat children with ALL; the combination of VM-26 and cytotosine arabinoside appears to be especially effective and may be a synergistic drug combination.

MECHANISM OF ACTION. The mechanism of action of these compounds is not clear; induction of single stranded breaks in DNA has been demonstrated in cells. One mechanism of resistance to etoposide in some cell lines is by increased expression of the P-glycoprotein found in the multidrug resistance (MDR) phenotype.

CLINICAL PHARMACOLOGY. Etoposide may be administered either orally or IV. The usual dose schedule for etoposide is 100–120 mg/sq m/day for 3 days, either consecutively or every other day. When administered orally, about 50% of the dose is absorbed; therefore, the dose should be increased twofold over the IV dosage.

After a single IV dose, the plasma half-levels are 2.8 and 15.1 hours. Approximately one half of the dosage is excreted in the urine; of this, one third is a metabolite. The remainder of the drug is excreted in the feces and further metabolized by the liver.

ADVERSE EFFECTS. When administered IV, both etoposide and VM-26 should be infused over a 30-minute period to avoid hypotensive episodes. The major toxicity of both these drugs is leukopenia, which is rapidly reversible. Thrombocytopenia may also occur, but it is much less common. Nausea and vomiting are common with IV drug administration. Alopecia may occur with both drugs, whereas other toxicities, such as fever, mild elevation of liver tests, or peripheral neuropathy, are relatively uncommon. Because the major toxicity of etoposide is limited to the marrow, this drug is under extensive investigation in high dose regimens followed by marrow transplantation.

Vinblastine causes leukopenia.

Etoposide has activity against Hodgkin's disease, lymphomas, leukemias, and testicular cancer.

Podophyllotoxin

R = CH₃ Etoposide (VP-16)

R = Teniposide (VM-26)

DRUGS THAT DAMAGE DNA

All the classes of drugs that are discussed in this section damage DNA by various mechanisms. Although the major mechanism of cytotoxicity is believed to occur as a consequence of this interaction, these agents usually have other sites of action and often react with other cellular targets, e.g., membranes. The classes of drugs that are discussed are alkylating agents, nitrosoureas, platinum compounds, and natural products or their derivatives, which include the anthracyclines, bleomycin, and actinomycin D.

The DNA-damaging agents are all capable of producing long-term toxicities because of their mutagenic properties. These are an increased risk of malignancy (usually acute leukemia 3–7 years after treatment) and gonadal damage that leads to infertility. They also are all potent inhibitors of bone marrow cell proliferation, and this is usually their dose-limiting toxicity.

> DNA-damaging agents all inhibit bone marrow cell proliferation. They also can cause second tumors and infertility.

The Alkylating Agents

These drugs are important in the treatment of malignancies, either as single agents or as components of effective combination regimens. In combination they may eradicate noncycling cells not killed by the cycle-active components of the treatment, and there appears to be little or no cross-resistance of alkylating agents with other classes of drugs. In this regard, it is of importance that some work has shown that a cell resistant to one alkylating agent may not be resistant to other alkylating agents. This has led to renewed interest in combinations of these agents, especially in preparative regimens for autologous bone marrow transplantation.

Nitrogen Mustards. The major cytotoxic and mutagenic effects of these agents are believed to result from their interactions with DNA. Alkylating agents are able to form positively charged carbonium ions, which react with nucleophilic groups, such as SH, PO_4, and NH_3, on nucleic acids, proteins, and smaller molecules. The N^7 atom of guanine is particularly susceptible to alkylation and is believed to be the major lesion in DNA. As a consequence of alkylation of DNA, cell damage may occur from single-strand breakage and cross-linking of DNA, thus interfering with cell division.

> Alkylating agents attack guanine residues in DNA, resulting in cross-linking of the DNA.

There are several drugs now on the market that are derivatives of the parent compound mechlorethamine.

Mechlorethamine (Mustagen). This nitrogen mustard is the most rapidly acting of this group of compounds and must be freshly prepared and administered into a rapidly flowing IV. If extravasated, it can cause severe local tissue damage.

This agent enters cells through a transport system in place for choline, and resistance to this drug has been attributed to a decrease in its uptake.

Cl—CH₂CH₂\
⟍\
N—CH₃\
⟋\
Cl—CH₂CH₂

Mechlorethamine (nitrogen mustard)

CLINICAL PHARMACOLOGY. This compound is administered IV, but may also be used intrapleurally for the control of effusions. It disappears rapidly from plasma. Its clinical use has been limited to the treatment of Hodgkin's disease, in which it is a component of MOPP (mechlorethamine, Oncovin® [vincristine], procarbazine, prednisone) chemotherapy. It is used topically to treat patients with mycosis fungoides, a T-cell lymphoma of skin.

> Nitrogen mustard is used for Hodgkin's disease.

ADVERSE REACTIONS. Like other alkylating agents, the dose-limiting toxicity to mechlorethamine is myelosuppression that may cause leukopenia and

Nitrogen mustard can cause local tissue damage as well as severe nausea and vomiting.

Cl—CH₂CH₂
Cl—CH₂CH₂
N—P=O
H
N
O

Cyclophosphamide

Cyclophosphamide must be activated by the P-450 system in the liver.

Cyclophosphamide has a wide spectrum of action.

Cyclophosphamide causes alopecia and hemorrhagic cystitis.

Cl—CH₂CH₂—N
Cl—CH₂CH₂—P=O
O

Ifosfamide

Ifosfamide must be activated by the P-450 system in the liver.

Dose-limiting toxicity, unlike most of the other DNA-damaging agents, is bladder toxicity. Mesna helps to control this.

thrombocytopenia, sometimes of several weeks' duration. Local tissue reactions due to extravasation should be treated immediately with administration of sodium thiosulfate and application of ice. Mechlorethamine also causes severe nausea and vomiting that occurs within the first hour or two after drug administration.

The major long-term toxicities of this drug, as with all alkylating agents, are gonadal damage, often leading to infertility, and an increased risk of secondary malignancies, in particular acute leukemia.

Cyclophosphamide. This nitrogen mustard was synthesized based on the rationale that it would be specifically cleaved and activated by tumor cells that contained an enzyme capable of cleaving the N-P bond in the molecule. Thus, the drug is relatively inert until activated by bond cleavage and may be administered orally. However, it is activated by the P-450 system in liver as well as in tumors; therefore, the basis of its selectivity is not clear.

PHARMACOLOGY. The half-life after IV administration is 6–7 hours. With time, the toxic metabolites phosphoramide mustard and acrolein are generated; the former compound is believed to be important in antitumor effects, and the latter compound responsible for bladder toxicity. After oral administration, peak levels are achieved in 1 hour.

CLINICAL USE. Cyclophosphamide, unlike nitrogen mustard, has a wide spectrum of antitumor and immunosuppressive activity. It is used as part of combination therapy regimens to treat lymphoma, breast cancer, bladder cancer, small cell lung cancer, ovarian cancer, and various childhood malignancies. It is used widely in high dose regimens with autologous marrow replacement to treat refractory lymphoma.

ADVERSE EFFECTS. Cyclophosphamide differs in certain ways from other nitrogen mustards. It is relatively "platelet sparing," i.e., there is less thrombocytopenia observed with this drug compared with other alkylating agents; there is more alopecia (hair loss); and sterile hemorrhagic cystitis is seen in 5–10% of patients treated with high doses unless vigorous hydration and bladder emptying are employed. Long-term toxicity that includes sterility and carcinogenesis is also noted with this agent.

Ifosfamide. This compound has been approved for use in the United States. It differs from cyclophosphamide only in the location of a chlorethyl moiety.

MECHANISM OF ACTION AND CLINICAL PHARMACOLOGY. Activation of ifosfamide, like cyclophosphamide, also occurs predominantly in liver by the P-450 mixed function oxidase system. Ifosforamide mustard, the active compound, is generated. Acrolein and chloroacetic acid are the principal toxic metabolites. The plasma disappearance of ifosfamide is slightly longer than cyclophosphamide, and some of the compound is excreted unchanged in the urine.

ADVERSE REACTIONS. The dose-limiting toxicity of this drug is bladder toxicity, presumably due to accumulation of acrolein and chloroacetic acid in the bladder. Dose fractionation and vigorous hydration with diuretics will decrease this toxic effect. Mesna, a thiol that is excreted in the urine, is now used routinely in ifosfamide-containing regimens because of its ability to inactivate the toxic metabolites of ifosfamide in the bladder. Mesna is generally well tolerated but may cause some nausea and vomiting. The nausea and vomiting produced by ifosfamide are less than that observed with large doses of cyclophosphamide, as is the degree of myelosuppression. Central nervous system (CNS) toxicity is occasionally seen in patients treated with high doses of ifosfamide/mesna and is manifested by changes in mental status, cerebellar dysfunction, and even seizures.

CLINICAL USE. Ifosfamide, like cyclophosphamide, has a broad spectrum of activity. Antitumor effects are seen in patients with lymphomas, ovarian cancer, testicular cancer, and in various solid tumors. Its role in combination therapy is still under investigation.

Phenylalanine Mustard. The rationale for synthesis of phenylalanine mustard (melphalan) was based on the premise that certain tumors, in particular myeloma and melanoma, might preferentially accumulate compounds that were analogs of phenylalanine or tyrosine.

CLINICAL PHARMACOLOGY. Phenylalanine mustard is well absorbed orally and, unlike mechlorethamine, reacts slowly with nucleophiles. It enters cells through the L-amino acid transport system through an active transport process. The half-life of this drug administered orally is approximately 90 minutes, and 10–15% is excreted unchanged in the urine.

CLINICAL USE. The major use of this agent has been in the treatment of multiple myeloma, usually in combination with prednisone. It has also been used to treat breast cancer and melanoma, but it has been supplanted by other drugs in the treatment of these diseases.

ADVERSE EFFECTS. Nausea and vomiting are infrequent with this agent, as is hair loss. The major toxicities are similar to those of other alkylating agents: marrow suppression and similar late effects.

Chlorambucil. Chlorambucil, like melphalan, is a slow-acting nitrogen mustard. It was synthesized with the hope that it would penetrate tumor tissue readily and slowly react with DNA.

PHARMACOLOGY. This drug is administered orally, and it is absorbed well. It is metabolized completely, and little or no free drug is found in the urine.

CLINICAL USE. Chlorambucil is used primarily to treat patients with chronic lymphocytic leukemia and low-grade lymphomas, in particular, follicular lymphomas and Waldenstrom's lymphoma.

ADVERSE REACTIONS. Chlorambucil is well tolerated, and usually does not cause nausea or vomiting. Its cytotoxicity is similar to phenylalanine mustard.

Ethylenimines and Methyl Melamines

- *Triethylenemelamine* (TEM). This compound was first synthesized by chemists for use in industry. Because of the ethylenimine group in its structure and the recognition that it was an alkylating agent, it was studied as an anticancer drug. Currently it is not used in the clinic except for the treatment of retinoblastoma.
- *Thio-TEPA.* This compound was introduced into the clinic in 1953. There has been a resurgence of interest in this compound for use in autologous marrow transplant regimens.
- *Hexamethylmelamine.* This drug has activity in ovarian cancer when used in combination.

Melphalan

Chlorambucil

Chlorambucil is used for chronic lymphocytic leukemia and lymphomas.

TEM is used for retinoblastoma.

Thio-TEPA

Busulfan

BCNU

CCNU

Methyl CCNU

BCNU and CCNU are used for lymphomas and brain tumors.

Alkylsulfonates. Structure activity studies with this group of drugs showed that the optimal length of the methylene bridge for activity and the highest therapeutic index was $n = 4-5$. Busulfan causes predominantly myelosuppression, with little other pharmacological action. It is used exclusively to treat chronic myelocytic leukemia.

PHARMACOLOGY. This agent is well absorbed orally, and virtually 100% is excreted in the urine as methane sulfonic acid.

ADVERSE EFFECTS. The drug has some unusual side effects in addition to its myelosuppressive activity. It may cause generalized skin pigmentation, gynecomastia, and pulmonary fibrosis.

The Nitrosoureas

Carmustine and Lomustine

HISTORY. Carmustine (BCNU, bischloroethylnitrosourea) was the first of the nitrosourea compounds in clinical trial to receive extensive clinical evaluation. An unusual feature of these highly reactive compounds is their lipid solubility and, thus, their ability to cross the blood-brain barrier.

Lomustine (CCNU, 1-(2-chlorethyl)-3-cyclohexyl-1-nitrosourea) is similar to carmustine in its mechanism of action and clinical activity. It is administered orally and is rapidly absorbed and biotransformed.

MECHANISM OF ACTION. The nitrosoureas, in particular carmustine and lomustine, have been extensively studied in animal tumor models and in the clinic. The nitrosoureas show some degree of cross-resistance with other alkylating agents, and more recent studies indicate that these compounds are primarily alkylating agents. A base-catalyzed decomposition of these compounds generates the alkylating chlorethyldiazonium hydroxide entity.

CLINICAL PHARMACOLOGY. After IV administration, carmustine disappears from plasma with an initial half-life of 6 minutes and a half-life β of 68 minutes.

TOXICITY. The nitrosoureas, like other alkylating agents, are potent bone marrow toxins. However, the hematopoietic depression produced by the nitrosoureas occurs later than that seen with other alkylating agents. Leukocyte and platelet nadirs occur 4–5 weeks after drug administration. Thus, the nitrosoureas appear to damage a primitive stem cell. The late marrow depression and cumulative toxicity make these drugs difficult to use clinically. Nausea and vomiting occur frequently with the nitrosoureas. Nephrotoxicity may also result from nitrosourea treatment. Both drugs may produce hepatotoxicity; this side effect is less common with lomustine. A large adjuvant study of lomustine with 5-FU by the GI cancer group has shown that treatment with this combination was associated with an increased incidence of acute leukemia, presumably attributable to the nitrosourea.

THERAPEUTIC USES. Nitrosoureas have a reasonably broad spectrum of activity; currently, they are used in the treatment of lymphoma as well as certain solid tumors, in particular brain tumors. Their use in the treatment of GI cancer has been diminishing.

Streptozocin

INTRODUCTION. Streptozocin is a nitrosourea that has been in clinical trial since 1967.

MECHANISM OF ACTION AND CLINICAL PHARMACOLOGY. Like the other nitrosoureas, this drug functions as an alkylating agent. The plasma half-life is short (35 minutes), and the drug is excreted in the urine as metabolites. This drug selectively destroys β islet cells of the pancreas and causes diabetes in animals.

Streptozocin

ADVERSE EFFECTS. Unlike carmustine and lomustine, the dose-limiting side effect of streptozocin is nephrotoxicity. Diabetes is not seen in humans, but mild glucose intolerance may occur as a result of its use. Similar to the other nitrosoureas, nausea and vomiting may be severe. Unlike carmustine and lomustine, little or no bone marrow depression is seen with this drug, thus allowing it to be used in combinations.

CLINICAL USE. The major use for streptozocin is in the treatment of carcinoid and islet cell tumors. It has also been used in combinations to treat Hodgkin's disease and colon cancer, but its contribution to the antitumor effects seen is not well defined.

Platinum Compounds

Cisplatin

HISTORY. Cisplatin (diamino-dichloro-platinum, DDP) is a platinum coordination complex that has broad-spectrum antitumor activity in humans. The story of its discovery is one of serendipity and the prepared scientific mind.

CIS-P (II) (cisplatin)

Dr. I. Rosenberg noted that in experiments with bacteria, a toxic substance was being produced by platinum electrodes. He found this material to be the platinum coordination complex, cisdiaminodichloroplatinum. He subsequently investigated its cytotoxic effects on bacteria as well as mammalian tumor cells. These results prompted a clinical trial in humans, and despite some antitumor activity in early Phase I trials, further trials were stopped because of renal toxicity. The drug was then found to be relatively safe when administered with forced hydration.

MECHANISM OF ACTION. Cisplatin is a reactive molecule and is able to form inter- and intrastrand links with DNA to cross-link proteins with DNA.

Cisplatin cross-links DNA.

Drug-resistant cell lines have been produced, and resistance has been attributed to various mechanisms, including decreased uptake, an increase in repair of DNA lesions, and an increase of the metal-binding protein metallothionine.

CLINICAL PHARMACOLOGY. Cisplatin is administered IV with forced hydration. Following drug administration, the drug is rapidly bound to protein and persists in serum for long periods of time, with only 20–40% excreted in the urine within the first few days following drug administration. High concentrations of platinum, as measured by atomic absorption, persist in liver, intestines, and kidney.

ADVERSE EFFECTS. The dose-limiting toxicity of cisplatin is nephrotoxicity due to tubular injury. This complication may be largely, but not completely,

Cisplatin causes kidney damage.

avoided by vigorous hydration before and after cisplatin administration. The use of 3% sodium chloride may allow for even higher doses to be safely administered, because chloride ion may decrease activation of this compound and renal injury. Hypomagnesemia may also result from tubular damage.

Severe nausea and vomiting are noted with this drug; only more recently has antiemetic therapy been shown to control this problem. Myelosuppression is not a major problem, although anemia has been noted frequently in patients receiving multiple courses of this drug. Neurotoxicity is a problem with patients receiving multiple courses; this includes peripheral neuropathy and ototoxicity, especially high frequency hearing loss. Rarely, Ig-mediated hypersensitivity reactions have occurred.

Cisplatin is used for a variety of solid tumors. Its use in combination with other agents results in a synergistic effect.

THERAPEUTIC USES. Cisplatin has significant antitumor effects in ovarian, testicular, lung, and head and neck carcinomas. Of great importance is the ability of cisplatin, when used in combination, to give additive or synergistic activity. The use of cisplatin with vinblastine and bleomycin, or more recently with etoposide, has led to a high cure rate (77%) in patients with advanced testicular cancer. In combination with cyclophosphamide, it is the treatment of choice in the treatment of ovarian cancer, leading to a high response rate (70%), and some cures (about 10%). Cisplatin and 5-FU infusions also are highly effective in causing tumor regressions in patients with squamous cell carcinoma of the head and neck, although the remissions produced are only temporary.

CBDCA (carboplatin)

Carboplatin. This platinum complex has been approved by the FDA for the treatment of ovarian cancer. It has the same mechanism of action as cisplatin, and there is some cross-resistance between it and cisplatin. A major advantage of carboplatin over cisplatin is its lack of nephrotoxicity; it may be administered without the need for hydration. The limiting toxicity is bone marrow depression.

Triazenes

Dacarbazine

Although dacarbazine (DTIC, ditriazenoimidazolecarboxamide) is structurally similar to the purine precursor 5-aminoimidazole-4-carboxamide, this compound acts primarily as an alkylating agent.

Dacarbazine and procarbazine require activation by the liver's P-450 system.

MECHANISM OF ACTION AND CLINICAL PHARMACOLOGY. Dacarbazine is activated by the hepatic cytochrome P-450 system, and an alkylating moiety is generated. The half-time for excretion is about 5 hours, and the drug is excreted in the urine, about half as unchanged drug and the rest as metabolites.

Dacarbazine

ADVERSE REACTIONS. Severe nausea and vomiting occur with therapeutic dosages of this drug. Myelosuppression is uncommon with the usual dosages but occasionally can be severe. Other toxic effects are a flu-like syndrome and facial flushing. Hepatotoxicity has occasionally been noted. Dacarbazine may cause severe pain and tissue necrosis if infiltration occurs.

Dacarbazine is used in combination to treat Hodgkin's disease.

CLINICAL USE. Dacarbazine is used in combination with doxorubicin, bleomycin, and vinblastine to treat Hodgkin's disease (ABVD), and is also used to treat soft tissue sarcoma and malignant melanoma.

Procarbazine. This drug appears to require activation by the P-450 cytochrome system in liver to produce several active metabolites that produce effects on DNA similar to that of classic alkylating agents.

CLINICAL PHARMACOLOGY AND ADVERSE EFFECTS. Procarbazine is administered orally and is well absorbed. The drug equilibrates rapidly between plasma and CSF. The half-life of the parent compound is 10 minutes, and the drug is excreted mainly in the urine in the form of metabolites. Nausea and vomiting commonly occur with the use of this drug, but tolerance develops to this side effect rapidly. The major toxic effect is myelosuppression that is dose-related. Foods with a high tyramine content may precipitate a reaction that includes severe headache, because this drug is a weak monoamine oxidase inhibitor. Interaction with sympathomimetic amines, tricyclic antidepressants, and alcohol have also been reported. Neurotoxicities that include dizziness, ataxia, paresthesia, headache, insomnia, and nightmares have also been reported, especially in patients receiving CNS drugs.

CLINICAL USE. The major indication for procarbazine use is in the MOPP regimen for the treatment of Hodgkin's disease. Procarbazine also has activity in other neoplasms, including non-Hodgkin's lymphoma, lung cancer, and brain tumors.

Procarbazine is used in the MOPP regimen.

ANTITUMOR ANTIBIOTICS

Anthracyclines

The three anthracyclines approved for clinical use are doxorubicin, daunorubicin, and mitoxantrone. The former two compounds are alkaloids produced by various *Streptomyces* species, whereas mitoxantrone is a synthetic compound, not containing a sugar moiety. Doxorubicin is a drug with a broad spectrum of activity *versus* neoplastic disease and is an important drug in the treatment of hematological malignancies, especially ALL, Hodgkin's disease, and the non-Hodgkin's lymphomas. Daunomycin is used almost exclusively in the treatment of AML. Mitoxantrone has been approved for the treatment of AML.

Doxorubicin is used to treat both solid and hematologic tumors.

Daunorubicin is used for acute myelocytic leukemia.

These drugs appear to exert their effects by binding to DNA and intercalation. In addition, doxorubicin and daunorubicin also affect preribosomal RNA synthesis and membranes.

These drugs intercalate into DNA.

Because of their clinical utility, a large number of analogs have been synthesized, and many are in clinical trial. The goal of analog development is to find drugs with decreased toxicity, in particular cardiac toxicity, or with improved therapeutic effects, or both.

The anthracyclines enter cells through a passive transport process and are pumped out of cells by the *p*-glycoprotein system that is increased in activity in MDR cells. Other mechanisms for anthracycline resistance have been reported, including increased metabolism and decreased binding to topoisomerase II.

R_1	
—CH₃	Daunomycin (daunorubicin)
—CH₂OH	Adriamycin (doxorubicin)

Mitoxantrone

CLINICAL PHARMACOLOGY. After an IV bolus of doxorubicin, the drug disappears in three phases: an initial rapid distribution phase lasts approximately 15 minutes; a second phase due to metabolism and elimination lasts several hours; and a prolonged third phase lasts 24–48 hours, which may represent release of the drug from binding sites. Both daunorubicin and doxorubicin are metabolized primarily in liver to daunomycinol or doxorubicinol respectively, compounds that are less toxic than the parent drugs. Dose modification has been recommended for patients with hepatic impairment, using bilirubin levels, but a firm basis for this recommendation has not been established.

The usual dose of doxorubicin used as a single agent is 60–75 mg/sq m given as a single dose every 3–4 weeks. There is some evidence to support the use of dose schedules employing more frequent, lower dose schedules, either weekly (15–25 mg/sq m) or by constant infusion over 48–96 hours; less cardiac toxicity may result by avoiding high peak plasma concentrations. When given in combination with other myelotoxic agents, such as cyclophosphamide, the dosage of doxorubicin is usually decreased by one third. Although daunorubicin has been used as the anthracycline of choice in the treatment of AML, usually in combination with cytosine arabinoside, evidence indicates that doxorubicin and mitoxantrone may be equally effective in this circumstance.

TOXICITY. Myelosuppression usually occurs with a nadir of 10 days after a single dose administration and recovers by 3 weeks. Other toxicities that are noted with these drugs are tissue necrosis, if the drug extravasates, and alopecia. Mitoxantrone usually does not cause these toxic effects and produces less nausea and vomiting than are seen with daunomycin or doxorubicin. Doxorubicin may cause mucositis, especially when used in maximally tolerated divided doses given over 2–3 days, or when used in combination with other drugs that cause mucositis. These drugs may cause a recall reaction in previously irradiated tissues, especially when the drug is administered just prior to (up to 3 weeks) or following irradiation.

Doxorubicin and daunorubicin cause myelosuppression and cardiac toxicity.

In addition to myelosuppression, the other significant toxic effect of doxorubicin and daunorubicin is cardiac toxicity. Both acute effects, manifested by arrhythmias and conduction abnormalities, and a pericarditis-myocarditis syndrome, as well as chronic effects may occur. Cardiac biopsy studies have shown a dose-dependent effect of doxorubicin on myocardial cell viability. The use of ejection fraction measurements has been extremely helpful as a noninvasive technique to demonstrate a decline in myocardial function and, thus, the need for cessation of anthracycline therapy. Most patients will tolerate doses of 450–550 mg/sq m of doxorubicin or daunorubicin before the risk of cardiac damage exceeds 5%. Once clinically overt cardiac toxicity occurs, usually manifested by congestive heart failure, the mortality rate may be as high as 48%. Congestive heart failure usually occurs during therapy or less than 1 month following cessation of therapy; rarely, heart failure may occur months to years later.

As mentioned, low-dose schedules may decrease cardiac toxicity. Monitoring of the ejection fraction is also important in patients after the cumulative dose of these drugs exceeds 250–300 mg/sq m. Other anthracycline analogs, such as mitoxantrone, may produce less cardiac toxicity, but the data with this drug are less complete.

Bleomycin

Bleomycin causes single- and double-strand breaks in DNA. There is little marrow toxicity.

Bleomycin can exert antitumor effects with little or no marrow toxicity. It has good clinical activity in lymphoma, and it is used as part of combination regimens to treat Hodgkin's disease (e.g., ABVD) or the high-grade non-Hodgkin's lymphomas. Bleomycin is a mixture of peptides produced by the fungus *Streptomyces verticillis*. The structure of bleomycin is shown in Figure 58–2.

Bleomycin A$_2$ R   NHCH$_2$CH$_2$CH$_2$S(CH$_3$)$_2$

Bleomycin B$_2$ NHCH$_2$CH$_2$CH$_2$CH$_2$NHC(=NH)NH$_2$

MECHANISM OF ACTION. Bleomycin has been shown to act by causing both single- and double-strand breaks in DNA as a consequence of production of a Fe (II) complex that generates free radicals. The reason for the tumor specificities of this drug, and the lack of toxicity of bleomycin to marrow and the GI tract, are not completely understood but may be due to the presence of a bleomycin-inactivating enzyme in these tissues. Of interest is the lack of activity of this enzyme in the lung and skin, two normal organs that are damaged by this drug. Cell killing is maximal in cells in the G$_2$ phase of the cell cycle.

CLINICAL PHARMACOLOGY. Bleomycin may be administered either IV or IM. Bleomycin may also be administered intrapleurally or intraperitoneally for control of malignant effusions. There is some preclinical data that supports the use of this drug as a continuous infusion, but definitive data on this point are lacking in humans. After a single IV injection, the drug disappears rapidly with over half of the dose excreted in the urine in 24 hours. The elimination half-life has been estimated to be about 2–3 hours.

Because this drug is primarily excreted by the kidney, bleomycin elimination may be markedly impaired in patients with poor renal function. Although exact guidelines for the use of this drug in patients with renal impairment are not available, dose reduction should be considered in these patients.

ADVERSE EFFECTS. As mentioned, bleomycin has little or no effect on normal marrow; however, in patients given other myelosuppressive drugs or recovering from marrow toxicity from these agents, additional mild myelosuppression may be observed.

The two major toxicities that may result from bleomycin administration are pulmonary fibrosis and skin changes. The risk of pulmonary toxicity is related to the cumulative dose administered, and the risk increases to 10% in patients administered more than 450 mg.

Bleomycin toxic effects on skin are also dose-related, and when the drug is given in conventional daily doses for longer than 2–3 weeks, erythema, hyperkeratosis, and even frank ulceration may be seen. Areas of

Bleomycin causes pulmonary fibrosis.

skin pressure, especially of the hands, fingers and joints, are initially affected. Nail changes and alopecia may occur with continued use of the drug. In combination regimens where bleomycin is used intermittently (e.g., ABVD), these skin toxicities are not usually seen.

Fever and malaise are common symptoms and may be alleviated with the use of acetoaminophen. Hypersensitivity reactions have been observed with bleomycin therapy. A peculiar type of idiosyncratic cardiovascular collapse has been rarely noted, particularly in lymphoma patients. A 1- or 2-mg–test dose in these patients may be useful in detecting patients who may have this problem.

Dactinomycin (Actinomycin D)

Dactinomycin is an antibiotic with antineoplastic activity; it is produced by *Streptomyces parvullus*. It is composed of a phenoxazone ring structure, to which two identical cyclic peptide chains are bound.

Dactinomycin intercalates into DNA.

Actinomycin D

Dactinomycin causes leukopenia and thrombocytopenia. It is used for Wilms' tumor, choriocarcinoma, and rhabdomyosarcoma.

MECHANISM OF ACTION. Dactinomycin bonds to DNA, with the polypeptide chains binding in the minor grove of the DNA helix. This intercalation is a result of a specific interaction between these chains and deoxyguanosine.

Little data are available on mechanisms of resistance to actinomycin D in patients or the basis for natural or inherent resistance or sensitivity to this drug. In experimental systems, actinomycin D participates in the MDR phenotype.

CLINICAL PHARMACOLOGY. The drug is rapidly cleared from the blood after an IV dose, and most of the drug is excreted unchanged in bile and urine. After an initial rapid plasma disappearance phase (minutes), a slow phase (36 hours) half-life occurs, presumably because of the slow release of drug from tissue and excretion into urine and bile.

ADVERSE EFFECTS. The major dose-limiting toxicities to this drug are leukopenia and thrombocytopenia. These effects reach a nadir 2–3 weeks after a course of therapy. Nausea and vomiting, common acute toxicities, begin within a few hours after treatment and may last as long as 24 hours. Other side effects noted with full doses of actinomycin D are stomatitis, cheilitis, glossitis, and proctitis. Actinomycin may cause radiation recall, i.e., cutaneous erythema, desquamation, and hyperpigmentation in previously irradiated areas. Cellulitis and pain can also result if the drug extravasates during IV administration. Alopecia and severe skin toxicity may occasionally be seen.

CLINICAL USE. Actinomycin D is used to treat Wilms' tumor, gestational choriocarcinoma, and embryonal rhabdomyosarcoma. Some regimens for osteosarcoma also include actinomycin D. Although this drug has a significant activity in the treatment of testicular cancer, it has been supplanted by other more effective drugs.

Mitomycin C

Mitomycin C is a quinone antibiotic, isolated from cultures of *Streptomyces caespitosus*. The drug requires reduction to produce an activated molecule that can cross-link DNA strands, similar to an alkylating agent.

CLINICAL PHARMACOLOGY. After IV administration there is a rapid half-life of distribution (2–10 minutes), followed by an elimination half-life of 25–90 minutes.

Mitomycin C

ADVERSE EFFECTS. In addition to nausea and vomiting that are commonly seen with drug administration, the major toxicity of mitomycin C is bone marrow suppression, usually cumulative. The nadir of blood element decrease is 3–5 weeks. Extravasation results in severe tissue damage. Less common side effects are the hemolytic uremic syndrome that may be fatal, interstitial pneumonitis, and cardiomyopathy.

CLINICAL USE. Mitomycin C is used in combination regimens in the treatment of lung and GI cancers.

Plycamycin (Mithramycin)

Mithramycin was isolated from *Streptomyces plicatus*. The major use for this drug is to treat hypercalcemia by malignancy. Although this drug was used to treat patients with embryonal carcinoma of the testis, other more effective and less toxic drugs have replaced it in the clinic.

MECHANISM OF ACTION. The precise mechanism of action of mithramycin is not fully worked out, but the drug has been shown to form complexes with DNA, with subsequent inhibition of DNA-dependent synthesis of RNA.

TOXICITY. Severe side effects were seen with doses of mithramycin used to treat patients with malignancy using daily dosing. Less toxicity was seen with an alternate-day regimen. A severe hemorrhagic syndrome associated with thrombocytopenia, prolonged clotting, and prothrombin times, in addition to hepatotoxicity and severe toxicity, were rather common with the daily high-dose regimen. Common side effects include nausea and vomiting. The severe side effects noted with the doses and schedules used to treat embryonal carcinoma are not seen with the doses used (15–25 μg/kg) at weekly intervals to treat hypercalcemia.

Mithramycin

MISCELLANEOUS DRUGS

Asparaginase

The enzyme L-asparaginase is used clinically in the treatment of lymphoid malignancies, in particular in null-cell ALL, T-cell leukemia, and lymphomas. This is one of the few circumstances in chemotherapy of malignant disease where a biochemical basis for selectivity is clear. These lymphoid malignancies require exogenous L-asparagine for growth. This is because of their lack of the enzyme L-asparagine synthetase; they obtain this amino acid from the circulating pool of amino acids generated by the liver primarily. The enzyme L-asparaginase that catalyzes the hydrolysis of asparagine to aspartic acid and ammonia is capable of rapidly depleting the serum level of L-asparagine and thus induces an asparagine deficiency in lymphoid malignant cells, which are incapable of synthesizing their own L-asparagine. The history of L-asparaginase as a therapeutic treatment is an interesting one; it first derived from an observation by Kidd, who in 1953 noted that the growth of certain transplantable lymphomas in the mouse were inhibited by guinea pig serum but not other mammalian sera. After intensive investigation, Bloom and coworkers in 1963 isolated the responsible factor for this antilymphoma activity and found it to be the enzyme L-asparaginase. There are two preparations of L-asparaginase now available for clinical use; one is from *Escherichia coli* and the other from *E. carotovora*.

Asparaginase depletes certain tumor cells that are incapable of synthesizing their own asparagine.

MECHANISM OF ACTION. The enzyme from *E. coli* has been utilized most widely in the clinical treatment of acute lymphocytic leukemia. As a consequence of the intracellular asparagine deficiency produced, there is a marked inhibition of protein synthesis, and the cytotoxicity of this enzyme correlates well with effects of this enzyme on protein synthesis.

CLINICAL PHARMACOLOGY. L-asparaginase is administered either IV or IM. The half-life of the enzyme in plasma is 14–24 hours.

> Asparaginase causes hypersensitivity reactions. It causes little marrow suppression.

TOXICITY. A major problem with administration of L-asparaginase is hypersensitivity reactions to this protein. Reactions to the first dose are uncommon, but after the second dose or more of the drug, hypersensitivity phenomena occur. These hypersensitivity reactions vary from urticarial to anaphylactic reactions, which include hypotension, laryngospasm, and cardiac arrest. Skin testing to predict allergic reactions are only partially helpful, and hypersensitive patients may have antibodies to L-asparaginase in serum. However, more than half of the patients with such antibodies will not display an allergic reaction to the drug clinically.

Patients who are treated with L-asparaginase should be watched carefully for several hours after the second or more doses, and epinephrine should be available if anaphylactic reactions occur. If an anaphylactic reaction occurs with the *E. coli* enzyme, the patient may still be treated with the enzyme from *E. carotovora*, because there is no cross-sensitivity to this L-asparaginase protein.

The other major toxic effects of L-asparaginase are due to the ability of this drug to transiently inhibit protein synthesis in normal tissues. Inhibition of protein synthesis in the liver will result in hypoalbuminemia, a decrease in clotting factors, and a decrease in serum lipoproteins. Inhibition of insulin production may lead to hypoglycemia. The clotting function abnormalities that are regularly observed as a consequence of L-asparaginase treatment include prolongation of the prothrombin time, partial thromboplastin time, and thrombin time. A marked fall in plasma fibrinogen and a decrease in clotting Factors IX and XI may also be observed. Other complications of L-asparaginase treatment when used in the high dose schedules are cerebral dysfunction, which may lead to confusion; stupor and coma; and acute pancreatitis, which in some patients may even progress to severe hemorrhagic pancreatitis.

> Asparaginase is used in combination with other drugs to treat acute leukemia.

USE IN COMBINATION CHEMOTHERAPY. Because L-asparaginase has no or little toxicity to bone marrow or GI mucosa, this drug has been used in combination with other drugs. Because L-asparaginase inhibits protein synthesis, it will ameliorate the toxic effects of drugs that inhibit DNA synthesis, such as methotrexate and cytosine arabinoside. This probably results from the inability of cells to enter the S phase because of the block of protein synthesis caused by this enzyme, making them less susceptible to the killing effects of S-phase specific agents. Based upon the observation that null-ALL cells and T cells are not rescued from methotrexate treatment by L-asparaginase, whereas normal stem cells are, a regimen in which the methotrexate is followed 24 hours later by L-asparaginase has been devised. This combination is effective even in acute leukemia refractory to conventional methotrexate doses. The interval of treatment of methotrexate followed by asparaginase is ideally 10–14 days, because as mentioned it takes 7–10 days for the asparagine levels of the blood to recover to normal after a single dose of L-asparaginase, at which time the leukemia cells begin to proliferate and may be more sensitive to a repeat of this treatment.

References

Allegra CJ: Antifolates. *In* Chabner BA, Collins JM (eds): Cancer Chemotherapy: Principles and Practice, 110–153. Philadelphia: JB Lippincott Co, 1990.

Bender RA, Hamel E, Hande KR: Plant alkaloids. *In* Chabner BA, Collins JM (eds): Cancer Chemotherapy: Principles and Practice, 253–275. Philadelphia: JB Lippincott Co, 1990.

Black DJ, Livingston RB: Antineoplastic drugs in 1990. Drugs 39:652–673, 1990.

Chabner BA: Clinical strategies for cancer treatment: The role of drugs. *In* Chabner BA, Collins JM (eds): Cancer Chemotherapy: Principles and Practice, 1–15. Philadelphia: JB Lippincott Co, 1990.

Chabner BA: Cytidine analogs. *In* Chabner BA, Collins JM (eds): Cancer Chemotherapy: Principles and Practice, 154–179. Philadelphia: JB Lippincott Co, 1990.

Chabner BA: Enzyme therapy: L-asparaginase. *In* Chabner BA, Collins JM (eds): Cancer Chemotherapy: Principles and Practice, 397–407. Philadelphia: JB Lippincott Co, 1990.

Clark PI, Slevin ML: The clinical pharmacology of etoposide and teniposide. Clin Pharmacokinet 12:223–252, 1987.

Colvin M, Chabner BA: Alkylating agents. *In* Chabner BA, Collins JM (eds): Cancer Chemotherapy: Principles and Practice, 276–313. Philadelphia: JB Lippincott Co, 1990.

Furner RL, Brown RK: L-phenylalanine mustard (L-PAM): The first 25 years. Cancer Treat Rep 64:559–574, 1980.

Grem JL: Fluorinated pyrimidines. *In* Chabner BA, Collins JM (eds): Cancer Chemotherapy: Principles and Practice, 180–224. Philadelphia: JB Lippincott Co, 1990.

McCormack JJ, Johns DG: Purine and purine nucleoside antimetabolites. *In* Chabner BA, Collins JM (eds): Cancer Chemotherapy: Principles and Practice, 234–252. Philadelphia: JB Lippincott Co, 1990.

Mihich E: Drug Resistance: Mechanism and Reverse. New York: John Libbey & Co, 1990.

Myers CE, Chabner BA: Anthracyclines. *In* Chabner BA, Collins JM (eds): Cancer Chemotherapy: Principles and Practice, 356–387. Philadelphia: JB Lippincott Co, 1990.

Reed E, Kohn KW: Platinum analogs. *In* Chabner BA, Collins JM (eds): Cancer Chemotherapy: Principles and Practice, 465–490. Philadelphia: JB Lippincott Co, 1990.

Schweitzer BA, Dicker AP, Bertino JR: Dihydrofolate as a therapeutic target. FASEB J 4:2441–2452, 1990.

Sobrero A, Bertino JR: Clinical Aspects of Drug Resistance. Cancer Surv 5:93–101, 1986.

Spivak SD: Procarbazine. Ann Int Med 81:795–800, 1974.

Vermeij J, den Nortigh J, Pinedo HM: Antitumor antibiotics. *In* Chabner BA, Collins JM (eds): Cancer Chemotherapy: Principles and Practice, 382–396. Philadelphia: JB Lippincott Co, 1990.

Weiss RB, Issell BF: The nitrosoureas: Carmustine (BCNU) and lomustine (CCNU). Cancer Treat Rev 9:313–330, 1982.

59

Immunopharmacology

Alan Winkelstein

Pharmacological agents capable of suppressing immune responses have assumed increasing importance in clinical medicine. These drugs are essential for inhibiting histoincompatible organ transplant rejection reactions. A second area of clinical importance is in the treatment of a spectrum of diseases thought to be due to aberrant immune responses. These disorders are believed to result from abnormalities of immune regulation in which this defense system loses its ability to discriminate between self and foreign. A consequence of this abnormality is the elaboration of immune responses directed at self-antigens. Immunosuppressive drugs serve to reduce the magnitude of these auto-directed reactions and thus are potentially able to prevent the resulting tissue damage.

Ideally, an immunosuppressant specifically inhibits one immune response without impairing any other reaction.

The ideal immunosuppressant would be an agent that selectively inhibits one specific immune response without impairing any other reaction. In addition, it would not be toxic for any other organ system. With the possible exception of RhoGAM, an antibody to the D antigen of the Rh system, none of the presently available immunosuppressants fulfills these criteria. Specifically, they do not selectively inhibit a single response; rather, all promote a state of generalized immune hyporeactivity. As a result of this global immune suppression, unwanted reactions are impaired. However, as a consequence of the immunosuppression, treated patients are more susceptible to infection and may have an increased risk of developing selected malignancies. Furthermore, all the available immunosuppressive drugs are highly toxic. In certain instances, their adverse effects may be more harmful to the patient than the underlying disease.

All available immunosuppressive drugs are highly toxic.

The major compounds used to suppress immune responses can be subdivided into several categories. Corticosteroids are the agents most widely used to suppress manifestations of potentially harmful immune responses. Certain drugs, classified as cytotoxins and initially developed for their antineoplastic properties, have been shown to exert profound immune inhibitory effects. More recently, a new class of immunosuppressants has been developed; these drugs appear to specifically interfere with selected functions of immunologically competent lymphocytes. The prototype for this group of agents is cyclosporine. As described later, this agent appears to selectively block essential functions of a subset of T lymphocytes that are required for cells to mount immune responses.

Corticosteroids

Drugs derived from the adrenal cortex glucocorticoid hormones are extensively used to suppress manifestations of many immune responses. Their effectiveness was first reported in 1949 when hydrocortisone (cortisol), the major corticosteroid secreted by the adrenal gland, was discovered to inhibit manifestations of rheumatoid arthritis, a presumed autoimmune disease. This was rapidly followed by successful clinical trials both in other connective tissue diseases and in many systemic autoimmune disorders. Because of hydrocortisone's potency as an inhibitor of both inflammatory and immune reactions, several synthetic steroid compounds were developed. These have distinct advantages over cortisol; they possess greater anti-inflammatory properties and have reduced salt-retaining activities. The synthetic compounds also differ from cortisol in their biological half-lives; their anti-inflammatory effects persist for longer periods. Despite these differences, all corticosteroid compounds exert their anti-inflammatory and immune-modulating activities by similar mechanisms.

Clinically, the most widely used steroid is the synthetic compound prednisone. This drug is generally used as the standard for comparing other steroid compounds. The major corticosteroid preparations used clinically and a comparison of their relative potencies are listed in Table 59 – 1.

Pharmacologically, all steroids exert their effects by a complex series of events that ultimately alter cellular metabolism. The drugs readily penetrate cell membranes, and in the cytoplasm, they bind to specific corticosteroid-binding proteins. The steroid-protein complexes are subsequently transported into the cell's nucleus, where they attach to discrete segments of the cell's DNA. The binding results in derepression of regulatory genes and the subsequent transcription of new mRNA. As a result, new regulatory proteins are formed; these variously act to either enhance or suppress specific cellular functions.

Clinical studies on the effects of steroids on lymphocytes have been confused by a failure to recognize that cells from different animal species vary in their susceptibility to drug-induced lysis. In mice, rats, and rabbits, corticosteroids are able to produce extensive lympholysis. By contrast, normal lymphocytes from guinea pigs, monkeys, and humans tend to be resistant to the destructive effects of these compounds. It should be noted that not all human lymphocytes are steroid-resistant; they will effectively kill acute lymphoblastic leukemic cells and are moderately cytolytic for neoplastic B cells in chronic lymphocytic leukemia and non-Hodgkin's lymphomas.

The anti-inflammatory and immunosuppressive activities of corticosteroids can be grouped conveniently into three general categories: the effects of these agents on leukocyte circulation, their ability to alter the functions of immunologically-related cells, and a series of miscellaneous anti-inflammatory properties.

Prednisone is used as the standard for comparing other steroids.

Table 59-1 CLINICAL PROPERTIES OF CORTICOSTEROID PREPARATIONS

Preparation	Anti-Inflammatory Potency	Equivalent Dose (mg)	Sodium-Retaining Potency	Approximate Plasma Half-Life (Minutes)
Hydrocortisone (cortisol)	1.0	20.00	2+	90
Cortisone	0.8	25.00	2+	30
Prednisone	4.0	5.00	1+	60
Prednisolone	4.0	5.00	1+	200
Methylprednisolone	5.0	4.00	0	180
Triamcinolone	5.0	4.00	0	300
Betamethasone	20 – 30	0.60	0	100 – 300
Dexamethasone	20 – 30	0.75	0	100 – 300

Adapted from Claman HN: Glucocorticosteroids II: The clinical response. Hosp Pract 18:144, 1983.

EFFECTS ON CELLULAR TRAFFIC

Corticosteroids transiently alter the number of circulating leukocytes.

One of the most important effects of corticosteroids is to transiently alter the number of circulating leukocytes. This is illustrated in Figure 59–1, which depicts the quantitative changes in each cell type following a single intravenous injection of a glucocorticoid. There is a prompt increase in the number of neutrophils and a concomitant decrease in the total number of lymphocytes, monocytes, eosinophils, and basophils. Maximal changes occur 4–6 hours after drug administration. In general, the amount of each cell type has returned to its baseline value within 24 hours.

The neutrophilia resulting from steroid administration appears to be due to at least two distinct pharmacological activities. Corticosteroids promote the rapid release of mature neutrophils from bone marrow reserves. Further, they reduce the ability of neutrophils to migrate from intravascular spaces into inflammatory exudates. This latter effect serves to increase the half-life of circulating neutrophils. It should be noted that the increase in the numbers of circulating neutrophils seen in patients receiving corticosteroids may, in fact, be a detrimental effect. Because these phagocytes are limited in their ability to migrate into extravascular sites of inflammation or infection, an important host defense mechanism is impaired.

Steroids reduce T cell population.

In contrast to the neutrophilia, steroids induce a striking reduction in the number of circulating lymphocytes. This is due primarily to the sequestration of recirculating lymphocytes into lymphoid tissues, including the bone marrow. With respect to lymphocyte subsets, it has been shown that the number of T (thymic-dependent) cells are markedly depressed. B (bone marrow–derived) lymphocytes are only modestly reduced, and the numbers of circulating null (non-T non-B) cells are not appreciably changed. Among the T lymphocyte subsets, T helper/inducer cells are decreased to a greater extent than T suppressor/cytotoxic lymphocytes.

Steroids induce a pronounced monocytopenia.

One of the important steroid-induced effects on circulating leukocytes is the induction of a pronounced monocytopenia. The numbers of these cells are reduced to a greater extent than any other type of leukocyte; monocyte counts frequently decline to almost undetectable levels. The decreased availability of monocytes has been postulated to be of prime importance in mediating steroid-induced anti-inflammatory activities. The numbers of eosinophils and basophils are also reduced; these effects are

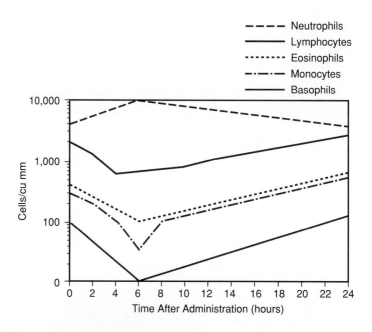

Figure 59–1

Quantitative changes in cell type following intravenous glucocorticoid injection. (Reprinted [adapted] with permission. Claman HN: Glucorticosteroids. I. Anti-inflammatory mechanisms. Hospital Practice Volume 18, issue 7, pages 123–134, 1983.)

also due to a redistribution of these cells. At present, the consequences of these latter activities are not known.

FUNCTIONAL CHANGE

In addition to affecting the distribution of leukocytes, corticosteroids alter important functional activities of both lymphocytes and monocytes. Neutrophilic activities, such as chemotaxis, are relatively resistant to steroids. Formerly, it was believed that steroids suppressed the release of neutrophilic lysosomal enzymes; this was postulated to inhibit manifestations of certain immune-induced injuries. However, some studies suggest that these neutrophilic activities are not significantly impaired. By contrast, the release of nonlysosomal proteolytic enzymes, such as collagenase and plasminogen activator, may be decreased by steroid therapy.

The functional activities of T lymphocytes are considerably altered by corticosteroids. One prominent manifestation is an inhibition of *in vitro* lymphoproliferative responses. This effect results, in part, from a reduction in the synthesis and secretion of an important lymphokine, interleukin-2 (IL-2). This is a lymphoid growth factor that is essential for the clonal expansion of activated lymphocytes (Fig. 59–2). The decreased availability of IL-2 is believed to be partially due to suppression of another interleukin, IL-1, which is primarily elaborated by monocytes. IL-1 serves to stimulate T helper lymphocytes to produce IL-2. By contrast, corticosteroids do not impair the ability of antigenic- or mitogenic-stimulated T cells to express IL-2 receptors. Thus, *in vitro*, the antiproliferative activities of corticosteroids can be overcome by exogenous IL-2. In other studies, steroids do not alter the release of two other lymphokines, interferon-γ and migration inhibition factor (MIF).

> T lymphocyte function is altered by corticosteroids.

> Migration inhibition factor (MIF)

Other studies show that corticosteroids can block the progression of phytohemagglutinin (PHA)–stimulated lymphocytes through the mitotic cycle (see later). They inhibit the entry of cells into the G_1 phase and arrest the progression of activated lymphocytes from G_1 to the S phase. In part, this arrest may be related to steroid effects on IL-2 production.

Corticosteroids have less effect on B lymphocytes. There is evidence that patients receiving moderate doses of prednisone are able to respond normally to test antigens. Nevertheless, short courses of high-dose corticosteroids modestly reduce the serum concentrations of IgG and IgA; there are only minimal effects on IgM levels. Decreased serum concentrations of these immunoglobulins are observed 2–3 weeks after a 5-day treatment course. In asthmatic children, the concentrations of IgE are also reduced. *In vitro* studies, using cultured spleen cells, indicate that steroids can impair

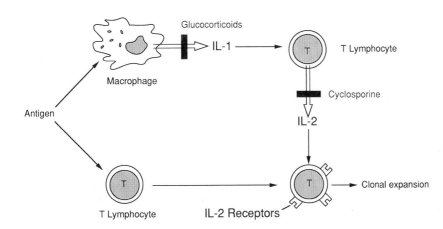

Figure 59–2

Clonal expansion of activated T lymphocytes and sites of inhibition by corticosteroids and cyclosporine.

Antibody-dependent cellular cytotoxicity (ADCC) reactions

the ability of B lymphocytes to synthesize IgG. Corticosteroids do not alter the activities of either natural killer (NK) cells or effectors of antibody-dependent cellular cytotoxicity (ADCC) reactions.

Paralleling the profound effects of corticosteroids on the number of circulating monocytes, this class of hormones induces striking impairment in monocyte/macrophage function. They suppress the bactericidal activities of these phagocytic cells; this can adversely affect resistance to infection. Steroids also interfere with the antigen-presenting function of monocytes; this is an essential initiating event in most immune responses. Other activities include reduced abilities of monocytes to undergo directed migration in response to chemotactic factors and decreased responses to the T cell cytokine MIF. Corticosteroids also appear able to block the differentiation of monocytes to macrophages; that is, to prevent cell activation. Furthermore, these agents decrease the capacity of monocytes to express Fc and complement receptors; the reduced numbers of these receptors appears to contribute to impaired phagocytic activities of these cells. An important effect is to inhibit synthesis and secretion of IL-1. This interleukin has numerous systemic effects; these include its ability to initiate T cell responses by inducing these lymphocytes to secrete IL-2.

In a closely related activity, *in vivo* administration of steroids results in decreased ability of reticuloendothelial cells to phagocytize antibody-coated cells. This effect correlates with *in vitro* studies indicating decreased binding of immune complexes to Fc and C3b membrane receptors. This impaired binding may account for the beneficial effects of steroids in diseases such as idiopathic thrombocytopenic purpura (ITP) and autoimmune hemolytic anemia (AIHA); treatment with these drugs acts primarily to reduce the phagocytosis and subsequent destruction of antibody-coated particles.

Delayed hypersensitivity skin tests are suppressed by prolonged treatment with corticosteroids. In general, these hormones must be administered for periods of 10–14 days before skin test reactivity is impaired. Loss of ability to mount cutaneous delayed hypersensitivity reactions is referred to as *anergy*.

Anergy is the loss of ability to mount cutaneous delayed hypersensitivity reactions.

OTHER EFFECTS

Steroids can also affect the production of soluble mediators that regulate both inflammatory and immune responses. An important activity is to inhibit the synthesis of prostaglandins and leukotrienes, potent mediators of inflammation. This suppression results from the synthesis of a new regulatory protein, lipomodulin. This protein specifically antagonizes the enzyme phospholipase A. The latter catalyzes the release of arachidonic acid from cell membranes. Free arachidonic acid serves as the precursor for both prostaglandins and leukotrienes.

Steroids also reduce the permeability of the vascular endothelium; this activity results in decreased fluid exudation and impairs the diapedesis of leukocytes. Another activity is to suppress IgE-mediated histamine release by basophils, an important component of certain allergic disorders.

CLINICAL USE OF CORTICOSTEROIDS

In pharmacological quantities, these hormones are effective, but nonspecific, inhibitors of numerous disorders of apparent immune pathogenesis. Typically, therapy is most effective in suppressing manifestations of acute inflammatory reactions. By contrast, they often do not prevent the long-term complications of chronic immunopathological processes. For example, they inhibit the acute inflammatory manifestations of diseases such as rheumatic fever and rheumatoid arthritis. However, they are of limited usefulness in preventing either chronic valvular heart disease or deforming arthritis.

Corticosteroids effectively suppress manifestations of acute inflammatory reactions.

There are no definite rules for steroid administration, but most protocols conform to one of three patterns. The first, often employed if these drugs are to be administered for extended time periods, entails the use of the minimal amount needed to partially suppress disease manifestations. An example of this is in the patient with rheumatoid arthritis receiving 7.5–10 mg of prednisone daily. The second approach uses larger doses in an attempt to both rapidly and completely suppress manifestations of an immunologically mediated disease. Quantities of 1–2 mg/kg prednisone are given daily, in one or divided doses. This type of therapy is often used in disorders that have a likelihood of causing the patient's death, such as AIHA, ITP, systemic lupus erythematosus (SLE), and immunologically induced acute glomerulonephritis.

The third pattern is the pulse administration of very high doses of an intravenous corticosteroid preparation (e.g., 10–30 mg/kg methylprednisolone). These ultra-large doses are usually reserved for "life-threatening" illnesses. They have also been used successfully in reversing acute allograft rejection reactions. Most studies suggest that the immunological effects of these massive-dose steroid protocols do not differ significantly from those resulting from more conventional doses. Although the therapeutic superiority of these regimens has not been proved in controlled trials, numerous reports imply effectiveness.

Prolonged therapy with corticosteroids is not innocuous; these drugs have numerous and potentially serious side effects. A full discussion of toxicities is beyond the scope of this section. However, it is important to recognize that chronic therapy with large doses of steroids may cause greater morbidity than that associated with the underlying disease.

Prolonged corticosteroid therapy has potentially serious side effects.

Cytotoxic Drugs

Cytotoxic drugs consist of a group of pharmacological agents that are able to kill cells capable of self-replication. In the process of responding to an antigen, immunologically competent lymphocytes are transformed from a resting or intermitotic (G_0) state to actively proliferating cells. Thus, these cells potentially constitute a susceptible cell population. Cytotoxic drugs were originally introduced into clinical medicine as anticancer agents. As extensions of their initial clinical trials, it was found that many also possessed important immunosuppressive activities. This resulted in a series of trials in which cytotoxic agents were used both to treat diseases due to aberrant immune responses and to inhibit transplant rejection reactions. Several agents proved highly active. At present, four cytotoxic drugs—cyclophosphamide, azathioprine, methotrexate, and chlorambucil—are commonly used for their clinical immunosuppressive activities.

Cytotoxic drugs kill cells capable of self-replication.

Although the antigen-specific lymphocytes responsible for the unwanted immune response are the targets for cytotoxic drugs, their inhibitory activities are not restricted to a single lymphocyte subset. In varying degrees, they affect all immunologically competent cells. Thus, therapy leads to a state of generalized immunosuppression; as a result, treated patients tend to be susceptible to both opportunistic infections and certain neoplastic diseases.

Furthermore, these drugs are not selectively toxic for lymphocytes; they can kill nonlymphoid proliferating cells, including hematopoietic precursors, gastrointestinal mucosal cells, and germ cells in the gonads. Thus, predictable side effects of all cytotoxic agents include bone marrow suppression, gastrointestinal complications, and reduced fertility.

The lymphocytotoxic activities of different cytotoxic drugs can be related to their toxicities for cells in specific phases of the mitotic cycle (Fig. 59–3). This cycle has been subdivided into four phases: G_1, or the pre– DNA-synthetic phase; S, the DNA synthetic phase; G_2, a premitotic phase; and the M phase, the actual mitosis. Cells in a prolonged intermitotic period are considered to be in G_0 phase. One group of drugs, including two that are widely used for immunosuppression, azathioprine and methotrexate, are considered to be *phase-specific*. These agents are cytotoxic to cells during a specific phase of the mitotic cycle. For example, both azathioprine and methotrexate kill cells that are in the S or DNA-synthetic phase of the mitotic cycle. Conversely, they are not toxic to cells that are not in this susceptible S phase.

Cyclophosphamide and chlorambucil are classified as *cycle-specific* agents. They are toxic for cells at all stages of the mitotic cycle, including intermitotic (G_0) lymphocytes. However, these drugs show differential cytotoxic activities; they are more effective in killing active-cycling than resting (G_0) cells. The third group, the *cycle-nonspecific* compounds, are equally cytotoxic for proliferating and intermitotic cells.

Based on animal experiments, certain principles have been formulated concerning the immunosuppressive activities of cytotoxic agents. By extension, these form the basis for many of their uses in clinical situations. These principles are summarized as follows:

- A primary immune response is more readily inhibited than a secondary or anamnestic reaction. Typically, cytotoxic drugs are highly effective in suppressing an immune response in an animal not previously immunized to a specific antigen. By contrast, these cytotoxins have only minimal inhibitory activities in a previously sensitized animal. The same effect is observed in humans. For example, the primary immune response elicited by a renal transplant is readily impaired by a combination of azathioprine and corticosteroids. However, if the recipient has been presensitized to donor histocompatibility antigens, this immunosuppressive regimen is relatively ineffective in inhibiting rejection reactions.
- The stages of an immune response differ markedly in their susceptibility to immunosuppressants. The cellular events associated with an antigenic

Azathioprine and methotrexate are phase-specific cytotoxic drugs.

Cycle-specific agents are more effective in killing active-cycling cells.

A primary immune response is more readily inhibited than a secondary reaction.

Figure 59–3

Mitotic cycle: Drugs that are selectively toxic for cells in a discrete phase of their cycle are designated *phase-specific agents:* Most exert their toxicity for cells in the S phase. *Cycle-specific agents* are toxic for both intermitotic and proliferating cells but show greater toxicity for those in active cycle. *Cycle-nonspecific agents* show equal toxicity for all cells regardless of the mitotic activity. (From Webb DR Jr, Winkelstein A: Immunosuppression, immunopotentiation, and anti-inflammatory drugs. *In* Stites DP, Stobo JD, Fudenberg HH, Wells JV [eds]: Basic and Clinical Immunology, 5th ed, 271–287. Los Altos, CA: Lange Medical Publications, 1984.)

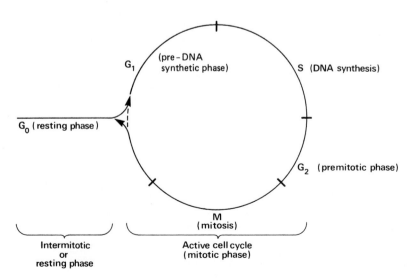

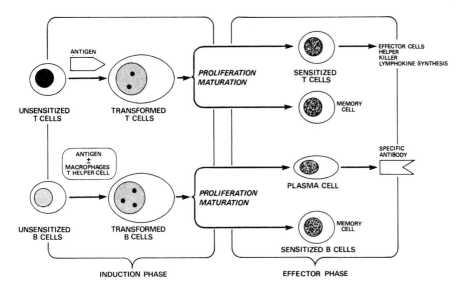

Figure 59-4

The development of an immune response. The period from antigenic challenge through the proliferative expansion of transformed lymphocytes is considered the *induction phase.* The period following cellular expansion is defined as the *established (effector) phase.* (From Webb DR Jr, Winkelstein A: Immunosuppression, immunopotentiation, and anti-inflammatory drugs. *In* Stites DP, Stobo JD, Fudenberg HH, Wells JV [eds]: Basic and Clinical Immunology, 5th ed, 271–287. Los Altos, CA: Lange Medical Publications, 1984.)

challenge can be subdivided into two phases, designated the *induction phase* and the *established* or *effector phase* (Fig. 59–4). The former is the interval between sensitization and generation of the final immune effectors; it is characterized by the rapid proliferative expansion of antigen-sensitive lymphocytes. Once the final effectors have been generated, the reaction is considered to have entered an established phase, and the vast majority of cells mediating the immune response are no longer in an active proliferative phase. This accounts for the observation that most cytotoxic drugs are maximally effective if the period of drug administration coincides with the induction phase. However, once the reaction has entered the established phase, cytotoxic agents are considerably less effective. Furthermore, once memory lymphocytes have been generated, it is almost impossible to erase immunological memory. Thus, if an animal has been presensitized to a specific antigen, it is exceedingly difficult to re-create a "tolerant" stage.

Cytotoxic agents are less effective once the reaction has reached the established phase.

■ The effectiveness of an immunosuppressive agent in a primary response is highly dependent on the timing of its administration relative to initial antigenic challenge. Based on their effective interval, immunosuppressive agents are divided into three groups: *Group I:* Agents that exert their maximal immunosuppressive activity when administered just prior to the antigen. These agents show reduced immunosuppressive activities if used in the period following antigenic challenge. Included in this group are corticosteroids, irradiation, and the cycle-nonspecific cytotoxin nitrogen mustard. *Group II:* Agents that show immunosuppressive properties only if administered in the period immediately following the immunological challenge. Specifically, these compounds do not inhibit responses if used prior to the antigen. Agents in this group are categorized as phase-specific drugs and include both azathioprine and methotrexate. *Group III:* Agents capable of inhibiting immune responses if administered either prior to or after antigenic stimulation. Comparatively, these drugs have their maximal suppressive activities if administered shortly after the immune challenge. Pharmacologically, these drugs are considered to be cycle-specific agents; cyclophosphamide is the most widely used drug in this group. The differential effects of timing of drug therapy on suppression of a test immune response are diagram-

Figure 59–5

Schematic representation of the effects of different classes of immunosuppressants on the numbers of antibody-producing cells. The *dotted lines* represent the effects of the drug given 24 hours before the antigen; the *solid lines* represent the effects of the drug given 24 hours after the antigen. (From Winkelstein A: Immune suppression resulting from various cytotoxic agents. Clin Immunol Allergy 4:295–315, 1984.)

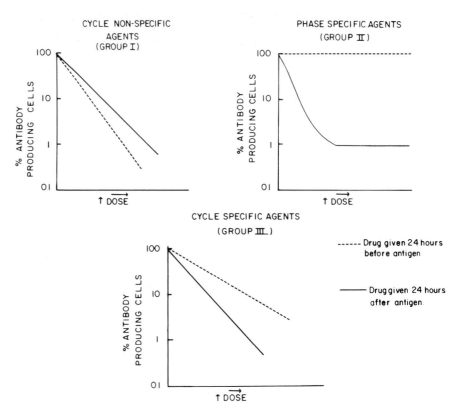

Immunosuppressive drugs can elicit a paradoxical effect, such as augmentation of a specific response.

matically depicted in Figure 59–5; this shows the response to sheep red cells in mice treated with an immunosuppressant either 24 hours before or 24 hours after antigenic challenge.

■ Immunosuppressive drugs may exert a differential toxicity for T and B lymphocytes. Cyclophosphamide appears to cause proportionately greater reduction in the number of B lymphocytes than in that of T cells. This observation correlates with its greater capacity to suppress humoral antibody responses compared with its activities against cell-mediated reactions. In clinical situations, cyclophosphamide is more effective in suppressing diseases of aberrant humoral immunity, such as ITP, than in inhibiting transplant rejection reactions. By contrast, azathioprine appears to be a more potent inhibitor of T cell–mediated responses.

■ In certain circumstances, a paradoxical effect may be elicited by an immunosuppressive drug; namely, augmentation of a specific response. It was noted originally that irradiation, administered several days before an antigenic challenge, led to a greater than normal antibody response. Similar effects were observed with 6-mercaptopurine (6-MP), the parent compound of azathioprine, when it was used prior to antigen challenge. With selected treatment protocols, cyclophosphamide can simultaneously suppress antibody responses and augment cell-mediated reactions to the same antigen. The heightened T cell responses have been attributed, in part, to this drug's toxicity for suppressor T lymphocytes.

■ In both animals and humans, the ability to inhibit manifestations of an immune response may result from pharmacological activities other than immunosuppression. Expression of most immune responses involves the participation of both immunologically competent lymphocytes and non-specific effectors, including neutrophils and monocytes. The numbers or functions of these phagocytic cells can be altered by immunosuppressive drugs, an effect which can modify or obliterate the expression of a particular response. Thus, apparent immunosuppression can result from the anti-inflammatory properties of a specific agent.

Table 59-2   SOME IMMUNOLOGICAL DISORDERS IN WHICH CYTOTOXIC DRUGS ARE EITHER EFFECTIVE OR PROBABLY EFFECTIVE

Rheumatoid arthritis
Systemic lupus erythematosus
Systemic vasculitis
Wegener's granulomatosis
Polymyositis
Membranous glomerulonephritis
Chronic active hepatitis
Primary biliary cirrhosis
Inflammatory bowel disease
Autoimmune hemolytic anemia
Immune thrombocytopenia
Circulating anticoagulants
Multiple sclerosis
Myasthenia gravis

CLINICAL USES OF CYTOTOXIC DRUGS

These agents are used to treat many autoimmune disorders. Table 59–2 is a partial list of disorders in which cytotoxic drugs have been reported to be effective.

Despite their clinical usage for more than a decade, it is still difficult to ascertain their true effectiveness in immunologically mediated diseases; there are only a few controlled clinical trials. In addition, many autoimmune diseases show unpredictable courses with both spontaneous remissions and exacerbations; thus, such claims of effectiveness must be interpreted cautiously. Despite these problems in data interpretation, it is almost universally accepted that cytotoxic immunosuppressants are potentially useful and, in some diseases, life-saving. One area in which cytotoxic drugs have been extensively employed is in the treatment of connective tissue diseases. Table 59–3 compares the activities of each of the commonly used cytotoxic immunosuppressants in these diseases.

Cytotoxic cells have been used extensively to treat connective tissue diseases.

Azathioprine

This compound, a nitroimidazole derivative of the purine antagonist 6-MP, is classified as a phase-specific drug. *In vivo,* it is rapidly converted to 6-MP. Although there are conflicting data, most investigators believe that the

Table 59-3   CLINICAL EFFICACY OF CYTOTOXIC DRUGS IN RHEUMATIC DISORDERS*

	Azathioprine	Chlorambucil	Cyclophosphamide	Methotrexate
Rheumatoid arthritis	++	+	++	++
Rheumatoid vasculitis	0	+	++	0
Systemic lupus erythematosus	+	+	+	0
Polyarteritis nodosa	+	0	++	0
Polymyositis	+	0	0	++
Psoriatic arthritis	0	0	0	+
Wegener's granulomatosis	+	+	++	0
Reiter's syndrome	0	0	0	+

Adapted from Nashel DJ: Mechanisms of action and clinical applications of cytotoxic drugs in rheumatic disorders. Med Clin North Am 69:832, 1985.
* ++ = substantial evidence of effectiveness; + = benefit suggested by some studies; 0 = not studied or benefit negligible.

Azathioprine and 6-MP impair DNA synthesis through competitive enzyme inhibition.

addition of the imidazole side chain both enhances its immunosuppressive potency and increases the therapeutic/toxic ratio.

Biochemically, both azathioprine and 6-MP are chemical analogs of physiologic purines—adenine, guanine, and hypoxanthine. Both drugs act by competitive enzyme inhibition to block synthesis of inosinic acid, the precursor of the purine compounds adenylic acid and guanylic acid. As a result, the major effect is to impair DNA synthesis; this results in a decreased rate of cell replication. Thus, this drug is classified as a phase-specific agent. A second and less important activity is to suppress RNA synthesis.

Comparatively, azathioprine appears to preferentially inhibit T cell responses compared with those resulting from activation of B lymphocytes. Nevertheless, both cell-mediated and humoral responses are suppressed. In addition, azathioprine appears to effectively reduce the numbers of circulating NK and K cells. The latter are responsible for ADCC reactions.

Prior to development of cyclosporine (see later), combinations of azathioprine and corticosteroids were standard therapy for inhibition of transplant rejection reactions. These two agents still maintain an important role in this area. In addition, azathioprine is used to treat many connective tissue diseases and other presumed immune-mediated disorders (Table 59–4). Extensive experience has been gained in patients with severe rheumatoid arthritis; this drug is classified as a *disease-remitting* agent. Beneficial effects have also been reported in patients with SLE, other connective tissue diseases, autoimmune blood dyscrasias, and immunologically mediated neurological diseases. This phase-specific drug may also permit the use of reduced amounts of corticosteroids in the treatment of primary biliary cirrhosis, chronic active hepatitis, and inflammatory bowel disease. Azathioprine is administered orally, and the maximal beneficial effects generally require continuous therapy for several weeks.

The primary lymphocytotoxic effects of azathioprine are directed against actively replicating cells; as such, short therapeutic courses do not reduce the numbers of T or B cells in the peripheral blood. They do decrease the number of large lymphocytes; these cells are believed to be transformed lymphocytes that have entered an active proliferative cycle following exposure to appropriate antigens. Immunoglobulin levels and titers of specific antibodies are not appreciably reduced by even chronic treatment with azathioprine. In a dose-dependent manner, this agent reduces the number of circulating neutrophils and monocytes. This effect results from its cytotoxic activities for hematopoietic precursors. Other adverse effects include transient liver function abnormalities and skin rashes.

Table 59–4   AZATHIOPRINE

Trade Name	Chemical Structure	Administration	Mechanism of Action	Major Indications	Toxicities
Imuran		Orally, 1.25–2.5 mg/kg/day	S phase toxin (phase-specific agent) Inhibits *de novo* purine synthesis	Transplant rejection reactions Chronic graft-versus-host disease Rheumatoid arthritis ? Systemic lupus erythematosus ? Vasculitis ? Other connective tissue diseases Inflammatory bowel disease Chronic active hepatitis/primary biliary cirrhosis ? Myasthenia gravis ? Multiple sclerosis	Bone marrow depression Gastrointestinal irritation Hepatotoxicity (rare) Infections Malignancies

Table 59-5 CYCLOPHOSPHAMIDE

Trade Name	Chemical Structure	Administration	Mechanism of Action	Major Indications	Toxicities
Cytoxan		Orally 1–3 mg/kg/day Intravenously 10–20 mg/kg/every 1–3 months	Cycle-specific agent Binds and cross-links DNA strands Effects B cells > T cells; T suppressors > T helpers	Rheumatoid arthritis and vasculitis Systemic lupus erythematosus Wegener's granulomatosis Systemic vasculitis Autoimmune blood dyscrasias Immune-mediated glomerulonephritis	Bone marrow depression Gastrointestinal reactions Sterility (may be permanent) Alopecia Hemorrhagic cystitis Opportunistic infections Neoplasms (lymphoma, bladder cancer, acute myelogenous leukemia) Goodpasture's syndrome

Cyclophosphamide

Both experimentally and clinically, this cycle-specific agent is an extremely potent immunosuppressant with a high therapeutic/toxic ratio (Table 59–5). Comparatively, cyclophosphamide has more sustained suppressive activities for humoral antibody responses than for those attributed to cellular reactions. This observation is in accord with its greater toxicities for B lymphocytes. Cyclophosphamide has a variable effect on cell-mediated responses; some reactions are inhibited, whereas others are augmented. The latter phenomenon has been attributed to the drug's effects on T suppressor lymphocytes.

Cyclophosphamide has been employed successfully in the treatment of numerous disorders believed to result from aberrant immunity. Beneficial effects have been documented in Wegener's granulomatosis, other forms of vasculitis, severe rheumatoid arthritis, the nephritis associated with SLE, autoimmune blood dyscrasias such as ITP, AIHA and pure red cell aplasia, Goodpasture's syndrome, and immune forms of glomerulonephritis.

Cyclophosphamide can be administered either orally or intravenously. The parent drug is inactive until metabolized by the enzymatic mixed-function oxidase system of the liver microsomes to 4-hydroxycyclophosphamide. The active moieties are present in the circulation for only a few hours; it is principally excreted in the urine. Cyclophosphamide exerts its cytotoxic properties by virtue of its ability to cross-link DNA chains. This effect may result in the immediate death of the target cell, or the cell may incur a lethal injury that is expressed during a subsequent mitotic division. Conversely, if the cell is capable of repairing the DNA injury, the cell survives normally (Fig. 59–6). In patients treated with cyclophosphamide there is a dose-related reduction in lymphocytes. Furthermore, residual cells show decreased *in vitro* proliferative responses following stimulation with antigens or nonspecific mitogens. Both T and B cells are susceptible to this alkylating agent. The drug's selectivity for B cells appears to result from a delay in the recovery of these lymphocytes. Studies in patients with connective tissue diseases indicate that extended therapy will reduce both immunoglobulin concentrations and autoantibody titers.

Although it is a potent immunosuppressant, cyclophosphamide is also a toxic drug. The immediate side effects include a dose-dependent suppression of hematopoiesis; gastrointestinal symptoms such as abdominal pain, nausea, and vomiting; and gonadal dysfunction. It has been reported

Cyclophosphamide inhibits some cell-mediated responses and augments others.

Cyclophosphamide is toxic and produces a variety of side effects.

Figure 59-6

The effect of cyclophosphamide on lymphocytes appears to be primarily due to cross-linking DNA strands. As shown, this can result in lympholysis and decreased in vitro proliferative response. In cells that are not extensively damaged, repair can occur and the lymphocyte regains its full proliferative capacity. Because of their slow rate of recovery, the effect on B cells is more pronounced than that on T cells. (From Webb DR Jr, Winkelstein A: Immunosuppression, immunopotentiation, and anti-inflammatory drugs. In Stites DP, Stobo JD, Fudenberg HH, Wells JV [eds]: Basic and Clinical Immunology, 5th ed, 271–287. Los Altos, CA: Lange Medical Publications, 1984.)

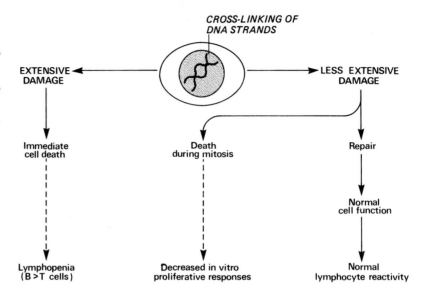

that cyclophosphamide is less toxic to platelets than are other alkylating agents. However, platelet counts can be significantly reduced by this drug. The gonadal dysfunction can lead to permanent sterility. The drug has teratogenic effects and should not be used in pregnant women.

In addition, this alkylating agent induces certain toxic manifestations not observed with other immunosuppressants; these include both hemorrhagic cystitis and alopecia. Sterile hemorrhagic cystitis occurs in up to 20% of treated patients; this complication can be severe or even fatal. It appears to be due to the chemical irritation of the bladder mucosa by active metabolites of cyclophosphamide that accumulate in concentrated urine. In most instances, the hematuria usually resolves within a few days but may persist for several months even after discontinuing therapy. Alopecia occurs in about one third of the treated patients and may have severe psychological effects.

The delayed toxicities include a higher than expected incidence of malignancies, specifically non-Hodgkin's lymphoma, bladder carcinoma, myelodysplastic syndromes, and acute myelogenous leukemia. In addition, patients treated with cyclophosphamide are at increased risk for developing opportunistic infections.

Methotrexate

Methotrexate is a phase-specific agent.

This drug is a reversible inhibitor of dihydrofolate reductase, an enzyme required for the conversion of folic acid to its active form, tetrahydrofolate (Fig. 59–7). The latter compound serves as a donor of one carbon fragment for the in vivo synthesis of thymidine. Thus, methotrexate serves as a potent inhibitor of DNA synthesis and is classified as a phase-specific agent. The toxic effects of methotrexate cannot be reversed by even large doses of folic acid. However, folinic acid (leucovorin factor), which is the tetrahydrofolate analog, can circumvent the enzymatic block.

Initial studies of methotrexate therapy showed a corresponding high incidence of hepatic fibrosis.

Methotrexate was one of the first anticancer drugs developed. Shortly after its introduction, it was found to be effective in the treatment of psoriasis. However, the initial trials had to be terminated because of a high incidence of hepatic fibrosis. Subsequently, investigators found that small quantities of this phase-specific agent were effective in controlling psoriatic manifestations. In these reduced amounts, methotrexate could be administered for extended periods without inducing hepatic injury. Concomi-

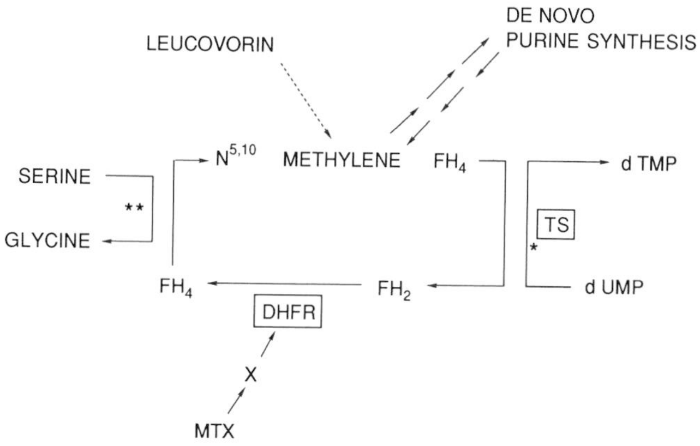

Figure 59–7

Conversion of dihydrofolate to its active form, tetrahydrofolate, is blocked by methotrexate's inhibition of the enzyme dihydrofolate reductase.

tantly, psoriatic patients with coexisting arthritis noted improvement in their articular manifestations.

These observations led several groups to evaluate methotrexate's activities in patients with rheumatoid arthritis (Table 59–6). Results of these studies indicated that approximately two thirds of the patients with severe rheumatoid arthritis achieved either partial or complete remissions. Other studies found that methotrexate effectively suppressed manifestations of polymyositis and Reiter's syndrome. This phase-specific agent is also of use in preventing graft-versus-host disease (GVHD) in patients undergoing allogeneic marrow transplants but not in suppressing manifestations of ongoing GVHD. However, because of its toxicities, it has largely been replaced in marrow transplant studies by cyclosporine.

A typical treatment regimen for rheumatic diseases consists of administering 2.5 mg of this drug every 12 hours for three doses; this course is repeated weekly. These doses are considerably less than those used in treating cancer patients. The major toxicity of methotrexate is hepatic fibrosis. This appears to be a dose-related matter; liver disease is rarely a problem until the total dose exceeds 1.5 g. Fibrosis can occur with normal liver function tests.

Another potential complication of methotrexate is pulmonary toxicities. This drug can induce a hypersensitivity pneumonitis; this is an idiosyncratic rather than a dose-related phenomenon. The clinical manifestations are often that of an acute fulminant and potentially life-threatening bilateral pneumonia. In other patients, the hypersensitivity reaction can result in slowly progressive pulmonary fibrosis. Other toxic manifestations include mucositis and megaloblastic anemia. These two complications are related to the drug's dose.

Table 59–6 METHOTREXATE

Chemical Structure	Administration	Mechanism of Action	Major Indications	Toxicities
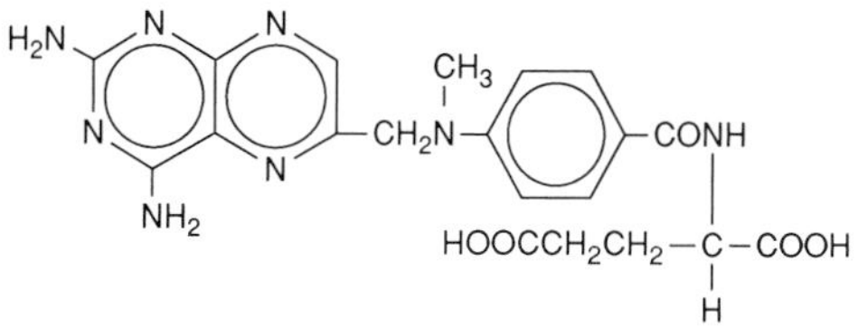	Orally, 2.5–5.0 mg every 12 hours for three doses, repeated weekly	S phase toxin (phase-specific) Competitively inhibits dihydrofolate reductase, thereby restricting synthesis of tetrahydrofolate. This is required for one-carbon transfer reactions involved in thymidine synthesis.	Rheumatoid arthritis Psoriasis and psoriatic arthritis Polymyositis/dermato-myositis Reiter's syndrome Prophylaxis for graft-versus-host disease in bone marrow transplants	Gastrointestinal — stomatitis, diarrhea, mucositis Bone marrow — megaloblastic anemia Hepatic fibrosis Pneumonitis Decreased fertility

Animal studies indicate that methotrexate is a potent immune inhibitor with a high therapeutic/toxic ratio. It suppresses both humoral and cellular responses. Short *in vivo* courses in guinea pigs do not reduce peripheral blood lymphocyte counts nor do they alter *in vitro* proliferative responses to either nonspecific mitogens or specific antigens. By contrast, the mechanisms by which methotrexate exerts its beneficial effects in rheumatic diseases are not well understood. In all probability, the small doses used to treat immunologically mediated diseases do not markedly inhibit immune responses.

Chlorambucil

Chlorambucil is an alkylating agent that has cytotoxic properties similar to those of cyclophosphamide. Comparatively, most studies suggest that it is less toxic than cyclophosphamide but lacks the latter's potency as an immunosuppressant.

Chlorambucil has been used extensively in Europe to treat immunologically mediated disease, and most reports suggest that it is effective in those disorders responsive to cyclophosphamide. These include rheumatoid arthritis, SLE, and Wegener's granulomatosis. It is the drug of choice for the treatment of idiopathic cold agglutinin hemolytic anemia and essential cryoglobulinemia.

Chlorambucil has advantages over cyclophosphamide; it does not cause alopecia or hemorrhagic cystitis and is less irritating to the gastrointestinal tract. Like cyclophosphamide, it causes marrow suppression and interferes with gonadal functions. Also, it is a fetal toxin. Furthermore, it increases the risk of both opportunistic infections and certain malignancies.

> Chlorambucil has been used extensively in Europe and has been shown to possess cytotoxic properties similar to those of cyclophosphamide.

Cyclosporine

> Cyclosporine selectively alters the immunological activities of T helper cells.

Cyclosporine is a novel immunosuppressant with activities distinct from all other agents. This drug is able to alter selectively the immunological activities of T helper/inducer cells. By contrast, it has minimal or no effect on T suppressor/cytotoxic cells, B lymphocytes, granulocytes, or macrophages. Furthermore, it impairs cell-mediated responses without killing the effector lymphocytes. One activity is to impair the maturation of precytotoxic T cells to competent killer cells. Because of its potency, it has become the agent of choice in allogeneic transplantation; most series indicate that it can inhibit rejection reactions more effectively than any other clinically available immunosuppressant. Trials using cyclosporine have been initiated for the treatment of several presumed immunologically mediated diseases.

Pharmacologically, cyclosporine is a unique nonpolar, cyclical undecapeptide, derived from the fermentation of certain soil fungi (Fig. 59–8).

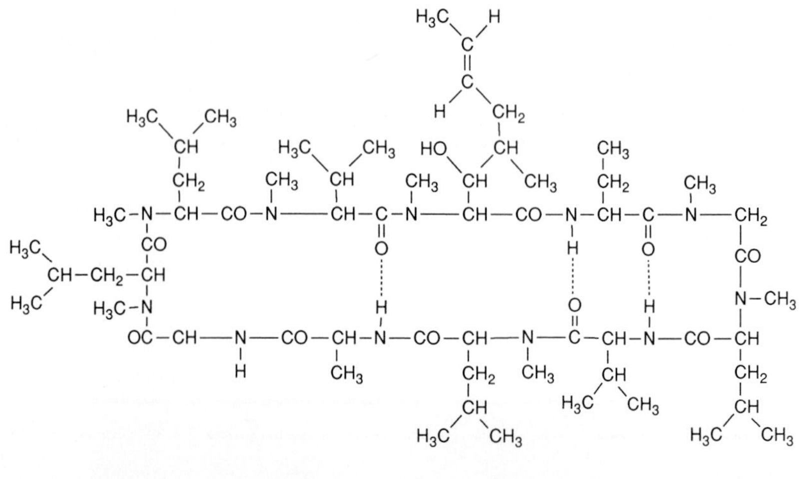

Figure 59–8

Chemical structure of cyclosporine.

The drug is not water-soluble, but it can be administered either orally or intramuscularly in a lipid vehicle. Immunologically, its effects are highly selective. It specifically inhibits the functions of T helper/inducer cells while sparing immunologically competent T suppressor/cytotoxic lymphocytes and B cells. Thus, it selectively blocks those immune responses that are dependent on T helper lymphocytes; these include the cells needed to effect allograft rejection reaction (precytotoxic T lymphocytes).

Cyclosporine acts at an early phase of a developing immune response. It appears to selectively and reversibly inhibit immunologically competent T helper/inducer cells in the G_0 or G_1 phase of the cell cycle. In contrast to cytotoxic drugs, immunosuppression is achieved without lympholysis. Its major activity appears to be an inhibition of IL-2 synthesis and secretion (see Fig. 59–2). As noted previously, this growth factor is required for the proliferative expansion of antigen-stimulated cells. In addition, cyclosporine also impairs the ability of activated T helper/inducer cells to respond to IL-2 by limiting expression of receptors for this growth factor.

Because of its ability to impair the function of T helper/inducer cells, cyclosporine can restrict the generation of antigen-specific T cytotoxic and T suppressor cells. Both these lymphoid subsets depend on the activities of T helper/inducer cells to mature from their immature pre–T cell stages to competent effectors. By contrast, it does not affect the activities of pre-formed killers or inhibitory cells. Thymic-dependent humoral responses are suppressed, whereas those that are independent of T helper/inducer cell function are not inhibited.

Clinically, cyclosporine has become the principal drug used to inhibit allograft rejection reactions (Table 59–7). Its development is one of the major reasons for the successful increase in all types of organ transplant surgery using kidneys, heart, heart-lungs, livers, and pancreas.

Cyclosporine inhibits allograft rejection reactions.

The effectiveness of this immunosuppressant may be increased by the simultaneous administration of moderate doses of corticosteroids. The two agents appear to act synergistically. Cyclosporine directly inhibits IL-2 production; steroids suppress indirectly the synthesis of this lymphoid growth factor by blocking monocyte-macrophage release of IL-1 (see Fig. 59–2).

Cyclosporine is also an effective means of preventing GVHD in histocompatibly matched allogeneic bone marrow transplants. By contrast, this drug is comparatively ineffective as a treatment for established GVHD.

Unlike cytotoxic drugs, cyclosporine is not myelotoxic and therefore does not inhibit bone marrow function. Renal failure is its major toxicity; this manifestation is both dose-dependent and generally reversible. Other important toxicities are hypertension, hyperkalemia, hyperuricemia, hypomagnesemia, and fluid retention. Reversible hepatotoxicity, with elevations of the serum bilirubin and transaminases, is also a common side effect.

Cyclosporine does not inhibit bone marrow function, unlike cytotoxic drugs.

Cyclosporine has been implicated in the development of lymphomas. In particular, it appears to permit development of B cell lymphoma due to

Table 59–7 CYCLOSPORINE

Administration	Mechanism of Action	Major Indications	Toxicities
Orally, intravenously Variable dosage, 5–20 mg/kg/day	Effects primarily limited to T helper cells; not cytotoxic Inhibits production of IL-2 ? Reduces expression of IL-2 receptors	Inhibition of transplant rejection reactions	Nephrotoxicity Hypertension Hepatotoxicity ? Epstein-Barr virus–induced lymphomas Hirsutism, gingival hyperplasia Neurotoxicity Hemolytic-uremic syndrome

Epstein-Barr virus (EBV). It has been postulated that the development of this tumor occurs because there is an escape from T cell surveillance, which is normally exerted over EBV-infected B cells. Nevertheless, the overall risk of lymphoma in cyclosporine-treated transplant patients appears to be similar to that of other immunosuppressive therapy. In parallel with other drugs, the immunosuppressive effects of cyclosporine can allow for the development of severe and fatal opportunistic infections.

There are additional side effects which can result from cyclosporine treatment. These include gingival hyperplasia, hirsutism, and central nervous system manifestations, including seizures. In marrow transplantation patients, cyclosporine may cause potentially either a fatal capillary leak syndrome or a hemolytic-uremic syndrome.

FK 506, a macrolipid antibiotic, functions similarly to cyclosporine.

A new compound designated FK 506 has been reported to have even greater immunosuppressive activities than those of cyclosporine. This macrolipid antibiotic is structurally unrelated to cyclosporine but appears to act by similar mechanisms. FK 506 both suppresses the production of IL-2 and inhibits stimulated T lymphocytes from expressing IL-2 receptors. Initial reports suggest that FK 506 may be less toxic than cyclosporine. Furthermore, its development may indicate that, in the near future, other and even more potent immunosuppressive compounds capable of specifically inhibiting discrete activities of selected lymphocyte subsets will be developed.

Intravenous Gammaglobulin

IV-IgG therapy has been effective in treating children with acute ITP.

Replacement therapy with intravenous gammaglobulin (IV-IgG) has become a standard treatment for severe humoral immunodeficiencies. Of particular interest, IV-IgG has also been found to influence the course of several autoimmune diseases, particularly ITP. IV-IgG has been highly effective in treating children with the acute forms of ITP. Although prolonged remissions in adults are rare, IV-IgG can often increase platelet counts transiently. This can be potentially life-saving in cases of bleeding diatheses resulting from severe thrombocytopenia. Although the mechanism of action is not fully known in ITP, IV-IgG appears to act primarily by blocking Fc receptors on reticuloendothelial cells. This serves to inhibit the phagocytosis of antibody-coated platelets. In some cases, IV-IgG may also displace platelet specific antibodies from the cell surface.

Based on the experience with ITP, several other immune-mediated diseases have been treated with IV-IgG. These include AIHA, autoimmune neutropenia, pure red cell aplasia due to an antibody mechanism, other platelet destructive diseases, autoantibodies against the blood clotting Factor VIII, myasthenia gravis, and Kawasaki's disease. With the exception of the latter, the accumulated experience is too small to determine the drug's true effectiveness.

Alternate mechanisms have been postulated to explain the immune-modulating activities of IV-IgG. It has been reported to nonspecifically augment T suppressor cell activities, to inhibit the activities of NK cells, and to reduce the synthesis of specific immunoglobulins. In addition, IV-IgG may contain anti-idiotypic antibodies, which will serve to inactivate autoantibodies.

RhoGAM, a human antibody, is the most specific immunosuppressive agent available.

RhoGAM, which is a human antibody directed at the D antigen of the Rh system, constitutes the most specific immunosuppressive agent currently available. This intramuscular preparation is used to prevent sensitization to this Rh antigen in an Rh-negative recipient of Rh-positive red cells. Its most important use is in pregnancy; it is effective for up to 72 hours after delivery in preventing maternal sensitization to Rh antigens. As such, it inhibits the development of Rh antibody–related diseases such as erythroblastosis fetalis during the next pregnancy. RhoGAM will not suppress antibody production if the mother has already been sensitized to Rh antigens. This preparation has also been used to prevent sensitization in individuals who received mismatched blood transfusions.

Antibodies to Lymphocytes

Heterologous antisera, reactive to lymphocyte membrane antigens, represent another mode of achieving nonspecific immunosuppression. These antibodies can be divided into two groups: polyclonal antisera that react with multiple membrane determinants, and monoclonal antibodies that are directed at only a single antigen.

POLYCLONAL ANTIBODIES

Polyclonal antibodies are generally prepared by immunizing animals with human lymphocyte suspensions. If cells from the thymus are used, the preparation is termed *antithymocyte serum (ATS)*; this is often further fractionated in order to obtain the globulin portion. This reagent is termed *antithymocyte globulin (ATG)*. Other antisera are prepared from thoracic duct lymphocytes, splenic cells, or peripheral blood lymphocytes obtained by leukophoresis. These antisera are referred to as either *antilymphocyte serum (ALS)* or *antilymphocyte globulin (ALG)*.

Polyclonal antibodies are prepared by immunizing animals with human lymphocyte suspensions.

Polyclonal antisera are effective immunosuppressants in animal studies. Their primary effect is to impair cell-mediated responses; this coincides with their specificities for T lymphocytes. However, the mechanisms responsible for their immunosuppressive activities are not fully understood. One *in vivo* effect is to cause lymphopenia. *In vitro*, they will lyse lymphocytes in the presence of complement; however, it has not been established that this occurs *in vivo*. Clinically, these antisera are used primarily to treat organ graft rejection reactions. More recently, they have been found to promote remissions in some patients with aplastic anemia and to treat patients with severe GVHD.

There are several major problems associated with the use of polyclonal antisera. First, the preparations are not standardized and there are no laboratory tests that measure the *in vivo* immunosuppressive activities of a particular preparation. Thus, the amount needed to achieve a specific *in vivo* immunosuppressive effect cannot be predetermined. Second, these reagents are not selective for T cells. They cross-react with other types of cells, including platelets, leading to a severe destructive thrombocytopenia. Third, these reagents are recognized as foreign proteins. As such, they elicit a humoral immune response that frequently causes serum sickness.

Problems with polyclonal antisera include difficulty in measuring doses, unselective reactions with other cells, including platelets, and possible serum sickness.

MONOCLONAL ANTIBODIES

Monoclonal antibodies, specific to lymphocyte membrane antigens, have several theoretical advantages over polyclonal ALS. They are highly selective in their reactivity—they do not cross-react with nonlymphoid cells. Furthermore, the amount of a specific antibody can be accurately quantitated; this allows for more precise administration.

Unlike polyclonal antisera, monoclonal antibodies can be precisely administered.

Two pan T cell monoclonal antibodies have been used to reverse transplant rejection reactions and to treat GVHD in allogeneic marrow transplants. One of the antibodies used therapeutically is anti CD3; this reacts with a determinant closely linked to the T cell antigen receptor. Thus, CD3 is expressed on all immunologically competent T cells. The other reacts with the T12 antigen, a membrane determinant also on most immunologically active T lymphocytes. Initial trials suggest that each of these monoclonal antisera has the ability to reverse some rejection reactions.

ACKNOWLEDGMENTS

The secretarial services of Miss Chris A. Chrzastek are most appreciated. This was supported by a grant from the National Cancer Institute, National Institutes of Health (CA 24429–17).

General References

Bach JF (ed): The Mode of Action of Immunosuppressive Agents. New York: Elsevier Science, 1975.

Ben-Yehuda O, Tomer Y, Shoenfeld Y: Advances in therapy of autoimmune diseases. Semin Arthritis Rheum 17:206–220, 1988.

Elion GB: Immunosuppressive agents. Transplant Proc 9:975–979, 1977.

Fahey JL, Sarna G, Gale RP, et al: Immune interventions in disease. Ann Intern Med 106:257–274, 1987.

Hazleman B: Incidence of neoplasms in patients with rheumatoid arthritis exposed to different treatment regimens. Am J Med 78(Suppl 1A):39–43, 1985.

Heppner GH, Calabressi P: Selective suppression of humoral immunity by antineoplastic drugs. Annu Rev Pharmacol Toxicol 16:367, 1976.

Mitchell MS, Fahey JL (eds): Immune Suppression and Modulation. Clin Immunol Allergy 4:197–451, 1984.

Penn I: The occurrence of malignant tumors in immunosuppressed states. Prog Allergy 37:259–300, 1986.

Schein PS, Winokur SH: Immunosuppressive and cytotoxic chemotherapy: Long-term complications. Ann Intern Med 82:84, 1975.

Spreafico F, Tagliabue A, Vecchi A: Chemical immunodepressants. *In* Sirois CP, Rola-Pleszczynski M (eds): Immunopharmacology, 315–345. New York: Elsevier Biomedical Press, 1982.

Strom TB: Immunosuppressive agents in renal transplantation. Kidney Int 26:353–365, 1984.

Tsokos GC: Immunomodulatory treatment in patients with rheumatic diseases: Mechanisms of action. Semin Arthritis Rheum 17:24–38, 1987.

Yunus MB: Investigational therapy in rheumatoid arthritis: A critical review. Semin Arthritis Rheum 17:163–184, 1988.

Corticosteroids

Claman HN: Glucocorticosteroids I: Anti-inflammatory mechanisms. Hosp Pract 18:123–134, 1983.

Claman HN: Glucocorticosteroids II: The clinical response. Hosp Pract 18:143–152, 1983.

Cupps TR, Fauci AS: Corticosteroid-mediated immunoregulation in man. Immunol Rev 65:133–155, 1982.

Meuleman J, Katz P: The immunologic effects, kinetics and use of glucocorticosteroids. Med Clin North Am 69:805–816, 1985.

Parrillo JE, Fauci AS: Mechanisms of glucocorticoid action on immune processes. Annu Rev Pharmacol Toxicol 19:179–201, 1979.

Zweiman B, Atkins PC, Bedard PM et al: Corticosteroid effects on circulating lymphocyte subset levels in normal humans. J Clin Immunol 4:151–155, 1984.

Cytotoxic Drugs

Ahmed AR, Hombal SM: Cyclophosphamide (Cytoxan). J Am Acad Dermatol 11:1115–1126, 1984.

Austin HA, Klippel JH, Balow JE, et al: Therapy of lupus nephritis. N Engl J Med 314:614–619, 1986.

Berd D, Mastrangelo MJ, Engstrom PF, et al: Augmentation of the human immune response by cyclophosphamide. Cancer Res 42:4862–4866, 1982.

Clements PJ, Davis J: Cytotoxic drugs: Their clinical application to the rheumatic diseases. Semin Arthritis Rheum 15:231–254, 1986.

Cupps TR, Edgar LC, Fauci AS: Suppression of human B lymphocyte function by cyclophosphamide. J Immunol 128:2453–2457, 1982.

Felson DT, Anderson J: Evidence for the superiority of immunosuppressive drugs and prednisone over prednisone alone in lupus nephritis. N Engl J Med 311:1528–1533, 1984.

Nashel DJ: Mechanisms of action and clinical applications of cytotoxic drugs in rheumatic disorders. Med Clin North Am 69:817–840, 1985.

Turk JL, Parker D: Effect of cyclophosphamide on immunological control mechanisms. Immunol Rev 65:99–113, 1982.

Winkelstein A: Effects of cytotoxic immunosuppressants on tuberculin-sensitive lymphocytes in guinea pigs. J Clin Invest 56:1587, 1975.

Winkelstein A: Effects of immunosuppressive drugs on T and B lymphocytes in guinea pigs. Blood 50:81, 1977.

Cyclosporine

Bennett WM, Norman DJ: Action and toxicity of cyclosporine. Annu Rev Med 37:215–224, 1986.

Cohen DJ, Loertscher R, Rubin MF, et al: Cyclosporine: A new immunosuppressive agent for organ transplantation. Ann Intern Med 101:667–682, 1984.

Antisera

Cosimi AB: Clinical development of orthoclone OKT3. Transplant Proc 19(Suppl 1):7–16, 1987.

Heyworth MF: Clinical experience with antilymphocyte serum. Immunol Rev 65:79–95, 1982.

Ortho Multicenter Transplant Study Group. A randomized clinical trial of OKT3 monoclonal antibody for acute rejection of cadaveric renal transplants. N Engl J Med 313:337–342, 1985.

Goldstein G: Overview of the development of orthoclone OKT3: Monoclonal antibody for therapeutic use in transplantation. Transplant Proc 19(Suppl 1):1–6, 1987.

Toxicology

Management of Acute Poisoning

60

Ralph J. Parod
Jill G. Dolgin

This chapter is divided into two parts. The first part reviews the epidemiological characteristics and general management of acutely poisoned patients. The final part reviews the clinical management of those toxins involved most frequently in fatalities.

Although several excellent texts contain valuable information on the toxicity and treatment of poisons (Dreisbach and Robertson, 1990; Klaasen et al, 1986), the most up-to-date information on both human and animal poisonings is provided by Poisindex (MICROMEDEX, Medical Information Systems, Denver). It contains data on the chemical composition, toxicity, and current medical management of over 750,000 drugs, household chemicals, industrial and environmental toxins, and biologicals (including plant and animal toxins). Poisindex also facilitates the identification of manufactured drugs by providing a visual reference of the symbols imprinted on tablets and capsules and of street drugs by indicating their slang terminology, color, and shape. Poisindex is reviewed and updated every 3 months.

Another valuable source of information is a regional poison control center. Currently there are over 100 regional poison control centers located throughout the United States; 36 have been certified by the American Association of Poison Control Centers (AAPCC). These centers provide around-the-clock information on poisons and patient care, collect and report poisoning data, and help educate both health professionals and the public.

GENERAL CHARACTERISTICS

A poison is a chemical substance that impairs the biochemical and physiological functions of an organism. Exposure to poisons continues to be a growing problem and challenge for the health care practitioner. Poisonings are the third leading cause of accidental death and the second leading cause of suicide (Centers for Disease Control, 1989). The AAPCC estimated 4.7 million poisonings occurred nationwide in 1988 (Litovitz et al, 1989). Of the 1.4 million poisonings reported to the AAPCC, 545 resulted in death. The majority of all poisonings occurred in the home and were managed without the need for emergency room referral (Tables 60-1 and 60-2). Nonpharmaceuticals were involved in 58% of all poisonings. In contrast, fatal poisonings most frequently involved pharmaceuticals (Table 60-3). Ingestion was the most common route of exposure (Table 60-4). Accidental poisonings are most common in children under 5 years of age and in the elderly. Intentional exposures (drug abuse and suicide attempts) are most common in adolescents (>14 years of age) and adults and are the most frequent cause of death (Tables 60-5 and 60-6).

Poisindex is a valuable source of poisoning information.

Table 60-1 DISTRIBUTION OF POISONING EXPOSURE SITES

Site	Percent
Residence	91.8
Workplace	2.6
School	0.9
Health Care Facility	0.6
Other/Unknown	4.1

Adapted from Litovitz TL, Schmitz BF, Holm, KC: 1988 annual report of the American Association of Poison Control Centers national data collection system. Am J Emerg Med 7:495–545, 1989.

The Poisoned Patient

Five million poisonings occur each year in the United States.

Table 60-2 DISTRIBUTION OF POISONING MANAGEMENT SITES	
Site	**Percent**
Non–Health Care Facility	72.6
Health Care Facility	25.3
Other/Unknown	2.1

Adapted from Litovitz TL, Schmitz BF, Holm, KC: 1988 annual report of the American Association of Poison Control Centers national data collection system. Am J Emerg Med 7:495–545, 1989.

Table 60-3 DISTRIBUTION OF EXPOSURE SUBSTANCES FOR ALL POISONINGS AND FATALITIES		
Substance	**All Cases (%)***	**Fatalities (%)***
Nonpharmaceuticals	836,021 (58.2)	172 (23.2)
Pharmaceuticals	601,096 (41.8)	569 (76.8)

Data from Litovitz TL, Schmitz BF, Holm, KC: 1988 annual report of the American Association of Poison Control Centers national data collection system. Am J Emerg Med 7:495–545, 1989.
* Percentages are based on the total number of known substances (1,437,117 and 741) rather than the total number of exposures (1,368,748 and 545).

PEDIATRIC POISONING

Most poisonings occur in children under 6 years old.

The 1988 AAPCC statistics show that 62% of all poisonings occurred in children under the age of 6; 46% involved children under the age of 3. Although child-resistant caps have reduced pediatric poisoning fatalities by 70% since their institution in 1972, the unintentional ingestion of drugs by children continues to result in significant morbidity, mortality, and consumption of health care resources (Centers for Disease Control, 1987). Most pediatric poisonings result from exposure to a variety of common household substances. Of all calls to regional poison control centers in 1988, cosmetics (8%) and plants (7%) were the causes of the poisonings reported most frequently. The majority of these poisonings involved children under the age of 6 and were safely handled at home. The more toxic household substances include soaps and detergents, drain and bathroom cleaners (caustics), plants, hydrocarbons, and insecticides/rodenticides. Some relatively nontoxic household substances are listed in Table 60–7.

Safety caps reduce the incidence of childhood poisoning.

Multiple factors contribute to the risk of accidental exposure of children to medications. These include their inability to recognize potential hazards, their curiosity about their environment, their tendency to put things in their mouth, and their access to easily reached medicinals in the kitchen and bedrooms. Other factors include ineffective and misused child-resistant closures as well as the failure of these items to function after continuous use. Public education and awareness efforts should be targeted at persons who have frequent contact with small children, including grandparents and those who may not be used to caring for children. Poison prevention advisements are listed in Table 60–8.

Table 60-4 DISTRIBUTION OF EXPOSURE ROUTE FOR ALL POISONINGS AND FATALITIES		
Route	**All Cases (%)***	**Fatalities (%)***
Ingestion	1,113,101 (77.9)	424 (75.6)
Dermal	97,631 (6.8)	4 (0.7)
Ophthalmic	83,885 (5.9)	0 (0.0)
Inhalation	76,592 (5.4)	72 (12.8)
Bites and stings	45,318 (3.2)	1 (0.2)
Parenteral	4258 (0.3)	31 (5.5)
Other/unknown	8979 (0.6)	29 (5.2)

From Litovitz TL, Schmitz BF, Holm, KC: 1988 annual report of the American Association of Poison Control Centers national data collection system. Am J Emerg Med 7:495–545, 1989.
* Multiple routes of exposure were sometimes observed. Percentages are based on the total number of exposure routes (1,429,764 for all cases and 561 for fatalities) rather than the total number of exposures (1,368,748) or fatalities (545).

Table 60-5   DISTRIBUTION OF REASON FOR EXPOSURE AND AGE FOR ALL POISONINGS

Reason	<6 Years	6-12 Years	13-17 Years	18-64 Years	>64 Years	Unknown	Total	(%)
Accidental	840,511	67,409	28,056	245,539	15,707	9774	1,206,996	(88.2)
Intentional	2556	3910	31,350	93,927	2138	2390	136,271	(10.0)
Adverse reaction	2151	1122	847	13,010	774	197	18,101	(1.3)
Unknown	572	406	1049	4599	295	459	7380	(0.5)
Total	845,790	72,847	61,302	357,075	18,914	12,280	1,368,748	
(%)	(61.8)	(5.3)	(4.5)	(26.1)	(1.4)	(0.9)	(100.0)	(100.0)

Adapted from Litovitz TL, Schmitz BF, Holm, KC: 1988 annual report of the American Association of Poison Control Centers national data collection system. Am J Emerg Med 7:495-545, 1989.

Table 60-6   DISTRIBUTION OF REASON FOR EXPOSURE AND AGE FOR FATALITIES

Reason	<6 Years	6-12 Years	13-17 Years	>17 Years	Total	(%)
Accidental	27	0	1	60	88	(16.1)
Intentional	1	2	38	385	426	(78.2)
Adverse reaction	0	0	0	3	3	(0.6)
Unknown	0	0	0	28	28	(5.1)
Total	28	2	39	476	545	(100.0)
(%)	(5.1)	(0.4)	(7.2)	(87.3)	(100.0)	

Adapted from Litovitz TL, Schmitz BF, Holm, KC: 1988 annual report of the American Association of Poison Control Centers national data collection system. Am J Emerg Med 7:495-545, 1989.

Table 60-7   NONTOXIC HOUSEHOLD SUBSTANCES

Adhesives	Matches
Antacids	Modeling clay
Antibiotics (oral and topical)	Pencils
Birth control pills	Petroleum jelly
Body lotions and conditioners	Play Dough
Candles	Shampoo
Chalk	Shaving cream/lotion
Cosmetics	Suntan preparations
Crayons	Sweetening agents
Desiccants	Thermometers
Deodorants	Toothpaste
Diaper rash lotions	Vitamins without iron or fluoride
Glues and pastes	Water-based paints
Hydrogen peroxide (3%)	Zinc oxide inks/markers

Adapted from Haddad LM: The emergency management of poisoning. Pediatr Ann 16:901, 1987.

Table 60-8   POISON PREVENTION ADVICE

1. Always keep medicines and household products in their original containers and out of reach of children, preferably in a locked cabinet.
2. Never call medicine "candy."
3. Always buy products with safety packages or child-resistant caps.
4. Never put chemicals in food containers.
5. Always read and follow label directions on all products.
6. Always keep ipecac syrup on hand at home and when traveling.
7. Always keep the phone number of the local poison control center on your telephone.

Most *fatal* poisonings occur in adults from intentional exposure.

Table 60–9 NUMBER OF SUBSTANCES INVOLVED IN ALL POISONINGS AND FATALITIES

Number of Substances	All Cases (%)	Fatalities (%)
1	1,284,991 (93.9)	346 (63.5)
2	62,474 (4.6)	128 (23.5)
3	13,690 (1.0)	70 (12.8)
≥4/unknown	7593 (0.5)	1 (0.2)

Adapted from Litovitz TL, Schmitz BF, Holm, KC: 1988 annual report of the American Association of Poison Control Centers national data collection system. Am J Emerg Med 7:495–545, 1989.

Alcohol is involved usually in suicide gestures.

Evaluating the Poisoned Patient

Supportive care is the mainstay of poisoning treatment.

Glucose and *naloxone* are given to patients with altered mental status.

A *history* and *physical examination* are keys to toxin identification.

ADOLESCENT-ADULT POISONING

Whereas pediatric poisonings make up the majority of calls received by poison control centers, adolescent and adult poisonings result more often in serious morbidity and mortality. A large percentage of these poisonings are due to drug abuse or suicide gestures. Men aged 20–39 accounted for 70% of all drug abuse emergency room visits and 65% of all drug abuse deaths in 1987. During the period 1980–1986, cocaine and heroin/morphine were involved in more than one-third of these deaths (Centers for Disease Control, 1989). Other commonly abused drugs include barbiturates, benzodiazepines, volatile inhalants such as isobutyl and amyl nitrate (Rush, Locker Room), typewriter correction fluid, trichloroethane, glues, over-the-counter (OTC) sedatives, and diet aids (legal stimulants) containing either phenylpropanolamine or ephedrine. Most suicide gestures involve drugs prescribed as therapy for the victim. Drugs commonly involved in these gestures include antidepressants, nonopioid analgesics, benzodiazepines and other sedative-hypnotics, psychotropics, central nervous system (CNS) stimulants, and cardiovascular/antihypertensive drugs. Polypharmacy in drug abuse and suicide gestures is common (Table 60–9). Alcohol is the second most commonly ingested substance. Owing to the alarming increase in drug abuse, suicidal intentions may be difficult to distinguish from recreational overdose. Many patients take overdoses as risk-taking behavior and have a history of prior treatment for psychiatric illness. These patients should receive psychiatric assessment before discharge.

STABILIZATION

Symptomatic medical care that supports vital functions is the mainstay of treatment because there is no antidote for the majority of poisons encountered in clinical toxicology. "Treat the patient, not the poison" remains the most basic tenet. Initial management requires establishing the *airway* as well as maintaining adequate *breathing* and *circulation*. Serial measurements of vital signs (i.e., blood pressure, heart rate, respiration, and core temperature), important reflexes, and acid-base status help to judge the progression of toxicity, response to therapy, and the need for additional treatment.

Generally, the use of drugs is limited to those required for resuscitation and antidotes. Patients who present with an altered mental status are an exception. These individuals should receive a diagnostic challenge with *glucose* (Adult: 50 ml of 50% dextrose intravenously [IV]; Pediatric: 1–2 ml/kg of 25% dextrose IV) to distinguish hypoglycemia from other etiologies as well as *naloxone* (2 mg for both adults and children as a starting dose), an opioid antagonist. Chronic narcotic users and victims of severe opiate overdoses may require at least 10 mg of naloxone, given in 1- to 2-mg increments, before a possible narcotic overdose can be excluded. Naloxone reverses the respiratory and CNS depression due to narcotics and may be useful in some cases of ethanol and sedative-hypnotic toxicity. Patients with a history of alcohol abuse should also receive 100 mg intramuscularly (IM) of *thiamine* to prevent Wernicke's encephalopathy.

HISTORY

Once vital functions have been stabilized, the diagnosis can be aided by a more detailed evaluation. This includes documenting any available history and performing a thorough physical examination. Historical information combined with the clinical findings may be quite accurate in predicting the toxins involved in the overdose patient. Family, friends, and paramedical personnel should be questioned about the environment in which the patient was found. Syringes and bottles of prescription and OTC preparations located in the vicinity of the patient should be brought to the emergency room.

PHYSICAL EXAMINATION

A toxicologically oriented physical examination emphasizes vital signs, eyes, mouth, skin, abdomen, and nervous system. The findings can suggest which toxin is involved as well as clinical interventions and laboratory tests that may confirm or quantitate its presence. A limited number of toxins produce no initial signs, symptoms, or routine laboratory abnormalities. The most important of these is acetaminophen. Serum acetaminophen levels should always be determined in patients with an unknown ingestion.

Blood Pressure and Heart Rate. Toxins that stimulate the sympathetic nervous system or block the parasympathetic system peripherally may cause hypertension and tachycardia. These findings are consistent with amphetamines, cocaine, and phencyclidine (PCP), as well as both anticholinergic (e.g., antihistamines, antispasmodics) and cholinergic (e.g., nicotine, physostigmine) drugs. In some cases the initial stimulation of vital signs is followed by a generalized depression (e.g., monoamine oxidase inhibitors, levodopa, bretylium). Hypotension and tachycardia are common with plant toxins (*Amanita* mushrooms), drugs that produce peripheral arteriolar dilatation with reflex compensation (antipsychotic agents, β_2-stimulants, theophylline), and toxin-induced tissue hypoxia (carbon monoxide, cyanide). Hypotension and bradycardia are characteristic features of narcotics, central α_2-agonists (e.g., clonidine), sedative-hypnotics, nicotine (late finding), β blockers, and calcium channel blockers.

Respiration. Both the rate and the depth of respiration may be increased by sympathomimetics, by drugs that stimulate the medullary respiratory center either directly (e.g., salicylates) or indirectly by causing cellular hypoxia (e.g., carbon monoxide, cyanide), and by metabolic acidosis. Respiration is depressed by opioids and sedative-hypnotics.

Core Temperature. Hyperthermia can be elicited by drugs that increase muscle activity or metabolic rate (e.g., salicylates, thyroid hormones, sympathomimetics, antimuscarinics) or by those that impair thermoregulation (e.g., anticholinergics, antidepressants, antipsychotics). Hypothermia is frequently caused by the inability of the body to respond to cool ambient temperatures. Alcohol, phenothiazines, narcotics, and sedative-hypnotics are examples of drugs that promote hypothermia by producing vasodilatation and inhibiting the shivering reflex. Sepsis, hypothyroidism, and hypoglycemia should be eliminated as non–drug-related causes of hypothermia.

Eyes. Constriction of the pupils (miosis) may be due to increased muscarinic tone (e.g., organophosphates, physostigmine), decreased sympathetic tone (e.g., narcotics, clonidine, phenothiazines, sedative-hypnotics), or brainstem injury. Dilatation of the pupils (mydriasis) may be due to increased sympathetic tone (e.g., lysergic acid diethylamide [LSD], cocaine, amphetamines) or muscarinic blockade (e.g., atropine, bethanechol). Hori-

Table 60–10 THERAPY PROVIDED IN POISON EXPOSURE CASES

Therapy	Number
Decrease Absorption	
Dilution	548,084
Irrigation/washing	250,513
Ipecac syrup	115,157
Activated charcoal	89,026
Cathartic	76,270
Gastric lavage	32,601
Other emetic	3282
Enhance Elimination	
Urinary alkalinization	4060
Hemodialysis	389
Forced diuresis	370
Hemoperfusion (charcoal)	108
Urinary acidification	47
Exchange transfusion	32
Peritoneal dialysis	30
Hemoperfusion (resin)	23
Antidotes	
Naloxone	5308
N-acetylcysteine	4935
Hydroxocobalamin	704
Atropine	620
Deferoxamine	594
Antivenin/Antitoxin	394
Ethanol	381
Fab fragments	331
Physostigmine	269
Pralidoxime (2-PAM)	157
Penicillamine	139
Dimercaprol (BAL)	138
Cyanide antidote kit	113
Pyridoxine	105
Methylene blue	66
EDTA	53

Adapted from Litovitz TL, Schmitz BF, Holm, KC: 1988 annual report of the American Association of Poison Control Centers national data collection system. Am J Emerg Med 7:495–545, 1989.

Toxicology screens are of limited value.

zontal nystagmus (e.g., phenytoin, ethanol, barbiturates) or vertical nystagmus (e.g., PCP) are also important findings. Ptosis (eyelid drooping) and ophthalmoplegia are features of botulism.

Mouth. The mouth should be inspected to determine whether the patient has a gag reflex and whether corrosives have caused ulceration in the mouth or pharynx. Some toxins result in detectable odors in the mouth, such as wintergreen (salicylates), acetone (isopropyl alcohol), almonds (cyanide), garlic (arsenic, organophosphates), alcohol, and petroleum distillates. Dry mucous membranes may indicate anticholinergic poisoning, whereas hypersalivation may suggest organophosphate poisoning.

Skin. The patient should be checked for needle tracks, burns or bruises, and abnormal skin temperature or color. Diaphoresis (sweating) may suggest an overdose with stimulants, salicylates, organophosphates, or nicotine. Extremely dry, *warm* skin may suggest an overdose wth anticholinergic drugs, whereas dry, *cool* skin may indicate sedative-hypnotic or barbiturate poisoning. Cutaneous bullae (skin blisters at pressure points) accompany sedative-hypnotic poisoning and are seen also in patients unconscious for prolonged periods of time. A cherry-red skin coloration (usually an autopsy finding) may suggest severe carbon monoxide poisoning.

Abdomen. Decreased or absent bowel sounds are typical findings in anticholinergic, narcotic, and sedative-hypnotic overdoses. Hyperactive bowel sounds, abdominal cramping, and diarrhea are common findings in poisonings with organophosphate and carbamate insecticides, iron and heavy metals, sympathomimetics, and Amanita *phalloides* mushrooms and in drug/alcohol withdrawal syndromes.

Nervous System. Ataxia and incoordination are symptoms of phenytoin, alcohol, barbiturate, and sedative-hypnotic intoxication. Muscle rigidity and hyperactivity suggest intoxication with sympathomimetic drugs, methaqualone, PCP, or haloperidol. Generalized seizures are often the result of severe intoxication from cyclic antidepressants, stimulants, isoniazid, and phenothiazines. Coma with absent reflexes and flaccid muscle activity may be present with narcotic and sedative-hypnotic drugs and may mimic brain death.

Toxicology Screen. Toxicology screens are often used to diagnose, assess prognosis in, and manage acute poisoning, particularly in comatose or uncooperative patients. However, toxicology screens are time-consuming, expensive, and often unreliable. Their reliability depends on (1) communication between the laboratory and the physician about drugs suspected to be involved, (2) correct sampling of appropriate biological fluids, (3) prompt reporting of the results, and (4) the number of substances listed on the drug analysis profile. Most laboratories limit screens to drugs commonly prescribed and to a few drugs of abuse.

Toxicology screens are no substitute for clinical judgment and should be ordered only in those few instances when the results obtained will influence the therapy provided. For example, plasma levels of a few toxins (e.g., acetaminophen, salicylates, lithium, carbon monoxide, theophylline, iron, ethylene glycol, methanol) may influence the course of therapy, whereas for many drugs (e.g., cyclic antidepressants) there is a poor correlation between plasma levels and toxicity. Interpretation of toxicological analyses must consider the clinical condition of the patient, the time elapsed since exposure, and the potential for delayed toxic effects. For example, therapeutic levels of acetaminophen (30 mcg/ml) 4–8 hours postingestion are associated with little risk of hepatotoxicity; the same level obtained more than 16 hours postingestion indicates a high risk of hepatotoxicity unless antidotal therapy is instituted immediately. Other considerations include the fact that toxic reactions may occur at therapeutic levels if the drug exacerbates an underlying pathology, the possibility of false negatives, and the realization that no assay or combination of assays can detect all possible poisons.

The three goals in treating acute poisoning are to (1) prevent absorption of the toxin, (2) enhance its elimination, and (3) reverse its toxicity by administering antidotes. Table 60–10 summarizes the therapies provided in intoxications reported to the AAPCC in 1988.

Treating the Poisoned Patient

DECREASE ABSORPTION

Irrigation-Washing. Decontamination of the skin, eyes, and gastrointestinal (GI) tract should be started after the initial diagnostic assessment and laboratory evaluation. Contaminated clothing should be removed once the patient is away from further exosure. The skin should be cleansed with copious amounts of soap and water to prevent further percutaneous absorption. The eyes should be irrigated with warm tap water or normal saline solution.

Dilution. Although diluting poisons within the GI tract with large volumes of water has been recommended in the past, the use of water may actually increase the acute toxicity of drugs by enhancing their dissolution and stimulating gastric emptying. The AAPCC has recommended that oral dilution with water be used only to minimize the risk of burns from caustic-type substances. Water can be given with ipecac syrup but is not required for its efficacy. Inhalation of humidified air or oxygen can dilute toxins in the nasal passages.

Emesis. Induction of vomiting with ipecac syrup is the preferred method for removing ingested substances from the stomach of patients with a gag reflex who are conscious and alert. It is most effective when initiated within 30 minutes of toxin ingestion. Recommended dosages and contraindications to emesis are listed on Table 60–11. Upon the advice of a physician or poison control center specialist, ipecac syrup can be used safely and effectively in the home. Other emetics such as lobeline injection, copper sulfate solution, salt water, and mustard powder have been abandoned because they are either impractical or ineffective or have a low margin of safety. Apomorphine is no longer used in humans owing to its side effects but is safely utilized in animals. A soapsuds solution (2–3 tablespoons of liquid dishwashing detergent, not automatic dishwasher detergent, in 6–8 ounces of water) is recommended as an emetic by some poison control centers in situations in which ipecac syrup is not available and a health care facility is greater than 30 miles away.

Activated Charcoal and Cathartics. Activated charcoal is the most efficacious procedure for preventing the absorption of drugs. Currently the use of activated charcoal alone, without prior ipecac-induced emesis or lavage, is favored, particularly in patients seen more than 1 hour postingestion. Optimal adsorption occurs when the dose of charcoal is at least ten-fold

Decreasing absorption is the most common form of poisoning therapy.

Ipecac syrup is the method of choice when emesis is indicated.

Table 60–11　IPECAC SYRUP

Administration

1. Carefully supervise all vomiting patients.
2. Administer ipecac syrup.

Age	Volume
6–12 months	10 ml–15 ml
1–5 yrs	15 ml–30 ml
>5 yrs	30 ml

3. Repeat dose if vomiting has not occurred within 20 minutes.
4. After vomiting has begun, give fluids (about 15–30 ml) until vomitus is clear.
5. Do not give food or drink for 1–2 hours to allow effects from ipecac to stop.
6. Keep patient in upright position or on side/stomach to prevent vomit aspiration.

Contraindications

1. Child less than 6 months of age unless in an emergency room.
2. Comatose patient or patient with altered level of consciousness.
3. Presence of seizures or expected onset of seizures owing to toxin involved.
4. Loss of gag reflex
5. Ingestion of sharp solid material.
6. Ingestion of caustics.
7. Nonaromatic and nonhalogenated hydrocarbons not containing other toxic agent.

Activated charcoal alone *is preferred for decontamination in the hospital setting.*

greater than the estimated dose of toxin. Charcoal does not adsorb iron salts, hydrocarbons, simple alcohols, boric acid, lithium, cyanide, and caustics. Thickening agents such as bentonite, 70% sorbitol, or 2% carboxymethylcellulose are effective in suspending charcoal without altering its adsorptive capacity. Flavoring agents such as jam, jelly, milk, cocoa powder, ice cream, and sherbet should be avoided because they compromise the efficacy of the charcoal. Administration of a cathartic with the activated charcoal hastens the removal of toxins from the GI tract and thereby reduces their systemic absorption. Sorbitol (40–70%) is the preferred cathartic agent if heart failure is not present. The use of sorbitol in the commercially available premixed activated charcoal preparations precludes the need for other cathartics. Magnesium or sodium sulfate and magnesium citrate can be used with the activated charcoal powder. Oil-based cathartics are of no value and are potentially harmful owing to the potential for lung aspiration. Table 60–12 lists usual dosages of common cathartics.

Table 60–12　ACTIVATED CHARCOAL AND CATHARTICS

Single-Dose Activated Charcoal

1. Administer 1.0 g/kg of activated charcoal mixed in water or 70% sorbitol.

Multiple-Dose Activated Charcoal

1. Administer one half of initial dose (without cathartic) every 2–6 hours until patient is asymptomatic.
2. Cathartic may be given every 8–12 hours if patient has not stooled.

Cathartics

1. Sorbitol (70%) is preferred (child: 1–2 ml/kg; adult: 100–150 ml).
2. Magnesium or sodium sulfate (10%); magnesium citrate (10%) (child: 4 ml/kg; adult: 150–250 ml).

Contraindications

1. Absence of bowel sounds.
2. Signs of intestinal obstruction, abdominal trauma, or GI bleeding.
3. Shock, poor tissue perfusion.
4. Use cautiously in patient with hematemesis.
5. Avoid magnesium cathartics in renal disease.
6. Avoid sodium cathartics in congestive heart failure.

Table 60–13 LAVAGE PROCEDURE

1. Protect the airway.
2. Patients in coma or without a gag reflex should receive nasotracheal or endotracheal (cuffed in patients >5 years old) intubation prior to lavage.
3. Place patient in lateral decubitus position.
4. Insert orogastric hose (child: 16–28 French; adult: 30–40 French).
5. Lavage until clear (child: 50–100 ml aliquots; adults: 200-ml aliquots).
6. Use orogastric or nasogastric hose to administer charcoal and a cathartic if indicated.

Gastric Lavage. Gastric lavage (Table 60–13) is used primarily in patients who are obtunded, comatose, or uncooperative. The most important factor in determining the efficacy of gastric lavage as well as ipecac-induced emesis appears to be the time elapsed between ingestion and implementation of the decontamination procedure. When either decontamination procedure is delayed more than 60 minutes postingestion, the amount of toxin recovered by gastric lavage and emesis is small and not significantly different. Gastric lavage performed more than 1 hour postingestion has shown no benefit over the administration of activated charcoal alone (Kulig et al, 1985). Epidemiological studies report that the mean time from ingestion to hospital presentation is 3.3 hours for adults and 68 minutes for children (Kulig et al, 1986; MacLean, 1973). Another important variable in determining the effectiveness of gastric lavage is the size of the tube. Decontamination with small-bore nasogastric tubes is inferior to ipecac-induced emesis. The larger orogastric tubes are more efficacious and can be used to introduce activated charcoal or a specific antidote. Contraindications for lavage are similar to those for emesis. Aspiration pneumonia, secondary to vomiting during the procedure, is the most common complication.

> Gastric lavage is no better than activated charcoal alone.

Whole Bowel Irrigation. Whole bowel irrigation is used primarily as a safe, precolonoscopy procedure. It involves the oral administration of large volumes of a polyethylene-glycol isosmotic electrolyte (GOLYTELY, COLYTE) solution that traverses the entire GI tract and is generally well tolerated. Although superior to gastric lavage and induced emesis, it is both labor-intensive and time-consuming. It should not be utilized routinely but may be promising for drugs that are not adsorbed by activated charcoal (e.g., iron, lithium) or for overdoses with delayed-release pharmaceuticals (Tenenbein, 1988).

ENHANCE ELIMINATION

Knowledge of basic concepts governing the pharmacokinetic or toxicokinetic (kinetics of a drug in overdose) properties of a drug can assist the clinician in deciding which therapies may accelerate the removal of the toxin and thus decrease morbidity and mortality. Procedures such as changing urinary pH (with or without diuresis, hemodialysis, or peritoneal dialysis), charcoal and resin hemoperfusion, exchange transfusion, repeated oral administration of activated charcoal, and plasmapheresis have all been used in attempts to hasten systemic elimination of drugs and poisons.

These therapies enhance the clearance of drugs but do not effect their volume of distribution (V_D). For drugs eliminated by first-order kinetics, both clearance and V_D are related to the half-life of the drug ($t_{1/2}$), the time necessary to eliminate one half the amount of drug in the body, by the following equation:

> Methods to enhance elimination are only useful for toxins with a small V_D.

$$CL = \frac{V_D \times C \times Wt \times 0.693}{t_{1/2}}$$

CL represents clearance (mg/minute); C is the plasma drug concentration (mg/l) and Wt is body mass (kg). Thus, for drugs with a large V_D, the $t_{1/2}$ is prolonged at any given clearance. Conversely, as clearance rate increases, the $t_{1/2}$ shortens for any given V_D. Generally methods to enhance elimination are clinically effective only for toxins with a V_D less than or equal to total body water, 0.6 l/kg. The degree of plasma protein binding also affects the efficacy of the treatment modality. Except for charcoal or resin hemoperfusion, therapies that enhance drug clearance primarily remove the free or unbound drug from the plasma compartment. Therefore, if a drug has a large V_D (e.g., cyclic antidepressants, digoxin), the removal of drug from plasma has minimal impact on the total amount of drug in the body. Plasma drug levels rebound to pretreatment levels as the drug exits tissue stores and re-equilibrates with plasma. In cases of massive overdose, elimination pathways that involve hepatic enzyme systems can become saturated. In these instances drug clearance remains constant and is concentration independent (zero-order kinetics). Drugs that exhibit zero-order kinetics in overdose include theophylline, salicylates, some barbiturates, chloral hydrate, ethchlorvynol, and acetaminophen. In these instances, utilizing methods to enhance drug elimination may contribute to total body clearance and may significantly improve the clinical outcome.

It is important to understand not only the toxicodynamic (injurious effects of toxins on vital functions) and toxicokinetic properties of toxins but also to be familiar with the risks versus the benefits of each technique. These methods should be considered only in those instances in which it has been shown to impact the clinical outcome or in high-risk patients who do not respond to traditional supportive care.

Forced Diuresis. Fluid loading and forced diuresis with furosemide or mannitol is one of the oldest techniques used to enhance drug elimination. Only drugs that are minimally protein-bound, eliminated primarily by renal excretion, and passively reabsorbed in the renal tubules are affected by diuresis. Forced diuresis may be useful in overdoses with bromides, phencyclidine, lithium, and amphetamines. Contraindications include renal or cardiac failure. Pulmonary edema and electrolyte imbalances are potential problems with diuresis.

Forced, acid, and alkaline diuresis are of limited value.

Acid-Alkaline Diuresis. Renal elimination of a few toxins is enhanced by alteration of urinary pH with or without forced diuresis. This technique takes advantage of the ionization properties (expressed as the negative log of their acid dissociation constant or pKa) of drugs that are weak acids and weak bases. Because the ionized forms of these drugs cannot diffuse through the cell membrane, they are trapped in compartments that promote their ionization. Acids (un-ionized when protonated) are trapped in alkaline compartments; bases (ionized when protonated) are trapped in acidic compartments. When the pH of the urine is altered appropriately, it can cause drugs contained within it to become ionized. In this form the drug is not reabsorbed by the renal tubules, and its excretion is hastened. Alkaline diuresis is a useful technique for weak acids such as salicylate (pKa = 3.0) and phenobarbital (pKa = 7.2). Acid diuresis has been advocated in strychnine (pKa = 8.0), PCP (pKa = 8.5), and amphetamine (pKa = 9.9) overdoses but does not appear to be clinically useful in most cases.

Dialysis. Dialysis refers to the diffusion of a toxin across a semipermeable membrane. Although it has been recommended for a variety of poisons, relatively few patients benefit from it. The physical characteristics of the drug are the major factors limiting its efficacy. The drug must have a small V_D, a molecular weight small enough (<500 daltons) to permit it to pass through the dialysis membrane, hydrophilicity, and low protein binding. *Hemodialysis* is indicated in renal failure secondary to toxin exposure, when the metabolism of a dialyzable drug is limited by saturation of liver enzymes, and in severe overdose with salicylates, lithium, ethylene glycol, or methanol. It is used also in the presence of fluid and electrolyte imbalances. *Peritoneal dialysis* is a relatively simple technique yet is only 10–25% as effective as hemodialysis and only slightly more effective than forced diuresis. It can be useful if short-term dialysis is required, as in salicylate or lithium overdoses.

Hemodialysis and hemoperfusion are used only in severe poisonings.

Charcoal-Resin Hemoperfusion. Hemoperfusion is a technique whereby blood is pumped through a cartridge containing either charcoal or an AMBERLITE resin. The affinity of the toxin for the adsorbent, the rate of blood flow through the cartridge, and the V_D of the toxin are the factors that contribute to the efficacy of hemoperfusion. Unlike dialysis, hemoperfusion is not limited to small, hydrophilic compounds and effectively extracts large, hydrophobic drugs exhibiting extensive protein binding. Charcoal removes both polar and nonpolar drugs, whereas the resin clears nonpolar drugs more effectively than does charcoal. It is the modality of choice in severe theophylline, paraquat, digitoxin, ethchlorvynol, phenytoin, and phenobarbital poisonings. It does not correct fluid and electrolyte imbalances or remove all toxic chemicals. Complications such as depletion of platelets and removal of plasma proteins and solutes have been minimized with increasing clinical experience and the advent of more adsorbent and coated cartridges.

Exchange Transfusion. Exchange transfusion is a technique in which blood of a poisoned patient is removed and replaced with fresh whole blood. Potentially its most effective applications are in patients with severe methemoglobinemia unresponsive to methylene blue and in severe iron poisoning.

Multiple-Dose Activated Charcoal. The oral administration of multiple doses of activated charcoal (MDAC), also called *gastrointestinal dialysis,* enhances drug elimination by (1) preventing the absorption of drugs from the GI tract, (2) adsorbing drugs that either diffuse or are transported back into the GI tract, and (3) adsorbing drugs that are excreted into the small intestine from the biliary tract (Levy, 1982; Watson, 1987). The ability of MDAC to remove drugs is influenced by the same pharmacokinetic principles that govern the effectiveness of hemodialysis and hemoperfusion. Drugs that undergo extensive enterogastric or enterohepatic recycling (e.g., digitoxin) may be removed more efficiently by MDAC. The efficacy of MDAC is affected also by the preparation and dose of charcoal, the time interval between drug intoxication and charcoal administration, the time interval between dosages of charcoal, and the severity of intoxication (Watson, 1987). Advantages of MDAC are that it can be initiated immediately in the primary care setting and that it is noninvasive, inexpensive, and generally well tolerated. Adverse effects include repeated emesis (especially after ipecac syrup), protracted diarrhea (owing to cathartic coadministration), aspiration, and GI obstruction. Although the plasma clearance of phenobarbital, theophylline, salicylates, and carbamazepine (Park et al, 1986; Tenenbein, 1986) is enhanced by MDAC, changes in morbidity and mortality have been demonstrated only for theophylline overdoses.

MDAC eliminates the need for more invasive and expensive techniques.

Plasmapheresis. Plasma exchange transfusion refers to the therapeutic removal of large volumes of plasma and its replacement with normal plasma or suitable colloid. It is most applicable to toxins that are highly protein bound, have a small V_D, and have a prolonged $t_{1/2}$ (e.g., phenytoin, digitoxin). Because hemodialysis and hemoperfusion clear larger plasma volumes at a faster rate, they should be considered first when supportive care is insufficient. As yet, owing to the multiple complications and costs involved, plasmapheresis should be considered an unproven and hazardous form of poisoning therapy.

ANTIDOTES

Antidotes antagonize the effects of toxins by inhibiting the binding of a toxin to its receptor (pharmacological antagonist), causing a physiological response that opposes the actions of a toxin (physiological antagonist), changing the chemical nature of a poison to a less toxic form (chemical antagonism), or decreasing the amount of toxin that reaches its site of action by either preventing its absorption or enhancing its elimination or metabolism (biochemical antagonism). Unfortunately, there are only a small number of toxins for which effective antidotes exist. Major antidotes

Antidotes are available for only a limited number of toxins.

Table 60–14 POISONS AND ANTIDOTES

Poison	Antidote	Dosage
Opiates	Naloxone (Narcan)	Adult and Ped: 2 mg IV Repeat with 1–2 mg to a maximum of 10 mg if no response
Acetaminophen	N-acetylcysteine (Mucomyst)	Load: 140 mg/kg orally Maintenance: 70 mg/kg every 4 hours for 17 dosages
Cyanide, nitroprusside	Hydroxocobalamine (vitamin B_{12a})	Load: 50 mg/kg IV Maintenance: 25 mg/hour
	Amyl nitrite, sodium nitrite, sodium thiosulfate (CN antidote kit)	1 ampule amyl nitrite inhaled 3 minutes until injection of sodium nitrite 300 mg at 2.5 ml–5 ml/minute, then inject 12.5 g of 25% sodium thiosulfate slowly
Organophosphates, carbamates	Atropine	Adult: 0.5–2 mg IV; Ped: 0.05 mg/kg IV Repeat dosage every 10 minutes until atropinized
	Pralidoxime (2-PAM) (organophosphates only)	Adult: 1 g over 30 minutes Ped: 25–50 mg/kg over 30 minutes
Iron	Deferoxamine (Desferal)	90 mg/kg IM to maximum 1 g Every 4–8 hours or 10–15 mg/kg/hour IV to maximum 6 g/24 hours
Ethylene glycol, methanol	Ethanol	Load: 7.6–10 ml/kg of 10% ethanol in D5W IV or orally Maintenance: 1.4 ml/kg/hour of 10% ethanol in D5W Maintain blood ethanol level 100–130 mg/dl
Digoxin	Fab fragments	Dose according to serum level or amount ingested
Atropine, anticholinergics	Physostigmine (Antilirium)	Adult: 0.5–2 mg IV; Ped: 0.5 mg (0.01 mg/kg) Repeat as required
Arsenic, lead, mercury	Dimercaprol (BAL in oil)	3–5 mg/kg dose IM every 4 hours for 48 hours, then 3 mg/kg/dose IM every 6 hours for 48 hours, then 3 mg/kg/dose every 12 hours for 7 days
	D-penicillamine	Adult: 250–500 mg every 6 hours for 5 days Ped: 4–10 mg/kg every 6 hours for 5 days to maximum of 250 mg/dose
Isoniazid	Pyridoxine (vitamin B_6)	5 g over 30–60 minutes Repeat to maximum 40 g adults; 20 g peds
Methemoglobinemia	Methylene blue	0.1–0.2 ml/kg of 1% solution
Lead	Ca EDTA (calcium disodium tetraacetic acid)	50–75 mg/kg/day deep IM or slow IV in 3–6 divided doses for 5 days
Warfarin	Phytonadione (vitamin K_1)	Adult: 10 mg IM: Ped: 1–5 mg IM

and dosages are listed in Table 60–14. These drugs are supplemented by immunological agents such as snake antivenins and bacterial antitoxins. Flumazenil and immunological agents are being evaluated currently as potential antidotes for benzodiazepine and tricyclic antidepressant poisonings respectively. Strong acids and bases are treated with water or milk. Neutralization of acids and bases with antacids or lemon juice, respectively, is no longer advocated owing to the exothermic reaction produced by these combinations.

Acute Poisons

The AAPCC began collecting data on human poisonings in 1983. Since that time it has been observed that more than 90% of the chemicals associated with fatalities are distributed among 13 generic classes of chemicals. Figure 60–1 depicts the rank of these classes according to the number of deaths with which they were associated in 1988. Although small changes in the relative order of these chemical classifications occur yearly, poisonings from chemicals within these classifications continue to be the major challenge to medical practitioners. The following text provides a general discussion of the toxicity and treatment for those chemicals within each category most frequently associated with fatality. More detailed discussions are available elsewhere (see Ellenhorn and Barceloux, 1991; Goldfrank, 1990; Gosselin et al, 1984; Haddad and Winchester, 1990; and Klaasen et al, 1986).

ANTIDEPRESSANTS

Antidepressants constitute the class of drugs found most commonly in deaths caused by acute poisoning. This observation is probably a reflection of their relatively low margin of safety as well as the fact that individuals taking them have a higher potential for suicide. Of the 741 poisons associated with fatality in 1988, 135 were antidepressants. The *cyclic antidepressants* were most frequently involved (125 deaths), followed by *monoamine oxidase (MAO) inhibitors* (4), *lithium salts* (4), and *trazodone* (1).

Antidepressants are the drug class involved most frequently in fatal poisonings.

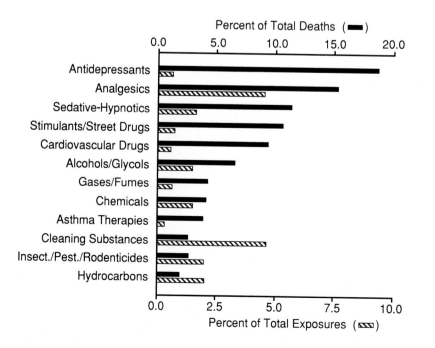

Figure 60–1

Distribution of deaths (*solid bars*) and exposures (*open bars*) among 12 categories of poisons. Percentages are based on the total number of poisons known to be involved in human fatalities (741) and exposures (1,437,117). Among the categories of poisons listed by the AAPCC, antidepressants were most frequently associated with fatalities (18.2%), whereas analgesics were most frequently involved in all cases of poisoning (10.0%). (Data from Litovitz, JL, Schmitz BF, Holm KC: 1988 annual report of the American Association of Poison Control Center national data collection system. Am J Emerg Med 7:495–545, 1989.)

Cyclic Antidepressants and Trazodone

Psychiatric depression is most often treated with the cyclic antidepressants, a group of structurally related drugs that share a characteristic three- or four-ring nucleus. *Amitriptyline* and *imipramine* are prototypical tricyclic antidepressants, whereas *amoxapine* and *maprotiline* are representative tetracyclic antidepressants. *Trazodone* as well as *fluoxetine* and *bupropion* are newer (second-generation) antidepressant drugs whose chemical structures differ from those of the cyclic antidepressants. To varying degrees, these compounds inhibit the reuptake of biogenic amines (particularly norepinephrine and serotonin) at nerve terminals, block the activation of muscarinic, α_1-adrenergic as well as H_1- and H_2-histaminergic receptors, and impair both cardiac conduction and contractility. Acute intoxication with these drugs begins usually with a brief phase of agitation and restlessness that may include tonic-clonic seizures. This may rapidly lead to coma with depressed tendon reflexes, depressed respiration, hypotension, and hypothermia. Antimuscarinic symptoms such as dry mouth, mydriasis, sinus tachycardia, the absence of bowel sounds, urinary retention, and a flushed, dry skin are also evident. Although sinus tachycardia is most common, a variety of cardiac conduction abnormalities and arrhythmias can also be observed. Amoxapine and maprotiline exhibit fewer cardiovascular effects but have a greater seizure potential than other cyclic antidepressants. Trazodone and fluoxetine exhibit less cardiotoxicity and neurotoxicity than the cyclic antidepressants and have weaker antimuscarinic properties. Overdoses with bupropion, a drug chemically related to amphetamine, commonly result in seizures.

The cyclic and second-generation antidepressants are pharmacokinetically similar. Most are absorbed incompletely and undergo significant first-pass metabolism. They are eliminated over the course of several days following their oxidation by hepatic microsomal enzymes and eventual conjugation with glucuronic acid. About 15% of the metabolized dose is excreted into the intestines through the bile and may remain biologically active. There are no antidotes for these drugs. Intoxications are best managed by supporting cardiac function and ventilation. The induction of emesis is contraindicated because it may precipitate seizures; gastric lavage is of limited benefit unless begun within 1 hour of exposure. Activated charcoal adsorbs these compounds and may be particularly efficacious in cases of overdose because their anticholinergic effects prolong their stay in the gut. Although MDAC can be given to interrupt the enterohepatic circulation of these drugs, the risk of bowel obstruction with MDAC outweighs its potential benefit in serious intoxications. The large volumes of distribution (V_D, 5–60 l/kg) exhibited by these drugs is a function of their lipophilicity and strong protein binding and may explain why attempts to enhance their elimination with dialysis and diuresis are of little clinical value. Because the $t_{1/2}$ of these antidepressants ranges from 8 to 100 hours, patients should be placed on a cardiac monitor for at least 24 hours following the resolution of CNS and cardiovascular symptoms.

There are no antidotes for cyclic antidepressant intoxication.

Monoamine Oxidase Inhibitors

Of this class of drugs, *isocarboxazid, phenelzine,* and *tranylcypromine* are the ones used currently in the United States for the treatment of depression. They share the ability to inhibit the oxidative deamination of monoamines (dopamine, norepinephrine, and serotonin). The disappointing results obtained with these drugs in early clinical trials and their relative toxicity compared with the cyclic antidepressants limited their use in depression to those cases that were refractory to treatment with cyclic antidepressants and electroconvulsive therapy. However, the use of MAO inhibitors appears to be increasing. More recent findings indicate that higher dosages of MAO inhibitors are as effective as the cyclic antidepressants in severe depression and that these drugs may be valuable in the treatment of phobias and neurotic illnesses with depressive features. Acute intoxications can result from either drug overdose or the interaction of MAO inhibitors with indirectly acting sympathomimetic agents. Toxic manifestations of drug overdose may be delayed 6–24 hours after ingestion and include restlessness, hypertension, hyperreflexia, mydriasis, sinus tachycardia, hyperpyrexia, diaphoresis, muscular rigidity, and coma. Hypertensive crisis is the primary complication resulting from the interaction between therapeutic dosages of MAO inhibitors and indirectly acting sympathomimetic drugs (amphetamine, ephedrine, phenylpropanolamine) and foods containing large amounts of tyramine (> 10 mg: e.g., aged cheeses, Chianti wine, and yeast-containing food supplements). Hypertension is accompanied usually by headache, hyperpyrexia, and tachycardia and may lead to cerebral hemorrhage and death. If MAO inhibitors are ingested alone, the late phases of severe intoxications (>4 mg/kg) may be associated with profound hypotension, bradycardia, and cardiac arrest.

> Hypertensive crisis is the primary complication of MAO intoxication.

MAO inhibitors are rapidly absorbed from the GI tract. Although little is known of their pharmacokinetics, MAO inhibitors are metabolized in the liver primarily by acetylation. About half the population in the United States and Europe are slow acetylators and are thus more susceptible to MAO toxicity. Because there is no antidote for MAO intoxication, treatment is supportive care. Particular attention should be given to assuring adequate ventilation and to controlling blood pressure, hyperthermia, excessive muscle rigidity, and seizures. Because isocarboxazid and phenelzine bind irreversibly with MAO, several weeks may be required to synthesize new enzyme and to restore monoamine metabolism to normal. Intoxications with tranylcypromine are reversed more rapidly, perhaps reflecting the reversible binding between the drug and MAO. Patients should be monitored in the intensive care unit until stable for 24 hours.

Lithium Salts

Although *lithium* is used primarily in the treatment of bipolar manic-depressive illness, it is sometimes used as an alternative or supplement to the cyclic antidepressants in severe depression. Recent studies indicate that therapeutic levels of lithium (0.6–1.2 mEq/l) may decrease the responsiveness of neurons and other cells to various neurotransmitters by lowering the content of phosphatidylinositides in their plasma membrane. However, the mechanism responsible for the therapeutic and toxic effects of lithium remains unclear. In patients on lithium therapy, toxicity is common at blood levels of 2 mEq/l; sustained levels of 4 mEq/l are often lethal. Higher levels may be tolerated in naive individuals. Although early signs of lithium overdose include nausea, diarrhea, and polyuria, neurological effects constitute the primary concern. These include mental confusion, drowsiness, dysarthria, blurred vision, tremor, fasciculations, myoclonus, and choreoathetosis and may progress to stupor, seizures, and coma. Renal and cardiac conduction abnormalities may be evident in severe cases.

> Lithium levels > 4 mEq/l may be lethal in patients on chronic therapy.

Lithium is well absorbed from the GI tract, is not bound by plasma proteins, and has a V_D (0.8 l/kg) that slightly exceeds total body water (0.6 l/kg). Although lithium quickly diffuses throughout the body's extracellular space, it crosses cell membranes slowly. This is particularly true in the

CNS, where equilibrium between plasma and brain takes from 8 to 10 days. This may explain why the toxic symptoms in patients who have not previously received lithium are sometimes limited to nausea and vomiting. Lithium is eliminated almost entirely by urinary excretion. Because there are no specific antidotes for lithium intoxication, treatment is primarily supportive. Emesis or lavage may be of value if initiated shortly after ingestion or when absorption is delayed as with sustained-release tablets. Sodium polystyrene sulfonate may bind lithium more effectively than activated charcoal, which is of dubious value.

Hemodialysis is the treatment of choice in severe intoxications. Hemodialysis markedly reduces serum lithium levels, although levels rise again following treatment owing to the redistribution of lithium from intracellular to extracellular sites. This observation may explain why, even with hemodialysis, recovery remains slow. Approximately 80% of the lithium filtered by the kidney is reabsorbed in the proximal tubule, where it competes with sodium for reabsorption. Thus, maintaining water and sodium balance is a major concern. Dehydration (vomiting, diarrhea) and hyponatremia (low salt; distal tubule diuretics, thiazides) can potentiate lithium toxicity by increasing its renal reabsorption. Forced diuresis with saline solution and osmotic diuretics (mannitol) can result in serious electrolyte imbalances and should not be used unless the glomerular filtration rate is below normal. Carbonic anhydrase inhibitors (acetazolamide) and urinary alkalinization have been reported to reduce plasma lithium levels, presumably through their effects on Na^+-H^+ exchange.

ANALGESICS

Analgesics made up 118 of the 741 fatal poisons reported to the AAPCC in 1988. Most of the analgesics associated with fatality could be classified as either *acetaminophen* (52 deaths), a *salicylate* (35), an *opioid* (24), or *ibuprofen* (3).

Acetaminophen

Acetaminophen has analgesic and antipyretic properties similar to those of the salicylates but does not possess their anti-inflammatory effects. Acetaminophen is becoming increasingly popular as a household analgesic because it lacks some of the side effects of aspirin. Acetaminophen does not cause gastric irritation, does not prolong the bleeding time, is not associated with Reye's syndrome in children, and is less likely to lead to an anaphylactic-type reaction (urticaria, bronchospasm, hypotension). Although acetaminophen is a weak inhibitor of prostaglandin synthesis, its mechanism of action is unclear. Acetaminophen poisoning is divided into four stages. The first (12–24 hours postexposure) is characterized by anorexia, nausea, vomiting, and diaphoresis. The second (1–2 days) is associated with clinical improvement. The prothrombin time and plasma levels of hepatic transaminases and bilirubin begin to increase. Hepatotoxicity, manifested by centrilobular necrosis, usually reaches its peak during the third stage (3–4 days). Mildly poisoned individuals enter stage four (5–7 days postexposure) and recover. Severe intoxications lead to hepatic encephalopathy that progresses from confusion to coma to death. Some patients also exhibit acute renal failure.

Acetaminophen is rapidly and completely absorbed from the GI tract. Therapeutic dosages are metabolized in the liver by conjugation to glucuronides (60%) and sulfates (35%). A small fraction (4%) is metabolized by the P-450 mixed-function oxidase system to a reactive intermediate, which is detoxified by glutathione to cysteine and mercapturic acid metabolites. At higher dosages, more acetaminophen is converted to the reactive intermediate because the conjugation pathways become saturated. As glutathione stores are depleted, the reactive intermediate binds to other cellular proteins and produces hepatic necrosis. Renal dysfunction has the same etiology. Acetaminophen intoxication is best treated by replenishing glutathione stores with *N-acetyl-L-cysteine* (NAC), a glutathione precursor. Emesis, lavage, and activated charcoal are also beneficial if initiated within 4–6 hours postexposure. However, in order to prevent hepatotoxicity following exposure, therapy with NAC should not be delayed more than 8–10 hours.

NAC is the antidote for acetaminophen intoxication.

Salicylates

Aspirin (acetylsalicylic acid) and other salicylates (sodium salicylate, salicylic acid, methyl salicylate) are nonsteroidal anti-inflammatory drugs (NSAIDs) found in hundreds of commercial products in the United States. All are effective analgesic, antipyretic, and anti-inflammatory agents whose therapeutic effects are mediated by the inhibition of prostaglandin synthesis. Aspirin alone inhibits platelet aggregation by virtue of its irreversible acetylation of platelet-prostaglandin synthetase.

Hundreds of commercial products contain salicylates.

Common features of acute salicylate poisoning involve the GI tract and the CNS. These include nausea and vomiting, tinnitus and hearing loss, as well as hyperventilation. Hyperventilation is mediated by the stimulatory effect of salicylates on the medullary respiratory center and by increased plasma CO_2 levels that result from the ability of salicylates to uncouple oxidative phosphorylation. The uncoupling of oxidative phosphorylation may be responsible also for the hyperpyrexia and sweating seen in cases of overdose. Acid-base imbalances are another important clinical manifestation of toxicity. Hyperventilation leads to respiratory alkalosis that is followed by the increased renal excretion of bicarbonate, potassium, and water. Severe salicylate intoxication is associated with a combination of respiratory alkalosis and metabolic acidosis. High dosages of salicylate depress respiration, which, in the presence of low plasma bicarbonate and the enhanced production of CO_2, results in respiratory acidosis. Salicylates produce metabolic acidosis by interfering with the citric acid cycle, which results in the accumulation of organic acids such as lactate, pyruvate, and acetoacetate. Severe intoxication may lead also to pulmonary edema, convulsions, and coma. These effects on the CNS may reflect a reduction in brain glucose levels as well as the shift of salicylates from the blood to the brain in acidemic patients owing to pH-partitioning.

Salicylates are rapidly and completely absorbed from the GI tract in therapeutic dosages. An acute overdose can result in the formation of drug concretions (bezoars) and delayed gastric emptying. Salicylic acid and methyl salicylate are well absorbed through the intact skin. Aspirin and methyl salicylate are rapidly hydrolyzed to salicylic acid by esterases in GI mucosa and liver. The plasma half-life of aspirin is 15–20 minutes, whereas the half-life of salicylic acid at therapeutic doses is approximately 3 hours. Salicylic acid is metabolized in the liver by conjugation with glycine to form salicyluric acid and with glucuronic acid to form salicylic phenolic and acyl glucuronides. A small portion is hydroxylated to gentisic acid. Because these metabolic pathways are quickly saturated at therapeutic dosages, the half-life of salicylate in cases of overdose can be as long as 36 hours. Salicylates are excreted primarily by the kidney as salicylic acid (10%), salicyluric acid (75%), phenolic (10%) and acyl (5%) glucuronides as well as gentisic acid (<1%). The salicylic acid content of urine is quite variable because it depends on both dosage and urinary pH.

The treatment for salicylate intoxication is primarily symptomatic. Particular attention should be given to correcting hyperpyrexia, dehydration, acid-base imbalances, and hypokalemia. CNS depression should be treated with IV glucose even when serum glucose levels are normal. Absorption from the GI tract can be prevented by emesis or gastric lavage within 2–4 hours of exposure or by activated charcoal alone up to 24 hours postexposure. MDAC may also enhance the elimination of absorbed drug. The elimination of aspirin (pKa = 3.5) and other salicylates can be enhanced by urinary alkalinization with sodium bicarbonate, hemodialysis, and hemoperfusion. Although the latter two treatments are equally effective in removing salicylates, hemodialysis is better able to control acid-base and electrolyte imbalances.

Opioids

Opioids are a class of drugs, natural *(morphine, codeine)*, semisynthetic *(heroin)* and synthetic *(propoxyphene, methadone, meperidine, pentazocine, fentanyl)*, that react with closely related receptors to produce morphine-like actions. Acute intoxication with opioids is associated with the triad of CNS depression (stupor, coma), respiratory depression, and pinpoint pupils (except meperidine). Opioids (except pentazocine) also produce peripheral vasodilation that, in the presence of hypoxia, may progress to shock. Seizures may be seen following overdoses with meperidine and propoxyphene. Cardiac arrhythmias are not uncommon in propoxyphene overdoses. Pulmonary edema is present in the majority of fatalities.

Following oral administration, opioids are readily absorbed in therapeutic doses from the GI tract and exhibit a significant but variable amount of first-pass biotransformation. They are metabolized primarily in the liver. Treatment of overdose begins with establishing adequate ventilation and circulation and is followed by the administration of *naloxone*, a pure opioid antagonist. Naloxone does not reverse cardiac arrhythmias seen with propoxyphene. The patient must be monitored carefully because the antagonistic effects of naloxone last for only a few minutes, whereas the toxic effects of long-acting opioids (methadone) may last several days. Induction of emesis is contraindicated unless initiated within 30 minutes postexposure; lavage may be effective within 1 hour postexposure. Activated charcoal alone may be effective any time postexposure owing to the decreased GI motility produced by opioids. Forced diuresis and dialysis are of no value owing to the large volumes of distribution and high degrees of protein binding exhibited by opioids. Also, forced diuresis may exacerbate pulmonary edema.

Naloxone is the antidote for opioid poisoning.

Ibuprofen

Ibuprofen poisoning is being encountered with increasing frequency.

Next to aspirin, ibuprofen is the most widely used NSAID in the United States. Owing to its more recent availability in OTC preparations, ibuprofen is being encountered with increasing frequency in poisonings. Like aspirin, ibuprofen probably acts by inhibiting the production of prostaglandins. Acute ibuprofen overdoses may result in mild GI symptoms such as nausea, vomiting, and epigastric pain. Peptic ulceration and hemorrhage are not common in acute overdoses. Other less commonly observed manifestations of ibuprofen toxicity include metabolic acidosis, hypotension, CNS depression, and renal dysfunction. Renal toxicity is thought to be due to the decreased production of intrarenal prostaglandins, which causes a decrease in both renal blood flow and glomerular filtration rate. In children, aspirin toxicity is associated with hyperventilation, whereas ibuprofen is more commonly associated with apnea.

Ibuprofen is rapidly absorbed from the GI tract. It is rapidly metabolized by the liver and has a half-life of about 2 hours. Only about 1% of the administered dose appears in the urine unchanged. Intoxications are treated with supportive care. Ipecac syrup may be of benefit if administered within 30 minutes of exposure. Activated charcoal alone may be of benefit any time postexposure because it adsorbs many other NSAIDs. Methods to enhance the elimination of ibuprofen are ineffective. There are no antidotes.

STIMULANTS AND STREET DRUGS

Of the fatalities reported to the AAPCC in 1988, 101 involved stimulants and street drugs. *Cocaine* was responsible for 63 deaths, followed by *amphetamines* (12), *heroin* (12), *caffeine* (5), *phencyclidine* (2), *phenylpropanolamine* (2) and *amyl/butyl nitrites* (1). The treatment for heroin (diacetylmorphine, which is rapidly deacetylated to morphine) and nitrite intoxication is presented under Opioids and Chemicals, respectively. Caffeine (1,3,7-trimethylxanthine) and theophylline (1,3-dimethylxanthine, discussed later under Asthma Therapies) intoxication are treated similarly.

Cocaine

Cocaine is a powerful CNS stimulant, local anesthetic, and sympathomimetic agent. In the periphery, it potentiates the actions of catecholamines by blocking their reuptake at adrenergic nerve terminals. Its effects on the CNS are probably mediated through a similar mechanism. The initial CNS effects (euphoria, garrulousness, restlessness) are due to cortical stimulation and are followed by effects (hyperventilation, tachycardia, hypertension, hyperthermia, emesis, tremor, convulsions) caused by the progressive involvement of lower brain centers. The central effects of cocaine on heart rate, blood pressure, and temperature are potentiated by its peripheral effects on the sympathetic nervous system. In high dosages, cocaine depresses the CNS as well as myocardial contractility and conduction. Death results from either respiratory failure or cardiac arrest.

Cocaine is well absorbed from nasal, respiratory, and GI mucosa. Following absorption, it is rapidly degraded by plasma and liver cholinesterases; only small amounts (10%) are excreted unchanged in the urine. Acute intoxications are best treated with supportive care. Particular attention should be given to controlling seizures, cardiac arrhythmias, and hyperthermia. Because cocaine is usually inhaled or injected, decontamination of the gut by lavage or emesis is frequently unwarranted. The short plasma $t_{1/2}$ (1 hour) and relatively large V_D (2 l/kg) of cocaine as well as the small fraction of cocaine excreted unchanged in the urine make attempts to enhance its elimination impractical. Diazepam can be used to control convulsions. The use of beta blockers and lidocaine should be reserved for patients with life-threatening cardiac arrhythmias.

Cocaine is well absorbed by all routes of administration.

Amphetamines and Phenylpropanolamine

Amphetamines refer to a class of drugs with similar pharmacological and toxicological properties. The amphetamines associated most frequently with fatality are *amphetamine* and two structural analogs, *methamphetamine* and *methylphenidate*. Smokable methamphetamine is called *ice.* Amphetamines are powerful CNS stimulants, anorectics, and sympathomimetic agents that act either by releasing norepinephrine and dopamine from their storage site in nerve terminals or by blocking neurotransmitter reuptake. The toxic manifestations of amphetamine overdose are similar to those described earlier for cocaine. *Phenylpropanolamine* (PPA) is an analog of amphetamine that is found in OTC preparations of nasal decongestants and diet aides. PPA is a less potent CNS stimulant than amphetamine and acts indirectly by releasing norepinephrine from sympathetic nerve terminals and directly as an α agonist. Hypertension is the most serious toxic effect of PPA. High doses of PPA have an effect on the CNS that is similar to that seen with cocaine.

Amphetamines and PPA are well absorbed from the GI tract. Although amphetamine, methamphetamine, and PPA are biotransformed in the liver, significant fractions of each are excreted in the urine unchanged. In contrast, most of the methylphenidate dose is de-esterified to an inactive metabolite; only 1% is excreted in the urine unchanged. Intoxication with these drugs is best treated with supportive care, with particular attention given to controlling hyperthermia, hypertension, and seizures. Although all these drugs delay gastric emptying, emesis is not recommended because it may provoke seizures, hypertensive hemorrhage, and cardiac complications. Activated charcoal and a cathartic are recommended. Because amphetamine ($pKa = 9.9$), methamphetamine ($pK_a = 10.1$), and PPA ($pKa = 9.4$) are weak bases, their elimination can be enhanced by urinary acidification. Acidification is contraindicated in the presence of rhabdomyolysis and myoglobinuria because myoglobin may precipitate in the renal tubules and damage the kidneys.

Phencyclidine

Although classified pharmacologically as a dissociative anesthetic, phencyclidine (PCP) is no longer used in humans owing to adverse reactions (delirium, seizures) seen postanesthesia. PCP produces a wide variety of physiological effects. Mild intoxications present with altered thought patterns, bizarre behavior, horizontal and vertical nystagmus, normal or pinpoint pupils, hyperthermia, hypertension, and tachycardia. Higher dosages result in convulsions, coma, respiratory depression, cardiac arrhythmias, and renal failure secondary to rhabdomyolysis. The psychoactive properties of PCP may be due to its interaction with dopamine (DA-2) and opioid (σ) receptors. PCP also inhibits the reuptake of dopamine, serotonin, and norepinephrine at presynaptic nerve terminals.

Amphetamines and PCP may provoke a severe hypertensive crisis.

PCP is a lipophilic drug that is well absorbed by the respiratory and GI tracts. Hydroxylation appears to be the primary route of biotransformation. The hydroxylated metabolites are excreted in the urine as conjugates of glucuronic acid; approximately 10% of the PCP dose appears in the urine unchanged. Most PCP fatalities are either homicidal or accidental. Intoxications are best treated by isolating the patient from unnecessary external stimuli to control self-destructive behavior and by supporting vital functions. Emesis and lavage are of questionable benefit because PCP is usually rapidly absorbed and these procedures may further agitate the patient. PCP is a weak base with a pKa of 8.5. Urinary acidification enhances PCP elimination but also increases the risk of renal failure in the presence of myoglobinuria. The large V_D of PCP (6.2 l/kg) may explain why acidification does not always lead to a significant clinical improvement. Activated charcoal may be useful to remove PCP trapped in the acidic environment of the stomach and to interrupt the enterogastric circulation of PCP.

SEDATIVE-HYPNOTICS

The category of drugs termed *sedative-hypnotics* ranked fourth (77 deaths) on the list of substances associated most frequently with fatality. Three classes of drugs, the *benzodiazepines* (42), *phenothiazines* (18), and *barbiturates* (8), were identified in the majority of fatal overdoses. Other drugs identified less frequently were *glutethimide, chloral hydrate, ethchlorvynol, diphenhydramine* (present in OTC sleep aides), and *meprobamate*. Although the spectrum of their effects varies, all these drugs depress the CNS. They are used clinically to induce drowsiness and promote sleep and as anxiolytics, muscle relaxants, anticonvulsants, and antipsychotic agents (phenothiazines). The toxic manifestations of these drugs are an increase in the depth of CNS depression (sedation, coma, respiratory depression) and cardiovascular instability (hypotension, decreased contractility, arrhythmias, pulmonary edema).

Sedative-hypnotics depress all vital functions.

The sedative-hypnotics share a similar pharmacological profile. They are lipophilic drugs that are well absorbed from the GI tract. They are extensively bound by plasma proteins and eliminated primarily by hepatic metabolism. Because there are no specific antidotes, acute intoxications are best treated with supportive care. This includes establishing a clear airway and maintaining adequate ventilation and cardiovascular function. Emesis or lavage should be initiated within 30 minutes of exposure to be effective. Activated charcoal may be of value 8–10 hours after exposure to sedative-hypnotics that delay gastric emptying (phenothiazines, barbiturates, glutethimide, meprobamate). Diuresis is generally ineffective because the kidney is not a significant elimination pathway; forced diuresis may exacerbate pulmonary edema. Alkalinization of the urine can increase the excretion of phenobarbital (pKa, 7.2) five- to tenfold. Resin hemoperfusion is generally accepted to be more beneficial than hemodialysis in those patients unresponsive to supportive care.

CARDIOVASCULAR DRUGS

In 1988, 65 fatalities were ascribed to cardiovascular drugs. *Cardiac glycosides* were responsible for 23 deaths, followed by *calcium channel blockers* (17), *β blockers* (80), *antiarrhythmics* (8), *antihypertensives* (7), and *vasodilators* (2).

Cardiac Glycosides

Digoxin was the drug involved in all cardiac glycoside fatalities. Digoxin is used to increase the force of myocardial contraction in congestive heart failure and to decrease the ventricular rate in atrial fibrillation. Cardiac glycosides produce these effects directly by inhibiting the Na^+-K^+ adenosine triphosphatase (ATPase) and indirectly by modifying the activity of the autonomic nervous system as well as the sensitivity of the heart to autonomic neurotransmitters. Nausea and vomiting are common symptoms of glycoside poisoning. Fatigue, mental confusion, and visual disturbances may be present also. Abnormalities in cardiac rhythm, particularly atrioventricular (A-V) block and ventricular tachycardia, are the usual cause of death. Acute intoxications are associated also with hyperkalemia, which may exacerbate dysrhythmias. Symptoms of toxicity may begin within 30 minutes; peak effects are noted between 3 and 12 hours.

The bioavailability of digoxin following oral administration ranges from 50 to 80%. The kidney excretes 60–80% of the drug unchanged. Decontamination of the GI tract with activated charcoal followed by a cathartic is beneficial. Emesis and lavage are not recommended because they may stimulate vagal reflexes and exacerbate bradyarrhythmias. The large V_D of digoxin (Table 60–15) limits the usefulness of diuresis, dialysis, and hemoperfusion. Hemodialysis may rectify hyperkalemia. Atropine is useful in managing A-V block; phenytoin effectively suppresses ventricu-

Table 60-15	PHARMACOKINETIC PROPERTIES OF CARDIOVASCULAR DRUGS				
	Acid	PK$_a$ Base	V$_D$ (l/kg)	Protein Binding (%)	Excreted in Urine Unchanged (%)
Cardiac Glycosides					
Digitoxin	—		0.6	95	33
Digoxin	—		7	25	60
Calcium Channel Blockers					
Diltiazem	—		5.3	78	<4
Nifedipine	—		1.2	98	≈0
Verapamil		8.8	4.0	90	<3
Beta Blockers					
Acebutolol		9.2	1.2	26	40
Atenolol		9.3	0.6	<5	85
Metoprolol		9.7	4.2	13	10
Propranolol		9.4	3.9	93	<0.5
Antiarrhythmics					
Disopyramide		8.4	0.6	30	55
Procainamide		9.2	1.9	16	67
Quinidine		4.2	2.7	90	18
		8.3			
Antihypertensives					
Captopril	3.7		0.7	30	50
	9.8				
Clonidine		8.2	2.1	—	62
Methyldopa	2.2		0.4	1–16	28
	10.4 (OH)				
	12.6 (OH)				
Vasodilators					
Diazoxide	8.5		0.2	94	35
Hydralazine		0.5	1.5	85	1–15
		7.1			
Minoxidil		4.6	12	0	12
Nitroprusside	—		—	—	—

Fab fragments of digoxin antibodies reverse digitalis toxicity.

lar arrhythmias and promotes A-V conduction. In severe intoxications, the IV administration of *Fab fragments* of immunoglobulins directed against digoxin (DIGIBIND) can rapidly reverse cardiac toxicity. The benefits of treatment with Fab fragments must be weighed against the possibility of hypersensitivity reactions and of precipitating congestive heart failure in severely diseased patients.

Calcium Channel Blockers

All three calcium channel antagonists available in the United States, *diltiazem, nifedipine,* and *verapamil,* have been associated with fatalities. They are used primarily in the treatment of supraventricular arrhythmias and angina. Calcium channel blockers are classified as Class IV antiarrhythmic agents and act by inhibiting the entry of calcium into cells or by inhibiting its release from intracellular stores. At therapeutic levels, verapamil and diltiazem, but not nifedipine, slow A-V node conduction. All three drugs produce vasodilatation. Manifestations of acute toxicity are exacerbations of these therapeutic effects. Bradycardia, conduction block, and hypotension are the major complications seen with verapamil and diltiazem; vasodilatation and tachycardia are the predominant features of intoxication with nifedipine.

Calcium channel antagonists are well absorbed following oral administration but undergo extensive first-pass metabolism in the liver. The amount of these drugs that appears in the urine unchanged is less than 4%. Decontamination of the stomach by the usual measures should be initiated. The pharmacokinetic characteristics of diltiazem, nifedipine, and verapamil (see Table 60–15) indicate that diuresis, hemodialysis, and hemoperfusion are impractical for these lipophilic drugs. Hypotension may be difficult to manage but usually responds to IV calcium and normal saline solution. Atropine, isoproterenol (or glucagon), and pacing can be used to treat bradycardia and A-V block.

Calcium can be used to manage overdoses with calcium channel blockers.

Beta Blockers

The nonselective (β_1 and β_2) adrenergic receptor antagonist *propranolol* and the selective (β_1) adrenergic receptor antagonists *metoprolol, acebutolol,* and *atenolol* were the β blockers identified in fatal overdoses. They are used to treat cardiovascular disorders such as hypertension, arrhythmias, and angina pectoris. Beta blockers are categorized as Class II antiarrhythmic drugs. Because the selectivity of the β_1 blockers is lost at high concentrations, the toxic effects of all β blockers are similar. These effects include bradycardia, depressed sinoatrial and A-V conduction, hypotension, and bronchospasm. Lipophilic β blockers like propranolol and, to a moderate degree, metoprolol can cause CNS depression, seizures, and sudden apnea.

Whereas β blockers are generally well absorbed from the GI tract, their bioavailability ranges between 30% and 90% owing to first-pass metabolism in the liver. Lipophilic β blockers are the primary targets of liver metabolism, whereas the hydrophilic β blockers like atenolol are excreted by the kidney largely unchanged. The first treatment in cases of overdose is to prevent further absorption with either lavage or charcoal followed by a cathartic. Emesis with ipecac may be contraindicated owing to the rapid onset of cardiovascular symptoms. Although hemodialysis and hemoperfusion are of no apparent benefit in overdoses with most β blockers, the pharmacokinetic properties of atenolol suggest that these procedures may enhance its elimination. Cardiovascular and CNS toxicity are treated symptomatically. Atropine can be used to reverse bradycardia. Conduction abnormalities usually respond to glucagon, which elevates cAMP through a β-adrenergic receptor-independent pathway, and to isoproterenol. Because isoproterenol is a nonselective β-adrenergic agonist, it often does not correct hypotension. Hypotension is best treated with glucagon or norepinephrine. Aminophylline or isoproterenol can alleviate bronchospasm. Seizures can be controlled with diazepam.

Antiarrhythmics

The drugs in this category associated most commonly with fatality are the Class 1A antiarrhythmics *disopyramide, procainamide,* and *quinidine.* These drugs decrease the conduction velocity of electrical impulses through the heart by interfering with sodium channel reactivation and are used primarily in the treatment of supraventricular and ventricular arrhythmias. Acute toxic effects are due to conduction delays (heart block, ventricular arrhythmias) and the depression of myocardial contractility. All three have anticholinergic properties. The negative inotropic and anticholinergic effects are more common with disopyramide. Hypotension may result from the α-adrenergic receptor blockade produced by quinidine. Procainamide and quinidine may produce CNS symptoms (confusion, convulsions, and coma).

Bioavailability of all three drugs is high (75–85%) following oral ad-

Depressed cardiac contractility is a major toxic effect of β blockers and antiarrhythmics.

ministration. The amount of drug excreted in the urine ranges between 20 and 60%; the remainder is metabolized by the liver. The anticholinergic properties of these drugs suggest that decontamination of the stomach (emesis within 30 minutes postexposure, lavage, and charcoal followed by catharsis) will be beneficial. Because disopyramide, procainamide, and quinidine are weak bases, they are concentrated in the acidic environment of the stomach. Repeated doses of activated charcoal (every 3–4 hours) may enhance their elimination. The pharmacokinetic properties of disopyramide (see Table 60–15) indicate that hemoperfusion and hemodialysis should effectively enhance its elimination. Unless renal failure is present, these techniques offer little benefit in intoxications with procainamide and quinidine. Ventricular arrhythmias can be successfully treated with phenytoin, isoproterenol, and overdrive pacing.

Antihypertensives

Drugs in this category associated with fatal poisonings are *captopril, clonidine,* and *methyldopa.* Captopril produces hypotension by inhibiting the enzyme that converts angiotensin I to the potent vasopressor angiotensin II. Clonidine, an α_2-adrenergic agonist, and methyldopa, which is metabolized to the α_2-adrenergic agonist α-methylnorepinephrine, act through central stimulation of presynaptic β_2-adrenergic receptors in the cardiovascular control centers. This stimulation decreases sympathetic outflow. Hypotension is the primary manifestation of overdose with all three agents. In severe overdose, clonidine and methyldopa may produce hypertension by stimulating peripheral α-adrenergic receptors. By decreasing sympathetic tone, clonidine and methyldopa can also produce dry mouth, bradycardia, and the impairment of A-V conduction. CNS symptoms of clonidine and methyldopa overdose include coma, hypothermia, miosis, and apnea.

Bioavailabilities of captopril, clonidine, and methyldopa following oral administration are 65%, 75%, and 25%, respectively. Significant amounts of these drugs appear in the urine unchanged (see Table 60–15). Overdoses are treated by removing these drugs from the stomach by either emesis or lavage and activated charcoal followed by a cathartic. Primary emphasis should be placed on treating hypotension by fluid infusion and vasopressor amines (dopamine, dobutamine, norepinephrine). Although supportive therapy is usually sufficient, the pharmacokinetic properties of captopril and methyldopa indicate that hemodialysis may be of benefit.

Vasodilators

Hydralazine, minoxidil, sodium nitroprusside, and *diazoxide* are peripheral vasodilating drugs sometimes associated with fatalities. All four agents cause a direct relaxation of vascular smooth muscle probably through the activation of guanylate cyclase. Acute intoxication with these agents leads to excessive vasodilatation and hypotension. The release of cyanide from sodium nitroprusside may also produce cyanide toxicity (see Chemicals). Hydralazine and minoxidil are well absorbed from the GI tract, although hydralazine is subject to extensive first-pass metabolism in the gut and liver. Sodium nitroprusside and diazoxide are administered by IV infusion. Management of toxicity is supportive and emphasizes treatment of hypotension. Hydralazine and minoxidil poisonings can be ameliorated by induction of emesis and gastric lavage. The pharmacokinetic properties of these drugs (see Table 60–15) indicate that methods to enhance their elimination are of little benefit. There are no antidotes for the hypotensive effects of these drugs.

ALCOHOLS AND GLYCOLS

Chemicals in this category were responsible for 46 fatalities in 1988. The chemicals involved were *ethanol* (36), *methanol* (4), *ethylene glycol* (4), and *isopropanol* (1).

Ethanol

Ethanol is a short-acting CNS depressant found in a variety of commercial products including beverages, medicinal liquids (some rubbing alcohols, cold/cough formulations), cosmetics (perfumes, aftershaves, colognes), mouthwashes, and liniments. Its depressant effects are probably due to an increase in the fluidity of neural cell membranes that disrupts the function of membrane-bound proteins. The reticular-activating system and portions of the cortex are most susceptible to ethanol toxicity. The suppression of inhibitory circuits in the cortex may account for the excitement seen at low doses. Higher doses affect the cerebellum and occipital lobe, leading to incoordination and visual disturbances. Severe intoxications produce a general CNS depression that may include hypothermia, coma, and respiratory failure. Hypoglycemia may be present also, especially in children.

Ethanol is well absorbed from the GI tract. The lung and kidney excrete 5–10% of the absorbed dose unchanged; the remainder is metabolized in the liver. Ethanol is first oxidized by alcohol dehydrogenase to acetaldehyde, which is oxidized then by aldehyde dehydrogenase to acetate. Because both oxidation reactions require nicotinamide-adenine dinucleotide (NAD), the hepatic NAD/NADH (nicotinamide-adenine dinucleotide [reduced form]) ratio is reduced. This reduction may decrease gluconeogenesis and explain the hypoglycemia associated with ethanol overdose. The rapid absorption of ethanol makes GI decontamination procedures of little benefit when they are initiated more than 1 hour postingestion. Activated charcoal does not bind alcohols in significant amounts. Most intoxications respond to supportive care that emphasizes maintaining adequate ventilation and body temperature as well as the IV administration of fluids to correct dehydration, acidosis, and hypoglycemia. Hemodialysis can enhance the elimination of ethanol (V_D of 0.6 l/kg and no protein binding) and is indicated when ethanol blood level exceeds 500 mg/dl and when hepatic function is compromised.

Ethanol is found in a variety of medicinals, cosmetics, and mouthwashes.

Methanol

Methanol is widely used as a solvent in shellacs, paints, varnishes, and paint removers. It is contained also in windshield washer fluid, gasoline antifreeze, and canned fuel (STERNO). Initially, methanol produces a mild CNS depression without the euphoria seen with ethanol. This is followed by an asymptomatic period that progresses within 6–30 hours to other signs of intoxication. These include GI disturbances (nausea, vomiting, abdominal pain), ocular abnormalities (blurred vision, hyperemia of the optic disk), and metabolic acidosis. The delayed symptoms are probably due to the accumulation of toxic metabolites, primarily formic acid, resulting from the oxidation of methanol. The pharmacokinetic properties of methanol and ethanol are similar. Methanol is metabolized by alcohol dehydrogenase to formaldehyde, which is oxidized by aldehyde dehydrogenase to formic acid. Formate is subsequently oxidized to carbon dioxide through a folate-dependent pathway. Mortality from methanol intoxication correlates best with serum formate levels. Treatment strategies emphasize supportive care (assuring adequate ventilation and circulation as well as controlling metabolic acidosis) and lowering serum formate levels.

The latter is accomplished by decreasing formate formation (emesis or lavage within 1 hour of exposure, administration of ethanol) and by increasing its elimination (hemodialysis, administration of folate). The benefits of ethanol are due to its tenfold greater affinity for alcohol dehydrogenase, which causes it to be oxidized by the enzyme in preference to methanol. (4-methylpyrazole [4MP], a potent inhibitor of *diphenylchlorarsine* (AD), is not a CNS depressant–osmotic diuretic, and coincident dehydration associated with it is currently being investigated as a substitute for ethanol, owing to its greater affinity for alcohol dehydrogenase and fewer side effects.)

Ethylene Glycol

In industry, *ethylene glycol* is used as a starting material in chemical syntheses; in the home it is found in radiator antifreeze and cosmetics. Intoxication occurs in three phases. In the first phase (1–12 hours) the patient appears inebriated without the odor of ethanol and may experience nausea and vomiting. Other symptoms includes acidosis, nystagmus, convulsions, and coma. The second phase (12–36 hours) is associated with hyperventilation, which may be indicative of metabolic acidosis or pulmonary edema, and tachycardia. The third stage (48–72 hours) is characterized by renal failure, which may be evidenced by lumbar pain, oliguria, and uremia. Calcium oxylate crystals in the urine are also indicative of ethylene glycol intoxication.

Ethylene glycol is well absorbed from the GI tract. The kidney excretes 20% of the absorbed dose unchanged; the remainder is metabolized in the liver. Alcohol dehydrogenase oxidizes ethylene glycol to glycoaldehyde. Both chemicals are thought to be responsible for the CNS depression seen during the first phase of ethylene glycol intoxication. Glycoaldehyde is oxidized to glycolate, which is primarily responsible for the metabolic acidosis seen in overdose. Glycolate can be oxidized further to oxalate, which chelates calcium. Tissue destruction induced by the deposition of calcium oxalate crystals is thought to result in the toxicity associated with the last two phases of intoxication. Supportive care should emphasize controlling acidemia with bicarbonate and maintaining urinary output. The acidic metabolites of ethylene glycol are more toxic than the parent compound. The accumulation of these metabolites can be inhibited by the administration of ethanol, which has a hundredfold greater affinity for alcohol dehydrogenase than does ethylene glycol. The elimination of these metabolites can be enhanced by hemodialysis and the administration of pyridoxine and thiamine, cofactors in the metabolism of glyoxalate.

Methanol and ethylene glycol toxicity are managed with ethanol and hemodialysis.

Isopropanol

Isopropanol is an industrial solvent that in the home is found primarily in rubbing alcohol, skin lotions, window cleaners, and gasoline antifreeze. Compared with ethanol, isopropanol is about twice as potent a CNS depressant and causes gastric distress (pain, nausea, vomiting) more frequently. Hypotension associated with severe intoxication is a poor prognostic indicator. Death is usually preceded by respiratory arrest in deep coma. Isopropanol is well absorbed from the GI tract; 20–50% of the absorbed dose is excreted unchanged. The remainder is oxidized in the liver, presumably by alcohol dehydrogenase, to acetone. Acetone, also a CNS depressant, is eliminated slowly by the lung and kidney and may be further oxidized to acetate and formate. The fact that isopropanol is metabolized more slowly than ethanol may explain the observation that toxic symptoms of isopropanol overdose last two to four times longer than those seen with ethanol. Treatment consists of gastric lavage or emesis within 1 hour of exposure followed by supportive care. The latter includes correcting hypotension and acidosis. Hemodialysis effectively enhances elimination. Ethanol is not used to treat isopropanol intoxication.

GASES, FUMES, AND VAPORS

As a category, gases, fumes (submicron particles, usually oxidized, produced during the heating or combustion of a solid), and vapors (gaseous phase of substances that are liquids or solids at room temperature and pressure) were responsible for 39 deaths in 1988. *Carbon monoxide* (CO, 27 deaths) and *hydrogen sulfide* (H_2S, 7 deaths) were the gases involved most frequently in fatalities. Other gases associated less frequently with fatality include *ammonia* (NH_3), *methane,* and *propane.* CO, H_2S, and NH_3 are chemical asphyxiants because they produce cellular hypoxia by interfering with oxygen transport and delivery to the tissues. In contrast, methane and propane are termed *simple asphyxiants* because they produce hypoxia by displacing oxygen from the respiratory environment. Hypoxia from simple asphyxiants is treated by resuscitation in air or with oxygen.

Chemical asphyxiants produce cellular hypoxia by interfering with tissue oxygenation.

Carbon Monoxide

Carbon monoxide is a colorless and odorless gas that is produced by the incomplete combustion of organic material. In the home it is a major component of the exhaust gases emanating from automobiles and heating equipment. Following its absorption through the lung, CO binds to hemoglobin with an affinity 250 times greater than oxygen to form carboxyhemoglobin (COHb). Hypoxia ensues because COHb carries less oxygen and has a greater affinity for the oxygen it does carry. Tissues with the greatest metabolic activity (e.g., brain, heart) are particularly vulnerable to hypoxia. Early symptoms include headache, weakness, irritability, and confusion. Moderate intoxications are associated with nausea and vomiting as well as increased respirations and tachycardia. Severe intoxications are manifested by coma, convulsions, and cardiopulmonary depression. Death results from respiratory failure. Treatment consists of moving the patient to an area without CO and administering oxygen to enhance its elimination. Pure oxygen (100%) reduces the $t_{1/2}$ of COHb from 5–6 hours to 0.5–1 hour; hyperbaric oxygen (3 atmospheric absolute [ATA]) reduces it to less than or equal to 0.5 hour.

Hydrogen Sulfide

Hydrogen sulfide is a colorless gas that has the smell of rotten eggs (0.3 ppm). It is found wherever the decay of sulfur compounds occurs and can reach lethal concentrations (500–700 ppm) in poorly ventilated spaces (sewers, liquid manure tanks). H_2S is associated also with a variety of industries, including petroleum, rubber, tanning, mining, and rayon manufacturing. At low concentrations (50–100 ppm) H_2S irritates the eyes and respiratory tract. Above 100 ppm, its odor becomes less intense owing to olfactory nerve paralysis; at 300–500 ppm pulmonary edema may become life-threatening. Severe systemic toxicity develops above 500 ppm (headache, vertigo, weakness, vomiting, confusion) and may lead to the rapid loss of consciousness, respiratory depression, and death within 30 minutes. The toxic effects of H_2S are probably due to its reversible inhibition of cytochrome oxidase a_3, the terminal enzyme in the electron transport chain, which results in the inhibition of aerobic metabolism. H_2S is absorbed primarily through the respiratory tract; it is thought to be eliminated by oxidation to sulfate, by methylation, and by reactions with metalloproteins and proteins containing disulfide bonds. Intoxications are treated by removing the patient from the contaminated area and establishing adequate ventilation with oxygen. *Nitrites* can be used to form methemoglobin, which binds H_2S and protects cytochrome oxidase. The subsequent administration of thiosulfate is not required because sulfmethemoglobin undergoes spontaneous detoxification in the body.

Ammonia

Ammonia is a colorless, water-soluble, alkaline gas that is commonly used as a fertilizer but is encountered also as an industrial refrigerant. It has a pungent odor at low concentrations (10 ppm) and causes a progressive irritation of the skin, eyes, and respiratory passages as its concentration begins to exceed 50 ppm. The liquefaction necrosis produced by NH_3 results in severe pulmonary dysfunction (dyspnea, laryngospasm, edema, pneumonitis) at concentrations near 1000 ppm; immediate death occurs at concentrations near 1500 ppm. Intoxications are treated by removing the patient from the contaminated area, irrigating the involved skin and eyes, and establishing adequate ventilation.

ASTHMA THERAPIES

Theophylline

Preparations of theophylline, a potent bronchodilating agent used in the treatment of asthma and chronic obstructive pulmonary disease, were responsible for 27 of the fatalities reported to the AAPCC in 1988. *Caffeine,* another methylxanthine-like theophylline, is found in a variety of OTC preparations used as analgesics and diet aids. The pharmacological and toxicological properties of theophylline and caffeine are similar. In addition to relaxing smooth muscle, both drugs stimulate the CNS and cardiac muscle and produce diuresis. At the cellular level the methylxanthines act as adenosine receptor antagonists, increase the concentration of the intracellular second messenger cyclic adenosine monophosphate (AMP) by inhibiting the enzyme responsible for its metabolism, and increase the circulating levels of catecholamines. The contribution of these actions to the therapeutic and toxic effects of the methylxanthines is unclear. Nausea and vomiting are the most common symptoms of methylxanthine overdose. Symptoms of CNS toxicity range from agitation to convulsions; symptoms of cardiovascular toxicity include tachycardia and arrhythmias. The hypokalemia that often accompanies acute intoxications may potentiate convulsions and arrhythmias.

Preparations of the methylxanthines are well absorbed from the GI tract. They rapidly distribute throughout the body, exhibiting a V_D of approximatey 0.6 l/kg. Metabolism occurs primarily in the liver; the kidney excretes only a small amount of theophylline (9%) and caffeine (1%) unchanged. Supportive care is the best treatment for methylxanthine intoxication, with emphasis placed on controlling convulsions and cardiovascular complications. Either emesis or lavage can remove methylxanthines from the stomach when initiated within 1 hour of exposure. Activated charcoal is effective any time postexposure. Because the methylxanthines are weak bases (pKa = 8.75), they will concentrate in the stomach owing to pH partitioning. Thus, multiple dosages of activated charcoal can reduce the serum $t_{1/2}$ of methylxanthines even when they are administered parenterally. Hemoperfusion is more effective than hemodialysis and is recommended in severe intoxications.

MDAC significantly shortens the $t_{1/2}$ of theophylline.

CHEMICALS

Cyanide was involved in 11 of the 24 fatalities caused by chemical toxicity in 1988. Chemicals associated less frequently with fatalities include nonautomotive *ethylene glycol, acids* and *alkali, methylene chloride,* as well as *nitrates* and *nitrites.* Ethylene glycol is discussed under Alcohols and Glycols; acids and alkali and methylene chloride are discussed under Cleaning Substances and Hydrocarbons, respectively.

Cyanide

Hydrogen cyanide (HCN) is an extremely volatile liquid that has the odor of bitter almonds. HCN and its common alkali salts (potassium, sodium, and calcium cyanide) are found in fumigants, metal polishes, electroplating solutions, and ore-extracting processes. Cyanogenic glycosides (e.g., amygdalin, the active ingredient of Laetrile) are found naturally in a variety of plants. Enzymes in the plants and the human GI tract hydrolyze the glycosides and release HCN. The toxic effects of cyanide are due to its reversible inhibition of aerobic metabolism. Cyanide blocks cellular respiration by binding to enzymes containing the ferric (3^+) ion, particularly cytochrome oxidase, which is involved in the last step of oxidative phosphorylation. Symptoms of cyanide poisoning that occur rapidly in succession include headache, dizziness, dyspnea, unconsciousness, convulsions, and respiratory arrest. Although the smell of bitter almonds can aide diagnosis, approximately one third of the population is genetically insensitive to the odor of cyanide.

The smell of bitter almonds can aid the diagnosis of cyanide poisoning.

Cyanides are rapidly absorbed from the skin and mucosal surfaces. Toxic symptoms may appear within seconds following the inhalation of HCN and within a few minutes following the ingestion of cyanide salts. Cyanide has a large V_D (1.5 l/kg) and exhibits significant (60%) binding to plasma proteins. Most of the absorbed cyanide (80%) is metabolized by the enzyme rhodanase that, in the presence of thiosulfate, converts cyanide to the relatively harmless thiocyanate ion that in turn is excreted by the kidney. Although rhodanase is found in a variety of tissues, particularly the liver, rhodanase activity is usually somewhat sluggish owing to the body's limited store of thiosulfate. Thus, one treatment in cases of overdose is the IV administration of *sodium thiosulfate* to enhance cyanide metabolism. To protect cells while this enzymatic transformation is occurring, a portion of the circulating hemoglobin is converted to methemoglobin by the administration of *amyl nitrite* (inhalation) or *sodium nitrite* (IV injection). The ferric ion of methemoglobin, like that of cytochrome oxidase, has a high affinity for cyanide. As the free cyanide concentration is reduced, cyanide is released from the cyanomethemoglobin complex and becomes available for enzymatic detoxification. Oxygen (100%) should be administered in conjunction with nitrite and thiosulfate therapy. *Hydroxycobalamine* (vitamin B_{12a}) is used also to treat cyanide toxicity. It combines with cyanide to form cyanocobalamin (vitamin B_{12}), which is excreted by the kidney. Owing to the rapidity by which symptoms appear, gastric lavage should be delayed until the treatments described earlier are initiated. Activated charcoal, hemodialysis, and hemoperfusion are ineffective.

Cyanide toxicity is reversed by thiosulfate and nitrite.

Nitrates and Nitrites

Nitrates ($-NO_3$) and nitrites ($-NO_2$) can be classified as either inorganic or organic. Inorganic nitrates are found in well water contaminated by runoff from various nitrogen sources (e.g., sewage treatment facilities, decaying matter, fertilizers) as well as certain plants (e.g., broccoli, cauliflower, spinach) and medicinals (e.g., diuretics, ammonium nitrate; antidiarrheal agents, bismuth subnitrate; topical burn treatments, silver nitrate). Inorganic nitrites are found also in well water owing to the reduction of nitrates to nitrites by bacteria. Organic nitrates and nitrites are used in the treatment of angina and congestive heart failure as well as in the manufacture of explosives. Organic nitrites are abused also as adjuncts to sexual intercourse. The toxicity of nitrates and nitrites is due to their ability to dilate smooth muscle and to oxidize hemoglobin to methemoglobin. Methemoglobin produces tissue hypoxia owing to its inability to transport and release oxygen. Because the nitrates are weaker oxidizers than nitrites, the nitrates are thus less likely to produce methemoglobinemia. The toxicity of dietary nitrates is primarily a consequence of their conversion to nitrites by bacteria residing in the GI tract. Compared with adults, infants are more susceptible to nitrate poisoning because their GI tracts contain more nitrate-reducing bacteria and because their hemoglobin is more susceptible to oxidation. Toxic symptoms include headache, dizziness, flushed skin, diaphoresis, hypotension, tachycardia, and particularly upon standing, syncope. Cyanosis may be one of the first symptoms owing to the dark brown color of methemoglobin.

Methemoglobinemia induced by nitrates and nitrites is reversed by methylene blue.

Organic nitrates and nitrites are well absorbed through the GI and respiratory tracts as well as the skin. The organic nitrates are hydrolyzed by the liver to inorganic nitrite and both partially and fully denitrated metabolites that may possess some of the vasodilatory activity of the parent compound. The metabolism of organic nitrites is unclear. Treatment of intoxications emphasizes establishing adequate tissue oxygenation (100% oxygen, IV *methylene blue*) and guarding against hypotension. In the presence of nicotinamide-adenine dinucleotide phosphate (reduced form) (NADPH), methylene blue acts as an exogenous cofactor that enhances the reduction of methemoglobin to hemoglobin by the relatively dormant methemoglobin reductase (diaphorase II) within the erythrocyte. Gastric decontamination may be of benefit also.

CLEANING SUBSTANCES

There were 19 deaths in 1988 attributable to chemicals used for cleaning. The majority were distributed among *acids* (9), *alkali* (5), and *detergents* (2).

Acids

Acids such as *chromic, hydrochloric, nitric, oxalic, phosphoric,* and *sulfuric* are found in a variety of household products, including toilet bowl cleaners, automobile batteries, metal cleaners, and soldering fluxes. These same chemicals as well as *hydrofluoric* acid are used industrially. Most fatalities result from the inhalation of acid vapors and the ingestion of strong acids. The inhalation of acid vapors and the aspiration of ingested acids produces a chemical pneumonitis that may progress to the acute respiratory distress syndrome. The ingestion of a strong acid is usually self-limiting owing to the intense pain it produces in the buccal cavity. Once swallowed, however, the acid causes a coagulation necrosis as it moves through the esophagus and along the lesser curvature of the stomach. When the acid reaches

Lung deposition of acids elicits a chemical pneumonitis and respiratory distress syndrome.

the pyloris and antrum, it induces spasms that trap the acid in the distal stomach where the greatest damage is produced. Death is usually the result of asphyxia owing to laryngeal or pulmonary edema, shock or peritonitis owing to gastric perforation, or in the more chronic phase of injury, pyloric stenosis. The toxicity of hydrofluoric acid is compounded by the release of fluoride that is itself toxic to the cardiovascular, neuromuscular, and central nervous systems. These effects may be due in part to the ability of fluoride to produce hypocalcemia.

Treatment for the inhalation and ingestion of acids emphasizes maintaining adequate ventilation and circulation. If the ingested acid is not concentrated, it is diluted with water or milk within 30 minutes. Fluids are limited to one or two glasses to avoid the induction of vomiting, which re-exposes the esophagus to the acid. Calcium gluconate is administered in cases of hydrofluoric acid poisoning. The removal of concentrated acids or hydrofluoric acid by lavage using a soft rubber catheter may outweigh the risk of perforation. Dilute bases are not administered as a neutralizing agent because they initiate an exothermic reaction that may exacerbate the injury. Bicarbonate is not administered because the release of carbon dioxide may lead to gastric distention and perforation.

Alkali

Fatalities in this category result usually from the ingestion of sodium, potassium, or ammonium *hydroxide,* which are contained in a variety of products including drain and oven cleaners, CLINITEST tablets used to test for urinary sugar, alkaline *button batteries,* and concentrated *ammonia* (> 6%). Alkali elicit a liquefaction necrosis that is more deeply penetrating than the coagulation necrosis seen with acids. The deeper burns produced by alkali result in greater scarring and stricture formation than that seen with acids. Solid alkali that adhere to the oral mucosa are associated usually with oropharyngeal and upper esophageal injuries; liquid alkali produce more distal esophageal injuries that may occur in the absence of oropharyngeal damage. Death may result from asphyxia owing to glottic or laryngeal edema, shock, perforation of the esophagus with mediastinitis, or in the more chronic stage of injury, to progressive dysphagia and anorexia owing to esophageal strictures. Gastric perforation is rare. Household ammonia rarely causes burns but may produce a chemical pneumonitis if aspirated. Button batteries produce burns by electrical discharge only if they become lodged in the esophagus or GI tract. Alkali and acid poisonings are treated similarly. Gastric lavage is not recommended for alkali ingestions.

Alkali elicit a liquefaction necrosis that is more deeply penetrating than the coagulation necrosis of acids.

Detergents

Detergents are composed of organic and, in many instances, inorganic ingredients. The primary organic ingredient is a synthetic surfactant (*surface active agent*) obtained from petrochemical precursors. Soaps differ from detergents in that the organic surfactants of soaps are salts of fatty acids obtained from animal and vegetable sources. Surfactants decrease the surface tension of water, which increases the wetting and emulsifying properties of the water-surfactant solution. Surfactants are classified by their electrical charge as either cationic, anionic, nonionic, or amphoteric. *Cationic surfactants* are the most toxic; fabric softeners are the primary household source. Household detergents usually contain the relatively nontoxic anionic and nonionic surfactants. The other primary ingredient of most detergents is a group of alkaline, inorganic salts called builders. Builders maintain the proper pH of the wash solution and inactivate cal-

Cationic detergents can cause esophageal and gastric burns.

cium and other minerals that may interfere with the actions of the surfactant. Builders are contained in heavy-duty laundry detergents and automatic dishwater detergents. High concentrations of cationic surfactants (> 7.5%) and builders are capable of causing esophageal and gastric burns, perforations, and peritonitis. Treatment is the same as that for acids and alkali.

INSECTICIDES, PESTICIDES, AND RODENTICIDES

The majority of the 14 fatalities owing to chemicals in this category were found among the *organophosphates* (9). Fatalities occurred less frequently in poisonings with *carbamates, anticoagulants,* and *strychnine.*

Organophosphates

Diazinon, malathion, and *parathion* are members of a group of organophosphate insecticides that have achieved great popularity owing to their effectiveness as insecticides and their relative lack of persistence in the environment compared with other insecticides like the organochlorines. The organophosphates inactivate acetylcholinesterase (AChE), the enzyme that hydrolyses acetylcholine at cholinergic (muscarinic and nicotinic) synapses in the periphery and CNS. The accumulation of acetylcholine leads to the stimulation and finally the paralysis of these synapses. The effects of organophosphate poisoning are listed in Table 60–16; the symptoms observed clinically are dependent on the balance between the stimulation and the blockade of both muscarinic and nicotinic synapses.

Atropine antagonizes the central and peripheral muscarinic effects of organophosphates.

Most organophosphates are well absorbed through the skin as well as the respiratory and GI tract. They are metabolized by the cytochrome P-450 system in the liver. In some instances, as in the case of the organophosphates listed earlier, the metabolites are more toxic than their parent. Initial treatment of poisonings emphasizes ensuring adequate oxygenation followed by *atropine* to noncompetitively antagonize the muscarinic and CNS effects of the organophosphates. It is usually recommended that ventilation be established prior to atropinization because failure to do so may precipitate ventricular fibrillation. However, clinical judgment is re-

Table 60–16 CLINICAL MANIFESTATIONS OF ORGANOPHOSPHATE POISONING

Muscarinic Synapses	Physiological Effects
Respiratory system	Wheezing, dyspnea, increased bronchial secretion
Cardiovascular system	Bradycardia, hypotension, ventricular tachycardia
Gastrointestinal system	Cramps, vomiting, diarrhea, tenesmus
Pupils	Miosis
Ciliary body	Blurred vision
Lacrimal glands	Increased lacrimation
Salivary glands	Increased salivation
Sweat glands	Increased perspiration
Bladder	Increased micturition, incontinence
Nicotinic Synapses	
Striated muscle	Cramps, fasciculations, twitching, paralysis
Sympathetic ganglia	Tachycardia, hypertension
Central Nervous System	Dizziness, anxiety, restlessness, confusion, insomnia, ataxia, coma, convulsions, absent reflexes, Cheyne-Stokes respiration, respiratory and circulatory depression

quired because the administration of atropine may alleviate respiratory distress by decreasing bronchial secretions and spasms. *Pralidoxime* (pyridine-2-aldoxime methochloride or 2-PAM) should be used in the presence of muscle fasciculations and muscular weakness to antagonize the toxicity of organophosphates on nicotinic synapses. Pralidoxime reactivates AChE if given within 24–48 hours of exposure. After that time, the organophosphate irreversibly destroys AChE. Should this occur, supportive care may be required for several weeks until the enzyme is resynthesized. Because organophosphates are absorbed through the skin, contaminated clothing is removed and the skin is washed with soap. Health personnel must avoid direct contact with all contaminated areas.

2-PAM reactivates AChE when given within 48 hours of exposure.

Gastric decontamination may be of value if initiated within 1 hour of exposure. Because antidotes are available, methods to enhance elimination are not required usually.

Carbamates

Aldicarb (TEMIK) and *propoxur* (BAYGON) are the two members of this category sometimes associated with fatality. Because the carbamates inactivate AChE, the toxic manifestations of carbamate poisoning mimic those seen with the organophosphates. There are two primary differences in toxicity between the two classes of insecticides. First, the symptoms of carbamate poisoning are less severe and of shorter duration because the carbamate-AChE complex, unlike the organophosphate-AChE complex, readily dissociates. Second, the carbamates produce only minor CNS effects because they poorly penetrate the blood-brain barrier. Like the organophosphates, the carbamates are well absorbed by all routes. Carbamate poisoning and organophosphate poisoning are treated similarly. The only exception is that pralidoxime is not indicated in carbamate poisoning because the effects of the carbamates are reversible. Pralidoxime should be considered in severe cases of AChE poisoning when the insecticide is unknown or contains an organophosphate.

2-PAM is not used in carbamate toxicity because it reversibly binds AChE.

Anticoagulants

The coumarin derivatives *warfarin* and *brodifacoum* are anticoagulants commonly found in commercial rodenticides. These anticoagulants antagonize the effects of vitamin K_1 (phytonadione), a cofactor in the postribosomal synthesis of clotting Factors II, VII, IX, and X. Brodifacoum is approximately 100 times more potent than warfarin and has a longer half-life (120 days *versus* 2 days). Hemorrhage is the primary toxic effect of these agents. Coumarin-derived anticoagulants are lipophilic compounds well absorbed from the GI tract. They are metabolized through hepatic cytochrome P-450 mixed-function oxidase enzymes; less than 2% of these compounds is excreted in the urine unchanged. Gastric decontamination may be of benefit if initiated within 1 hour postexposure. Lavage is usually preferred to the induction of emesis because the latter may provoke GI bleeding. Although warfarin is a weak acid (pKa = 5.0) with a small V_D (0.1 l/kg), diuresis and dialysis are of no benefit in warfarin toxicity owing to its extensive protein binding (99%). Other coumarin anticoagulants have similar pharmacokinetics. Cholestyramine, a high molecular weight anion exchange resin that is not absorbed from the GI tract, appears to be effective in the treatment of warfarin overdose, possibly by interrupting its enterohepatic circulation. Hemoperfusion and exchange transfusion have theoretical benefits. Phytonadione is an effective antidote that restores the prothrombin time and reduces bleeding.

Strychnine

Strychnine is a potent convulsant commonly used as a rodenticide. Strychnine competitively blocks the binding of glycine, an inhibitory neurotransmitter, to receptor sites located in the CNS. Although strychnine affects all levels of the CNS, its actions on the spinal cord predominate. Here it blocks the binding of glycine to motor neurons and leads to the uncontrolled excitation of skeletal muscles. Strychnine is well absorbed from the GI and nasal mucosa. Symptoms of strychnine poisoning usually appear within 10–20 minutes of exposure and include restlessness, apprehension, hyperreflexia, and muscle stiffness, particularly in the legs and face. Severe intoxications produce violent extensor convulsions that can be triggered by mild sensory stimuli. Seizures last from 1 to 2 minutes, occur at 5- to 15-minute intervals, and are separated by periods of complete recovery. Death is usually due to asphyxia from respiratory failure and commonly occurs within 3 hours of exposure. Treatment emphasizes maintaining adequate ventilation and controlling convulsions with diazepam. Neuromuscular blockade with succinylcholine may be required to prevent muscle spasms precipitated by endotracheal intubation. Diazepam noncompetitively antagonizes the effects of strychnine by potentiating the presynaptic inhibition of γ-aminobutyric acid on stimulatory neurons. Induction of emesis and gastric lavage are not recommended because they may induce convulsions. Activated charcoal followed by a cathartic may be of value to asymptomatic patients or symptomatic patients controlled with diazepam. There are no effective methods to enhance strychnine elimination. Although acid diuresis is theoretically advantageous (strychnine is a weak base, pKa = 8.0), the rapid onset of symptoms limits its use. Treatment is symptomatic and supportive.

> Death from strychnine commonly occurs within 3 hours of exposure.

ANTIHISTAMINES

Diphenhydramine was responsible for seven of the nine fatalities involving antihistamines in 1988. Diphenhydramine is a potent H_1 blocker noted for its antimuscarinic and sedative properties during both therapeutic use and overdose. Signs of peripheral anticholinergic toxicity include blurred vision, tachycardia, arrhythmias, decreased GI motility, urinary retention, and thickening of bronchial secretions. In children and young adults CNS toxicity is usually associated with stimulation; in adults toxicity is associated with CNS depression. Diphenhydramine is readily absorbed from the GI tract. Approximately 50% of the absorbed dose is metabolized on its first pass through the liver; 2% is excreted in the urine unchanged. The decreased GI motility associated with diphenhydramine overdose may increase the effectiveness of gut decontamination procedures initiated more than 1 hour postexposure. Activated charcoal effectively binds diphenhydramine. Methods to enhance its elimination are ineffective owing to its large V_D (6.5 l/kg) and significant protein binding (78%). *Physostigmine* may be given in life-threatening situations such as supraventricular tachycardia in the presence of coronary artery disease, hypertension, or severe agitation. Cardiac conduction delays contraindicate the use of physostigmine.

> Diphenhydramine has antimuscarinic and sedative properties at both therapeutic and toxic levels.

HYDROCARBONS

Hydrocarbons were responsible for eight fatalities in 1988. Half were due to *halogenated hydrocarbons; petroleum distillates* and *aromatic hydrocarbons* were associated with fatality less frequently.

Halogenated Hydrocarbons

Chemicals in this classification commonly associated with fatality include *carbon tetrachloride* (CCl_4), *chloroform* ($CHCl_3$), *trichloroethane* (CH_3CCl_3), and *methylene chloride* (CH_2Cl_2); they are volatile liquids that are used as solvents, aerosol propellants, and in the manufacture of FREON (i.e., CCl_4). They all depress the CNS, although CCl_4 is the most potent. They are well absorbed through the respiratory and GI tracts and slightly less so through the skin. The lung excretes most of the absorbed dose of these chemicals unchanged; the remainder is metabolized presumably through the hepatic cytochrome P-450 system.

Some of the metabolites are also toxic. CCl_4 is metabolized to free radicals and phosgene, which covalently bind to lipids and proteins and lead to fatty degeneration of the liver and hepatorenal necrosis. The metabolism of $CHCl_3$ is similar to CCl_4 except that $CHCl_3$ does not cause lipid peroxidation. CH_2Cl_2 is metabolized to carbon monoxide, which leads to the formation of carboxyhemoglobin, a result that may prove dangerous to individuals with impaired cardiovascular status. Halogenated hydrocarbons, particularly CCl_4, can cause cardiac dysrhythmias by sensitizing the myocardium to circulating catecholamines. CH_2Cl_2 is a potent irritant; prolonged contact (30 minutes) to high concentrations may cause chemical burns to the skin and mucosal surfaces. Symptoms of intoxication include headache, dizziness, fatigue, and nausea and may rapidly progress to unconsciousness. Treatment is supportive and includes removal from exposure (e.g., physical environment, clothing), administration of supplemental oxygen, and monitoring for dysrhythmias. Gastric decontamination (i.e., emesis, lavage, and charcoal) should be used following the ingestion of CCl_4 and may benefit ingestions of CH_2Cl_2 greater than a few swallows. The IV administration of *NAC* (see Acetaminophen, earlier) may reduce the hepatorenal toxicity owing to the depletion of glutathione stores by the reactive metabolites of CCl_4 and $CHCl_3$. There are no methods to enhance elimination.

> Halogenated hydrocarbons are potent skin irritants and cardiac sensitizers.

FREON is another chemical in this classification associated with fatalities. FREON refers to a group of fluorinated hydrocarbons that are used as aerosol propellants and refrigerants. FREONS are CNS depressants that generally have a lower systemic toxicity than their chlorinated hydrocarbon counterparts. Absorption of FREONS is approximately 40 times greater by inhalation than by ingestion. Concentrations above 5–15% may produce lightheadedness and altered consciousness. Higher concentrations of some FREONS, which may be achieved by their accidental or intentional discharge into enclosed spaces (e.g., plastic bags), can cause sinus bradycardia terminating in asystole. Like the chlorinated hydrocarbons, FREONS can produce cardiac dysrhythmias by sensitizing the heart to circulating catecholamines. Treatment is symptomatic and supportive.

> FREONS cause cardiac arrhythmias when inhaled in high concentrations.

Petroleum Distillates

Petroleum distillates are crude-oil byproducts that contain varying amounts of saturated and unsaturated aliphatic and aromatic hydrocarbons; the amount of each in any distillate depends on the manufacturing process involved (e.g., distillation, cracking). Petroleum distillates are responsible for the majority of all hydrocarbon exposures. Although turpentine is a distillate of pine resin, not petroleum, it is usually included in this classification because the presentation and treatment of turpentine and petroleum distillates are similar.

The primary concerns in petroleum distillate exposure are the respira-

Lung complications are the primary cause of death following hydrocarbon aspiration.

tory, central nervous, and GI systems. Deaths are almost always due to pulmonary complications initiated by aspiration of the distillate. These complications lead to hypoxemia and include the inhibition of pulmonary surfactant, bronchospasm, the displacement of alveolar oxygen by distillate vapors, and direct injury to alveolar parenchyma. In addition to volatility, viscosity is another property of the distillate that determines its aspiration hazard. Chemicals with a low viscosity (below 60 SSU) are more toxic because they are better able to reach distal airways. Distillates with a low viscosity include gasoline, kerosene, turpentine, mineral spirits, mineral seal oil (red furniture polish), various naphthas, as well as both halogenated and aromatic hydrocarbons. Chemicals with a high viscosity (above 100 SSU) have a minimal aspiration risk; they include motor and transmission oils, baby and suntan oils, fuel and diesel oils, grease, tar, petroleum jelly, and paraffin wax. Common symptoms of respiratory distress owing to aspiration include cough, choking, tachypnea, lethargy, and cyanosis.

CNS toxicity, with the exception of volatile aromatic hydrocarbons (e.g., benzene, toluene, xylene, turpentine), is usually the result of aspiration-induced hypoxemia, because the GI absorption of most petroleum distillates is poor. The major GI concern following ingestion is vomiting, because it increases the risk of aspiration. The treatment for petroleum distillate poisoning is supportive care. Gastric decontamination by the induction of emesis is an area of active controversy and requires that the potential toxicity of ingested petroleum distillates be weighed against their aspiration hazard. The induction of emesis is not recommended for highly viscous or highly volatile (e.g., mineral seal oil) petroleum distillates with limited GI absorption. Emesis is recommended in the alert patient for large ingestions (several ml/kg) of other petroleum distillates, the ingestion of chlorinated and aromatic hydrocarbons, as well as the ingestion of distillates containing highly toxic ingredients. Activated charcoal does not absorb most petroleum distillates but does bind significant amounts of kerosene and turpentine. Cathartics may be of benefit also. Avoid mineral oil cathartics because they increase the risk of aspiration and retard absorption. There are no antidotes or effective methods to enhance elimination.

Aromatic Hydrocarbons

The principal chemicals in this class include *benzene* (C_6H_6), the prototypical aromatic hydrocarbon, as well as *toluene* ($C_6H_5CH_3$) and *xylene* ($C_6H_4[CH_3]_2$). They are used as feedstock in chemical manufacturing, are excellent solvents for paints and glues, and are found in automotive and aviation fuels. In more recent years, household products containing benzene have been reformulated to contain toluene, a less toxic solvent. In 1986, all deaths from aromatic hydrocarbons were due to toluene. The primary effect of acute exposures is CNS depression. Symptoms include headache, drowsiness, nausea, and ataxia at low doses and confusion, respiratory depression, and coma at high doses. Severe inhalations may result in noncardiogenic pulmonary edema. Because they may also cause a feeling of euphoria, aromatic hydrocarbons, like the halogenated hydrocarbons, are also abused by sniffing. Aromatic hydrocarbons can also produce dysrhythmias by sensitizing the heart to circulating catecholamines. Aromatic hydrocarbons are generally well absorbed through the respiratory and GI tracts and slightly less so through the skin. Approximately 10% of the absorbed dose is exhaled through the lung unchanged. The remainder is biotransformed by the hepatic cytochrome P-450 system; toluene and xylene are also biotransformed by alcohol and aldehyde dehydrogenases. The metabolites of these pathways appear in the urine as

CNS depression is the primary toxic effect of aromatic hydrocarbons.

conjugates of glucuronic acid, glycine, and sulfate. Treatment is supportive and includes removal from exposure, administration of supplemental oxygen, and monitoring for dysrhythmias. Although emesis may be of value within 30 minutes of ingestion, the potential benefit must be weighed against the risk of aspiration.

References

Centers for Disease Control: Unintentional ingestions of prescription drugs in children under five years old. Morb Mort Week Rep 36:124, 1987.

Centers for Disease Control: Unintentional poisoning mortality—U.S. 1980–1986. Morb Mort Week Rep 38:153, 1989.

Dreisbach RH, Robertson WO: Handbook of Poisoning: Prevention, Diagnosis and Treatment, 15th ed. Norwalk: Appleton & Lange, 1990.

Ellenhorn MJ, Barceloux DG: Medical Toxicology: Diagnosis and Treatment of Human Poisoning, 2nd ed. New York: Elsevier, 1991.

Goldfrank LR: Toxicologic Emergencies, 4th ed. New York: Appleton-Century-Crofts, 1990.

Gosselin RE, Smith RP, Hodge HC: Clinical Toxicology of Commercial Products, 5th ed. Baltimore: Williams & Wilkins, 1984.

Haddad LM: The emergency management of poisoning. Pediatr Ann 16:901, 1987.

Haddad LM, Winchester JF: Clinical Management of Poisoning and Drug Overdose, 2nd ed. Philadelphia: WB Saunders, 1990.

Klaasen CD, Amders MO, Doull J: Casarett and Doull's Toxicology: The Basic Science of Poisons, 3rd ed. New York: MacMillan, 1986.

Kulig K, Bar-Or D, Cantrill SV, et al: Management of acutely poisoned patients without gastric emptying. Ann Emerg Med 14:562–567, 1985.

Levy G: Gastrointestinal clearance of drugs with activated charcoal. N Engl J Med 307:676, 1982.

Litovitz TL, Schmitz BF, Holm KC: 1988 annual report of the American Association of Poison Control Centers national data collection system. Am J Emerg Med 7:495–545, 1989.

MacLean WC Jr: A comparison of ipecac syrup and apomorphine in the immediate treatment of ingestion of poisons. J Pediatr 82:121, 1973.

Park GD, Spector R, Goldberg MJ, Johnson GF: Expanded role of chemical therapy in the poisoned and overdosed patient. Arch Intern Med 146:969–973, 1986.

Tenenbein M: Pediatric toxicology—current controversies and recent advances. Curr Probl Pediatr 16:218, 1986.

Tenenbein M: Whole bowel irrigation as a gastrointestinal decontamination procedure after acute poisoning. Med Tox 3:77, 1988.

Watson WA: Factors influencing the clinical efficacy of activated charcoal. Drug Intell Clin Pharm 21:160, 1987.

Selected Aspects of Therapeutics

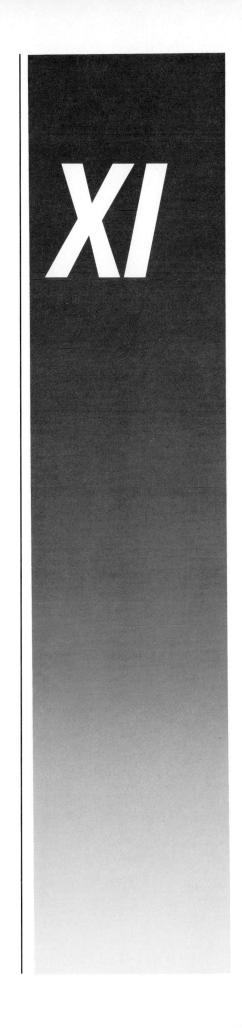

XI

Diagnostic Drugs

61

Edward A. Carr, Jr.

A drug is "any chemical compound that may be used on or administered to humans or animals as an aid in the diagnosis, treatment, or prevention of disease . . ." (Dorland's, 1988). Pharmacologists and clinicians are, quite properly, concerned chiefly with therapeutic and—as an even more desirable goal—preventive aspects of pharmacology. But several important groups of compounds aid in the diagnosis of disease. The common use of terms such as *diagnostic agents, contrast media,* or *imaging agents* to describe these compounds does not obviate the fact that they are drugs. Their administration must be justified by their efficacy, balanced against the risk of adverse effects. Diagnostic drugs come within the purview of regulatory agencies, and many are listed in official compendia such as the United States Pharmacopeia.

Many other substances used *in vitro* to measure various components of body fluids and tissues, e.g., antibodies for radioimmunoassay, are also termed *diagnostics,* but they are not used *in vivo.* Thus, they are laboratory reagents rather than drugs. They are not considered here.

Diagnostic drugs differ in several respects from other classes of drugs. Whereas the efficacy of prophylactic or therapeutic compounds is judged by the outcome they prevent or produce, respectively, diagnostic drugs are judged by the outcome they predict. The value of a test employing a diagnostic drug is judged by the same criteria as any other type of diagnostic test, i.e., its sensitivity, specificity, positive and negative predictive values, and overall accuracy. Although data permitting such calculations are absent for many tests and the tests continue to be used because accumulated clinical experience has shown their value, such data should be sought whenever possible. A consideration implicit in all diagnostic studies utilizing any type of recording instrument is that the test's accuracy depends *inter alia* upon the performance of the recording instrument.

> Diagnostic drugs differ from other classes of drugs in the criteria used to judge their effectiveness.

Whereas therapeutic use of a drug implies by definition that a patient is already sick, diagnostic drugs are often administered to individuals who eventually prove to have no disease at all. Thus a high degree of safety, while important for all classes of drugs, is especially necessary for diagnostic drugs. Most diagnostic drugs are used almost exclusively by physicians in a given specialty. Nevertheless, any physician who requests the performance of a diagnostic test involving the administration of a drug should have knowledge of the probable value of the test and the likelihood of adverse effects. The physician incurs significant responsibility by initiating the request. It is also reasonable for patients to ask their physician questions as they would about any other proposed administration of a drug.

> A high degree of safety is especially necessary for diagnostic drugs.

Some drugs are used exclusively for diagnosis, e.g., most compounds

Table 61-1   DIAGNOSTIC (INFORMATIONAL) DRUGS

Class	Examples	Use		
		To Support the Diagnosis of	To Determine	To Aid in Imaging of
1. Antigens	Benzylpenicilloyl polylysine (PPL)*	Allergy to penicillin G		
	Tuberculin purified protein derivative (PPD)	*M. tuberculosis* infection†		
2. Markers (tracers) to measure a compartment or function without altering it	Iodinated I 125 albumin		Plasma volume	
	Sodium *p*-aminohippurate (PAH)		Renal plasma flow	
3. Stimulating or inhibiting drugs	Edrophonium chloride (Tensilon)	Myasthenia gravis		
	Pentagastrin		Gastric acid– secreting ability	
	Dexamethasone	Cushing's syndrome		
4. Drugs used with imaging procedures				
a. Radiographic contrast agents	Iopanoic acid (Telepaque)			Gallbladder
b. Radiopharmaceuticals for scintigraphy	Sodium pertechnetate Tc 99m			Thyroid gland Salivary gland
c. Magnetic resonance imaging (MRI) contrast agents	Gadolinium diethylene-triaminepentaacetate meglumine (gadopentetate dimeglumine; Gd DTPA)			Kidney Lesions of brain and spinal cord Lesions of other organs‡

* PPL is able to elicit a reaction in sensitized individuals but is itself a poor antigen for sensitizing.
† A positive test does not necessarily indicate *active* infection.
‡ See text.

used in association with imaging procedures. Other drugs, although used largely for diagnosis, occasionally may be employed therapeutically, e.g., [¹³¹I]m-iodobenzylguanidine(MIBG), which is used chiefly for diagnosis of pheochromocytomas but occasionally for their therapy. Still other drugs, although used chiefly for therapeutic purposes, also have certain diagnostic uses, e.g., dexamethasone.

Four main groups of diagnostic drugs are described.

Diagnostic drugs may be classified in four main groups: (1) those that aid in assessing the allergic or immune status of a patient; (2) those used as markers (tracers) *in vivo* to measure a compartment or function without altering it; (3) those that stimulate or inhibit some function and, in so doing, provide diagnostic information; (4) those used in association with imaging procedures. Examples are given in Table 61–1. These and other selected examples are discussed later, but no attempt is made to list all, or even the majority, of the available diagnostic drugs within the confines of this chapter. Even if such a complete list were attempted, it would soon be outdated.

Note to the Student or Young Physician Reader

A convenient way to read this chapter is to use one strategy for the sections describing the first three classes of diagnostic drugs and a different strategy for the fourth. For the first three classes a single careful reading should give the reader not only information on the relatively few examples given, but also an opportunity to correlate this material with appropriate sections of other chapters. Thus, skin testing for penicillin allergy, the diagnostic uses of edrophonium, and the metyrapone test should be reviewed in connection with the appropriate sections, elsewhere in this book, on drug allergy, cholinesterase inhibitors and adrenal cortical hormones, respectively. But the most convenient way to study the fourth class is to read the section once to obtain an overview without dwelling on the details and then to re-read it, concentrating on certain points as suggested at the end of this chapter.

Certain substances are used to test for previous exposure to a given microorganism or to test for anergy. Examples of such preparations are tuberculin, histoplasmin, and mumps skin test antigen.

A number of antibody preparations are used to induce passive immunity and prevent or treat infection (e.g., specific hyperimmune human γ globulin preparations against tetanus, pertussis, vaccinia, or rabies; botulism antitoxin) or poisoning by venoms (e.g., polyvalent antivenin [Crotalidae]). Whenever such antibodies have been raised in animals and thus contain nonhuman protein, it is necessary to precede their clinical use by using them diagnostically in appropriate skin tests to determine whether the patient is allergic to the preparation. Positive tests make it necessary to carry out temporary hyposensitization of the patient before systemic administration of such a preparation is undertaken.

Skin testing for allergy to any drug is obviously a diagnostic use. This procedure and its limitations are discussed in Chapter 64.

Assessment of Allergic or Immune Status

Materials derived from microorganisms or antibodies from nonhuman sources are sometimes used to test a patient's sensitivity to them, e.g., by a skin test.

Plasma volume and circulating red cell volume, respectively, may be measured by the method of isotope dilution. If a labeled substance is injected directly into a body compartment and reaches equilibrium without leaving that compartment, it is possible to calculate from the change in specific activity of the injected material the volume into which it has been distributed. Iodinated I 125 albumin injection, a solution of human serum albumin labeled with ^{125}I, is used to measure plasma volume.* At 10, 20, and 30 minutes, respectively, after injection of the labeled albumin a blood specimen is withdrawn and the plasma radioactivity determined:

Measurement of a Compartment or Function Without Altering It

Radioactive-labeled serum albumin or erythrocytes may be used to measure plasma or red cell volume, respectively, by isotope dilution.

Total dose injected (counts/minute) =
    Concentration (counts/minute/ml) $\times$ volume (ml) injected

Plasma volume (ml) =
$$\frac{\text{Total dose injected (counts/minute)}}{\text{Concentration (counts/minute/ml) in plasma sample}}$$

To correct for leakage of albumin from the vascular space during the period of equilibration, the three values are plotted against time in a semilogarithmic graph, and the resulting line is extrapolated back to time zero.

For determination of circulating red cell volume by isotope dilution the patient's own red cells are labeled. A blood sample is withdrawn, the red cells are labeled *in vitro* by incubation with ^{51}Cr in the form of sodium chromate, and reinjected then into the patient. After time to permit equilibrium has elapsed, a single blood sample is withdrawn. Although the calculation of red cell volume is, in principle, similar to that of plasma volume, the determination of red cell volume requires measurement of whole blood radioactivity, plasma radioactivity, and hematocrit in both the injected blood and the sample withdrawn.

---

* In current usage, the radionuclide in a radiopharmaceutical is written in the superscript form, e.g., ^{125}I, if no generic name has been officially assigned to that radiopharmaceutical. If a generic name has been assigned, the superscript form is not used, e.g., iodohippurate sodium I 123.

Certain stable (i.e., nonradioactive) compounds are used to measure important physiological functions.

An example of a stable compound used to measure a physiological function is aminohippurate sodium injection. It is excreted by glomerular filtration and by transport across the renal tubules. The tubular transport is through a carrier mechanism for weak organic acids. When this compound is administered intravenously (IV) at a rate that does not exceed the tubular transfer maximum, the rate-limiting step in its clearance is the delivery of the compound to the kidney by the blood. Therefore, under these conditions the clearance is a measure of renal plasma flow. On the other hand, inulin is excreted solely by glomerular filtration, and its clearance is a measure of glomerular filtration rate.

Stimulation or Inhibition of a Function for Diagnostic Purposes

Provocative diagnostic tests are sometimes dangerous.

When stimulated either by histamine or glucagon, a pheochromocytoma characteristically releases a significantly larger amount of catecholamines than the normal adrenal medulla. Therefore, appropriate measurements made before and after the injection of histamine or glucagon may aid in the diagnosis of pheochromocytoma. But the release of excessive amounts of catecholamines may be dangerous to the patient. Purely provocative tests for any disease are likely to be uncomfortable at best and dangerous at worst. Therefore, they are not widely used. Skin tests for systemic allergy may be considered a mild type of provocative test. But in this instance the aim is to produce a mild reaction in the skin rather than to provoke the more serious type of allergic reaction, such as asthma, for which the patient is under investigation. Even in skin testing, a scratch test is usually performed before an intradermal injection in order to decrease the likelihood of a dangerous systemic reaction.

Edrophonium is useful in the diagnosis of myasthenia gravis and also in distinguishing between overtreatment and undertreatment of this disease.

Edrophonium chloride (TENSILON), a short-acting cholinesterase inhibitor, is useful in the diagnosis of untreated myasthenia gravis, because it alleviates rather than provokes a pathological state. Improvement in muscle strength within 1–3 minutes after a small (e.g., 2 mg) IV dose is strong evidence in favor of the diagnosis of myasthenia gravis. If this dose causes no change in muscle strength, a second, larger dose (e.g., 8 mg) is administered. If this dose fails to increase strength also, the test is considered negative. Edrophonium is useful also in patients who are receiving chronic anticholinesterase treatment for myasthenia gravis but fail to maintain satisfactory muscle strength despite this treatment. An obvious possible reason for the unsatisfactory result is that the patient is receiving too low a dose of the drug used for chronic therapy, e.g., pyridostigmine. On the other hand, overdosage with cholinesterase inhibitors can also lead to weakness by permitting excessive concentrations of acetylcholine to accumulate at the motor end-plate, preventing repolarization and thus interfering with muscle contraction. Weakness resulting from such overtreatment may become severe (cholinergic crisis). A clinician whose myasthenic patient remains weak despite apparently adequate therapy is faced with the dilemma of deciding whether to increase or decrease the dosage. Administration of edrophonium may resolve the issue, for an undertreated patient usually responds with an increase in muscle strength after edrophonium, whereas an overtreated patient is likely to note an increase in weakness. When used to distinguish between over- and undertreatment, the initial dose of edrophonium should be 1 mg. If this dose produces no change in muscle strength, a second dose of 1 mg may be given after approximately 1 minute. As the use of edrophonium to distinguish between under- and overtreatment represents one situation in which this diagnostic drug can, in some patients, provoke a worsening of the abnormal state, the drug's short duration of action is an important advantage. Nevertheless, facilities for artificial respiration should be at hand when this test is performed.

Less dramatic functional changes are measured sometimes to provide diagnostic information. Achylia gastrica, loss of the stomach's ability to secrete hydrochloric acid, is characteristic of pernicious anemia. Absence of gastric acidity even after stimulation by an H_2 agonist is supporting evidence for the diagnosis of pernicious anemia. Although histamine itself can be used in this test, betazole hydrochloride (HISTALOG), an analog of histamine and an H_2 agonist, is preferable to histamine because it has fewer side effects. Even betazole may cause significant gastrointestinal (GI) and circulatory side effects. Pentagastrin (PEPTAVLON), a pentapeptide in which four of the amino acids are homologous with those in the NH_2-terminal of gastrin, is an effective stimulant of gastric acid secretion also and causes less discomfort than betazole. Betazole is given either subcutaneously or intramuscularly (IM); pentagastrin is given subcutaneously.

The field of endocrinology is rich in diagnostic tests. The use of dexamethasone in a suppression test in the diagnosis of Cushing's syndrome is a classical example. Liddle (1956, 1960) showed that 0.5 mg dexamethasone given orally every 6 hours suppressed adrenal cortical secretion of cortisol, as measured by its principal urinary metabolites, on the second test day in normal individuals but not in patients with Cushing's syndrome. Patients whose hypercorticism was due to bilateral adrenal cortical hyperplasia secondary to excessive pituitary adrenocorticotropic hormone (ACTH) secretion did show suppression, however, when the dosage of dexamethasone was increased to 2 mg every 6 hours. Patients whose hypercorticism was due to cortical neoplasm showed no such suppression even with the higher dosage. Although additional methods of distinguishing among the various causes of Cushing's syndrome have been developed since this test, the dexamethasone suppression test continues to be useful.

The dexamethasone suppression test is useful in the diagnosis of Cushing's syndrome.

The aforementioned uses of betazole (or pentagastrin), dexamethasone, and edrophonium exemplify three different strategies in obtaining diagnostic information. Although gastric acid secretion can be quantified, clinicians testing for ability to secrete gastric acid usually seek a yes/no answer. But the dexamethasone suppression test utilizes a dose-response curve to permit not only distinction between normal and abnormal, but also, in case of an abnormal response, to provide quantitative information that suggests the specific nature of the abnormality. When the edrophonium test is used to determine the cause of weakness in a myasthenic patient already under chronic treatment with another cholinesterase inhibitor, a qualitative difference in response (increased or decreased weakness) provides information on the nature of the abnormality (over- or undertreatment, respectively).

Metyrapone (METOPIRONE) is used to test the ability of the pituitary to increase its secretion of ACTH in response to an abrupt decrease in the plasma cortisol concentration. Metyrapone inhibits the 11-β-hydroxylation of 11-desoxycortisol to cortisol in the adrenal cortex. Therefore, in a patient with a normal pituitary-adrenal axis, administration of metyrapone causes a decrease in adrenal cortisol secretion and an increase in pituitary ACTH secretion. The latter results in increased production of 11-desoxycortisol, which cannot be converted to cortisol because of the metyrapone-induced block in its further metabolism. The diagnostic *information* in this test is provided by the *stimulation* that results indirectly from the metyrapone-induced block, i.e., the increased ACTH and 11-desoxycortisol are evidence that the axis is behaving normally. Therefore, the test is invalid if the adrenal cortex is hypofunctioning and unable to produce a significant amount of cortisol even in the absence of metyrapone. The *risk* of the test comes from the temporary *inhibition* of cortisol synthesis. If a patient already has a hypofunctioning adrenal cortex even before the test, the test

Metyrapone may be used to test the normality of the pituitary-adrenal axis.

itself may precipitate acute adrenal insufficiency. For both of these reasons, an ACTH stimulation test of cortical function (see Chapter 43) should precede the metyrapone test, and the latter should not be conducted if cortical function is subnormal.

Drugs Used to Permit or Improve Diagnostic Imaging Procedures

This large group may be subdivided into the radiopaque contrast agents (contrast media) used in radiography, the radiopharmaceuticals (imaging agents) used in nuclear medicine, and the more recently developed compounds used to improve contrast in magnetic resonance imaging (MRI).

RADIOGRAPHIC CONTRAST AGENTS

These compounds are administered to patients prior to radiographic procedures in order to block the transmission of x-rays and thus outline the cavity or tissue space containing the radiopaque substance. If one wishes to study radiographically an organ, vessel, or cavity that is not well visualized in the absence of contrast agent, an obvious strategy is to obtain a high concentration of contrast agent in that organ, vessel, or cavity and thus improve its visualization. Barium (atomic weight 137) and iodine (atomic weight 127) are the elements commonly used to confer radiopacity on compounds containing them.

Barium and iodine are the elements used to confer radiopacity on contrast agents used in radiography.

Suspensions of barium sulfate are used chiefly to outline the GI tract after direct introduction as a barium meal or barium enema. Barium ions are too toxic to permit the systemic use of soluble barium salts, and the safety of barium sulfate for GI studies depends upon its insolubility and consequent lack of systemic absorption. Although a barium enema is often an uncomfortable procedure, barium sulfate itself, when used by experienced radiologists, has few adverse effects in the GI tract except for a mild constipating effect in some individuals. However, severe allergic reactions to the cuffed enema tip inserted to permit a barium enema have occasionally occurred in patients allergic to latex.

Iodized fatty acids and oils can be introduced directly into various body cavities and in the past were frequently used for such procedures as myelography, sialography, bronchography, and hysterosalpingography. However, improvements in diagnosis following the introduction of computed tomography (CT), the availability of water-soluble nonionic compounds for myelography, and the advent of MRI have led to a sharp decrease in the use of iodized fatty acids and oils. Even for hysterosalpingography, where CT and MRI have not replaced the older radiographic procedure, water-soluble contrast agents are now used instead of fatty acids or oils.

The radiographic contrast agents administered systemically are water-soluble, iodine-containing compounds.

Soluble iodine-containing compounds are widely used for *intravascular* administration, either to visualize the lumen of blood vessels (angiography) or for urography. They can be given IV or intra-arterially. Diatrizoate and iothalamate salts, which are useful urographic contrast agents also, are employed in angiography because their relatively low toxicity permits rapid injection of highly concentrated solutions into blood vessels in order to opacify the lumen. Diatrizoate meglumine injection, diatrizoate sodium injection, as well as diatrizoate meglumine and diatrizoate sodium injection are examples of radiopaque compounds for intravascular use. The analogous meglumine, sodium, and meglumine plus sodium salts of iothalamic acid have similiar use. Although the differences between the diatrizoates and iothalamates are not striking, the latter are preferred for neuroangiography, because they appear to be somewhat less neurotoxic than the former, and meglumine salts are preferable to sodium salts, because they are somewhat less toxic to neural tissue and to vascular endothelium. For the latter reason meglumine salts are also preferable for phlebography (venography) (Dawkins, 1989). Sodium salts, which contain relatively more iodine per molecule than their meglumine counterparts, are slightly more radiopaque than the latter at equal concentrations. Sodium salts are also somewhat less viscous than the meglumine salts. The latter are more soluble in water than their sodium counterparts. In coronary angiography either pure sodium or pure meglumine salts cause a higher risk of ventricular fibrillation than a mixture of the two salts. Therefore, mixtures were used in coronary angiography until they were supplanted by low osmolality contrast agents.

Angiographic procedures utilizing soluble iodine-containing compounds include angiocardiography; aortography; and cerebral, coronary, renal, or other selective angiography. IV injection permits phlebography.

Diatrizoate and iothalamate salts, administered IV, are also useful urographic contrast agents because they are rapidly excreted by glomerular filtration. They are not significantly secreted or absorbed by the renal tubules. But tubular absorption of water greatly increases the concentration of contrast agent in the proximal and distal nephron, an important factor in opacification. Some of this advantage is lost, however, because the ionic nature of the diatrizoate and iothalamate salts causes them to function as osmotic diuretics and partially interferes with the tubular reabsorption of water. The nonionic agents discussed later do not have this disadvantage.

> Rapid renal excretion of diatrizoates and iothalamates permits their use in urography.

Urographic contrast agents may also be used for cystourethrography and retrograde pyelography following their installation into the lower urinary tract by catheter.

Iothalamate and diatrizoate salts may be injected directly into the biliary tract to outline the bile ducts (cholangiography), e.g., through a T tube or transhepatically. The bile ducts may also be visualized after IV administration of iodipamide meglumine, but such IV cholangiography has been largely supplanted by ultrasonic or scintigraphic procedures or by percutaneous transhepatic cholangiography.

For visualization of the gallbladder (cholecystography) after oral administration of a radiopaque compound, iopanoic acid tablets, ipodate calcium for oral suspension, and ipodate sodium capsules are available. After their absorption from the intestine, a process greatly aided by the solubilizing action of bile salts, these biliary contrast agents circulate in the blood, largely but reversibly bound to albumin. They are subsequently eliminated by the same pathway as bilirubin; they are taken up by hepatocytes, converted to the more water-soluble glucuronides, and excreted into the biliary passages. Ipodate, but not iopanoic acid, is itself choleretic. The normal gallbladder absorbs water, heavily concentrating the bile contained in the bladder. The highly ionized glucuronides of the biliary contrast agents present in the bile are not absorbed by the gallbladder. The consequent increased concentration of contrast agent in the gallbladder permits opacification. Although formerly widely used, especially to detect calculi in the gallbladder, cholecystography has now been largely supplanted by other modalities, e.g., ultrasound when calculi are suspected and scintigraphy when acute cholecystitis is suspected. It should be noted that hepatobiliary disease may interfere with opacification of the gallbladder in several ways. If obstruction of the biliary tract prevents bile salts from entering the intestine, absorption of the contrast agent from the intestine is hindered. Liver disease may result in decreased ability of hepatocytes to take up the contrast agent from the blood. Moreover, if the concentration of bilirubin in the blood is increased, competition between bilirubin and contrast agent for hepatic excretion occurs. Finally, if the gallbladder is diseased, the

> A different class of iodinated compounds permits hepatobiliary radiographic studies.

normal selective absorption of water by the gallbladder may not occur, and the contrast agent in the gallbladder may not achieve sufficient concentration to permit visualization.

Hepatobiliary contrast agents are not used in angiography because they are more toxic than the diatrizoates and iothalamates. When iopanoic acid or ipodate salts are given for cholecystography, however, severe systemic reactions are rare, because high concentrations are not achieved in the blood. The doses used, under normal circumstances, permit absorption of sufficient compound to produce opacification of the gallbladder *after* uptake by the liver and concentration by the gallbladder, but the concentration in the blood is too low to permit angiography.

Whereas the usefulness of cholecystographic compounds is due to their excretion by hepatocytes into the biliary tree, renal excretion also occurs. Renal effects of these compounds are discussed later.

The advent of CT has modified the use of radiopaque compounds in three different ways. First, some imaging procedures that required the use of contrast agents before CT became available can now be successfully carried out by CT without contrast agents. Second, when radiopaque compounds are used with CT, the contrast agents may be employed in a somewhat different way than in other radiographic techniques. In the radiographic techniques available prior to the development of CT, contrast agents are used to improve visualization of the cavity, lumen, or organ in which they are concentrated, e.g., barium sulfate is placed in the stomach to improve visualization of the stomach. But in CT, ingestion of a barium sulfate suspension or a dilute solution of diatrizoate salts may facilitate, for example, examination of abdominal organs *other than* the stomach and intestines. By increasing the radiodensity of the gut the contrast agent may improve delineation between the gut and the pancreas, thus permitting better study of the latter. Usually a positive contrast agent, i.e., one that increases radiodensity, is employed in this strategy. But negative contrast agents, which decrease radiodensity, may also be used. For negative contrast, carbon dioxide may be used, ingested in the form of preparations that release the gas after ingestion, effervescent preparations, or even soft drinks.

The third and most extensive use of contrast agents in CT is in the enhancement of contrast by IV administration of diatrizoates, iothalamates, or nonionic contrast agents. The positive contrast provided by these agents permits rapid identification of landmark vascular structures after administration, followed by increased opacification of various tissues as the contrast agent reaches them through their blood supply and diffuses into the extravascular compartment. If all structures showed equal increases in radiodensity simultaneously, there would of course be no advantage. But CT enhancement is valuable because differences in rate and degree of opacification occur among various tissues, since tissues differ from one another in the richness of their blood supply. Moreover, the rate of leakage of the contrast agent from the blood compartment into the extravascular space may be more rapid at one site, e.g., a lesion, than in the surrounding tissue.

Adverse Effects. These may result from oral administration of contrast agents, e.g., diarrhea after ingestion of an iodinated contrast agent for CT or (seldom severe) GI irritation after ingestion of a cholecystographic contrast agent. Direct introduction of an iodinated contrast agent into a tissue space, e.g., into a joint cavity for arthrography, may lead to discomfort or to exacerbation of any baseline discomfort that had preceded the injection. The pressure necessary to deliver contrast material to the desired site, e.g.,

Visualization of structures in computer-assisted tomography may be improved by using radiopaque compounds to enhance contrast.

to the colon in a barium enema, may produce discomfort also. Allergic reactions, such as urticaria, angioedema and so forth, occasionally occur following oral administration or local injection of contrast agents.

But adverse effects are more common after *intravascular* administration of radiopaque compounds than after oral administration or local injection. Severe adverse effects are fortunately uncommon, even after intravascular administration, but their occurrence is a sobering reminder that reasonable caution must be exercised in requesting such diagnostic procedures. A study of 112,000 patients receiving these compounds intravascularly showed that 4.95% had some type of adverse effect, but the majority of these were not severe. The fatality rate was approximately 1 in 10,000 in this study (Shehadi, 1975). Ansell and associates (1980) conducted a survey of excretory urographic procedures in a large number of hospitals during two different 1-week periods and obtained data on 6500 cases. The reported incidence of minor, intermediate, and severe reactions was 8.1%, 1.7%, and 0.2%, respectively, during the first week; the corresponding figures during the second week were 5.7%, 0.9%, and 0.1%, respectively. Hartmann and colleagues (1982) reported four deaths due to excretory urography in 300,000 patients undergoing this procedure at the Mayo Clinic over an 18-year period, an incidence of 1.3 deaths per 100,000 procedures.

Adverse effects of intravascular contrast agents are not uncommon. The majority of these effects are mild. Rarely, dangerous reactions occur.

Four types of adverse effect may occur after intravascular administration of these compounds: discomfort, sudden severe anaphylactoid reactions, direct toxic effects, and hemodynamic effects.

Discomfort. This category includes vascular pain at the site of injection, an uncomfortable sensation of warmth or burning, flushing, headache, dizziness, faintness, unpleasant taste, nausea, and vomiting.

Anaphylactoid Reactions. These include urticaria, angioedema (which may be laryngeal), hypotension, or even cardiac and respiratory arrest. The term *anaphylactoid* accurately conveys our present uncertainty about the mechanism of these reactions. Manifestations such as urticaria and angioedema suggest allergic responses. Patients with a history of other allergies, e.g., food allergies, were about twice as likely to sustain some type of adverse effect from intravascular radiopaque compounds in Shehadi's series as patients without such a history; patients who had a history of a reaction in a previous procedure involving contrast media were three times as likely to suffer some type of adverse effect when they again underwent the procedure as were patients without such a history. In the series of Ansell and associates a history of allergy increased the risk of a severe reaction fourfold and a specific history of asthma increased it fivefold; a history of previous reaction to contrast media increased the risk of severe reaction elevenfold. All four deaths in the series of Hartman and colleagues occurred in patients with a history of allergy.

The mechanism of anaphylactoid reactions to contrast agents is still under debate.

On the other hand, the majority of patients who sustain an anaphylactoid reaction experience this reaction the first time they receive a radiopaque compound. None of the patients who suffered fatal reactions in the series of Hartman and colleagues (1982) had ever received intravascular contrast agents in the past. It is difficult to invoke an allergic mechanism to explain a phenomenon in which the history of a previous exposure that might act as a sensitizing dose is conspicuous by its absence in the majority of cases. Moreover, despite the aforementioned increased risk in patients who have had a previous reaction to one of these compounds, many patients with such a history do not suffer any adverse effects from re-administration (Shehadi, 1975). The use of a test dose, i.e., a small amount of the compound injected intravascularly with close observation of the patient, before deciding whether to proceed with the full dose did not appear useful in Shehadi's series. Each of the four patients in Hartman's series who died had received a test dose without demonstrating any reaction. Skin testing has proven of no value in predicting reactions to these compounds.

Prevention of anaphylactoid reactions by the use of antihistamines or corticosteroids is controversial. Lasser and associates (1987) showed, in a large series of patients, that two doses of methylprednisolone, given 12 and 2 hours, respectively, before administration of the contrast agent, significantly decreased the overall incidence of adverse effects. But in Shehadi's series those patients who had received premedication with corticosteroid or antihistaminic drugs did not have a significantly lower incidence of adverse effects than other patients. The routine use of such a prophylactic measure for all patients who are to receive intravascular contrast media has not been widely adopted and does not appear practical. For those patients whose history suggests high risk of a serious reaction, it is best to avoid iodinated contrast agents altogether by choosing some other diagnostic approach, i.e., a different imaging modality. However, if this is not feasible and the use of an iodinated contrast agent is imperative, then the use of such premedication, especially a corticosteroid drug, may be advisable. But even more important is the use of a nonionic agent, as discussed later.

Given the importance of radiographic diagnosis in many patients, these procedures will continue to be widely used. But resuscitative equipment should always be at hand when any of these compounds is injected by any route. Hartman and colleagues, while demonstrating the death rate for excretory urography quoted earlier, also reported an incidence of life-threatening reactions of about 1/3000 excretory urographic procedures. Thus, resuscitative measures were successful in approximately 96% of those sustaining a life-threatening reaction.

Direct Toxic Effects. These may involve any organ with which the radiopaque compounds come in contact, e.g., chemical pneumonitis, but the most important target organs are the kidney and heart. The reported incidence of adverse effect on the kidney ranges from 1 to 2% (Parfrey et al, 1989; Brezis and Epstein, 1989) to 40 to 100% (Brezis and Epstein), depending on the definition of adverse effect and the patient population. A mild transient increase in serum creatinine concentration is common, but precipitation of acute renal failure is rare. The most reliable predictor of nephrotoxic effect from radiopaque compounds is significant pre-existing renal disease. Decreased extracellular fluid volume from dehydration or other causes clearly increases the risk also. If careful weighing of risk and potential benefit leads to the conclusion that use of an intravascular contrast agent is indicated in a patient with high renal risk, coexisting abnormalities should be corrected if possible first, and concomitant administration of other potentially nephrotoxic drugs should be avoided.

As noted earlier, compounds administered orally for cholecystography are excreted in part by the kidney. Their administration may cause further decrease in renal function in patients who already have severe renal disease. Because of the possibility of additive adverse effect on the kidney, it is inadvisable to perform both cholecystography and urography within the same short period of time in any patient.

Adverse effects on the heart include arrhythmias, conduction defects, negative inotropic effect, and even asystole or ventricular fibrillation. In procedures such as coronary angiography where administration of a radiopaque compound is combined with cardiac catheterization, both the procedure itself and the compound contribute to the risk.

Pre-existing renal disease increases the risk of significant nephrotoxic effects from contrast agents.

Hemodynamic Effects. These occur as the result of a bolus injection of a foreign compound in a solution of high osmolality into the circulatory system. After IV injection there is temporary expansion of the blood volume; increased pulmonary artery pressure, systemic hypotension, and reflex tachycardia may occur. Injection into the right heart or pulmonary artery may cause additional changes (Fischer, 1989).

Nonionic Compounds

The iothalamates and diatrizoates used in roentgenography are fully substituted triiodinated compounds. In aqueous solutions they are ionized. The iodine atoms in the organic anion are solely responsible for the radiopacity of these compounds, but a sodium or meglumine cation is introduced into the circulation with every anion. Thus, for every three atoms of iodine administered, two osmotically active particles—the triiodinated anion and the cation—must be injected. An attractive alternative is the use of water-soluble but nonionic compounds (Almen, 1969). Metrizamide (AMIPAQUE), the first nonionic iodinated contrast agent to undergo clinical testing, proved superior to oily agents and water-soluble ionic agents for *myelography* and *cerebral ventriculography*. Metrizamide led to the study of other nonionic compounds, which in turn proved superior to it. Although MRI has now greatly decreased the use of myelography and ventriculography, several of the nonionic contrast agents introduced after metrizamide have become important as contrast agents for intravascular use.

Nonionic radiopaque compounds approved (as of 1990) in the United States for intravascular use are iopamidol injection (ISOVUE), iohexol (OMNIPAQUE), and ioversol (OPTIRAY). They provide images equal in quality to those given by ionic compounds but have significantly *lower osmolality* than the latter, because only one osmotically active particle is administered for every three iodine atoms. A related contrast agent approved in the United States for intravascular use, ioxaglate (HEXABRIX), is ionic but has the same advantage of low osmolality as the nonionic compounds because it is a dimer with only one ionizable group and hence only one cation. For every six atoms of iodine (triiodinated dimer), only two osmotically active particles (the dimer and the single cation) are injected, thus achieving the same 3:1 ratio as iopamidol, iohexol, and ioversol. All these compounds are significantly more expensive than the older, ionic compounds.

An early study (Ingstrup and Hauge, 1982), in which the two types of compound were compared with each other in the same radiographic procedures and at dosages that produced equally satisfactory images, showed that the nonionic compounds caused less discomfort than the ionic compounds. In a comparison of 7100 patients who received iohexol with 6000 historical controls who had received ionic agents, Wolf and colleagues (1989) stratified adverse effects into mild, moderate, and severe; in each category the nonionic compounds caused fewer reactions than the ionic compounds. A review by Kinnison and colleagues (1989) of reports of 100 randomized controlled trials found no differences in incidence of urticarial reactions between the two types of compound. But prospective multicenter studies have convincingly established the greater overall safety of nonionic compounds. In a study of 109,000 patients, Palmer (1988) found highly significant differences in the incidence of total adverse reactions (3.8% with ionic, 1.2% with nonionic compounds) and of severe adverse reactions (0.09% and 0.02%, respectively). The differences were especially striking in high-risk patients, in whom the incidence was 10.3% and 1.3%, respectively, for total reactions; for severe reactions, the incidence was 0.36% and 0.03%, respectively.

Some water-soluble iodinated contrast agents are nonionic. Their lower osmolality makes them superior to the older ionic compounds for many clinical uses.

In 1990, Katayama and associates reported on 337,000 patients and found a total incidence of adverse reactions of 12.66% associated with ionic and 3.13% with nonionic compounds. Although differences in the definition of adverse reactions may have accounted for the higher overall frequency of reactions in this study than in previous studies, the significant advantage of nonionic compounds was confirmed. This Japanese study reported an incidence of severe reactions of 0.22% and 0.04% with ionic and nonionic compounds, respectively. Ionic compounds caused four times as many severe reactions as the nonionic compounds in patients with a history of a previous reaction to a contrast agent and five times as many severe reactions as nonionic compounds in patients with a history of allergy.

Nonionic compounds are clearly safer than high osmolality ionic compounds in cardiac studies such as coronary arteriography and ventriculography (Benotti, 1988; Davidson et al, 1989). The exact status of ioxaglate relative to nonionic compounds in coronary arteriography is still uncertain, but initial comparisons of ioxaglate with iopamidol have suggested approximately equal safety in this procedure insofar as cardiac toxicity is concerned. However, Vacek and associates (1990) in a retrospective study found that 11% of 324 patients receiving ioxaglate experienced nausea, vomiting, or allergic reactions, as compared with 3% of 205 patients receiving iohexol (p<.005). Despite their potential advantage for renal imaging, nonionic compounds have *not* been found less nephrotoxic than ionic compounds (Parfrey et al, 1989; Davidson et al, 1989).

Both types of compound have an anticoagulant effect that is usually transient and not clinically significant, except for the possibility of additive effect in patients whose coagulation is already impaired. The effect is weaker with nonionic than with ionic compounds. The appearance of red cell aggregates, or at times clots, in syringes where blood comes in contact with nonionic compounds has even raised concern about their possible thrombogenic effect. But the risk of *in vivo* thrombosis from nonionic compounds appears low (Bettman, 1988).

DIAGNOSTIC RADIOPHARMACEUTICALS FOR NUCLEAR MEDICINE PROCEDURES

Diagnostic studies in nuclear medicine are of three types. In *kinetic studies* the uptake or disappearance of an administered radionuclide by some compartment, tissue, or organ is measured. Thus, the uptake of iodine by the thyroid gland may be measured after administration of a suitable radioisotope of iodine, e.g., ^{123}I, ^{125}I, or ^{131}I, in the form of sodium iodide. Capsules and solutions of sodium salts of each of these three radioisotopes are listed in the United States Pharmacopeia. Similarly, external counting over the kidney area after administration of iodohippurate sodium I 123 injection or its ^{131}I analog permits construction of a time-radioactivity curve providing information about the kidney's ability to excrete this compound.

A much more common type of study, *scintigraphy*, utilizes a gamma camera to produce an image of an organ, tissue, or compartment of interest, i.e., a scintigram, after administration (usually IV injection) of a radioactive imaging agent. This second type of study may be considered an extension of the first type except that spatial information is obtained. Thus, a scintigram of the thyroid after administration of radioactive iodine may be considered an uptake study with a pictorial read-out. Even when scintigraphy is used simply to demonstrate a lesion, its fundamental difference from radiography should be noted. X-ray images are based on anatomical structures, whereas scintigraphic images are based on organ or tissue function,

The primary basis of roentgenographic (x-ray) images is anatomical *structure*; the primary basis for scintigraphic images is *function*, i.e., uptake of radiopharmaceuticals.

because they depend on uptake and distribution processes. Because radiographic and magnetic resonance images are much superior to scintigrams in resolution, the clinical value of scintigraphy may lie increasingly in showing changes in function (blood flow, transport, receptor status, and so forth).

A third type of *in vivo* study, which depends upon the principle of *isotope dilution*, is described earlier.

Among drugs that currently have wide, established clinical use, no other group—diagnostic or therapeutic—is regularly administered systemically in such small dosages as are radiopharmaceuticals. A dose of 2 mCi (74 MBq) ^{201}Tl, given as TlCl for myocardial scintigraphy, contains approximately 9.4 ng ^{201}Tl, plus $\leq$0.2 ng contaminating ^{202}Tl or about 11.3 ng (48 picamols) thallium chloride. Even those radiopharmaceuticals that contain the stable compound in addition to the radioactive compound can be obtained now in such high specific activity that the amount of stable compound injected is very low. Thus, the risk of toxic effects is negligible. However, because of the absorbed radiation dose to the patient, administration of radiopharmaceuticals is not totally innocuous.

In vivo distribution is an important consideration in the pharmacology of any systemically administered drug, but the clinical relevance of *in vivo* distribution is more obvious for radioactive imaging agents than for any other class of drugs. The special pharmacological interest of most of these agents lies in the fact that they must be designed to achieve selective concentration (localization) in the target organ or tissue in order to provide a satisfactory image. ^{99m}Tc is by far the most commonly used radionuclide for scintigraphy, because the energy of its γ emission is in the optimum range for currently available gamma cameras. Its short (6 hour) physical half-life is also an advantage from the standpoint of absorbed radiation dose to the patient. A variety of kits are available to permit rapid incorporation of ^{99m}Tc into a given radiopharmaceutical just before administration to a patient. Several radioisotopes of iodine have been incorporated also into various imaging agents; ^{123}I has favorable emission characteristics and a half-life of 13 hours. When radio-iodinated compounds are administered, subsequent deiodination *in vivo* may release iodide ion, which is taken up by the thyroid. To prevent unnecessary irradiation of the thyroid, especially when ^{125}I or ^{131}I is used, stable iodine, e.g., as Lugol's solution, is usually administered orally beforehand to saturate the thyroid's uptake process and prevent entry of the radioactive isotope.

In vivo localization of a radionuclide *depends upon the chemical form in which it is administered.* Thus, radioactive iodine given as sodium iodide localizes in the thyroid gland, which builds it into thyroid hormone, and in the kidney, which excretes the iodide ion. But localization of radioactive iodine given in the form of N-isopropyl-iodoamphetamine (IMP), iodocholesterol, and m-iodobenzylguanidine (MIBG) is in the brain, adrenal cortex, and adrenal medulla, respectively. Selective concentration in the target of interest is achieved by designing radiopharmaceuticals to utilize one or more *mechanisms of localization.* For most radiopharmaceuticals it is convenient to consider a simple two-compartment model, with the plasma as the first compartment and the tissues as the second. The chief mechanisms of localization currently exploited are as follows.

Mechanisms of Localization

Distribution in the First Compartment. This is the simplest mechanism. For example, determination of the cardiac ejection fraction by scintigraphy requires satisfactory labeling of the intravascular space in order that the

^{99m}Tc and certain isotopes of iodine are the most common radionuclides used in scintigraphy. They are targeted toward specific organs or tissues by incorporation into appropriate compounds.

Clinically useful radiopharmaceuticals exploit various mechanisms of localization to obtain selective high concentrations in target organs or tissues.

cardiac blood pool may be visualized in systole and diastole. Although labeled serum albumin could be used for this purpose, a more satisfactory visualization of the cardiac blood pool is obtained with erythrocytes labeled with ^{99m}Tc. The red cells are labeled *in vivo* by IV administration of sodium pertechnetate Tc 99m injection after a preceding injection of the reducing agent stannous pyrophosphate.

Several auxiliary mechanisms permit the distribution of radiopharmaceuticals in subdivisions of the blood compartment. After IV administration of gallium citrate Ga 67 injection, the radionuclide binds to transferrin, thus labeling the plasma. Imaging of abscesses after injection of this radiopharmaceutical is due, in part, to the vasodilation and hyperemia that develops around an abscess. However, other mechanisms, not clearly understood, also favor localization of gallium in both leukocytes and certain neoplastic cells, making gallium a somewhat nonspecific and unsatisfactory imaging agent.

But currently the most important use of a radiopharmaceutical for imaging a subdivision of the vascular compartment is in pulmonary scintigraphy. If human serum albumin is denatured *in vitro* to produce aggregates of controlled particle size (10–30 micra) and is labeled with ^{99m}Tc, these particles will be trapped by a subdivision of the vascular compartment, the pulmonary capillary bed, after IV injection. Thus, a *perfusion scintigram* of the lung can be obtained. The aggregated albumin breaks down subsequently into particles of smaller size and leaves the lung to be phagocytosed eventually by the reticuloendothelial system. In a different technique the inhalation of radioactive xenon (^{133}Xe) permits an *inhalation scintigram* of the lung. In this instance the air spaces of the lung represent the first compartment into which the imaging agent is introduced directly. A comparison of a scintigram of the lung after inhalation of xenon Xe 133 with a perfusion scintigram obtained by IV administration of technetium Tc 99m albumin aggregated injection is useful in the diagnosis of pulmonary embolism. A mismatch between the two scintigrams, in which a well-ventilated area, as shown by ^{133}Xe, is not well perfused, as shown by the labeled albumin aggregates, is strongly suggestive of embolism.

Comparison of perfusion and inhalation scintigrams of the lung, using two different radiopharmaceuticals, provides diagnostic information beyond that given by either one alone.

Diffusion. If ^{99m}Tc in the form of a diethylenetriamine pentaacetate (DTPA) chelate (technetium Tc 99m pentetate injection) is injected IV, little will diffuse normally into the brain. If, however, a lesion such as a brain tumor causes a breakdown of the blood-brain barrier, extracellular fluid accumulates around the lesion, and the labeled chelate diffuses into this area. Although the vascular compartment remains labeled also, elimination of the labeled chelate by the kidney lowers the concentration in the vascular compartment more rapidly than the concentration in the lesion. Eventually back diffusion from the lesion into the vascular compartment will restore equilibrium, but this process takes time. Thus, there is a critical period of time in which the lesion has a higher concentration of the labeled chelate than does the blood and can be imaged clearly. CT and MRI have largely superseded scintigraphy in diagnosis of brain tumors, but the principle discussed here is also applicable to MRI.

However, the blood-brain barrier does not prevent rapid diffusion of highly lipid-soluble compounds from the blood into the brain, provided the compound is not highly bound to plasma proteins and is not highly ionized at body pH. The rate of uptake of such lipophilic compounds is not limited by the rate of their diffusion into the brain but by the rate of their delivery to the brain, i.e., their uptake is perfusion-limited. Therefore, scintigraphy after IV administration of such compounds permits estimation of regional cerebral blood flow. These compounds include iofetamine hydrochloride

Certain lipid-soluble radiopharmaceuticals diffuse so easily into the brain that their uptake is limited by perfusion.

I 123 injection (IMP), an amphetamine derivative; technetium Tc 99m exametazime injection (hexamethyl propyleneamine oxime, HM-PAO); and a ^{123}I-labeled propanediamine derivative, HIPDM. Although additional mechanisms of localization may exist for these compounds, e.g., binding of the amphetamine derivative to synaptosomes or ionic trapping of HIPDM as a result of differences between intracellular and extracellular pH, their lipophilicity is their most important characteristic. Their uptake is not limited to the brain, e.g., iofetamine is also widely taken up by liver and lung. Iofetamine also differs from most radiopharmaceuticals in that the amount of stable compound in the injected preparation may be sufficient occasionally to have a pharmacological effect, in this instance mild elevation of blood pressure (McAfee, 1989).

Phagocytosis. If ^{99m}Tc is given IV in colloidal form, e.g., technetium Tc 99m sulphur colloid injection, the reticuloendothelial cells of the liver and spleen take up the colloidal particles and permit imaging of these organs, especially the liver.

Active Transport. Several important imaging agents are actively transported into their target organs. When radiopharmaceuticals of high specific activity are used, saturation of the transport systems is not achieved, and high selective concentrations can be obtained in target organs. The active transport system that concentrates iodide ion in the thyroid gland can be utilized not only to localize radioactive iodine in the gland but also to permit imaging of the thyroid after IV administration of sodium pertechnetate Tc 99m injection, because the pertechnetate ion is actively transported by the same thyroidal system. However, unlike iodine, pertechnetate does not enter into the chain of biochemical reactions involved in synthesis of thyroid hormones. Therefore, pertechnetate leaves the gland more rapidly than iodine.

Active transport mechanisms permit localization of radiopharmaceuticals at many sites, e.g. the thyroid gland, myocardium, adrenal medulla and hepatobiliary system.

The Na, K-activated ATPase system that achieves a high myocardial concentration of potassium also permits localization of certain other monovalent cations in the myocardium. Following the demonstration that ^{131}Cs permits imaging of myocardial infarcts, a number of radioisotopes of K, Rb, and Cs were studied in an attempt to find a radionuclide with better physical characteristics than ^{131}Cs. None of these cations proved as satisfactory as the thallous ion. Although ^{201}Tl permits scintigraphic imaging of myocardial infarcts, its principal value is in the diagnosis of coronary artery disease. The active transport system for the cation is so efficient that its uptake by myocardium is perfusion-limited in most instances. In the ^{201}Tl stress test the patient exercises directly after IV administration of ^{201}Tl. Regions of compromised coronary blood flow may show decreased uptake in this situation of high myocardial demand, whereas a second scintigram, taken at rest a few hours later, may show apparent redistribution of the radionuclide back into the previously hypoperfused area. This apparent redistribution is due to the fact that the normally perfused area, having a higher initial uptake than the ischemic area, also loses the ^{201}Tl faster than the latter, and the difference in uptake between the two areas is therefore not seen in the second scintigram. Regions of scarring usually show decreased uptake in both scintigrams. For patients unable to perform vigorous exercise, an alternative way to obtain the necessary vasodilation in the ^{201}Tl test is to administer dipyridamole.

Unlike ^{201}Tl, certain other perfusion-limited radiopharmaceuticals remain at their site of myocardial uptake with only very slow washout, e.g., the ^{99m}Tc-isonitriles. Their uptakes at rest and during exercise can be compared by giving two separate injections at the appropriate times. The isonitriles have proved useful in a variety of cardiac studies. Thus technetium Tc 99m sestamibi, a methoxyisobutyl isonitrile, permits simultaneous measurements of ejection fraction, segmental motion of the myocardium, and myocardial perfusion (Wackers et al, 1989). The very slow washout of the sestamibi has several advantages. Coupled with the favorable physical characteristics of ^{99m}Tc, it permits single photon emission CT (SPECT) images of high quality. In patients with acute myocardial infarction this imaging agent has been used not only to estimate the exent of myocardium at risk but also to study the effect of acute reperfusion therapy (thrombolysis or coronary angioplasty) without the need to delay therapy in order to perform scintigraphy. In this strategy the imaging agent is injected just *prior to* the reperfusion therapy, but the scintigram is postponed until a few hours *after* completion of the therapy. This scintigram will still reveal the ^{99m}Tc distribution that resulted from the original injection, i.e., the pretherapy status of the myocardium. At a later time, after the ^{99m}Tc has largely decayed, a second injection can be given and a new scintigram obtained to determine the effect of therapy (Pellikka et al, 1990). Although this isonitrile is listed for convenience in the same subsection of this chapter as the thallous ion and is a monovalent cation like the thallous ion, the myocardial uptake of the two does not appear to be by the same mechanism. The lipophilic nature of the isonitrile may be partly responsible for its uptake, but metabolic inhibitors depress myocardial uptake of the compound. The uptake may be governed by plasma and mitochondrial membrane potentials.

Active transport of ^{99m}Tc-labeled iminodiacetic (IDA) derivatives by hepatocytes permits scintigraphic imaging of the bile ducts and gallbladder. In this instance the system may be considered to have three compartments: plasma, hepatocytes, and biliary passages. Technetium Tc 99m disofenin (diisopropyl IDA) is an example of this class of imaging agents.

The scintigraphic diagnosis of pheochromocytoma by [^{131}I]-MIBG is noted earlier. Its mechanism of localization, at least in part, is the active transport system that is responsible for uptake of catecholamines by sympathetic neurons and adrenal medullary tissue, commonly termed *neuronal uptake* or *uptake₁*. Therefore, this compound is useful also in the scintigraphic diagnosis of neuroblastoma.

Special Mechanisms of Retention in the Second Compartment. A number of mechanisms trap radiopharmaceuticals after their entry into certain tissues and permit high selective concentrations.

1. Entry of iodine into the synthetic chain for thyroid hormone is noted earlier. Because cholesterol is the raw material for synthesis of steroid hormones by the adrenal cortex, [^{131}I]-19-iodocholesterol was synthesized by Counsell and colleagues (1970) and used to visualize the adrenal cortex scintigraphically by Beierwaltes and associates (1971). A later derivative, [^{131}I]-6-iodomethyl 19-norcholesterol, proved superior and is useful in the scintigraphic diagnosis of various lesions of the adrenal cortex, including hyperplasia and neoplasms.

2. A simple but highly effective mechanism of localization permits imaging of bone after administration of a number of phosphorus-containing compounds, e.g., technetium Tc 99m pyrophosphate injection or technetium Tc 99m etidronate injection, a diphosphonate. Localization depends upon the binding of the phosphorus-containing moiety to the calcium phosphate of bone, especially at bone surfaces. When bone turnover is active, as in metastases, fractures or other lesions, more bone surface is exposed and a "hot area" appears on the scintigram. Although the ability of such bone-seeking compounds to permit scintigraphic diagnosis of an-

other lesion, acute myocardial infarction, appears at first glance to make little sense, the underlying mechanism of localization is the same for infarcts as for bone. As they lose their viability, damaged myocytes are unable to prevent excessive accumulation of calcium ions intracellularly. Therefore, myocardial infarcts of sufficient size may be imaged with the labeled pyrophosphate or diphosphonate compounds.

Why should an imaging agent for bone also localize in myocardial infarcts?

3. The imaging of various tumors by radioimmunoconjugates, i.e., labeled monoclonal antibodies (or their Fab fragments) to tumors, is under active investigation. The possibility of achieving sufficiently intense localization to permit therapeutic irradiation of tumors adds further interest to this field. But this mechanism of localization is not limited to tumors. Monoclonal antimyosin antibody (Fab fragment) labeled with ^{111}In does not bind extensively to normal myocardium. But when myocytes are damaged, as in myocardial infarction or rejection of a cardiac transplant, breakdown of sarcolemmal integrity permits access of the antibody to myosin. Significant binding occurs and permits imaging. Antigranulocyte monoclonal antibodies labeled with ^{99m}Tc permit imaging of foci of infection, but labeled *nonspecific* poly-clonal immunoglobulin (IgG) also localizes at such foci by means that are still unclear; here the Fc fragment is important.

Labeled antibodies and labeled compounds with high affinity for specific receptors are currently under active investigation as imaging agents.

4. Binding to receptors is exemplified by quinuclidinyl iodobenzilate (IQNB) labeled with ^{123}I, which binds to muscarinic cholinergic receptors and permits imaging of their distribution in the human brain, i.e., relatively high concentration in the cerebrum but not in the cerebellum. Other ^{123}I-labeled receptor ligands are under investigation in humans for imaging D_2 dopamine receptors and benzodiazepine receptors.

Miscellaneous Mechanisms

RENAL. The DTPA chelate of ^{99m}Tc, discussed earlier as an imaging agent for brain lesions, is excreted by glomerular filtration and thus may be used to image the kidney. However, both this compound and the iodohippurate discussed earlier are rapidly excreted by the kidney, making them useful in dynamic studies but unsatisfactory for imaging of renal morphology and lesions. Technetium Tc 99m gluceptate injection, a labeled glucoheptonate, is retained longer by renal tubules and permits better imaging of the kidney, but the mechanism of this compound's localization in the tubules is still uncertain.

An example of the use of ^{99m}Tc-DTPA and of labeled iodohippurate in a dynamic study is the renogram, i.e., continuous recording of radioactivity over the renal areas after IV injection of a radiopharmaceutical, in hypertensive patients suspected of having unilateral renal artery stenosis (RAS). The angiotensin-converting enzyme inhibitor, captopril, causes vasodilation of renal efferent arterioles more than the afferent arterioles, leading to a fall in intraglomerular pressure and glomerular filtration rate. This fall is exaggerated in kidneys with RAS. As ^{99m}Tc-DTPA is excreted by glomerular filtration, renal uptake of this compound may be markedly *depressed* after captopril in RAS. If renograms performed before and after captopril administration show a striking difference in one kidney as compared with the contralateral kidney, this finding is strongly suggestive of RAS on the side showing marked captopril effect.

But labeled iodohippurate is excreted primarily by tubular secretion and to a lesser extent by glomerular filtration. The decreased filtration caused by captopril in kidneys with RAS *increases* the availability of iodohippurate to the renal tubules. But, as urine flow decreases, the compound accumulates in the renal cortex. Thus, the effect of captopril is to *delay* the time of *peak* radioactivity in the affected kidney as compared with the contralateral kidney. Although captopril-induced changes in the renogram are at times more dramatic with ^{99m}Tc-DTPA than with labeled iodohippurate, the reliability of the test is higher with the latter (Sfakianakis et al, 1987). A ^{99m}Tc-containing compound would be preferable to iodohippurate. Technetium Tc 99m mertialide (^{99m}Tc-mercaptoacetyltriglycine) is excreted in the same manner as iodohippurate, provides scintigrams of high quality, and thus is very promising as a replacement for iodohippurate (Muller-Suur et al, 1990).

FOCI OF INFLAMMATION. The use of ^{67}Ga has been described earlier. But a different approach to imaging sites uses *cellular sequestration*. The patient's own leukocytes, obtained from a blood sample, are labeled with ^{111}In *in vitro* and then reinjected. Their localization at foci of inflammation permits imaging.

RADIOPHARMACEUTICALS USED IN POSITRON EMISSION TOMOGRAPHY

The radiopharmaceuticals discussed earlier are used in SPECT. But positron emission tomography (PET) permits much more accurate localization of the source of each count recorded, i.e., the position of the atom whose disintegration resulted in a given signal is more precisely established with PET than with SPECT. An additional advantage of PET is that positron-emitting isotopes of carbon, oxygen, and nitrogen exist. As there are no radioisotopes of these elements available for SPECT, most biologically important amino acids, carbohydrates, and fatty acids must be altered by addition of some foreign element, e.g., iodine or technetium, to permit their imaging by SPECT. But PET permits noninvasive *in vivo* studies of the metabolism of unaltered amino acids, carbohydrates and fatty acids, labeled at appropriate carbon, oxygen, or nitrogen sites.

PET has special advantages for metabolic and receptor studies, but the short half-life of important positron-emitting nuclides poses a problem.

Especially important in pharmacology is the ability of PET to provide images of the *in vivo* distribution of receptors after administration of ^{11}C-labeled compounds, e.g., dopamine and serotonin receptors after administration of ^{11}C-labeled methylspiperone, and opioid receptors after administration of ^{11}C-labeled carfentanil. More recently individualization of therapy has been greatly advanced by the ability to measure the concentration of many drugs in the plasma, which provides more useful information than obtained by simply knowing the dose administered to the patient. If we can obtain noninvasive information about actual occupancy of appropriate receptors by a drug in any given patient, the information should be even more useful in adjusting therapy (Wagner, 1985). However, there are serious practical obstacles to reaching this goal. For example, the half-life of ^{11}C is 20 minutes, and its use requires a cyclotron in close proximity to the imaging facilities. Thus, the increasing availability of ^{123}I-labeled receptor ligands for SPECT imaging, noted earlier, is potentially very important for improving the understanding of neurological and psychological disorders (Wagner, 1990).

[^{18}F]-fluorodeoxyglucose has already proved useful in clinical studies.

But the half-life of the positron emitter, ^{18}F, is 107 minutes. [^{18}F]-fluorestradiol has permitted imaging of estrogen receptors in breast cancers. A compound of particular importance is [^{18}F]-fluorodeoxyglucose (FDG), which permits evaluation of the metabolic state of various regions of the brain by PET. The mechanism of localization is entry into a metabolic pathway. Although deoxyglucose, after uptake by cells, follows the same initial metabolic step as glucose, i.e., conversion to the 6-phosphate, deoxyglucose does not proceed further along the glucose-metabolizing pathway. Thus, in contrast to the rapid metabolism and disappearance of glucose, labeled deoxyglucose remains at its site of uptake longer and permits PET imaging. Identification of epileptogenic foci, areas of cell dropout in Huntington's disease, and other regional brain abnormalities can be visualized. Brunetti and associates (1989) have used FDG to show reversal of brain abnormalities following treatment of acquired immunodeficiency syndrome (AIDS) dementia with zidovudine. FDG is useful also in evaluating the metabolic state of the myocardium. When combined with another tracer such as ^{13}N ammonia to estimate blood flow, FDG accurately predicts whether regions of a poorly contractile left ventricle will show improvement after coronary bypass surgery.

Several positron-emitting radionuclides with very short half-lives are potentially useful because they can be obtained from generators available at the site of clinical use, e.g., ^{82}Rb (half-life, 74 seconds) from a generator containing ^{82}Sr (half-life, 25 days). As the myocardium takes up Rb$^+$ by the same active transport mechanism as K$^+$ and Tl$^+$, Rb$^+$ permits cardiac imaging by PET.

CONTRAST AGENTS FOR MAGNETIC RESONANCE IMAGING

MRI, unlike scintigraphy, does not require administration of any exogenous compound. The vast majority of clinical MR images obtained at present are based on proton resonance, especially the protons of tissue water, and many structures are imaged well without the need for contrast enhancement. But significantly better images of some organs or lesions can be obtained when an appropriate compound is administered to enhance contrast. Two types of compound are potentially useful. First, compounds containing ^{19}F or ^{13}C, nuclides that have satisfactory nuclear magnetic resonance (NMR) sensitivities and occur in normal tissues only in low concentration, are of interest because the ^{19}F or ^{13}C signal obtained after administration of the respective compounds comes largely from the exogenous nuclide. Therefore, the distribution of the contrast agent containing that nuclide can be imaged. Second, compounds containing paramagnetic elements, such as gadolinium and manganese, are useful because paramagnetic substances affect the intensity of the MR image indirectly by their effect on relaxation times. Gd- or Mn-containing compounds, if concentrated selectively by some organ or tissue, shorten the T_1 relaxation time of protons at that site and increase the intensity of the image. This second type of MRI contrast agent appears more promising than the first.

Gadolinium increases intensity in MRI by shortening T_1 relaxation time.

The most widely used compound at present is gadopentetate dimeglumine injection (MAGNEVIST), the meglumine salt of the gadolinium complex of DTPA. It has found its most extensive use in enhancing contrast of lesions in the central nervous system (CNS). After IV injection this compound enters the edema fluid around brain tumors in the same manner as the similar chelate of ^{99m}Tc used in nuclear medicine. Thus, the gadopentetate permits separation of the area of edema around the tumor from the tumor itself on an MR image. This contrast agent is not equally useful in the diagnosis of all brain tumors, as recognized early by Felix and colleagues (1985). With diagnostic drugs as with therapeutic drugs, early expectations may not be entirely fulfilled by later experience, and the experience of Brant-Zawadzki and associates (1986) and Berry and coworkers (1986) suggests somewhat more limited usefulness of this compound in the diagnosis of brain lesions than the early studies of Carr and associates (1984a, 1984b) and Felix and colleagues (1985). The probable explanation is not that the early studies were wrong in any way, but simply the fact that radiologists subsequently accumulated more experience in reading MR

The first contrast agent to achieve wide clinical use in MRI is gadopentetate, a chelate of gadolinium.

images and became increasingly competent in making diagnoses in the absence of enhancement by the contrast agent. Although somewhat less important in the diagnosis of axial lesions of the brain, "judicious use of Gd-DTPA should improve ability of MR to detect extra-axial lesions, delineate their extent and characterize their perfusion" (Berry et al, 1986). Many studies have shown the usefulness of gadopentetate in the diagnosis of spinal cord lesions.

It is likely that, at least in selected instances, gadopentetate will find clinical use also in imaging of other organs, e.g., the liver and kidney, but further experience is needed to evaluate these uses. Unlike the previously noted development of brain imaging with gadopentetate, the compound's usefulness in demonstrating liver lesions was less apparent in the earliest clinical studies than in later studies. The explanation lies in the more recent development of faster MRI methods, which enable better detection of events that occur promptly after IV injection of the contrast agent. The diagnostic drug did not change, but the recording methods improved.

Under certain circumstances MRI agents may show a negative concentration-intensity curve, i.e., image intensity may *decrease* as the concentration of contrast agent at a given site *increases*. Paramagnetic contrast agents increase intensity by shortening T_1 relaxation time. However, they also shorten T_2 relaxation time, and shortening of the latter increases the rate of signal decay, thus decreasing image intensity. With the dose of gadopentetate used clinically, the effect on T_1 relaxation time usually predominates, and image intensity increases at most sites of gadopentetate accumulation. However, the chelate is excreted so effectively by the normal kidney that very high gadopentetate concentrations appear in the renal pelvis, and the T_2 effect becomes significant, causing a decrease in image intensity in that area (Kikinis et al, 1987).

Side effects from administration of gadopentetate do not occur in the majority of patients, but about 10% report headache, with nausea and vomiting in a smaller number, and hypotension in occasional patients. The compound causes alterations in red cell membranes, the clinical significance of which is still uncertain, and serum iron concentrations increase in some patients receiving it. The safety of gadopentetate administration in patients with sickle cell disease or hemolytic anemia is still undetermined.

Other MRI contrast agents, able perhaps to exploit some of the more sophisticated mechanisms of localization that radiopharmaceuticals already use, are likely to be developed in the future.

Note to the Student or Young Physician Reader

Students and young physicians face a bewildering array of brand names for radiographic contrast agents, often with a variety of numbers indicating concentration or osmolality. The futility of attempting to learn all these names and the specific uses of each preparation, unless one plans to specialize in radiology, has led many students and young physicians to dismiss the whole area from their minds. Such a know-nothing attitude is not the most responsible way for a physician to deal with the problems of judiciously requesting imaging procedures.

The first question in requesting an imaging procedure should be: if there are several possible procedures, which is the first choice for this patient? For example, the thallium stress test is usually preferable to coronary arteriography as a screening procedure because the thallium test is noninvasive. But if one is already convinced that a patient has significant coronary disease and wishes to know the precise sites and extent of coronary narrowing, arteriography with a radiopaque contrast agent is necessary. In the diagnosis of skeletal lesions most bony metastases result in positive scintigrams, using one of the ^{99m}Tc-labeled phosphorus compounds, earlier than the lesion can be shown by x-ray. The increased bone *turnover* in the metastasis, which makes more bone surface available for deposition of the labeled phosphorus compound and thus leads to a positive scintigram, occurs early but the *net loss* of calcium from the metastatic site, which must occur to a significant degree before it is detectable by x-ray, takes longer to develop. On the other hand, a positive scintigram does not distinguish between a traumatic fracture and a metastasis, whereas x-ray, with its much superior resolution, usually permits the distinction. Specialists in radiology are not only important consultants in the interpretation of various studies but also in their selection.

As these important clinical details are beyond the scope of a pharmacology text, the student or young physician is advised at this point to reread the section on radiopaque compounds, bearing in mind the following points. The compounds used to visualize the gallbladder, iopanoic acid (TELEPAQUE) and the ipodates (OROGRAFIN), and biliary passages are somewhat different from those used for intravascular studies. Intravascular studies employ the salts of diatrizoic (HYPAQUE, RENOGRAFIN) and iothalamic (CONRAY) acids, or are members of the newer nonionic and low-osmolality family of compounds. The reader should review the various types of adverse effect of intravascular radiopaque compounds, both the fairly common mild effects and the less common dangerous reactions. The factors predisposing a patient to the dangerous effects should be noted.

The subsection on radiopharmaceuticals is best reviewed in a different way. As the noninvasive nature of scintigraphy depends in the first instance on the relation between chemical structure and distribution — the pharmacological basis of noninvasiveness — the student or young physician is faced with a large and constantly changing set of compounds, many with complex chemical structures. The abbreviations commonly used for these structures are often little help to the learner. The reader is advised, therefore, to review now the mechanisms of localization discussed earlier and, where several agents have been given as important examples of one mechanism, to remember at least a single example for each mechanism in order to reinforce understanding. Subsequently, in the clinic each time a scintigram is performed in one of the student's or physician's patients, the radiopharmaceutical used should be identified. Its mechanism of localization should be briefly reviewed then and the clinical significance of the findings considered in the light of this background information.

It is important also to recognize that many of the radiopharmaceuticals used currently to exploit a given mechanism of uptake are by no means ideal and may be replaced subsequently by compounds that utilize that mechanism more effectively. New radiopharmaceuticals, whether developed initially in the United States or abroad, often enter clinical use in other countries earlier than in the United States, chiefly because the approval policies of the United States Food and Drug Administration (FDA) tend to be more conservative than those of other countries (McAfee, 1989). Several promising compounds, already in clinical use elsewhere but omitted from this chapter because of their current unavailability in the United States, are likely to appear in American clinics at a later time.

References

Almen T: Contrast agent design. Some aspects of the synthesis of water soluble contrast agents of low osmolality. J Theor Biol 24:216–226, 1969.

Ansell G, Tweedie MCK, West CR, et al: The current status of reactions to intravenous contrast media. Invest Radiol 15:S32–S39, 1980.

Beierwaltes WH, Lieberman LG, Ansari AN, Nishiyama H: Visualization of human adrenal glands in vivo by scintillation scanning. JAMA 216:275–277, 1971.

Benotti JR: The comparative effects of ionic versus non-ionic agents in cardiac catheterization. Invest Radiol 23(Suppl 2):S366–S373, 1988.

Berry I, Brant-Zawadzki M, Osaki L, et al: Gd-DTPA in clinical MR of the brain. 2. Extraaxial lesions and normal structures. AJR 147:1231–1235, 1986.

Bettman M: Clinical summary and conclusions. Ionic versus nonionic contrast agents and their effects on blood coagulation. Invest Radiol 23(Suppl 2):S378–S380, 1988.

Brant-Zawadzki M, Berry I, Osaki L, et al: Gd-DTPA in clinical MR of the brain. 1. Intraaxial lesions. AJR 147:1223–1230, 1986.

Brezis M, Epstein FH: A closer look at radiocontrast-induced nephropathy. N Eng J Med 320:179–181, 1989.

Brunetti A, Berg G, Dichiro G, et al: Reversal of brain metabolic abnormalities following treatment of AIDS dementia complex with 3′-azido-2, 3′-dideoxythymidine (AZT, Zidovudine): A PET: FDG study. J Nucl Med 30:581–590, 1989.

Carr DH, Brown J, Bydder GM, et al: Gadolinium-DTPA as a contrast agent in MRI. Initial clinical experience in 20 patients. AJR 143:215–224, 1984a.

Carr DH, Brown J, Bydder GM, et al: Intravenous chelated gadolinium as a contrast agent in NMR imaging of cerebral tumours. Lancet 1:484–486, 1984b.

Counsell RE, Ranade VV, Blair RJ, et al: Tumor localizing agents: IX Radioiodinated cholesterol. Steroids 16:317–328, 1970.

Davidson CJ, Hlatky M, Morris KG, et al: Cardiovascular and renal toxicity of a nonionic radiographic contrast agent after cardiac catheterization. A prospective trial. Ann Int Med 110:119–124, 1989.

Dawkins P: Conventional angiography. *In* Skucas J (ed): Radiographic Contrast Agents, 162. Rockville, MD: Aspen Publications, 1989.

Dorland's Illustrated Medical Dictionary. 27th ed, 510. Philadelphia: WB Saunders, 1988.

Felix R, Schorner W, Laniado M, et al: Brain tumors: MR imaging with gadolinium-DTPA. Radiology 156:681–688, 1985.

Fischer HW: Idiosyncratic reactions. *In* Skucas J (ed): Radiographic Contrast Agents, 145. Rockville, MD: Aspen Publications, 1989.

Hartman GW, Hattery RR, Witten DM, Williamson B Jr: Mortality during excretory urography. Mayo Clinic experience. AJR 139:919–922, 1982.

Ingstrup HM, Hauge P: Clinical testing of iohexol, Conray meglumine and Amipaque in cerebral angiography. Neuroradiology 23:75–79, 1982.

Katayama H, Yamaguchi K, Kozoka T, et al: Adverse reactions to ionic and nonionic contrast media. A report from the Japanese Committee on the Safety of Contrast Media. Radiology 175:621–628, 1990.

Kikinis R, VonSchulthess GK, Jager P, et al: Normal and hydronephrotic kidney: Evaluation of renal function with contrast-enhanced MRI imaging. Radiology 165:837–842, 1987.

Kinnison ML, Powe NR, Steinberg EP: Results of randomized controlled trials of low- versus high-osmolality contrast media. Radiology 170:381–389, 1989.

Lasser EC, Berry CC, Talner LB, et al: Pretreatment with corticosteroids to alleviate reactions to intravenous contrast material. N Eng J Med 317:845–855, 1987.

Liddle GW: Δ',9α-fluorohydrocortisone. A new investigative tool in adrenal physiology. J Clin Endocrinol Metab 16:557–559, 1956.

Liddle GW: Tests of pituitary-adrenal suppressibility in the diagnosis of Cushing's syndrome. J Clin Endocrinol Metab 20:1539–1560, 1960.

Muller-Suur R, Bois-Svensson I, Mesko L: A comparative study of renal scintigraphy and clearance with technetium-99m-MAG$_3$, and iodine-123-hippurate in patients with renal disorders. J Nucl Med 31:1811–1817, 1990.

McAfee JG: Update on radiopharmaceuticals for medical imaging. Radiology 171:593–601, 1989.

Palmer FJ: The RACR survey of intravenous contrast media reactions. Australas Radiol 32:426–428, 1988.

Parfrey PS, Griffiths SM, Barrett BJ, et al: Contrast material-induced renal failure in patients with diabetes mellitus, renal insufficiency or both. A prospective controlled study. N Eng J Med 320:143–148, 1989.

Pellikka PA, Behrenbeck T, Verani MS, et al: Serial changes in myocardial perfusion using tomographic technetium-99m-hexakis-2-methoxy-2-methylpropyl-isonitrile imaging following reperfusion therapy of myocadial infarction. J Nucl Med 31:1269–1275, 1990.

Sfakianakis GN, Bourgoignie JJ, Jaffe D, et al: Single-dose captopril scintigraphy in the diagnosis of renovascular hypertension. J Nucl Med 28:1383–1392, 1987.

Shehadi WH: Adverse reactions to intravascularly administered contrast media: A comprehensive study based on a prospective survey. Am J Roentgenol Radium Ther Nucl Med 124:145–152, 1975.

Vacek JL, Gersema L, Woods M, et al: Frequencies of reactions to iohexol versus ioxaglate. Am J Cardiol 66:1277–1278, 1990.

Wackers FJT, Berman DS, Maddami J, et al: Technetium-99m-hexakis-2-methoxyisobutyl isonitrile: Human biodistribution, safety and preliminary comparison to thallium-201 for myocardial perfusion imaging. J Nucl Med 30:301–311, 1989.

Wagner HN Jr: Nuclear medicine in the 1990s: The challenge of change—SNM scientific meeting highlights. J Nucl Med 26:679–686, 1985.

Wagner HN Jr: Scientific highlights 1990: The universe within. J Nucl Med 31:17A–26A, 1990.

Wolf GL, Arenson RL, Cross AP: A prospective trial of ionic vs. nonionic contrast agents in routine clinical practice. Comparison of adverse effects. AJR 152:939–944, 1989.

Drug Therapy of Asthma

62

Peter S. Creticos

The therapy of allergic respiratory tract disease is based on several important concepts (Table 62–1). The IgE-mediated allergic process is now recognized as the basis not only for the immediate phase of the asthmatic patient's clinical reaction with shortness of breath, cough, chest tightness, and wheezing on exposure to a relevant allergen but also for a late allergic phase consisting of a smoldering persistence of clinical symptoms. This late phase can evolve into exaggerated nonspecific bronchial reactivity. The key to successful therapy is the prevention or suppression of these allergic and inflammatory processes.

Asthma is a heterogeneous disease process with multiple triggering factors (Table 62–2). The precipitating factors in allergic asthma include protein components of airborne allergens such as pollens, mold spores, house dust mites, cockroach- and insect-related allergens, and animal proteins (Kaliner et al, 1987; Creticos, 1989).

The precipitating factors in allergic asthma include perennial as well as seasonal allergens (Table 62–3). Several of these allergens induce perennial allergic symptoms as a result of their persistence in the indoor environment. Dust mites feed off dried skin debris and represent a significant indoor allergen burden in the home. These insects accumulate in mattresses, box springs, feather pillows, stuffed animals, carpeting, upholstery, and clothes (especially wool materials). Although they have a rather specific growth season, which is relatively dependent on an optimal temperature (60–80°F) and humidity (55–85%), they represent a significant perennial indoor burden because of our typical airtight homes with central heating and air conditioning systems that continue to circulate the allergens through the indoor air. This material is typically 5–20 μ in diameter and composed of fecal particles and decaying body parts. Those particles <10 μm can easily reach the lower respiratory tract, inducing asthma (Creticos, 1989).

Other important indoor allergens are cockroaches and other insects. Decaying body parts, salivary protein, and emanations appear to be the important allergic materials. Insects are most prominent in geographical niches close to sea level and humid and damp locations, as well as in older dwellings. Again, the small particle size of the allergic material is easily circulated through the indoor ventilation system (Platts-Mills et al, 1986).

Animals represent an important source of allergens. Not only domesticated cats and dogs but also rodents may be introduced into the house as pets (e.g., mice or hamsters) or may reflect poor living conditions. The

---

Table 62–1 COMPONENTS OF ALLERGIC ASTHMA

Relevant allergens
Immediate-phase reaction
Late-phase reaction
Inflammation
Nonspecific bronchial reactivity

Relevant Allergens

Pollens, mold spores, and house dust mites are among the many triggering factors of asthma.

Table 62–2 TRIGGERS OF ASTHMA

Allergy
Infection
Industrial/environmental exposure
Chemical/drug ingestion
(e.g., aspirin, indomethacin, or food additives)
Exercise
Vasculitis
Idiopathic

Table 62–3 RELEVANT ALLERGENS

Pollen grains
Mold spores
Dust mites
Cockroaches/insects
Animals

---

allergen load actually involves three different protein sources — the saliva, the urine, and the dander of the animal. For instance, a cat constantly licks its fur, depositing salivary protein on the fur, which as the hair sheds, disperses this protein material onto the floor. As it dries, this 3–5 μm allergenic particle easily becomes airborne through the indoor ventilation system. Furthermore, not only is urinary protein important with cats (cat litter box) but it is also the major allergen source from laboratory animals and rodents. These nocturnal animals scurry around in their cages, adding dander and urinary protein to the air (Kaliner et al, 1987; Creticos, 1989).

Therefore, it is apparent that a significant allergen burden can easily accumulate in the bedroom of a child who is exposed nightly to allergen from a pet sleeping in his or her arms, from dust mite material in the mattress, or from urinary protein from the hamster's cage.

Whether pollens and mold spores can induce asthma is an interesting question inasmuch as pollen grains are too large to reach the lower airways (e.g., ragweed 23 μm in diameter), but a significant amount of total allergenic activity reflects not only intact pollen grains but also pollen fragments (3–7 μm in diameter) and microaerosol suspensions of specific ragweed protein (e.g., ragweed antigen E, 3–7 μm) (Agarwal et al, 1983). A single ragweed plant produces a million grains of pollen in 1 day. As these pollen grains are deposited on the ground, humidity, dew, and rainfall extract the relevant protein from the grains, and this then becomes airborne as microaerosol particles and droplets (Fig. 62–1). A similar phenomenon occurs with mold spores, with the dispersion into the air of not only mold spores but also mycelial elements and distinct soluble protein from these mold components.

If intact pollen grains (23 μm) are blown directly into the nose, they can trigger a typical allergic reaction, consisting of sneezing and mediator release. However, when these same intact pollen grains are inhaled, there is no allergic reaction because the particles are too large to reach the lower airways. But, if fragments of pollen or an extract of the pollen is inhaled into

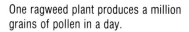

One ragweed plant produces a million grains of pollen in a day.

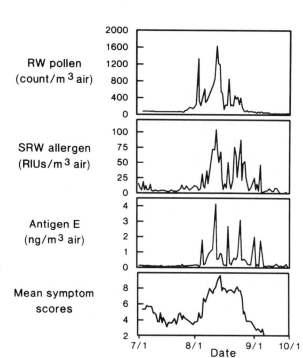

Figure 62–1

Atmospheric ragweed (RW) pollen counts, short ragweed (SRW) allergenic activity, antigen E content, and average symptom scores of SRW-sensitive individuals — results of 24-hour samples from July 1 to October 1, 1980. (RIU = radioallergosorbent test [RAST] inhibition unit.) (From Agarwal MK, Swanson MC, Reed CE, Yunginger JW: Immunochemical quantitation of airborne short ragweed, *Alternaria*, antigen E, and Alt-I allergens: A two-year prospective study. J Allergy Clin Immunol 72:40–45, 1983.)

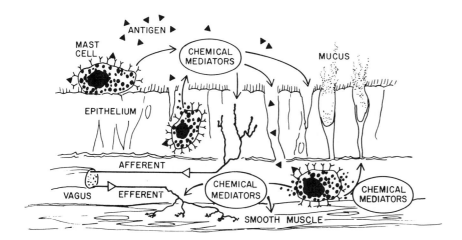

Figure 62-2

The acute response to antigen challenge: Cellular, chemical, and neural interactions. (From Schleimer RP: Mechanisms of anti-inflammatory steroid action in allergic diseases. Annu Rev Pharmacol Toxicol 25:381, 1985; as modified from Pare PO, Hogg JC: Topical Steroid Treatment for Asthma and Rhinitis, pp. 12–21. London: Bailliere Tindall, 1980. Reproduced, with permission, from the Annual Review of Pharmacology and Toxicology, Vol. 25, © 1985 by Annual Reviews, Inc.)

the lower airways, it readily produces a classic allergic asthmatic response.

The hallmark of asthma has always been reversible airway obstruction; however, asthma is also an inflammatory process involving mucosal edema, mucus production, and increased vascular permeability (Djukanovic et al, 1990). In this diathesis, the mast cell and surface basophils are the pivotal cells in the immediate phase, which is the result of the interaction of a specific allergen with IgE antibodies bound to receptors on these cell surfaces. Bridging of IgE receptors leads to modification of the receptor and results in a complex sequence of biochemical events, resulting in cellular activation, arachidonic acid metabolism, and mediator release (Fig. 62–2). The biochemical mediators so far identified include preformed mediators such as histamine, a variety of enzymes, and chemotactic factors (important in the subsequent late phase), as well as newly generated mediators of the arachidonic acid pathway—prostaglandins (PGD_2), leukotrienes (LTC_4, LTD_4, LTE_4), and platelet-activating factor (Table 62–4) (Creticos et al, 1984).

When nasal provocation is used to challenge a patient with a specific allergen, clinical symptoms such as sneezing correlate with the initial appearance of inflammatory mediators, and both the clinical symptoms and the mediator release increase in a dose-response fashion to greater pollen challenge (Fig. 62–3).

The late-phase component of the allergic reaction can be observed in both the upper and the lower airways. Typically, this late phase appears 4–10 hours after allergen exposure and results in a recrudescence of symptoms accompanied by the generation of a second wave of inflammatory mediators (Fig. 62–4). The chemotactic factors, such as eosinophil chemotactic factor of anaphylaxis, neutrophil chemotactic factor, and leukotriene B_4, are released during the immediate phase from mast cells, macrophages, and various lymphocytes, and these, in turn, are responsible for recruiting neutrophils, eosinophils, and basophils into the inflammatory site, where they "set up shop" and begin to release specific mediators, resulting in a smoldering late-phase reaction of mucosal and bronchial hyperreactivity. Bronchoalveolar lavage studies demonstrate that eosinophils represent the most prominent inflammatory cells present in this late phase, and evidence suggests that major basic protein and eosinophil cationic protein result in epithelial damage (Gleich et al, 1988; Venge et al, 1987). Furthermore,

Pathophysiology

Table 62-4 MAST CELL-DERIVED MEDIATORS

Preformed Rapidly Released Under Physiological Conditions

Histamine
Eosinophil chemotactic factors of anaphylaxis
Neutrophil chemotactic factors
Kininogenase
Arylsulfatase A
Serotonin*
Exoglycosidases* (β-hexosaminidase, β-D-galactosidase, β-glucuronidase)

Secondary or Newly Generated Mediators

Superoxide and other reactive oxygen species
Leukotrienes C_4, D_4, E_4 (previously known as SRS-A)
Prostaglandins
Monohydroxyeicosatetraenoic acids
Hydroperoxyeicosatetraenoic acids
Hydroxyheptadecatrienoic acid
Thromboxanes
Prostaglandin-generating factor of anaphylaxis
Adenosine
Bradykinin
Platelet-activating factor*

Granule-Associated Mediators

Heparin or other proteoglycans
Tryptase
Chymotryptic proteinase
Arylsulfatase B
Inflammatory factors of anaphylaxis*
Peroxidase*
Buperoxide diamulase*

From Kaliner M, Eggleston PA, Mathews KP: Primer on allergic and immunologic diseases, Chapter 3: Rhinitis and asthma. JAMA 258:2851–2873, 1987. Copyright 1987, American Medical Association.
* Demonstrated in nonhuman mast cells.

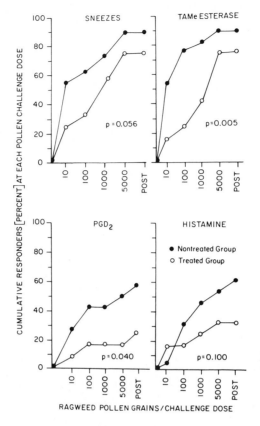

Figure 62-3

Response to pollen challenge; effects of immunotherapy. Comparison of the nontreated (n = 26) (●) and treated (n = 12) (○) groups of patients based on cumulative percentage (%) of patients sneezing or demonstrating mediator release at each respective pollen challenge dose. Statistical comparison made on the threshold dose of pollen required to provoke a significant response (employing the Mann-Whitney test). (From Creticos PS, Adkinson MF Jr, Kagey-Sobotka A, et al: Nasal challenge with ragweed pollen in hay fever patients. Reproduced from the Journal of Experimental Medicine, 1985, Vol. 76, pp. 2247–2253, by copyright permission of the Rockefeller University Press.)

Late-phase symptoms occur 4–10 hours after allergen exposure.

neutrophil products such as reactive oxidants and enzymes may also contribute to this inflammatory damage in the airways (Zweiman, 1988). The development of nonspecific bronchial reactivity in patients as they proceed through a specific allergen season has been demonstrated.

DIAGNOSTIC APPROACH

The evaluation of the patient with asthma should include a thorough patient history that focuses on environmental factors that could be important in the disease process. Present data would support an allergic evaluation for practically every patient with asthma so that appropriate environmental control measures and proper therapeutic management to suppress the inflammatory component can be employed effectively (Creticos, 1990). It is one disease in which identification of specific triggering factors and environmental manipulation can have a dramatic impact. This diagnostic approach is effectively based on a skin test evaluation, which provides accurate data on the degree of clinical sensitivity. However, radioallergosorbent testing can also provide useful data in selected individuals (Baer et al, 1988; Ellis, 1988).

Identification of triggering factors and environmental manipulation are important aspects in controlling the inflammatory response.

Treatment Strategies

In view of the pathophysiology, the management of allergic asthma has evolved into the strategy of "preventive" therapy (Table 62–5).

PATIENT EDUCATION

Patient education is an important component of preventive therapy.

Once the allergic component in a patient's disease process has been established, patient education is the first crucial step in patient care, although

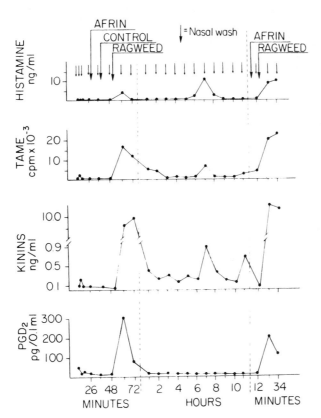

Figure 62–4

Mediators in nasal secretions during early, late, and rechallenge responses of an allergic subject to nasal challenge with ragweed extract. The *vertical dashed lines* represent changes in the time units; minutes are expressed from the beginning of the interval, and hours represent time elapsed from the first challenge. *Large arrows* indicate administration of the specified material, and small arrows indicate performance of nasal lavage. (PGD_2 = prostaglandin D_2; TAME = tosyl-L-arginine methyl ester; AFRIN = oxymetazoline.) (From Naclerio RM, Proud D, Togias AG, et al: Inflammatory mediators in late antigen-induced rhinitis. Reproduced by permission of The New England Journal of Medicine 313:65–70, 1985.)

this is an often neglected area of patient management. Asthma is a chronic disease process with periods of waxing and waning symptoms often directly related to environmental influences. Such patients have inherited the ability to become atopic and develop the propensity to respond abnormally to allergens and irritants ("twitchy airways"); nevertheless, the environmental exposure ("environmental load") determines how affected a patient will be. Thus, simple environmental measures to reduce the allergen burden in a given patient's setting can have a dramatic effect on a patient's disease state. For example, removing an offending animal from a cat-sensitive patient's home or employing strict "dust-control" measures in a home can significantly influence an asthmatic patient's condition. But even more to the point, patient educators need to work with patients so that they understand the reasoning behind the prophylactic use of medication and learn to adjust their medications on a daily basis to control minor "breakthrough flares" and prevent occurrence of a more aggressive process. By using peak flow meters, patients can interpret their daily fluctuations and be better able to make adjustments in medications, in a manner similar to that of a diabetic adjusting insulin dosage prior to a meal based on blood sugar levels. Obviously, the key to this successful management is a close interaction between patient and physician so that changes in regimen or medication can be made in a facile manner as indicated by the clinical picture (Weinstein, 1987).

PREVENTIVE PHARMACOTHERAPY

The concept of *preventive therapy* encompasses the use of specific pharmacotherapeutic agents capable not only of ablating the immediate phase of the allergic asthmatic reaction but also of suppressing the ensuing late-phase inflammatory component. Specifically, pharmacotherapy emphasizes the use of cromolyn or topical corticosteroids in the management of

Table 62–5 APPROACH TO PATIENT MANAGEMENT

Patient education
Environmental control
Preventive pharmacotherapy
Cromolyn
Topical inhaled corticosteroids
Breakthrough bronchodilator therapy
Inhaled β-adrenergic agonists
Theophylline preparations
Ipratropium
Immunotherapy

Table 62-6 INDICATIONS FOR CROMOLYN SODIUM

Seasonal allergic asthma
Perennial allergic asthma
Exercise-induced asthma
Irritant-induced asthma
Occupational asthma

Cromolyn has been used successfully to treat several types of asthma.

allergic asthma. For "breakthrough" symptoms these agents should be supplemented as necessary with bronchodilator agents (β-adrenergic agonists or theophylline).

CROMOLYN

Cromolyn sodium has been shown to be clinically effective in the prophylactic management of seasonal allergic asthma, perennial allergic asthma, animal-induced asthma, exercise-induced asthma, occupational asthma, and irritant-induced asthma (Table 62–6) (Murphy, 1989; Petty et al, 1989). The mechanism of its actions is not completely understood, but it may stabilize mast cell membranes, preventing mast cell degranulation and mediator release. It modifies both the immediate and the late phases of bronchial reactivity, as evidenced by its block of both phases of allergen-induced bronchoconstriction (Fig. 62–5) (Cockcroft and Murdock, 1987). Cromolyn can also interrupt the migration of eosinophils into the inflammatory site and decrease the number of eosinophils or eosinophil products in bronchoalveolar lavage fluid of asthmatics treated with cromolyn (Fig. 62–6). Moreover, it can abort or prevent exercise-induced asthma or reactivity to animals when given before exercise or animal exposure, pointing to as yet unelucidated mechanisms.

The key to successful therapy with cromolyn is to employ the drug prophylactically (7–10 days) prior to the anticipated allergen season or allergen exposure. An aggressive approach to treatment can usually be utilized because

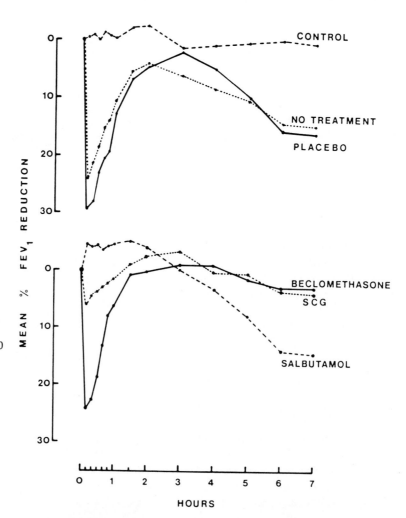

Figure 62-5

Forced expiratory volume in 1 second (FEV$_1$) in response to allergen challenge at 0 time. Cromolyn (SCG, sodium cromoglycate) pretreatment blocked early and late response to allergen challenge. Albuterol blocked only the early response, whereas beclomethasone blocked only the late response. (From Cockcroft DW, Murdock KY: Comparative effects of inhaled salbutamol, sodium cromoglycate, and beclomethasone dipropionate on allergen-induced early asthmatic responses, late asthmatic responses, and increased bronchial responsiveness to histamine. J Allergy Clin Immunol 79:734–740, 1987.)

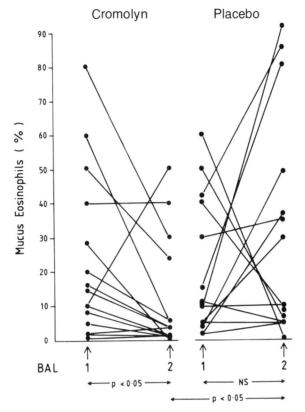

Figure 62-6

Cromolyn therapy for 4 weeks led to a significant decrease in numbers of eosinophils recovered by bronchoalveolar lavage (BAL). *Arrows* indicate BAL measurements before and after therapy. (NS = not significant.) (From Diaz P, Galleguillos FR, Gonzalez MC, et al: Bronchoalveolar lavage in asthma: The effect of disodium cromoglycate (cromolyn) on leukocyte counts, immunoglobulins, and complement. J Allergy Clin Immunol 74:41–48, 1984.)

of the safety of the drug, with an initial dose of 2 puffs four times a day from a metered-dose inhaler (Blumenthal et al, 1988). This approach requires patient compliance; with adequate patient education and compliance this early phase can be followed by subsequent tapering of the drug to a more convenient regimen of two or three doses a day if this continues to achieve sustained control (Table 62–7).

In patients already symptomatic, it is even more important to emphasize aggressive use of the drug; it may be necessary to double the dose to 2–4 puffs four times a day during the initial 1–2 weeks of therapy to obtain adequate control of symptoms. Furthermore, it may be necessary to extend treatment for 2–4 weeks before optimal efficacy is noted. Once satisfactory control is achieved, a tapering of the drug to a dose still clinically effective should be attempted in order to maintain patient compliance.

Studies employing the metered-dose inhaler have consistently shown improvements in overall asthma scores, cough, nighttime asthma, peak expiratory flow rate (PEFR) readings, pulmonary function tests (forced expiratory volume in 1 second, FEV_1), forced vital capacity (FVC), and use of concomitant medications (Murphy, 1989; Petty et al, 1989). Comparative studies have shown cromolyn to be as efficacious as the bronchodilating agents in the management of asthma. In comparison with theophylline, both drugs demonstrate a reduction in clinical symptoms (cough, tightness, wheeze, acute asthma), nocturnal symptoms, missed school days, spirometric measurements (FEV, FVC, forced expiratory flow 25–75%, PEFR), and ancillary β-adrenergic agonist usage. The combination of the two drugs has been shown to be beneficial. Furthermore, the low frequency of adverse effects associated with cromolyn represents a significant advantage. However, studies suggest that adverse effects on learning and behavior may be associated with theophylline therapy (Rachelefsky et al, 1986; Furukawa et al, 1984). *Cromolyn has demonstrated better asthma control than*

Table 62-7 CROMOLYN SODIUM

Prophylactic Therapy

Start 5–10 days prior to seasonal allergen exposure

2 puffs q.i.d.* by metered dose inhaler/spacer

Symptomatic Therapy

2–4 puffs q.i.d.* by metered-dose inhaler/spacer to bring symptoms under control

Once symptoms stabilized (1–3 weeks) then "back off" to a more patient-compliant dosage of two to four times a day

* q.i.d. = four times a day.

The combination of cromolyn and a β_2-adrenergic agonist provides better symptom control than the use of cromolyn alone.

a β₂-adrenergic agonist alone, although the combination of the two provides the best symptom control (Shapiro et al, 1986).

The use of a spacer with an inhaler can further improve drug delivery and clinical response in certain patients, and this should be the first manipulation attempted in patients not demonstrating satisfactory results before adding an additional agent. The spacer can be particularly helpful in patients complaining of cough with cromolyn powder or the metered-dose inhaler. Likewise, the nebulized formulation of cromolyn can be employed effectively in patients unable to use the metered-dose inhaler or to maintain therapeutic levels when a metered-dose inhaler cannot be continued (e.g., in young children; in patients with severe upper airway inflammation such as that caused by bronchitis or respiratory infection, which makes an aerosol intolerable; in patients with intolerance to the aerosol propellent or spinhaler powder) (Shapiro et al, 1986).

In summary, cromolyn can have a profound influence in 60–75% of patients with mild to moderate asthma. It should be viewed as first-line therapy in the prophylaxis and suppression of allergen-induced bronchospasm but is not useful for alleviation of the acute attack. Furthermore, cromolyn may be useful in preventing exercise-induced asthma and blocking irritant/nonallergic asthma triggers in certain patients (Murphy, 1989; Petty et al, 1989).

TOPICAL STEROIDS

Topical inhaled steroid preparations remain the "gold standard" for suppressing IgE-mediated inflammation. Corticosteroids may act through several different mechanisms including

- inhibition of release of mediators;
- inhibition of synthesis of mediators or arachidonic acid metabolites;
- inhibition of leukocyte migration;
- restoration of β-adrenergic agonist receptor responsiveness or influences on cholinergic pathways (Fig. 62–7).

The same concepts previously discussed with cromolyn are also important for success with corticosteroid therapy. Prophylactic use of topical corticosteroids provides the best chance to prevent the development of the inflammation, bronchial hyperresponsiveness, and nonspecific bronchial reactivity. Topical steroids need to be administered prophylactically for approximately 7 days prior to allergen exposure to be therapeutically efficacious. Studies of rhinitis suggest that topical (not systemic) steroids may prevent the immediate as well as the late components of bronchial reactivity to allergen challenge (Pipkorn et al, 1987).

To be effective, topical steroids must be administered in a dose adequate to bring symptoms under control and then tapered as tolerated to the lowest effective dose to maintain symptom control during the maintenance phase of therapy (Table 62–8). Studies suggest that doses of 800–1500 μg/day of beclomethasone are far superior to the previously suggested lower doses of 300–400 μg/day in bringing asthma symptoms under control (Baer et al, 1988). Other topical corticosteroid drugs available include triamcinolone and flunisolide (see Chapter 43).

As with cromolyn, the key to successful therapy with topical steroids is patient compliance. Thus, the dosing frequency and the number of doses required to achieve therapeutic efficacy become important factors. Some studies suggest that twice-a-day dosing of beclomethasone (Pauwels et al, 1985; Baker et al, 1988) may be as effective as four-times-a-day dosing (Joad et al, 1987; Creticos and Norman, 1987). Certainly, this would im-

Topical steroids should be administered 7 days prior to allergen exposure to achieve maximal effectiveness.

Pathologic Observation	Effect of Steroids
1. Increased mast cell numbers	Reduce mast cell numbers
2. Leukocyte infiltrate with elevated eosinophil MBP in sputum	Reduce leukocyte numbers, MBP
3. Decreased β adrenergic tone	Restore β adrenergic responses
4. Epithelial shedding	Protect epithelium
5. Bronchial hyperreactivity	Reduce airway reactivity
6. Increased mucous secretion	Reduce mucous secretion
7. Bronchial edema (increased edema mediators)	Decrease vascular permeability (decrease mediators)

Figure 62–7

Diagram of a small airway and summary of pathologic observations and beneficial effects of glucocorticoids in asthma. (MBP = major basic protein.) (This figure has been reproduced with the permission of Hans Huber Publishers, 14 Bruce Park Avenue, Toronto, Ontario M4P 2S3, from the article by R. P. Schleimer: Mechanisms underlying the beneficial effects of glucocorticosteroids in asthma, published in Allergy and Clinical Immunology News, Volume 2, issue 2, 1990. Copyright © 1990 by Hans Huber Publishers.)

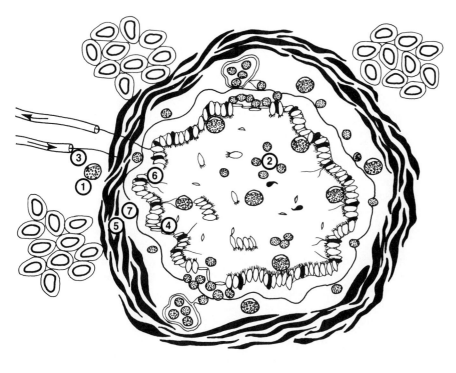

prove patient compliance. However, therapy should be individualized based on the patient's appreciation of symptom control, daily PEFR readings, and periodic spirometry measurements.

Unfortunately, at the present time it requires numerous puffs (16–40 puffs) to achieve a dose of 800–1500 μg of beclomethasone. It is anticipated that delivery systems capable of delivering larger doses per actuation (250 μg versus 42 μg), which are available in Europe and Canada, will soon be commercially available in the United States.

The question of the safety of topical corticosteroids becomes a relevant issue, especially if higher-dose therapy is advocated. Systemic side effects of adrenal axis suppression, growth retardation, osteoporosis, and cataracts

Table 62–8   STEROIDS FOR INHALATION

Drug	Usual Dosage	Total Dose
Beclomethasone (Beclovent/Vanceril, 42 μg/puff)	2 puffs every 6 hours (84 μg q.i.d.)	336 μg/day
Flunisolide (Aerobid, 250 μg/puff)	2 puffs every 12 hours (500 μg b.i.d.)	1000 μg/day
Triamcinolone (Azmacort, 200 μg/puff)	2 puffs every 6 hours (400 μg q.i.d.)	1600 μg/day

Table 62–9   SYSTEMIC SIDE EFFECTS OF CORTICOSTEROIDS*

	Adrenal Suppression	Growth Retardation	Osteoporosis	Cataracts	Hematologic Changes	Weight Gain	Hypertension
Daily systemic steroids	++	+++	+++	+++	+	+++	++
Alternate-day systemic steroids	+	++	++	++	+	++	++
Inhaled steroids	±†	±	+‡	±	+	0	0

From König P: Inhaled Corticosteroids—their present and future role in the management of asthma. J Allergy Clin Immunol 82:297–306, 1988.
* 0 = None; ± = contradictory data; + = statistically significant, but not clinically important; ++ = clinically relevant; +++ = clinically serious.
† Probably only at doses of >500 μg in children and >1000 μg in adults.
‡ Only one study published.

have all been reported with daily oral prednisone and alternate-day oral prednisone (Table 62–9; see Chapter 43). The relevant question is how likely are these effects to occur with topical inhaled therapy? Adrenal axis suppression is not consistently seen in adults until a maintenance dose of 1600 μg/day is employed. Studies in children suggest the critical dose is approximately 500–800 μg/day.

More subtle markers such as effects on growth or osteoporosis require long-term studies. Several 1- to 5-year studies in children have not shown an effect on growth with inhaled doses of up to 800 μg of beclomethasone. However, in a study of rheumatoid arthritis, a reduction in Ca^{2+} (8.8%) was seen in patients on inhaled beclomethasone 400 μg/day (Reid et al, 1986).

A few reported cases of posterior, subcapsular cataracts have been reported in patients on inhaled steroids, but this risk appears to be minimal compared with the 20%–30% incidence in patients on oral corticosteroids (see Table 62–9).

Local side effects due to topical steroid therapy include oral candidiasis (13% of patients) and hoarseness/dysphonia (5–50%). Both are minimized by the use of a spacer device in the inhaler.

In summary, topical steroid therapy can be dramatically successful in the treatment of mild to severe asthma. Our approach has been to employ cromolyn first, based on its safety and efficacy, and then in a logical step-wise fashion to proceed to topical steroid therapy early in the course of treatment in an unresponsive asthmatic patient in an attempt to either prevent or suppress the underlying inflammatory process. Obviously, the risks versus benefits need to be weighed in the use of inhaled steroid therapy, but it is apparent that aggressive high-dose therapy is significantly safer than either oral daily or alternate-day therapy. Furthermore, the therapeutic efficacy of inhaled corticosteroids appears to be superior to that of oral steroids (Siegel, 1985; Toogood et al, 1984).

BRONCHODILATOR THERAPY

Preventive therapy is the desirable approach to management of asthma; however, asthmatic symptoms can occur acutely as "breakthrough asthmatic" symptoms in those being treated. Bronchodilator agents are important adjunctive medications for control of these breakthrough asthmatic symptoms.

β-Adrenergic Agonist Therapy

Sympathomimetic bronchodilators have become a mainstay in the therapeutic approach in the treatment of asthma. Table 62–10 lists the various

Table 62–10 β-ADRENERGIC AGONISTS FOR INHALATION

Drug*†	Selectivity‡	Onset of Action (Minutes)	Peak Action (Minutes)	Duration (Hours)
Catecholamines				
Epinephrine (Primatene, 0.2 mg/p)	$\alpha_1 \beta_1 \beta_2$	2–7	15–20	0.5
Isoproterenol (Isuprel, 0.125 mg/p)	$\beta_1 \beta_2$	2–5	5	1.5–2
Isoetharine (Bronkometer, 0.34 mg/p)	β_2	2–5	15	1.5–2
Noncatecholamines				
Bitolterol (Tornalate, 0.37 mg/p)	β_2+	3–5	30–60	4–8
Metaproterenol (Alupent, 0.65 mg/p)	β_2++	5–10	120–180	3–4
Terbutaline (Brethaire, 0.25 mg/p)	β_2+++	5–10	90–120	3–4
Albuterol (Proventil/Ventolin, 0.09 mg/p)	β_2+++	5–15	60–90	4–6
Pirbuterol (Maxair, 0.2 mg/p)	β_2+++	3–5	30–60	4–6

* p = puff.
† Usual doses are 1–2 p every 4–6 hours; bitolterol, 2–3 p every 6–8 hours; metaproterenol, 2–3 p every 4 hours.
‡ + = low selectivity; ++ = moderate selectivity; +++ = high selectivity.

catecholamine and noncatecholamine compounds that are available. Improved B$_2$ selectivity as well as increased duration of action is seen with the majority of noncatecholamines (see Chapter 14).

Therapeutic effects of β-adrenergic agonist therapy include (1) bronchodilation as a result of actuation of the cell membrane's adenylcyclase enzyme, which converts adenosine triphosphate to cyclic adenosine monophosphate with its inherent ability to relax smooth muscle, (2) increased ciliary movement, which should improve secretion clearance, and (3) effects on the mast cell to decrease mediator release (Nelson, 1989). Challenge studies demonstrate that β-adrenergic agonists can effectively ablate the immediate asthmatic (bronchospastic) response but have no effect on the late-phase asthmatic response (see Fig. 62–5).

The aerosol adrenergic agonists are potent bronchodilators that can be used alone for the treatment of mild, intermittent asthma or to prevent or reverse exercise-induced asthma (Newhouse and Dolovich, 1986). They demonstrate bronchodilatory properties over a wide range of doses, up to 720 µg of albuterol (8 puffs). Furthermore, they effect a rapid reversal of acute asthmatic symptoms within minutes (Nelson, 1989).

In general, β-adrenergic agonists provide better bronchodilatation than that of theophylline products in both acute and chronic therapy. Furthermore, the addition of aminophylline to maximal-dose inhaled β-sympathomimetic therapy does not improve the bronchodilator response.

However, in chronic therapy, receptor subsensitivity can develop to β-adrenergic agonist therapy. This tolerance can occur with both oral and inhaled formulations and is currently managed by a short course of oral prednisone that appears to restore β-receptor sensitivity. In contrast, subsensitivity or tachyphylaxis does not occur with chronic theophylline therapy (Nelson, 1989).

Aerosol adrenergic agonists effect a rapid reversal of acute asthmatic symptoms.

Proper administration of the aerosol preparation is crucial to its success.

The proper method of administration of the aerosol is critical. Careful demonstration of inhaler technique by the physician, nurse, or patient educator is mandatory and often requires repeated reinforcement. Several techniques are satisfactory, but most investigators would suggest discharging the inhaler while it is about 1–1½ inches away from the open mouth. The patient should then take a slow, deep inspiration (from functional residual capacity to total lung capacity), and then hold the breath for 10 seconds (Newhouse and Dolovich, 1986). Utilizing this technique improves medication deposition and can result in twice as much medication (13–20%) reaching the lower respiratory tract. This can be further improved by employing a spacer for optimal aerosol delivery (20–40% deposition). Typically, 2–3 minutes should lapse between the first and the second puffs, such that the maximal bronchodilating effect of the first puff allows better penetration of the second puff. A dry powder formulation of albuterol has also been made available and may provide an advantage for patients prone to irritant effects of a freon-metered device or who cannot use the pressurized aerosol properly. However, an irritant cough reflex can be associated with the powder.

An important point to emphasize is that if the patient is apparently not responding to a β-adrenergic agonist, the key is to employ proper techniques to ensure adequate delivery of the medication before adding a second or third drug for control.

In certain instances, nebulization of a β-adrenergic agonist solution can be an effective means of delivering a drug to the lower airways. This can be particularly useful in the face of a viral infection in which the irritation of the airways may preclude the frequent use of an aerosol inhaler. In this manner, the β-adrenergic agonist as well as cromolyn can be easily delivered and not cause interruption or loss of the long-term therapeutic benefits of cromolyn.

Oral β-adrenergic agonist preparations are available, but inhalation administration delivers more of the active drug directly to the mucosal surface and at the same time minimizes side effects. Oral therapy may be useful in situations in which intense irritation prohibits the facile use of an inhaled agent. Side effects associated with β-adrenergic agonist therapy include tremor and, with higher doses of even the selective β_2 agents, tachycardia or palpitations (see Chapter 14).

Clinical studies have conclusively demonstrated the utility of selective β_2 sympathomimetic therapy in the treatment of intermittent asthma, seasonal or perennial allergic asthma, and exercise-induced asthma. These agents are the logical adjunctive medications to employ in combination with inhaled cromolyn or inhaled corticosteroids in the management of chronic asthma.

ANTICHOLINERGIC AGENTS

The parasympathetic nervous system appears to play a prominent role in the bronchoconstriction pathway in human airways. Parasympathetic activity may be particularly relevant in cold air–induced asthma, SO_2–induced asthma, and histamine-induced asthma; this may reflect the interplay between neural mechanisms and inflammatory mediators or simply reflex cholinergic bronchoconstriction.

Ipratropium is an anticholinergic agent used to treat asthma.

Ipratropium can reduce the cholinergic hyperreactivity present in many patients with chronic bronchitis, emphysema, and asthma. This agent can be useful alone or, more typically, in combination with a selective β_2 sympathomimetic, with which a synergistic effect may be produced

(Newhouse and Dolovich, 1986). It is administered as a metered-dose inhalation of 2 puffs every 6 hours.

THEOPHYLLINE

Theophylline therapy has been a cornerstone of asthma therapy through the years. As with β-adrenergic sympathomimetic agents, theophylline appears to exert its primary influence through relaxation of smooth muscle of the bronchial tree. It does this through its inhibition of the breakdown enzyme phosphodiesterase with a resultant increase in cAMP concentrations, which results in smooth muscle cell relaxation (Kaliner et al, 1987; Nelson, 1989).

The current approach to the treatment of asthma involves the aggressive use of inhaled preventive therapeutic agents. As a result, theophylline therapy is now viewed as an adjunctive, albeit important, therapeutic agent in those asthmatic patients whose condition is not easily controlled by the use of inhaled cromolyn or inhaled corticosteroids supplemented by an inhaled β_2-selective sympathomimetic agent. This current strategy reflects not only the appreciated superior anti-inflammatory properties of these "preventive" inhaled agents but also the toxic effects associated with theophylline therapy. In addition to producing bronchodilatation, theophylline improves diaphragmatic excursion and ciliary transport and stabilizes the mast cell. This last effect is particularly important because it relates to theophylline's anti-inflammatory properties that are manifested by inhibition of mediator release from the mast cell with a reduction in the accompanying mediator-induced vascular permeability, vasodilatation, and mucus production (Kaliner et al, 1987; Nelson, 1989; Persson, 1988). In addition, theophylline attenuates the late-phase asthmatic response to allergen challenge (Pauwels et al, 1985).

To be most effective, theophylline must be used judiciously with careful attention paid to blood level monitoring. Typically, a serum theophylline concentration of 10–20 μg/ml correlates with optimal effectiveness. As dosage is increased, side effects become more problematic and toxicity may present. Appetite loss, nausea, vomiting, headache, palpitations, tachycardia, nervousness, insomnia, anxiety, and seizures may be manifestations of toxicity in both adults and children. Overt overdoses can result in arrhythmias, coma, or death. Table 62–11 lists some of the many factors that can affect the serum theophylline clearance and have an impact on the blood level (Kaliner et al, 1987). Caffeine, a closely related xanthine, shares many of the pharmacological properties of theophylline, including bronchodilatation; however, it is not therapeutically useful by itself.

In view of the very small margin between therapeutic effects and toxicity, individualization of dose is mandatory with theophylline therapy. The use of sustained-release long-acting (every 12 hours) preparations has improved this aspect of care because of the more consistent theophylline-release characteristics, which provide more constant plasma concentration with less-marked peak-trough variation. In this regard, it is important to not switch among various preparations as significant differences in serum blood levels may result because of the differences in absorption characteristics between preparations from different manufacturers (Kaliner et al, 1987; Baker et al, 1988).

In management of combinations, it is better to "push" the dose of the preventive therapeutic agent (cromolyn, topical corticosteroids) than to further increase the theophylline dosage. The newer once-a-day sustained-release products may be the most useful in the subset of asthmatics with nocturnal symptoms who otherwise find it difficult to sleep through

Xanthine

Caffeine

Theophylline

Caffeine is the most widely known xanthine agent.

Table 62–11 FACTORS AFFECTING THEOPHYLLINE BLOOD LEVELS

Conditions Increasing Theophylline Blood Levels

Older age (> 50 years)
Obesity
Liver disease
Congestive heart failure
Chronic obstructive pulmonary disease
Acute viral infections
High-carbohydrate, low-protein diet
Influenza A vaccine
Drug use
    Troleandomycin
    Erythromycin preparations
    Allopurinol
    Cimetidine
    Propranolol hydrochloride

Conditions Decreasing Theophylline Blood Levels

Young age (1–16 years)
Cigarette smoking
Eating charcoal-broiled meat
Low-carbohydrate, high-protein diet
Drug use
    Phenobarbital
    Phenytoins
    Isoproterenol hydrochloride

From Kaliner M, Eggleston PA, Mathews KP: Primer on allergic and immunologic diseases, Chapter 3: Rhinitis and asthma. JAMA 258:2851–2873, 1987. Copyright 1987, American Medical Association.

Figure 62–8

Immunotherapy in cat-induced asthma: Bronchial inhalation challenge with cat pelt extract. Provocative dose in breath units that resulted in a 20% drop in forced expiratory volume in 1 second ($PD_{20} - FEV_{1.0}$) is indicated on vertical axis (log scale). Mean $PD_{20} - FEV_{1.0}$ for placebo subjects was 294 and 56 breath units before and after cat pelt immunotherapy, respectively. This was not a significant change. Mean $PD_{20} - FEV_{1.0}$ for subjects who received cat pelt extract was 51 and 2354 breath units before and after therapy ($p < 0.01$). (From Taylor WW, Ohman JL Jr, Lowell FC: Immunotherapy in cat-induced asthma. Double-blind trial with evaluation of bronchial responses to cat allergen and histamine. J Allergy Clin Immunol 61:283, 1978.)

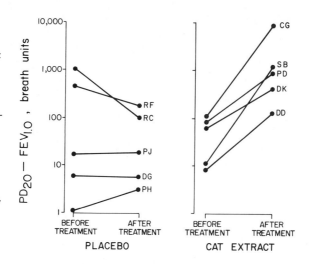

Immunotherapy can result in a life-saving form of treatment in sting-allergic patients.

the night because of the short duration of activity of other sympathomimetic agents (Joad et al, 1987).

IMMUNOTHERAPY

When incremental doses of a specific allergenic extract known to produce allergic symptoms in an individual patient on natural exposure are administered over a certain time period, that patient's tolerance to these allergens can be expected to increase as reflected by significantly reduced or ameliorated symptoms with subsequent natural exposure. Numerous studies with pollens (weeds, grasses, trees), animal allergens, and dust mites support the efficacy of immunotherapy in treating allergic rhinitis (Creticos, 1989; Creticos and Norman, 1987). In insect-sting–allergic patients, specific venom immunotherapy (yellow jacket, hornet, wasp, honeybee) can result in a life-saving form of preventive therapy. However, only a few, well-controlled studies evaluating the role of immunotherapy in treating patients with allergic asthma have been carried out.

Improvements in subjective clinical response, bronchial hyperactivity, or late phase of bronchial reactivity have been reported with dust extract, dust mite, or cat pelt immunotherapy (Fig. 62–8). At present, two major immunotherapy studies are under way in children and in adults, attempting to measure subjective as well as objective parameters to further elucidate the role of immunotherapy in asthma. In the childhood study, multiple allergen therapy is being employed, whereas in the adult study, specific immunotherapy to either dust mites or ragweed is being investigated. In the adult immunotherapy study, the patients have been thoroughly characterized by clinical history, symptom diary scores through the respective season, and bronchial challenge to a specific antigen (ragweed or dust mite) as well as a nonspecific substance (methacholine); they were then randomized to specific immunotherapy. After treatment for 2–3 years, repeat immunological measurements, bronchial challenges, and clinical assessments should provide further information regarding the efficacy of immunotherapy.

Summary

In patients with only occasional episodes of bronchospasm or those with exercise-induced asthma, a simple aerosolized selective β_2-adrenergic agonist is the drug of choice. However, in those patients who have practically daily symptoms or who need medications on a daily or practically daily basis, then therapy with a preventive therapeutic agent such as inhaled cromolyn or an inhaled topical corticosteroid is the therapy of choice; the objective of such therapy is the suppression of the inflammatory process that would otherwise culminate in a clinical picture of smoldering chronic asthma. In many patients, adjunctive therapy with β_2-adrenergic agents, anticholinergic agents, or theophylline compounds may be necessary in order to control "breakthrough" symptoms. A trial of immunotherapy is indicated for those allergic asthmatic patients who demonstrate a clinically relevant allergic component, and who have had an inadequate response to pharmacotherapy, troublesome side effects associated with medical therapy, or persistent disease.

General References

Agarwal MK, Swanson MC, Reed CE, Yunginger JW: Immunochemical quantitation of airborne short ragweed, *Alternaria* antigen E, and Alt-1 allergens: A two-year prospective study. J Allergy Clin Immunol 72:40–45, 1983.

Baer H, Anderson MC, Turkeltaub PC: Allergenic extracts. *In* Middleton, E Jr, Ellis EF, Adkinson NF, Yunginger J (eds): Allergy Principles and Practice, 3rd ed, Vol 1, 373–401. St. Louis: CV Mosby Co, 1988.

Baker JR, Moessner H, Gonzales U, et al: Clinical relevance of the substitution of different brands of sustained-release theophylline. J Allergy Clin Immunol 81:664–673, 1988.

Barnes PJ: A new approach to the treatment of asthma. N Engl J Med 321:1517–1526, 1989.

Benowitz NL: Clinical pharmacology of caffeine. Annu Rev Med 41:277–288, 1991.

Blumenthal R, Selcow J, Spector S, et al: A multicenter evaluation of the clinical benefits of cromolyn sodium aerosol by metered-dose inhaler in the treatment of asthma. J Allergy Clin Immunol 81:681–687, 1988.

Cockcroft DW: The bronchial late response in the pathogenesis of asthma and its modulation by therapy. Ann Allergy 55:857, 1985.

Cockcroft DW, Murdock KY: Comparative effects of inhaled salbutamol, sodium cromoglycate, and beclomethasone dipropionate on allergen-induced early asthmatic responses, late asthmatic responses, and increased bronchial responsiveness to histamine. J Allergy Clin Immunol 79:734–740, 1987.

Creticos PS: The clinical implications of the inflammatory component of allergic respiratory tract disease: A case study. ACI News 2:50–53, 1990.

Creticos PS: Immunotherapy in asthma. J Allergy Clin Immunol 83:554–562, 1989.

Creticos PS, Adkinson NF Jr, Kagey-Sobotka A, et al: Nasal challenge with ragweed pollen in hay fever patients. J Clin Invest 76:2247–2253, 1985.

Creticos PS, Marsh DG, Adkinson NF Jr, et al: Demonstration of peptide-leukotriene release following nasal antigen challenge in vivo. N Engl J Med 310:1626–1630, 1984.

Creticos PS, Norman PS: Immunotherapy with allergens. JAMA 258:2874–2880, 1987.

Djukanovic R, Roche WR, Wilson JW, et al: State of the art—mucosal inflammation in asthma. Am Rev Respir Dis 142:434–457, 1990.

Ellis EF: Asthma in infancy and childhood. *In* Middleton, E Jr, Ellis EF, Adkinson NF, Yunginger J (eds): Allergy Principles and Practice, 3rd ed, Vol 2, 1037–1062. St. Louis: CV Mosby Co, 1988.

Furukawa CT, Shapiro GG, Duttamel T, et al: Learning and behavioral problems associated with theophylline therapy. (Letter) Lancet 1:621, 1984.

Gleich GJ, Flavahan NA, Fujisawa T, et al: The eosinophil as a mediator of damage to respiratory epithelium: A model for bronchial hyperreactivity. J Allergy Clin Immunol 81:776–781, 1988.

Joad JP, Ahrens RC, Lindgren SD, et al: Relative efficacy of maintenance therapy with theophylline, inhaled albuterol and the combination, for chronic asthma. J Allergy Clin Immunol 79:78–85, 1987.

Kaliner M, Eggleston PA, Mathews KP: Primer on allergic and immunologic diseases; Chapter 3: Rhinitis and asthma. JAMA 258:2851–2873, 1987.

Konig P: Inhaled corticosteroids — Their present and future role in the management of asthma. J Allergy Clin Immunol 82:297–306, 1988.

Murphy S: The role of cromolyn sodium in the treatment of asthma. J Respir Dis (Suppl):S66–S70, 1989.

Naclerio RM, Proud D, Togias AG, et al: Inflammatory mediators in late antigen-induced rhinitis. N Engl J Med 313:65–70, 1985.

Nelson HS: Bronchodilator therapy for reversible obstructive airway disease. J Respir Dis (Suppl):S58–S65, 1989.

Newhouse MT, Dolovich MB: Control of asthma by aerosols. N Engl J Med 315:870–874, 1986.

Pauwels R, Van Renterghem D, Van Der Straeten M, et al: The effect of theophylline and enprofylline on allergen-induced bronchoconstriction. J Allergy Clin Immunol 76:583–590, 1985.

Persson CGA: Xanthines as airway inflammatory drugs. J Allergy Clin Immunol 81:615–617, 1988.

Petty TL, Rollins DR, Christopher K, et al: Cromolyn sodium is effective in adult chronic asthmatics. Am Rev Respir Dis 139:694–701, 1989.

Pipkorn U, Proud D, Lichtenstein LM, et al: Inhibition of mediator release in allergic rhinitis by pretreatment with glucocorticosteroids. N Engl J Med 316:1506–1510, 1987.

Platts-Mills TAE, Heymann PW, Chapman MD, et al: Immunologic triggers in asthma. The Proceedings of the XII International Congress of Allergology and Clinical Immunology. July 1986:214–220, 1986.

Rachelefsky GS, Wo J, Adelson J, et al: Behavior abnormalities and poor school performance due to oral theophylline use. Pediatrics 78:1133–1138, 1986.

Reid DM, Nicoll JJ, Smith MA, et al: Corticosteroids and bone mass in asthma: Comparisons with rheumatoid arthritis and polymyalgia rheumatica. Br Med J 293:1463–1465, 1986.

Schleimer RP: Mechanisms underlying the beneficial effects of glucocorticosteroids in asthma. ACI News 2:54–57, 1990.

Shapiro G, Furukawa C, Pierson W, et al: Double-blind crossover study of nebulized cromolyn, terbutaline and the combination in asthmatic children. [Abstract] J Allergy Clin Immunol 77:184, 1986.

Siegel SC: Corticosteroid agents: Overview of corticosteroid therapy. J Allergy Clin Immunol 76:312–320, 1985.

Toogood JH, Jennings B, Baskerville J, Lefcoe NM: Personal observations on the use of inhaled corticosteroid drugs for chronic asthma. Eur J Respir Dis 65:321–338, 1984.

Venge P, Hakansson L, Peterson CGB: Eosinophil activation in allergic disease. Int Arch Allergy Appl Immunol 82:333–337, 1987.

Weinstein AM: Asthma: The Complete Guide to Self-Management of Asthma and Allergies for Patients and Their Families. New York: McGraw-Hill Book Co, 1987.

Zweiman B: Mediator of allergic inflammation in the skin. Clin Allergy 18:419–433, 1988.

63

Vitamins As Therapeutic Agents

Peter J. Horvath

The science and research of vitamins is relatively new, but the therapeutic use of foods that are good sources of certain vitamins is ancient. Vitamins are organic compounds that cannot be synthesized by an organism and are required for proper functioning of the body. Humans have specific vitamin requirements; most of these are also required by all other mammals. Some are unique to only a few animals, such as ascorbic acid. Humans have a wide range of individual requirements that change with age, state of health, types of activity, and many other factors. The wide range in the present-day recommendations points to this fact. The requirements listed in Table 63–1 were developed to provide the vast majority of people with the amounts required to meet certain criteria. These criteria and objectives are to maintain adequate stores of the vitamins, to prevent the occurrence of disease with periods of stress or low intake, to maintain maximal stores without toxicity, or to provide enough of a vitamin to maintain growth and prevent the occurrence of specific diseases. The variability in human biochemistry must be kept in mind when considering the effectiveness of vitamin treatments.

The vitamins have been historically and biochemically divided by their solubility — fat- and water-soluble. This division is still useful, but it is not as clear-cut as in the past with the advent of water-soluble forms of the classic fat-soluble vitamins. For uniformity, this chapter is divided by solubility.

VITAMIN A, THE RETINOIDS AND CAROTENOIDS

There are ancient historical records in China and Egypt of the use of foods rich in vitamin A or its precursors to cure night blindness. It was not until 1909 that Strep showed that a fat-soluble material in egg yolk was essential for life. In 1913 two groups reported on a similar compound: McCollum and Davis found a fat-soluble factor in butter/egg yolk that was necessary for rat growth; Osborn and Mendel showed butter and cod liver oil promoted growth and cured an "eye disease." It was not until the 1930s that the structure of β retinol and associated compounds were determined.

Vitamin A is actually a group of retinoids and carotenoids. One of the key features of the vitamin A group is the presence of conjugated double bonds, making them easily oxidized, isomerized, and polymerized in light and acid in dilute concentrations, with the retinoids being more stable than carotenoids. They are fairly stable as crystals and as the acyl ester.

There are over 400 naturally occurring carotenoids, making them the most prevalent pigment in nature. They are the colored compounds in

Vitamin deficiencies are ancient diseases with many folk medicines.

Fat-Soluble Vitamins

1067

Table 63-1 FOOD AND NUTRITION BOARD, NATIONAL ACADEMY OF SCIENCES—NATIONAL RESEARCH COUNCIL RECOMMENDED DIETARY ALLOWANCES*
(Designed for the maintenance of good nutrition of practically all healthy people in the United States)

Category or Condition	Age (Years)	Weight (kg)	Weight (lb)	Height (cm)	Height (in)	Protein (g)	Fat-Soluble Vitamins — Vitamin A (μg RE)‡	Vitamin D (μg)§	Vitamin E (mg α-TE)‖	Vitamin K (μg)	Water-Soluble Vitamins — Vitamin C (mg)	Thiamin (mg)	Riboflavin (mg)	Niacin (mg NE)¶	Vitamin B6 (mg)	Folate (μg)	Vitamin B12 (μg)	Minerals — Calcium (mg)	Phosphorus (mg)	Magnesium (mg)	Iron (mg)	Zinc (mg)	Iodine (μg)	Selenium (μg)
Infants	0.0-0.5	6	13	60	24	13	375	7.5	3	5	30	0.3	0.4	5	0.3	25	0.3	400	300	40	6	5	40	10
	0.5-1.0	9	20	71	28	14	375	10	4	10	35	0.4	0.5	6	0.6	35	0.5	600	500	60	10	5	50	15
Children	1-3	13	29	90	35	16	400	10	6	15	40	0.7	0.8	9	1.0	50	0.7	800	800	80	10	10	70	20
	4-6	20	44	112	44	24	500	10	7	20	45	0.9	1.1	12	1.1	75	1.0	800	800	120	10	10	90	20
	7-10	28	62	132	52	28	700	10	7	30	45	1.0	1.2	13	1.4	100	1.4	800	800	170	10	10	120	30
Males	11-14	45	99	157	62	45	1000	10	10	45	50	1.3	1.5	17	1.7	150	2.0	1200	1200	270	12	15	150	40
	15-18	66	145	176	69	59	1000	10	10	65	60	1.5	1.8	20	2.0	200	2.0	1200	1200	400	12	15	150	50
	19-24	72	160	177	70	58	1000	10	10	70	60	1.5	1.7	19	2.0	200	2.0	1200	1200	350	10	15	150	70
	25-50	79	174	176	70	63	1000	5	10	80	60	1.5	1.7	19	2.0	200	2.0	800	800	350	10	15	150	70
	51+	77	170	173	68	63	1000	5	10	80	60	1.2	1.4	15	2.0	200	2.0	800	800	350	10	15	150	70
Females	11-14	46	101	157	62	46	800	10	8	45	50	1.1	1.3	15	1.4	150	2.0	1200	1200	280	15	12	150	45
	15-18	55	120	163	64	44	800	10	8	55	60	1.1	1.3	15	1.5	180	2.0	1200	1200	300	15	12	150	50
	19-24	58	128	164	65	46	800	10	8	60	60	1.1	1.3	15	1.6	180	2.0	1200	1200	280	15	12	150	55
	25-50	63	138	163	64	50	800	5	8	65	60	1.0	1.2	15	1.6	180	2.0	800	800	280	15	12	150	55
	51+	65	143	160	63	50	800	5	8	65	60	1.0	1.2	13	1.6	180	2.0	800	800	280	10	12	150	55
Pregnant						60	800	10	10	65	70	1.5	1.6	17	2.2	400	2.2	1200	1200	320	30	15	175	65
Lactating	1st 6 months					65	1300	10	12	65	95	1.6	1.8	20	2.1	280	2.6	1200	1200	355	15	19	200	75
	2nd 6 months					62	1200	10	11	65	90	1.6	1.7	20	2.1	260	2.6	1200	1200	340	15	16	200	75

From Food and Nutrition Board: Recommended Dietary Allowances. 10th ed. Washington, DC: National Academy of Sciences, National Research Council, 1989.

* The allowances, expressed as average daily intakes over time, are intended to provide for individual variations among most normal persons as they live in the United States under usual environmental stresses. Diets should be based on a variety of common foods in order to provide other nutrients for which human requirements have been less well defined. See text for detailed discussion of allowances and of nutrients not tabulated.

† Weights and heights of Reference Adults are actual medians for the U.S. population of the designated age, as reported by National Health and Nutrition Survey (NHANES) II. The median weights and heights of those under 19 years of age were taken from Hamill et al (1979) (see pp. 16-17). The use of these figures does not imply that the height-to-weight ratios are ideal.

‡ Retinol equivalents. 1 retinol equivalent = μg retinol or 6 μg β-carotene. See text for calculation of vitamin A activity of diets as retinol equivalents.

§ As cholecalciferol. 10 μg cholecalciferol = 400 IU of vitamin D.

‖ α-Tocopherol equivalents. 1 mg d-α tocopherol = 1 α-TE. See text for variation in allowances and calculation of vitamin E activity of the diet as α-tocopherol equivalents.

¶ 1 NE (niacin equivalent) is equal to 1 mg of niacin or 60 mg of dietary tryptophan.

plants, salmon, lobster, bird feathers, and in many other species. Many of the carotenoids, termed *provitamin A,* have vitamin A activity. Some carotenoids have biological actions independent of their vitamin A activity.

Retinoids usually contain five *trans* double bonds with different functional groups at carbon 15, usually either an alcohol, an aldehyde, or an acid. The retinol may be esterified with palmitate, acetate, or propionate. The unit of measurement is based on all-*trans* retinol with 1 μg equal to 1 RE (retinol equivalent). The older system of units equated 0.3 μg of all-*trans* retinol to 1 international unit (IU). 3-dehydroretinol (A_2) has a biological activity of 0.4 RE. Retinoic acid itself has activity only for some functions, such as growth, and some aspects of reproduction.

The carotenoids have widely varying activity with β carotene being the highest. Theoretically, β carotene can be split into two retinols, but considering the variability of absorption and incomplete conversion, 1 mg of β carotene is equivalent to 1/6 RE. Most other carotenoids are at most half as potent; moreover, some have no vitamin A activity.

Absorption. For absorption of the vitamin A group, fat must be present in the meal (except with the synthetic water-soluble forms). In some cases the vitamin has to be released from proteins by digestion. The fat is necessary for the release of bile and pancreatic enzymes, and bile acids and phospholipids are required for micelle formation (without micelles the fat is poorly absorbed, as are the fat-soluble vitamins). Provitamin A carotenoids, carotenoids, vitamin A and esters remain in the micelle. The retinol esters are hydrolyzed by a specific esterase; the ester is poorly absorbed. Retinol may be absorbed by a carrier-mediated mechanism at low concentrations and by passive cellular diffusion at higher concentrations. The absorption of β carotene is much lower than that of the retinoids. Before transport from intestine, some β carotene may be cleaved by carotenoid 15-15' dioxygenase to retinal. The retinal is reduced to retinol by alcohol dehydrogenases and esterified with palmitate. Chylomicrons carry mostly retinylester, with retinoic acid going into the portal vein.

In the liver, hepatocytes continue the β carotene cleavage with eventual formation of additional retinyl palmitate. PreapoRBP (retinol-binding protein) made in the hepatocyte is converted to apoRBP and combined with retinol to form holoRBP (40–50 μg/ml in blood) in a 1:1 ratio. HoloRBP in plasma combines with prealbumin. By being combined with prealbumin, holoRBP avoids excretion into the urine. There are holoRBP receptors in the intestine, the Ito cells in the liver, the retina, and many other tissues; these receptors internalize the retinol and bind it to intracellular RBPs. Altered apoRBP is released into plasma and is catabolized by the kidney. The liver can further metabolize retinol to retinoic acid; this process is irreversible. The retinoic acid can be glycosylated to β glucuronide and is secreted into bile and eventually to the feces; the glucuronide pathway may represent 67% of retinoic acid excretion, with the kidney excreting the remainder as retinoic acid and its metabolites. The Ito cells in the liver store most of the vitamin A in the human, whereas adipocytes are the primary storage area for carotenoids. The presence of the carotenoids provides a yellowish tint to fatty tissue. An excess of carotenoids may appear as jaundice, but the eyes do not change color.

Functions. The function of retinol and retinal in vision is well-known. Retinoic acid cannot be used for this function. In the retina, retinol is transferred to the rods or cones where it performs one of its key functions. Retinol isomerase converts all-*trans* to 11-*cis* retinol, then retinol dehydrogenase forms 11-*cis* retinal. In the rods, 11-*cis* retinal is bonded with a

Vitamin A (all-*trans*)

R =

Retinol

Retinal

Retinoic acid

β carotene

lysine in opsin to form rhodopsin and in the cones to form three different iodopsins for blue, green, and red light absorption. Photons cause the conversion of 11-*cis* retinal to all-*trans* retinal, which separates from opsin. Retinene isomerase converts the all-*trans* retinal to the 11-*cis* form in the dark, or alcohol dehydrogenase converts the all-*trans* retinal to all-*trans* retinol, which can be acted on then by retinol isomerase and retinol dehydrogenase.

Vitamin A also plays a key role in differentiation, and in this case retinoic acid may be the most important. The mechanism of the effect of vitamin A on gene expression involves retinoic acid and retinol binding to chromatin through the supersteroid receptor family. With a vitamin A deficiency, columnar epithelial and mucus cells change to a keratin-type of cell. Vitamin A also causes differentiation of carcinoma cells, perhaps because vitamin A can control fibronectin release or the release of surface and extracellular proteins. There are glycoprotein characteristics that change with vitamin A deficiency. They involve retinyl-mannoside, possibly through the dolichol phosphate mannose pathway with dolichol pyrophosphate (DPP)–oligosaccharide being elongated with saccharides and the addition to asparagine residue. Retinyl-mannoside adds to the protein directly after DPP.

The effects of a vitamin A deficiency on reproduction are not permanent and can be reversed. Retinoic acid is not useful for this purpose. The deficiency syndrome is characterized by the replacement of normally functioning squamous cells with cornified vaginal tissue. The columnar cells are required for the maintenance of the placenta. They are required also for the development of testes and the maintenance of germinal epithelium, with a vitamin A deficiency leading to a failure of spermatogenesis. There are questions whether these results are specific or an expression of the lack of cellular differentiation.

The importance of vitamin A group and other carotenoids in immunological processes has come to the forefront of research. Vitamin A is necessary for lysosome production in saliva, tears, and sweat, having an important antibacterial function. Beta carotene may have its own effects by increasing natural killer cell activity, increasing T cell and B cell proliferation, and inhibiting the proliferation of neoplastic cells. Cancer risk may be decreased by an increase in differentiation and by the antioxidant function of β carotene.

Deficiency. Deficiency can be caused by a low intake or by fat malabsorption due to cystic fibrosis, cholestasis, pancreatic insufficiency, or chronic diarrhea. Alcohol consumption may decrease the storage in liver by the Ito cells. Kidney disease can lead to a tubular reabsorption decrease. Total parenteral nutrition (TPN) solutions may also be low in vitamin A resulting from adsorption to intravenous (IV) tubing.

Sign and symptoms of vitamin A deficiency may include xerophthalmia and keratomalacia with the clinical signs being conjunctival xerosis, Bitot's spot, and corneal xerosis. The mechanisms underlying these signs are the degradation of the mucus cells of the cornea leading to leukocyte invasion of the corneal stroma with proteases hydrolyzing collagen and other connective tissue, with eventual tissue collapse and perforation. The dryness of the eye is due to an alteration of the glycoprotein in tears that reduces the ability of tears to keep the eyes moist. Another important sign of vitamin A deficiency is night blindness. The health and integrity of the skin is also decreased with vitamin A deficiency.

There are two levels of vitamin A deficiency defined by tissue levels of vitamin A. One is *frank deficiency* with plasma levels less than 10 μg/dl and liver levels less than 5 μg/g. The other is termed *marginal deficiency* with

Retinoic acid is an extremely potent differentiation agent.

plasma levels between 10 and 20 μg/dl and liver levels between 5 and 20 μg/g. Another good measure of vitamin A nutriture based on the response to a supplement is the relative dose response. Plasma levels are measured before a dose and 5 hours after a 450 μg dose. If the percent increase in plasma level is greater than 50%, the patient is considered deficient but marginal. If the increase is between 15 and 20%, it falls into the category of correctable night blindness. The relative dose technique is based on the theory that at low levels of vitamin A, not resulting from protein malnutrition, the apoRBP stored in hepatocytes is released quickly with vitamin A addition.

VITAMIN D

The history of vitamin D started in 1809 with Bardsley, who found that cod liver oil could cure rickets. The relationship between sunlight and rickets was recognized in 1890 by Palm. The great expansion in the understanding of vitamin D occurred in the late 1910s and early 1920s with experimental rickets (Sir Mellanby, 1919), teeth development (Lady Mellanby, 1918), and its distinction from vitamin A due to its stability (McCollum et al, 1922).

Sources. Vitamin D is a sterol that is acid- and light-unstable. The two major vitamin D compounds are D_2 from ergosterol in plants, yeast, and fungi and D_3 from 7-dehydrocholesterol from animal sources. Hydroxylation can occur at three positions: 1, 24, and 25 as a 25 monohydroxy; 1,25 or 24,25 dihydroxy; or 1,24,25 trihydroxy. (In terms of activity in rats D_3 and D_2 are equal, but not in chickens, where D_2 is ten times more potent.) The 25 hydroxylated vitamin D is between two and five times as effective as the unhydroxylated form and 1,25 $(OH)_2$ vitamin D is an order of magnitude more potent.

Aside from the dietary sources, sunlight exposure can produce vitamin D by photobiogenesis. 7-dehydrocholesterol is converted in the skin to previtamin D_3 producing 10 μg within 10–15 minutes' exposure of hands and face by ultraviolet (UV) at 282 nm. Photobiogenesis is not controlled except that less previtamin D is produced by tanned or pigmented skin. Perhaps the production of melanin acts as a protective agent against vitamin D toxicity. Prolonged light exposure can result in the production of other metabolites such as lumisterol.

Absorption. As with vitamin A, fat digestion products are required for optimal intestinal absorption of vitamin D because bile acids are required for micelle formation. Absorption probably occurs in both the jejunum and ileum. It is transported then in chylomicrons to the liver and fat tissue and stored with DBP (vitamin D–binding protein) in the liver. Subsequent transport from the liver or skin uses α_2-globulin DBP as a carrier, except previtamin D. The first major step in vitamin D metabolism is 25 hydroxylation in the hepatocytes; it may also occur in lung, kidney, and intestine. This may increase with deficiency. The second important step is 1 α hydroxylation by the kidney and placenta, a step tightly regulated by hormones. Low serum calcium causes release of parathyroid hormone (PTH), which lowers intracellular phosphate and in turn stimulates 1 α hydroxylation of 25 vitamin D. It is suppressed also by 1,25 $(OH)_2$ vitamin D and serum calcium. 24 hydroxylation, which probably occurs in the kidney, is regulated also but opposite to 1 α hydroxylation in relation to 1,25 vitamin D levels. 24 hydroxylation is a preliminary step to biliary excretion, which is the major pathway. Chronic alcohol consumption can cause an increased loss of 25 vitamin D into bile.

1,25 (OH)$_2$ vitamin D$_3$ is a key hormone in calcium homeostasis.

Functions. The active form of vitamin D is the metabolite 1,25 (OH)$_2$ vitamin D, which acts as a hormone controlling calcium and phosphorus homeostasis. Calcium absorption is increased by 1,25 vitamin D. 1,25 vitamin D binds to a cytosol receptor protein (RP) that is similar to the other steroid receptors. RP with 1,25 vitamin D binds to DNA causing mRNA transcription for calcium-binding protein (CaBP). This process is inhibited by glucocorticoids, which are useful therefore in the therapy for hypervitaminosis D. Phosphorus absorption is increased by 1,25 vitamin D also. Renal reabsorption of calcium by the distal kidney tubule and bone mobilization of calcium is stimulated by PTH with existing 1,25 vitamin D. Calcitonin from thyroid blocks the action of vitamin D and is useful also in the therapy for hypervitaminosis D (see also Chapter 31).

Bone formation is another important function of 1,25 vitamin D, which can increase receptors for epidermal growth factor and stimulate transforming-growth factor β (TGF β). TGF β stimulates bone resorption and cartilage induction.

Vitamin D also affects differentiation of some cells, i.e., myleocytes to monocytes or macrophages. It inhibits the growth of some carcinomas, especially breast cancer and malignant melanoma, exhibiting a biphasic effect, stimulating replication at low physiological levels, and inhibiting at higher levels.

Deficiency. Deficiency is indicated at serum levels of 25 OH vitamin D of less than 7 ng/ml. Infants, especially breast-fed, and the elderly are at risk. Breast-fed infants may have a dietary deficiency that may be exacerbated by lack of sunlight exposure. The elderly may be at risk for a vitamin D deficiency also because of a decreased 1,25 vitamin D synthesis, decreased milk intake, decreased light exposure (especially during bad weather), and decreased 7-dehydrocholesterol in the skin. Renal failure can also result in a deficiency in 1,25 vitamin D due to a lack of synthesis resulting in low serum calcium and high serum phosphorus; hypoparathyroidism and estrogen administration can result in decreased parathyroid hormone (PTH) levels and have similar effects. There is an inborn error of metabolism that affects 1,25 vitamin D status, familial hypophosphatemia. There are significant drug interactions with the anticonvulsive drugs phenytoin and phenobarbital. These drugs may induce hepatic 25 hydroxylation and kidney 1 α hydroxylation, which induces further metabolism and may increase inactive vitamin D metabolite excretion in the bile (possibly as 24,25 vitamin D). Finally, fat malabsorption and alcohol consumption may result in deficiency. Alcohol consumption may cause pancreatic and bile acid deficiency, and 25 hydroxylation may result from hepatocyte failure.

The classical deficiency syndromes of vitamin D are rickets and osteomalacia; *rickets* comes from the Old English *wrikken* meaning bend or twist. The sequence of events are decreased calcium absorption; low calcium levels; hyperparathyroidism with PTH release; PTH elevates serum calcium from bones and causes phosphaturia; low serum P$_1$; and finally, bone disease and lack of mineralization. The treatment consists of 1.25–2.5 mg of vitamin D daily.

Osteoporosis may be caused by the result of estrogen-induced release of bone calcium, which decreases PTH release and 1,25 vitamin D synthesis; in the face of no increase in calcium absorption there is subsequent bone loss. Hypocalcemic tetany can also be the result of vitamin D deficiency.

VITAMIN K

In 1929, Dam and associates reported hemorrhages in chickens fed a low-fat diet in a study of cholesterol metabolism. They found a delay in coagulation due to an effect on prothrombin time. Six years later Dam named the factor required to cure this disease *vitamin K* (Koagulation factor). Four years later it was isolated from alfalfa by Doisey and from putrefied fish meal by Dam.

Vitamin K is a quinone derivative, labile to alkali and light. A key function of vitamin K involves its capacity to form a stable free radical (quinol). Vitamin K_1, phylloquinone, is from plants. K_2, menaquinone, with unsaturated side chains of various numbers of prenyl units, usually 7 through 13, is derived from bacterial sources. Menaquinone-4 is the most biologically active form; there is lessened activity observed with compounds with longer or shorter side chains, reaching a low with menaquinone (no side chain and 1/120 the activity). K_3, menadione, is a synthetic that can be elongated by alkylation with digeranyl pyrophosphate to form menaquinone-4.

Absorption. The absorption of vitamin K requires bile and pancreatic juices and probably occurs by a passive mechanism, but K_1 may also have an active transport process in the distal small intestine. Vitamin K is transported from the intestine to the rest of the body in chylomicrons and later in very low density lipoproteins (VLDL) and low-density lipoproteins (LDL). The highest concentrations occur in the liver, spleen, and lungs, but even with a lower concentration the muscle is the largest storage site. Vitamin K has a short half-life, 2–3 hours, excreted primarily as lactones and glucuronides in the feces through bile with a much smaller amount appearing in the urine.

Functions. The primary function of vitamin K is in the posttranslational modification of glutamate (Glu) to γ carboxyglutamate (Gla). This carboxylase-epoxidase system requires a peptide substrate, Mg^{2+}, O_2, CO_2, and nicotinamide-adenine dinucleotide (reduced form) (NADH) or nicotinamide-adenide dinucleotide phosphate (oxidized form) (NADPH), but the mechanism is unclear. The vitamin K cycle for this conversion occurs by at least two pathways with dithiol (warfarin sensitive) or with NADH (or NADPH, which is much less active) for the reduction of vitamin K to the dihydroxyl hydroquinone, which is the active form for the carboxylation reaction. The carboxylation of Glu results in a 2,3 epoxide that is reduced by dithiol epoxidase reductase to vitamin K, the quinone. This reaction is also warfarin-sensitive. Warfarin is used as an oral anticoagulant, for prevention of thrombosis, and as rat poison. Warfarin is also teratogenic. A similar compound, dicoumarol, found in fermented clover can also inhibit this cycle.

Coagulation occurs through the clotting factor cascade, with many factors involved with vitamin K. The major factor is prothrombin, which is synthesized in the liver with amino acids 7,8,15,17,20,21,27,30,33 being γ carboxyglutamate. Factors VII, IX, and X are in this clotting factor cascade. Other factors are C and S (anticoagulants) and M and Z (stimulate platelet activity).

Another γ-carboxyglutamate protein is found in the bone, Bone-Gla protein (BGP) or osteocalcin, which makes up 1% of total bone protein and is regulated by 1,25 vitamin D_3. Osteocalcin binds Ca^{2+} and hydroxyapatite. Other possible effects of vitamin K relate to anti-inflammatory actions and rheumatoid arthritis. Vitamin K inhibits the rise in intracellular calcium that stimulates leukocyte function. This may be through the reduction in glutathione, which is used to protect the macrophage from its own superoxide that is stimulated by vitamin K.

Deficiency. Few people develop vitamin K deficiency because of its common occurrence and microbial production. However, drug therapy with

Phylloquinone (vitamin K_1)

Menaquinone-n (MK-n, vitamin K_2)

A major portion of the vitamin K needs are produced by the intestinal microflora.

anticoagulants (warfarin), anticonvulsants (hydantoins), and antibiotics (neomycin, moxalactam), especially when used in patients undergoing surgery and maintained on TPN, may result in a vitamin K deficiency. Adult TPN solutions do not contain vitamin K. Newborns, especially premature or home births, are at risk because of the low amount of vitamin K in breast milk and low intestinal synthesis. Fat malabsorption resulting from ingestion of mineral oil and other unabsorbed lipids, low fat intake, bile acid deficiency caused by biliary obstruction, cystic fibrosis, or chronic liver disease, or megadoses of vitamin E can exacerbate marginal situations. The primary symptom of vitamin K deficiency is a lengthened prothrombin time (see also Chapter 46).

VITAMIN E: TOCOPHEROLS AND TOCOTRIENOLS

The history of vitamin E and the tocopherols started with an observation that has yet to be found in humans. Evans and Bishop in 1922 showed that a fat-soluble substance prevented fetal death in rats when the diet contained rancid lard. They named it *tocopherol* ("to bring forth offspring"). Two years later, Sure named it vitamin E. It was not until 1968 that the National Academy of Sciences (NAS) established a Recommended Dietary Allowance (RDA) (see Table 63–1).

There are many stereo isomers of vitamin E. All are labile to light (important in using TPN solutions), oxygen, peroxides (e.g., as occurs in rancid fat), $FeCl_3$, and heating at high temperature. Therefore, most vitamin E in oils and fried frozen foods is lost. Two thirds of that in the germ of grains can be lost in processing the oil and most is lost in white bread by the removal of the germ and bleaching.

The tocopherols differ only in the methylation on the benzene ring, but they have different activities. All are alcohols, which can be esterified; the acetate ester is the most water-soluble. All must be de-esterified to be biologically active. The reactive hydroxyl groups that can form free radicals are crucial to the functional action of vitamin E. Alpha tocopherol is the most abundant with the d form the one present in foods and the most potent. Synthetic α tocopherol has eight epimers and is less potent. Beta tocopherol with one less methyl is at least half as potent as the α form and is found in high quantities in wheat. Gamma tocopherol is much less potent than either but is present in much higher concentrations in oils, especially corn and soybean and also in margarines, depending on the oil used. Gamma also has one less methyl than the α. Delta tocopherol, which is high in some oils like safflower and has two less methyls than α, has almost no biological activity. Another group of vitamin E compounds, the tocotrienols, have many double bonds, similar to vitamin K, with intermediate biological activities. Biological activity is measured in IU, which are equal to 1 mg of d,l α tocopherol-acetate.

Absorption. Fat digestion products are important in the absorption of the vitamin Es, the amount absorbed being proportional to the amount of lipids in the diet. The percent absorption can range from 10 to 70%. Absorption is also inversely proportional to the amount of vitamin E in the diet, with about 10% at 200 mg/day. The absorbed vitamin E is transported from intestine in chylomicrons; one of its storage sites are Ito cells in the liver. Further transport to most other tissues occurs by way of the lipoproteins, VLDL and LDL. There are many distribution pools with various biological half-lives, a relatively short-term pool in the plasma and liver, and a longer one in adipocytes (a major storage site) and muscle. The isomers have varying half-lives, with the α isomer lasting much longer than the γ. The major excretory route is through the bile in the feces.

The various forms of vitamin E have widely different bioactivities.

Naturally occurring vitamin E compounds

α tocopherol

β tocopherol

γ tocopherol

δ tocopherol

α tocotrienol

Functions. An important function of vitamin E is as a biological antioxidant acting in concert with the enzymes glutathione peroxidase, superoxide dismutase, and catalase. Vitamin E prevents peroxidation by stopping a chain reaction between free radicals and other compounds (especially polyunsaturated fatty acids). Vitamin E does this by reacting with the free radical and becoming a semiquinone with subsequent conversion to a quinone or a hydroquinone.

Vitamin E also prevents the formation of ceroid pigments (lipofuscin), pigment granules in soft tissue resulting from oxidized unmetabolizable lipids cross-linked with proteins. The amount of lipofuscin present appears to be a function of age.

The reproductive function of vitamin E, which brought about its discovery, has not been demonstrated in humans. In many mammals, other than humans, there is a degeneration of seminiferous tubule epithelium in males, and lack of uterine function in females associated with resorption of the fetus with a diet deficient in vitamin E.

Other functions and properties include decreased fecal mutagens (50–100 IU/day with vitamin C 120 mg), decreased prostaglandin and thromboxane synthesis (PGI_2, which promotes platelet aggregation and is low in diabetics; this may be correctable with additional vitamin E), increased blood circulation in elderly (300–600 mg/day for 3 months), increased esterification and decreased de-esterification of vitamin A in the liver, and protection of the lung from air pollutants such as nitrogen dioxide and ozone.

Deficiency. Deficiency of vitamin E can occur in humans with fat malabsorption from pancreatic disease, biliary obstruction, cystic fibrosis, cirrhosis of the liver, or enteritis. Premature infants are at risk of vitamin E deficiency because of the low storage of vitamin E resulting from low transplacental delivery, low body fat, poor fat absorption, and rapid growth. Patients with abetalipoproteinemia, being unable to synthesize apoprotein B, may develop symptoms of vitamin E deficiency. Two good tests for low levels of vitamin E nutriture are peroxide hemolysis and blood analysis. It is important to express plasma levels in relationship to lipids (deficient being less than 0.5 mg/g total plasma lipids). It may be useful also to do an isomer analysis. The symptoms of vitamin E deficiency include hemolysis, anemia, neural degeneration, and perhaps retrolental fibroplasia (neonatal infants with low vitamin E and oxygen toxicity) and abnormal lung development.

VITAMIN C, ASCORBIC ACID

Vitamin C deficiency states, like those of vitamin A, have a long history, with many folk remedies and a long history of treatments. Vitamin C became especially important when long sea voyages became common, with perhaps more sailors dying of scurvy than any other single cause. In the 1500s, Hawkins prescribed oranges and lemons for long sailing voyages. Possibly the first controlled clinical trial was done by Lind in 1742 using citrus fruits as a preventive for scurvy. An important breakthrough in vitamin C research occurred when Holst and Frölich accidentally found that guinea pigs required this factor. Three years later, Zilva in 1910 isolated ascorbic acid. Two decades later Szent-Györgyi characterized hexuronic acid and identified it as vitamin C, for which he received the Nobel Prize.

Vitamin C exists as either L-ascorbic acid or dehydroascorbic acid; both forms are water-soluble. L-ascorbic acid is oxidized easily in water with O_2

Water-Soluble Vitamins

Ascorbic acid is the most labile of all vitamins.

to dehydroascorbic. L-ascorbic acid has a half-life of less than 2 minutes in water at pH 6 and 158° F. It is sensitive to heat with metals such as iron and copper acting as catalysts, being unstable in TPN solutions because of the cupric ion and O_2. In general, it is the most easily lost of all vitamins. There is a significant seasonal variation in the daily intake, with citrus juice and potatoes being the main sources in American diets. Of the ascorbic acid in orange juice, 75% may be lost in 3 weeks even when stored in the refrigerator in paper containers (breathable). Potatoes retain 75% of the ascorbic acid after being fried, but within 1–2 hours of slicing 30–50% of the vitamin C can be lost by oxidation.

Absorption, Metabolism, Excretion. Absorption occurs by two mechanisms. Both forms can be absorbed by passive diffusion, but only ascorbic acid is absorbed by a sodium-dependent carrier-mediated mechanism. In guinea pigs, one of the few animals that require vitamin C, most absorption occurs in the ileum. The percent absorption decreases with increasing intake, ranging from 90 to 20%, with the maximal percent absorption occurring at amounts below 180 mg and the lowest at levels at or above 2 g.

Vitamin C is stored in all tissues, with the highest concentrations in the adrenal and pituitary glands, and lower levels in the liver, spleen, and brain. Humans have about 100 days of storage, but this can change with the season, being lower in the winter.

Ascorbic acid is reversibly converted to dehydroascorbic acid using glutatione with niacin and riboflavin. Further oxidation to diketo-L-gulonic acid can occur, but the reaction is irreversible and the activity is lost. This enzyme is missing in humans, guinea pigs, primates, and some other species that require ascorbic acid as a nutrient. Further metabolism results in oxalate and threonic acid. 5-keto acids, L-lyxonic, and L-xylonic acid are also formed. Ascorbic acid is not metabolized to CO_2 in humans (although this is a major pathway in guinea pigs). In humans, vitamin C can be excreted in the urine without being metabolized; renal reabsorption of L-ascorbic acid occurs using a sodium-dependent mechanism. The amount in the urine is usually less than 3 mg/day at low intakes (~30 mg/day), but levels increase with increasing intakes. Metabolites are excreted also in the urine with oxalate being prominent at low intakes; small amounts of 2,3 diketo-L-gulonate, ascorbate-2-sulfate, L-xylonic, and L-lyxonic acids also appear. At megadose levels (over 1000 mg) some ascorbic acid is excreted in the feces, and oxalate is not prominent. Thus, oxalate kidney stones with megadoses of vitamin C may not be a problem.

Functions. Vitamin C has many important functions. A crucial feature of vitamin C is its antioxidant properties. It can reduce ferrous iron to ferric iron with the promotion of nonheme iron absorption. Other aspects of iron metabolism are also related to vitamin C, such as the transfer of plasma iron to the liver and into ferritin for storage and for transfer between iron-binding proteins. It acts as a protective agent with enzyme reactions. As a hydroxylation enzyme cofactor, it is essential for collagen formation. Without vitamin C, protocollagen does not cross-link properly, which leads to impaired wound healing and bone formation and weakened capillary walls. This defect in collagen formation involves the enzymes proline prohydroxylase for the triple helix of collagen, and lysyl hydroxylase for glycosylation linkage.

The carrier for activated fatty acid into mitochondria for β oxidation, carnitine, can come from the diet or be synthesized. Its synthesis from lysine and methionine by some dioxygenases requires vitamin C. Biogenic amine synthesis requires a reducing agent, vitamin C, for the oxygenase. Two important examples are the conversion of dopamine to norepinephrine and tyrosine to epinephrine (see Chapter 14).

Many hormones undergo α amidation with the addition of an amide on the carboxyl end of the peptide. This monooxygenase uses vitamin C, copper, and O_2. Hydroxylations also employ vitamin C for cholesterol degradation with 7α hydroxylation, which is the first step in bile acid synthesis and for drug metabolism by the cytochrome P-450–dependent mixed-function oxidases (MFO) in mitochondria.

Toxicity. At large doses of at least 1 g/day, there are effects on immunological functions and cancer. Vitamin C (50 mg/kg/day) can increase the chemotaxis of neutrophils in chronic granulomatous disease, a genetic disorder of leukocyte function, leading to a reduction in a number of infections in this condition. Cancer treatment with vitamin C is still controversial and is based on the observations that vitamin C alters certain immunological functions. The type of cancer may be crucial. Earlier studies examined vitamin C effects on cancer in general, whereas cancer in the stomach and uterus may be more responsive. Some of the possible actions in preventing cancer may be due to the effect of vitamin C on nitrosamine protection or a possible reduction in the occurrence of mutagens in feces that is seen with increases in vitamin E. Nitrosamines are powerful cancer-causing agents, especially in the stomach and colon. They can be produced by the conversion of nitrates to nitrites with the nitrites going to nitrosonium ion, which then reacts with amines or amides. Vitamin C reacts with nitrites to reduce this conversion. Nitrate intake can be quite high, 75–100 mg/day, with vegetarians taking in about 250 mg/day owing to the higher consumption of vegetables. Nitrites, which are more potent, are consumed usually in amounts less than 1 mg/day, but a high intake of cured meat intake can increase this up to 2 mg/day. The amount of vitamin C that has been demonstrated to reduce the conversion of nitrates to nitrosamine is rather large, some 4 g/day.

Other possible health effects of vitamin C in high doses include a lowering of hyperlipidemia and protection from heavy-metal toxicity. The reduction in hexavalent chromium to trivalent chromium, which is much less toxic, may be helpful in those exposed. There is also a reduction in the toxicity of cadmium, vanadium, nickel, and lead.

Deficiency. The main cause for marginal vitamin C deficiency is an increased requirement combined with a low intake. Increased requirements may be due to many causes: disease (such as cancer and rheumatoid disease that result in increased turnover), oral contraceptives (progesterones increase MFO), stress (such as burns and infection), and smoking. In addition, the elderly may have an increased requirement. Low intake can occur most easily in the winter, in association with a lower intake of fresh vegetables. A mild deficiency may be exacerbated by the low vitamin C reserves in some people during the winter. It can be affected also by decreased absorption with diarrhea or ethanol consumption. Chronic heavy alcohol consumption may be associated with both a low intake and altered liver metabolism.

Early marginal deficiency is manifested by either normal or lowered plasma ascorbic acid levels, with the next stage exhibiting not only a decrease in plasma levels but also decreases in leukocyte and urine levels. There are also biochemical changes with vitamin C deficiency with an increase in proline/hydroxyproline ratio and a decrease in serum carnitine. A marginal vitamin C deficiency might contribute also to general symptoms of ill health, including fatigue, poor wound healing, increased susceptibility to bruising, loss of appetite, and reduced immune responses.

Clinical (scorbutic) deficiency occurs when plasma levels are less than 0.2 mg/l plasma. Scurvy presents with red, swollen, and bleeding gums; perifolliculosis; increased capillary fragility; subcutaneous hemorrhages; and swollen joints. Long-term, untreated vitamin C deficiency can result in sudden death.

VITAMIN B₁, THIAMIN

The deficiency disease of thiamin (vitamin B_1) is an ancient disease that has become more apparent with the widespread consumption of polished rice. In the 1880s Takaki used dietary supplements of meat and grains to cure sailors of the Japanese navy of shipboard beriberi. Ten years later, Eijkman developed an animal model for beriberi in chickens, which Grijns showed subsequently was due to their diet of polished rice. The first use of the term *vitamine*, an amine vital to life, was used by Funk in the 1910s for the factor he isolated that cured beriberi. This factor was found to be a water-soluble pyrimidyl with a thiazole ring existing either free, as a hydrochloride, as the coenzyme thiamin pyrophosphate (TPP), or as a triphosphate (TTP). The coenzyme is heat-stable; all the forms are destroyed by alkalis, including phenobarbital, but are stable at a pH less than 5.5. Because they are water-soluble, they are lost in cooking water when it is thrown away.

Absorption. Some antinutrients to thiamin exist. The most important antithiamin is the enzyme thiaminase that is found in some raw fish and in tea, coffee, blueberries, brussels sprouts, and red cabbage. Tannins found in tea and red wine may also destroy thiamin.

Thiamin can be absorbed passively in the small intestine at high levels (less than 5 mg/day) and by an active carrier-mediated mechanism probably in the jejunum. The large intestine may absorb thiamin also by a passive pathway. In the intestine, thiamin is phosphorylated by thiaminokinase to TPP and secreted into the portal blood. It is in this form (TPP) that most of the thiamin is stored with about one half in muscle and one tenth in the brain (as TTP). The pool in the brain is slow to turn over, being metabolized to thiamin monophosphate. Most of the thiamin in the plasma is free as the alcohol. Many thiamin metabolites are excreted in the urine.

Functions. The primary function of thiamin is to act in the transfer of an aldehyde. There are three important enzymes where it is a cofactor, the oxidative decarboxylases of α keto acids and transketolase (TK) for formation of α ketols. TK in the cytosol is part of the pentose phosphate shunt that serves as a source of ribose and NADPH. NADPH is required for fatty acid biosynthesis. Pyruvate decarboxylase of the mitochondria is essential for acetyl-CoA formation and for the tricarboxylic acid (TCA) cycle, being part of the pyruvate dehydrogenase complex. As a cofactor for α-ketogluterate decarboxylase it is involved with branched chain amino acid catabolism and another part of the Krebs cycle.

Deficiency. Thiamin deficiency can be assumed with either less than 27 μg of thiamin per gram creatinine in the urine or as a response of greater than 20% in plasma TPP activity with an additional dose of TPP. Rice-eating populations are at risk of becoming deficient in thiamin, especially in Southeast Asia. Unenriched white bread is also low in thiamin. Excess excretion caused by heavy alcohol consumption or by renal disease (renal dialysis) can increase the risk for thiamin deficiency. Elderly are also at risk because of a low intake and low absorption. There are some inborn errors in metabolism that are associated with thiamin : lactic acidosis associated with low levels of pyruvate decarboxylase and branched chain ketoaciduria.

Symptoms of thiamin deficiency include mental confusion and anorexia. Beriberi can take two forms: dry beriberi (muscle wasting) with peripheral neuropathy, especially in limbs that are used frequently; and wet beriberi (edema) with cardiovascular effects frequently associated with a high carbohydrate diet or exercise leading to a retention of sodium. Wernicke's encephalopathy and Korsakoff's psychosis (amnesic disorder) are examples of dry beriberi that may be the consequence of disturbed carbohydrate metabolism in the neurons with a lack of the triphosphate form. A deficiency can be corrected with 1–2 mg/day oral (3 μg/IU) given adequate intestinal absorption; the inborn errors can be alleviated with 5–20 mg/day. The thiamin deficiency syndromes of Wernicke's encephalopathy and Korsakoff's psychosis are irreversible if not treated promptly. The most common occurrence of these syndromes is with individuals who are acutely hospitalized and given IV carbohydrates. (The presence of prior heavy alcohol consumption is frequently not clinically apparent.) The combination of marginal thiamin deficiency consequent to possible heavy alcohol consumption and the infusion of glucose requires parenteral administration (usually IM) of thiamin (e.g., 100 mg or more daily). (The susceptibility to Wernicke's encephalopathy may be associated with a genetic difference in the transketolase enzyme system.)

> Acute hospitalization with IV glucose administration can precipitate potentially irreversible Wernicke's encephalopathy or Korsakoff's psychosis.

VITAMIN B₂, RIBOFLAVIN

Riboflavin was part of the complex antiberiberi factor with niacin, vitamin B$_6$ and pantothenic acid. Riboflavin was separated from thiamin by McCollum based on its stability to heating. The name *riboflavin* is partially derived from the ribitol portion of the vitamin, which also contains an isoalloxazine ring. Riboflavin exists free but is usually as riboflavin-phosphoric acid, flavin mononucleotide (FMN), or flavin adenine dinucleotide (FAD) (combined with ribose and adenine). It is only slightly soluble in water. It is heat-stable but is light-sensitive.

Absorption. Before absorption, riboflavin must be released from dietary protein by acidic gastric conditions, and phosphatases are required for its release from the covalently linked forms. It is absorbed by a passive and active mechanism that is saturated at consumptions of 25 mg/day. There is little storage of riboflavin, and this occurs mainly in the plasma complexed with proteins (for transport) and intracellularly with flavoprotein complexes and covalent flavoproteins. The amount of riboflavin excreted in the urine provides a fairly accurate measure of riboflavin intake.

Functions. The primary function of riboflavin is in oxidation/reduction reaction for metabolism and respiration (oxidative phosphorylation). It acts as a direct link between the Krebs cycle and the respiratory chain during the conversion of succinate to fumarate. It is involved also in fatty acid synthesis and oxidation, amino acid oxidation, xanthine oxidase, glutathione reductase, lactic acid dehydrogenase, and ferridoxin. FAD, a stronger oxidizing agent than NAD, is used by cytochrome c reductase for NAD$^+$ reduction.

Deficiency. Riboflavin deficiency is usually present when there is urinary excretion of less than 27 μg riboflavin per gram creatinine. The symptoms are vascularization of cornea, sore throat, fissures at the side of the mouth, and a magenta-colored tongue. Riboflavin deficiency can be precipitated by general malnourishment and malabsorption associated with lactose malabsorption, diarrhea, and the irritable bowel syndrome. Deficiency resulting from chronic low intake can occur also with amounts less than 0.3 mg/kcal. Increased requirement for riboflavin because of protein wasting, or increased excretion associated with phenothiazine administration, exacerbates a mild deficiency. Therapy for riboflavin deficiency is either 6 mg/day oral or 25 mg/day IM.

NIACIN

Niacin deficiency was first described by Casal in 1735 as the *Mal de la Rosa* disease, sickness of the rose, because of the skin roughness and color. This disease was the result of the corn brought from the New World for the masses in Europe. In the 1910s and 1920s the cause of the disease *pellagra* (Latin: *pelle*, skin + *agra*, rough) was disputed, some claiming that it was infectious. Sandwich (1913) suggested that it was due to a tryptophan deficiency, and a year later Voegtlin proved it to be a deficiency disease by feeding two contrasting diets to pellagra patients. Still, the belief that it was infectious continued until elegant studies by Goldberger and associates proved that it was a deficiency, again by feeding various diets to inmates at state asylums and orphanages in South Carolina, Georgia, and Mississippi. It was not until 1937 that Elvehjem and associates showed that nicotinic acid could also cure pellagra in the animal model of black tongue in dogs.

There are two active forms of niacin: nicotinic acid (niacin) and nicotinic acid amide (nicotinamide) and four derivatives: NMN (nicotinic acid mononucleotide), NaMN (nicotinic acid amide mononucleotide, a tryptophan metabolite), NAD, and NADP (phosphate on the ribose). Nicotinic acid is a pyridine-3-carboxylic acid; the reduced form is labile to acid, and the oxidized form is labile to alkali. Both are stable to heat and are stable as solids. Tryptophan can be converted to niacin with an efficiency of about 60 tryptophan molecules for 1 niacin molecule. This ratio varies with individuals and certain conditions (e.g., estrogen administration increases the efficiency of conversion).

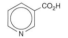

Nicotinic acid (niacin)

Nicotinamide (niacinamide)

Absorption, Metabolism. Nicotinic acid is absorbed passively in the intestine after hydrolysis of either the protein or the nucleotide and coenzymes, but nicotinamide is not readily absorbed. The storage of niacin occurs in all tissues, but the total is low. The usually storage forms are NAD or NADP, but some is stored in the liver as niacin. The liver is also the primary site of nicotinic acid formation from tryptophan. Tryptophan is converted to quinolinate and then to NaMN.

NaMN and NMN are metabolized eventually by different routes to NAD and then to NADP. Nicotinamide is converted to nicotinic acid after conversion to NAD with the production of adenosine-5′-pyrophospho-5-ribose (ADPR). With a normal intake of niacin, most of the metabolites are excreted in the urine as 1-methyl-nicotinamide (20–30%) and 1-methyl-3-caroxamido-6-pyridone (40–60%). These metabolites are made in the liver through a pathway that utilizes methionine. A high intake of nicotinic acid results in an increase in the 1-methyl and glycine conjugates, whereas a high intake of nicotinamide increases the excretion of unmetabolized nicotinamide.

Functions. As with riboflavin, the main function of niacin is in oxidation/reduction reactions using NAD or NADP. It is essential for many dehydrogenases in the Krebs cycle, such as pyruvate and α ketoglutarate and with alcohol dehydrogenase. It is also part of anaerobic carbohydrate metabolism with triose-P-dehydrogenase (NAD), glucose-6-P-dehydrogenase (NADP) and 6-phosphogluconate dehydrogenase (NADP). Its involvement in lipid metabolism is crucial, being part of glycerol synthesis and breakdown (NAD), fatty acid oxidation, fatty acid, and steroid synthesis (NADP). Protein metabolism requires niacin also. Electron transport needs niacin through FMN to CoQ to the cytochromes. There are other less defined functions of niacin involving with ADPR transferase, as a hypocholesterolemic agent (see Chapter 37), and in association with chromium and the glucose tolerance factor.

Deficiency. At high risk for niacin deficiency are individuals with Hartnup's disease, which involves disturbed amino acid absorption leading to a low absorption of tryptophan. The absorption of tryptophan is also lowered in certain foods, such as corn, in which tryptophan is bound to the epsilon amide of lysine. Corn is also low in niacin. Therefore, the undernourished populations of the world for whom corn is the major protein source are at risk of developing niacin deficiency. Tryptophan can be released with alkali treatment of the corn, which is used traditionally in the Mexican diet; the corn for tortillas is soaked in lime water. Therefore, even though corn is low in niacin and tryptophan, what is present is available.

Tryptophan metabolism is altered by carcinoid disease or a high intake of leucine, and both decrease the conversion of tryptophan to niacin. Therapy for Hartnup's or carcinoid involves 40–200 mg of niacin equivalent/day.

Symptoms of pellagra are the 3 Ds: *d*ermatitis, *d*ementia, and *d*iarrhea. The dermatitis is erythematous, especially on sun-exposed areas. The dementia involves fatigue, insomnia, apathy, with confusion leading to psychoses. The diarrhea is due to inflammation of intestinal epithelium and may also include vomiting and dysphagia. A fourth D can occur—*d*eath. Laboratory signs of niacin deficiency include the development of a urinary pyridone: methyl metabolite ratio of less than one.

VITAMIN B$_6$, PYRIDOXINE, PYRIDOXAMINE, PYRIDOXAL

Early in the history of vitamin B$_6$, there was confusion between pellagra based on the rat pellagra factor and vitamin B$_6$ deficiency. The rush to isolate the rat pellagra factor resulted in five laboratories reporting its isolation in 1938. A year later, pyridoxine was separated from pantothenic acid by chromatography. In 1950, Snyderman and associates and Mueller and Vilter showed that vitamin B$_6$ was required by humans.

Vitamin B$_6$ is basically a 4-substituted-2-methyl-3-hydroxyl-5-hydroxymethyl-pyridine. Pyridoxine is an alcohol, pyridoxamine an amine, and pyridoxal an aldehyde. The 5' phosphate esters of all three are found in nature: pyridoxal phosphate (PLP) is the most common coenzyme in animals; pyridoxamine phosphate is used for transamination in animals; and pyridoxine phosphate is used in plants. All are water-soluble and sensitive to light and alkali, and PLP is subject to thermal degradation. During pasteurization of milk, there is a 20–40% loss in vitamin B$_6$ activity.

Absorption. After ingestion, the unphosphorylated forms are absorbed by passive diffusion, and the phosphorylated forms, after they are hydrolyzed

Free and phosphorylated forms of vitamin B$_6$

$$R =$$

$$-CH_2OH$$

Pyridoxine

$$-CH_2NH_2$$

Pyridoxamine

$$-CHO$$

Pyridoxal

from esters by phosphorylases in the lumen of the intestine. Pyridoxine is transported as the free vitamin bound to albumin. Pyridoxine is converted to pyridoxal in the liver. After pyridoxal is formed, it is phosphorylated by pyridoxal kinase to PLP with adenosine triphosphate (ATP) to adenosine diphosphate (ADP). PLP is also formed from the phosphate of pyridoxal or pyridoxamine by a riboflavin (FMN) dependent oxidase. PLP is the active form that binds to enzymes. Most of the body's store of vitamin B_6, approximately 25 mg, is as PLP with glycogen phosphorylase. Excretion of vitamin B_6 occurs through the urine as pyridoxic acid from pyridoxal oxidized with NAD.

Functions. Vitamin B_6 functions with at least 60 known enzymatic reactions: tryptophan metabolism to niacin; transamination (e.g., L-alanine and α ketoglutarate to pyruvate and L-glutamate); deamination (serine and threonine); decarboxylation for the formation of epinephrine, norepinephrine, serotonin, and γ aminobutyrate (GABA); the formation of taurine from cysteine, which can be used as a clinical test for vitamin B_6 deficiency (this enzyme has the lowest affinity for B_6 with low levels of taurine being a sign of deficiency); carbon side-chain transfer (serine to glycine with transformation of tetrahydrofolic acid (THFA) to $N^{5,10}$ methylene THFA); amine oxidation (histamine breakdown); desulfuration of amino acids; amino acid absorption; heme formation; glycogen phosphorylase in skeletal muscle for glycogen degradation; sphingolipid formation; and antibody production (which is reduced with a deficiency).

Deficiency. A common test for deficiency involves administration of a 2–5 g tryptophan load; greater than 250 mg/l xanthurenate (XA) in urine is indicative of a vitamin B_6 deficiency. However, this test may not have clinical significance and may only represent a stress response. Elevated levels of kynurenic acid (KN) and hydroxykynurenic acid can also be used, but KN levels increase with estrogen, pregnancy, and oral contraceptives because of the inhibition of kynureninase. Other measures include less than 20 μg B_6/g creatinine; less than 8 mg/l pyridoxic acid; 5 ng/ml PLP in plasma as measured by tyrosine decarboxylation with apodecarboxylase; and less than 50% increase in erythrocyte aminotransferases with PLP addition. Plasma levels by themselves are not useful because they may be elevated in a variety of diseases. Deficiency is uncommon all by itself, although the elderly and people with heavy alcohol consumption are at some risk. There are some genetic disorders that may be responsive to additional vitamin B_6: homocystinuria; primary cystathioninuria; xanthurenic aciduria; and infant convulsions. Vitamin B_6 nutriture can also be affected by drug interactions with penicillamine (see Chapter 60, heavy-metal poisoning antidote and Wilson's disease), isoniazid (see Chapter 53, a tuberculostatic), and oral contraceptives (see Chapter 42). Indicators of vitamin B_6 deficiency may include decreases in serum PLP, B_6 urinary metabolite levels, and transaminases. Convulsions can result from glutamate decarboxylase inactivity or γ aminobutyrate deficiency; also, dermatitis can occur. Therapeutic dosages of 2–6 g/day may be useful for carpal tunnel syndrome and pre-eclampsic edema; paradoxically, long-term excessive dosages of vitamin B_6 can result in peripheral neuritis.

PANTOTHENIC ACID

Pantothenic acid is a relative late-comer to the vitamin field; in the 1930s it was distinguished and isolated, and a deficiency disease was identified (chicken dermatitis). It is an acidic compound with widespread occurrence (hence its name, *pan*, found everywhere). Lipmann and Kaplan showed in 1946 that it functions as coenzyme for the acetylation of sulfanilamide, named *CoA* for coenzyme of acetylation for which they received the Nobel Prize. Pantothenic acid is made up of pantoic acid linked to β alanine by an amide bond. It is water-soluble and labile to acid, alkali, and heat. Much of its activity is lost during cooking (33% in meat, especially if it is hot and long, but much less in vegetables). Processing also removes pantothenate with milling of wheat, accounting for a loss of 57%.

Absorption. Absorption is almost complete at normal intakes with subsequent transport from intestine through the portal vein as the free vitamin. Most of the pantothenic acid is stored as CoA (80%), with the highest levels found in the liver. Excretion in the urine is as pantothenate.

Functions. The active forms of pantothenic acid are CoA and acyl carrier protein (ACP). 4'-phosphopantetheine is the building block for both, being phosphorylated pantothenic acid with a decarboxylated cysteine linked to the β-alanine moiety. CoA is made by the addition of 3'-phospho-ribosyl-adeninylate, and ACP is derived from CoA. CoA is a part of more than 70 enzymes with the major function being the formation of thio esters of acyls, also called Co-A·SH. The importance of this bond is that little energy is lost in its formation. The α carbon can form carbonyl and enolate ions for condensation reactions, e.g., acetyl CoA with oxalacetate to form citrate, acetyl CoA with choline to form acetylcholine, and acetoacetate formation in liver. CoA is crucial for carbohydrates and ketogenic amino acids catabolism, especially branched chain amino acids. Entry into the citric acid cycle requires CoA with acetyl CoA. It is involved also in cholesterol and steroid synthesis from acetyl CoA and bile acid conjugation. Its importance is shown by the necrosis of the adrenal gland that occurs in deficient animals. Anemia is also common in deficient animals, because it is needed for heme synthesis, with condensation of succinyl CoA and glycine being the first step. CoA is used also in xenobiotic metabolism for acetylation before excretion. ACP is used for lipid synthesis and catabolism: synthesis by elongation with ACP as acceptor for malonyl from malonyl CoA, and catabolism by β oxidation with the thiolytic reaction used for the second CoA after acetyl CoA is formed.

Pantothenic acid, part of CoA

Deficiency. A pantothenic acid deficiency has not been clinically recognized because pantothenic acid is so common in foods, but patients with liver disease and alcoholics may be at risk for developing a deficiency. A test for deficiency includes whole blood levels less than 100 μg/dl and urine excretion of less than 1 mg/day. Symptoms include irritability, hypotension, rapid heart rate with exertion, and numbing and tingling of feet and hands. Therapeutic dosages fall in the range of 10–100 mg/day.

BIOTIN

A group of growth factors for yeast were isolated by Wilder in 1901. These were Bios I, which is inositol, and Bios II, a collection including biotin. Factor X, biotin, was found by Boas (1927) to be able to counteract a toxin in egg white. In 1936 biotin was named and isolated from egg yolk by Kogl and Tonnis. About 4 years later, Gyorgy, who was involved in vitamin B_6 research, showed that egg white toxin dermatitis could be cured by a vitamin H. Within a year all these factors, vitamins, and coenzyme R were shown to be the same substance, biotin, by du Vigneaud and colleagues. Lardy and Peanasky in 1953 demonstrated that it was involved with carboxylation during leucine degradation. Its importance in fatty acid biosynthesis as the functional moiety of acetyl-CoA carboxylase was reported by Wakil and associates in 1960.

Sources, Absorption. Biotin as the acid is only slightly soluble in water, but as a salt it is water-soluble. It is stable and oxidized in hot alkali. There are four chiral carbons resulting in eight stereoisomers, but only d-biotin is biologically active. There are some biologically active analogs; oxybiotin having an oxygen instead of a sulfur, dethiobiotin with a reduced sulfur, and the sulfoxide form with SO instead of S. The sulfoxide is converted slowly to biotin. Biotin is linked to the ϵ amide of lysine of a protein with the proteolytic product of digestion being ϵ-N-biotinyl-L-lysine, biocytin. Microflora in the intestine can provide enough biotin to meet the human requirement, with fecal output being many times greater than the usual intake. Digestion of the enzyme with biotin to biocytin occurs except when avidin, the toxin in egg white, forms a complex. Absorption is rapid and active in the upper small intestine and at least passive in the large intestine.

There is little storage of biotin, about 1 mg total, probably mostly in the liver as cytoplasm and mitochondrial carboxylases. It is excreted in the urine as biotin.

Functions. Biotin is involved in the functioning of only a few enzymes. It is most important as a carboxylase reacting with carbonylphosphate forming inorganic phosphate with the addition of the carboxyl to biotin N-1 with aldehyde formation. The first step, though, is the phosphorylation of bicarbonate to carbonylphosphate with ATP to ADP. It is involved in fatty acid synthesis with the conversion of acetyl CoA to malonyl CoA in the cytosol. The metabolism of propionyl CoA to methylmalonyl CoA for odd chain fatty acid catabolism, leucine catabolism, and succinyl formation and propionate use biotin also. The conversion of leucine to isovalerate to β methylcrotonyl in the liver is crucial for branched chain amino acid catabolism. Finally, it is used in the metabolism of pyruvate to oxalacetate in the mitochondria to provide the carbon for gluconeogenesis. There are also other possible decarboxylases and transcarboxylases that utilize biotin as the cofactor. Brain function has been shown to be related to biotin, inasmuch as biotin deficient rats learn slower. This may be due to the fact that glucose is important for brain metabolism, and therefore, it is the organ to show an effect of deficiency.

Deficiency. The major possible causes of biotin deficiency include long-term TPN and antibiotic treatment; infants and alcoholic patients are at the most risk. Deficiency has been observed with a large dose of 6 g of streptomycin for 10–20 days. The avidin in raw egg whites can cause a deficiency if it is consumed in large amounts, especially by infants. There are some inborn errors of metabolism involving the carboxylases. Symptoms of deficiency include anorexia, nausea, vomiting, glossitis, pallor, depression, general lassitude, and a dry dermatitis.

Therapy for a biotin deficiency requires 150–300 μg/day for 3–5 days. Larger dosages of 5 mg/day for 2–3 weeks may be useful for seborrheic dermatitis and Leiner's disease.

VITAMIN B₁₂, COBALAMINS

Vitamin B₁₂ and folate, a tightly linked pair

The history of vitamin B_{12} has long been intermingled with folic acid and the disease pernicious anemia. In the 1820s, Combe described an anemia associated with a digestive or absorptive failure that resulted from a degeneration of glands in the stomach observed by Flint 40 years later. Minot and Murphy (1926) received a Nobel Prize for showing that injections of raw liver could cure pernicious anemia. This, combined with the work of Castle and associates in 1929 showing that an "intrinsic factor" in gastric secretions combines with vitamin B_{12} in food, forms the basis of the understanding that pernicious anemia is due to the lack of the intrinsic factor. Another Nobel Prize was given for work in this area to Hodgkin for her work establishing the structure of vitamin B_{12} using x-ray diffraction. Work on the structure first required the isolation of the vitamin. A ton of liver was used to produce only 20 mg of vitamin B_{12}. This was done in the late 1940s by Smith and Parker and by Rickes and colleagues.

Sources, Absorption, Storage. The cobalamins are both a complex group and the most complex vitamin, but only a small part of the molecule varies from one analog to the next. The basic structure of vitamin B_{12} consists of a planar corrin nucleus linked to a nucleotide (ribose and dimethylbenzimidazole) through a D-l-amino-2-propanol with a cobalt bound to a nitrogen on the nucleotide and to four of the corrin nuclei. The synthetic cyanocobalamin is the oxidized form with the last coordination site of the cobalt bound to the carbon of a cyano group. The cyanide (CN) is removed from cynanocobalamin enzymatically and converted to coenzymes in the epithelial cells. The vitamin B_{12} coenzyme form is methylcobalamin (methyl B_{12}) with a methyl group instead of CN; this is a common form for transportation in the body. It may also be the most active. Coenzyme B_{12} has a 5' deoxyadenosyl instead of CN and is the storage form. Hydroxycobalamin is found in foods. There are also inactive analogs such as pseudo B_{12} (adenylcobalamide cyanide). The active enzyme form is reduced and conjugated with peptides. The different analogs have varying stability. Cyanocobalamin is labile to heavy metals and strong reducing/oxidizing agents (i.e., vitamin C) forming new analogs (usually antivitamins). It is stable and soluble in water. The methyl and 5' deoxyadenosyl forms are labile to light but fairly stable to heat at pH 4–5.

The physiological absorption of vitamin B_{12} is a complicated process. Large oral doses of vitamin B_{12} are taken up by a passive mechanism that may account for 1% of the total absorption at normal intakes. Initially, if the vitamin is not linked to a protein, it is bound to a salivary protein. If it is attached to a protein hydrolysis of the peptide, linkages occur through acid denaturation and proteases, primarily pepsin, and then it is bound to the salivary protein. B_{12} is then freed from salivary protein by trypsin and the neutral pH of the small intestine where it binds in a 2:1 ratio with intrinsic factor (IF). IF is released by the parietal cells in the fundus of the stomach; it has a higher affinity for true B_{12} than for some of the inactive analogs. This complex of vitamin B_{12} and IF then binds to receptors in the ileum, requiring calcium and a pH more than 6 and is taken into the cell.

From the intestinal cells, vitamin B_{12} is transported to other tissues bound to transcobalamin II (TC II), a protein that is made in the liver. TC II is usually free for binding and may be elevated in autoimmune diseases. After transport, vitamin B_{12} is stored with TC I and TC III, glycoproteins that are also called R proteins. They are made by primarily granulocytes and salivary glands. These glycoproteins are present in plasma and secretions from salivary and bile, with plasma levels increasing with increases in neutrophils. The TBBC (total vitamin B_{12}–binding capacity) of the plasma is between 1 and 1.8 ng/ml and is usually 60–75% saturated. The difference is UBBC (unsaturated vitamin B_{12}–binding capacity), which is mainly composed of unsaturated TC II. These three binding proteins have various biological half-lives with TC III (minutes) $\ll$ TC II $\ll$ TC I; nevertheless, there is a 0.1–0.2% turnover regardless of nutrient state. The storage of vitamin B_{12} is rather large in relationship to its requirement, being between 2 and 10 mg mostly in the liver at 1 $\mu g/g$ in the form of coenzyme B_{12}. This amount can last for up to 3–6 years, but with the efficient reabsorption of vitamin B_{12} it may be decades before a deficiency develops with a sustained low intake of vitamin B_{12}.

The bile is the main pathway for excretion of the unmetabolized vitamin B_{12}. Bile also has a high amount of metabolic analogs. The biliary vitamin B_{12} can be reabsorbed, and the feces have a higher concentration in vitamin B_{12} analog because true B_{12} is absorbed better, and some analogs are produced in the large intestine. Urine has significant amounts only when intakes are excessive.

Functions. There are only two known systems that use vitamin B_{12}: methylmalonyl-CoA isomerase for the conversion of methylmalonate to succinate from propionate and folate regeneration. The involvement of vitamin B_{12} with l-C metabolism and its interaction with folate may explain how B_{12} deficiency is associated with impaired DNA synthesis. $N^{5,10}$ methylene THFA is used to methylate deoxyuridylate to form thymidylate for DNA synthesis. THFA is used to form $N^{5,10}$ methylene THFA. THFA has to be regenerated from N^5 methyl THFA, and the major pathway utilizes B_{12} with a methyl group from N^5 methyl THFA added to homocysteine to form methionine.

Vitamin B_{12} may be involved with folate transport and storage. A yet to be defined relationship between vitamin B_{12} and myelin synthesis may be the origin of the neurological effects of B_{12} deficiency. This could be a result of a build-up of methylmalonate with subsequent competitive inhibition of malonyl CoA, through the incorporation of branched chain fatty acids or glutathione reduction.

Deficiency. Deficiency of vitamin B_{12} is associated with plasma levels of less than 80 pg/ml, with the normal between 200 and 900 pg/ml; however, these levels may vary as much as 80 pg/ml within a day, and a small number of patients with clinical disease responsive to parenteral vitamin B_{12} can have false normal plasma levels. Excess urinary methylmalonic acid can be used also as a measure of vitamin B_{12} deficiency. Patients with achlorhydria, stomach, ileum, or pancreas dysfunction or following gastrointestinal (GI) resection for problems associated with diseases such as Crohn's disease may become deficient because of a low absorption of vitamin B_{12}. This can occur also with the genetic pernicious anemia characterized by the lack of IF. Fish tape worm infection and the use of H_2 blockers such as cimetidine at dosages of 1 g/day can also lead to a decreased absorption of vitamin B_{12}. Bacterial overgrowth due to the blind loop syndrome with bacterial utilization of vitamin B_{12} is another cause of deficiency. Furthermore, low intake owing to a strict vegan diet without special sources of B_{12} can result in deficiency. This low intake of true vitamin B_{12} may be combined with the higher intake of analogs that can occur in special food sources. The use of nitrous oxide as an anesthetic can produce excessive analog formation with the development of a functional B_{12} deficiency (see Chapters 16 and 46).

Vitamin B_{12} deficiency can present as a psychiatric, neurological, or hematological disease.

Symptoms of a B_{12} deficiency are pernicious anemia (megaloblastic-enlarged red cells and marrow reticulocytes), numbness and tingling in extremities, poor musculature coordination, ataxia, bilateral vision failure, and mental changes (moodiness, poor memory, depression, delusions, or psychosis). As discussed in Chapter 46, pernicious anemia can present as a psychiatric, neurological or hematological disease, or as a combination. The therapy for B_{12} deficiency differs if it results from nutritional causes or from impaired absorption: for a nutritional deficiency, 0.05 mg IM weekly for 2 weeks followed by 1 μg/day oral, for vegetarians or B_{12} rich food; for deficiency caused by impaired absorption, 100 μg IM monthly, or at least every 3 months. Vitamin B_{12} has a large safety margin, so therapy can employ dosages beyond the recommended daily requirement. For many pernicious anemia patients, oral doses of vitamin B_{12} of 1000 μg a day avoids IM injections and is effective, as well as practical and inexpensive (Lederle, 1991; Hathcock and Troendle, 1991).

FOLIC ACID

Channing in 1824 identified an anemia associated with pregnancy and the puerperium that was fatal when combined with nutritional stress of repeated pregnancies. Osler in 1919 showed that this anemia was different from the one caused by B_{12} deficiency. The turning point in the study of folic acid research was when Lucy Wills and colleagues in 1937 cured, by feeding autolyzed yeast, the *tropical macrocytic anemia* that was associated with pregnancy and a diet of primarily white rice and bread. Later, Wills developed an animal model with monkeys of an anemia that could be cured with a crude but not purified extract of liver. The factor present in the crude extract was named the Will's factor. The term *folic acid* was coined by Mitchell and associates in 1941, because this factor was obtained from more than 10 tons of spinach (Latin: *folium*, leaf). Within 5 years, pteroylglutamic acid (pteGlu) was purified (Stokstad, 1943), crytallized (Pfiffner, 1943), and synthesized (Angier, 1946).

PteGlu as such is not found in foods; it is prepared synthetically. It is made up of a pterin moiety, 2,4 substituted (xanthoxine), paraaminobenzoic acid (PABA), and glutamic acid. The disodium salt is slightly water-soluble. There are many forms of folic acid, mainly reduced forms such as THFA (FH_4) with four hydrogens at positions 5 through 8, dihydrofolate (7,8), and with R groups linkages occurring through N 5 or N 10, or both. The N-linked compounds include N^5 formyl THFA, N^{10} formyl THFA, N^5 formimino THFA, $N^{5,10}$ methenyl, $N^{5,10}$ methylene, and N^5 methyl THFA. They may all have glutamate residues through a peptide linkage on the γ carboxyl ranging from 1 to 11 with the average being 7 or 3. The THFAs are unstable in light, and THFA is labile to oxidation. PteGlu, the oxidized form, is more stable but is labile at pH less than 4. Because of the labile nature of folic acid, most of it is lost with long cooking and canning.

Absorption, Metabolism, Excretion. There is a brush border conjugase that hydrolyzes the glutamate tail of folic acids in foods. Like vitamin B_{12}, the ileum is the primary site of absorption, being both passive and facilitated, probably actively with sodium. The percentage absorbed with the diet can be high, up to 90%, but is usually lower, around 50%.

Transport from the intestine, at low physiological levels, occurs after it is converted to N^5 methyl THFA. At high levels of intake milligrams it may get into blood as unmethylated THFA. The amount of folic acid stored by the human is intermediate from 2 to 10 mg, lasting 3–6 months with no intake; about half of this is in the liver as polyglutamates, which are bigger and have a greater charge. It is transported as the free acid, competitively bound to plasma proteins with a low affinity and on high affinity–binding proteins. Although these high affinity–binding proteins are present in low concentrations, carrying about 5% of the serum folate, they may have an important function in the transport of folic acid from cerebrospinal fluid.

Further metabolism occurs after cellular uptake by active mechanisms. There are polyglutamate synthetases that add glutamates, and conjugases that remove glutamates from the tail for its release from cells; both may be related to activity and storage. The formation of THFA requires vitamin C and NADPH for both formation of DHFA and THFA. The conversion of THFA to $N^{5,10}$ methylene and back involves the conversion of serine to glycine and requires vitamin B_6. THFA can go also to N^5 formimino THFA with the conversion of N formimino-L-glutamate to glutamate. Then N^5 formimino THFA can be metabolized to $N^{5,10}$ methenyl THFA with deamination, which can go to either THFA for nucleotide synthesis or $N^{5,10}$ methylene using NADPH. $N^{5,10}$ methylene can be converted to N^5 methyl with $FADH_2$. N^5 methyl THFA is a storage form that has to be converted to THFA and then to other forms for functioning; this requires B_{12}. Without vitamin B_{12}, THFA that enters the metabolic pool may not be regenerated and thus may explain some of the effects of B_{12} deficiency.

Folic acid is excreted mainly in the bile with 0.1 mg/day reabsorbed. The amount excreted is increased with liver disease. It is excreted also in the urine as a metabolite after 9–10 oxidation and acetylation in liver, as acetamidobenzoylglutamate. Also filtered by the kidney is N^5 methyl THFA, but most is reabsorbed.

Functions. The primary function of folic acid is as a methyl group donor. One specific involvement is in the synthesis of thymidylate for DNA. $N^{5,10}$ methylene THFA supplies a methyl group to form thymidylate from deoxyuridylate. This process is the rate-limiting step in DNA formation. The result of folic acid deficiency is megaloblastosis (see Chapter 46) in association with bone-marrow pancytopenia (anemia and leukopenia). Megaloblastosis occurs also in the rest of the body, including the GI tract. Another key function of folic acid is for purine synthesis using $N^{5,10}$ methenyl THFA to N^{10} formyl THFA, which involves formate incorporation. Folic acid is involved also in amino acid conversions: serine to glycine and back; homocysteine to methionine, which also requires vitamin B_6; and histidine to glutamic acid. N^{10} formyl THFA incorporation into choline is crucial to initiation of protein synthesis and methylation of transfer RNA by either transmethylation with methionine or methylation of ethanolamine to choline.

Deficiency. Normal plasma levels of folic acid are 5–16 ng/ml with marginal deficiency defined as less than 3 ng/ml. Normal red blood cell (RBC) levels are greater than 200 ng/ml, and deficient individuals usually have less than 160 ng/ml. Deficiency can be detected also by using tests for defective DNA synthesis and by measuring urinary excretion of formiminoglutamate (FIGLU), urocanate, formate, or amino-imidazole carboxamhistidine (AIC, which may occur also with B_{12} deficiency). Pregnant women are likely to be deficient; in fact, up to one third of pregnant women may exhibit a deficiency. Alcoholic patients are also at risk because of increased loss of folic acid metabolites in the bile. Increased mean corpuscular value (MCV) is one of the common laboratory findings in alcoholism. Increased excretion of folic acid occurs with dialysis also. Diets high in glycine or methionine increase the need for folic acid. There are significant drug interactions with phenytoin, barbiturates, antimalarial drugs, methotrexate (an analog), aminopterin (an analog that interferes with dihydrofolic reductase), and oral contraceptives (that interfere with polyglutamate tail metabolism and decrease absorption by 50%; see Chapters 42 and 58).

Signs and symptoms of deficiency are wasting of body tissue, diarrhea, and macrocytic anemia. The deficiency associated with pregnancy can be prevented by folate supplements. Folate deficiency can be corrected with

Folate deficiency and macrocytic anemia are common in pregnant women and alcoholic patients.

15 mg IM followed by 5 mg/day orally for a month with 100 μg/day for 1–4 months or one serving of fresh fruit or vegetable a day.

General References

Alhadeff LC, Gualtieri T, Lipton M: Toxic effects of water-soluble vitamins. Nutr Rev 42:33–40, 1984.

Briggs M (ed): Vitamins in Human Biology and Medicine. Boca Raton, FL: CRC Press, 1981.

Brown ML (ed): Present Knowledge in Nutrition. 6th ed. Washington, DC: The Nutrition Foundation, 1990.

England S, Seiffer S: The biological functions of ascorbic acid. Annu Rev Nutr 6:365–406, 1986.

Food and Nutrition Board: Recommended Dietary Allowances. 10th ed. Washington, DC: National Academy of Sciences, National Research Council, 1989.

Hathcock JN, Troendle GJ: Oral cobalamin for treatment of pernicious anemia. JAMA 265:96–97, 1991.

Hunt SM, Groff JL: Advanced Nutrition and Human Metabolism. New York: West Publishing Company, 1990.

Lederle, FA: Oral cobalamin for pernicious anemia—Medicine's best-kept secret. JAMA 265:94–95, 1991.

Machlin LJ (ed): Handbook of Vitamins. New York: Marcel Dekker, 1990.

Plesofsky-Vig N, Brambl R: Pantothenic acid and coenzyme A in cellular modification of proteins. Annu Rev Nutr 8:461–482, 1988.

Sauberlich HE: Bioavailability of vitamins. Prog Food Nutr Sci 9:1–33, 1985.

Shane B, Stokstad ELR: Vitamin B_{12}-folate interrelations. Annu Rev Nutr 5:115–141, 1985.

Shils ME, Young VR (eds): Modern Nutrition in Health and Disease. 7th ed. Philadelphia: Lea & Febiger, 1988.

Winter J: True Nutrition, True Fitness. Clifton, NJ: Humana Press, 1991.

64

Interactions: Drug Allergy; Drug-Drug; Drug-Food

Roger K. Cunningham
Cedric M. Smith

Untoward reactions to drugs are not always allergic.

Untoward reactions to drugs can occur for essentially four reasons: allergy, intolerance, idiosyncrasy, or adverse drug interaction. Thus, in any given case of suspected untoward reaction to a drug, it is important to recognize the exact nature of the underlying cause.

Intolerance to a given drug occurs when side effects occur at doses tolerated by most individuals. In other words, there is a quantitative difference in the response to the drug. The condition is sometimes referred to as *metareaction.* An example would be severe respiratory depression occurring in a patient given a fraction of the usual analgesic dose of morphine. The underlying basis for intolerance is poorly understood, but probably reflects one extreme of a gaussian distribution of responses in the population.

Idiosyncrasy, in contrast, is used most often to describe a state of altered drug metabolism. An example would be the development of hemolytic anemia in individuals deficient in glucose-6-phosphate dehydrogenase who are given primaquine. The underlying basis for this state is clearly genetic, and the nature of the untoward response is qualitative.

Adverse drug interactions are examined in detail in later sections of this chapter.

Allergy and Drugs

Each of these states must be distinguished from *allergy,* or hypersensitivity. Allergy to a drug must be developed, in contrast to intolerance and idiosyncrasy, which are both pre-existing states. The capacity to develop an allergy pre-exists, but for the allergic state to develop an individual must have prior exposure. Thus, to understand allergy, one must understand the underlying immunological principles that govern both the development of the condition and the production of symptoms.

IMMUNE RESPONSE

Allergy is the result of an immune response.

Allergy or hypersensitivity is the result of an immune response to a drug or preparation. As in any immune response, the substance is recognized by the immune system as foreign. That is, the compound is seen as antigenic. Once this occurs, a portion of the drug becomes sequestered into the lymphatics of the host, is processed immunologically, and evokes the production of two types of effectors—specific antibodies will be produced against the antigen by B lymphocytes, and specifically sensitized effector cells (T lymphocytes) will be elaborated in large numbers. Both the B and the T lymphocytes are precommitted to the structure on the drug molecule with which they react. In the case of a large complex molecule, as many drugs are, several different structures may be recognized by different precommitted T and B cells. The point is that as many different structures as possible are detected as foreign, and hence the response is polyclonal. More than one precommitted precursor cell can respond to different parts of the molecule, each capable of reaction with one small portion of the foreign molecule. That is, a normal immune response has multiple specificities within it. The antigen, in turn, is a mosaic of different substructures that give rise to a spectrum of specificities. The word *epitope* has been coined to describe each individual structure that has been identified. The totality of the epitopes make up the antigen.

During a normal immune response, both humoral (antibody-mediated) and cellular immunity are evoked. This is also the case with allergy. After exposure to the antigen (allergen), a period ensues during which an immune response is being mounted but no symptoms appear (the lag period). After this time, IgM antibodies begin to appear in the serum of the individual. These are soon replaced by antibodies of the same specificity but of different chain structure. The cells producing antibody undergo what is known as a *switch* from IgM to the other classes of antibody: IgG, IgA, and IgE. It is the IgE that is involved in allergy for reasons that are described later. None of the other antibody classes has been shown to be responsible for allergy.

Molecules below a certain size are generally not recognized by the immune system as foreign. For example, proteins with molecular weights below approximately 10,000 do not evoke an immune response. Yet many drugs are recognized as foreign even though their molecules are quite small. This phenomenon is due to what is known as the *hapten effect.* Many drugs have the capacity to bind to constituents of the blood. For example, penicillin binds to human serum albumin and erythrocytes. By so binding, the penicillin, in some individuals, causes a distortion of the normal structure of albumin or the erythrocyte membrane, or both. The distorted albumin or membrane is now recognized by the recipient as foreign and no longer *self.* During the immune response that follows, the penicillin forms an epitope on the larger structure and antibodies are produced both to the penicillin and to the altered host component. The altered host component has become a *carrier* for the hapten penicillin. The important point here is that after antibody has once been formed, the carrier is not required for reaction of the antipenicillin antibodies with penicillin to occur.

Some drugs are haptens.

Some drugs are antigenic by themselves. As might be expected, these are usually large molecules. In general, the more complex the molecule, the more readily it will evoke an immune response. In addition, although any drug can be responsible for evoking allergy, some drugs have a much higher propensity to produce hypersensitivity than others. Drugs that are chemically reactive are more likely to sensitize a person than those that are less reactive.

THE PATIENT'S ROLE IN HYPERSENSITIVITY

The other side of hypersensitivity is the patient. Some individuals are much more likely to develop allergy than others. Such persons are said to be

Individuals vary in the tendency to become allergic.

atopic, and their condition is termed *atopy.* As a rule, individuals with many known allergies are more likely to develop allergies to drugs than are those who have no such history. Such individuals can be detected only by a careful history. The importance of a thorough history cannot be overstated.

In passing, it should be noted that in spite of careful questioning of patients, sometimes the person will deny sensitivity to a substance that is, in fact, responsible for the allergic attack. For example, a patient develops an untoward reaction to injected penicillin, yet denies ever having received the drug. There may be several explanations for this: (1) The drug was administered at an early age and the person was not informed. (2) Many food animals are routinely fed rations containing prophylactic antibiotics. Milk that contains penicillin is produced by cows that are treated for mastitis with the drug.

Patient history is essential but may not be accurate.

IMMEDIATE AND DELAYED HYPERSENSITIVITY

Hypersensitivity is divided into two types: immediate and delayed. *Immediate hypersensitivity* is so called because the reaction occurs within a period of minutes to hours. The state is due to IgE antibodies that have been produced through prior exposure to the allergen. *Delayed hypersensitivity,* sometimes referred to as *cell-mediated hypersensitivity,* is mediated by T lymphocytes and normally requires 36–48 hours to develop. The classic model for delayed hypersensitivity is the tuberculin response, which requires 2–3 days to develop a skin lesion after challenge with purified protein derivative (PPD).

Immediate hypersensitivity is due to IgE.

Immediate Hypersensitivity

Immediate hypersensitivity can manifest itself in many forms. The most severe form is a complete collapse of a patient into shock within minutes of administration of the drug (anaphylaxis). This usually occurs with administration of the drug by a route that maximizes the uptake of the drug, such as intravenously or by inhalation. Fortunately, anaphylaxis is a relatively uncommon event. Hypersensitivity is manifested more generally in organ systems other than the vascular compartment. Rashes, urticaria (giant hives), wheezing, photosensitivity, and gastrointestinal symptoms are the more common manifestations of allergy. Fever may accompany the administration of an offending drug. The so-called drug fever is typically a low-grade fever that waxes and wanes in synchrony with taking the drug. The fever may not develop for several days, but when it appears it may increase incrementally as more drug is taken. Cessation of a low-grade fever following discontinuation of a drug is good evidence that allergy is involved.

The role of IgE antibodies in immediate hypersensitivity is certain. The role of other antibodies is highly doubtful. From time to time, a role for some subclasses of IgG has been postulated, but evidence is lacking. IgE antibodies are known to bind to mast cells and circulating basophilic granulocytes. They do so by virtue of a receptor on these cells that specifically binds to the Fc portion of the IgE antibody molecule. This leaves each mast cell with a bound layer of IgE antibodies oriented with the Fc bound to the membrane and the Fab portion of the antibody free to react with allergen (epitope). Each mast cell carries IgE antibodies of all the specificities present in a given individual. That is, a statistical representation of antibodies to all the substances that an individual is allergic to are distributed among her or his mast cells.

Mast cells are involved in immediate hypersensitivity.

The atopic individual, then, after becoming immunized, carries IgE antibodies bound to mast cells. At low concentrations of IgE, there is little problem, even when the allergen is introduced into the patient. However, as exposure to the allergen continues, the amount of IgE increases, just as in any other immune response. At a certain critical concentration, when an allergen encounters a mast cell, it is able to react with the Fab portion of two IgE molecules that are side by side on the cell surface, both having specificity for that particular allergen. When this occurs, a signal is transduced through the membrane, causing the mast cell to degranulate. Degranulation in turn leads to the release of pharmacologically active compounds that produce the symptoms of the allergic reaction.

The list of mediators released by mast cells is prodigious and continues to grow. The major mediators are histamine, eosinophil chemotactic factor (ECF), slow-reacting substance of anaphylaxis (SRS-A), platelet-activating factor (PAF), and heparin. Secondarily, serotonin, prostaglandins, and kinins of many specificities are elaborated. The net effect of these mediators is the induction of smooth muscle contraction, increased vascular permeability, hypersecretion of glands, and alterations in blood coagulability. Subsequently, physiological alterations result that include hypoxia, necrosis, hemorrhage, and shock. The exact symptoms exhibited by the patient depend on the organ in which the release has occurred. In humans, most organs are rich in mast cells; thus, the so-called shock organ can be almost any organ. The route of exposure often determines which organ will manifest allergic symptoms. The term *shock organ* simply refers to that organ in which the allergic reaction occurs for a given species of animal. For example, the bronchioles of the lung in a guinea pig are more richly endowed with mast cells than is any other organ of the animal. When challenged, an allergic guinea pig will exhibit pulmonary distress. A dog will show liver failure. Humans have rich accumulations of mast cells in virtually every major organ, and almost any one can be the shock organ.

Mast cells release mediators.

Delayed Hypersensitivity

The other type of hypersensitivity is delayed hypersensitivity. This limb of the immune response is due to T lymphocytes that are specific for the allergen. As in humoral hypersensitivity, precommitted T cells undergo a clonal expansion caused by exposure to the allergen. These cells are then distributed throughout the lymphatics. When allergen is introduced into a hypersensitized individual, the T cells, through a poorly understood signaling system, migrate to the area where the allergen is located. Here, they react with the allergen by means of a specific receptor and begin to secrete a series of mediators collectively known as *lymphokines*. The lymphokines have an effect on both tissue and circulating cells. As a result of their release, inflammation ensues. The delay in reaction is due to the time required for the T cells to migrate into the offending area of allergen. It is important to realize that in a given individual both immediate and delayed hypersensitivity may occur sequentially.

Delayed hypersensitivity is due to T cells.

DIAGNOSIS

The diagnosis of allergy can be difficult. The concentration of IgE in an individual's serum can be helpful, but often is uninformative. More difficult still can be the identification of the offending substance. Patients may be taking more than one drug. They may be taking a drug that they do not

Diagnosis can be difficult.

report. There are a few testing methods: Skin testing by challenging is commonly used as a screening method. Weak dilutions of common or suspected allergens are placed on the skin, and a needle is used to scratch the skin beneath the drop of allergen solution. If IgE antibodies to the allergen are bound to the mast cells in the individual's skin, a *wheal and flare* reaction will occur within a few minutes. This is typically a reddening of the skin and induration at the site of challenge.

Tests are available.

Tests for specific IgE are now available. The most widely used is the radioallergosorbent test (RAST). In this assay, the serum of the patient is mixed with allergen in a test tube. The allergen is usually bound to a particle or is otherwise made insoluble. If antibody is present, it will bind to the allergen. Note that both IgE and IgG are bound by this procedure. The bead is then washed to remove unbound protein, and the amount of IgE present is estimated by treating with a radiolabeled antibody to human IgE that does not cross-react with IgG. Such examinations are usually made against large panels of known allergens and require only small amounts of a patient's serum.

The classic method of demonstrating allergy, no longer in use, was the Prausnitz-Küstner (PK) reaction, in which the serum of an atopic individual was injected intradermally into the skin of a normal individual at many sites. Twenty-four to 48 hours later, individual suspected allergens were injected into each site, which was then observed for a wheal and flare reaction.

TREATMENT

What should be done if one suspects that a patient is allergic to a drug? If the patient is currently taking the drug, it should be immediately discontinued until evidence is available that the drug is not an allergen to this individual. If the history suggests that the person is allergic to a drug, change to a different drug. The use of any drug should be balanced against its potential for harm. Once a patient is hypersensitive, he or she should be considered hypersensitive for life. There is at present no method for reversing hypersensitivity in any individual. In general, the reactions begin as mild skin manifestations, but they grow progressively more severe with continued challenge.

In specific situations, desensitization can help.

In particular situations — for example, a construction worker who has become severely allergic to wasp venom — attempts can be made to *desensitize* the individual. This is done by repeated injections of venom into the individual, beginning with a highly diluted preparation that evokes no untoward reaction. Over time, the injections are continued using increasing concentrations of venom, until such time that an undiluted injection is tolerated, at least reasonably well. It might seem paradoxical that to extinguish an allergy, injections of the offending allergen are used, but some amount of success has been achieved with this method. Why the method works is difficult to explain. The commonest, and probably most accepted, explanation maintains that the secondary IgE response is feeble and the bulk of antibodies produced are IgG. Thus, the idea is to take advantage of the brisk secondary production of IgG, which then competes for the allergen before it can reach the IgE bound to mast cells (see Chapter 62).

HEMOLYTIC ANEMIA

Some drugs can cause anemia.

There remains an additional topic that should be mentioned in discussing immunological reactions to drugs — hemolytic anemia. Although this is not strictly an allergic response, this phenomenon is another manifestation of antibodies produced against a given drug. The antibodies in these cases are not IgE but rather IgG and IgM. The drug binds to the patient's erythrocytes and serum proteins as described previously. Antibodies that can react with the erythrocyte-bound drug are then evoked. Complement may be activated as well. In either case the presence of immunoglobulin or complement components causes a shortened life-span of the antibody-coated cells, which are prematurely removed by the reticuloendothelial system. Antibodies specific for red cell antigens may also be evoked.

Only a proportion of patients with antibody to drugs will develop a hemolytic anemia severe enough to require treatment, and the condition may be entirely overlooked in the absence of symptoms. In fact, the majority of patients who develop a positive antiglobulin test do not have decreased red cell survival times. When the condition is suspected, however, the diagnostic test of choice is a direct Coombs (antiglobulin) test on the patient's erythrocytes. A positive direct Coombs test is highly correlated with hemolytic anemia caused by drugs but is not associated invariably with it. For example, methadone may cause the development of a positive Coombs test but is not associated with hemolytic anemia. Table 64–1 lists some drugs that cause positive direct antiglobulin tests and that are also associated with hemolytic anemia. This table lists only the most well-documented offenders.

Most cases of drug-induced, antibody-mediated hemolytic anemia can be resolved by merely discontinuing the drug. In some instances, however, when the drug is stopped the hemolytic episode persists, even after the drug is undetectable. The reasons for this are not entirely clear, but it is postulated that these patients represent those in whom autoantibodies have been made to the patient's own red cells directed against normal antigens of the cell.

Table 64–1 SOME DRUGS THAT CAUSE POSITIVE DIRECT ANTIGLOBULIN TESTS AND THAT ARE ASSOCIATED WITH HEMOLYTIC ANEMIA	
α-methyldopa	p-aminosalicylate
Cephalothin	Penicillin
Chlorpromazine	Phenacetin
Chlorpropamide	Aminopyrine
Dipyrone	Quinidine
Insulin	Quinine
Isoniazid	Stibophen
Mefenamic acid	Streptomycin
Melphalan	Sulfonamides

Drug-Drug and Drug-Food Interactions

Drug-drug and drug-food interactions may involve diagnostic, prophylactic, or therapeutic drugs. Moreover, some drugs may interfere with diagnostic tests. Although some drug interactions are deliberately sought by the physician because they are advantageous, such as in the use of antagonists in poisonings, the majority of drug interactions are unplanned, and most (but certainly not all) drug interactions are disadvantageous. When a disadvantageous, or adverse, drug interaction has occurred or is likely to occur, the physician may choose to (1) discontinue one (or both) of the drugs; (2) modify the dose of one (or both) of the drugs; or (3) continue without change, despite the potential or actual interaction, *if the benefit clearly outweighs the risk.*

Although an adverse drug interaction is potentially a problem whenever any two drugs are given in close time proximity, situations in which the probability of important interactions are likely to occur or be unappreciated are (1) *whenever starting or changing therapy,* (2) *whenever a new physician takes over responsibility for a patient,* and (3) *whenever a therapeutic regimen is unexpectedly disappointing in that it fails to have an expected beneficial effect or has resulted in an unexpected adverse effect.*

Drug interactions are the rule for most patients.

Expect drug interactions — beneficial and adverse.

TYPES AND MECHANISMS OF DRUG-DRUG INTERACTIONS

Since the number of possible drug-drug and drug-food interactions is astronomical, the only practical way to deal with the potentially frequent problems are the following:

Computer-based advice on potential interactions is now available for every medication order.

■ *Have immediately available for consultation a resource that lists all the known interactions (see Chapter 68).*

■ *Possess an understanding of the main types and mechanisms of drug interactions.*

The different types and mechanisms of interactions are presented in relation to the time course of events following the administration of a drug. Each of these types is illustrated by a few of many possible examples.

Incompatibilities in Intravenous Solutions. Examples: Mixing tetracyclines and sulfonamides may cause the latter to precipitate. Methicillin and ampicillin are easily degraded in the presence of drugs affecting the pH, whereas chloramphenicol and tetracyclines often inactivate other drugs in the intravenous (IV) solution. Carbenicillin and gentamicin interact in the IV solution with loss of activity (direct chemical reaction between the two drugs). Among the general caveats is the undesirability of mixing solutions containing proteins with other solutions. Therefore, before modifying any IV solutions, consult a definitive, up-to-date manual on IV solutions and compatibilities, such as the Handbook of Injectable Drugs (Trissel, 1990).

Foods and nutrition increase, decrease, or have no effect on a given drug's actions.

Interaction in the Gastrointestinal Tract. Examples: Foods in the gastrointestinal tract may increase, decrease, or have no effect on the absorption of specific drugs (Table 64–2).

Table 64–2 EXAMPLES OF REPORTED FOOD EFFECTS ON ABSORPTION OF DRUGS FROM THE GASTROINTESTINAL TRACT (Selected Drugs)*

	Some Drugs Whose Absorption Is:		
Decreased by Food	*Increased by Food*	*Not Affected by Food*	*Increased or Decreased, Depending on Preparation*
Alcohol	Carbamazepine	Prednisone	Theophylline and erythromycin
Aspirin	Phenytoin	Procainamide	
Ibuprofen	Diazepam	Verapamil	
Diclofenac	Dicoumarol		
Piroxicam	Diftalone		
Cimetidine	Erythromycin estolate		
Digoxin	Erythromycin ethylsuccinate		
Hydrocortisone	Erythromycin stearate		
Levodopa	Nitrofurantoin		
Methyldopa	Griseofulvin		
Metronidazole	Hydralazine		
Nafcillin	8-methoxsalen		
Penicillin G	Metoprolol		
Penicillin V	Labetalol		
Ampicillin	Propranolol		
Amoxicillin	Spironolactone		
Isoniazid	Chlorothiazide		
Rifampin			
Cefaclor			
Cephalexin			
Ketoconazole			
Sulfonamides			
Tetracycline			
Doxycycline			
Erythromycin stearate (film-coated tablets)			
Sotalol			
Atenolol			

* See also Winstanley PA, Orme ML: The effects of food on drug bioavailability. Br J Clin Pharmacol 28:621–628, 1989.

A constipating or laxative drug may increase or decrease, respectively, absorption of another drug. Some antibiotics alter vitamin K synthesis by gut flora, which can result in an increase in the effect of oral anticoagulants (see Table 64–4). Some antibiotics, especially erythromycin, alter the bacterial degradation of digoxin. Cholestyramine can bind a variety of acidic drugs and thus interfere with their absorption.

Direct Interaction in the Blood and Adjacent Compartments. Examples: Neutralization of a venin by an antivenin. Antagonism of heparin by protamine by direct chemical reaction.

Examples illustrate the variety of the potential interactions.

Interactions Involving Plasma Proteins. Examples: Warfarin and phenylbutazone are both largely bound to albumin in the plasma. Phenylbutazone can therefore displace warfarin from its binding sites and increase warfarin's effect. Other examples of displacement reactions identify some important displacers — phenylbutazone, indomethacin, tolbutamide. Among important displacees are warfarin, phenytoin, tolbutamide.

Interference With the Distribution or Storage of One Drug by Another. Examples: A decrease in uptake of ^{131}I by the thyroid gland in the presence of large doses of stable iodine or iodine-containing contrast media. The quinidine-induced decreased binding of digoxin in peripheral tissues such that digoxin levels in plasma increase.

Interaction at the Receptor. Examples: Competitive and allosteric antagonism at the receptor, such as the antagonism of the effect of morphine by naloxone. Potassium depletion (corticosteroids, diuretics, amphotericin B, diarrhea, poor potassium intake, and so on) increases the reactivity to cardiac glycosides and to neuromuscular blocking agents, an effect probably mediated by interactions at their receptors. Halogenated hydrocarbon anesthetics may increase the cardiac arrhythmic effects of catecholamines.

Modification of the Metabolism of One Drug by Another. Examples: Alcohol-disulfiram (ANTABUSE) reaction. Disulfiram inhibits the metabolism of ethanol such that acetaldehyde levels rise to levels that cause a number of unpleasant and undesirable symptoms. (A variety of drugs other than disulfiram, including metronidazole and some cephalosporins, may cause this reaction.)

Examples of other potential interactions are the following:

Enzyme Induction. Example: Barbiturates or a diet rich in Brussels sprouts increases the hepatic metabolism of warfarin. In addition many drugs are inducers of drug metabolism, and many drugs besides warfarin are affected.

Interactions in relation to absorption, distribution, metabolism, excretion, and effect

Inhibition of Metabolism. Examples: Isoniazid inhibits metabolism of phenytoin. Allopurinol inhibits metabolism of azathioprine and 6-mercaptopurine. Ethanol inhibits the metabolism of diazepam. Caffeine inhibits the metabolism of phenylpropanolamine (PPA). Cimetidine inhibits the metabolism of warfarin, diazepam, theophylline, and other drugs.

Modification of the Excretion of One Drug By Another. Examples: Increased excretion of phenobarbital after administration of a systemic alkalinizing drug because of ionic trapping. Probenecid competes with penicillin for renal excretion. Cimetidine competes with procainamide for renal excretion. Quinidine decreases renal clearance of digoxin.

Addition of Effects or Side Effects of Each Drug. Examples: Additive central nervous system depression in a patient who takes a benzodiazepine while consuming alcohol. These additive effects can be illustrated by a number of drug effects, such as the additive effects on anticoagulation by aspirin plus warfarin; the potential heart block with verapamil plus a β-adrenergic blocking drug; hypotension produced by enalapril or captopril plus a vasodilating drug; the additional chemotherapeutic effects that may be achieved with penicillin plus an aminoglycoside against steptococcal infections; the increased neuromuscular block produced by a curarizing drug by an aminoglycoside; the increased risk of ototoxicity with ethacrynic acid plus an aminoglycoside.

Subtraction in Drug Effects. Examples: Preservation of normal serum potassium concentration in the presence of a potassium-losing diuretic by the simultaneous administration of a potassium-sparing diuretic. The anticoagulant effects with an oral contraceptive with warfarin. The decrease in the emetic effects of cisplatin by metoclopramide.

Cross-reactions

Cross-tolerance, addition, potentiation.

- *Allergic cross-reactions* were discussed earlier in this chapter. Some examples are allergic cross-reactions to thiazide diuretics—furosemide or sulfonylureas—in a patient allergic to sulfonamides or the cross-reaction of a patient *allergic* to penicillin to a chemically similar compound such as a cephalosporin.
- *Pharmacological cross-reactions.* Examples: a patient *hyperreactive* or *intolerant* to morphine is at risk of having a cross-reaction to a *pharmacologically* similar compound such as meperidine.

Cross-tolerance. Examples: Tolerance to meperidine in a patient tolerant to morphine or any morphine agonist. Cross-tolerance among benzodiazepines and to benzodiazepines in those who consume large quantities of alcohol.

The antagonistic aspects of many drug interactions constitute the basis for many of the treatments of poisonings and overdoses. These are covered in Chapter 60 on toxicology and poisoning.

DRUG-FOOD INTERACTIONS

Drug-food and food-drug interactions.

The effects of foods on drug absorption have been discussed briefly earlier (see Table 64–2). Looked at from the other direction, drugs can interact with foods and nutrition along the analogous dimensions as drug-drug interactions. In addition, drugs can alter the nutritional effects of a variety of foods including vitamins; some of these kinds of interactions are mentioned in Chapter 63.

Not only can drugs interact in terms of drug actions and nutrition but drugs can also alter food palatability, appetite, and consumption. Some drugs directly affect taste, whereas others appear to influence appetite and consumption—either to increase or to decrease (Table 64–3). These effects have been used in therapy, for example to induce anorexia in obesity. However, of more widespread concern are the undesirable side effects on appetite and consumption of therapeutic drugs, for example the weight gain that antipsychotic or antidepressant agents can produce. A number of the more well established of these effects on appetite are listed in Table 64–3, and those affecting taste are discussed in detail in Chapter 26. Note that some drugs appear to cause an increased appetite in some patients and a decreased appetite in others.

Consideration of the material summarized in Tables 64–4 to 64–6 illustrates the importance of a full dietary history in most diagnostic work-ups and prior to initiation of drug therapy—all diagnostic histories should include information about the previous few days as well as the intake in relation to medications. Such a diet history should include all intake—including multivitamins (see Table 64–4), aspirin, laxatives, snacks of all kinds, alcoholic beverages, beverages—and the pattern and variability in eating habits.

Unfortunately, there are few pertinent, useful generalizations regarding the interactions of foods and drugs except that they do occur, that they can be clinically significant, and that individuals vary in terms of their responses to specific doses of specific drugs and in terms of the impact of food and its consumption on drug effects and conversely (see Table 64–5).

Careful attention to potential interactions among foods and drugs is especially warranted when (1) consumption is characterized by any large excesses, (2) there is a marked change in intake, or (3) any nutrient or class of nutrients is absent from the diet.

Taste, appetite, consumption, choice, and effects.

Dietary history as an essential part of the clinical history.

The major generalization: drug-food interactions occur.

Alcohol-food-drug interactions necessitate precise patient information and compliance.

Table 64–3 DRUGS THAT MODIFY APPETITE AND FOOD INTAKE

Suppress	Stimulate
Numerous drugs that evoke nausea or vomiting (~75% of all oral agents)	Androgens
Amphetamines*	Antihistamines and antiserotoninergic agents
Anticonvulsants	Benzodiazepines
Antineoplastic agents	Corticosteroids
Carbonic anhydrase inhibitors	Hypoglycemic agents
Diethylproprion*	Lithium
Digitalis glycosides	Oral contraceptives
Estrogens	Antipsychotic—phenothiazines and related agents
Fenfluramine*	Tricyclic antidepressants
Flurazepam	Marijuana
Indomethacin	
Levodopa	
Lithium salts	
Mazindol*	
Metronidazole	
MAO inhibitors	
Phenmetrazine*	
Phenteramine*	
Procainamide	
Tetracyclines	
Thiazide	
Tolazamide	
Also, experimentally, opioids, inosine, cholecystokinin	

* Drugs that have had some use in the treatment of obesity.

Table 64-4 DRUG-VITAMIN INTERACTIONS

Drug	Vitamin	Possible Mechanism	Possible Manifestation
Antibiotics, sulfa drugs, PABA	Vitamin K	Decreased vitamin K from intestinal bacterial metabolism	Hypoprothrombinemia
Anticonvulsants	Folic acid	Decreased absorption of folacin; competitive inhibition of dehydrofolate reductase; enzyme reduction	Megaloblastic anemia
	Vitamin D	Enzyme induction	Rickets; osteomalacia
	Vitamin K	Enzyme induction	Neonatal hemorrhage
Cholestyramine	Folic acid	Complexing of the vitamin	
	Vitamin B_{12}	Inhibition of intrinsic factor function	
	Vitamin A	Binding of bile salts	Osteomalacia
	Vitamin D	Binding of bile salts	Osteomalacia
	Vitamin K	Binding of bile salts	Osteomalacia
Colchicine	Vitamin B_{12}	Malabsorption of B_{12}	
Coumarin anticoagulants	Vitamin K	Antagonism	Hemorrhage
Estrogen-containing oral contraceptives	Folic acid	Inhibition of absorption of folic acid; increased synthesis of folate-binding macroglobulin;	Megaloblastic anemia
	Vitamin B_{12}	Enzyme induction	
	Vitamin B_6	Pyridoxine deficiency; competition for vitamin-binding sites	Depression
	Riboflavin		Deficiency
	Thiamin		Deficiency
	Vitamin C	Decreased absorption	Scurvy symptoms
Hydralazine	Vitamin B_6	Increased excretion of vitamin-drug complex	Peripheral neuropathy
Irritant cathartics	Vitamin D	Increased peristalsis; damage to the intestinal wall	Osteomalacia
Isoniazid	Vitamin B_6	Increased excretion of vitamin-drug complex; clinically effective antagonist of isoniazid toxicity	Peripheral neuropathy; generalized convulsion (infants); anemia
	Niacin	Competitive inhibition of vitamin coenzymes; secondary to vitamin B_6 deficiency	Pellagra
Levodopa	Pyridoxine	Antagonism by increasing rate of amino acid decarboxylation; note that carbidopa, as in Sinemet, inhibits this action of pyridoxine	Levodopa ineffective
Methotrexate	Folate	Inhibition of dihydrofolate reductase enzyme	Megaloblastic anemia
Mineral oil	Vitamin A	Lipid solvent	Rickets; osteomalacia in elderly
	Vitamin D	Lipid solvent	
	Vitamin K	Lipid solvent	
Neomycin	Vitamin B_{12}	Damage to the intestinal wall; inhibition of intrinsic factor function	
	Vitamin A	Damage to the intestinal wall; inhibition of pancreatic lipase; binding of bile salts	
Nitrous oxide (chronic)	Vitamin B_{12}	Block of B_{12} action	Megaloblastic anemia, blood dyscrasias
Potassium chloride	Vitamin B_{12}	Decreased ileal pH	
Pyrimethamine	Folic acid	Inhibition of dihydrofolate reductase enzyme	Megaloblastic anemia
Salicylates	Folic acid	Decreased protein binding of folate	Deficiency
	Vitamin C	Decreased tissue uptake	Deficiency
	Vitamin K	Antagonism	Increased bleeding
Sulfasalazine	Folic acid	Decreased absorption of folic acid	
Tetracycline	Vitamin C	Decreased tissue levels of vitamin C	
	Niacin	Decreased absorption with deficiency of niacin	
Triamterene	Folic acid	Inhibition of dihydrofolate reductase	Megaloblastic anemia
Trimethoprim	Folic acid	Inhibition of dihydrofolate reductase	Megaloblastic anemia

Table 64-5 SOME SELECTED DRUG-FOOD INTERACTIONS

Drug	Food	Adverse Interaction
MAO inhibitors	Foods containing tyramine (liver, pickled herring, cheese, bananas, avocados, soup, beer, wine, yogurt, sour cream, yeast, nuts)	Palpitations, headache, hypertensive crises
Digitalis	Licorice	Digitalis toxicity
Griseofulvin	Fatty foods	Increased blood levels of griseofulvin
Timed-release drug preparations	Alcoholic beverages	Increased rate of release for some
Lithium	Decreased sodium intake	Lithium toxicity
Quinidine	Antacids and alkaline diet (alkaline urine)	Quinidine toxicity
Thiazide diuretics	Carbohydrates	Elevated blood sugar
Tetracyclines	Dairy products high in calcium; ferrous sulfate; or antacids	Impaired absorption of tetracycline
Vitamin B_{12} (cyanocobalamin)	Vitamin C — large doses	Precipitate B_{12} deficiency
Fenfluramine	Vitamin C addition	Antagonism of antiobesity effect of fenfluramine
Thiamine	Blueberries, fish Alcohol	Foods containing thiaminases Decreased intake, absorption, utilization
Benzodiazepines	Caffeine	Antagonism of antianxiety action

Table 64-6 SUMMARY OF ADVERSE INTERACTIONS OF DRUGS WITH ALCOHOLIC BEVERAGES

Drug	Adverse Effect With Alcohol
Anesthetics, antihistamines, barbiturates, benzodiazepines, chloral hydrate, meprobamate, narcotics, phenothiazines, tricyclic antidepressants	1. Increased central nervous system depression due to additive effects 2. Decreased sedative or anesthetic effects with chronic use due to tolerance
Phenothiazines	Increased extrapyramidal effects, drug-induced parkinsonism
Diazepam (Valium)	Increased diazepam blood levels, varying with beverage
Acetaminophen (Tylenol)	Hepatotoxicity
Anticoagulants	Chronic — decreased anticoagulant effect Acute — increased anticoagulant effect
Bromocriptine	Nausea, abdominal pain (due to increased dopamine-receptor sensitivity?)
Disulfiram (Antabuse), chloramphenicol, oral hypoglycemics, cephalosporins, metronidazole, quinacrine, moxalactam	Disulfiram-alcohol syndrome reactions
Cycloserine	Increased seizures with chronic use
Imipramine	Lower blood level in alcoholic patients
Isoniazid	Increased hepatitis incidence, decreased isoniazid effects in chronic alcohol use due to increased metabolism
Propranolol (Inderal)	Decreased tremor of alcohol withdrawal; decreased propranolol blood levels
Sotalol	Increased sotalol blood levels
Phenytoin (Dilantin)	Decreased metabolism with acute combination with alcohol; but increased metabolism with chronic alcohol consumption; increased risk of folate deficiency
Nonsteroidal anti-inflammatory agents (aspirin and related)	Increased gastrointestinal bleeding

Alcoholic beverages: food or drug?

    Some view alcoholic beverages as a food, others emphasize that alcohol is a drug. From either point of view, alcohol consumption has a number of important interactions with drugs (see Table 64–6).

General References

Allergy and Drugs

Graziano FM, Lemanske RF Jr (eds): Clinical Immunology. Baltimore: Williams & Wilkins, 1989.

IgE, Mast Cells and the Allergic Response. Ciba Found Symp 147. New York: John Wiley & Sons, 1989.

Middleton E Jr, Reed CE, Ellis EF, et al (eds): Allergy: Principles and Practice. 3rd ed, 2 vols. St. Louis: CV Mosby, 1988.

Sampter M, Talmadge DW, Frank MM, et al (eds): Immunological Diseases. 4th ed, 2 vols. Boston: Little, Brown, 1989.

Drug-Drug and Drug-Food Interactions

Books and computer-based information sources for drug interactions and drug-food interactions are cited in the references for Chapter 68.

Carr CJ: Food and drug interactions. Annu Rev Pharmacol Toxicol 22:19–29, 1982.

Carrato PL: Drugs and food: When the dangers increase. RN 51:65–67, 1988.

Drug Interactions and Side Effects Index. (Current edition.) Oradell, NJ: Medical Economics Company.

Drug-Nutrient Interactions (Journal)

Food interacting with MAO inhibitors. Med Lett Drugs Ther 31:11–12, 1989.

Halsted CH, Heise C: Ethanol and vitamin metabolism. Pharmacol Ther 34:453–464, 1987.

Hamberg O, Ovesen L, Dorfeldt A, et al: The effect of dietary energy and protein deficiency on drug metabolism. Eur J Clin Pharmacol 38:567–570, 1990.

Interactions of drugs with alcohol. Med Lett Drugs Ther 23:33–34, 1981.

Levitsky DA: Drugs, appetite, and body weight. In Roe DA, Campbell TC (eds): Drugs and Nutrients: The Interactive Effects, 375–408. New York: Marcel Dekker, 1984.

Linnoila M, Mattila MJ, Kitchell BS: Drug interactions with alcohol. Drugs 18:299–311, 1979.

Melander A, Lalka D, McLean A: Influence of food on the presystemic clearance of drugs. Pharmacol Ther 38:253–267, 1988.

Ovesen L, Lyduch S, Idorn ML: The effect of a diet rich in Brussels sprouts on warfarin pharmacokinetics. Eur J Clin Pharmacol 34:521–523, 1988.

Ovesen L: Drugs and vitamin deficiency. Drugs 18:278–298, 1979.

Peterkin K, Black DV (eds): Directory of On-line Healthcare Databases, 5th ed. Oak Park, IL: Medical Data Exchange, Alpine Guild, 1990.

Powers D et al: Food-Medication Interactions, 6th ed. Tempe AZ: Food-Medication Interactions, 1988.

Rizach MA, Hillman CDM: The Medical Letter Handbook of Adverse Drug Interactions. New Rochelle, NY: The Medical Letter, 1989 and subsequent editions.

Roe DA: Drug-induced Nutritional Deficiencies, 2nd ed. New York: AVI, 1985.

Roe DA: Geriatric nutrition. Clin Geriatr Med 6:319–334, 1990.

Roe DA: Handbook on Drug and Nutrient Interactions: A Problem-Oriented Reference Guide, 4th ed. Chicago: American Dietetic Association, 1989.

Roe DA: Nutrient and drug interactions. Nutr Rev 42:141–154, 1984.

Roe DA: Therapeutic significance of drug-nutrient interactions in the elderly. Pharmacol Rev 36:109S–122S, 1984.

Smith C, Bidlack W: Dietary concerns associated with the use of medications. J Am Diet Assoc 84:901–914, 1984.

Spiller GA (ed): Nutritional Pharmacology. New York: AR Liss, 1981.

Trissel LA: Handbook of Injectable Drugs, 6th ed. Bethesda, MD: American Society of Hospital Pharmacists.

Weiner M, Bernstein IL: Adverse Reactions to Drug Formulation Agents: A Handbook of Excipients. New York: Marcel Dekker, 1989.

Welling P: Nutrient effects on drug metabolism and action in the elderly. Drug-Nutr Interact 4:173–207, 1985.

Winick M: Control of Appetite. New York: John Wiley & Sons, 1988.

Winstanley PA, Orme ML: The effects of food on drug bioavailability. Br J Clin Pharmacol 28:621–628, 1989.

Yue QY, Svensson JO, Alm C, et al: Interindividual and interethnic differences in the demethylation and glucuronidation of codeine. Br J Clin Pharmacol 28:629–637, 1989.

65

Histamine and H₁-Receptor Antagonists

F. Estelle R. Simons
Keith J. Simons

Histamine

Preformed histamine is stored in cytoplasmic granules of tissue mast cells and blood basophils.

Synthesis and Storage

Histamine is formed from the decarboxylation of the amino acid histidine by the enzyme L-histidine decarboxylase. Most histamine is stored preformed in cytoplasmic granules of tissue mast cells and blood basophils, in close association with proteoglycans such as heparin or chondroitin 4-sulfates that make up the granule matrix. In humans, mast cells are found in the loose connective tissue of all organs, especially around blood vessels, nerves, and lymphatics of the skin, upper and lower respiratory tract, and gastrointestinal mucosa. Non–mast cell sites of histamine formation and storage include epidermal cells, gastric mucosa, central nervous system (CNS) neurons, and regenerating or rapidly growing tissue.

Histamine plays a central role in the immediate hypersensitivity and allergic responses, in gastrointestinal secretion, and in neurotransmission.

Release

Histamine is released from mast cells and basophils by antigens and by numerous nonantigenic factors.

Activation of human mast cells and basophils by antigen bridging of membrane-bound immunoglobulin E (IgE) aggregates IgE receptors and initiates a cascade of metabolic events in the membrane, leading to opening of calcium channels and release of secretory granules containing histamine and other preformed pharmacologically active chemicals.

Some substances stimulate release of histamine from mast cells and basophils directly and without prior sensitization. These include clinically useful materials such as morphine, succinylcholine, tubocurarine, and radiocontrast media; and nontherapeutic substances such as the polypeptides in stinging insect venoms, low-molecular-weight peptides cleaved from complement, basic polypeptides such as bradykinin and substance P, cytokines, histamine-releasing factors from a variety of cells, and polybasic materials such as compound 48/80. Nonspecific tissue injury produced by scratching or by physical factors such as cold can also stimulate release of histamine from mast cells directly.

Once released, histamine diffuses rapidly into the surrounding tissues and appears in the blood within minutes. Histamine concentrations in plasma are normally very low, but transient elevations of plasma histamine are found after experimental challenge with antigen or with physical factors such as exercise in patients with asthma and after challenge with physical factors such as cold, vibration, or pressure in patients with urticaria.

Metabolism and Excretion

Although the turnover of histamine in secretory granules in mast cells and basophils is very slow, epidermal cells, gastric mucosa, CNS neurons, and any tissues undergoing growth or regeneration synthesize and metabolize histamine at a rapid rate.

Only 2 or 3% of histamine is excreted unchanged in the urine. Most is metabolized to *N*-methylhistamine by *N*-methyltransferase (50–70%) or to imidazoleacetic acid by diamine oxidase (histaminase) (30–45%).

Histamine Receptors

The types of histamine receptors described to date include: H_1-receptors, which play an extremely important role in allergic disorders; H_2-receptors, which are important in gastric acid secretion, in immune system down-regulation, and in feedback control of histamine release; H_3-receptors, which are involved in modulation of cholinergic neurotransmission in human airways, also in CNS functioning, and in the feedback control of histamine synthesis and release; and low-affinity non–H_1-, non–H_2-, and non–H_3-receptors, which may be involved in histamine's role as an intracellular messenger. Histamine receptors have been defined pharmacologically for many years, but their actual structure and method of signal transduction by G proteins are now being elucidated. The gene for the H_2-receptor was cloned in 1991; the genes for the H_1- and H_3-receptors have not yet been cloned.

> There are at least three types of histamine receptors.

Pharmacological Actions

Histamine, through its action on H_1-receptors, produces contraction of vascular and bronchial smooth muscle, causes pruritus, increases cyclic guanosine monophosphate (GMP), increases prostaglandin generation, decreases atrioventricular node conduction time, activates airway vagal afferent nerves, and stimulates cough receptors.

Histamine works on both H_1- and H_2-receptors to increase the amount (H_2) and the viscosity (H_1) of mucous glycoprotein secretion from goblet cells and bronchial glands in the respiratory epithelium and to increase vascular endothelial permeability, thereby decreasing the blood pressure and causing flushing, headache, and tachycardia.

Histamine, through its action on H_2-receptors, increases gastric acid secretion and increases the permeability of the respiratory epithelium. It inhibits histamine release from basophils, inhibits chemotaxis of basophils, eosinophils, and neutrophils, and elevates cyclic adenosine monophosphate (AMP) in eosinophils. It induces a lymphocyte suppressor factor, activates suppressor T cells, and reduces cytolytic ability, lymphocyte proliferation, immunoglobulin production, and lymphokine production. In monocytes it inhibits secretion of complement proteins, and in neutrophils it inhibits lysosome release as well as superoxide and peroxide production.

Use in Clinical Medicine

The histamine-induced wheal-and-flare response in the skin is widely used in clinical trials to assess the efficacy of H_1-receptor antagonists. When a dilute solution of histamine is introduced into the epicutaneous region or injected intradermally, a characteristic sequence of events known as the *triple response of Lewis* occurs. At the injection site, a small, localized red area appears within minutes, becoming maximal in 1 minute. A wheal then

> Histamine elicits a wheal-and-flare response in the skin.

replaces the original red area at the injection site, becoming maximal in 10 minutes. A brighter red flush or flare develops beyond the wheal, also becoming maximal in 10 minutes. The initial red area is due to the direct vasodilator effect of histamine, the wheal reflects histamine's capacity to cause edema, and the flare is due to histamine-induced stimulation of local axon reflexes causing vasodilatation indirectly.

Histamine, in a weak isotonic solution administered by inhalation, is used in pulmonary function testing to assess bronchial hyperreactivity in patients with clinically stable chronic asthma.

Histamine is no longer used to test parietal cell function and gastric acid secretion because, in the dose required parenterally for this purpose, it causes flushing and warmth of the skin, a decrease in systolic blood pressure, acceleration of heart rate, headache, and other distressing side effects.

Antihistamines: History

Terfenadine, the first relatively nonsedating H_1-receptor antagonist, was introduced in the late 1970s.

Antihistamines have been widely used in clinical medicine since the early 1940s, when phenbenzamine, pyrilamine, diphenhydramine, and tripelennamine were synthesized. In the early 1970s, antihistamines with a gastric antisecretory effect were developed; subsequently H_2-receptor antagonists such as cimetidine, ranitidine, and famotidine have revolutionized the treatment of peptic ulcer and related gastric hypersecretory states (see Chapter 45). In the late 1970s, the introduction of the first relatively nonsedating H_1-receptor antagonist, terfenadine, was another important milestone in antihistamine research. Recently, the era of H_3-receptor antagonist investigation has begun.

H_1-Receptor Antagonists

Table 65-1 PHARMACOLOGICAL ACTIONS OF H_1-RECEPTOR ANTAGONISTS

Relax vascular and bronchial smooth muscle
↓ Pruritus
↓ Cyclic GMP
↓ Prostaglandin generation
↑ Atrioventricular node conduction time
Inhibit activation of airway vagal afferent nerves
↓ Cough receptor stimulation
↓ Amount and viscosity of mucous glycoprotein secretion in respiratory epithelium*
↓ Vascular permeability*
↓ Hypotension*
↓ Flushing*
↓ Headache*
↓ Tachycardia*
↓ Release of mediators of inflammation†
↓ Recruitment of inflammatory cells†
↓ Early and late response to antigen†

* These are also H_2-receptor antagonist effects.
† Some, but not all, H_1-receptor antagonists have these effects.

BASIC PHARMACOLOGY

Structure and Classification

H_1-receptor antagonists bear some structural resemblance to histamine; and, like histamine, they contain an ethylamine group. The traditional classification of H_1-receptor antagonists according to chemical structure (e.g., ethanolamine, ethylene diamine, alkylamine, piperazine, piperidine, and phenothiazine) is becoming anachronistic, because some of the second-generation H_1-receptor antagonists, such as terfenadine, astemizole, and azelastine, do not fit readily into the old classification system. Cetirizine, a piperazine, is the carboxylic acid metabolite of the first-generation H_1-receptor antagonist hydroxyzine (Fig. 65-1).

Pharmacological Activities

At low concentrations, H_1-receptor antagonists are reversible, competitive antagonists of the actions of histamine on H_1-receptors. The principal pharmacological actions of H_1-receptor antagonists are to relax vascular and bronchial smooth muscle, decrease pruritus, decrease cyclic GMP, decrease prostaglandin generation, increase atrioventricular node conduction time, inhibit activation of airway vagal afferent nerves, and decrease cough receptor stimulation. Like the H_2-receptor antagonists, they also decrease glycoprotein secretion in the respiratory epithelium and decrease vascular endothelium permeability, hypotension, flushing, headache, and tachycardia (Table 65-1).

In addition to their H_1-blocking activity, some of the new H_1-receptor

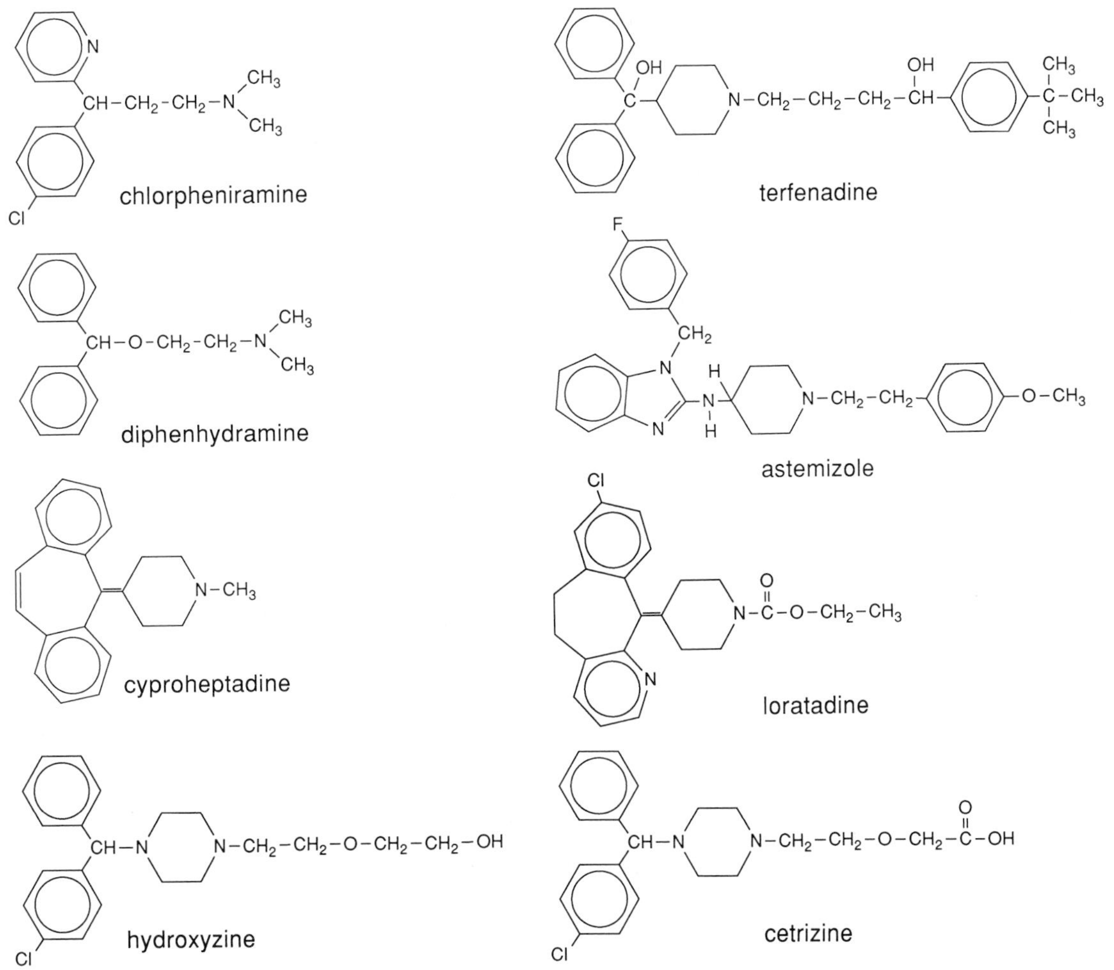

Figure 65-1

Chemical formulas of some representative first-generation H₁-receptor antagonists: chlorphen-iramine, an alkylamine; diphenhydramine, an ethanolamine; cyproheptadine, a piperidine; and hydroxyzine, a piperazine; and the second-generation H₁-receptor antagonists, terfenadine, astemizole, loratadine, and cetirizine, a piperazine.

antagonists such as terfenadine, loratadine, cetirizine, and azelastine have antiallergic properties; that is, they inhibit release of mediators of inflammation such as histamine and prostaglandin D_2 from mast cells and basophils. This effect occurs *in vitro* at "physiological" concentrations of the H₁-receptor antagonists and also *in vivo,* after usual therapeutic doses. Cetirizine also has an anti-inflammatory effect and inhibits recruitment of inflammatory cells, including eosinophils, neutrophils, and basophils, to the site of an immediate (type 1) hypersensitivity reaction (see Table 65–1; see also Chapter 28).

> Some of the new H₁-receptor antagonists have antiallergic properties.

Drowsiness from antihistamines has been attributed to inhibition of histamine *N*-methyltransferase with consequent elevations of CNS histamine concentrations and blockade of central histaminergic receptors. Antagonism of other CNS receptor sites, such as those for serotonin (5-hydroxytryptamine), acetylcholine, and α-adrenergic stimulation, may also be involved. The *second-generation* H₁-receptor antagonists, terfenadine, astemizole, loratadine, cetirizine, and azelastine, are relatively lipophobic and do not penetrate into the CNS as well as the first-generation H₁-receptor antagonists do. Furthermore, the second-generation H₁-receptor antag-

> Second-generation H₁-receptors do not penetrate into the CNS as well as the first-generation H₁-receptors do.

onists bind preferentially to peripheral H_1-receptors rather than to CNS H_1-receptors. Also, they are relatively free from antiserotonin effects, anticholinergic effects, and α-adrenergic blocking activity.

CLINICAL PHARMACOLOGY

Pharmacokinetics

H₁-receptor antagonists are reasonably well absorbed when administered orally.

H_1-receptor antagonists are reasonably well absorbed when administered by mouth, with peak serum concentrations reached approximately 2 hours after dosing. All the first-generation H_1-receptor antagonists and most of the second-generation H_1-receptor antagonists available currently are metabolized by the hepatic cytochrome P-450 system. Clearance rates and β-phase serum elimination half-life values are extremely variable, with half-life values ranging from approximately 24 hours or less for chlorpheniramine, brompheniramine, hydroxyzine, terfenadine, loratadine, and azelastine, to 9.5 days for astemizole and its active metabolites. Apparent volumes of distribution tend to be large. They are usually uncorrected for bioavailability because intravenous formulations are available for comparison with oral formulations for only two H_1-receptor antagonists—chlorpheniramine and diphenhydramine (Table 65–2).

Children have shorter serum elimination half-life values for H_1-receptor antagonists than adults do, and the elderly may have prolonged values compared with those of young adults. Serum elimination half-life values of H_1-receptor antagonists generally increase with the increasing age of the patient. The serum elimination half-life of most H_1-receptor antagonists is prolonged in patients with severe hepatic dysfunction.

Cetirizine, the relatively nonsedating carboxylic acid metabolite of hydroxyzine, has unique pharmacokinetic properties. Unlike other H_1-receptor antagonists, it is not extensively metabolized by the hepatic cy-

Table 65–2 PHARMACOKINETICS AND PHARMACODYNAMICS OF H_1-RECEPTOR ANTAGONISTS

H_1-Receptor Antagonist	β-Phase Serum Elimination Half-Life (Hours)	Significant Wheal Suppression After a Single Dose (Hours)*
First-Generation		
Chlorpheniramine	24.4 (11.0)‖	24
Brompheniramine	24.9	9
Triprolidine	2.1	—
Diphenhydramine	9.2 (5.4)‖	10
Hydroxyzine	20.0 (7.1)‖	36
Second-Generation		
Terfenadine†	17.0	12–24
Astemizole	9.5 days‡	§
Cetirizine	6.6–10.6 (7.0)‖	24
Loratadine	11.0	12–24
Azelastine	25	12–24

* Dose-dependent; see specific references for doses used.
† Terfenadine metabolite I.
‡ Includes $t_{1/2}$ of hydroxylated metabolites.
§ A single dose of astemizole does not suppress the wheal and flare very well, but after a short course of treatment (7 days) suppression may last for weeks.
‖ Serum elimination half-life in children.

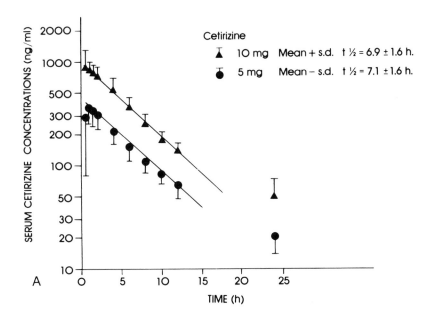

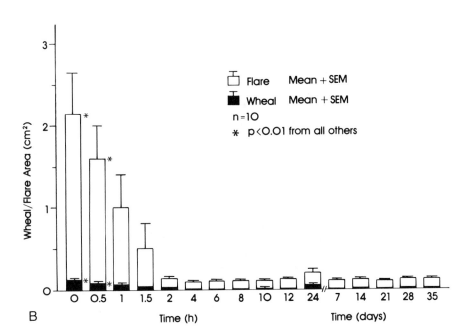

Figure 65-2

A, In a double-blind, parallel-group study of a single oral dose of cetirizine 5 mg in 10 children with allergic rhinitis versus a single oral dose of cetirizine 10 mg in 9 children with allergic rhinitis, the serum elimination half-life of cetirizine was approximately 6.9–7.1 hours. *B,* A single-dose of cetirizine 5 mg in children significantly suppressed the mean histamine-induced wheal-and-flare areas resulting from epicutaneous tests with histamine phosphate, 1 mg/ml, from 1 to 24 hours postdose. During the subsequent 5 weeks, the wheal-and-flare suppression 12 hours after the cetirizine dose did not differ significantly on days 7, 14, 21, 28, and 35. (From Watson WT, Simons KJ, Chen XY, Simons FE: Cetirizine: A pharmacokinetic and pharmacodynamic evaluation in children with seasonal allergic rhinitis. J Allergy Clin Immunol 84:457–464, 1989.)

tochrome system; rather, 70% of a dose of cetirizine appears as unchanged drug in the urine within 72 hours. It has a mean serum elimination half-life value of 6.6–10.6 hours in adults and 7 hours in children (Fig. 65–2A). However, in adults with decreased renal function, the half-life may be increased to 18 hours.

Breast milk concentration versus time curves parallel serum concentration versus time curves in single-dose studies of H_1-receptor antagonists.

Pharmacodynamics: Relationship of Efficacy to Serum Concentrations

Maximal antihistaminic effects of the H_1-receptor antagonists occur several hours after peak serum concentrations have passed and persist even when serum concentrations of the parent compound have declined to the lowest limits of analytical detection. H_1-receptor antagonists should therefore be

Figure 65 – 3

In a single-dose, double-blind, seven-way cross-over study in 20 healthy male adults, chlorpheniramine 4 mg, astemizole 10 mg, loratadine 10 mg, terfenadine 60 mg, terfenadine 120 mg, cetirizine 10 mg, and placebo differed significantly in their suppressive effect on the histamine-induced wheal. The rank order of suppression was placebo (*least* suppressive), chlorpheniramine 4 mg, astemizole 10 mg, loratadine 10 mg, terfenadine 60 mg, terfenadine 120 mg, and cetirizine 10 mg (*most* suppressive). (From Simons FE, McMillan JL, Simons KJ: A double-blind, single-dose, cross-over comparison of cetirizine, terfenadine, loratadine, astemiozole, and chlorpheniramine versus placebo: Suppressive effect on histamine-induced wheals and flares during 24 hours in normal subjects. J Allergy Clin Immunol 86:540–547, 1990.)

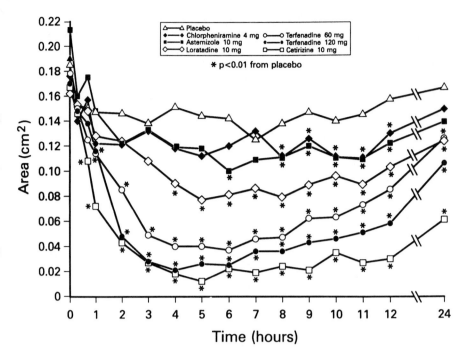

To achieve maximal efficacy, H_1-receptor antagonists should be given before an anticipated allergic reaction.

given *before* an anticipated allergic reaction, if possible, in order to achieve maximal efficacy. The duration of action of these medications, as assessed objectively by suppression of the histamine- or allergen-induced wheal and flare in the skin or subjectively by suppression of symptoms of, for example, rhinoconjunctivitis or urticaria, is much more prolonged than might be expected from consideration of the serum elimination half-life values (Fig. 65–3; see also Fig. 65–2).

The degree and duration of wheal-and-flare suppression relate to H_1-receptor antagonist dose as well as to the serum elimination half-life of the drug. Some first-generation H_1-receptor antagonists, such as tripelennamine and triprolidine, in manufacturers' recommended doses, are not very potent in suppressing the wheal and flare. Others, such as chlorpheniramine and hydroxyzine, are relatively potent and should not yet be discarded from therapeutic use; a single-dose of chlorpheniramine or hydroxyzine suppresses the histamine-induced wheal and flare for 24 hours.

A single dose of the second-generation H_1-receptor antagonist loratadine (10 mg) suppresses the histamine-induced wheal and flare for 12–24 hours. A single dose of terfenadine (60–120 mg) or cetirizine (10 mg) significantly suppresses the wheal-and-flare response to histamine for 24 hours. A single dose of astemizole (10 mg) is not very effective in suppressing the histamine-induced wheal and flare, but after a short course of astemizole (10 mg daily) has been discontinued, the histamine-induced wheal and flare may remain suppressed for 6 or 8 weeks (see Table 65–2 and Fig. 65–3).

Lack of Subsensitivity

Long-term administration of first-generation H_1-receptor antagonists may be associated with an *apparent* decrease in efficacy. This phenomenon has been attributed to autoinduction of hepatic metabolism and increased hepatic clearance of the H_1-receptor antagonist, with consequent lower serum and, presumably, lower tissue concentrations of the medication. Support for this concept was based on limited data obtained in dogs administered diphenhydramine or chlorcyclizine by mouth for a few weeks. In a study designed to reexamine this issue, however, dogs administered hydroxyzine daily for 150 days (21 weeks), intramuscularly to ensure compliance, had somewhat higher mean serum hydroxyzine concentrations at the end of the treatment course than on the first day of treatment, significantly slower mean clearance rates, and longer mean serum half-life values on days 30, 60, 120, and 150 than after the first dose of hydroxyzine on day 1. No evidence of autoinduction of metabolism was found.

Furthermore, humans do not eliminate chlorpheniramine or terfenadine more rapidly during long-term dosing than during short-term dosing, and the efficacy of chlorpheniramine, loratadine, terfenadine, or cetirizine in suppressing skin tests to histamine or in relieving rhinoconjunctivitis symptoms does not diminish over a period of 4 – 12 weeks, as demonstrated in studies in which compliance was monitored rigorously (Fig. 65 – 2B). The apparent subsensitivity reported years ago with the first-generation H$_1$-receptor antagonists may have been due, at least in part, to poor compliance because of sedation or lack of efficacy.

EFFICACY IN TREATMENT OF ALLERGIC DISORDERS

H$_1$-receptor antagonists provide relief of allergic rhinoconjunctivitis symptoms. They have a modest bronchodilator effect in patients with asthma. They effectively relieve pruritus, new wheal formation, and duration of whealing in patients with urticaria; and first-generation H$_1$-receptor antagonists effectively relieve pruritus in patients with atopic dermatitis. The effectiveness of H$_1$-receptor antagonists in treatment of upper respiratory tract infections and in otitis media is controversial. Formulations and recommended dosages of representative H$_1$-receptor antagonists are listed in Table 65 – 3.

Table 65 – 3 FORMULATIONS AND DOSAGES OF REPRESENTATIVE H$_1$-RECEPTOR ANTAGONISTS

Generic (Trade Name)	Formulation	Recommended Dose
First-Generation		
Chlorpheniramine maleate (many named products)	Syrup, 2.5 mg/5 ml; tablets, 4 mg; time-release, 8, 12 mg; parenteral solution, 10 mg/ml	Pediatric,* 0.35 g/kg/24 hours; adult, 8 – 12 mg b.i.d.‡
Diphenhydramine hydrochloride (Benadryl)	Children's liquid, 6.25 mg/5 ml; elixir, 12.5 mg/5 ml; capsules, 25 or 50 mg; parenteral solution, 50 mg/ml	Pediatric,* 2.5 mg/kg/24 hours; adult, 25 – 50 mg t.i.d.‡
Hydroxyzine hydrochloride (Atarax)	Syrup, 10 mg/5 ml; capsules, 10, 25, 50 mg	Pediatric,* 2 mg/kg/24 hours; adult, 25 – 50 mg o.d. (h.s.) *or* b.i.d.‡
Second-Generation (Relatively Nonsedating)		
Terfenadine (Seldane)	Suspension, 30 mg/5 ml;† tablet, 60 mg, 120 mg†	Pediatric, 3 – 6 years old: 15 mg b.i.d., 7 – 12 years old: 30 mg b.i.d.; adult, 60 mg b.i.d. *or* 120 mg o.d.‡
Astemizole (Hismanal)	Suspension, 10 mg/5 ml;† tablet, 10 mg	Pediatric,* 0.2 mg/kg/24 hours; adult, 10 mg o.d.‡
Loratadine (Claritin)	Tablet, 10 mg†	Adult, 10 mg o.d.‡
Cetirizine (Reactine)	Tablet, 10 mg†	Adult, 10 mg o.d.‡
Azelastine (Astelin)	Tablet, 2 mg†	Adult, 2 mg b.i.d.‡

Note: To minimize the potential central nervous system depressive effects of the first-generation H$_1$-receptor antagonists listed in this table, many physicians now try to give as much as possible of the daily dose h.s.
* For patients weighing ≤ 40 kg.
† Not available in the United States at the time of publication.
‡ b.i.d. = twice a day; t.i.d. = three times a day; o.d. = once a day; h.s. = at bedtime.

Allergic Rhinoconjunctivitis

In patients with allergic rhinitis, histamine released in the immediate (type 1) hypersensitivity response binds to H_1-receptors on the blood vessels in the nasal mucosa, submucosa, and lamina propria. Histamine produces symptoms by inducing vasodilation through a direct effect on relaxation of the vascular smooth muscle and by increasing secretion from the submucous glands through a vagal reflex.

In studies in which patients with allergic rhinitis are challenged intranasally with antigens to which they are sensitized, H_1-receptor antagonists given by mouth relieve the sneezing, itching, and nasal discharge of the immediate reaction to allergen. Some second-generation H_1-receptor antagonists decrease release of mediators of inflammation such as histamine in nasal secretions.

In numerous placebo-controlled studies in which patients have recorded symptom scores over weeks or months, H_1-receptor antagonists have proved to be useful in ameliorating sneezing, itching, and nasal discharge and also for relief of ocular symptoms such as itching, tearing, and erythema (Fig. 65–4). They are not as effective in relieving congestion; hence, decongestants such as pseudoephedrine are sometimes added to the H_1-receptor antagonists in order to provide relief of congestion.

In randomized, prospective, double-blind studies in patients with seasonal or perennial rhinitis, the second-generation H_1-receptor antagonists have been generally found to be superior to placebo and comparable to a first-generation H_1-receptor antagonist such as chlorpheniramine. The second-generation H_1-receptor antagonists are used increasingly for the treatment of allergic rhinoconjunctivitis because they are relatively nonsedating. Terfenadine, 60 mg twice daily or 120 mg once daily, astemizole 10 mg daily, loratadine 10 mg daily, cetirizine 10 mg daily, and azelastine 2 mg twice daily are the doses recommended by the manufacturers as providing optimal efficacy with minimal likelihood of causing sedation or other adverse effects (see Table 65–3). Terfenadine seems to provide faster onset of symptom relief than that of astemizole, but in long-term studies, astemizole provides greater overall symptom relief than that obtained with

> H_1-receptor antagonists are useful in relieving sneezing, itching, and sneezing symptoms in patients with allergic rhinoconjunctivitis.

> Second-generation H_1-receptor antagonists are used increasingly for the treatment of allergic rhinoconjunctivitis because they are relatively nonsedating, unlike their first-generation counterparts.

Figure 65–4

Efficacy of terfenadine and chlorpheniramine versus placebo in patients with allergic rhinoconjunctivitis. Both H_1-receptor antagonists were effective in reducing sneezing and rhinorrhea but were not significantly more effective than placebo in relieving nasal congestion. The incidence of sedation in the terfenadine-treated group (7.6%) and in the placebo-treated group (2.4%) did not differ significantly. The incidence of sedation in the chlorpheniramine-treated group was 19%, significantly higher than in either the terfenadine- or the placebo-treated group. The physicians' pretreatment severity scores are presented in the upper left corners of each plot because no pretreatment severity of symptoms was obtained from the patients' diaries. (From Kemp JP, Buckley CE, Gershwin ME, et al: Multicenter, double-blind, placebo-controlled trials of terfenadine in seasonal allergic rhinitis and conjunctivitis. Ann Allergy 54:502–509, 1985.)

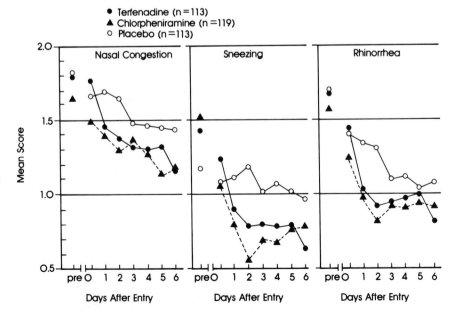

terfenadine. Terfenadine and loratadine appear to be comparable in onset of action and potency of allergic rhinoconjunctivitis symptom relief. Terfenadine may be slightly less potent than cetirizine.

Although H_1-receptor antagonists are extremely useful in the treatment of mild or moderate allergic rhinoconjunctivitis, other chemical mediators contribute to the inflammation in the nasal and conjunctival mucosa in this disorder, and these mediators are not blocked by H_1-receptor antagonists. Patients with severe allergic rhinoconjunctivitis generally require a topical intranasal corticosteroid for complete relief of symptoms.

Asthma

Histamine is an important mediator of asthma symptoms. Most of the histamine in the lungs is located in the secretory granules of mast cells in the airway. Specific challenge with allergen or nonspecific challenge with exercise or cold air stimulates the release of this preformed mediator of inflammation and contributes to airflow obstruction. Plasma histamine concentrations increase transiently after bronchoprovocation with inhaled allergen and in association with spontaneous acute asthma episodes. Histamine produces asthma symptoms by numerous mechanisms of action: causing bronchoconstriction and stimulation of cough receptors via H_1-receptors, causing increased permeability of the vascular endothelium and increased amount and viscosity of mucous glycoprotein secretion from bronchial glands and goblet cells via H_1- and H_2-receptors, and causing increased permeability of the respiratory endothelium via H_2-receptors.

The *first-generation* H_1-receptor antagonists chlorpheniramine, diphenhydramine, and hydroxyzine have some bronchodilator effect, but in clinically useful antiasthma doses they cause sedation and other adverse effects. The *second-generation* H_1-receptor antagonists terfenadine, astemizole, loratadine, cetirizine, and azelastine clearly have dose-related bronchodilator activity and a protective effect against histamine-, allergen-, exercise-, hyperventilation-, and cold, dry air–induced bronchospasm; like their predecessors, they do not protect against methacholine-induced bronchospasm. These medications provide relief from mild seasonal or chronic asthma symptoms when taken over weeks or months (see Chapter 62).

H_1-receptor antagonists are not drugs of first choice for asthma; however, patients with asthma who require H_1-receptor antagonists for treatment of concurrent rhinoconjunctivitis or urticaria will not be harmed by H_1-receptor antagonist treatment and may benefit from the antiasthma effect of the H_1-receptor antagonist.

H_1-receptor antagonists have a modest bronchodilator effect in asthmatic patients, although they are not drugs of first choice for asthma.

Chronic Urticaria

In prospective, controlled, double-blind studies in adults with chronic idiopathic urticaria, the first-generation H_1-receptor antagonists hydroxyzine, chlorpheniramine, and diphenhydramine and the second-generation H_1-receptor antagonists terfenadine, astemizole, cetirizine, and loratadine result in significant remission of symptoms compared with the relief provided by placebo. They reduce pruritus and the number, size, and duration of urticarial lesions. In chronic urticaria treatment, use of first-generation H_1-receptor antagonists is declining in comparison to the use of the second-generation H_1-receptor antagonists, which have an enhanced safety profile. Terfenadine and astemizole have been compared directly in patients with chronic urticaria, and astemizole seems to be the more potent of these two medications, although it may have a slower onset of action.

Anaphylaxis

Second-generation H$_1$-receptor antagonists are useful for control of itching in patients with urticaria.

In patients with anaphylaxis, for whom, of course, *treatment of first choice is epinephrine,* first-generation H$_1$-receptor antagonists such as chlorpheniramine and diphenhydramine, which are available in formulations for intravenous administration, are useful adjunctive treatment for control of pruritus, rhinorrhea, and other symptoms. Second-generation H$_1$-receptor antagonists are not currently recommended for use in anaphylaxis because they are not available in formulations for intravenous administration and there are no published studies of their efficacy in anaphylaxis.

Atopic Dermatitis

The mechanism of itching associated with atopic dermatitis remains unknown, but histamine is almost certainly involved to some extent because histamine concentrations are increased in the skin and in the plasma of patients with this disorder. First-generation H$_1$-receptor antagonists, which may have a CNS sedative effect, seem to relieve itching in atopic dermatitis better than second-generation H$_1$-receptor antagonists do, leading some investigators to conclude that the second-generation H$_1$-receptor antagonists should not replace the first-generation H$_1$-receptor antagonists in the treatment of this condition.

Other

H$_1$-receptor antagonists are widely used for symptomatic treatment of upper respiratory tract infections, although there is limited evidence from double-blind, placebo-controlled studies to support this practice. Similarly, H$_1$-receptor antagonists have been widely prescribed for patients with acute otitis media and for those with chronic otitis media with effusion, despite studies demonstrating that these medications do not significantly hasten the resolution of otitis media. The second-generation H$_1$-receptor antagonists have not been adequately studied in otitis media.

The first-generation H$_1$-receptor antagonists dimenhydrinate and promethazine are still used for prophylaxis in treatment of motion sickness; dimenhydrinate is also used in patients with vestibular disturbances. Second-generation H$_1$-receptor antagonists, acting either at the peripheral vestibular end-organ or at CNS structures *outside* the blood-brain barrier, may also be effective in the treatment of patients with these disorders. Terfenadine in a 300-mg dose gives some protection against motion sickness, and astemizole is effective in the treatment of chronic vertigo.

ADVERSE EFFECTS

First-Generation H$_1$-Receptor Antagonists

The elderly and patients with hepatic dysfunction are particularly prone to the adverse effects of first-generation H$_1$-receptor antagonists.

First-generation H$_1$-receptor antagonists may cause sedation, impairment of cognitive function, diminished alertness, slowed reaction times, confusion, dizziness, and tinnitus or anticholinergic effects such as dry mouth, blurred vision, and urinary retention. These symptoms, to which elderly patients and patients with hepatic dysfunction are particularly prone, correlate with peak serum concentrations. Some first-generation H$_1$-receptor antagonists, such as diphenhydramine, in ordinary therapeutic doses occasionally cause unusual adverse effects such as dystonic reactions. (Paradoxically, diphenhydramine may produce dramatic relief of acute dystonic reactions produced by antipsychotic drugs [see Chapter 21].)

Fatal or near fatal intoxication has been reported rarely following ingestion of massive overdoses of first-generation H_1-receptor antagonists such as tripelennamine, chlorpheniramine, cyproheptadine, dimenhydrinate, diphenhydramine, and hydroxyzine. Toxic encephalopathy or psychosis may occur and has even been reported after topical application of an H_1-receptor antagonist such as diphenhydramine; patients with epidermal breakdown are particularly susceptible to this adverse effect. Adults usually manifest lethargy, extreme drowsiness, or coma after first-generation H_1-receptor antagonist overdose, but young children may suffer from excitation, irritability, hyperactivity, insomnia, visual hallucinations, and seizures. Patients generally exhibit anticholinergic effects such as dryness of the mucous membranes, fever, flushed facies, pupillary dilatation, urinary retention, decreased gastrointestinal motility, and hypotension. Tachycardia, conduction disturbances, dysrhythmias, and occasionally, myocardial depression refractory to vasopressor support have been reported. Cardiorespiratory arrest and death may occur.

Treatment of a patient who has overdosed on a first-generation H_1-receptor antagonist consists of general supportive measures, such as evacuation of stomach contents, use of anticonvulsants, and hemodialysis. Shortly after ingestion of an H_1-receptor antagonist with strong antiemetic effects, gastric lavage may be more effective than a centrally acting emetic such as ipecac. There are no specific antidotes for H_1-receptor antagonist poisoning. Histamine itself is not helpful because the signs and symptoms of an H_1-receptor antagonist overdose are *not* related to histamine H_1-receptor blockade.

> There are no specific antidotes for H_1-receptor antagonist poisoning.

Second-Generation H_1-Receptor Antagonists

Although many of the *first-generation* H_1-receptor antagonists produce sedation or other CNS system symptoms in approximately 20% of users, the incidence of sedation or other CNS impairment in patients receiving a *second-generation* H_1-receptor antagonist such as terfenadine, astemizole, loratadine, cetirizine, or azelastine, in manufacturers' recommended doses, is comparable to the incidence of sedation in patients receiving placebo and is not clinically important in most patients (Fig. 65–5). The incidence of sedation is not zero, however; therefore, from time to time, physicians may encounter patients who complain of sedation after ingestion of a second-generation H_1-receptor antagonist. Also, when manufacturers' recommended doses of these medications are exceeded, the frequency of sedation may increase.

The relative lack of sedation produced by the new H_1-receptor antago-

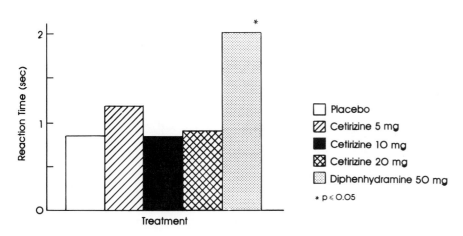

Figure 65–5

Double-blind, five-way cross-over study in 15 male volunteers, mean age 23.8 years, who ingested placebo, cetirizine 5, 10, or 20 mg, and diphenhydramine 50 mg. Numerous subjective measurements of drowsiness and objective measurements of mental performance were made 2 hours after dosing. During simulated accident avoidance in a simulated automobile-driving situation, diphenhydramine 50 mg slowed the reaction time significantly compared with placebo and with cetirizine 5, 10, and 20 mg. (From Gengo FM, Gabos C, Mechtler L: Quantitative effect of cetirizine and diphenhydramine on mental performance measured using an automobile driving simulator. Ann Allergy 64:520–526, 1990.)

Table 65-4 SOME TESTS USED FOR ASSESSMENT OF SEDATION AND OTHER CENTRAL NERVOUS SYSTEM ADVERSE EFFECTS OF H₁-RECEPTOR ANTAGONISTS

Subjective

Diary cards to record daytime sleepiness
Visual analog scales to record daytime sleepiness
Self-rating of sleepiness, impairment, and fatigue, using Stanford Sleepiness Scale or Profile-of-Moods
   questionnaire

Objective

Multiple sleep-latency test
Latency of P3 evoked electroencephalographic potentials (measure of sustained attention and cerebral
   processing speed)
Dynamic visual acuity
Pupillary light responses
Critical flicker fusion
Simple reaction time
Choice reaction time
Digit-symbol substitution
Monitoring of computer-simulated driving errors
Monitoring of actual driving errors

nists has been documented in numerous double-blind, placebo-controlled studies. Methods of assessment of sedation have been subjective (e.g., a diary card on which the patient records daytime sleepiness) and objective (e.g., multiple sleep-latency tests, in which the investigator obtains an electroencephalographic record of the length of time a patient takes to fall asleep during the day, under standardized conditions). Some of the different types of tests used for assessment of sedation and other CNS adverse effects of H₁-receptor antagonists are summarized in Table 65–4.

Investigators do not always find a strong correlation between subjective symptoms of sleepiness and objective measurements of CNS dysfunction such as prolongation of reaction time, indicating that patients may not necessarily recognize reduction in alertness and functioning produced by H₁-receptor antagonist ingestion.

Fixed-dose combinations of second-generation H₁-receptor antagonists with decongestants such as pseudoephedrine are associated with a higher incidence of insomnia and other CNS adverse effects than first-generation H₁-receptor antagonist/decongestant fixed-dose combinations, in which the CNS stimulation of the decongestant is counteracted by the sedation produced by the H₁-receptor antagonist.

Other adverse effects of second-generation H₁-receptor antagonists have been reported. Astemizole may cause appetite stimulation and inappropriate weight gain. A few patients receiving astemizole, most of whom have admitted to taking an overdose, have had prolonged QT intervals and the ventricular arrhythmia known as *torsade de pointes,* accompanied by syncope and cardiac arrest. Terfenadine, in very high doses, or when ingested by patients who are concomitantly taking ketoconazole or other cytochrome P-450 inhibitors, may also have cardiotoxic effects. Azelastine may alter taste perception and has been described as causing a metallic or bitter taste several hours after ingestion of liquids.

High doses of terfenadine or astemizole may have cardiotoxic effects.

Interaction of Second-Generation H₁-Receptor Antagonists With Central Nervous System–Active Substances

The first-generation H₁-receptor antagonists enhance the adverse psychomotor effects of ethanol, diazepam, and other CNS-active chemicals. The second-generation H₁-receptor antagonists, in manufacturers' recommended doses, have not been found to potentiate the CNS effects of these substances.

Safety in Pregnancy and Lactation

Although teratogenic effects of first-generation H₁-receptor antagonists (piperazines) have been noted in animals, fetal anomalies in humans have not been proved to be due to any H₁-receptor antagonists. A neonatal withdrawal syndrome has been described in infants born to mothers receiving large therapeutic doses of hydroxyzine or diphenhydramine immediately before parturition.

Embryo toxicity, fetal wastage, fetal anomalies, or other problems in pregnancy in humans have not been attributed to any of the second-generation H₁-receptor antagonists to date. The number of pregnant patients who have received these medications is small, however; and in most countries they are classified as Schedule C drugs or equivalent—that is, although there is no evidence that they are unsafe, they should be used only if expected benefits outweigh the unknown potential risks of toxicity. H₁-receptor antagonists are excreted in breast milk.

Summary

H₁-receptor antagonists differ considerably from one another in some aspects of basic pharmacology and in pharmacokinetics and pharmacodynamics. An understanding of these differences will facilitate their optimal clinical usage.

The second-generation H₁-receptor antagonists do not penetrate into the CNS as readily as the first-generation H₁-receptor antagonists do. They bind preferentially to peripheral rather than central H₁-receptors. In manufacturers' recommended doses, they cause no more sedation than a placebo does.

Because of their more favorable benefit/risk ratio, the second-generation H₁-receptor antagonists are replacing the first-generation H₁-receptor antagonists in the symptomatic treatment of allergic rhinoconjunctivitis and in relieving pruritus in patients with urticaria. They have a mild beneficial effect in patients with chronic asthma. They have *not* supplanted the first-generation H₁-receptor antagonists in atopic dermatitis treatment or as adjunctive treatment of pruritus and other symptoms in patients with anaphylaxis.

General References

Arrang JM, Garbarg M, Lancelot JC, et al: Highly potent and selective ligands for histamine H₃-receptors. Nature 327:117–123, 1987.

Birnbaumer L, Brown AM: G proteins and the mechanism of action of hormones, neurotransmitters, and autocrine and paracrine regulatory factors. Am Rev Respir Dis 141:S106–S114, 1990.

Campoli-Richards DM, Buckley MMT, Fitton A: Cetirizine: A review of its pharmacological properties and clinical potential in allergic rhinitis, pollen-induced asthma, and chronic urticaria. Drugs 40:762–781, 1990.

Clissold SP, Sorkin EM, Goa KL: Loratadine. A preliminary review of its pharmacodynamic properties and therapeutic efficacy. Drugs 37:42–57, 1989.

Gantz I, Schaffer M, DelValle J, et al: Molecular cloning of a gene encoding the histamine H₂-receptor. Proc Natl Acad Sci 88:429, 1991.

Garrison JC: Histamine, bradykinin, 5-hydroxytryptamine, and their antagonists. *In* Gilman AG, Rall TW, Nies AS, Taylor P (eds): Goodman and Gilman's The Pharmacological Basis of Therapeutics, 8th ed, 575–588. New York: Pergamon Press, 1990.

Gengo FM, Gabos C, Mechtler L: Quantitative effects of cetirizine and diphenhydramine on mental performance measured using an automobile driving simulator. Ann Allergy 64:520–526, 1990.

Howarth PH: Histamine and asthma: An appraisal based on specific H_1-receptor antagonism. Clin Exp Allergy 20:31–41, 1990.

Ichinose M, Barnes PJ: Inhibitory histamine H_3-receptors on cholinergic nerves in human airways. Eur J Pharmacol 163:383–386, 1989.

Kemp JP, Buckley CE, Gershwin ME, et al: Multicenter, double-blind, placebo-controlled trial of terfenadine in seasonal allergic rhinitis and conjunctivitis. Ann Allergy 54:502–509, 1985.

McTavish D, Goa KL, Ferrill M: Terfenadine: An updated review of its pharmacological properties and therapeutic efficacy. Drugs 39:552–574, 1990.

McTavish D, Sorkin EM: Azelastine. A review of its pharmacodynamic and pharmacokinetic properties, and therapeutic potential. Drugs 38:778–800, 1989.

Meltzer EO: Antihistamine- and decongestant-induced performance decrements. J Occup Med 32:327–334, 1990.

Richards DM, Brogden RN, Heel RC, et al: Astemizole. A review of its pharmacodynamic properties and therapeutic efficacy. Drugs 28:38–61, 1984.

Rimmer SJ, Church MK: The pharmacology and mechanisms of action of histamine H_1-antagonists. Clin Exp Allergy 20:3–17, 1990.

Saxena SP, Brandes LJ, Becker AB, et al: Histamine is an intracellular messenger mediating platelet aggregation. Science 243:1596–1599, 1989.

Simons FER: H_1-receptor antagonists: Clinical pharmacology and therapeutics. J Allergy Clin Immunol 84:845–861, 1989.

Simons FER: Loratadine, a non-sedating H_1-receptor antagonist (antihistamine). Ann Allergy 63:266–268, 1989.

Simons FER, McMillan JL, Simons KJ: A double-blind, single-dose, cross-over comparison of cetirizine, terfenadine, loratadine, astemizole, and chlorpheniramine versus placebo: Suppressive effects on histamine-induced wheals and flares during 24 hours in normal subjects. J Allergy Clin Immunol 86:540–547, 1990.

Simons FER, Simons KJ: Second-generation H_1-receptor antagonists. Ann Allergy 66:5–19, 1991.

Watson WTA, Simons KJ, Chen XY, Simons FER: Cetirizine: A pharmacokinetic and pharmacodynamic evaluation in children with seasonal allergic rhinitis. J Allergy Clin Immunol 84:457–464, 1989.

66

Legal Aspects of Drug Prescribing

Robert M. Cooper

This chapter is designed to provide the reader with a basic understanding of the legal aspects of drug prescribing. Because of the distribution of this text, this chapter deals primarily with federal law. The reader must keep in mind, however, that state law may at one extreme be stricter than federal law, and at the other, not even deal with a particular issue. Throughout the chapter, reference is made to examples of state requirements. Remember that stricter law always applies and that practitioners need to know the law in the state in which they practice.

Classification of Drugs

The 1951 Durham-Humphrey Amendment to the Federal Food Drug and Cosmetic Act established two major drug classifications:

1. Drugs sold only by prescription, known as *legend* or prescription drugs.
2. Drugs sold without prescription, otherwise known as nonlegend or over-the-counter (OTC) drugs.

Prescription drugs are defined as hypnotic or habit-forming drugs; drugs not safe for self-medication; and drugs classified as "new drugs." They require the use of the Rx legend, "CAUTION: Federal Law Prohibits Dispensing Without Prescription" on the manufacturer's label. Hence the term *legend drug*. The legend status of a drug is determined by the United States Food and Drug Administration (FDA).

OTC drugs are those that the FDA has approved for specific uses and in specific dosage and determined to be safe for a layman to use in self-medication. The drug must bear adequate directions for safe and effective use and provide warnings against misuse by the layman.

> The two major drug classifications are prescription drugs and over-the-counter drugs.

Who May Legally Prescribe?

It is up to the states to determine who may legally issue a prescription. States have indicated clearly that a licensed physician, dentist, and veterinarian may prescribe. Others may be able to do so also with full or qualified privileges (e.g., no controlled substance prescriptions, special training, and so forth), including podiatrists, osteopathic physicians, physician's assistants, and nurse practitioners. Throughout this chapter, the term *practitioner* is used to denote the persons authorized by a state to prescribe. Consult state law to determine who can prescribe and what qualifications might apply in your state.

When a practitioner is licensed by a state, it is done with regard to the areas of the practitioner's specific training and practice as set forth in the

> The states determine who can prescribe medication.

States Practice Act. For example, a veterinarian cannot practice on humans. In addition, a practitioner may prescribe only in the specific area of licensure. For example, a podiatrist may only write prescriptions for drugs used in the treatment of problems associated with the human foot.

Whereas a practitioner may be licensed to practice and write prescriptions in a state, in order to prescribe controlled substances (narcotic, stimulant, depressant, and hallucinogenic substances) the practitioner must register and obtain a Federal Drug Enforcement Administration registration number as well. The procedure is discussed later.

> Any practitioner who prescribes controlled substances must have a registration number from the Federal Drug Enforcement Administration.

Prescription Blanks

Whereas some states may require that a prescription blank be presented graphically in a certain way, or that various statements be printed on the blank, usually in conjunction with state drug product selection laws, federal law does not require a particular form for the prescription. Some states do require special blanks (duplicate or triplicate prescription blanks) for some or all controlled substances.

Practitioners should use one prescription pad at a time and keep blanks in a safe place to reduce the possibility of the blanks being stolen. Blanks should be used only for writing prescription orders. Never sign prescription blanks in advance. Prior to printing blanks, consult state laws and consider practical considerations such as size of the blank, amount of space provided to clearly indicate the drug and amount prescribed, placement of refill instructions, and so forth.

> Prescription blanks should never be signed in advance.

Written Prescriptions

The information that must be indicated by the prescriber on a written prescription depends on whether the drug prescribed is classified as a controlled or noncontrolled prescription drug. Controlled drug status is established by federal and state law. Prescription regulations pertaining to controlled substances are stricter.

Although federal law does not clearly and unambiguously spell out what information must be written on a prescription for a noncontrolled prescription drug, labeling requirements identify the following information that should appear:

> *name* of the *patient*
> *date* prescription written
> *name* of the *drug*
> *strength* of drug, if applicable
> *quantity* to be dispensed
> *directions* for use
> *prescriber's name*
> *prescriber's signature*

Often state laws require additional information for a written prescription, including the patient's address and age, and the prescriber's address, telephone number, profession, and so forth.

In addition, many states require that the pharmacist label the prescription "as to content" (e.g., tetracycline HCl 250 mg) unless the practitioner indicates otherwise somewhere or in some way on the prescription. The procedure may be as simple as checking a box or may require the prescriber to indicate such in their own handwriting. Federal law does not require the automatic labeling of a prescription "as to content."

In the case of prescriptions for controlled drugs, federal law requires the practitioner to indicate the following information:

> Many states require the pharmacist to label the prescription "as to content."

name of the *patient*
address of the *patient*
date prescription signed by practitioner
name of the *drug*
strength of drug, if applicable
quantity to be dispensed
directions for use
name of the *prescriber*
prescriber's address
DEA registration number of the prescriber
signature of the *prescriber*

Also states may require the patient's age, sex, practitioner's telephone number, specific directions for use, designation of the practitioner's profession, and instructions for labeling "as to content."

Prescribers must write prescriptions in ink, indelible pencil, or they may be typewritten. Written prescriptions must be signed by the prescriber. A stamped signature is not valid. Federal law indicates that erasable pens may not be used to write and sign prescriptions for controlled substances. Because the ink in such pens does not become permanent for 3 days, prescription information could be altered without detection.

In some states, practitioners may write only one prescription per blank. Preprinted prescription blanks may be illegal also. A preprinted blank is one where the name, strength, amount and directions for use of a drug, or some combination of same, are preprinted on the blank.

Federal law allows a nurse or secretary to prepare prescription orders (including controlled substances) for the signature of the practitioner. The prescriber is responsible for making sure the prescription conforms in all essential respects to the law and regulations. State law may not allow such a practice. Practitioners should be aware also that the pharmacist has an equal responsibility with the practitioner to make sure the prescription meets all legal requirements.

When writing a prescription, practitioners should be sure to write clearly, avoid writing for a larger quantity of a drug than is necessary, provide for specific and clear directions for use, and meet all legal requirements.

> The prescriber must sign the prescription; stamped signatures are not valid.

> The practitioner and the pharmacist share responsibility in ensuring that the prescription meets all legal requirements.

Oral Prescriptions

The Durham-Humphrey Amendment to the Federal Food Drug and Cosmetic Act established the legality of filling an oral order to dispense medication. Federal law provides that oral orders must be reduced promptly to writing and filed by the pharmacist. Oral prescriptions must indicate the same information described in the discussion under written prescriptions, except for the practitioner's signature.

However, not all drugs may be prescribed by giving an oral order. Certain controlled substances may be dispensed only pursuant to a written prescription. Exceptions may be made in some cases for an emergency situation, as discussed later. Requirements for controlled drugs vary from state to state.

> Not all drugs can be prescribed orally.

Oral Authorization of Refills

Federal law allows pharmacists to take oral authorization for refills for noncontrolled drugs and some controlled substances, as noted later. The Durham-Humphrey Amendment specifies that refill instructions may be entered by the pharmacist on the oral instruction of the practitioner or a legally authorized representative.

Refills may be authorized orally by the practitioner or a legally authorized representative.

A legally authorized representative may be an employee or agent of the practitioner, most likely a nurse or secretary. A patient is not recognized as an authorized representative. Because the practitioner may not delegate authority to make decisions to someone else, the agent may only *communicate* or transmit the prescriber's decision or instruction to the pharmacist. Agents may not issue prescriptions or authorize refills. Again, note that state law may not allow such a procedure.

Federal law also allows for the oral authorization of refills for Schedule III and IV controlled substance prescriptions. Refer to the section on controlled substances for details.

Expiration of Prescriptions

States have established time limits for prescription filling; New York requires controlled substance prescriptions must be filled within 30 days of the order.

Federal law does not establish any legal time by which a patient must have a prescription filled after having been written by a practitioner. Some states have established time limits, particularly for controlled drugs. New York, for example, only allows a controlled substance prescription to be filled by the pharmacist within 30 days of the date the prescription was written by the practitioner.

Although noncontrolled prescriptions do not have to be filled within any particular time limit, patients should present prescriptions within a reasonable period of time. The pharmacist should question and the practitioner should be concerned about patients presenting prescriptions written some time prior to the presentation. Pharmacists should consult with the practitioner in such cases. Of course, there may be good reason for such a prescription, such as a chronic condition, being away from home, and the nature of the drug.

Prescriptions for controlled substances authorizing refills must be refilled within a specified period of time, which is discussed under refill instructions.

Refill Instructions

Practitioners must indicate whether the prescription can be refilled.

The Durham-Humphrey Amendment legalized the refilling of written and oral prescriptions as long as the refilling was authorized by the prescriber either in the original prescription or by oral order.

In the case of a written prescription, it is up to the practitioner to indicate clearly whether or not the prescription is to be refilled. The best and clearest method is to indicate a specific number of times a prescription may be refilled. Most prescription blanks are printed with a space for the practitioner to indicate the number of refills. It can be as simple as

refill: _____ times,

or a series of numbers that can be circled, such as

refill: 0   1   2   3   4   5   times.

If no refills will be allowed, the practitioner should indicate "none," "zero," or "0" in the refill space. The absence of any refill instruction on the prescription means no refills are allowed.

The FDA discourages the use of prn for refills.

Again, if refills are to be allowed, a specific number is desirable. However, some practitioners use the designation "prn" *(pro re nata)* meaning to refill "as needed" or "as necessary." Over the years the FDA has discouraged the use of prn, indicating that the physician cannot delegate his or her authority to someone else. In other words, it is not up to the pharmacist to decide the number of times the prescription should be refilled. In *The Rx*

Legend, the FDA recommends that a pharmacist receiving a prn prescription

1. use care and professional judgment in handling it;
2. refill it only with a frequency consistent with the directions for use;
3. check with the practitioner after a reasonable time to make sure the medication is to be continued.

Pharmacists are encouraged also to urge the prescriber to indicate the number of refills on the prescription.

Whereas the federal law reluctantly allows the practitioner to use prn, states may not allow the use of prn to indicate refills, claiming that it is not a specific instruction. At least one state indicates that using prn means the prescription can be refilled only once.

A variation, prn with some time limit (e.g., prn — 1 year), may be seen. In this case there is a limit to the number of refills. "Prn — 1 year" would mean, refill this prescription for 1 year from the date of writing consistent with the directions for use. Controlled substance regulations would not allow the use of prn or any variation.

Lastly, instructions such as refill for lifetime are clearly unreasonable. Federal law limits the number of refills for Schedule III and IV controlled drugs to five times or 6 months, whichever comes first.

A question is asked often about whether or not a prescription may be refilled if the practitioner who wrote the prescription dies. The FDA has stated that once a physician-patient relationship is broken, the prescription is no longer valid because the physician is no longer available to that patient to oversee the patient's use of the prescribed medication.

> The FDA has stated that prescriptions are not valid after a physician-patient relationship has been broken.

Prescription Labeling

Specific legal requirements affecting the labeling of prescription drugs have been established by the Federal Food, Drug and Cosmetic Act, the Federal Controlled Substances Act, and various state acts. Requirements are discussed for noncontrolled and controlled drugs.

For noncontrolled drugs, federal law requires that the pharmacist indicate the following information on a prescription label:

> *name* and *address* of the pharmacy
> *prescription number*
> *name* of the *patient* (if stated in the prescription)
> *name* of the *practitioner*
> *date* the prescription was filled or refilled
> *directions* for use
> *caution/warning* statements

In addition, states may require such information as the patient's name and address; labeling "as to content;" the dispensing pharmacist's name or initials; lot numbers; expiration dates; the name of the drug manufacturer/ distributor; and the telephone number of the pharmacy.

Federal law requires the following information on a controlled substance prescription label:

> *name* and *address* of the pharmacy
> *prescription number*
> *name* of the *patient*
> *name* of the prescribing *practitioner*
> *date* the prescription was filled or refilled
> *directions* for use
> *caution/warning* statements

federal warning statement for Schedules I–IV controlled substances, which reads: "Caution: Federal law prohibits the transfer of this drug to any person other than the patient for whom it was prescribed"

In addition, states may require the items listed under noncontrolled prescription labeling as well as additional legends, the practitioner's DEA (Drug Enforcement Administration) number, and the pharmacy DEA number. Some states may require the label to be of a specific color. For example, New York requires an orange-colored controlled substance label.

Practitioners dispensing medication to patients may be subject to any or all of the labeling requirements mentioned. Consult your state law.

Drug Product Selection Laws

Most states have legalized the substitution of generic products by the pharmacist as long as she or he has authorization from the practitioner.

Most states have enacted legislation that, under a specific set of circumstances, allows the pharmacist to substitute a different brand or a generic drug product for the drug product prescribed by the practitioner on the prescription.

The substitution must be authorized by the practitioner. Various mechanisms are employed by states to indicate authorization, including a designated signature line(s) or box that must be checked, or the use of a specific statement or abbreviation.

The substituted drug must be of the same chemical entity and dosage form as the drug prescribed. Many states have established a formulary system to help professionals in the selection process. Some may be of the positive type, indicating drugs that may be substituted, whereas others are of the negative type, indicating drugs that may not be substituted. Consult your state law.

Copies of Prescriptions

Patients have a right to obtain a prescription copy from the pharmacist, but the copy cannot be used to refill the prescription.

In general, a patient has a right to get a copy of a prescription from a pharmacy. However, some states may limit the patient's possession to noncontrolled prescriptions. In such a case, the patient may request that a copy of a controlled drug prescription be sent to the patient's practitioner.

Copies have no legal status as valid prescriptions; they cannot be filled or refilled. They are a source of information only and must be so-worded. Some states require the pharmacist to indicate a specific statement, such as "COPY—FOR INFORMATION ONLY," on the copy of the prescription or indicate "COPY" or a specified statement in a color, red for example. Other states do not require a specific statement.

The FDA has indicated that copies are not valid prescriptions because there is no assurance

1. that it is an accurate or valid prescription;
2. that other copies have not been delivered to other pharmacies;
3. that the original prescription will not be recognized for the remaining refills.

Pharmacists receiving such prescriptions must call the practitioner for authorization to refill (fill) the prescription.

Federal regulations allow for the transfer of original prescription information between pharmacies for the dispensing of refills of controlled substances in Schedules III, IV, and V. State law may not allow for such a procedure.

Out-of-State Prescriptions

Practitioners cannot write prescriptions in states in which they are not licensed.

Practitioners may legally write prescriptions only in the states in which they are licensed to practice. In any other state they are considered a layperson. A practitioner who is a federal employee must be licensed in at least one state to have prescription-writing authority in any federal facility.

Can a pharmacist fill a prescription written by a practitioner licensed in another state? The answer depends on state law. Some do not address the problem. Others indicate a limited filling of such prescriptions, allowing them to be filled by practitioners of neighboring states or border communities. Some limit the filling to noncontrolled drugs.

The FDA has indicated that there is no federal requirement that a prescriber be licensed in the state where the prescription is filled, provided the prescription was valid where written. Consult your state law for particulars.

Safety Packaging

The Poison Prevention Packaging Act of 1970 was enacted to provide special packaging to protect children from serious personal injury and illness from ingesting, handling, or using household substances. The Act is administered by the Federal Consumer Product Safety Commission (CPSC).

Products covered by the Act include human prescription drugs in oral dosage forms, all controlled drugs (whether prescription or not), aspirin, acetaminophen, and a host of household products. Some prescription and OTC products are exempt from the Act. Examples include sublingual dosage forms of nitroglycerin and specific aspirin-containing products.

Normally it is the pharmacist who is responsible for making the appropriate decision as to whether or not a prescription must be dispensed using a child-resistant container. However, practitioners dispensing medication directly to the patient are also responsible for dispensing drugs in packaging that complies with the requirements of the Act. Child-resistant containers are available in a wide variety of formats.

Pharmacists are generally responsible for assigning child-resistant containers to prescriptions.

The law makes provision for waiving the safety packaging requirements of the Act. For example, patients may request that a prescription medication be dispensed in a noncomplying container. Also, a patient may ask the pharmacy for a blanket waiver for all the medication they have dispensed at a particular pharmacy. A practitioner may request a waiver for the patient on a single prescription-by-prescription basis. However, practitioners may not request blanket waivers for patients.

Whereas the federal law does not require that a request for noncomplying packaging be in writing, some states do require written documentation. Pharmacists and practitioners are encouraged to get the waiver in writing from the patient.

Practitioners should note that federal law indicates that the container cannot be reused, because the closure may lose its child-resistant properties after continued use. In the case where a plastic container has been used, the cap and container must be replaced. Where glass is used, only a new cap is required. State law may modify these requirements.

Under federal law, child-resistant containers cannot be reused.

It should be noted that provisions of the Poison Prevention Packaging Act do not apply to inpatient situations.

Syringes and Needles

Federal law does not make any provision for the sale or prescribing of hypodermic syringes and needles. However, state laws may restrict sales to pharmacies or require dispensing only by prescription. Consult your state law.

Prescriptions for Over-the-Counter Medication

A practitioner may decide that a medication normally available OTC without a prescription should be provided to the patient only on the basis of a prescription. This is likely to occur when the dosage regimen requires supervision or there is the possibility of a drug interaction.

In this case the practitioner should provide the patient with a prescription that is legally complete (e.g., name, address, and so forth). Simply writing the name of the medication on a prescription blank may not clearly convey the practitioner's intentions.

If refills have been indicated, they should be handled in the same manner as the original filling of the prescription.

Controlled Substances

REGISTRATION

Practitioners who wish to administer, prescribe, or dispense any controlled substance must be registered with the Federal Drug Enforcement Administration.

Practitioners are required to register with the Drug Enforcement Administration, Registration Unit, P.O. Box 28083, Central Station, Washington, D.C. 20005 by applying on Form DEA–224, available through the Unit or DEA Field Office.

A certificate of registration is required to administer, prescribe, or dispense controlled substances.

Once an application is approved, a certificate of registration is issued to the practitioner. Valid for a period of 3 years, the certificate must be maintained at the registered location and be made available for official inspection. A practitioner who has more than one office in which controlled substances are administered or dispensed is required to register for each office.

According to the DEA, any physician who is an intern, resident, foreign physician, or physician on the staff of a Veterans Administration facility (exempted from registration) may dispense, administer, and prescribe controlled substances under the registration of the hospital or other institution in which the physician is employed, provided that

1. the dispensing, administering, or prescribing is in the usual course of professional practice;
2. the physician is authorized or permitted to do so by the state where practicing;
3. the hospital or institution has verified that the physician is permitted to dispense, administer, or prescribe drugs within the state;
4. the physician acts only within the scope of employment in the hospital or institution;
5. the hospital or other institution authorizes him to dispense or prescribe under its registration and assigns a specific internal code number for each physician so authorized (an example would be BD1234567–08, where the "–08" represents the practitioner's hospital code number, and the other numbers represent the hospital DEA number—the code number must be included on all prescriptions issued by the physician);
6. a current list of internal codes and the corresponding individual practitioners is kept by the hospital or other institution and is made available at all times to other registrants and law enforcement agencies upon request for purpose of verifying the authority of the prescribing physician.

In addition, each written prescription must have the name of the physician stamped, typed or handprinted on it, as well as the signature of the physician.

SCHEDULES OF CONTROLLED SUBSTANCES

The drugs and drug products covered under the Federal Controlled Substances Act are divided into five schedules. Schedules are indicated by roman numerals, with Schedule I having the strictest control, decreasing to Schedule V, having the least control. A definition and examples for each

Table 66-1 SCHEDULES AND EXAMPLES OF CONTROLLED SUBSTANCES

Schedule I

These drugs have no currently accepted medical use in treatment in the United States and have a high potential for abuse.

Examples: opiates; opium derivatives, including heroin; hallucinogenic substances, including LSD and marijuana; depressants, including methaqualone; and certain stimulants

Schedule II

These drugs have a high potential for abuse and have a currently accepted medical use in treatment in the United States or a currently accepted medical use with severe restrictions.

Examples: opium derivates, including extracts and tincture of opium; morphine; codeine; hydromorphone (Dilaudid); oxycodone (Percodan); cocaine; meperidine (Demerol); amphetamines; phenmetrazine (Preludin); methylphenidate (Ritalin); amobarbital (Amytal); pentobarbital (Nembutal); and secobarbital (Seconal). Some forms of codeine and amo-, pento-, and secobarbital appear in other Schedules.

Schedule III

These drugs have a potential for abuse less than the drugs in Schedules I and II and have a currently accepted medical use in the United States.

Examples: some derivatives of barbituric acid (Butisol); paregoric; APC with codeine; Empirin with codeine; Fiorinal with codeine; Tylenol with codeine; Tussionex; and suppository forms of amo-, pento-, and secobarbital; substances classified as "anabolic steroids" under federal law, such as methyltestosterone and fluoxymesterone. See also Schedules II and V for other codeine preparations.

Schedule IV

These drugs have a low potential for abuse relative to the drugs in Schedule III with a currently accepted medical use in the United States.

Examples: phenobarbital; chloral hydrate (Noctec); meprobamate; paraldehyde; pentazocine (Talwin); dextropropoxyphene (Darvon); benzodiazepines, including alprazolam (Xanax), chlordiazepoxide (Librium), clorazepate (Tranxene), diazepam (Valium), flurazepam (Dalmane), lorazepam (Ativan), oxazepam (Serax), and triazolam (Halcion); diethylpropion (Tenuate); and phentermine (Ionamin).

Schedule V

These drugs have a low potential for abuse relative to the drugs in Schedule IV with a currently accepted medical use in the United States.

Examples: codeine-containing cough preparations such as elixir of terpin hydrate and codeine, Robitussin A-C, and Triaminic Expectorant with codeine; Lomotil; and Parepectolin.

---

schedule are indicated in Table 66-1. A complete list of drugs covered under the Act can be obtained from the Drug Enforcement Administration.

The reader should keep in mind that states also have regulations governing controlled substances and may assign a drug to a different schedule than the federal law. In such a case, the strictest law applies. Check your state law.

PRESCRIBING REQUIREMENTS FOR SCHEDULE I-V DRUGS

Prescription orders must be prepared in the manner described for controlled substances earlier in this chapter. Prior to writing a prescription, a practitioner must understand the rules that apply to each drug.

Schedule I

Under normal circumstances, practitioners cannot write for nor can pharmacists fill prescriptions for Schedule I drugs. Consult the DEA and your state agency with responsibility for controlled substances for specific requirements that must be met to prescribe and write prescriptions for drugs in Schedule I.

Normally, Schedule I drugs cannot be prescribed by a practitioner or filled by a pharmacist.

Schedule II

Schedule II drugs require written prescriptions and cannot be refilled.

The Federal Controlled Substances Act requires a written prescription for the dispensing of substances listed in Schedule II. Such prescriptions may not be refilled. Several states require the use of a special triplicate prescription form to dispense Schedule II and sometimes other scheduled drugs.

The federal law makes a provision for an Emergency Telephone Prescription Order for Schedule II controlled substances. In such an emergency, a practitioner may telephone a prescription order for a Schedule II controlled substance to a pharmacist. An emergency means that the immediate administration of the drug is necessary for proper treatment, that no alternative treatment is available, and that it is not possible for the physician to provide a written prescription order for the drug at that time.

In such an emergency, the amount furnished on the order is limited to that needed to treat the patient during the emergency period. Within 72 hours of the emergency order, the practitioner must furnish the pharmacy with a written, signed prescription for the controlled substance prescribed. If the pharmacist does not receive the written prescription within the 72-hour period, the pharmacist is required by law to notify the DEA of the fact. States may have stricter requirements.

Schedules III and IV

Schedules III and IV drugs can be prescribed in writing or orally and, if authorized, be refilled up to five times within 6 months of the date of issue.

Prescription orders for substances in Schedules III and IV may be issued in writing or given orally to the pharmacist. If authorized on the prescription, orders may be refilled up to five times within 6 months of the date of issue. A new prescription would be required then.

Federal law allows for the oral authorization of *additional refills* to the original prescription for Schedules III and IV controlled substances, provided the following provisions are met:

1. The *total quantity* of the drug authorized (including the amount of the original prescription) does not exceed five refills nor extend beyond 6 months from the date of issue of the original prescription;

2. The quantity of each additional refill authorized is equal to or less than the quantity authorized for the initial filling of the original prescription;

3. The prescribing practitioner must execute a new and separate prescription for any additional quantities beyond the five-refills, 6-months' limitation.

For example, the practitioner who had provided a written prescription for 100 tablets and two refills could telephone the pharmacist and authorize a maximum of three additional refills of the prescription of no more than 100 tablets per refill.

Schedule V

Schedule V drugs are not required to be prescribed by federal law.

The Federal Controlled Substances Act does not require Schedule V drugs to be prescribed by prescription. Such drugs may only be purchased from a pharmacy by a person 18 years or older, in limited quantities (e.g., 4 fl oz), and only after 48 hours has elapsed since a previous purchase. Pharmacists are required to indicate certain information about the sale in a register designated for the purpose. Some states require that Schedule V drugs be dispensed only on prescription.

SECURITY REQUIREMENTS

Practitioners who store controlled substances in their office must keep them in a securely locked, substantially constructed cabinet or safe. The

DEA recommends that controlled substance stock be kept to a minimum. If larger quantities are needed, the DEA encourages practitioners to have a security system that exceeds the minimum requirements, such as a safe and alarm system. Access to controlled substance storage areas should be restricted to a minimum number of employees.

Practitioners must notify the nearest DEA field office and local police department upon discovering any loss or theft of controlled substances.

Ordering Drugs

How do practitioners obtain drugs for office or medical use? The most appropriate method is to establish an account with a local wholesaler or by using direct order privileges with a pharmaceutical manufacturer. Controlled substances may be ordered only from a pharmacy that is registered as a wholesaler.

Schedule II controlled substances must be obtained through the use of a federal order form (not to be confused with the duplicate or triplicate prescription blanks used in some states).

ORDER FORMS FOR SCHEDULES I AND II CONTROLLED SUBSTANCES

Federal order forms are triplicate forms produced in sets of seven forms per book. They may be obtained at the time of initial registration (by marking

Figure 66-1

Sample order form for DEA Schedules I and II drugs. (Courtesy of the United States Drug Enforcement Administration.)

See Reverse of PURCHASER'S Copy for Instructions	No order form may be issued for Schedules I and II substances unless a completed application form has been received (21 CFR 1305.04).	OMB APPROVAL No. 1117-0010

TO: *(Name of Supplier)* | STREET ADDRESS

CITY AND STATE | DATE | TO BE FILLED IN BY SUPPLIER | SUPPLIER'S DEA REGISTRATION No.

LINE No	No. of Packages	Size of Package	Name of Item	National Drug Code	Packages Shipped	Date Shipped
	TO BE FILLED IN BY PURCHASER					
1						
2						
3						
4						
5						
6						
7						
8						
9						
10						

◀ NO. OF LINES COMPLETED | SIGNATURE OF PURCHASER OR HIS ATTORNEY OR AGENT

Date Issued	DEA Registration No.	Name and Address of Registrant
Schedules		
Registered as a	No. of this Order Form	

DEA Form -222 (Jun. 1983)

U.S. OFFICIAL ORDER FORMS - SCHEDULES I & II
DRUG ENFORCEMENT ADMINISTRATION
SUPPLIER'S COPY 1

sample

Federal order forms are needed to obtain Schedule II controlled substances.

the appropriate space on form DEA–224) or using a separate form DEA–222A thereafter. No charge is made for the order forms. Directions for completing the forms are indicated on the reverse side of the purchaser's copy. Figure 66–1 indicates a sample order form.

Record-Keeping Requirements — Controlled Substances

The Federal Controlled Substances Act requires that certain practitioners keep records of drugs purchased, distributed, and dispensed. The scope of a practitioner's activities determines what records must be kept.

Prescribing. Practitioners involved in the prescribing of Schedules II, III, IV, and V controlled substances in the course of their professional practice are not required to keep records of the transactions. This requirement should not be confused with any medical practice requirements that should be indicated in the patients' medical records.

Dispensing. Practitioners who dispense controlled substances as a part of their medical practice are required to keep a record of each transaction.

Physicians must keep a record of all transactions when dispensing a controlled substance from the same inventory.

Administration. The DEA Physician's Manual indicates that a physician who regularly engages in the administration of controlled substances in Schedules II, III, IV, and V is required to keep records if patients are charged for drugs either separately or with other patient services. When a physician dispenses a controlled substance and administers this substance occasionally or regularly from the same inventory, he or she must keep a record of all transactions. A physician who occasionally administers a controlled substance and does not dispense the controlled substance from the same inventory is not required to keep records of these transactions.

INVENTORIES

Practitioners who are required to maintain records must take an inventory of all stocks of the substance on hand every 2 years. An initial inventory must be taken on the date the practitioner first engages in such activity. Thereafter, a biennial inventory must be taken. Specific requirements for taking the inventory may be found in the DEA Physician's Manual or from a DEA field office.

NARCOTIC TREATMENT

The DEA Physician's Manual indicates that records are required for controlled substances prescribed, dispensed, or administered for maintenance or detoxification treatment. A physician is required to be registered as a narcotic treatment program to conduct these activities.

All controlled substance records and inventories must be filed in a readily retrievable manner from all other business documents and retained for 2 years. Schedule II records must be maintained separately from all other records. Schedules III, IV, and V records must be maintained separately or be kept in such a way that they are readily retrievable from the ordinary professional and business records of the practitioner.

The DEA Physician's Manual indicates that all records, including controlled substance records maintained as part of a patient's file, shall be available for inspection and copying by duly authorized officials of the DEA.

A practitioner who is registered with the DEA and wishes to dispose of excess or undesirable controlled substances should request DEA Form 41. The form should be completed as directed and submitted to the DEA regional director. State law may dictate disposal procedures also.

Disposal of Controlled Substances

A question arises as to whether or not a practitioner or pharmacist may give a patient a drug product package insert. Such inserts are provided with the product as part of its labeling for use by professionals. The FDA has stated that there is no regulation that prevents the practitioner or pharmacist from providing the patient with the package insert. Practitioners should use caution, because such inserts are written for professionals using language and providing information that may not be understood by the patient.

FDA has required that the manufacturers of several drug products prepare and provide *patient* package inserts for dispensing to the patient whenever a prescription for the drug is filled by the pharmacist. Patient package inserts are written at a patient level of understanding and provide information regarding the appropriate use of the drug, methods of administration, and possible side effects. Current examples include the oral contraceptives, estrogenic drug products, and intrauterine devices.

Package Inserts

Patient package inserts are required for oral contraceptives, estrogenic drug products, and intrauterine devices.

The 1987 Prescription Drug Marketing Act amended the Federal Food Drug and Cosmetic Act for various purposes, including the placing of restrictions on the distribution of drug samples. Specifically, the law defines a drug sample as a unit of a drug subject to the act that is not intended to be sold and is intended to promote the sale of the drug.

Licensed practitioners who desire drug samples must make a written request of a manufacturer or distributor on a form that provides the following information:

name
address
professional designation
signature of the practitioner making the request
identity of the drug sample requested
quantity requested
name of the manufacturer of the drug sample
date of the request

Once the sample is received, the practitioner must execute a written receipt and return it to the manufacturer or distributor of the sample drug.

Drug Samples

Generally, the requirements listed in this chapter can be applied also to hospitals, nursing homes, and so forth. However, states may have established additional or substitute regulations that pertain specifically to institutions. Consult your state law.

Institutional Requirements

References

Approved Prescription Drug Products With Therapeutic Equivalence Evaluations, 8th ed. Washington, DC: U.S. Department of Health and Human Services, 1988.

Code of Federal Regulations, Title 21, 1300. Superintendent of Documents, U.S. Government Printing Office, Washington, DC 20402.

Drug Enforcement Administration: Physician's Manual. Washington, DC: Drug Enforcement Administration.

The Rx Legend — An FDA Manual for Pharmacists. Rockville, MD: U.S. Food and Drug Administration.

67

Substance Abuse Treatment

Peter K. Gessner

That people use and abuse a substance, in the final analysis, must depend in some part on pharmacological properties such a substance possesses. Substance abuse is, however, a complex phenomenon that also involves human behavior and learning as well as the impact of society on the abuser. Detailed knowledge of all the pharmacological and toxic properties of each of the various classes of agents that are abused is both to a degree redundant and, in itself, not sufficient to achieve an understanding of the substance abuse phenomenon. Accordingly, while maintaining a pharmacological perspective, an effort is made in this chapter to identify and to discuss the crucial aspects that govern substance abuse generally. Sections devoted to the more important individual classes of abused drugs address primarily abuse-relevant characteristics that are unique to those classes of agents.

Definitions

Substance abuse and *addiction* are societally, not scientifically, defined terms.

Substance abuse is a term used in our culture for the self-administration of pharmacologically active substances for nonmedical purposes, generally pleasure or recreation, in spite of society having proscribed either the substance altogether (e.g., lysergic acid diethylamide, LSD) or its use to this end (e.g., morphine). Society sanctions the recreational use of some substances (e.g., ethanol), but only within defined bounds of context, amount, frequency, and so on. The use of these substances outside such bounds is also viewed as abuse. These definitions are social rather than scientific or medical. They reflect society's perception of the adverse consequences of such use to the individual, to society, or to both. These perceptions are based, to a degree, on scientific evidence and can therefore change as new toxicological information becomes available.

Addiction is a term used for the perseverance by individuals in their substance use in spite of societal strictures, medical or other consequences (whether personally or vicariously experienced), and frequently, the users' own professed resolve and better judgment. This again is a social definition and, as such, one that can change as more information becomes available. A case in point is cigarette smoking, which used to be viewed as a habit but which came to be considered an addiction as the broad range of its toxic consequences became well documented. A broader and more generic term is *addictive behaviors.* It encompasses gluttony and gambling in addition to substance abuse and refers to behaviors indulged in habitually for the gain of short-term pleasure at the expense of long-term adverse consequences. *Craving,* when used in a scientific sense, is a variable quantifiable in terms of the effort a human, or an animal, will expend to secure additional doses of the substance. Thus it is an objective measure of the behavioral drive induced by a given substance and under specified conditions.

Many substances that are abused possess the ability to induce tolerance and physical dependence. *Physical dependence* is the phenomenon whereby with chronic use of a substance, stopping its use gives rise to signs and symptoms of a pathological nature, collectively called the *withdrawal syndrome*. By definition, the *status quo ante* can be restored (e.g., the syndrome can be terminated by administration of the substance). The degree of deviation from normality induced by the withdrawal of the substance, that is, the intensity of a withdrawal syndrome, can be quantitated, and thereby so too can the degree of physical dependence that induced it. The terms *physical dependence* and *withdrawal syndrome* are therefore scientific ones. Although physical dependence and a desire to avoid withdrawal may result in some drug-seeking behavior, they are not essential corollaries of addiction and craving. That is made apparent, on the one hand, by agents such as phencyclidine (PCP) that are abused yet do not induce physical dependence, and on the other hand, by agents such as propranolol that induce physical dependence but are not abused. Papering over this lack of correspondence by introduction of terms such as *psychic dependence* or *psychological dependence* is unhelpful, since these are neither equatable to craving nor variables that can be independently quantitated. To add to the confusion the term *dependence*, when either employed by itself or modified by the name of a substance or group of substances, as in *alcohol dependence* or *narcotic dependence*, is commonly used as synonymous with *addiction*.

Cross *physical dependence* is the ability of substances to mutually terminate each other's withdrawal syndromes. Its occurrence is considered to indicate that substances sharing this property induce physical dependence by mechanisms that are at least partially common. This has led to the classification of substances of abuse into pharmacologically distinct groups.

Tolerance is a phenomenon whereby, with repeated use, a substance becomes less effective, so that to obtain a given effect it becomes necessary to increase the dose. Several mechanisms are considered as potentially able to contribute to the phenomenon of tolerance. *Pharmacokinetic, dispositional,* or *metabolic tolerance* is the ability of the organism chronically exposed to a xenobiotic to eliminate it at a rate faster than previously; quantitatively this usually represents a modest contribution to overall tolerance. *Pharmacodynamic* or *functional tolerance* is the lessening of sensitivity of the target tissue, owing to changes induced at the neuropharmacological level, to a given level of the agent in contact with it. It makes by far the largest contribution to overall tolerance. *Behavioral tolerance* is the ability of the individual, through learning, to compensate for impairment in some modalities of function by utilization of other modalities. *Conditioned tolerance* is a classic learned conditioning response that tends to compensate for the effect of the drug by eliciting the opposite actions.

Substance abuse may cause individuals to require medical assistance for a variety of reasons. (1) The degree to which the substance available illicitly has been "cut" with inert material varies as does the dosing sophistication of the users. As a result, the presentation of overdose toxicity (e.g., a opiate overdose resulting in severe depression of respiration) is a common occurrence. (2) For some agents the effects experienced, even in the absence of an overdose, can be quite alarming and rather different from those sought by users (e.g., LSD-induced panic reaction), leading them to seek medical assistance. (3) Individuals often present with pathologies resultant not

Physical dependence is defined by the occurrence of a withdrawal syndrome upon cessation of the use of a substance.

There are several types of tolerance: pharmacokinetic, pharmacodynamic, behavioral, and conditioned.

Contingencies Requiring Medical Intervention

Abuse-engendered problems requiring medical intervention include acute and overdose toxicities, drug-induced organ pathologies, and withdrawal management.

from the pharmacological effect of the substance but rather from the manner of self-administration, which permits the introduction of vectors of infection (e.g., human immunodeficiency virus, HIV) or other foreign matter parenterally. (4) Many of the substances of abuse are inherently toxic and in the long run cause organ toxicities (e.g., lung cancer in cigarette smokers). (5) Physicians are frequently called on to medically manage withdrawal syndromes. Untreated, the withdrawal from some substances (e.g., ethanol) can be both miserable and life-threatening. The goal of such treatment is both to alleviate the acute syndrome and to withdraw individuals from the substance so that they can function normally in its absence.

The medical ministrations mentioned in the preceding paragraph are likely to prove no more than palliative if substance abuse recurs. Even in the absence of medical consequences, cessation of abuse is frequently essential for legal, economic, occupational, or other reasons. Society, faced with individuals who persistently and recurringly engage in addictive behavior, is forced to suppose such individuals are unable to cease the behavior of their own volition. In such instances, society usually concludes that the intervention of some outside agency is required to bring the behavior to an end or, failing that, to institute *maintenance* of the individual on a drug analogous to that abused, but judged by society to have less adverse consequences. The societal agency called on depends on the *construct* adopted in seeking to explain the abuser's inability to stop the recurrent behavior. The preponderant current construct is that of the *medical model*, which views the addictive behavior not to be the result of demonic possession, lack of moral fiber, or of some inherent property of the abused substance, but rather as a *malady* or illness. Nominally, therefore, treatment of alcohol, opiate, and other dependencies is seen as a responsibility of the medical profession. In reality, however, the bulk of treatment facilities that offer such care are staffed by non–medically trained substance abuse and alcoholism counselors. Physician participation in substance abuse treatment tends to be rather limited, particularly if the treatment is drug-free.

Pharmacological treatment of dependence by blocking, aversion, or maintenance therapy

Physicians can play an important role in primary and secondary prevention of substance abuse among their patients. They are in a better position than almost anyone else with whom their patients are likely to come into contact to detect developing or established substance abuse among their patients. They are also uniquely able to convincingly document to such individuals the overt or incipient pathophysiology resulting from their substance abuse. Both of these are important aspects of secondary prevention because a necessary first step for individuals to alter their pattern of substance abuse is a realization that they are indeed engaging in such behavior and that it is injurious to them. With respect to primary prevention, ascertaining the absence of substance abuse by one on one questioning during an office visit and the sharing, in this context, of information regarding the health consequences of such use is very effective in changing patient attitudes, particularly among the young.

Classification of Abused Substances

Cross-tolerance and cross physical dependence help classify abused drugs into categories.

Grouping of abused substances is useful if their properties are sufficiently similar that phenomena associated with the use of one substance are predictive of those attendant on the use of another. The criteria used in arriving at such groupings are, first, the existence of cross physical dependence. The reciprocal ability of two agents to terminate each other's withdrawal syndrome is strong evidence that they induce some of the same pharmacological effects. Second, a reciprocal inability to distinguish between two substances by experienced substance abusers and animals trained to react to the administration of a given substance is suggestive that the subjective effects these substances have (i.e., the effects that are sought by the abuser) are very similar. A third and weaker criterion is a similarity in the objective effects of the two agents.

If, in the listing of classes of abused substances, importance were to be gauged by the morbidity and mortality resultant from such abuse, cigarette smoking—the elimination of which would reduce overall mortality by 25%—would head the list. Instead, most such lists are headed by opiates, that is, agents such as heroin, morphine, and meperidine. This is due to the high frequency with which abusers of this class of agents require medical intervention, by the acute nature of much of the morbidity associated with their use, and probably also by the high correlation between their use and participation by users in criminal activity. Second in importance are probably central nervous system (CNS) depressants of the ethanol-barbiturate type, their high placement being attributable to ethanol and the wide extent to which it is abused. Third come stimulants of the cocaine-amphetamine type. Nicotine-containing products, PCP (a dissociative agent), LSD-type hallucinogens, marijuana, atropine-related deliriants, and anabolic steroids would follow in such a list.

Characteristics of Abused Substances

A discussion of substance abuse in a pharmacological context necessarily must focus on what properties such substances share that causes them to have a high abuse potential.

REINFORCING PROPERTIES

Abused substances are said to induce hedonistic or euphoric effects, that is, effects that are inherently pleasurable or that the individual has been socialized to regard as desirable. The effects are thereby considered as rewarding. Since the satisfaction gained by use of the substance increases the probability that the individual will use it again, such substances are termed *reinforcers.* Most reinforcing are substances that act on the CNS. The reinforcing properties of most naturally occurring substances can be ascribed, principally, to the pharmacological action of specific components —morphine in opium, cocaine in coca leaves, and nicotine in tobacco. Chemical technology allows isolation of the active ingredients in a more or less pure form. As a rule, self-administration of the active ingredients is much more reinforcing than the parent substance: it obviates coadministration of other potentially noxious components of the original substance, reduces the bulk, and permits the user to employ parenteral routes of administration and to increase the dose.

Study of the behavior of animals allowed to self-inject abused substances makes it evident just how reinforcing such substances are. Monkeys who discover that pressing a lever will result in the intravenous injection of an opiate or cocaine, will do so repeatedly, increasing the frequency of self-administration so as to overcome tolerance and continuing with the behavior in preference to such instinctive drives as satisfaction of thirst, hunger, or sexual need. Nor will having to perform substantial work in order to be rewarded deter them: monkeys have been observed to emit as many as 13,000 bar-pressing responses to obtain just one dose of cocaine. It is noteworthy that all monkeys tested respond in a similar fashion, indicating the behavior to be a normal response rather than the result of some pathological process.

Although human drug-taking behavior confirms abused substances to be potent reinforcers, the patterns of behavior actually observed depend to

Abused drugs are potent reinforcers.

a large extent on the reinforcement contingencies (i.e., what action is necessary to get more drug) in which individuals find themselves. Using opiates as an example, the pattern of human responses makes it evident such substances are potent reinforcers, although the nature of the pattern elicited depends on the reinforcement contingency.

When free access to a opiate (morphine) was provided to a drug-free,

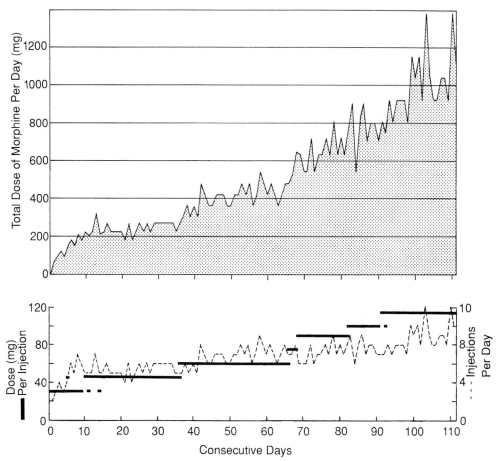

Figure 67–1

The subject, a previously narcotic-dependent individual who volunteered for the experiment, was advised that, for an unspecified period of time (the duration of which would be communicated to him a month before its end), he could have any drug, in any amount, by any route, and as often as he liked. He was also told that he would not be required to work during this period and that he need not become physically dependent unless he wanted to. He appeared elated and asked for and received 30 mg of morphine intravenously. Immediately after the injection, his skin was flushed, he rubbed his nose and appeared very happy. The flush subsided in a few seconds. On interrogation, he said the sensation was comparable with sexual orgasm. This lasted only a few seconds and was followed by a feeling similar to that he would have experienced if he had had one or two drinks of whiskey, but better because it lasted for hours. A few hours later, he was much more loquacious. He said he now had "pep" and could do anything he wanted—go to a show, go for a walk, or go to sleep. Over the period of the next 3 months the patient increased his daily consumption of morphine to as much as 1400 mg *(top panel)*. He spontaneously compared the feeling, before the next "shot" was due, with hunger, and the satisfaction afterward to satiation of hunger. He gradually increased the dose per injection to 115 mg *(lower panel)* because he was not getting the "hold" long enough. On the other hand, since he developed tolerance, he was able to get 6 or 8, and on occasion as many as 12, orgasm-like "thrills" a day. In this respect, being physically dependent was an advantage. He recalled that after he had once become physically dependent, he always felt as if some dear friend were missing during periods when he was not taking drugs at all. (Data from Wikler A: Psychodynamic study of patient during experimental self-regulated re-addiction to morphine. Psychiatric Quart 26:270–293, 1952.)

previously opiate-dependent individual, the pattern of drug-taking behavior observed (Fig. 67–1) proved very similar to that observed in monkeys. Over a period of months the subject continued to increase the frequency and quantity of morphine administered until, at a peak, he was receiving a dose of 115 mg up to 12 times a day and his cumulative 24-hour morphine dosage exceeded 23-fold that which satisfied him in the initial 24-hour period.

Given the opportunity to work for either money or opiate (heroin), the behavior (Fig. 67–2) of another previously opiate-dependent individual makes it very clear that his drive for opiate exceeded that for money, even when the opiate thus earned would not be available to him for another 48 hours. The work task consisted of pressing a button at intervals of 1 second or more on a hand-held device. The subject worked for as long as 10 hours/day, performing the task as many as 30,000 times/day in the process. He continued doing so even when dosed with 40 mg of heroin/day (the maximum permitted under the experimental protocol), making it evident the drug did not impair his ability to do so. Nor was his ability to work, this time for money, impaired during a 5-day methadone-moderated withdrawal period.

Moderate doses of narcotics do not impair an individual's ability to work for a reward.

In the real world, opiate abusers tend not to maintain a steady dosing

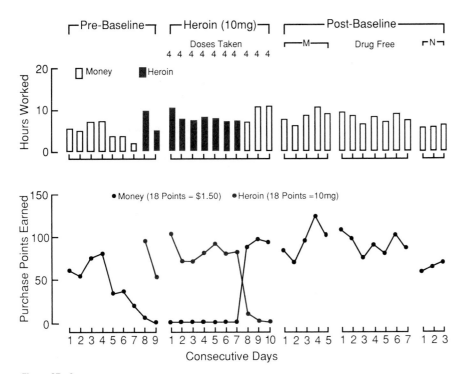

Figure 67–2

The subject, a drug-free but previously narcotic-dependent individual allowed to volunteer for the experiment, remained drug-free on the prebaseline days. Throughout the duration of the experiment he was given the opportunity to work for "points" that were exchangeable for money at the rate of $1.50/18 points, each point being earned by pressing a response button on a hand-held device 300 times. On the last two prebaseline days and during the "heroin" period, he had the opportunity to work for heroin points. These were exchangeable, although only during the heroin period, for IV heroin at the rate of 10 mg/18 points, up to a maximum of 40 mg on any one day. During the five postbaseline days, the subject was detoxed by being given 25 mg of methadone on the first day, and the dose was decreased decrementally by 5 mg/day on each day thereafter. (From Mello NK, Mendelson JH, Kuehnle JC, Sellers MS: Operant analysis of human heroin self-administration and the effects of naltrexone. J Pharmacol Exp Ther 216(1):45–54, 1981, © by American Society for Pharmacology and Experimental Therapeutics.)

Figure 67-3

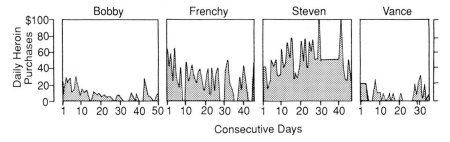

The subjects were residents of the Harlem section of New York City who considered themselves to be narcotic addicts. For a daily monetary reward ($5–$10) they agreed to report daily on their activities, including their purchases of heroin. Their heroin use is recorded in dollar units. With the exception of Steven, all the other 30 subjects in the study had heroin-free days alternating with days of heroin use. None reported withdrawal syndromes, however, implying an absence of physical dependence. The source of the subjects' income was 46% from crime, 11% from the drug business, and 14% from employment. (Redrawn from Johnson BD, Goldstein PJ, Duchaine MA: What is an addict? Empirical patterns and concepts of addiction. Paper read at the Society for the Study of Social Problems, Boston, MA, August 1979.)

schedule. In Figure 67–3, the daily heroin purchases of four opiate addicts are reported in dollars expended. It is evident that many opiate addicts purchase opiate only intermittently and experience therefore many abstinent days. Nonetheless they continue to use opiates. Similar use patterns are observed among alcoholics who, by pressing a button of a hand-held device, can work for alcohol and use it immediately or retain it for later consumption (Fig. 67–4).

Although opiates have a reputation for being particularly addictive, there exists among opiate abusers a small subset of individuals who use these drugs only occasionally and in a manner that minimizes the impact such use has on their lives. Such *chippers,* who are distinguished by maintaining a pattern of more or less controlled use for long periods of time, have been found to impose a significant number of self-made rules on their use of opiates. These can include setting up special times for such use (e.g., only on Saturdays), limiting the amount of opiates on hand, and never using them alone or with strangers. Even when opiates are used in intermittent fashion, they are apparently powerfully rewarding.

Figure 67-4

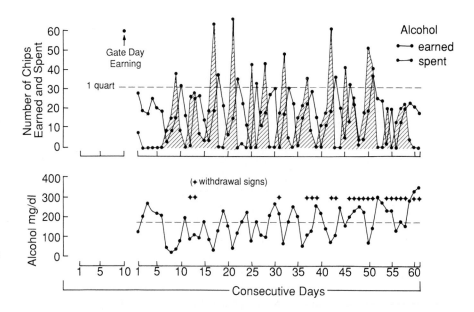

The subject was a male alcoholic who volunteered for the experiment and had been abstinent for at least 7 days previously. He was given the opportunity to work for cigarette tokens throughout the experiment (data not shown) and for bourbon tokens on the last prealcohol day (gate day) and during the alcohol phase of the experiment. Bourbon could be purchased at a rate of 30 ml of 100-proof Hiram Walker Ten High for each token from a dispenser on the wall of one of the rooms. Tokens were earned by pressing a response button on a hand-held device 1000 times for each one, and the payout occurred the following day at 8:00 A.M. The pattern of tokens earned (black graph) and spent (colored graph) is shown in the top panel. The daily mean ethanol blood level, based on three daily measurements, and the average blood ethanol level maintained throughout the drinking period *(horizontal line)* are shown in the bottom panel. The occurrence of withdrawal signs during this period is shown. (From Mello NK, Mendelson JH: Drinking patterns during work contingent and non-contingent alcohol acquisition. *In* Mello NK, Mendelson JH (eds): Recent Advances in Studies of Alcoholism, 647–686. Rockville, MD: National Institute of Alcohol Abuse and Alcoholism, 1971.)

POTENTIAL FOR RAPID DELIVERY TO THE CENTRAL NERVOUS SYSTEM

The passage of substances from the blood to the brain is impeded by the existence of the blood-brain barrier, which, functionally, behaves as a lipid layer. Although some molecular species enter the brain as the result of active transport, this is not the case for any abused substance. Accordingly, such substances must possess significant lipid solubility and must be mostly un-ionized at physiological pH. Blood, on the other hand, although it comprises many colloids as well as cells, is primarily aqueous in nature. When highly lipid-soluble agents with very low aqueous solubility are added to blood they tend to become adsorbed on lipoproteins, and their concentration in the aqueous phase may be so low as to significantly impede their reaching the blood vessel wall. Accordingly, the relationship between the lipid solubility (which can be measured in terms of the distribution ratio of an agent between a water and a lipid such as olive oil) and the uptake of an agent from blood into brain is a parabolic one. Uptake into the brain during one pass of the blood through the cerebral circulation initially increases with increasing lipid solubility, but beyond a certain value of the latter, the brain uptake starts to decrease. Heroin is found near the maximum of the curve for this relationship; so is cocaine.

The route and manner of administration constitutes another important factor in determining how rapid is the onset of action following dosing. Introduction of the agent directly into the bloodstream, as by intravenous injection, is an obvious way to speed the process. Inhalation of the substance in smoke, however, is an even more effective manner of administration in this respect. This is so because material introduced intravenously must first return to the right side of the heart, but that adsorbed at the alveolar surface returns directly to the left side of the heart and this reduces the duration of transit between the site of entry and the brain from 30 seconds to 7. For this latter route of administration to be effective, the substance in question must be both volatile and resistant to pyrolysis, properties shared, for instance, by nicotine and cocaine base (crack), but not by cocaine hydrochloride. Additionally, pulmonary inhalation is relatively easy if the smoke is acidic, as is true of cigarette-derived smoke. The alveolar lung surface is very extensive and possesses a large buffering capacity. As a result absorption at this surface is virtually instantaneous. Pipe and tobacco smoke, on the other hand, are alkaline, and most people find these too irritating to inhale. The absorption of nicotine from such smoke takes place at the mucosal surfaces in the oral-pharyngeal cavity and is a much slower process. This renders cigarette smoking more addictive than either cigar or pipe smoking. Smoking is regularly used for the self-administration of marijuana, and by some users also for that of cocaine, heroin, and PCP.

Although the onset of action of ingested substances is almost invariably slower than that observed following administration by inhalation or the intravenous route, enough of the substance may enter the systemic circulation by the oral route—i.e., it may have sufficient "oral availability"—to result in its having a significant abuse potential. Whether this is so is determined by a number of factors: (1) the substance either must be stable in the gastrointestinal tract or the breakdown product must be active. Heroin is an example of the latter, for although it is quickly hydrolyzed in the stomach, the product of the hydrolysis is morphine. (2) The substance must be readily absorbed from the gut. (3) Because absorption from the upper gastrointestinal track is into the portal circulation, the agent must be sufficiently resistant to hepatic degradation to survive the passage

The rapidity of onset is an important factor determining how reinforcing a substance is.

Substances that are smoked reach the brain faster than those that are injected.

Table 67–1 ORAL AVAILABILITY AND HALF-LIVES OF DRUGS COMMONLY ABUSED

Drug	Oral Availability (%)	Half-life (Hours)	References‡
Morphine	24	2	3
Codeine	50	3	6, 7
Meperidine	56	5	1
Methadone	90	23	3, 8
Buprenorphine	14*	7	2, 4
Naloxone	Minimal	1	5
Naltrexone	High†	10	9

* Sublingual: 58%.
† If calculated in terms of its active metabolite.
‡ References
  1. Edwards DJ, Svensson CK, Visco JP, Lalka D: Clinical pharmacokinetics of pethidine [meperidine]. Clin Pharmacokinet 7:421–433, 1982.
  2. Hand CW, Sear JW, Uppington J, et al: Buprenorphine disposition in patients with renal impairment: Single and continuous dosing, with special reference to metabolites. Br J Anaesth 64:276–282, 1990.
  3. Hoskin PJ, Hanks GW, Aherne GW, et al: The bioavailability and pharmacokinetics of morphine after intravenous, oral and buccal administration in healthy volunteers. Br J Clin Pharmacol 27:499–505, 1989.
  3. Inturrisi CE, Colburn WA, Kaiko RF, et al: Pharmacokinetics and pharmacodynamics of methadone in patients with chronic pain. Clin Pharmacol 41:392–401, 1987.
  4. McQuay H, Moore RA, Bullingham RES: Buprenorphine kinetics. In Foley KM, Inturrisi CE (eds): Advances in Pain Research and Therapy, vol 6, pp 271–278. New York: Raven Press, 1986.
  5. Ngai SH, Berkowitz BA, Yang JC, et al: Pharmacokinetics of naloxone in rats and in man: Basis for its potency and short duration of action. Anesthesiology 44:398–401, 1976.
  6. Quinding H, Anderson P, Bondesson U, et al: Plasma concentrations of codeine and its metabolite, morphine, after single and repeated oral administration. Eur J Clin Pharmacol 30:673–677, 1986.
  7. Rogers JF, Findley JWA, Hull JH, et al: Codeine disposition in smokers and nonsmokers. Clin Pharmacol Ther 32:218–227, 1982.
  8. Sawe J: High-dose morphine and methadone in cancer patients. Clinical pharmacokinetic considerations of oral treatment. Clin Pharmacokinet 11:87–106, 1986.
  9. Wall ME, Brine DR, Perez-Reyes M: Metabolism and disposition of naltrexone in man after oral and intravenous administration. Clin Pharmacol Ther 46:226–233, 1981.

of the portal blood through the liver (first-pass metabolism). Morphine, for instance, is much less effective orally because much of it is eliminated during first-pass metabolism. Its oral availability (Table 67–1) is sufficient, however, so that if it is ingested in sufficient quantity it is pharmacologically effective.

POTENTIAL FOR DOSE TITRATION

Whether the use of a substance is reinforcing can be very dependent on dose. Too low a dose may have no effect, too high a dose may induce unpleasant effects. Therefore, being able to titrate the amount employed against the effect induced in order to administer the optimally rewarding amount can be all-important. A case in point is that of PCP. When first tested in clinical trials as an anesthetic, it was used in a dose that caused effects so unpleasant that it was considered totally devoid of abuse potential. Even after it became available on the illicit market (in the form of a pill), its use spread very slowly until users discovered that adding the powdered material to marijuana cigarettes permitted both much faster delivery of the agent to the CNS and exquisitely sensitive, puff by puff, control of the dose.

For substances whose onset of action is not immediate, self-titration also requires learning to recognize *symptom hierarchies.* Continuation of self-administration of such a substance until optimally rewarding effects are achieved is likely to result—by the time the effects of the drug become eventually fully manifest—in an unintended level of intoxication, undesirable side effects, or frank toxicity. Users of such agents must therefore learn, by experience, to recognize a hierarchy of symptoms so as to know at which point to stop further self-administration in order to assure that a rewarding and satisfactory maximum ensues when the effects of the drug become fully manifest. Ceremonial or quasi-ceremonial use of moderate

With slowly acting agents, there is a propensity for users to obtain a greater than desired effect because self-titration is difficult.

amounts of alcoholic beverages within the family context (e.g., in Jewish households) has been claimed, for instance, to provide training for neophyte drinkers in recognition of the hierarchy of alcohol-induced symptoms. Individuals brought up in such households tend to have low rates of alcohol abuse.

POTENTIAL FOR FREQUENT REINFORCEMENT

Self-administration is a form of operant conditioning: every response, that is each act of self-administration, results in a reinforcement that renders the occurrence of the response more likely, and the behavior becomes conditioned by the reinforcing stimuli. From animal studies it is known that the strength of the conditioning, measured in terms of the number of unreinforced responses necessary to extinguish the behavior, is a function of the number of responses that have been reinforced. Obviously, the longer a substance has been used, the harder it will be to give it up. Additionally, however, the shorter the duration of action of a substance, the more frequent can be its use and the larger the total number of reinforcements per unit time. In particular, the number of reinforcements rises dramatically if the reinforcements are delivered rapidly without satiating the subject, as in smoking, where each inhalation results in a separate reinforcement. It is a method of delivery that is being used for cocaine and heroin as well as nicotine.

> The more times an individual has experienced the reinforcing effects of a substance, the stronger will be the resulting habit.

Lipid-solubility characteristics that permit rapid entry of a substance into the CNS will assure its equally rapid passage back into the blood, once the blood has been cleared of the substance. Two processes are responsible for such clearing. The first of these is redistribution to other tissues. The brain, which is approximately 2% of body weight, receives about 20% of the cardiac output. Accordingly, following bolus intravenous administration of a substance, the amount initially presented to the brain is much larger, per unit mass, than that presented to other tissues. The capacity of the latter to clear the blood of the substance is therefore significantly higher than that of the brain, and these tissues can thereby act as a rather effective sink for the substance.

The second mechanism whereby the substance is cleared from the blood is by its elimination from the body through metabolism and, to a lesser extent, excretion. In either event the process is much slower.

Generally, abusers prefer agents with a shorter half-life to those with a longer one, for instance, morphine over methadone (half-lives of 3 and 30 hours, respectively; see Table 67–1). Heroin is a special case. It has a very short half-life in blood, although long enough for much of it to reach the brain. Heroin is also subject to rapid hydrolysis within the CNS; however, 6-acetylmorphine and morphine, the products formed thereby, are more active at the receptor than heroin itself. Thus the main result of the acetylation of morphine to heroin is a substance rapidly delivered to the brain.

Facilitation of Substance Use by Substance-Unrelated Factors

Both genetic and environmental factors may predispose individuals to substance use. Experimentation with recreational drug use has been found to be correlated with sensation-seeking, a human trait defined by a desire or need for varied, novel, and complex situations or experiences and the willingness to take physical and social risks to achieve this end. Originally measured by choices respondents made among 40 dichotomous statements, the trait has been found to be highly heritable (70% of variance genetic in origin) and to be significantly correlated with a number of physiologically relevant biochemical determinants. Thus it is negatively correlated with platelet monoamine oxidase, with cerebrospinal fluid (CSF) norepinephrine and endorphin levels, and with plasma dopamine-β-hy-

Figure 67-5

Substance use by adults as a function of its use by significant others. Census track respondents were asked for each of the three substances whether they were using it and whether any or all of three categories of their significant others, namely, their parents, their past friends, and their current friends, had used or were using the substance. The percentage of use of the substance by the respondents was then plotted as a function of the number of categories of significant others they reported to be using it. The area of each point is proportional to the number of respondents that cluster on it. The overall mean percentage of use of each substance by the responents as a group is given by a horizontal line. (Data from Apsler R, Blackman C: Adults' drug use: Relationship to perceived drug use of parents, friends while growing up, and present friends. Am J Drug Alcohol Abuse 6:291–300, 1979.)

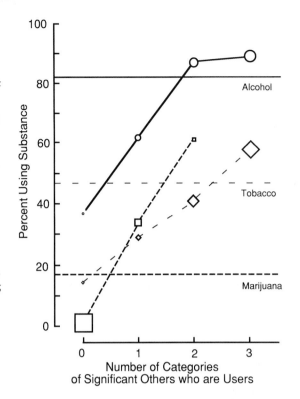

droxylase levels, and positively correlated with those of plasma androgens and estrogens.

The most potent environmental factor facilitating substance use is probably the substance-using behavior of people in one's own current and past environment. Individuals whose parents, and past and present friends, all used a given substance are much more likely to be using it themselves than are those whose friends and parents did not (Fig. 67–5). It is also known that it is much more difficult for individuals to abstain from the abuse of a substance if those around them continue to use it. This presumably is a factor that leads to the formation of self-help groups such as Alcoholics Anonymous.

Effect of substance use by family and peers

Substance-Induced Changes That Maintain Substance Use

PHYSICAL DEPENDENCE

Many, but not all, abused substances induce physical dependence; the intensity of the withdrawal syndrome that follows cessation of use of the substance is characteristically a function of the duration and level of its use prior to cessation. In some instances, as with ethanol, the syndrome can evolve into a life-threatening condition. In other instances, as with opiates, although the syndrome is not life-threatening it can be very unpleasant. Individuals physically dependent on a substance will expend significant effort to secure additional supplies to either prevent or reverse withdrawal symptoms. Physical dependence therefore plays a role in maintenance of substance-abusing behavior. It is not, however, a central one. Over the period of a couple of weeks, individuals can be pharmacologically managed through the withdrawal to the point at which all the symptoms disappear. Nonetheless, as a rule, the individual so detoxified resumes sooner or later, and frequently sooner, the abuse of the substance. Even among individuals who enter special treatment programs, the failure to maintain abstinence is high. Nor is this phenomenon substance-specific: it is possible to find treatment programs for alcohol, heroin, and tobacco dependence (really addiction) that have analogous relapse rates (Fig. 67–6).

Role of physical dependence in promoting addictive behaviors

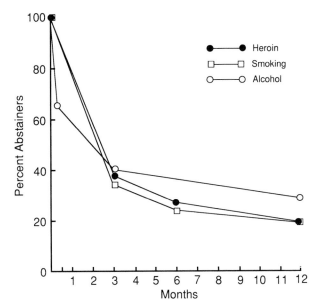

Figure 67-6

Relapse rate. Comparison of the fraction of patients enrolled in three treatment programs (for ethanol, heroin, and cigarette smoking, respectively) who relapsed as a function of time. (From Hunt WA, Barnett LW, Branch LG: Relapse rates in addiction programs. J Clin Psychol 27:455–456, 1971. Reprinted with permission of Clinical Psychology Publishing Co., Inc. Brandon, VT 05733.)

PROTRACTED WITHDRAWAL SYNDROME

Exposure to substantial levels of an opiate for a period of time can lead to subtle changes in systemic physiological functioning that last in excess of half a year. These changes, which in the case of morphine involve lowered body temperature, a raised respiratory rate, and a decreased pupillary diameter (Fig. 67–7), are collectively termed the *protracted withdrawal* (or *protracted abstinence*) syndrome. These changes, although too small to be readily evident upon inspection of a single individual, indicate nonetheless long-term alterations in homeostatic mechanisms. Concurrently, the autonomic system is more labile to stress, and the individual is prone to subjective symptoms of chronic fatigue and dysphoria, symptoms that opiate abusers know from experience are countered by opiates. Similarly, subtle long-term changes in function can occur following abuse of substances that belong to other pharmacological classes, e.g., ethanol and cocaine.

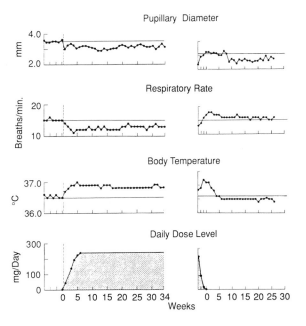

Figure 67-7

Effects of morphine on some physiological parameters when administered for a prolonged time. Data in the left-hand column are based on seven subjects, those in the right-hand column on six subjects, one subject having developed cholecystitis. (From Martin WR, Jasinski DR: Physiological parameters of morphine dependence in man—Tolerance, early abstinence, protracted abstinence. J Psychiat Res 7:9–17, 1969.)

Figure 67–8

Rating of successive IV self-administrations of saline placebo in an environment similar to that in which the previously dependent individual has self-administered narcotics in the past. (Courtesy of O'Brien CP.)

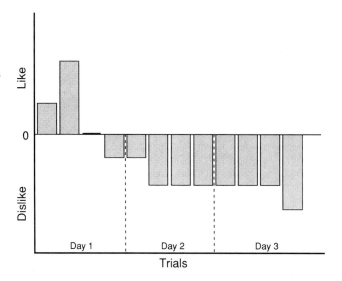

Long-term abuse of either PCP or ethanol results in development of chronic deficits in cognitive and memory functions. With abstinence and in time, such effects are partly reversible. In the case of ethanol, this phenomenon is accompanied by an enlargement of the cerebral ventricles, i.e., a shrinkage of brain mass. This too is partly reversible. Since the life of an alcoholic becomes centered on alcohol, maintenance of abstinence demands adoption of a radically different lifestyle, and that requires much learning. Acquisition of the necessary new behaviors is difficult for individuals in the presence of these deficits, so much so that one of the best predictors of success in therapy is a test of cognitive function.

CONDITIONED RESPONSES AND CONDITIONED WITHDRAWAL

The repeated pairing of substance self-administration and its pharmacological effects leads to the development of classic conditioned responses that mimic some of the pharmacological effects. Detoxified opiate users allowed to prepare ("cook-up") a syringe full of heroin in a naturalistic setting (e.g., one reminiscent of that in which such activities are usually carried out) and, following a surreptitious exchange of syringes, to inject themselves intravenously with saline solution, experience a rewarding opiate effect almost as strong as that of the opiate (Fig. 67–8). When the procedure is repeated several times, the effect ceases to be rewarding and becomes quite aversive. Yawning, tearing, runny nose, and other signs of opiate withdrawal are observed. The phenomenon is termed the *conditioned withdrawal*. The conditioning in question is considered to result from the fact that some opiate abusers frequently self-administer heroin when experiencing withdrawal, and thus the administration procedure and the environment in which it occurs are paired repeatedly with the withdrawal symptoms. In this view the conditioned, drug-like response is much more easily extinguished than the conditioned withdrawal. Accordingly, upon repeated presentations of the conditioned stimuli, the latter response becomes dominant. The phenomenon can be viewed alternatively as an example of conditioned tolerance. Either way, a former opiate abuser experiencing such symptoms would know from experience that administration of an opiate would terminate them.

Protracted and conditioned withdrawals as contributors to continued addictive behavior

Substance Abuse Attendant Toxicity

Certain principles apply to the toxic effects of abused substances generally. First, toxicity and intoxication are somewhat relative concepts that can vary with the expectations of the user. What may be acceptable to or even sought by an experienced user may be alarming to a neophyte and result in the seeking of medical assistance. Some of the disorienting effects of LSD, for instance, can cause panic reactions in users who neither have experienced them previously nor have been warned of them by those who have. The level of intoxication sought by the user is frequently defined by cultural norms. Richard and Eva Blum observed a striking example of this in Greece at a new-wine festival involving free wine and 10,000 or so celebrants. Only 2 men had to be carried out drunk: both wore the United States Navy uniform. An example of the opposite extreme is furnished by some users of PCP who seek levels of intoxication verging on the catatonic. These effects do not appear to be rewarding *per se,* but rather provide an opportunity for users to prove to their peers their toughness by "riding out" the drug's effect. Needless to say, under such circumstance the dividing line between the desired dose and that which may bring the individual to the attention of the health professional may be very narrow indeed.

What users consider an untoward effect may depend on their expectations.

Second, pathologies associated with substance abuse are frequently due not to the pharmacological properties of the substance, but rather to the manner in which it is merchandised and the unhygienic conditions used in its administration. Subcutaneous injections ("skin popping"), particularly popular among women because they leave no tell-tale tracts, lead to abscesses, pyogenic sepsis, and tetanus. Sharing of needles, endemic among opiate users, has become the most prevalent method of HIV transmission in the United States. Infectious endocarditis, hepatitis, syphilis, and tuberculosis are all also transmitted in this manner. At one time, so was malaria, but the quinine used in cutting the opiate kills the parasites in the solution to be injected. Additionally, because the injected material may contain insoluble foreign matter, intravenous-drug users are also prone to develop pulmonary fibrosis and granulomas. As for smoking, carcinogenic polynuclear hydrocarbons are produced in the combustion process and inhaled regardless of what vegetable matter (tobacco, marijuana, and so on) is used to support the combustion.

Toxicities associated with mode of use and administration

Last, epidemiological identification of organ pathologies associated with or caused by long-term abuse of a given substance is important from a public health point of view and because it allows the health professional to inform and warn the substance abuser of the consequences of continued abuse. Identification of such pathologies is easiest if they have a very low natural incidence rather than a moderate one. A case in point is the correlation between increases in cigarette consumption and those in mortality

Occurrence and identification of organ pathologies

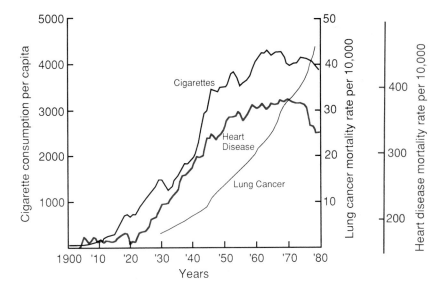

Figure 67-9

Historical trends in cigarette smoking and mortality from lung cancer and from cardiac disease in the United States in the period 1900–1985.

Figure 67 – 10

International correlation between per capita manufactured cigarette consumption among adults and the lung cancer rates in the mid-1970s among those who were entering adulthood around 1950. (From Doll R, Peto R: The causes of cancer: Quantitative estimates of avoidable risks of cancer in the United States today. J Natl Cancer Inst 66:1191–1308, 1981.)

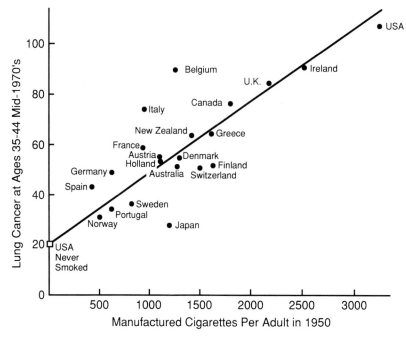

from lung cancer on one hand and from heart disease on the other. Historically, both have risen concurrently with increases in cigarette consumption, although that from lung cancer has a 20-year time lag (Fig. 67–9). Moreover, in absolute terms the rise in excess mortality from heart disease has been five times as large as that from lung cancer. Nevertheless, because the percentage increase in lung cancer deaths was so dramatic, this pathology was identified much earlier as being correlated with cigarette smoking than was the cardiac pathology. The correlations evident in Figure 67-9 are suggestive, but little more. The association is strengthened on consideration of data derived from different venues (Fig. 67–10). In establishing causality, however, dose-response relationships have proved the most convincing to date. For instance, the fact that lung cancer incidence was found to be a function of (1) the number of cigarettes smoked per day, (2) the number of years the individual had smoked, and (3) whether the individual inhaled the cigarette smoke or not was the most compelling evidence that led the United States Surgeon General to conclude in 1964 that cigarette smoking caused lung cancer.

Opiates

Morphine

OH

CH₃O

Codeine

OH

The opium poppy, particularly its seed pod, contains morphine and its phenolic methyl ether, codeine. Incisions of the seed pod result in an exudate. This, allowed to dry and then collected, is opium; accordingly, morphine and codeine as well as compounds derived from them are called *opiates*. This includes heroin, which is obtained by acetylating morphine. Strictly speaking, synthetic compounds that possess morphine-like properties but lack the opiate structure are called *opioids*. *Narcotics* is a term applied to all agents with morphine-like actions. Use of the term *narcotic* at various times with reference to agents that induce sleep and benumb and at other times to identify drugs subject to certain laws has resulted in some ambiguity regarding its exact meaning (see Chapter 18).

REINFORCING PROPERTIES

Although in therapeutics the powerful analgesic effects of opiates are the most important, in the context of substance abuse it is their potent reinforcing properties that are most salient. Foremost among the reinforcing properties is elevation of mood, which, regardless of route of administration is a longer-lasting effect than their analgesic action. The feelings of repose, tranquility, and unconcern that opiates induce were fully appreciated even in the times of Homer, as evidenced by the following passage from The Odyssey

Those who partook of it did not shed a tear the whole day long even though their father or mother were dead, even though a brother or beloved son had been killed before their eyes.

Second, on intravenous administration an immediate orgasmic, thrill-like, transient but extremely pleasurable sensation is experienced. The development of tolerance to opiates does not prevent the occurrence of this effect; on the contrary, tolerance permits more doses of the opiate to be used per day and thus more frequent evocation of the experience. Lastly, opiate users indicate that they feel energized by the drug.

Morphine and opioids exert their reinforcing actions by acting on μ receptors. In order to have high affinity for this receptor, opioids must possess a phenolic ring and a piperidine nitrogen. For high intrinsic activity an aliphatic side chain on the piperidine nitrogen is required. Substitution at this site with either an allyl or a cyclopropyl side chain reduces intrinsic activity markedly, leading to compounds that have either a very low intrinsic activity (buprenorphine) or none at all (naloxone, naltrexone). Because such compounds nonetheless occupy the receptor, they block the reinforcing actions of opioids and act as either partial or pure antagonists (see Chapter 18).

Experimental evidence obtained using animals trained to self-administer opioids suggests that receptors both in the ventral tegmental area and in the nucleus accumbens mediate their reinforcing effects.

TOLERANCE

Marked tolerance develops to many actions of opioids. There are large differences, however, in the speed and completeness of tolerance development for different opioid actions. Thus, complete tolerance develops rapidly to the ability of opioids to induce vomiting, although this tolerance is lost if the user becomes abstinent for a period of time. Tolerance to some effects, such as analgesia and constipation, occurs quite gradually. (Individuals on methadone maintenance are troubled by constipation for the better part of a year.) Although tolerance to depression of respiratory rate, pupillary constriction, and body temperature elevation (hence sweating) develops rapidly at first, it then increases very slowly and may never be complete.

THE ACUTE WITHDRAWAL SYNDROME

The intensity of the acute withdrawal syndrome is proportional to the habit size that precedes it. This can be documented by scoring the intensity of the various symptoms associated with it on arbitrary scales and comparing the totals obtained with the quantity of opiate used during the dependence phase (Fig. 67–11). If the degree of dependence is low, the withdrawal may never progress beyond the early flu-like signs of yawning, rhinorrhea (runny nose), lacrimation, sweating, and tossing ("yen") sleep. More severe withdrawal (Fig. 67–12) is accompanied by an elevation in body temperature. This results in chills and piloerection, or gooseflesh, a reaction to the chills that is the origin of *cold turkey*, a vernacular term for withdrawal. Anorexia, coupled with nausea and vomiting, leads to a marked decrease in caloric intake. These manifestations, together with the intestinal spasms

Heroin

Opioid structure-activity relationships

Buprenorphine

Naloxone

Naltrexone

Methadone

The acute opioid withdrawal syndrome

Figure 67-11

Intensity of morphine withdrawal in subjects dependent on different doses of morphine per day. The points represent mean total responses for 11 hourly observations from the 14th through the 24th hours of withdrawal. The abstinence score is based on deviations of blood pressure, rectal temperature, pulse rate, respiratory rate, and pupil size from the values obtained when the subjects were stabilized on morphine and on the presence of lacrimation, rhinorrhea, perspiration, yawning, tremor, piloerection, restlessness, and emesis. (From Jasinski DR: Assessment of the abuse potential of morphinelike drugs [methods used in man]. *In* Martin WR [ed]: Drug Addiction I: Morphine, Sedative/Hypnotic and Alcohol Dependence, 197–258. Berlin: Springer-Verlag, 1977.)

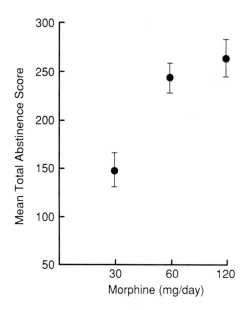

and diarrhea induced by the withdrawal, can result in dehydration and an electrolyte imbalance as well as a significant weight loss. Additionally, the subject is likely to experience bone and muscle pains, abdominal cramps, and muscle spasms of the lower extremities, the latter giving rise to the expression *kicking the habit,* another vernacular term for withdrawal. Two other concomitants of opiate withdrawal are ketosis and leukocytosis. The withdrawal peaks in intensity at 48–72 hours following cessation of opiate use and is considered to dissipate over a 2-week period.

The intensity of the acute withdrawal syndrome also depends in part

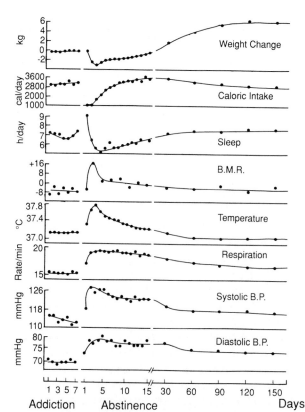

Figure 67-12

Abstinence correlates in opiate-dependent patients stabilized on morphine (N = 11) or morphine congeners (N = 10) and then withdrawn from it. *Abscissa*: Patients stabilized on opiate for 8 days, then withdrawn from it and followed daily for 150 days. *Ordinate*: Changes in a number of physiological variables. (From Himmelsbach CK: Clinical studies of drug addiction: Physical dependence, withdrawal and recovery. Arch Intern Med 69:766–772, 1942.)

on the speed with which the action of the opiate is terminated or reversed. It is greater, therefore, for morphine, which has a short half-life, than for methadone, whose half-life is ten times longer. Also, the withdrawal precipitated by the administration of an opiate antagonist is intense.

The intensity of withdrawal syndromes seen currently among opiate users is typically much milder than that described. This is ascribed to the very low heroin content of material that is sold as heroin. Even the administration of naloxone fails to precipitate withdrawal in a significant proportion of applicants to methadone treatment programs who claim to be heroin addicts and whose urines contain quinine (a common dilutent of illicit heroin).

THERAPY OF THE OPIOID WITHDRAWAL SYNDROME

The opioid withdrawal syndrome is not a life-threatening condition, but it is very unpleasant and can be treated. The classic method of detoxication is based on the concept that the withdrawal should be terminated first by administration of an orally effective, long-acting opiate, namely methadone, and that, having established the level of the subject's dependence, the daily methadone dose is incrementally decreased over a period of 2–3 weeks. To establish the level of dependence, the patient is given 10 mg doses of methadone at 2-hour intervals until the symptoms of withdrawal disappear. Since methadone is not a fast-acting drug, more frequent administration could lead to the patient being overdosed.

Part of the symptoms of the opioid withdrawal syndrome are mediated by the cells of the locus ceruleus, a structure with a large collection of noradrenergic neurons. These cells are inhibited by stimulation of their μ opiate receptors, usually by endogenous opiates (e.g., β endorphin). In the chronic opiate user, this function is taken over by the administered opiate, with a resultant down-regulation of endogenous opiate synthesis and consequent noradrenergic overactivity on opioid withdrawal. These cells are also inhibited by stimulation of their α_2 adrenergic receptors by clonidine, an α_2 adrenergic agonist (Chapter 14). Clonidine is also considered to attenuate the noradrenergic activity during withdrawal by acting at postsynaptic α_2 adrenergic receptors. Accordingly, an alternate method of detoxication is administration of clonidine. The method involves sudden discontinuation of the opiate and administration of clonidine every 4–6 hours, a larger dose being administered at bedtime. As a rule, lethargy, dizziness, sleepiness, and hypotension are the only side effects. Because the hypotension can be marked, the procedure is usually carried out on an inpatient basis. After 10–15 days on clonidine, a naloxone challenge is used to determine whether the opiate detoxication is complete. Once this has been ascertained, clonidine is discontinued and the patient can be placed directly on *naltrexone*, a long-acting opiate antagonist.

Clonidine, although not an opioid, is effective in the treatment of the opioid withdrawal syndrome.

During a period of high-level opiate use, the suppression of central noradrenergic activity leads to development of supersensitivity at postsynaptic sites resulting from an up-regulation of adrenergic receptors. Opiate antagonists rapidly reverse this up-regulation and supersensitivity. Accordingly, administration of naltrexone would be expected both to intensify and to shorten the duration of the withdrawal syndrome. Taking advantage of the ability of clonidine to mitigate the withdrawal, a third and accelerated method of detoxication from opiate dependence has been developed. The method is employed primarily with patients who need to be removed from methadone maintenance. Within 24 hours of their last methadone dose, these patients are started on clonidine and then are given naltrexone. The more or less concurrent administration of these two agents

Role of naltrexone in the treatment of the opioid withdrawal syndrome is then continued on a frequent schedule (varying, during daylight hours, from every 6 hours to every 90 minutes), titrating, in effect, the withdrawal suppressing and eliciting effects of these drugs against each other. The starting clonidine dose used is relatively high and that of naltrexone relatively low. During the 3–5 days of therapy the dose of naltrexone is escalated so that from a starting dose of 1 mg it is increased at the end to as much as 50 mg, whereas the clonidine requirement is found to diminish. In the more rapid version of this approach, patients are also given diazepam to further mitigate the symptoms of withdrawal induced by naltrexone.

TOXICITY

Opiate addicts suffer from a large excess morbidity and mortality, much of it due to the unhygienic conditions and the less than pure products used.

Overdose toxicity is a frequent medical problem. Its occurrence is abetted by the variability in the opiate content of illicit heroin, which is usually quite low but not predictably so. Diagnostically, the classic triad of signs of opiate overdose are coma, miosis, and depressed respiration. However, mydriasis does not rule out the diagnosis because hypoxia may cause it. Hypotension may also be present. Pulmonary edema of rapid onset is sometimes a complicating feature. It is characterized by a frothy sputum that may be bloody. The treatment of choice for opiate-induced coma is the intravenous administration of naloxone every 5 minutes until the coma is reversed. Because vomiting may occur, comatose patients should be intubated to prevent aspiration. An excess of naloxone will precipitate withdrawal in the dependent individual. Also, the half-life of naloxone is shorter even than that of morphine. Accordingly, the patient has to be closely monitored lest the depressant effects of the opiate return.

The potent analgesic actions of opiates contribute to two conditions seen in opiate addicts. Protected against the pain, addicts tend to ignore gastric ulcers, allowing these to exacerbate to the point of perforation. Because of the analgesia they also fail to react in a timely fashion to the ischemic pain resulting from limb compression induced by postures they may assume in a stuporous state. In the ensuing crush syndrome, myolysis can follow and result in the release of myoglobin into the bloodstream. The latter can cause renal impairment. Yet another syndrome associated with opiate addiction is heroin nephropathy, which progresses to end-stage renal disease (ESRD) necessitating chronic dialysis treatment. The mechanism responsible for precipitating this condition is unknown, but the condition is encountered disproportionately often among black users of heroin. Finally, intravenous street heroin users are immunosuppressed, but individuals on methadone maintenance are much less so. Although opiates have immunosuppressant effects in experimental animals, the role they play in inducing immunosuppression clinically remains unclear.

The analgesic effects of opiates cause opiate abusers to ignore painful symptoms of various pathologies.

TREATMENT OF OPIATE DEPENDENCE

The primary challenge that the treatment of opiate dependence presents is not achieving abstinence but rather maintaining it. The vast majority of detoxified opiate abusers return rapidly to using opiates. Longitudinal statistics gathered among opiate addicts in a period in which this was the only treatment offered, indicate that only 7% of them gave up the addiction each year; that is, the addiction had a half-life of 24 years.

Methadone maintenance is by far the most widely used medical response to this challenge. Paradoxically, it is a response that jettisons abstinence as a goal, adopting instead the strategy of replacing illicit opiates with an institutionally dispensed one. The goals of this strategy are to reduce the need for illicit opiates and the associated criminal activity; to increase the health, self-esteem, and employability of the addict; and to improve family and community functioning of these individuals. In the original program, individuals were to receive increasing daily doses of methadone so that, as tolerance developed, they would become refractory to the acute effects of heroin self-administration and would then be maintained on this dose. In reality, intravenously administered heroin can produce some rewarding effects no matter how high the methadone dose. Nonetheless, even relatively low daily doses of methadone have been found to relieve the dependent user's craving for opiates and to lead to a significant decrease in heroin use and associated criminality.

Methadone maintenance

Since methadone maintenance renders the patient physically dependent on opiates, a preliminary requirement to induction into such a program is administration of a test dose of naloxone to check, by the precipitation of a withdrawal syndrome, that the patient is already dependent on opiates. Induced patients are started on a low dose of methadone, which is increased gradually to 40–100 mg/day. Once the desired dose is achieved, patients are asked to return to the clinic daily to receive (ingest) the methadone and to donate a urine sample, which is checked for morphine. In some jurisdictions, patients are allowed to return to the clinic less often and are given a supply of methadone to take on the intervening days. Diversion of dispensed methadone to an illicit market, driven by the fact that abusers find the intravenous administration of methadone to be rather reinforcing, is a problem. It is lessened by the dispensation of the methadone in orange juice and also by it being dispensed as a mixture with naloxone. The latter, having an extremely low oral availability, has no effect on ingested methadone but effectively antagonizes it if the mixture is injected.

There is a 2-year statutory limit, frequently extended, on how long a patient can be maintained on methadone. Discontinuation involves reducing the daily dose incrementally, at first by 5 mg/week and, after it has declined to 25 mg/day, even more gradually. Alternatively, clonidine detoxication can be performed.

Methadone maintenance treatment has high continuation rates, and the pharmacological side effects are relatively few and benign. Although in the first year of maintenance, patients experience increased sweating, constipation, and more rarely, decreased libido and insomnia, generally all other aspects of the patients' health improve owing to better nutrition and cessation of unhygienic self-administration practices. Infants born to women on methadone maintenance have significant body burdens of methadone, which in the neonate has a half-life seven times longer than in the adult. Such infants are physically dependent, and maternal preparturition maintenance has to be restricted to 25 mg/day, otherwise an unacceptable incidence of neonatal mortality occurs. Physically dependent neonates can be treated using phenobarbital to prevent convulsions and paregoric (tincture of opium) to control gastrointestinal symptoms; withdrawn neonates prosper, and no teratogenic effects have been noted.

Opiate blockade with naltrexone (TREXAN), a long-lasting opiate antagonist, represents the best alternative strategy currently employed for the treatment of opiate dependence. Administered two to three times per week, it has no discernible effect of its own but effectively blocks the actions of any opiate the patient might self-administer. However, opiate addicts do not find taking it reinforcing, and as a consequence, their dropout rate from this treatment is very high. On the other hand, health professionals and business executives, who are highly motivated because their employment

Use of blocking drugs in the treatment of opiate dependence

depends on continued opiate abstinence, have high continuation rates and opiate-free urines. Likewise, inmates of correctional institutions, whose participation in work-release programs depends on supervised compliance, do well in such programs.

Partial opiate agonist/antagonists such as buprenorphine (BUPRENEX), an agent currently marketed for the relief of moderate to severe pain, show promise as alternatives to naltrexone. Unlike naltrexone, buprenorphine has a significant, although limited, morphine-like effect. From preliminary studies it appears to be reinforcing to the opiate addict, yet, like naltrexone, it blocks the actions of other opiates. Such drugs, however, have significant market potential as legitimate, nonaddicting analgesics. The latter market dwarfs that for the treatment of opiate dependence. A long history of false starts (heroin was first marketed as a cure for morphinism, meperidine was first marketed as "nonaddicting," as was later also pentazocine) renders manufacturers wary of the possible merchandising consequences of also entering the opiate-maintenance market with such drugs. Buprenorphine itself also has the disadvantages of a fairly low oral availability (although it is relatively well absorbed sublingually); although its half-life is significantly shorter than that of methadone, its analgesic effects are longer lasting.

Cocaine and Amphetamines

Cocaine

Amphetamine

D-amphetamine has much greater effect on the CNS than does L-amphetamine.

Methamphetamine

Cocaine is an alkaloid ester with a rigid structure that is present in a 1% concentration in the leaves of a shrub that grows at elevations between 2000 and 8000 feet in the Andes Mountains. It can be liberated therefrom by maceration with alkali. Since Inca times, chewing of coca leaves with lime (calcium hydroxide) or ash (source of potassium hydroxide) has been a custom of the high Andean region, particularly at altitudes above 10,000 feet where the thin air leads to easy fatigue. Cocaine hydrochloride ("crystal," "snow") used to be the mainstay of the illicit cocaine market. It is a white crystalline powder that abusers snort, usually in "lines" of 5–10 mg or more as tolerance permits. Being readily soluble in water, it can also be injected intravenously. It is not, however, suitable for smoking because, although it melts at 187°C, it decomposes before reaching a boiling point. The free cocaine base, on the other hand, melts at 98°C and boils at 250°C, allowing it to be smoked. It is also very lipid soluble and therefore passes more rapidly across mucous membranes, such as those in oral-pharyngeal cavity. *Free-basing* involves dissolution of street cocaine hydrochloride in alkali, extraction with ether, and evaporation of the latter. More simply, solid free base ("crack," or "rock") is produced by boiling the hydrochloride with a solution of sodium bicarbonate and filtering the precipitated free base. Much of street cocaine is now merchandised as crack.

Amphetamines are synthetic phenylamines with an unsubstituted phenyl ring and an ethylamine side chain that has an alkyl substituent on the alpha carbon; that is, the carbon next to the amine nitrogen. Many of the amphetamines exist in dextrorotatory and levorotatory forms: D-amphetamine possess fourfold greater central nervous activity than the L-form. On the other hand, L-amphetamine has more potent cardiovascular effects. Prior to 1972 D-amphetamine sulfate was widely used in the United States. In 1966 eight billion tablets were produced; of these about half were diverted to the illicit market, with long-distance truck drivers as major consumers. Because it was judged a drug of limited medical usefulness and one of great abuse potential, its legitimate production has since been markedly curtailed. Some of the better known amphetamines are: D-amphetamine, methamphetamine, methylphenidate (RITALIN), diethylpropion (TENUATE), and phenmetrazine (PRELUDIN).

REINFORCING PROPERTIES

The central effects of cocaine and D-amphetamine are very reinforcing and quite similar; users are unable to distinguish intravenous injections of D-amphetamine from those of cocaine. The intensity and nature of the effects are very much a function of dose. Both agents have significant effects on mood, performance, judgment, and appetite. The effects on mood result in significant changes in self-descriptors. Respondents report that they perceive themselves as more talkative, good-natured, energetic, clearheaded, effective, self-confident, happy, elated, impulsive, boastful, and restless. The effects of increasing doses of cocaine are illustrated in passages written by individuals who self-administered it soon after its isolation, and who thus presumably had no preconceived notions regarding what its effects ought to be.

Methylphenidate

65–130 mg PO (by mouth)	One is simply normal, and soon finds it hard to believe that one is under the influence of any drug. . . . Long-lasting, intensive mental or physical work can be performed without any fatigue; it is as though the need for food and sleep were completely banished. SIGMUND FREUD, UEBER COCA, ZENTRALBLATT GES THERAP 2:289–314, 1884
65 mg SC (subcutaneously)	A sense of exhilaration and an increase of mental activity that were well marked. I was writing at the time and I found that my thoughts flowed with increased freedom and were unusually well expressed. . . .
130 mg SC	A similar exhilaration . . . a great desire to write . . . did so with a freedom and apparent clearness that astonished me. The following morning, when I came to read it over, . . . it was entirely coherent, logical, and as good if not better as anything I had previously written. . . .
260 mg SC	Effects were similar, except that they were much more intense. I wrote page after page, throwing the sheets on the floor without stopping to gather them together. The following morning, I found that I had written a series of high-flown sentences altogether different from my usual style, and bearing upon matters in which I was not the least interested.
780 mg SC	I was conscious of a tendency to talk, and as far as my recollection extends, I believe I made a long speech on some subject of which I have no remembrance the next day.
1370 mg SC	I felt my mind was passing beyond my control. I was in such a frame of mind as to be utterly regardless of any calamity or danger. I lost consciousness of all my acts within, I think, half an hour after administration. Next day when I came downstairs I found the floor of my library strewn with encyclopedias, dictionaries and other books of reference and one or two chairs overturned. . . . WA HAMMOND, COCA: Its preparations and their therapeutic qualities, with some remarks on the so-called cocaine habit. TRANS MED SOC VIRG 1887:212–226

As dose is escalated, the perception of effectiveness and sagacity is replaced by disorganization.

Amphetamine has been shown to have a significant enhancing effect on athletic performance, whether in swimming, track, or field events. Although the magnitude of the effect is small, it is large enough to make a decisive difference in competitive sport. Amphetamines have also been found to enhance performance of simple repetitive tasks that easily induce fatigue, for instance in a coding task requiring the subject to cross each uppercase letter and circle each lowercase vowel in many lines of material such as

4 d P q r M d B 7 W b J p 6 E m N a 5 z v p

Performance on intellectually challenging tasks, on the other hand, is not enhanced. Thus, for instance, the performance of Massachusetts Institute of Technology (MIT) students on a calculus examination was unaffected by administration of amphetamine. Judgment is affected: when the selfsame MIT students were asked to give estimates of their exam scores, those given amphetamine overestimated them more than did students given placebo. Both agents have anorectic effects. Rapid intravenous administration induces a *rush,* an intense, orgasm-like sensation.

Cocaine and amphetamine have multiple actions on CNS monoamine neurotransmitters, namely norepinephrine, dopamine, and serotonin. The reinforcing properties of cocaine are specifically mediated by inhibition of the reuptake of dopamine. Those of amphetamine are mediated primarily by its enhancement of the release of dopamine from its storage sites. In both instances this results in higher concentration of dopamine at its synaptic receptor as well as at the site of its enzymatic deactivation. Although this leads to an enhanced response to dopaminergic stimulation, it also causes depletion of dopamine stores.

The onset of cocaine's action is fastest following smoking of the free base. Intravenous administration of the hydrochloride and intranasal administration are other favored routes. Cocaine has a high oral availability. The blood levels that are reached after oral administration are comparable to those seen after intranasal administration, although with a 30-minute delay. Once in the systemic circulation, cocaine, having a lipid solubility intermediate between that of heroin and that of methadone, crosses the blood-brain barrier rapidly. The biological half-life of cocaine is short, 0.7–1.5 hours; its action is mostly terminated by metabolism. Some (2–6%) is converted by N-demethylation to norcocaine, which is also active, but the bulk undergoes hydrolysis to inactive metabolites through the action of blood pseudocholinesterases and hepatic esterases.

The oral bioavailability of amphetamine is also high, the substitution on the α carbon protects the molecule from first-pass metabolism. The half-life of amphetamine is 4–20 hours. It is mostly eliminated by urinary excretion. Since it is a strong base, its half-life is therefore a function of urinary pH (Fig. 67–13). Methamphetamine is more lipid-soluble and

Mechanism of action

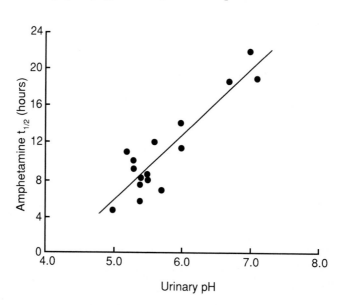

Figure 67–13

Half-life of amphetamine as a function of urinary pH. (From Änggärd E, Gunne LM, Jönsson LE, Niklasson F: Pharmacokinetic and clinical studies on amphetamine-dependent subjects. Eur J Clin Pharmacol 3:3–11, 1970.)

enters the brain more rapidly than D-amphetamine to which it is demethylated.

TOLERANCE

Cocaine or amphetamine use is associated with atypical tolerance and withdrawal phenomena. High-level use of these substances is characterized by episodes ("runs") of repetitive self-administration that may last many hours or days, during which time the user remains continually awake, and typically continue until supplies are exhausted. Monkeys allowed to self-administer cocaine at will continue to do so until they die. In humans the symptoms observed during the run include touching and picking of the face and extremities, fascination with philosophical concerns ("meanings," "essence"), and perseveration in stereotypic behavior (e.g., repeatedly taking apart and putting together some gadget). During a run, the reinforcing effects of the substance become increasingly attenuated. Some chronic tolerance does build up in time to the euphoriogenic, cardiovascular, and hyperthermic effects, but so does kindling, a phenomenon whereby the threshold for seizures is lowered following repeated cocaine exposure.

THE ACUTE WITHDRAWAL SYNDROME

Cessation of amphetamine or cocaine use has been known for some time to be followed, first, by increased hunger and prolonged sleep, and second, by depression, general fatigue, and a marked increase in REM (rapid eye movement) sleep. These effects are reversed by administration of either cocaine or amphetamine. Because the withdrawal does not result in major, grossly observable physiological disruption, however, there was initially some reluctance to accept this phenomena as a withdrawal syndrome.

Naturalistic evaluation of psychic symptoms that follow cocaine runs has led to conceptualization of a three-phase sequence of post–cocaine abuse abstinence symptoms. The first phase, or "crash," begins within 15–30 minutes following the last dose of cocaine and lasts from 3 to 6 days. It is heralded by rapidly mounting depression and characterized by anhedonia, insomnia, irritability, anxiety, and suicidal ideation. The craving for cocaine gradually diminishes, and after 2–5 hours the individual refuses cocaine even if offered. Gradually, lethargy and somnolence become apparent and eventually lead to a long sleep, occasionally interrupted by bouts of eating. The second phase, which can last from 1 to 10 weeks, begins with negligible cocaine craving and near normal mood and functioning. In due course dysphoria, joylessness, and a perception of intense boredom develop and are accompanied by increasing craving for cocaine, by memories of the reinforcing effects of the drug, by increasing anxiety, and by efforts to arrange for supplies. During the third phase that follows, the affective state returns to near-normal levels and craving is episodic, but extreme when triggered by environmental clues such as friends who previously shared in cocaine use or the sight of venipuncture. Such episodes suggest conditioned tolerance as the responsible mechanism. This phase can last for months.

The withdrawal syndrome is characterized by three phases.

TOXICITY

Both cocaine and the amphetamines potentiate the peripheral effects of sympathomimetic innervation, causing vasoconstriction. Applied to the nasal mucosa, these agents are therefore effective decongestants. At one time, over-the-counter amphetamine (BENZEDRINE) nasal inhalers were

Toxic effects of cocaine on nasal tissues

widely used. Earlier, during the last two decades of the nineteenth century and at a time when the ability of cocaine to cross mucosal membranes was not appreciated, topical application of cocaine was used for the treatment of acute coryza and hay fever. Relief was only temporary, with rebound rhinitis and, on chronic use, local necrosis caused by the ischemia. Freud, for instance, wrote that in 1895, "I was making frequent use of cocaine to reduce some troublesome nasal swellings, . . . and one of the women patients who followed my example had developed an extensive necrosis of the nasal mucous membrane." Perforated nasal septa began to be observed clinically with the resurgence of cocaine use in the 1970s, with at least one report of a nasal drip of cerebrospinal fluid secondary to a perforation. At the time, cocaine was very expensive, and nasal pathology constituted the main toxic manifestation of its use; it has been said of that period that the user was protected by "the limitations of his pocketbook and of his nasal mucosa."

In large doses cocaine causes cardiovascular and central nervous system toxicity.

In large doses the adrenergic effects include marked tachycardia, extreme vasoconstriction and blood pressure increases, hyperpyrexia, anxiety, paranoia, and generalized convulsions. The ready availability of cocaine in the form of crack and the use of administration routes selected for maximal speed of onset have resulted in much more extreme adrenergic effects and severe toxic reactions. In many of these, sudden extreme surges in blood pressure, closely temporally associated with cocaine self-administration, are the central component and lead to myocardial infarctions, cerebrovascular accidents, ruptured aortas, and abruptio placentae in pregnant women. Arrhythmias, in many instances, occur in young adults with no pre-existing conditions and are seen following not only intravenous and inhalation dosing but also intranasal administration. Postmortem examination of heart sections indicates the presence of contraction bands. Such bands are known to occur as a consequence of catecholamine-induced cardiac damage and represent a disruption of intracellular calcium homeostasis.

Ingestion of large doses of cocaine can result in intestinal ischemia secondary to intense mesenteric vasoconstriction; untreated, it can lead to gangrene. The effects of maternal cocaine use on the fetus include smaller birth weight and length for gestational period, smaller head circumference, a fourfold greater incidence of congenital malformations, and an 8% stillbirth rate owing to abruptio placentae.

Chronic cocaine or amphetamine abuse is correlated with toxic paranoid-schizophrenia–like reaction characterized by vivid hallucinations (visual, auditory, tactile), paranoid ideation, and changes in affect. All these symptoms occur with a clear sensorium and, if there is no continued use of the agent, resolve in a week or so.

TREATMENT OF COCAINE DEPENDENCE

Elimination of craving is the goal of cocaine dependence treatment.

The pharmacological treatment of the various phases of amphetamine and cocaine abuse and withdrawal is an area of intense clinical investigation. To date, the most promising results have been obtained with desipramine. When it is administered to cocaine abusers, it significantly reduces both cocaine use and cocaine craving and has been found to remain effective for at least 6 weeks. Its main disadvantage is that the reduction in craving develops slowly over 7–14 days. It has been proposed that the mode of action of desipramine is to reverse a dopaminergic inhibitory autoreceptor supersensitivity induced by the stimulant and thus to reduce the depression and anhedonia characteristic of withdrawal from these substances. The long delay in the onset of craving reduction by desipramine poses a problem because, among outpatients, resumption of cocaine use in the interim is frequent. Preliminary studies suggest that administration of a depot form of flupenthixol, a neuroleptic agent that in low doses has a rapid antidepressant activity and the action of which lasts for 2–4 weeks, may prove useful. Flupenthixol is considered to block dopamine receptors, including the inhibitory autoreceptors. Clinically, it decreases cocaine craving and increases retention of patients in treatment.

Based on the premise that the reinforcing effect of cocaine, and thereby also cocaine craving, is mediated by dopaminergic mechanisms, the effects of bromocriptine, a dopaminergic agonist, have been investigated clinically. This agent does suppress cocaine craving; however, the effect wanes when the agent is used for a week or more. Also, the agent sustains self-administration, and patients taken off bromocriptine suffer a craving rebound. Amantadine, an agent known to release dopamine and norepinephrine from their storage sites and to retard their reuptake, also initially suppresses cocaine craving, but like bromocriptine, it loses efficacy after about 2 weeks of use.

Behavioral treatment of cocaine abuse has proved effective for a certain class of individuals—that is, those who seek treatment out of concern for the losses they might sustain as a consequence of continued use. The strategy employed is to utilize such concerns to create motivation for day-by-day abstinence. The patient's concerns are explored, and the patient is asked to write a letter, addressed to an appropriate authority, identifying him or her as a cocaine addict and surrendering the instruments (certification, license, and so on) that allow the individual to practice a profession, craft, and the like. The patient and the treatment facility then enter into a written contract whereby the patient agrees to donate urine samples for a chemical screen on a random biweekly basis and instructs the treatment facility to formally transmit the letter to the addressee in the event that the urine samples reveal cocaine use. This approach has proved highly successful with select professional groups, such as physicians.

Depressants

The pharmacological effects of barbiturates and other nonbenzodiazepine sedative-hypnotic drugs—namely, chloral hydrate, paraldehyde, gluthethimide, meprobamate, methyprylon, ethinamate, and ethchlorvynol—are similar to those of ethanol. A marked similarity also exists with respect to the tolerance, dependence, and withdrawal phenomena seen when these substances or ethanol are abused. Pharmacologically all these agents are classified, therefore, as belonging to the same category of substances, namely CNS depressants of the alcohol-barbiturate type. The benzodiazepines also share many but not all the properties and problems of these substances. Accordingly, the focus of this section is on the similarities and differences between the abuse characteristics of these various agents and those of ethanol.

> Pharmacologically, most CNS depressants have central effects similar to those of ethanol.

REINFORCING PROPERTIES

The reinforcing properties of barbiturates, benzodiazepines, and other CNS depressants of this type are qualitatively similar to those of ethanol. The abuse potential of such agents tends to be determined primarily by how rapid is the onset of their action, this in turn being a function of the lipid solubility and route of administration of these drugs.

TOLERANCE AND PHYSICAL DEPENDENCE

Both functional and metabolic tolerance tend to develop to the agents in this class, the former predominating. Although tolerance develops even when only small amounts of barbiturates or other nonbenzodiazepine sedative-hypnotics are used, physical dependence does not if the dose used is not increased above that initially necessary to induce significant pharmacological effects. This is not the case with diazepam and alprazolam, however; physical dependence had been observed in some individuals who had used only therapeutic doses of these agents.

THE ACUTE WITHDRAWAL SYNDROME

In those physically dependent on depressants, the rapidity with which symptoms of withdrawal appear is a function of the half-life of the drug. The withdrawal syndrome from barbiturates of intermediate duration (e.g., pentobarbital, secobarbital) bears a striking similarity to that from ethanol (Table 67–2). As with ethanol, the severity of the withdrawal is correlated with the dose to which individuals are dependent. Among the minor signs and symptoms are coarse tremor, progressive weakness, insomnia, anorexia, nausea, and vomiting. More serious symptoms are hallucinations and grand mal–type seizures. Untreated, some of the individuals dependent on 1.0 g/day or more of the barbiturate progress to develop hyperthermia and a delirium analogous to delirium tremens. The similarity between the withdrawal phenomena from these barbiturates and those from ethanol is underlined by the ability of the two sets of agents to terminate each other's withdrawal syndrome (although not the delirium). The withdrawal phenomena from the other nonbenzodiazepine sedative-hypnotics are quite similar. The withdrawal syndrome from barbiturates with a longer half-life (e.g., phenobarbital) is generally milder and more prolonged.

Based on clinical case reports, it is clear that upon discontinuation of benzodiazepines, even when taken in therapeutic doses, withdrawal syndromes do develop. Moreover, the severity of the withdrawal syndrome is not necessarily proportional to the size of the dose employed and, in the case of diazepam, is usually seen only after use of the agent for a much longer time, stretching into many months. Additionally, although the var-

The severity of the withdrawal syndrome from diazepam is not proportional to the dose employed.

Table 67–2 WITHDRAWAL REACTION SEVERITY AS A FUNCTION OF PRECEDING EXPOSURE TO A DEPRESSANT

Period of Maximal Exposure			Incidence of Withdrawal Signs and Symptoms					
			Minor		Major			
Daily Amount	Duration	Number	TREMOR (%)	OTHER (%)	HALLUCI-NATIONS (%)	SEIZURES (%)	DELIRIUM TREMENS (%)	FEVER (%)
Ethanol								
Drinks*	Days							
30	52	6	100	100	60	33	33	100
23	23	10	80	80	50	0	0	10
26	10	4	100	100	0	0	0	0
19	3	8	100	†	0	0	0	0
Barbiturate								
Doses*	Days							
9–22	90	18	100	100	67	78	39	†
8	90	8	†	100	26	13	0	†
6	90	18	†	50	0	14	0	†
4	90	18	†	6	0	0	0	†

From Gessner PK: Drug therapy of the alcohol withdrawal syndrome. *In* Majchrowicz E, Noble EP (eds): Biochemistry and Pharmacology of Ethanol, vol 2, 375–435. New York: Plenum Press, 1979.
* Dose units: ethanol drink—15 ml ethanol; barbiturate—100 mg secobarbital or pentobarbital.
† Data not available.

ious signs and symptoms of alcohol/barbiturate withdrawal have all been seen also in diazepam and alprazolam withdrawal, there are a number of signs and symptoms that are unique to these agents as well—paranoia, blurring of vision, headache, and for diazepam also facial numbness and cramps. For alprazolam, which has a half-life of 12–15 hours, the withdrawal syndrome emerges in 18–48 hours. With agents with long half-lives, such as diazepam, withdrawal, on the other hand, is much delayed and its course is prolonged. If seizures occur, for instance, they are typically seen on the eighth to tenth days. Some of the peculiar features of the diazepam withdrawal syndrome may be related to its very long half-life and the fact that it forms active metabolites with even longer half-lives and a tendency to accumulate. Finally, the inability of diazepam to control, in a number of instances, the alprazolam withdrawal syndrome suggests that these agents may be acting on different populations of receptors (see Chapter 20).

Nicotine and Cigarette Smoking

Nicotine is an alkaloid present exclusively in the tobacco plant indigenous to the American continent. Both the plant products and the methodology for self-administration by smoking were brought back to Europe in the 1600s by the early explorers. There tobacco met both enthusiastic adoption and fervent opposition. The alkaline nature of the smoke derived from air-dried pipe and cigar tobacco generally prevents its inhalation, delays the onset of action of the nicotine in the smoke, and curbs the extent of its use. The discovery at the turn of the nineteenth century that flue-dried tobacco gives an acid smoke that can be inhaled much more readily led to the introduction of cigarettes and a marked escalation in the proportion of the population using tobacco.

Cigarette smoking is more reinforcing than either cigar or pipe smoking.

REINFORCING PROPERTIES

The smoking habit is so old, commonplace, and currently enjoys so little status that appreciation of its considerable reinforcing properties is jaded. The words of an earlier writer may serve to correct this.

> This precious herbe, Tobacco, most divine
> Then which nere Greece, nere Italy did list
> A flower more fragrant to the Muses shrine
> A purer sacrifice did nere adorne
> Apollos altars, then this Indian fire,
> The pipe, thy head: the flame to make it burne
> The furie, which the Muses doe inspire:
>   O sacred smoke, that doth from hence arise
>   The authors winged praise, which beats upon the skies.
>
> Sir John Beaumont, 1602
> The Metamorphosis of Tobacco

TOLERANCE AND PHYSICAL DEPENDENCE

In naive subjects, nicotine induces nausea and vomiting, but tolerance to this and its other effects develops rapidly. Both functional and metabolic tolerance are observed. Smokers seek to maintain certain nicotine blood levels. Administration of ammonium chloride, which leads to acidification of the urine and more rapid nicotine elimination, results in an increase in the number of cigarettes smoked. Upon sudden cessation of smoking, individuals who smoke 20 or more cigarettes a day develop an abstinence syndrome. This includes a lower diastolic blood pressure, bradycardia, palpitations, gastric disorders, irritability, difficulties in concentrating, anxiety, and restlessness. During withdrawal, craving for cigarettes may be

Tobacco dependence is as enduring as that to agents more commonly considered addictive.

intense and persistent; it can last many months. As a consequence, over half of the cigarette smokers who seek treatment for alcohol and drug dependence identify quitting cigarette smoking as harder than stopping the use of the substance for which they seek treatment. Also, in populations exposed to life-terminating starvation (e.g., in concentration camps in Nazi Germany during World War II) trading of cigarettes for food was common. At an earlier time, before cigarettes were widely used, individuals smoking pipes or cigars also found quitting very hard. Freud, for instance, continued his cigar habit (20/day) until death, in spite of an endless series of operations for mouth and jaw cancer (the jaw was eventually totally removed), persistent heart problems that were exacerbated by smoking, and numerous attempts at quitting.

THERAPY OF NICOTINE DEPENDENCE

In efforts to relieve the craving for cigarettes, products have been developed that provide nicotine without combustion. Of these the best known is nicotine chewing gum (NICORETTE). This releases nicotine gradually upon chewing and at a rate calculated to decrease the probability of dependence.

An alternative therapeutic strategy is the use of low-dose clonidine (200 μg/day). This reduces withdrawal symptoms and craving in heavy cigarette smokers and doubles (from 30 to 60%) the number who remain abstinent for 6 months or more. Individuals with a history of major depression (although no current symptoms) are only half as likely to succeed in quitting to smoke. Although individuals with such a history do have a higher quitting rate if receiving clonidine rather than placebo, in both groups the rate is lower than among individuals with no such history.

TOXICITY

The morbidity associated with cigarette smoking is very high.

Cigarette smoking is the single major cause of cancer mortality. In addition to cancers of the lung, the larynx, and the oral cavity, cigarette smoking has been found to be a factor in the genesis of numerous other neoplasms, including cancers of the bladder, kidney, esophagus, pancreas, stomach, and uterus. It is also a major cause of cardiovascular mortality, causing coronary heart disease, and a significant factor in sudden cardiac death and stroke. Additionally, cigarette smoking is the major cause of obstructive lung disease, thus chronic bronchitis and emphysema. Babies born to women smokers are small for their gestational age. Also, at age 11 such children are significantly shorter in stature and lower in mathematical ability and reading comprehension than children of nonsmokers.

Phencyclidine

The principal effects of PCP are dissociative.

PCP, an agent with a chemical structure similar to the anesthetic ketamine (Chapter 16), was developed in 1957 by Parke-Davis, a pharmaceutical company, as a dissociative anesthetic. The vivid dreams patients, particularly young males, experience during emergence from anesthesia and the confused and irrational behavior manifested by them led the company to restrict the use of the agent after 1962 to veterinary medicine. Illicit use of the substance spread rapidly after 1972, once users realized that the substance could be inhaled in smoke.

REINFORCING PROPERTIES

Several effects of PCP appear to be rewarding in the sense that users find them worth evoking. It produces spatial distortions and a dissociation from

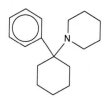

Phencyclidine

current concerns, from the environment, and from the body. It causes decreased touch (two-point discrimination), pain, and position sense. Also, thresholds to audiometry and visual perimetry are increased, causing a dissociation between sensory and motor functioning. In the words of one user

> I felt a little drunk and had some trouble walking around the apartment. Objects appeared either very far or very close and I could not judge distance at all. I liked being apart from things, and felt outside my body for most of the trip. That was fun.
>
> RK Siegel, Phencyclidine and ketamine intoxication: A study of four populations of recreational users. NIDA Res Monog 21:119–143, 1978

PCP has been shown to have affinity for two receptors in the CNS. One of these is what used to be termed the σ *opiate receptor*, but it is now referred to simply as the σ *receptor* because opiate antagonists such as naloxone do not displace agonists from it, although haloperidol does. The other is referred to as the *PCP receptor*, and haloperidol does not displace agonists from it. The respective role of these receptors in mediating the effects of PCP is not yet clear.

The lipid solubility of phencyclidine is high (the brain/plasma ratio is between 6 and 9) and so it has a rapid onset. Thus, following its inhalation in smoke, the effects are evident in 1–5 minutes. Following ingestion the onset occurs in 15–30 minutes, with peak blood levels being observed at 2 hours.

The duration of action is 4–6 hours, but it can be much longer depending on dose. The high lipid solubility renders redistribution an important mechanism in the termination of its action. The half-life of the compound is 21 hours. Because about 10% of the substance is excreted unchanged in the urine, the half-life is dependent on urinary pH.

TOLERANCE AND PHYSICAL DEPENDENCE

Chronic PCP users report that gradual tolerance develops to the psychic effects of low doses. This forces users to take larger amounts, but that, in turn, is correlated with increasingly dysphoric experiences. Such experiences are reported by three quarters of the users, and many feel trapped by the drug. In animals, tolerance to the anesthetic effects of PCP is observed following repeated administration over a period of weeks or months.

Animals will maintain themselves on PCP. Withdrawal of monkeys after 10 days on the drug produces a syndrome marked by emesis, anorexia, tremors, and contact avoidance, fighting, and restlessness. No description of a well-characterized withdrawal syndrome in humans is available.

TOXICITY

The acute effects of PCP change, as the dose is increased, from a mild euphoria and stimulation (which does not interfere with normal functioning) to a body-wide anesthetic effect (legs and feet especially) that makes coordination difficult, produces slurred speech, and may involve an out-of-body experience. This can lead to bizarre behavior, unresponsiveness, combativeness, and with higher doses, to catatonia as the individual becomes incoherent and immobile, although conscious. With further increases in dose, convulsions (diazepam has been used for these) and coma ensue. The intoxication is characterized by nystagmus, which in 90% of patients is both horizontal and vertical, by ataxia, and by hyperreflexia. Other clinical correlates of the intoxication are an elevation of systolic and diastolic pressure (potentially controlled by diazoxide), hyperthermia (potentially controlled by naloxone), and oliguria. The latter is accompanied by elevated serum creatinine phosphokinase activity and serum uric acid, as well as myoglobinuria. It is indicative of rhabdomyolysis. The possibility of the latter renders acidification of the urine, which would speed the renal elimination of PCP, hazardous because myoglobin is more likely to cause renal damage under such circumstances.

The effects of PCP on the psyche include unique and profound alterations of thought, gross changes in body image, loss of ego boundary, depersonalization, estrangement, and isolation. Patients may have religious ideation, feelings of God-like power, perceptions of superhuman strength (local anesthetic effects permit behavior that would otherwise be too painful) and invulnerability, as well as a pathological preoccupation with death (meditatio mortis). Behavior is extremely unpredictable, the patients being cooperative one minute and violently assaultive the next. Patients present an immediate danger to others merely on the basis of their misperceptions, paranoia, and hostility. This threat is compounded by their confusion and their inability to cooperate. Patients are ambivalent and unpredictable even toward their close friends and relatives (see also descriptions in Chapter 27).

The PCP overdose syndrome is frequently indistinguishable from schizophrenia.

Following PCP self-administration, patients may present with psychoses indistinguishable clinically from schizophrenia. Haloperidol may be useful in alleviating the symptoms. As the body burdens of PCP are cleared, the psychoses resolve in most patients. In some, however, they persist for weeks or months. In schizophrenic patients, PCP brings about a rapid and extreme exacerbation of psychoses.

Chronic PCP use causes long-lasting difficulties with mentation.

Following prolonged use of PCP, users develop persistent speech difficulties (stuttering, blocking), an inability to think clearly, problems with recent memory, incoherency, and unreliability. They also appear to undergo personality changes and to develop severe depression and social withdrawal. Recovery is slow, the effects lasting 6 months to a year. (Clonidine has been reported to alleviate the depression.)

Hallucinogens

Lysergic acid diethylamide (LSD) was discovered by Hofmann, a chemist with the Swiss pharmaceutical company Sandoz, in the early 1940s, while he was trying to develop an analeptic. Noting that he was experiencing marked mental changes after handling the drug, Hofmann concluded that this was likely to be due to his having inhaled or ingested some of the substance accidentally. To confirm this, he deliberately self-administered a very small quantity of LSD and experienced rather dramatic effects.

Other hallucinogens in this group include mescaline (3,4,5-trimethoxyphenyl-ethylamine, found in a Mexican cactus the dried top of which is called *peyote* or *mescal*), N,N-dimethyltryptamine and 5-methoxy-N,N-dimethyltryptamine (both present in snuffs of plants origin used by natives of the Caribbean and Amazon basin areas, respectively), psilocin and psilocybin (4-hydroxytryptamine and its phosphate ester, respectively; found in psilocybe mushrooms native to Mexico), and a number of substituted amphetamines, including 2,5-dimethoxy-4-methylamphetamine (MDA, STP) and 2,5-dimethoxyamphetamine (DMA). In the 1960s taking LSD became a fashionable component of the hippie lifestyle and LSD was used with considerable frequency. Although the actions of the other hallucinogens in this group are similar to those of LSD, these latter agents never achieved widespread use. Accordingly, knowledge of the toxic and other properties of this group of substances derives primarily from the clinical experience with LSD.

REINFORCING PROPERTIES

Perception and interpretation of both external and internal sensory stimuli are altered by LSD. Although visual perception is the modality most obviously affected (objects assume great plasticity: walls, faces, and so on recede, advance, change shape and color, and acquire halos and new qualities), other senses are also affected (e.g., touch: clothes may feel velvety one moment, gritty the next). So is proprioception, with resulting distortions of body image, out-of-body sensations, and depersonalization. Fragments of the perceptual field are perceived out of context with the usual frame of reference. Background stimuli, normally ignored (the sound of a breeze, the drip of a tap), compel attention. Unusual associations come to mind and stimulate each other. The drug is a potent enhancer of suggestibility, exceeding in this respect the effects of hypnosis. It has major effects on mood. Objects seen and events occurring are felt to have great portentousness. Feelings of insight and unity with the universe, with humankind, and so on are experienced. Chains of thought are less subject to critical review and appear to take command, resulting in thinking that is more innovative, but also more tangential. LSD-induced feelings of greatly enhanced creativity, insight, and so on cannot be either verbalized or otherwise recorded.

The onset of central effects of LSD is relatively slow — during the first 30 minutes only somatic effects (weakness, tremor, occasionally parasthesias, sometimes muscle cramps, and nausea) are perceived. Thereafter the central effects become rapidly manifest and reach a peak at about 3 hours. The following day the individual feels fatigued and depressed. The other hallucinogens act more rapidly and for a shorter time.

Most hallucinogens act more rapidly and for shorter periods of time than does LSD.

TOLERANCE

Tolerance develops if LSD is taken repeatedly in a short period of time: the effects become less and less. Also there is cross tolerance to other hallucinogens (e.g., psilocybin). On the other hand, no withdrawal phenomena from LSD have been observed in humans or animals.

TOXIC EFFECTS

LSD users usually retain enough insight to know that the mental changes and hallucinations are consequences of ingestion of the hallucinogen. Nonetheless, sometimes they act out their illusions with potentially catastrophic effects (e.g., deciding to fly off a building). Sometimes, anxiety, fear of the unknown, perhaps of losing one's mind, become intense enough that frank panic occurs, requiring hospitalization. In individuals unaware of having ingested a hallucinogen, such fears have resulted in suicide.

Some fraction of the LSD-induced experiences are sufficiently dysphoric ("bad trips") for users to seek medical assistance. The user's expectations regarding the effects of the drug (the "set"), the "setting," and the presence of an experienced user, or "sitter," who can lead and reassure the neophyte, decrease, to a degree, the probability of a dysphoric experience, but even seasoned users have some occasionally. Some LSD users may seek medical assistance because of the recurrence of the hallucinogenic experience at a later date and in the absence of the ingestion of a hallucinogen. To some, this can be extremely distressing. The most serious, although relatively rare, toxic effect of LSD is the induction of psychoses in previously normal individuals. Such psychoses do not always respond to treatment and can be long-lasting (weeks, months).

Some fraction of LSD users experience long-lasting psychotic breaks.

Chlorpromazine decreases the intensity of the effects of LSD and has been used in the treatment of dysphoric experiences. Diazepam can be used to relieve anxiety. Additionally, the patient needs continued reassurance or "talking down."

Ecstasy and Eve

3,4-methylenedioxymethamphetamine (MDMA, Ecstasy, Adam) and its homolog, 3,4-methylenedioxyethamphetamine (MDEA, Eve) are ring-substituted amphetamines that became popular on college campuses in the 1980s as recreational drugs. During this period, MDMA was also used as an adjunct to psychotherapy by some psychiatrists. The drug causes irreversible neurotoxicity in experimental animals, and the possibility that it may do so also in humans has led the drug to be placed on the list of Schedule I substances by the United States Food and Drug Administration. MDEA is said to have effects similar to MDMA, although they are milder.

REINFORCING PROPERTIES

Upon first-time use, most MDMA users experience a pleasant mood change without hallucinations. The effects range from a lowering of interpersonal anxiety and defenses, greater closeness with others, and increased communication and sociability to a visionary experience of a mystical nature inducing a sense of wholeness, connectedness, or enlightenment.

The onset occurs in about 30 minutes following oral ingestion. Somatic effects include some tingling and spasmodic jerking as well as a sensation of coldness. The acute effects peak after a couple of hours and wane by 6 hours.

TOXIC EFFECTS

Jaw clenching, teeth grinding, muscle aches, difficulty concentrating, fatigue, and depression are reported in the days immediately following MDMA use. Upon repeated use of the drug, the pleasurable effects are much diminished and the side effects enhanced; this is true even when long periods of time elapse in the interim.

In the rat, both racemic MDMA (the substance in illicit trade) and each of the enantiomers cause an acute depletion of brain 5-hydroxytryptamine (serotonin, 5-HT), with recovery to control levels within 12 hours. Animals given either the racemic MDMA or the (+) enantiomer suffer a secondary depletion of 5-HT 7 days later, although this is not seen with the (−) enantiomer. Repeated injections of MDMA destroy serotoninergic neurons in rats and monkeys, the latter species being much more sensitive. Such monkeys become extremely passive and insomniac. The increase in serum prolactin concentrations seen following L-tryptophan infusion appears to be blunted in human MDMA users. Since the rise in serum prolactin is a response mediated by 5-HT synthesis and release, this finding has raised concerns that MDMA may cause long-term loss of 5-HT neurons in human users also.

Destruction of serotoninergic neurons by ecstasy has been observed in animals.

Atropine-Type Deliriants

The use of atropine and other atropine-type drugs to cause out-of-body experiences and deliria has a long history in Western civilization.

The belladonna alkaloids, atropine, scopolamine, and hyoscine, as well as plant materials containing them (e.g., *Datura stramonium*, jimsonweed) have a long history of use to induce mental effects. This history includes application of salves containing them to skin or mucosal surfaces by witches in the Middle Ages. Although these agents were never widely used as recreational substances in this century, isolated instances of such use continue to be encountered.

TOXIC PROPERTIES AND TREATMENT

These substances are classic muscarinic cholinergic-blocking agents. They cause dry mouth, inability to swallow, dilated pupils and blurred vision, hyperthermia, tachycardia, and urinary retention. Toxic manifestations include disorientation, irrationality, amnesia, and a delirium characterized by hallucinations and loss of insight (see also Chapter 27). Physostigmine, infused slowly, reverses the delirium; in its absence, diazepam can be used to control the excitement and alcohol or sponge baths to lower body temperature.

General References

Benowitz NL: Pharmacological aspects of cigarette smoking and nicotine addiction. N Engl J Med 319:1318–1330, 1988.

Brewer C, Rezae H, Baily C: Opioid withdrawal and naltrexone induction in 48–72 hours with minimal drop-out, using a modification of the naltrexone-clonidine technique. Br J Psychiat 153:340–343, 1988.

Busto U, Bendayan R, Sellers EM: Clinical pharmacokinetics on non-opiate abused drugs. Clin Pharmacokinet 16:1–26, 1989.

Carroll ME: PCP and hallucinogens. Adv Alcohol Subst Abuse 9:167–190, 1990.

Compton DR, Dewey WL, Martin BR: Cannabis dependence and tolerance production. Adv Alcohol Subst Abuse 9:129–147, 1990.

Gawin FH, Ellinwood EH Jr: Cocaine and other stimulants: Actions, abuse and treatment. N Engl J Med 318:1173–1182, 1988.

Glassman AH, Stetner F, et al: Heavy smokers, smoking cessation, and clonidine: Results of a double-blind, randomized trial. JAMA 259:2863–2866, 1988.

Gossop M: Clonidine and the treatment of the opiate withdrawal syndrome. Drug Alcohol Depend 21:253–259, 1988.

Griffiths R, Woodson P: Caffeine physical dependence. Psychopharmacology 94:437–451, 1988.

Jaffe JH: Drug addiction and drug abuse. In Gilman AG, Rall TW, Nies AS, Taylor P (eds): Goodman and Gilman's Pharmacological Basis of Therapeutics, 8th ed, 522–573. New York: Pergamon Press, 1990.

Koob GF, Bloom FE: Cellular and molecular mechanisms of drug dependence. Science 242:715–723, 1988.

Mello NK, Mendelson JH, Kuehnle JC, Sellers MS: Operant analysis of human heroin self-administration and the effects of naltrexone. J Pharmacol Exp Ther 216:45–54, 1981.

Miller NS, Millman RB, Gold MS: Amphetamines: Pharmacology, abuse and addiction. Adv Alcohol Subst Abuse 8:53–69, 1988.

Oates JA, Wood AJJ: Pharmacological aspects of cigarette smoking and nicotine addiction. N Engl J Med 319:1318–1330, 1988.

Report of the Surgeon General: The health consequences of smoking: Nicotine addiction. Washington, DC: U.S. Department of Health and Human Services, 1988.

Rickels K, Schweizer E, Case WG, Greenblatt, DJ: Long-term therapeutic use of benzodiazepines. I. Effects of abrupt discontinuation. Arch Gen Psychiatry 47:899–907, 1990.

Salzman C (Task Force Chair): Benzodiazepine Dependence, Toxicity, and Abuse. A Task Force Report of the American Psychiatric Association. Washington, DC: American Psychiatric Press, 1990.

Schmidt CJ: Neurotoxicity of the psychedelic amphetamine, methylenedioxymethamphetamine. J Pharmacol Exp Ther 240:1–7, 1987.

Schweizer E, Rickels K, Case WG, Greenblatt DJ: Long-term therapeutic use of benzodiazepines. II. Effects of gradual taper. Arch Gen Psychiatry 47:908–915, 1990.

Woods JH, Katz JL, Winger G: Use and abuse of benzodiazepines: Issues relevant to prescribing. JAMA 260:3476–3480, 1988.

Zweben JE, Payte JT: Methadone maintenance in the treatment of opioid dependence: A current perspective. West J Med 152:588–599, 1990.

68

Information and Learning Resources in Pharmacology

Alan M. Reynard
Cedric M. Smith

Need for information about drugs.

The rapidly growing knowledge base about drugs creates the necessity of having available a variety of accurate, up-to-date reference sources. This is true not only for the medical student but also for the house officer and for the experienced practitioner. This chapter developed in response to the realization that not only did students beginning their study of drugs need a guide to teaching and learning resources but they also needed such a guide in their unfolding careers. Thus, we have attempted to provide descriptions and advice regarding the effective and rational utilization of these resources. Because these lists of available materials will soon become incomplete, new, potentially useful sources are appearing almost every day.

The Association for Medical School Pharmacology, composed of the chairpersons of all the departments of pharmacology in schools of medicine, has published a consensus document, Medical Knowledge Objectives in Pharmacology (Fisher, 2nd ed, 1990). This has proved useful for the design of learning programs, for review, and for the development of questions for certification examinations. The editors used these essential knowledge objectives in the planning of the present book. In addition, the National Boards of Medical Examiners use these objectives as a knowledge base for the National Board examinations.

There is a general problem in preparing "core" or "minimal essential information." In trying to be succinct there is the serious risk of misleading oversimplification inherent in presenting limited, and therefore at least partially inaccurate, information. In view of the fact that no one can really know and apply all the relevant information about a drug, a disease, and a patient, the more physicians know about the principles of drug actions and side effects, the more patients will be benefited and the fewer harmed. In truth, those who prescribe and receive medications can never know too much about medications' actions and possible harmful side effects.

One can never know too much about the potential good and bad effects drugs can produce.

Information Sources

Students and practitioners need immediately available, accurate, comprehensive information about drugs.

Table 68–1 presents suggestions for the "compleat" physician's reference and learning resources, listed by primary use, starting with readily accessible textbooks and reference sources familiar to most readers. The references have been prepared to provide a wide variety, albeit not exhaustive, of choices. The following text serves to illustrate and explain the material in the tables and references.

Table 68-1 LEARNING RESOURCES—THE COMPLEAT PHYSICIAN'S BOOKSHELF	
Source	**Some Selected Examples**
Comprehensive textbooks	Gilman et al, 1990, *or* DE Drug Evaluations subscription Facts and Comparisons

Shorter textbooks	This book, or the books by Craig and Stitzel, 1989; Katzung,
	    1987; Clark and colleagues, 1988; or Kalant and Roschlau,
	    1989

Comprehensive information	Package inserts for each drug United States Pharmacopeia Drug Information Facts and Comparisons Computer Databases such as RxTRIAGE, DRUGDEX, AHFS DIF Nonprescription drug information such as the American Pharmaceutical Association Handbook

Therapeutics manuals	Textbooks of medicine such as Cecil Essentials of Medicine
	    (Andreoli et al, 1990) or the comprehensive two-volume
	    Cecil Textbook of Medicine (Wyngaarden and Smith, 1988)
	Dunagan and Ridner, 1989
	Larson and Ramsey, 1989
	Therapeutic manuals for medical specialties

Adverse drug reactions and interactions	Drug Interaction Facts from Facts and Comparisons Handbook
	    of Adverse Drug Interactions
	Drug Interactions Handbook from the Medical Letter
	RxTRIAGE
	Meyler's Side Effects of Drugs (Dukes MNG, ed)
	Drug Interactions Decision Support Tables (Hansten PD)
	MEDI-SPAN Drug Therapy Monitoring System (DTMS)
	MEDICOM Drug interaction Database (MEDICOM Clinical
	    Laboratory Test Interference Database and Parenteral
	    Admixture Incompatability Database, Drug to Food
	    Interaction Module (DFIM)

Poisoning and toxicology	Doull et al, 1990 Ellenhorn and Barceloux, 1988
General principles of drug action	Pratt and Taylor, 1990
Governmental and hospital formularies	
Convenient access to medical literature	MEDLINE via modem, medical library
Information for patients	USP Drug Information AMA Patient Information Sheets RxTRIAGE
Computer-assisted instruction	HyperPharm MacPharmacology MICAL, PSYCAL, ENDOCAL (see References and Directories)

TEXTBOOKS, DRUG INDEXES, AND DIRECTORIES

The package insert item is the legally required labeling information for all drugs mandated by the Food and Drug Laws; this is included with every legally available drug. With every order or prescription of a drug the physician, resident, or clerk needs to review the package insert. The content of the package inserts is agreed upon after negotiation between the manufacturer and the United States Food and Drug Administration (FDA). They contain *indications* that range from medicines that are truly indicated for a given disease state (for example, penicillin for streptococcal infections) to medicines that might have some efficacy in treatment (for example, a benzodiazepine for mild insomnia). This information is often ambiguous and should be used with caution.

More important than the indications section is the list of potential side effects and adverse drug interactions. Inasmuch as the benefit/risk decision of taking or not taking a drug is not only the physician's but also the

The package insert is the full label for the drug.

In the package insert "Indications" does *not* mean that the drug is *indicated*, only that it *may* have some use.

patient's and patient's significant others, the prescriber is obliged, both ethically and legally, to inform the patient not only of the benefits but also of the risks.

Many of the package inserts are included in the Physicians' Desk Reference (PDR), which is published each year by the Medical Economics Company from material provided by pharmaceutical manufacturers. It is thus incumbent on all prescribers to review either the package insert or a *current* PDR (also available on CD-ROM and hand-held computer).

Out-of-date PDRs may contain erroneous, potentially harmful, or inadequate information.

The single, most comprehensive source for resources about drug information is the compact, exhaustive compilation of Snow (1988). A number of the clinically useful drug directories are listed in the References. Noteworthy are standard reference textbooks, Drug Evaluations, Facts and Comparisons, United States Pharmacopeia, and the computer-based databases such as RxTRIAGE and DRUGDEX. Also useful are the American Society of Hospital Pharmacists AHFS Drug Information and the Handbook on Injectable Drugs available in print form and on-line as Drug Information Fulltext (DIF).

ADVERSE DRUG REACTIONS AND INTERACTIONS

Resources of information about adverse drug actions and interactions are also listed in a section of the References. The Medical Letter and RxTRIAGE systems are recommended because they facilitate keeping essential records of drugs that individual patients are or have been receiving. RxTRIAGE and PDR CD-ROM also provide ready access to monographs on each drug as well as patient information sheets.

Using up-to-date information on potential adverse drug reactions and interactions can avoid harm and pain on the part of both patients and doctors.

Although the choice of therapy rests, according to law and by medical ethics, with both the physician and the patient, the physician is in the position of the most information. Nevertheless, most practitioners are not aware of how frequently they make egregious and potentially harmful errors (of commitment or omission). A study of one university-affiliated teaching hospital documented significant risks to patients with errors in prescribing at a rate of more than 3 per 1000 prescriptions, with almost 2 out of 3 judged as being significantly hazardous (Lesar et al, 1990); not included were errors of omission, diagnosis, and work-up or errors actually detected and corrected by other staff. Moreover, a large percentage of all the medical staff were responsible for the errors; of 580 detected errors in a series, 170 different prescribers were responsible, ranging from first-year house officers to attendings, with 1 to 12 errors per prescriber.

Drugs should *never* be prescribed or administered without knowing what other drugs the patient has taken or might take.

Computer-accessible databases can now easily provide essentially all that is possible to know about a drug or toxic agent.

The challenge is the effective utilization of available information.

Improvement in detection and awareness has been demonstrated (Scott et al, 1990). A subscription to an adverse drug reaction and interaction database is a practical way to keep abreast of all the new reports on such adverse reactions. A number of sources are available as presented in both Table 68 – 1 and in the Reference lists. In this connection it should be obvious that every practitioner should be aware of all drugs a patient is, or potentially could be, receiving.

The physician treats the patient only with the patient's consent.

ADVERSE FOOD REACTIONS

These are now available for computer access, such as WellAware: Food Sensitivity (reviewed by Podolsky, 1990). Programs such as this provide a computer-based method of recording and cataloging every item a patient ingests and then correlating foods, ingredients, and symptoms. This program is useful for physicians, dieticians, and other health providers as well as patients to keep track of all possible symptoms related to an allergic response to foods. Another example is Nutri-Calc HD (1990), a nutritional food database and nutritional values from the 10th edition of Recommended Dietary Allowances; it will prepare weight gain/loss dietary plans based on food intake and activity.

FORMULARIES

Most medical practice is in group clinics, health maintenance organizations (HMOs), or hospital settings, and these usually have associated pharmacies with formularies that include only a selected list of drugs. In some states, such as New York, the department of health mandates the prescribing and filling of prescriptions with generic agents unless otherwise specifically requested by the doctor in writing on each prescription.

POISONING AND TOXICOLOGY

Useful information is available from poison control centers. POISONDEX and TOXLINE are two extensive computer-accessible toxicology databases covering medicinal, commercial, industrial, and botanical sources.

PRESCRIBING PRINCIPLES AND MANAGEMENT SYSTEMS

A number of systems are now available for recording of patient data, clinical laboratory findings, diagnosis, progress notes, medication, and treatment records. These range from very primitive to very complete. For management of patients' medication, we have found the RxTRIAGE system comprehensive, accurate, and very easy to use. Other examples are Dr. Smartkey, a macro-writing program and macro editor designed for use with WordPerfect for progress notes, using templates for illnesses or drugs frequently encountered as well as patient data, telephone dialers, and the like. A number of systems are now available, and many more will be appearing in the near future. Some available materials are listed in the References and a detailed compilation appears in an annual issue of M.D. Computing magazine.

PATIENT INFORMATION

The United States Pharmacopeia (USP) and the American Medical Association (AMA) have pioneered the preparation and use of printed materials on specific drugs or drug classes written in a language suitable for the general public. The USP sheets are titled USP-DI (Drug Information) and the AMA's as Patient Management Information Sheets. Both provide spaces for the physician to insert specific information for a given patient.

The best patient is an informed patient.

Such patient information materials are now available on personal computer disks for direct use by patients or as templates that can be edited by the physician for individual patients. In addition some medical specialties such as psychiatry have developed videotapes for viewing by patients that explain the uses, side effects, and precautions for psychotropic agents.

Accurate patient-oriented information, as monographs and books, are now widely available.

Medical Informatics

Medical Informatics is a discipline emerging in medical schools, health care institutions, and libraries; it focuses on the management of information

A new medical specialty, Medical Informatics.

used to support education and decision making in patient diagnosis and management, research, and communication (Greenes and Shortliffe, 1990; Shortliffe et al, 1990). The American Medical Informatics Association (AMIA) sponsors two major conferences each year. In the fall is the Symposium on Computer Applications in Medical Care (SCAMC) on the east coast (usually Washington, D.C.) and in the spring on the west coast. These conferences include presentations of submitted papers and workshops. Attendees are clinicians, researchers, and educators from all the health sciences.

The establishment in medical institutions of academic and service units that deal with Medical Informatics is being seriously advocated. Among the interests of this field are medical education, patient management, coping with new technology, and development and utilization of electronic knowledge resources (e.g., hypertext, hypermedia, on-line textbooks, bibliographical databases, clinical case simulations, educational testing, and decision aids).

Learning Resources

Questioning is the beginning of knowledge.

Trying to answer pertinent questions about drugs, how they act, and what hazards they may present remains the essential component of learning.

Studying questions from old examinations is useful for mentally active review, for testing one's knowledge, and for identifying areas of ignorance as well as of knowledge.

QUESTION BANKS

A number of computer-based question banks are available on computer disk, some of which are devoted to pharmacology. Since the 1950s the editors' department, like many departments of pharmacology, has made available copies of the examinations to students as learning aids. More recently, copies of examinations used in the past 3 – 5 years have been made available from a copy service. The students are encouraged to use these questions in planning their studying, for review, and to test their knowledge.

Computer-based versions of question banks have an appreciably greater potential for learning as well as for testing. Prime among these has been the pioneering efforts of Walaszek and colleagues. Their system involves 240 lessons of 4 different types: review questions, self-study, case histories, and laboratory exercises. Examinations are drawn from a question bank of 14,000 items (Walaszek and Doull, 1985; Doull and Walaszek, 1990; BASIC SCIENCES: UMKC Software Series). Others are listed in the different References lists (e.g., Katzung and Trevor, 1990; Hyperpharm, Aronow and Moore, 1990; MacPharmacology, Eisenberg et al, 1990; Emmett-Oglesby and Yorio, 1985; Elliott, 1987; Goldstein, 1990). Most of these contain at least some programs or text that comments on the reasons why a particular item selected is either correct or incorrect. One of the textbooks in pharmacology, Bevan and Thompson, unfortunately now out of print, included questions at the end of each chapter plus advice on how to use the book for self-study.

The use of computer-based questions can facilitate active problem-based learning.

Almost uniformly these pharmacology question banks are limited by the fact that they use, almost exclusively, the standard multiple-choice formats that stress recognition (or at least potentially can be answered using straight recall or recognition) as opposed to the "real world" context that requires uncued recall, synthesis of diverse pieces of information, or problem solving. Even the case management questions designed as "problems" are often trivial or can be answered correctly using some simple recall strategies and recognition knowledge.

In contrast, the more open-ended questions, such as those used in the Nierenberg and Smith book (1989), are at the same time more similar to the clinical situation as well as encouraging (or least permitting) more detailed recall and reconstruction of existing knowledge to address the problems presented by the clinical cases.

PATIENT-ORIENTED PROBLEM SESSIONS (POPS)

The POPS units in pharmacology have been developed to encourage and stimulate problem solving by groups of students, with a focus on the patient, disease process, and specific drug classes (Burford et al, 1990). Experiences with these POPS sessions in a basic pharmacology course for medical and graduate students found that some students use them enthusiastically whereas others participate only reluctantly (Lathers and Smith, 1989). The POPS provide efficient learning of relevant material. However, it will be necessary to update certain sections in light of new information. Currently available are sessions on pharmacokinetics, theophylline, drug therapy of hypertension and congestive heart failure, antiarrhythmic drugs, toxicity of analgesic agents, and treatment of poisoning.

PROGRAMMED AND CASE-RELATED TEXTS

A unique review text by Neal (1987) has a number of interesting summaries and presentations. Case-related, problem-oriented textbooks can be quite useful, especially for review. Among the more useful are Nierenberg and Smith (1989) and Sweeney (1990). Both of these use selected cases to illustrate basic drug actions, uses, and principles of drug therapy.

COMPUTER-ASSISTED INSTRUCTION

It is abundantly clear that computer systems are tremendously and uniquely useful in the management, storage, and ready retrieval of vast amounts of information on medical topics including drugs. A few of these resources have been discussed. Under development are practical and feasible use of computers for clinical decision making in addition to more useful and readily available computer-accessible databases and knowledge databases. The drug interaction databases (such as those in RxTRIAGE and the Medical Letter programs) are good examples of a functionally operational systems that are relatively inexpensive, readily available, and clinically extremely important. Some computer-based diagnostic systems are also clinically very useful.

> CAI will only increase in availability and efficiency in the future.

> Answering new clinical therapeutic problems is now possible with the readily accessible information databases.

To date there are no comprehensive interactive computer-assisted instruction (CAI) programs focusing on medical students learning pharmacology for the first time. There are, nevertheless, programs available that feature limited aspects of pharmacology. These are described here. For all of them it appears that students will use them only to the extent that the CAI is integrated with other components of the course and curriculum (Keith Killam, personal communication; Garrett et al, 1987). In addition to education itself, computer systems are being implemented for curricular tracking, scheduling, and a variety of testing and evaluations (Wigton, 1990).

> A number of well-designed CAI programs are useful for efficient learning.

One area of pharmacology, pharmacokinetics, lends itself to computer-based instruction as well as practical application in designing drug-dosing regimens (Feldman et al, 1989). Among the many programs available are PCNONLIN, PHARMKIN (Neubig, 1987), MINSQ, MacKinetics (Aronow and Moore, 1990), and BASIC PRINCIPLES OF THERAPEUTIC DRUG MONITORING. Each of these seeks to assist the user to develop practical (and intuitive) knowledge of therapeutics by providing hands-on exposure to dosage selection and monitoring, using simulation of plasma concentrations as a function of dosing and time. Most of these are relatively rudimentary although suitable for sophomore medical students; however, some provide a detailed simulation potential and regime design

> The available effective CAI programs demonstrate the practicality and potential for future programs.

> Especially useful are programs dealing with dynamic processes, such as pharmacokinetics, and massive databases for adverse drug reactions.

(e.g., Washington et al, 1990); others include Pharmcokinetics (USC PC-PACK by Jelliffe and colleagues, listed in the Wisc-Ware catalog of more than 200 MS DOS – based instructional software programs).

Gas Man: Understanding Anesthesia Uptake and Distribution is a computer simulation program that illustrates the principles of anesthetic gas uptake and distribution. The program displays the information for several anesthetics graphically. It permits reviewing of current clinical situations as well as testing theories by simulation. This program has a superb reputation for learning by residents in anesthesia and could be employed in the pharmacology curriculum.

MICAL (Upjohn) presents a series of patients and questions regarding choice of diagnosis of an infection, initial choice of an antibiotic, and how the medication should be managed. Students find the cases and program interesting, a glimpse of the practical and useful for review and learning.

PSYCAL (Upjohn), although focused on psychiatric diagnosis and not therapy, is well edited and contains pertinent information. It has been judged by a small group of students as one of the best of a number of software programs; this series was characterized as providing more feedback and control than most (Xakellis and Gjerde, 1990).

ENDOCAL (Upjohn) is another in the series that provides good user control and feedback. The focus is on endocrinology rather than therapeutics.

CAI programs in a number of other medical areas related to pharmacology are now being developed. The report of Hutcheon and El-Gawly (1991) illustrates how microcomputer technology can provide new ways of incorporating problem-based learning procedures using both analog and digital systems. They describe a model system of four problem-oriented exercises that require the student to interpret electrocardiograms and the drug-induced changes in cardiac rhythm. Students obtain an understanding of the electrophysiological basis for managing cardiac arrhythmias in clinical practice that supplements and expands laboratory and conference sessions. In practice the exercise can be run as an individual student or a group activity.

Hybrid systems allow use of different modeling and demonstration techniques.

INTERACTIVE VIDEO

Interactive video is currently the most powerful technique for learning.

Interactive video is considered the best computer-based way currently available to deliver didactic information to students.

An interactive video system is one that can deliver images (and text) to an individual who can interact with the system to evoke responses. This can be accomplished in several ways. Currently the most popular way is to combine a video disk player with a computer, so that images from the player appear on the screen, sometimes overlayed with text or graphics from the computer. The presentation of the images is controlled by a program running on the computer. The user can interact with the system with a keyboard, a mouse, a light pen, or by touching the screen (if the system has a touch-sensitive screen).

Interactive implies the control by the user's interactions with the various media.

There is much effort under way to find efficient ways to store the images digitally on a computer's hard disk rather than on a video disk. A few such systems are currently in development but not yet commercially available. In summary, this type of delivery system consists of a computer, a method of delivering images such as a disk player, a disk, and a computer program. A video disk can hold 54,000 still images, 30 minutes of motion video, or a combination of both.

An example of its use is the presentation of the image of a cell on the screen, with an arrow pointing to a structure in the cell and a corner of the screen devoted to a multiple-choice question that the user can answer. The computer program determines which image and question are put on the screen, monitors the user's response, and provides feedback to the user.

There are no interactive video programs available exclusively for pharmacology. However, several programs/disks involve pharmacology while dealing with other areas of medicine; most of the pharmacology relates to treatment. These are listed here.

The *DxTER series* of disks on emergency medicine was developed by Intelligent Images. In these the student manages a patient in real time using images displayed from the video disk. The computer program tracks decisions made by the student and calculates care costs.

CBT are computer-based examinations produced by the National Board of Medical Examiners use images from a video disk. These programs are currently being tested in a number of medical schools.

OTHER

The CYBERLOG system from Cardinal Health Systems is a hybrid system covering 16 topics dealing with clinical management. Some are concerned in detail with pharmacological matters; one focuses on clinical pharmacology and pharmacokinetics; others focus on specific clinical syndromes — hypertension, diabetes, coronary artery disease, arthritis, infectious diseases, cardiac arrhythmias, thyroid diseases, and gastrointestinal diseases. Each of these programs includes a general text, explicit objectives, tutorials, sample clinical case studies, and reference "tools" such as tables of established values, nomograms, and drug formularies. An illustrated text and computer disks are provided. For the most part this system is programmed learning with some question-and-answer format. The didactic material is accessible by computer read-out or printed text.

Up-to-date authoritative information is essential for today's practice of medicine. Keeping informed and aware of information pertinent to one's practice presents a persistent challenge. Table 68–2 lists many of the more useful journals in the area of therapeutics and pharmacology.

There are literally thousands of reputable medical journals publishing mostly articles that have received rigorous peer review. Each specialty has its own journal(s); major journals are found among the national and international medical organizations — for example, the New England Journal of Medicine, Journal of the American Medical Association (JAMA), British Medical Journal, and Lancet. In relation specifically to therapeutics, the Medical Letter on Drugs and Therapeutics is among the more accessible sources of consistently high quality; this newsletter also includes a Continuing Medical Education (CME) program. The regular perusing of the Medical Letter and following CME are potentially very effective ways to learn and keep up to date with important drug use and toxicity.

ACCESS TO MEDICAL LITERATURE

Perhaps almost important as having these references is knowing where and how to obtain answers to new questions regarding drug uses or effects. To

Stunning visual displays are available for thousands of images, coupled with easy access and control.

Keeping Current

All the learning in medical school is only the foundation and prelude to life-long learning from patients and from colleagues.

Using available learning resources rests on routine habits of seeking out and using the most accurate and valid information.

Access to relevant information is now a critical component of every medical practice.

Table 68-2 SOME MAJOR JOURNALS THAT PUBLISH ARTICLES THAT EVALUATE BASIC AND CLINICAL PHARMACOLOGY AND THERAPEUTICS

Annals of Internal Medicine
Annual Review of Pharmacology and Toxicology
Archives of Internal Medicine
Biochemical Pharmacology
Clinical Pharmacology and Therapeutics
Drugs
JAMA
Journal of Clinical Pharmacology
Journal of Pharmacology and Experimental Therapeutics
The Medical Letter on Drugs and Therapeutics
Molecular Pharmacology
New England Journal of Medicine
Pharmacological Reviews
Postgraduate Medicine
Toxicology and Applied Pharmacology
Toxicon
Trends in Pharmacological Sciences, including toxicological sciences
Yearbook of Drug Therapy

obtain answers to this class of question, the most useful resource is MEDLINE, the National Library of Medicine's on-line index of medical journals —available directly or through GRATEFUL MED, SILVER PLATTER, or other computer/modem connections, such as DIALOG. An abbreviated version of MEDLINE is available in many institutions, frequently designated as MINIMEDLINE. For all patient-related and research-related questions, the full search capability of MEDLINE should be used.

A glimpse of the future for most specialties is the problem-oriented information retrieval system in clinical neurosciences, Nervline: A Microcomputer Information Retrieval System in the Clinical Neurosciences (Finelli, 1988). This system provides a focused neurological reference and keyword system that accesses citations chosen by the author in 20 commonly available journals that is searchable by subject, signs or symptoms, or author (reviewed by Steiner, 1990).

SOURCES OF INFORMATION ABOUT COMPUTER SOFTWARE AND HARDWARE

The magazine M.D. Computing has many articles of interest. Especially useful are the Buyer's Guide issues that lists thousands of information and software packages, instruments, and manufacturers. The National Library of Medicine's (NLM) Audiovisuals Catalog and AudioVisuals onLine (AVLINE) provides bibliographical citations for all audiovisuals and software catalog by NLM since 1975. Other directories are the Medical Disc Directory and the Medical and Health Information Directory.

CONTINUING MEDICAL EDUCATION

Relevant information includes patient data, disease/symptom data, laboratory findings, medication information, adverse reaction, procedures; the records must document patient, doctor, and staff time and effort for billing, insurance, peer review, and fiscal management.

There is currently a wealth of educational materials and programs available under continuing medical education (CME) auspices. Each medical school and most major medical institutions have ongoing medical education programs. Of more general accessibility are the many television video presentations. Many of these present focused clinical pharmacology instruction. As just one example, an AMA Videoclinic presented Common Arrhythmias: New Concepts for the Selection of Antiarrhythmic Agents, including illustrated EKGs and current approaches to therapy. A tremendously important limitation to CME programs, including the video clinics, is the fact that most, if not all, receive major support from pharmaceutical and medical industries. Granted, some of the programs are exemplary in the balance of their discussions; however, drug industry expenditures are based on a variety of potential benefits to the industry involved. Those interests or industry objectives may not be readily apparent, and thus an industry's influence may not even be recognized, let alone compensated for, by the physician or student participant.

The References section also lists sources of reliable information about drugs, suitable for patients. Noteworthy among these, as mentioned earlier, are the USP-DI and the AMA Patient Information Management Sheets that provide succinct, well-written summaries of information about specific drugs or drug classes that can be given to patients or modified by the doctor for a specific patient's management. Software packages, such as RxTRIAGE, also have the capability of printing out patient and drug information from the computer; these sheets can be edited and modified by the physician for the given patient or for the drug information itself.

An interesting application of interactive video was made in evaluating the usefulness of prostatectomy when it was discovered that patients' knowledge of the benefits and risks made them unable to help with the decision of whether or not to operate (Lyon et al, 1990). A video disk was prepared to deliver the requisite information to patients, whereby the patients were able to participate more actively in the decision-making process.

Patient Education

Patient compliance and cooperation in therapy depends, ultimately, on the patient's truly informed consent.

Selected References and Directories

Listed under three headings: Teaching About Drugs, Drug Indexes, and Databases; Poisoning, Toxicology, and Interactions; Examples of Learning Resources

Teaching About Drugs, Drug Indexes, and Databases

Aarons L, Foster RW, Hollingsworth M, et al: Computer-assisted learning lessons in drug disposition and pharmacokinetics. J Pharmacol Methods 20:109–123, 1988.

Ackerman MJ: New media in medical education. Methods Inf Med 28:327–331, 1989.

AMA DE Drug Evaluations: Subscription (or book) published quarterly by the Division of Drugs and Toxicology, American Medical Association, Chicago. annual, 1990.

American Medical Association guide to prescription and over-the-counter drugs, Clayman CB (ed). New York: Random House, 1988.

Andreoli TE, Carpenter CCJ, Plum F, Smith LH Jr: Cecil Essentials of Medicine, 2nd ed. Philadelphia: WB Saunders Co, 1990.

ASHP Drug Information and the Handbook on Injectable Drugs: Drug Information Fulltext (DIF) and Consumer Drug Information (CDIF). American Society of Hospital Pharmacists, ASHP Database Services, Bethesda, MD.

Audiovisuals Catalogue Quarterly: National Library of Medicine (NML). Washington, DC: Superintendent of Documents, US Government Printing Office.

AVLINE: Bibliographical citations to all audiovisuals and computer software cataloged by the National Library of Medicine (NLM), Bethesda, MD 20894.

Barnett GO: Information technology and undergraduate medical education. Acad Med 64:187–190, 1989.

Barnett O: Computers in medicine. JAMA 263:2631–2633, 1990.

Baselt RC: Disposition of Toxic Drugs and Chemicals in Man, 3rd ed. Chicago: Year Book Medical Publishers, 1990.

Beck JR, Shultz EK, Edwards BR: Medical informatics for the other ninety percent: The Dartmouth experience. Acad Med 65:298–301, 1990.

Bevan JA, Thompson JH: Essentials of Pharmacology, 3rd ed. Philadelphia: JB Lippincott Co, 1983.

Bogner PH: Handbook of Pharmacologic Therapeutics — A Disease-Oriented Review. Boston: Little Brown & Co, 1988.

Brater DC: Pocket Manual of Drug Use in Clinical Medicine, 4th ed. Toronto and Philadelphia: BC Decker, 1989.

Brater DC, Nierenberg DW: Medical student education in clinical pharmacology and therapeutics. Ann Intern Med 108:136–138, 1988.

Burford HJ, Ingenito AJ, Williams PB: Development and evaluation of patient-oriented problem solving materials in pharmacology. Acad Med 65:689, 1990.

Charles SC: Malpractice. JAMA 264:528, 1990. (Book review of Edwards, 1989.)

Clark WG, Brater DC, Johanson AR (eds): Goth's Medical Pharmacology, 12th ed. St Louis: CV Mosby Co, 1988.

Clyman SG, Orr NA: Status report on the NBME's computer-based testing. Acad Med 65:235–241, 1990.

Conn PM, Gebhart GF (eds): Essentials of Pharmacology. Philadelphia: FA Davis Co, 1989.

Conn's Current Therapy (see Rakel RE, 1991).

Consumer Reports Books: The Complete Drug Reference. New York: Consumer Reports Books, 1991.

Craig CR, Stitzel RE (eds): Modern Pharmacology, 3rd ed. Boston: Little Brown & Co, 1989.

Crawford S, Evens RG: Medical school libraries in the United States: Evolution to information management. Pharos 53:38–41, 1990.

CYBERLOG: The Library of Applied Medical Software: Perspectives in Rational Management. Diskettes, documentation, and manuals on 16 topics. Cardinal Health Systems, Edina, MN, 1989.

DIALOG: Provides via modem on-line or CD-ROM information from more than 320 databases including all major medical and health care reference sources. Dialog Information Services, Inc.

Dietary Analysis Program (USDA). US Department of Commerce, National Technical Information Service, Springfield, VA 22161. (Cited in Consumer Reports Health Letter 2:24, March 1990.)

DiPalma JR, DiGregorio GJ: Basic Pharmacology in Medicine, 3rd ed. New York: McGraw-Hill Publishing Co, 1990.

Dr. Smartkey — A macro-writing program and macro editor for progress notes, patient data, telephone dialers, and so on. Professional Health Systems, Honolulu.

DRUG THERAPY SCREENING SYSTEM (DTSS): A variety of drug therapy monitoring and reporting databases, including drug-drug, drug-food, and adverse reactions. Medi-Span, Indianapolis.

Dunagan WC, Ridner ML (eds): Manual of Medical Therapeutics. St Louis: Department of Medicine, Washington University, 1989.

Edwards FJ: Medical Malpractice: Solving the Crisis. New York: Henry Holt & Co, 1989.

Electronic Drug Reference, Version 3.0. Computer-based information on 3500 drugs, extracted from the USP DI, Facts and Comparisons, Facts and Comparisons Drug Newsletter, Drug Interaction Facts, Medical Newsletter, PDR, and other sources. Clinical Reference Systems, Ltd.

Encyclopedia of Health Information Sources, 1st ed. Detroit: Gale Research, 1987.

Facts and Comparisons and Facts and Comparisons Drug Newsletter, Drug Interaction Facts. Facts and Comparisons Division. Tatro DS (ed). Philadelphia: JB Lippincott Co, 1990 and later editions.

Feldman RD, Schoenwald R, Kane J: Development of a computer-based instructional system in pharmacokinetics: Efficacy in clinical pharmacology teaching for senior medical students. J Clin Pharmacol 29:158–161, 1989.

Finelli PF: Nervline: Microcomputer Information Retrieval System in the Clinical Neurosciences (version 1.3, 3 floppy disks for the IBM PC/KT AT, or MS-DOS compatible). Stoneham, MA: Butterworths, distributor, 1988.

Fisher JW, Gourley DRH, Greenbaum LM: Knowledge objectives in medical pharmacology. Pharmacologist 27:73–78, 1985. 2nd ed. (1990) prepared by Association for Medical School Pharmacology, Committee on Essential Knowledge Base in Pharmacology. Fisher JW, Chairman.

Garrett TJ, Ashford AR, Savage DG: A comparison of computer-assisted instruction and tutorials in hematology and oncology. J Med Educ 62:918–922, 1987.

Gilman AB, Rall TW, Nies AS, Taylor P (eds): Goodman and Gilman's The Pharmacological Basis of Therapeutics, 8th ed. Elmsford, NY: Pergamon Press plc, 1990.

GRATEFUL MED: A user-friendly software package providing access via modem to the computer files of the National Library of Medicine that includes MEDLINE, AIDSLINE, CANCERLINE, PDQ, HEALTH, TOXLINE, TOXLIT, and others. US Department of Commerce, National Technical Information Service, Springfield, VA 22161.

Green M, Andrews LG, Faich GA: Physician reporting of adverse drug reactions. JAMA 263:1785–1788, 1990.

Greenes RA, Shortliffe EH: Medical informatics—An emerging academic discipline and institutional priority. JAMA 263:1114–1120, 1990.

Hollister LE, Csernansky JG: Clinical Pharmacology of Psychotherapeutic Drugs, 3rd ed. New York: Churchill Livingstone, 1990.

Hussar DA (ed): Modell's Drugs in Current Use and New Drugs. New York: Springer Pub Co, 1990.

Index Nominum: International Drug Directory 1990/1991. Medpharm European Scientific Publishers. Boca Raton, FL: CRC Press, 1991.

Ingenito AJ, Lathers CM, Burford HJ: Instruction in clinical pharmacology: Changes in the wind. J Clin Pharmacol 29:7–17, 1989.

IPA (International Pharmaceutical Abstracts). Abstracts of literature dealing with pharmacy or drugs. Available through on-line database hosts such as DIALOG, Datastar, MEDLARS (TOXLINE).

Kalant H, Roschlau WHE: Principles of Medical Pharmacology. Toronto and Philadelphia: BC Decker, 1989.

Katzung BG (ed): Basic and Clinical Pharmacology, 5th ed. Norwalk, CT: Appleton & Lange, 1990.

Katzung BG, Trevor AJ: Pharmacology Examination and Board Review, 2nd ed. Norwalk, CT: Appleton & Lange, 1990.

Larson EB, Ramsey PG (eds): Medical Therapeutics. A Pocket Companion. Philadelphia: WB Saunders Co, 1989.

Lathers CM, Smith CM: Teaching clinical pharmacology: Coordination with medical pharmacology courses. J Clin Pharmacol 29:581–597, 1989.

Lesar TS, Briceland LL, Delcoure K, et al: Medication prescribing errors in a teaching hospital. JAMA 263:2329–2334, 1990.

Lyon HC, Henderson JV, Beck JR, et al: A multipurpose interactive videodisk with ethical, legal, medical, educational, and research implications: The informed patient decision-making procedure. *In* Kingsland LC (ed): Proceedings of the 13th Annual Symposium on Computer Applications in Medical Care, 1989, 1043–1045. Washington, DC: IEEE Computer Society Press, 1989.

McArthur JR, Bolles JR, Fine J, et al: Interactive computer-video modules for health sciences education. Methods Inf Med 28:360–363, 1989.

M.D. Computing. Springer-Verlag, New York.

Medical and Health Information Directory, 5th ed., 1989. Contains a wealth of information on medical and research organizations as well as chapters on computerized information systems and services and audiovisual producers and services. Gale Research, Detroit, MI 48232.

The Medical Letter for Drugs and Therapeutics. New Rochelle, NY. (Also Continuing Medical Education Program, handbooks on different drug topics, e.g., Handbook of Antimicrobial Therapy, Handbook of Adverse Drug Interactions, Drugs of Choice.)

MEDICATION ADVISOR, Version 2.0. Software program that provides 1 page of patient advice for each of over 5000 drugs. Clinical Reference Systems, Englewood, CO.

Medication Manager: Medication database manager; generates prescriptions, patient medication, and allergy listings, and reports including patient medication history. Clinician's Software, San Diego, CA.

Medication Profile and Prescription Form. Provides analysis of patient medication usage, diagnosis, and patient information. C&S Research Corporation, King of Prussia, PA.

MEDICOM Drug Interaction Database. Professional Drug Systems, St Louis.

MEDLINE: National Library of Medicine (NLM) index of the biomedical literature.

MEDTEACH: Software program that includes the contents of the ASHP's Medication Teaching Manual for patient education. American Society of Hospital Pharmacists. Bethesda, MD 20814.

National Library of Medicine (NLM): MEDLINE, AVLINE, TOXLINE, and other databases, and the Audiovisuals Catalogue Quarterly. Superintendent of Documents, US Government Printing Office, Washington, DC 20402. (See GRATEFUL MED.)

Neal MJ: Medical Pharmacology at a Glance. Boston: Blackwell Scientific, 1987.

Nierenberg DW, Smith RP: Clinical Problems in Basic Pharmacology. St Louis: CV Mosby Co, 1989.

Nutri-Calc HD: Nutritional food database, recommended daily allowances, prepares weight gain/loss dietary plans based on food intake, activity. Tempe, AZ: Camde Corp, 1990.

PATIENT EDUCATION SYSTEM. Management Solutions International, Health Industry Division, Jerico, NY.

Peterkin K, Black CF: Directory of on-line healthcare databases, 5th ed. Oak Park, IL: Medical Data Exchange, Alpine Guild, 1990.

Physicians' Desk Reference (PDR): Oradell, NJ: Medical Economics Co. Also available on CD-ROM, which includes generic drugs, drug interactions, adverse drug effects, and drug "indications"; based on the package inserts and labeling required by the Food and Drug Administration.

Physician's 1990 Drug Handbook. Springhouse, PA: Springhouse Corp, 1990. (Loeb S, executive director, Editorial.)

Pratt WB, Taylor P: Principles of Drug Action. The Basis of Pharmacology (3rd ed is update of Goldstein, Kalman, Aronow's 2nd ed). New York: Churchill Livingstone, 1990.

Rakel RE (ed): Conn's Current Therapy 1991. Philadelphia: WB Saunders Co, 1991. (Updated annually.)

Recommended Dietary Allowances, 10th ed. National Research Council Subcommittee on the Tenth Edition of the RDAs, National Academy Press, Washington DC 1989.

Reid JL, Rubin PC, Whiting B: Lecture Notes on Clinical Pharmacology, 3rd ed. Chicago: Mosby Year Book, 1989.

RxDx: Computer software series from Williams & Wilkins, Baltimore; topics range from abdominal pain to management of hypertension.

RxTRIAGE: A drug interactions and decision support software subscription service, drug and drug-food interactions, clinical information, patient information, duplicate therapy checking. San Bruno, CA: First DataBank, 1990.

Schatzberg AF, Cole JO: Manual of Clinical Psychopharmacology, 2nd ed. Washington, DC: American Psychiatric Press, 1991.

Scott HD, Thacher-Renshaw A, Rosenbaum SE, et al: Physician reporting of adverse drug reactions. JAMA 263:1785–1788, 1990.

Shannon JD: Small-group interactive computer-assisted teaching. Med Educ 24:148–150, 1990.

Shortliffe EH, Perrault L, Widerhold G, Fagen LM (eds): Medical Informatics: Computer Applications in Health Care. Menlo Park, CA: Addison-Wesley Publishing Co, 1990.

SILVER PLATTER: Information retrieval system CD-ROM (Compact Disk Read Only Memory) for all major medical databases including MEDLINE, TOXLINE, Excerpta Medica, Drugs and Pharmacology and many others. Silver Platter Information, Inc., Newton Lower Falls, MA 02162.

Smith CM, Reynard AM: Resources for teaching of pharmacology. Draft text and extensive bibliography available from the authors. Unpublished data, 1991. Buffalo, NY 14214.

Snow B: Drug Information: A Guide to Current Resources. Chicago: Medical Library Association, 1989.

Stair TO, Corn M, Broering NC: First year's experience of the MAClinical computer workstations project. Acad Med 65:20–22, 1990.

Stevens RH, Kwak AR, McCoy JM: Evaluating preclinical medical students by using computer-based problem-solving examinations. Acad Med 64:685–687, 1989.

Sweeney G: Clinical Pharmacology—A Conceptual Approach. New York: Churchill Livingstone, 1990.

TOXLINE. Toxicology information on-line. National Library of Medicine On-line Service, Bethesda, MD.

United States Pharmacopeia Drug Information (USP DI): Vol 1, Drug Information for the Health Care Professional; vol 2, Advice for the Patient; vol 3, Approved Drug Products and Legal Requirements Review, USAN and USP Dictionary of Drug Names. USP Leaflet Diskette for patient information. The United States Pharmacopeial Convention, Rockville, MD.

Walaszek ED, Doull J: Use of computers in the teaching of pharmacology, toxicology and therapeutics. Physiologist 28:419–421, 1985.

Walaszek ED, Doull J: Use of computers in the teaching of pharmacology. FASEB J 4:A1236, 1990.

Washington University Manual of Medical Therapeutics. Boston: Little Brown & Co. Also available on CD-ROM from MAXX (Maximum Access to Diagnosis and Therapy).

Wigton R: Computers in medical education: What next? Seventh National Symposium on Computers in Medical Education, Omaha, Nebraska, 1990.

Williams RL, Brater DC, Mordenti J: Rational Therapeutics: A Clinical Pharmacological Guide for the Health Professional. New York: Marcel Dekker, 1990.

Wyngaarden JB, Smith LH Jr (eds): Cecil Textbook of Medicine, vol 1 and 2, 18th ed. Philadelphia: WB Saunders Co, 1988.

Xakellis, GC, Gjerde C: Evaluation by second-year medical students of their computer-aided instruction. Acad Med 65:23–26, 1990.

Yearbook of Drug Therapy, Hollister LE, Lasagna L (eds). Chicago: Year Book Medical Publishers, 1991 and prior years. Abstracts of articles of general interest in the practice of medicine.

Poisoning, Toxicology, and Interactions (see also Chapter 64)

Amdur MO, Doull J, Klaassen CD (eds): Casarett and Doull's Toxicology. The Basic Science of Poisons, 4th Ed. New York: Pergamon Press plc, 1991.

Borin SM, Smith WH, Hansten PD, Horn JR: Hansten and Horn's drug interaction program, Version 2.0, 1990. Philadelphia: Lea & Febiger, 1990.

Ciraulo DA, Shader RI, Greenblatt DJ, Creelman W (eds): Drug Interactions in Psychiatry. Baltimore: Williams & Wilkins, 1989.

Diet Analyst: Database of nutrient content of foods; diet and exercise monitor. Parsons Technology, Cedar Rapids, IA 52406.

Diet Helper, Executive; Menu Planner, Weight Loss Planner. Columbus: Ohio Distinctive Software, 1990.

Drug Interaction Facts. Facts and Comparisons Division, Tatro DS (ed). Philadelphia: JB Lippincott Co, 1988 and later editions.

Drug Interactions and Side Effects Index. Oradell, NJ: Medical Economics Co, 1990 and later by year.

DRUG MASTER and DRUG MASTER PLUS. Drug-drug, drug-food, drug-alcohol interactions plus patient education information. Medical Software Consortium, St Peters, MO.

DrugNews. A daily updated clinical news service including Inpharm (global drug reactions weekly review) and Reactions (alerts to reports of adverse effects, drug interactions, poisoning, overdosing, and drug abuse). Available on-line on Data-Star. ADIS Press International, Langhorne, PA 19047.

DRUG TO FOOD INTERACTION MODULE (DFIM). Computer-based alert system of potential interactions between drugs and food components (designed as a stand-alone system for pharmacy-system environment). First DataBank, San Bruno, CA.

Dukes MNG (ed): Meyler's Side Effects of Drugs, Vol 1 (1977) through vol 13 (1989). Amsterdam: Excerpta Medica; New York: Elsevier/North Holland.

Ellenhorn MJ, Barceloux DG: Medical Toxicology—Diagnosis and Treatment of Human Poisoning. New York: Elsevier, 1988.

Handbook of Adverse Drug Interactions. New Rochelle, NY: The Medical Letter. Latest edition, 1991.

Hansten PB: Drug Interactions Decision Support Tables. Spokane, WA: Applied Therapeutics, 1987.

Hansten PB, Horn JR: Drug Interactions, 6th ed. Philadelphia: Lea & Febiger, 1990.

MEDICOM DRUG INTERACTION DATABASE. Professional Drug Systems, St Louis, MO 63146.

MEDI-SPAN Drug Therapy Monitoring System (DTMS). Knowledge Bases on drug-drug and drug-food interactions. Indianapolis, IN 46268.

Olson KR (ed): Poisoning and Drug Overdose. Norwalk, CT: Appleton & Lange, 1990.

PDR's Drug Interactions and Side Effects Index. (See Drug Interactions and Side Effects Index.)

POISONDEX: Toxicology database on commercial, industrial, pharmaceutical, and botanical substances, including treatment and management protocols. MICRO-MEDEX, Medical Information systems, Denver, CO.

Rizack MA, Hillman CDM: The Medical Letter Handbook of Adverse Drug Interactions 1989. New Rochelle, NY: The Medical Letter.

Roe DA: Diet and Drug Interactions. New York: Van Nostrand Reinhold, 1989.

Roe DA: Drug-nutrient interactions in the elderly. *In* Munro HN, Danford DE (eds): Nutrition, Aging and the Elderly, 363–384, New York: Plenum Press, 1989.

Rogers AS: Adverse drug events: Identification and attribution. Drug Intell Clin Pharm 21:915–920, 1987.

Scott HD, Thacher-Renshaw A, Rosenbaum SE, et al: Physician reporting of adverse drug reactions. JAMA 263:1785–1788, 1990.

S-O-A-P Drug Interaction Program for Drug-, food-, disease-drug interactions and side effects of 2500 drugs. Brownfield, TX: Patient Medical Records, 1990.

Swiney MF, Cacace L: Book review of PDR Drug Interactions and Side Effects Diskettes. JAMA 264:97–98, 1990.

WellAware: Food Sensitivity: Computer-based analysis of foods and symptoms. Monterey, CA: 1989. (Reviewed by Podolsky ML: Software. JAMA 263:2376, 1990.)

Examples of Learning Resources

Aronow L, Moore K: Q/Bank—A Macintosh-based question review system. FASEB J 4:A1237, 1990. (Department of Pharmacology, Uniformed Services University of Health Sciences, and Henry M. Jackson Foundation for the Advancement of Military Medicine, Rockville, MD 20852.)

BASIC PRINCIPLES OF THERAPEUTIC DRUG MONITORING. Computer program for learning about drug administration, absorption, distribution, metabolism, elimination, and pharmacokinetics using animated graphics and tutorial exercises. Baltimore: Williams & Wilkins.

BASIC SCIENCES. Self-assessment in basic medical sciences including pharmacology. System provides correct and incorrect responses, flags the correct answer, supplies a reference, and keeps a percentage score. UMKC Software Series (2411 Holmes Street, Kansas City, MO 64108–2792).

Cardiolab. Program simulating cardiovascular pharmacology experiments in vivo. Miltown, NJ: Biosoft.

Cardiovascular Software Directory. Compiled by the American College of Cardiology, Bethesda, MD: Computer Applications Committee, 1988.

CBT: Computer-Based Testing Project, Version 2.0. Philadelphia: National Board of Medical Examiners, 1989.

CYBERLOG: The Library of Applied Medical Software: Perspectives in Rational Management. Diskettes, documentation, and manuals includes 16 topics in a subscription series. Edina, MN: Cardinal Health Systems, 1989.

Digitalis Pharmacology and Clinical Use: Basic and Clinical Pharmacology of Digitalis Medications. Massachusetts General Hospital Laboratory of Computer Science. Baltimore: Williams & Wilkins, 1987.

DiPalma JR, Barbieri EJ, DiGregorio GJ, et al: Pharmacology: PreTest Self-Assessment and Review, 5th ed. New York: McGraw-Hill Book Company, 1988.

Drug Therapy for the 1990s: Clinical Pharmacology—Therapeutics and Toxicity. (A home-study course.) Forum Medicum, and the American College of Clinical Pharmacology, Philadelphia, PA 19103.

DxTER Series. Intelligent Images, a division of DAROX Corp, San Diego, CA.

Eisenberg RM, Wallace KB, Trachte GJ: MacPharmacology: Cardiovascular pharmacology study/review program. FASEB J 4:A1236, 1990.

Elliott HL: Self-Assessment in Clinical Pharmacology. Blackwell Scientific Publications. Distributed in the USA and Canada by Blackwell/Year Book Medical Publishers, Chicago, 1987.

Emmett-Oglesby MW, Yorio T: Pharmacology Computer-Assisted Instruction Package. Ft Worth, TX, 1985.

Friedman CP, Twarog RG, File DD, et al: Computer databases as an educational tool in the basic sciences. Acad Med 65:15–16, 1990.

Gas Man: Understanding Anesthesia Uptake and Distribution. Med Man Simulations, PO Box 67–160, Chestnut Hill, MA 02167.

Goldstein DB: Teaching pharmacology on the Macintosh. FASEB J 4:A1237, 1990.

Hanes DP, Tallarida RJ: Computer-assisted instruction in pharmacokinetics for second-year students. J Med Educ 63:336–338, 1988.

Hughes I: Cardiolab, A program simulating cardiovascular pharmacology experiments in vivo, for IBM PC, Apple II and BBC B. Cambridge, MA: Elsevier-Biosoft.

Hughes I: ILEUM. Simulation of laboratory experiments investigating effects of drugs on the in vitro guinea-pig ileum (Apple II; IBM PC and BBC B). Cambridge, MA: Elsevier-Biosoft.

Hutcheon DE, El-Gawly HW: A computer-based, problem-solving system of instruction in clinical pharmacology. J Clin Pharmacol 31:198–204, 1991.

HyperPharm and HyperPharm/DOS. (See Aronow and Moore, 1990.)

Johnson Gordon E: Pharmacology PDQ series. Philadelphia: BC Decker, 1988.

Katzung BG, Trevor AJ: Pharmacology Examination and Board Review, 2nd ed. Norwalk, CT: Appleton & Lange, 1990.

KINCALC. Computer program that simulates first-order chemical kinetics. Biosoft, Miltown, NJ.

Large BAJ, Hughes IE: Learning Pharmacology through MCQ, 2nd ed. London: John Wiley & Sons, 1990.

Learning Resources Center: Software for Health Sciences Education: An Interactive Resource, 2nd ed. 1989. (Learning Resources Center, University of Michigan Medical Center, 1135 East Catherine, Ann Arbor, 48109–0726.)

McArthur JR, Bolles JR, Fine J, et al: Interactive computer-video modules for health sciences education. Methods Inf Med 28:360–365, 1989.

MacPharmacology: Pharmacology Study/Review Program, Eisenberg R (ed). Minnesota Medical Edu-ware, Duluth, MN.

MEDI-SPAN: Drug Therapy Monitoring System (DTMS). Knowledge Bases on drug-drug and drug-food interactions. Medi-Span, Inc., Indianapolis, IN 46268.

MEDITEXT INTERACTIVE LEARNING PROGRAMS. Interactive review system for course or comprehensive board review; includes pharmacology. Interactive Teleducation Corporation, Medford, NJ.

MICAL: Microbiology Computer-Assisted Learning software on chemotherapy. Educational Services, The Upjohn Company, Kalamazoo, MI 49001. (Also available: PSYCAL, dealing with psychiatry, and ENDOCAL, dealing with endocrinology.)

MINSQ. Pharmacokinetics Library, MicroMath, Salt Lake City, Utah, 1990.

Moore L, Waechter D, Aronow L: Assessing the effectiveness of computer-assisted instruction in a pharmacology course. Acad Med 66:194–196, 1991.

Neubig RR: PHARMKIN. A Pharmacokinetics Teaching Simulation GraphPAD Software. San Diego, 1987. University of Michigan Software, Ann Arbor, MI. (Reviewed in FASEB J 4:A1237, 1990.)

Patient Care Flowcharts: The magazine Patient Care publishes clinical cases for CME in a flowchart algorithm format available for interactive computer programs. Ten clinical problems from acute abdomen to rheumatoid arthritis are currently available.

PCNONLIN 3.0. Pharmcokinetic modeling program for IBM PC compatible computer. Statistical Consultants, Lexington, KY.

PHARMACOKINETICS/DOS. Available from Dr. Leon Moore at Uniformed Services University, Bethesda, MD 20814.

Rose KM, Rosenfeld GC, Loose-Mitchell DS: Board Review Series, Pharmacology. Baltimore: Williams & Wilkins, 1989.

Washington C, Washington W, Wilson CG: Pharmacokinetic modeling using STELLA on the Apple MacIntosh. New York: Prentice Hall, 1990.

Waterman RE, Duban SL, Mennin SP, et al: Clinical Problem-Based Learning: A Workbook for Integrating Basic and Clinical Science. Albuquerque: University of New Mexico Press, 1988. (Reviewed by Verghese A: JAMA 261:3036–3037, 1989.)

Index

Note: Page numbers in *italics* refer to illustrations; page numbers followed by t refer to tables.